Pediatric ICD-10-CM 2025

A Manual for Provider-Based Coding

American Academy of Pediatrics

DEDICATED TO THE HEALTH OF ALL CHILDREN®

American Academy of Pediatrics Publishing Staff

Mary Lou White, *Chief Product and Services Officer/SVP, Membership, Marketing, and Publishing*

Mark Grimes, *Vice President, Publishing*

Mary Kelly, *Senior Editor, Professional/Clinical Publishing*

Laura Underhile, *Editor, Professional/Clinical Publishing*

Jason Crase, *Senior Manager, Production and Editorial Services*

Leesa Levin-Doroba, *Production Manager, Practice Management*

Peg Mulcahy, *Manager, Art Direction and Production*

Mary Louise Carr, MBA, *Marketing Manager, Clinical Publications*

Published by the American Academy of Pediatrics
345 Park Blvd
Itasca, IL 60143
Telephone: 630/626-6000
Facsimile: 847/434-8000
www.aap.org

The American Academy of Pediatrics is an organization of 67,000 primary care pediatricians, pediatric medical subspecialists, and pediatric surgical specialists dedicated to the health, safety, and well-being of all infants, children, adolescents, and young adults.

While every effort has been made to ensure the accuracy of this publication, the American Academy of Pediatrics (AAP) does not guarantee that it is accurate, complete, or without error.

Any websites, brand names, products, or manufacturers are mentioned for informational and identification purposes only and do not imply an endorsement by the American Academy of Pediatrics (AAP). The AAP is not responsible for the content of external resources. Information was current at the time of publication.

This publication has been developed by the American Academy of Pediatrics. The contributors are expert authorities in the field of pediatrics. No commercial involvement of any kind has been solicited or accepted in development of the content of this publication. Disclosure: Dr Parsi disclosed an ownership and consulting relationship with The PEDS MD Company and is part of the Mead Johnson Speaker Bureau.

Visit www.aap.org/errata for an up-to-date list of any applicable errata for this publication.

Special discounts are available for bulk purchases of this publication. Email Special Sales at nationalaccounts@aap.org for more information.

© 2025 American Academy of Pediatrics

All rights reserved. No part of this publication may be reproduced, stored in a retrieval system, or transmitted in any form or by any means—electronic, mechanical, photocopying, recording, or otherwise—without prior written permission from the publisher (locate title at https://publications.aap.org/aapbooks and click on © Get Permissions; you may also fax the permissions editor at 847/434-8780 or email permissions@aap.org). First edition published 2015; 10th, 2025.

Printed in the United States of America.

11-114I   1 2 3 4 5 6 7 8 9 10

MA1151

ISBN: 978-1-61002-751-9
eBook: 978-1-61002-752-6
Print ISSN: 2475-9708
Online ISSN: 2475-9716

2024–2025 Committee on Coding and Nomenclature

Eileen D. Brewer, MD, FAAP, Chairperson
Margie C. Andreae, MD, FAAP
Suzanne K. Berman, MD, FAAP
Kimberly Brennan, MBA, CMPE
Mark Joseph, MD, FAAP
David M. Kanter, MD, MBA, CPC, FAAP, Immediate Past Chairperson
Steven E. Krug, MD, FAAP
Kathryn B. Lalor, MD, FAAP
Edward A. Liechty, MD, FAAP
Jeffrey F. Linzer Sr, MD, FAAP
Sheri L. Nemerofsky, MD, FAAP
Linda D. Parsi, MD, MBA, CPEDC, FAAP
Benjamin Shain, MD, PhD
Renee F. Slade, MD, FAAP
Mark C. Smith, MD, FAAP
Samuel D. Smith, MD, FAAP

2023–2024 AAP Coding Publications Editorial Advisory Board

Linda D. Parsi, MD, MBA, CPEDC, FAAP, Editor in Chief
Greg Barabell, MD, CPC, FAAP
Vita Boyar, MD, FAAP
Timothy Ryan Hensley, MD, CPC, CPEDC, FAAP
David M. Kanter, MD, MBA, CPC, FAAP
Steven E. Krug, MD, FAAP
Kathryn B. Lalor, MD, FAAP, Associate Editor
Edward A. Liechty, MD, FAAP
Jeffrey F. Linzer Sr, MD, FAAP
Richard A. Molteni, MD, FAAP
Karen Nauman, MD, FAAP
Sheri L. Nemerofsky, MD, FAAP, Associate Editor
Julia M. Pillsbury, DO, FAAP
Renee F. Slade, MD, FAAP
Karla Nickolas Swatski, MD, FAAP
Sanjeev Y. Tuli, MD, FAAP

AAP Staff

Stefanie Muntean-Turner, CPC, CPMA

Consulting Editor

Cindy Hughes, CPC, CFPC

Disclaimer

Every effort has been made to include all pediatric-relevant *International Classification of Diseases, 10th Revision, Clinical Modification* (*ICD-10-CM*) codes and their respective guidelines. It is the responsibility of the reader to use this manual as a companion to the official *ICD-10-CM* publication. Do not report new or revised *ICD-10-CM* codes until their published implementation date, at time of publication set for October 1, 2024. Readers are encouraged to visit www.aap.org/errata routinely to find any corrections due to errata in the published version.

Equity, Diversity, and Inclusion Statement

The American Academy of Pediatrics is committed to principles of equity, diversity, and inclusion in its publishing program. Editorial boards, author selections, and author transitions (publication succession plans) are designed to include diverse voices that reflect society as a whole. Editor and author teams are encouraged to actively seek out diverse authors and reviewers at all stages of the editorial process. Publishing staff are committed to promoting equity, diversity, and inclusion in all aspects of publication writing, review, and production. Likewise, it is the intent of the authors and publishing team to use visual representations of the diverse range of patients seen in medical settings where children are evaluated and treated.

Contents

Foreword VII

Acknowledgments VIII

Introduction IX

Quick Reference to 2025 *ICD-10-CM* Pediatric Code Changes XI

How to Use This Manual XVI

ICD-10-CM Official Guidelines for Coding and Reporting FY 2025 XVIII

Alphabetic Index 1

Tabular List

Chapter 1. Certain infectious and parasitic diseases (A00–B99) 131

Chapter 2. Neoplasms (C00–D49) 145

Chapter 3. Diseases of the blood and blood-forming organs and certain disorders involving the immune mechanism (D50–D89) 157

Chapter 4. Endocrine, nutritional and metabolic diseases (E00–E89) 167

Chapter 5. Mental, behavioral, and neurodevelopmental disorders (F01–F99) 181

Chapter 6. Diseases of the nervous system (G00–G99) 193

Chapter 7. Diseases of the eye and adnexa (H00–H59) 207

Chapter 8. Diseases of the ear and mastoid process (H60–H95) 215

Chapter 9. Diseases of the circulatory system (I00–I99) 221

Chapter 10. Diseases of the respiratory system (J00–J99) 231

Chapter 11. Diseases of the digestive system (K00–K95) 241

Chapter 12. Diseases of the skin and subcutaneous tissue (L00–L99) 255

Chapter 13. Diseases of the musculoskeletal system and connective tissue (M00–M99) 265

Chapter 14. Diseases of the genitourinary system (N00–N99) 283

Chapter 15. Pregnancy, childbirth and the puerperium (O00–O9A) 293

Chapter 16. Certain conditions originating in the perinatal period (P00–P96) 301

Chapter 17. Congenital malformations, deformations and chromosomal abnormalities (Q00–Q99) 313

Chapter 18. Symptoms, signs, and abnormal clinical and laboratory findings, not elsewhere classified (R00–R99) 327

Chapter 19. Injury, poisoning and certain other consequences of external causes (S00–T88) 341

Chapter 20. External causes of morbidity (V00–Y99) 425

Chapter 21. Factors influencing health status and contact with health services (Z00–Z99) 457

Chapter 22. Codes for special purposes (U00–U85) 481

ICD-10-CM External Cause of Injuries Due to Collisions Table 483

ICD-10-CM External Cause of Injuries Index 489

Table of Drugs and Chemicals 513

Foreword

The American Academy of Pediatrics (AAP) is pleased to publish this 10th edition of *Pediatric ICD-10-CM: A Manual for Provider-Based Coding*, a pediatric version of the *International Classification of Diseases, 10th Revision, Clinical Modification* (*ICD-10-CM*) manual. The AAP believes it is vital to publish an *ICD-10-CM* manual that is designed for pediatric providers. The expansive nature of the code set from *International Classification of Diseases, Ninth Revision, Clinical Modification* to *ICD-10-CM* overwhelmed many physicians, providers, and coders, so we condensed the code set to focus on pediatric-relevant diagnoses and their corresponding codes. When needed, additional codes can be located in the larger *ICD-10-CM* manual. We also reduced the guidelines so that only those applicable to the physician or provider are included, while those only relevant to facilities are removed. Lastly, guidelines for topic-specific chapters or specific codes can be found in their respective tabular chapter or right where the specific code is listed. This aids the user in identifying any chapter- or code-specific guidelines where they are needed most. This should assist in reducing any coding errors caused by reporting services that go against the guidelines that were once solely kept in the front of the manual, away from applicable codes.

The AAP is committed to the clinical modification of the *ICD* code set and, for the past several years, has sent an AAP liaison to the *ICD* Coordination and Maintenance Committee Meeting. We are especially grateful to Edward A. Liechty, MD, FAAP, and Jeffrey F. Linzer Sr, MD, FAAP, our appointed liaisons. The *ICD* Coordination and Maintenance Meeting is the semiannual meeting where all new *ICD* codes are presented, as well as revisions to the tabular list, index, and guidelines. Having dedicated expert liaisons aids in presenting pediatric and perinatal issues at the meeting. The AAP is also very pleased to continue its work with the *ICD* Editorial Advisory Board for *Coding Clinic for ICD-10-CM and ICD-10-PCS*. *Coding Clinic* is responsible for publishing *ICD* coding guidance and clarifications to supplement the *ICD-10-CM* manual. Dr Linzer sits on the Editorial Advisory Board, and Dr Liechty is our alternate. They represent pediatric issues, and both are experts on all *ICD-10-CM* matters.

The AAP will continue to support its members on issues regarding coding, and the AAP Pediatric Health Care Systems and Finance Transformation staff at the AAP headquarters stands ready to assist with problem areas not adequately covered in this manual. The AAP Coding Hotline can be accessed at https://form.jotform.com/Subspecialty/aapcodinghotline.

Acknowledgments

Pediatric ICD-10-CM: A Manual for Provider-Based Coding is the product of the efforts of many dedicated individuals. First and foremost, we must thank the members of the American Academy of Pediatrics (AAP) Committee on Coding and Nomenclature, past and present, and the AAP Coding Publications Editorial Advisory Board. They support all coding efforts here at the AAP. These members contribute extensive time to reviewing and editing coding content for the AAP.

We would also like to extend a very special thank-you to members of various subspecialty sections of the AAP who contributed their expertise and knowledge to the development of the original manual.

Lastly, we would like to acknowledge the tireless work of Jeffrey F. Linzer Sr, MD, FAAP, and Edward A. Liechty, MD, FAAP. Both Dr Liechty and Dr Linzer are advocates for pediatrics and neonatology and ensure that our issues are heard. They advocate for all pediatric patients in helping establish codes for conditions that need to be tracked for purposes of research and quality. They both keep the AAP and pediatric issues at the forefront of diagnostic coding, and we are very grateful for their time and expertise!

Introduction

The Basics of *ICD-10-CM*

The *International Classification of Diseases (ICD)* is published by the World Health Organization (WHO) for epidemiologic tracking and collection of mortality statistical data worldwide. The *ICD* is currently in its 11th revision. On October 1, 2015, the United States adopted a clinical modification of *ICD-10* called *International Classification of Diseases, 10th Revision, Clinical Modification (ICD-10-CM).* However, even as the United States was adopting *ICD-10-CM* for reporting morbidity data, the WHO was developing *ICD-11.* It is not known when the United States will adopt *ICD-11.*

ICD-10-CM diagnosis codes are used to communicate the following:

- Why the patient sought care
- The clinical indications for services provided
- The current status of chronic or recurring conditions, manifestations of underlying disease, and current stage of management of an injury
- The patient's personal or family history that affected patient management
- External factors that provide detail on how and where an illness or injury occurred
- External factors that impacted decisions for management (eg, social determinants of health)
- Reasons the recommended care was not provided (eg, patient/caregiver refusal, patient allergy)

How are *ICD-10-CM* codes added?

The National Center for Health Statistics (NCHS), a division of the Centers for Disease Control and Prevention, is responsible for adding new *ICD-10-CM* codes annually or as needed to improve epidemiologic and statistical tracking. Additionally, payers in the United States use the codes as part of their determination for payment. Adding a code isn't a simple process, however, and can take between 1 and 5 years. The American Academy of Pediatrics (AAP) has 2 members with *ICD-10-CM* expertise who sit on the NCHS Editorial Advisory Board (EAB). The NCHS EAB consists of *ICD-10-CM* experts across all medical specialty associations who offer medical and coding guidance that helps determine if a code/code set should be added, removed, or expanded.

Adding *ICD-10-CM* codes helps to increase the granularity of reporting. This, in turn, improves

- Demonstration of disease severity
- Measurement of health care services and quality metrics
- Identification of health care risks
- Identification of fraud and abuse

The codes also support improved public health surveillance and epidemiological research.

How do payers use *ICD-10-CM* codes?

ICD-10-CM is used by payers to

- Calculate hierarchical condition category.
- Justify evaluation and management (E/M) code levels.
- Necessitate clinical services.
- Develop quality measures.

When the diagnoses documented and/or the codes reported do not reflect the nature of the presenting problem or reason for encounter, the following may result:

- Delays in prior authorization for medically necessary services
- Claim denials or down-coding
- Inaccurate prediction of a patient's cost of care (risk adjustment) potentially causing lower payment for care
- Audit of medical records

Payers are increasingly down-coding E/M services based solely on the diagnosis codes reported (ie, not requesting medical records for the encounter). Accurate diagnosis codes may protect revenue and prevent claims audits.

ICD-10-CM Code Structure

Codes in *ICD-10-CM* begin with a letter. For codes that extend beyond 3 characters, the first 3 characters are found to the left of a decimal with the remaining characters to the right.

Pattern: XXX.XXXX

Although typically illustrated in capital letters, the alphabetic characters are not case sensitive. Each 3-character code category may then be further expanded with etiology, severity, site, manifestations, or intent within the fourth through sixth characters. When required, a seventh character is an extension to further define the episode of care, status of fracture healing, number of the fetus in obstetric conditions, or site of recording of the Glasgow Coma Scale.

Examples of complete codes include

Z23	Encounter for immunization
J06.9	Acute upper respiratory infection
H65.04	Acute recurrent serous otitis media, right ear
Z00.129	Encounter routine child health examination without abnormal findings
W07.XXXA	Fall from chair, initial encounter

Note the letter **X** is used as a placeholder in code **W07.XXXA**. The tabular listing for this code is **W07** with no further subcategories but with an instruction that the appropriate seventh character **A**, **D**, or **S** must be added to code **W07** to indicate the initial encounter, subsequent encounter, or encounter for a sequela of the fall from chair. The placeholder must be used to complete the code so the seventh character is in the appropriate position. If **W07.A** were submitted, the associated claim would likely be rejected because this is not a valid *ICD-10-CM* code. The letter **X** is also embedded in some codes to provide for future expansion of a code category (eg, **H60.8X1**, other otitis externa of the right ear).

Quick Reference to 2025 *ICD-10-CM* Pediatric Code Changes

This list does not include all changes made to *International Classification of Diseases, 10th Revision, Clinical Modification* (*ICD-10-CM*). Every effort has been made to include the diagnosis code changes that most apply to pediatric practices. Revisions and/or additional codes may have been published after the date of this printing. Always begin in the *ICD-10-CM* Alphabetic Index to locate the code most specific to the condition or other reason for encounter. Codes are valid as of October 1, 2024.

Quick Reference to 2025 *ICD-10-CM* Pediatric Code Changes

Anal fistula

Code	Description
●K60.30	Anal fistula, unspecified
●K60.31	Anal fistula, simple
●K60.311	Anal fistula, simple, initial
●K60.312	Anal fistula, simple, persistent
●K60.313	Anal fistula, simple, recurrent
●K60.319	Anal fistula, simple, unspecified
●K60.32	Anal fistula, complex
●K60.321	Anal fistula, complex, initial
●K60.322	Anal fistula, complex, persistent
●K60.323	Anal fistula, complex, recurrent
●K60.329	Anal fistula, complex, unspecified
●K60.40	Rectal fistula, unspecified
●K60.41	Rectal fistula, simple
●K60.411	Rectal fistula, simple, initial
●K60.412	Rectal fistula, simple, persistent
●K60.413	Rectal fistula, simple, recurrent
●K60.419	Rectal fistula, simple, unspecified
●K60.42	Rectal fistula, complex
●K60.421	Rectal fistula, complex, initial
●K60.422	Rectal fistula, complex, persistent
●K60.423	Rectal fistula, complex, recurrent
●K60.429	Rectal fistula, complex, unspecified

Blood type

Code	Description
●Z67.A	Duffy phenotype
●Z67.A1	Duffy null
●Z67.A2	Duffy a positive
●Z67.A3	Dufy b positive
●Z67.A4	Duffy a and b positive

Body mass index

Code	Description
▲Z68.54	Body mass index [BMI] pediatric, 95th percentile for age to less than 120% of the 95th percentile for age
●Z68.55	Body mass index [BMI] pediatric, 120th percentile for age to less than 140% of the 95th percentile for age
●Z68.56	Body mass index [BMI] pediatric, greater than or equal to 140% of the 95th percentile for age

Congenital malformations of anterior segment of eye

Code	Description
▲Q13.81	Rieger anomaly

Congenital malformations of aortic and mitral valves

Code	Description
●Q23.81	Bicuspid aortic valve
●Q23.82	Congenital mitral valve cleft leaflet
●Q23.88	Other congenital malformations of aortic and mitral valves

continued

Disorders of autonomic nervous system

Code	Description
•G90.81	Serotonin syndrome
•G90.89	Other disorders of autonomic nervous system

Eating disorders

Code	Description
•F50.010	Anorexia nervosa, restricting type, mild
•F50.011	Anorexia nervosa, restricting type, moderate
•F50.012	Anorexia nervosa, restricting type, severe
•F50.013	Anorexia nervosa, restricting type, extreme
•F50.014	Anorexia nervosa, restricting type, in remission
•F50.019	Anorexia nervosa, restricting type, unspecified
•F50.020	Anorexia nervosa, binge eating/purging type, mild
•F50.021	Anorexia nervosa, binge eating/purging type, moderate
•F50.022	Anorexia nervosa, binge eating/purging type, severe
•F50.023	Anorexia nervosa, binge eating/purging type, extreme
•F50.024	Anorexia nervosa, binge eating/purging type, in remission
•F50.029	Anorexia nervosa, binge eating/purging type, unspecified
•F50.20	Bulimia nervosa, unspecified
•F50.21	Bulimia nervosa, mild
•F50.22	Bulimia nervosa, moderate
•F50.23	Bulimia nervosa, severe
•F50.24	Bulimia nervosa, extreme
•F50.25	Bulimia nervosa, in remission
•F50.810	Binge eating disorder, mild
•F50.811	Binge eating disorder, moderate
•F50.812	Binge eating disorder, severe
•F50.813	Binge eating disorder, extreme
•F50.814	Binge eating disorder, in remission
•F50.819	Binge eating disorder, unspecified
•F50.83	Pica in adults
•F50.84	Rumination disorder in adults

Encounter for other aftercare and medical care

Code	Description
•Z51.A	Encounter for sepsis aftercare

Epilepsy and recurrent seizures

Code	Description
•G40.84	KCNQ2-related epilepsy
•G40.841	KCNQ2-related epilepsy, not intractable, with status epilepticus
•G40.842	KCNQ2-related epilepsy, not intractable, without status epilepticus
•G40.843	KCNQ2-related epilepsy, intractable, with status epilepticus
•G40.844	KCNQ2-related epilepsy, intractable, without status epilepticus

Family history of other specific diseases

Code	Description
•Z83.72	Family history of familial adenomatous polyposis

Follicular lymphoma

Code	Description
•C82.0A	Follicular lymphoma grade I, in remission
•C82.1A	Follicular lymphoma grade II, in remission
•C82.2A	Follicular lymphoma grade III, unspecified, in remission
•C82.3A	Follicular lymphoma grade IIIa, in remission
•C82.4A	Follicular lymphoma grade IIIb, in remission
•C82.5A	Diffuse follicle center lymphoma, in remission
•C82.9A	Follicular lymphoma, unspecified, in remission

continued

Genetic susceptibility to disease	
●Z15.1	Genetic susceptibility to epilepsy and neurodevelopmental disorders
●Z15.2	Genetic susceptibility to obesity
Hepatosplenic T-cell lymphoma	
●C86.10	Hepatosplenic T-cell lymphoma not having achieved remission
●C86.11	Hepatosplenic T-cell lymphoma, in remission
Hodgkin lymphoma	
●C81.0A	Nodular lymphocyte predominant Hodgkin lymphoma, in remission
●C81.1A	Nodular sclerosis Hodgkin lymphoma, in remission
●C81.2A	Mixed cellularity Hodgkin lymphoma, in remission
●C81.3A	Lymphocyte depleted Hodgkin lymphoma, in remission
●C81.9A	Hodgkin lymphoma, unspecified, in remission
Irritable bowel syndrome	
▲K58.9	Irritable bowel syndrome, unspecified
Malignant immunoproliferative diseases and certain other B-cell lymphomas	
●C88.20	Heavy chain disease not having achieved remission
●C88.21	Heavy chain disease, in remission
Mature T/NK-cell lymphomas	
●C84.0A	Mycosis fungoides, in remission
●C84.4A	Peripheral T-cell lymphoma, not elsewhere classified, in remission
●C84.6A	Anaplastic large cell lymphoma, ALK-positive, in remission
●C84.ZA	Other mature T/NK-cell lymphomas, in remission
Non-follicular lymphoma	
●C83.0A	Small cell B-cell lymphoma, in remission
●C83.390	Primary central nervous system lymphoma
●C83.398	Diffuse large B-cell lymphoma of extranodal and solid organ sites
●C83.3A	Diffuse large B-cell lymphoma, in remission
●C83.7A	Burkitt lymphoma, in remission
●C83.8A	Other non-follicular lymphoma, in remission
●C83.9A	Non-follicular (diffuse) lymphoma, unspecified, in remission
Other and unspecified disorders of nose and nasal sinuses	
●J34.82	Nasal valve collapse
●J34.820	Internal nasal valve collapse
●J34.8200	Internal nasal valve collapse, unspecified
●J34.8201	Internal nasal valve collapse, static
●J34.8202	Internal nasal valve collapse, dynamic
●J34.821	External nasal valve collapse
●J34.8210	External nasal valve collapse, unspecified
●J34.8211	External nasal valve collapse, static
●J34.8212	External nasal valve collapse, dynamic
●J34.829	Nasal valve collapse, unspecified

continued

	Other aplastic anemias and other bone marrow failure syndromes
•D61.03	Fanconi anemia

	Other disorders of brain
▲G93.42	Megalencephalic leukoencephalopathy with subcortical cysts
•G93.45	Developmental and epileptic encephalopathy

	Other disorders of carbohydrate metabolism
•E74.82	Disorders of citrate metabolism
•E74.820	SLC13A5 Citrate Transporter Disorder
•E74.829	Other disorders of citrate metabolism

	Other disorders of muscle
•M62.85	Dysfunction of the multifidus muscles, lumbar region

	Other disorders of pancreatic internal secretion
•E16.A	Hypoglycemia level
•E16.A1	Hypoglycemia level 1
•E16.A2	Hypoglycemia level 2
•E16.A3	Hypoglycemia level 3

	Other endocrine disorders
•E34.00	Carcinoid syndrome, unspecified
•E34.01	Carcinoid heart syndrome
•E34.09	Other carcinoid syndrome

	Other specified and unspecified types of non-Hodgkin lymphoma
•C85.9A	Non-Hodgkin lymphoma, unspecified, in remission

	Other specified congenital malformation syndromes affecting multiple systems
•Q87.86	Kleefstra syndrome

	Other symptoms and signs involving cognitive functions and awareness
•R41.85	Anosognosia

	Overweight and obesity
•E66.81	Obesity class
•E66.811	Obesity, class 1
•E66.812	Obesity, class 2
•E66.813	Obesity, class 3
•E66.89	Other obesity not elsewhere classified

	Personal history of drug therapy
•Z92.26	Personal history of immune checkpoint inhibitor therapy

	Problems related to housing and economic circumstances
•◻Z59.71	Insufficient health insurance coverage
•◻Z59.72	Insufficient welfare support

	Pruritus
•L29.81	Cholestatic pruritus
•L29.89	Other pruritus

	Spotted fever
▲A77.41	Ehrlichiosis chaffeensis [E. chaffeensis]

continued

Synovitis and tenosynovitis

Code	Description
•M65.90	Unspecified synovitis and tenosynovitis, unspecified site
•M65.91	Unspecified synovitis and tenosynovitis, shoulder
•M65.911	Unspecified synovitis and tenosynovitis, right shoulder
•M65.912	Unspecified synovitis and tenosynovitis, left shoulder
•M65.919	Unspecified synovitis and tenosynovitis, unspecified shoulder
•M65.92	Unspecified synovitis and tenosynovitis, upper arm
•M65.921	Unspecified synovitis and tenosynovitis, right upper arm
•M65.922	Unspecified synovitis and tenosynovitis, left upper arm
•M65.929	Unspecified synovitis and tenosynovitis, unspecified upper arm
•M65.93	Unspecified synovitis and tenosynovitis, forearm
•M65.931	Unspecified synovitis and tenosynovitis, right forearm
•M65.932	Unspecified synovitis and tenosynovitis, left forearm
•M65.939	Unspecified synovitis and tenosynovitis, unspecified forearm
•M65.94	Unspecified synovitis and tenosynovitis, hand
•M65.941	Unspecified synovitis and tenosynovitis, right hand
•M65.942	Unspecified synovitis and tenosynovitis, left hand
•M65.949	Unspecified synovitis and tenosynovitis, unspecified hand
•M65.95	Unspecified synovitis and tenosynovitis, thigh
•M65.951	Unspecified synovitis and tenosynovitis, right thigh
•M65.952	Unspecified synovitis and tenosynovitis, left thigh
•M65.959	Unspecified synovitis and tenosynovitis, unspecified thigh
•M65.96	Unspecified synovitis and tenosynovitis, lower leg
•M65.961	Unspecified synovitis and tenosynovitis, right lower leg
•M65.962	Unspecified synovitis and tenosynovitis, left lower leg
•M65.969	Unspecified synovitis and tenosynovitis, unspecified lower leg
•M65.97	Unspecified synovitis and tenosynovitis, ankle and foot
•M65.971	Unspecified synovitis and tenosynovitis, right ankle and foot
•M65.972	Unspecified synovitis and tenosynovitis, left ankle and foot
•M65.979	Unspecified synovitis and tenosynovitis, unspecified ankle and foot
•M65.98	Unspecified synovitis and tenosynovitis, other site
•M65.99	Unspecified synovitis and tenosynovitis, multiple sites

Type 1 diabetes mellitus

Code	Description
•E10.A	Type 1 diabetes mellitus, presymptomatic
•E10.A0	Type 1 diabetes mellitus, presymptomatic, unspecified
•E10.A1	Type 1 diabetes mellitus, presymptomatic, Stage 1
•E10.A2	Type 1 diabetes mellitus, presymptomatic, Stage 2

How to Use This Manual

HOW TO USE THIS MANUAL

While attempting to stay true to the complete *International Classification of Diseases, 10th Revision, Clinical Modification* (*ICD-10-CM*) manual, *Pediatric ICD-10-CM: A Manual for Provider-Based Coding* only includes conditions more commonly seen in pediatrics. We have attempted to remove all adult-only conditions, as well as conditions not typically found in the United States. Because *ICD* classification is used worldwide, many conditions listed in the official manual are not found in this part of the world.

Some codes are included under *Excludes* notes in the Tabular List for reference purposes only and to be consistent with the coding guidance. However, not every code included under *Excludes* will be found in the Tabular List if the condition is not specific to US pediatric health care. Again, these conditions are not commonly found in US pediatric health care, and the codes are included in the Alphabetic Index for reference purposes only. These conditions can be found in the larger Tabular List on the National Center for Health Statistics website (www.cdc.gov/nchs/icd/icd-10-cm/files.html).

Guidelines

Guidelines relevant to all pediatric codes are included. Note that some chapter-specific guidelines will appear at the beginning of the related chapter when they apply to most of that chapter. However, chapter-specific guidelines that are relevant only at specific category or code levels can be found at those category or code levels. The beginning of each chapter will reference the category(ies) or code(s) where the guidelines can be found. Guidelines that are **bold** have been revised or added for 2025. Guideline updates for the current year in the front matter and chapter-specific guidelines are printed in **bold.**

Abbreviations

We use our own abbreviations throughout that may not appear in *ICD-10-CM*; however, all abbreviations are defined on the inside front cover for easy access as you navigate through the manual.

Unspecified Laterality

While unspecified codes can still be found throughout and in certain instances will be the most appropriate code, we have removed nearly every code that uses unspecified laterality. We feel it is important that laterality is documented in nearly all conditions. You will see a footnote in those chapters where we have specifically left out laterality in nearly all conditions. If you need to report unspecified laterality for a condition and it is not listed in the chapter, refer to the full *ICD-10-CM* manual. Those codes will typically have a final character of 0 (zero) or 9.

Three-Character Codes

Three-character codes still exist in *ICD-10-CM*. Those will be noted specifically throughout the chapters as well.

E15 NONDIABETIC HYPOGLYCEMIC COMA

☑ *Includes:* drug-induced insulin coma in nondiabetic
hyperinsulinism with hypoglycemic coma
hypoglycemic coma NOS

Abbreviated Code Descriptors

To help keep the size of the manual manageable, some codes are only written out fully at the category or subcategory level. The category or subcategory will be notated with a semicolon (;) and the code will begin with a lowercase letter. For example,

A37.0 Whooping cough due to Bordetella pertussis;
A37.00 without pneumonia
A37.01 with pneumonia

At the subcategory level (**A37.0**) you see the semicolon (;), and at the code levels (**A37.00** and **A37.01**), the codes begin with a lowercase letter. Therefore, code **A37.00** reads, "Whooping cough due to Bordetella pertussis without pneumonia."

Symbols

The following symbols are used throughout the text:

- ● Identifies new codes
- ▲ Identifies revised codes
- ◻ Identifies codes linked to social determinants of health

ICD-10-CM Official Guidelines for Coding and Reporting FY 2025

Narrative changes appear in bold text

Items underlined have been moved within the guidelines since the FY 2024 version

Italics are used to indicate revisions to heading changes

The Centers for Medicare and Medicaid Services (CMS) and the National Center for Health Statistics (NCHS), two departments within the U.S. federal government's Department of Health and Human Services (DHHS), provide the following guidelines for coding and reporting by using the *International Classification of Diseases, 10th Revision, Clinical Modification* (*ICD-10-CM*). These guidelines should be used as a companion document to the official version of the *ICD-10-CM* as published on the NCHS website. The *ICD-10-CM* is a morbidity classification published by the United States for classifying diagnoses and reason for visits in all health care settings. The *ICD-10-CM* is based on the *ICD-10*, the statistical classification of disease published by the World Health Organization (WHO).

These guidelines have been approved by the four organizations that make up the Cooperating Parties for the *ICD-10-CM*: the American Hospital Association (AHA), the American Health Information Management Association (AHIMA), CMS, and NCHS.

These guidelines are a set of rules that have been developed to accompany and complement the official conventions and instructions provided within the *ICD-10-CM* itself. The instructions and conventions of the classification take precedence over guidelines. These guidelines are based on the coding and sequencing instructions in the Tabular List and Alphabetic Index of *ICD-10-CM*, but provide additional instruction. Adherence to these guidelines when assigning *ICD-10-CM* diagnosis codes is required under the Health Insurance Portability and Accountability Act (HIPAA). The diagnosis codes (Tabular List and Alphabetic Index) have been adopted under HIPAA for all healthcare settings. A joint effort between the healthcare provider and the coder is essential to achieve complete and accurate documentation, code assignment, and reporting of diagnoses and procedures. These guidelines have been developed to assist both the healthcare provider and the coder in identifying those diagnoses that are to be reported. The importance of consistent, complete documentation in the medical record cannot be overemphasized. Without such documentation, accurate coding cannot be achieved. The entire record should be reviewed to determine the specific reason for the encounter and the conditions treated.

The term encounter is used for all settings, including hospital admissions. In the context of these guidelines, the term provider is used throughout the guidelines to mean physician or any qualified health care practitioner who is legally accountable for establishing the patient's diagnosis. Only this set of guidelines, approved by the Cooperating Parties, is official.

The guidelines are organized into sections. Section I includes the structure and conventions of the classification and general guidelines that apply to the entire classification, and chapter-specific guidelines that correspond to the chapters as they are arranged in the classification. Section II includes guidelines for selection of principal diagnosis for non-outpatient settings. Section III includes guidelines for reporting additional diagnoses in non-outpatient settings. Section IV is for outpatient coding and reporting. It is necessary to review all sections of the guidelines to fully understand all the rules and instructions needed to code properly.

Section I. Conventions, general coding guidelines, and chapter-specific guidelines XIX

- A. Conventions for the *ICD-10-CM* XIX
   1. The Alphabetic Index and Tabular List XIX
   2. Format and Structure XIX
   3. Use of codes for reporting purposes XIX
   4. Placeholder character XX
   5. 7th Characters.. XX
   6. Abbreviations XX
      - a. Alphabetic Index abbreviations XX
      - b. Tabular List abbreviations XX
   7. Punctuation XX
   8. Use of "and" XX
   9. Other and Unspecified codes XX
      - a. "Other" codes XX
      - b. "Unspecified" codes XX
   10. Includes Notes XX
   11. Inclusion terms XX
   12. Excludes Notes XX
       - a. Excludes1 XX
       - b. Excludes2 XXI
   13. Etiology/manifestation convention ("code first," "use additional code," and "in diseases classified elsewhere" notes) XXI
   14. "And" XXI
   15. "With" XXI
   16. "See" and "See Also" XXII
   17. "Code also" note XXII
   18. Default codes XXII
   19. Code assignment and Clinical Criteria..........................XXII
- B. General Coding Guidelines XXII
   1. Locating a code in the *ICD-10-CM* XXII
   2. Level of Detail in Coding XXII
   3. Code or codes from A00.0 through T88.9, Z00–Z99.8, U00-U85 XXII
   4. Signs and symptoms XXII

5. Conditions that are an integral part of a disease process XXII
6. Conditions that are not an integral part of a disease process XXII
7. Multiple coding for a single condition XXII
8. Acute and Chronic Conditions XXIII
9. Combination Code XXIII
10. Sequela (Late Effects) XXIII
11. Impending or Threatened Condition XXIII
12. Reporting Same Diagnosis Code More Than Once XXIII
13. Laterality XXIV
14. Documentation by Clinicians Other Than the Patient's Provider XXIV
15. Syndromes XXIV
16. Documentation of Complications of Care XXIV
17. Borderline Diagnosis XXV
18. Use of Sign/Symptom/Unspecified Codes XXV
19. Coding for Healthcare Encounters in Hurricane Aftermath XXV
    a. Use of External Cause of Morbidity Codes XXV
    b. Sequencing of External Causes of Morbidity Codes..XXV
    c. Other External Causes of Morbidity Code Issues XXVI
    d. Use of Z codes XXVI

C. Chapter-Specific Coding Guidelines XXVI

Section II. Selection of Principal Diagnosis XXVI

Section III. Reporting Additional Diagnoses XXVI

Section IV. Diagnostic Coding and Reporting Guidelines for Outpatient Services XXVI

A. Selection of first-listed condition XXVII
   1. Outpatient Surgery XXVII
   2. Observation Stay XXVII
B. Codes from A00.0 through T88.9, Z00–Z99, U00–U85 XXVII
C. Accurate reporting of *ICD-10-CM* diagnosis codes XXVII
D. Codes that describe symptoms and signs XXVII
E. Encounters for circumstances other than a disease or injury XXVII
F. Level of Detail in Coding XXVII
   1. *ICD-10-CM* codes with 3, 4, 5, 6, or 7 characters XXVII
   2. Use of full number of characters required for a code .XXVII
   3. Highest level of specificity XXVII
G. *ICD-10-CM* code for the diagnosis, condition, problem, or other reason for encounter/visit XXVII
H. Uncertain diagnosis XXVII
I. Chronic diseases XXVIII
J. Code all documented conditions that coexist XXVIII
K. Patients receiving diagnostic services only XXVIII
L. Patients receiving therapeutic services only XXVIII

M. Patients receiving preoperative evaluations only XXVIII
N. Ambulatory surgery XXVIII
O. Routine outpatient prenatal visits XXVIII
P. Encounters for general medical examinations with abnormal findings XXVIII
Q. Encounters for routine health screenings XXVIII

Section I. Conventions, general coding guidelines, and chapter-specific guidelines

The conventions, general guidelines, and chapter-specific guidelines are applicable to all health care settings unless otherwise indicated. The conventions and instructions of the classification take precedence over guidelines.

A. Conventions for the *ICD-10-CM*

The conventions for the *ICD-10-CM* are the general rules for use of the classification independent of the guidelines. These conventions are incorporated within the Alphabetic Index and Tabular List of the *ICD-10-CM* as instructional notes.

1. The Alphabetic Index and Tabular List

The *ICD-10-CM* is divided into the Alphabetic Index, an alphabetical list of terms and their corresponding code, and the Tabular List, a structured list of codes divided into chapters based on body system or condition. The Alphabetic Index consists of the following parts: the Index of Diseases and Injury, the Index of External Causes of Injury, the Table of Neoplasms, and the Table of Drugs and Chemicals.

See Chapter 2, Neoplasms

See Chapter 19, Adverse effects, poisoning, underdosing and toxic effects

2. Format and Structure

The *ICD-10-CM* Tabular List contains categories, subcategories, and codes. Characters for categories, subcategories, and codes may be either a letter or a number. All categories are 3 characters. A three-character category that has no further subdivision is equivalent to a code. Subcategories are either 4 or 5 characters. Codes may be 3, 4, 5, 6, or 7 characters. That is, each level of subdivision after a category is a subcategory. The final level of subdivision is a code. Codes that have applicable 7th characters are still referred to as codes, not subcategories. A code that has an applicable 7th character is considered invalid without the 7th character.

The *ICD-10-CM* uses an indented format for ease in reference.

3. Use of codes for reporting purposes

For reporting purposes only codes are permissible, not categories or subcategories, and any applicable 7th character is required.

4. Placeholder character

The *ICD-10-CM* utilizes a placeholder character "X." The "X" is used as a placeholder at certain codes to allow for future expansion. An example of this is at the poisoning, adverse effect and underdosing codes, categories T36-T50. Where a placeholder exists, the X must be used in order for the code to be considered a valid code.

5. 7th Characters

Certain *ICD-10-CM* categories have applicable 7th characters. The applicable 7th character is required for all codes within the category, or as the notes in the Tabular List instruct. The 7th character must always be the 7th character in the data field. If a code that requires a 7th character is not 6 characters, a placeholder X must be used to fill in the empty characters.

6. Abbreviations

a. Alphabetic Index abbreviations

NEC "Not elsewhere classifiable": This abbreviation in the Alphabetic Index represents "other specified." When a specific code is not available for a condition, the Alphabetic Index directs the coder to the "other specified" code in the Tabular List.

NOS "Not otherwise specified": This abbreviation is the equivalent of unspecified.

b. Tabular List abbreviations

NEC "Not elsewhere classifiable": This abbreviation in the Tabular List represents "other specified." When a specific code is not available for a condition, the Tabular List includes an NEC entry under a code to identify the code as the "other specified" code.

NOS "Not otherwise specified": This abbreviation is the equivalent of unspecified.

7. Punctuation

[ ] Brackets are used in the Tabular List to enclose synonyms, alternative wording, or explanatory phrases. Brackets are used in the Alphabetic Index to identify manifestation codes.

( ) Parentheses are used in both the Alphabetic Index and Tabular List to enclose supplementary words that may be present or absent in the statement of a disease or procedure without affecting the code number to which it is assigned. The terms within the parentheses are referred to as *nonessential modifiers.* The nonessential modifiers in the Alphabetic Index to Diseases apply to subterms following a main term, except when a nonessential modifier and a subentry are mutually exclusive, in which case the subentry takes precedence. For example, in the *ICD-10-CM* Alphabetic Index under the main term *Enteritis,* "acute"

is a nonessential modifier and "chronic" is a subentry. In this case, the nonessential modifier "acute" does not apply to the subentry "chronic."

: Colons are used in the Tabular List after an incomplete term, which needs one or more of the modifiers following the colon to make it assignable to a given category.

8. Use of "and"

See Section I.A.14 , "And"

9. Other and Unspecified codes

a. "Other" codes

Codes titled "other" or "other specified" are for use when the information in the medical record provides detail for which a specific code does not exist. Alphabetic Index entries with NEC in the line designate "other" codes in the Tabular List. These Alphabetic Index entries represent specific disease entities for which no specific code exists, so the term is included within an "other" code.

b. "Unspecified" codes

Codes titled "unspecified" are for use when the information in the medical record is insufficient to assign a more specific code. For those categories for which an unspecified code is not provided, the "other specified" code may represent both other and unspecified.

See Section I.B. 18, "Use of Sign/Symptom/ Unspecified Codes"

10. Includes Notes

This note appears immediately under a three-character code title to further define, or give examples of, the content of the category.

11. Inclusion terms

List of terms is included under some codes. These terms are the conditions for which that code is to be used. The terms may be synonyms of the code title, or, in the case of "other specified" codes, the terms are a list of the various conditions assigned to that code. The inclusion terms are not necessarily exhaustive. Additional terms found only in the Alphabetic Index may also be assigned to a code.

12. Excludes Notes

The *ICD-10-CM* has two types of excludes notes. Each type of note has a different definition for use, but they are all similar in that they indicate that codes excluded from each other are independent of each other.

a. Excludes1

A type 1 Excludes note is a pure excludes note. It means "NOT CODED HERE!" An Excludes1 note indicates that the code excluded should never be used at the same time as the code above the Excludes1 note. An Excludes1 is used when two conditions cannot occur together, such as a congenital form versus an acquired form of the same condition.

An exception to the Excludes1 definition is the circumstance when the two conditions are unrelated to each other. If it is not clear whether the two conditions involving an Excludes1 note are related or not, query the provider. For example, code F45.8, Other somatoform disorders, has an Excludes1 note for "sleep related teeth grinding (G47.63)," because "teeth grinding" is an inclusion term under F45.8. Only one of these two codes should be assigned for teeth grinding. However psychogenic dysmenorrhea is also an inclusion term under F45.8, and a patient could have both this condition and sleep related teeth grinding. In this case, the two conditions are clearly unrelated to each other, and so it would be appropriate to report F45.8 and G47.63 together.

b. Excludes2

A type 2 Excludes note represents "Not included here." An Excludes2 note indicates that the condition excluded is not part of the condition represented by the code, but a patient may have both conditions at the same time. When an Excludes2 note appears under a code, it is acceptable to use both the code and the excluded code together, when appropriate.

13. Etiology/manifestation convention ("code first," "use additional code," and "in diseases classified elsewhere" notes)

Certain conditions have both an underlying etiology and multiple body system manifestations due to the underlying etiology. For such conditions, the *ICD-10-CM* has a coding convention that requires the underlying condition be sequenced first, if applicable, followed by the manifestation. Wherever such a combination exists, there is a "use additional code" note at the etiology code and a "code first" note at the manifestation code. These instructional notes indicate the proper sequencing order of the codes, etiology followed by manifestation.

In most cases the manifestation codes will have in the code title, "in diseases classified elsewhere." Codes with this title are a component of the etiology/ manifestation convention. The code title indicates that it is a manifestation code. "In diseases classified elsewhere" codes are never permitted to be used as first listed or principal diagnosis codes. They must be used in conjunction with an underlying condition code and they must be listed following the underlying condition. See category F02, Dementia in other diseases

classified elsewhere, for an example of this convention.

There are manifestation codes that do not have "in diseases classified elsewhere" in the title. For such codes, there is a "use additional code" note at the etiology code and a "code first" note at the manifestation code, and the rules for sequencing apply.

In addition to the notes in the Tabular List, these conditions also have a specific Alphabetic Index entry structure. In the Alphabetic Index both conditions are listed together with the etiology code first, followed by the manifestation codes in brackets. The code in brackets is always to be sequenced second.

An example of the etiology/manifestation convention is dementia with Parkinson's disease. In the Alphabetic Index, code G20 is listed first, followed by code F02.80 or F02.81- in brackets. Code G20 represents the underlying etiology, Parkinson's disease, and must be sequenced first, whereas codes F02.80 and F02.81- represent the manifestation of dementia in diseases classified elsewhere, with or without behavioral disturbance.

"Code first" and "Use additional code" notes are also used as sequencing rules in the classification for certain codes that are not part of an etiology/manifestation combination.

See Section I.B.7., "Multiple coding for a single condition."

14. "And"

The word "and" should be interpreted to mean either "and" or "or" when it appears in a title.

For example, cases of "tuberculosis of bones," "tuberculosis of joints," and "tuberculosis of bones and joints" are classified to subcategory A18.0, Tuberculosis of bones and joints.

15. "With"

The word "with" or "in" should be interpreted to mean "associated with" or "due to" when it appears in a code title, the Alphabetic Index (either under a main term or subterm), or an instructional note in the Tabular List. The classification presumes a causal relationship between the two conditions linked by these terms in the Alphabetic Index or Tabular List. These conditions should be coded as related even in the absence of provider documentation explicitly linking them, unless the documentation clearly states the conditions are unrelated or when another guideline exists that specifically requires a documented linkage between two conditions (e.g., sepsis guideline for "acute organ dysfunction that is not clearly associated with the sepsis"). For conditions not specifically linked by these relational terms in the classification or when a guideline requires that a linkage between two conditions be explicitly documented, provider documentation must link the conditions in order to code them as related.

The word "with" in the Alphabetic Index is sequenced immediately following the main term or subterm, not in alphabetical order.

16. "See" and "See Also"

The "see" instruction following a main term in the Alphabetic Index indicates that another term should be referenced. It is necessary to go to the main term referenced with the "see" note to locate the correct code.

A "see also" instruction following a main term in the Alphabetic Index instructs that there is another main term that may also be referenced that may provide additional Alphabetic Index entries that may be useful. It is not necessary to follow the "see also" note when the original main term provides the necessary code.

17. "Code also" note

A "code also" note instructs that two codes may be required to fully describe a condition, but this note does not provide sequencing direction. The sequencing depends on the circumstances of the encounter.

18. Default codes

A code listed next to a main term in the *ICD-10-CM* Alphabetic Index is referred to as a default code. The default code represents that condition that is most commonly associated with the main term or is the unspecified code for the condition. If a condition is documented in a medical record (for example, appendicitis) without any additional information, such as acute or chronic, the default code should be assigned.

19. Code assignment and Clinical Criteria

The assignment of a diagnosis code is based on the provider's diagnostic statement that the condition exists. The provider's statement that the patient has a particular condition is sufficient. Code assignment is not based on clinical criteria used by the provider to establish the diagnosis. If there is conflicting medical record documentation, query the provider.

B. General Coding Guidelines

1. Locating a code in the *ICD-10-CM*

To select a code in the classification that corresponds to a diagnosis or reason for visit documented in a medical record, first locate the term in the Alphabetic Index, and then verify the code in the Tabular List. Read and be guided by instructional notations that appear in both the Alphabetic Index and the Tabular List.

It is essential to use both the Alphabetic Index and Tabular List when locating and assigning a code. The Alphabetic Index does not always provide the full

code. Selection of the full code, including laterality and any applicable 7th character, can only be done in the Tabular List. A dash (-) at the end of an Alphabetic Index entry indicates that additional characters are required. Even if a dash is not included at the Alphabetic Index entry, it is necessary to refer to the Tabular List to verify that no 7th character is required.

2. Level of Detail in Coding

Diagnosis codes are to be used and reported at their highest number of characters available and to the highest level of specificity documented in the medical record.

ICD-10-CM diagnosis codes are composed of codes with 3, 4, 5, 6, or 7 characters. Codes with three characters are included in *ICD-10-CM* as the heading of a category of codes that may be further subdivided by the use of fourth and/or fifth characters and/or sixth characters, which provide greater detail.

A three-character code is to be used only if it is not further subdivided. A code is invalid if it has not been coded to the full number of characters required for that code, including the 7th character, if applicable.

3. Code or codes from A00.0 through T88.9, Z00–Z99.8, U00-U85

The appropriate code or codes from A00.0 through T88.9, Z00–Z99.8 and U00–U85 must be used to identify diagnoses, symptoms, conditions, problems, complaints, or other reason(s) for the encounter/visit.

4. Signs and symptoms

Codes that describe symptoms and signs, as opposed to diagnoses, are acceptable for reporting purposes when a related definitive diagnosis has not been established (confirmed) by the provider. Chapter 18 of *ICD-10-CM*, Symptoms, Signs, and Abnormal Clinical and Laboratory Findings, Not Elsewhere Classified (codes R00.0 – R99), contains many but not all codes for symptoms.

See Section I.B.18., "Use of Signs/Symptom/ Unspecified Codes"

5. Conditions that are an integral part of a disease process

Signs and symptoms that are associated routinely with a disease process should not be assigned as additional codes, unless otherwise instructed by the classification.

6. Conditions that are not an integral part of a disease process

Additional signs and symptoms that may not be associated routinely with a disease process should be coded when present.

7. Multiple coding for a single condition

In addition to the etiology/manifestation convention that requires two codes to fully describe a single condition that affects multiple body systems, there are other single conditions that also require more than one code. "Use additional code" notes are found in the Tabular List at codes that are not part of an etiology/ manifestation pair where a secondary code is useful to fully describe a condition. The sequencing rule is the same as the etiology/manifestation pair; "use additional code" indicates that a secondary code should be added, if known.

For example, for bacterial infections that are not included in Chapter 1, a secondary code from category B95, Streptococcus, Staphylococcus, and Enterococcus, as the cause of diseases classified elsewhere, or B96, Other bacterial agents as the cause of diseases classified elsewhere, may be required to identify the bacterial organism causing the infection. A "use additional code" note will normally be found at the infectious disease code, indicating a need for the organism code to be added as a secondary code.

"Code first" notes are also under certain codes that are not specifically manifestation codes but may be due to an underlying cause. When there is a "code first" note and an underlying condition is present, the underlying condition should be sequenced first, if known.

"Code, if applicable, any causal condition first" notes indicate that this code may be assigned as a principal diagnosis when the causal condition is unknown or not applicable. If a causal condition is known, then the code for that condition should be sequenced as the principal or first-listed diagnosis.

Multiple codes may be needed for sequela, complication codes, and obstetric codes to more fully describe a condition. See the specific guidelines for these conditions for further instruction.

8. Acute and Chronic Conditions

If the same condition is described as both acute (subacute) and chronic, and separate subentries exist in the Alphabetic Index at the same indentation level, code both and sequence the acute (subacute) code first.

9. Combination Code

A combination code is a single code used to classify:

Two diagnoses, or

A diagnosis with an associated secondary process (manifestation)

A diagnosis with an associated complication

Combination codes are identified by referring to subterm entries in the Alphabetic Index and by reading the inclusion and exclusion notes in the Tabular List.

Assign only the combination code when that code fully identifies the diagnostic conditions involved

or when the Alphabetic Index so directs. Multiple coding should not be used when the classification provides a combination code that clearly identifies all of the elements documented in the diagnosis. When the combination code lacks necessary specificity in describing the manifestation or complication, an additional code should be used as a secondary code.

10. Sequela (Late Effects)

A sequela is the residual effect (condition produced) after the acute phase of an illness or injury has terminated. There is no time limit on when a sequela code can be used. The residual may be apparent early, such as in cerebral infarction, or it may occur months or years later, such as that due to a previous injury. Examples of sequela include: scar formation resulting from a burn, deviated septum due to a nasal fracture, and infertility due to tubal occlusion from old tuberculosis. Coding of sequela generally requires two codes sequenced in the following order: the condition or nature of the sequela is sequenced first. The sequela code is sequenced second.

· An exception to the above guidelines are those instances where the code for the sequela is followed by a manifestation code identified in the Tabular List and title, or the sequela code has been expanded (at the fourth, fifth or sixth character levels) to include the manifestation(s). The code for the acute phase of an illness or injury that led to the sequela is never used with a code for the late effect.

See Chapter 19, "Application of 7th Characters in Chapter 19"

11. Impending or Threatened Condition

Code any condition described at the time of discharge as "impending" or "threatened" as follows:

If it did occur, code as confirmed diagnosis. If it did not occur, reference the Alphabetic Index to determine if the condition has a subentry term for "impending" or "threatened" and also reference main term entries for "Impending" and for "Threatened." If the subterms are listed, assign the given code. If the subterms are not listed, code the existing underlying condition(s) and not the condition described as impending or threatened.

12. Reporting Same Diagnosis Code More Than Once

Each unique *ICD-10-CM* diagnosis code may be reported only once for an encounter. This applies to bilateral conditions when there are no distinct codes identifying laterality or two different conditions classified to the same *ICD-10-CM* diagnosis code.

13. Laterality

Some *ICD-10-CM* codes indicate laterality, specifying whether the condition occurs on the left, right or is bilateral. If no bilateral code is provided and the condition is bilateral, assign separate codes for both the left and right side. If the side is not identified in the medical record, assign the code for the unspecified side.

When a patient has a bilateral condition and each side is treated during separate encounters, assign the "bilateral" code (as the condition still exists on both sides), including for the encounter to treat the first side. For the second encounter for treatment after one side has previously been treated and the condition no longer exists on that side, assign the appropriate unilateral code for the side where the condition still exists (e.g., cataract surgery performed on each eye in separate encounters). The bilateral code would not be assigned for the subsequent encounter, as the patient no longer has the condition in the previously-treated site. If the treatment on the first side did not completely resolve the condition, then the bilateral code would still be appropriate.

When laterality is not documented by the patient's provider, code assignment for the affected side may be based on medical record documentation from other clinicians. If there is conflicting medical record documentation regarding the affected side, the patient's attending provider should be queried for clarification. Codes for "unspecified" side should rarely be used, such as when the documentation in the record is insufficient to determine the affected side and it is not possible to obtain clarification.

14. Documentation by Clinicians Other Than the Patient's Provider

Code assignment is based on the documentation by the patient's provider (i.e., physician or other qualified healthcare practitioner legally accountable for establishing the patient's diagnosis). There are a few exceptions when code assignment may be based on medical record documentation from clinicians who are not the patient's provider (ie, physician or other qualified healthcare practitioner legally accountable for establishing the patient's diagnosis). In this context, "clinicians" other than the patient's provider refer to healthcare professionals permitted, based on regulatory or accreditation requirements or internal hospital policies, to document in a patient's official medical record.

These exceptions include codes for:

- Body Mass Index (BMI)
- Depth of non-pressure chronic ulcers
- Pressure ulcer stage
- Coma scale
- NIH stroke scale (NIHSS)
- Social determinants of health (SDOH) classified to Chapter 21
- Laterality
- Blood alcohol level
- Underimmunization status

This information is typically, or may be, documented by other clinicians involved in the care of the patient (e.g., a dietitian often documents the BMI, a nurse often documents the pressure ulcer stages, and an emergency medical technician often documents the coma scale). However, the associated diagnosis (such as overweight, obesity, acute stroke, pressure ulcer, or a condition classifiable to category F10, Alcohol related disorders) must be documented by the patient's provider. If there is conflicting medical record documentation, either from the same clinician or different clinicians, the patient's attending provider should be queried for clarification.

The BMI, coma scale, NIHSS, blood alcohol level codes, codes for social determinants of health and underimmunization status should only be reported as secondary diagnoses.

See Section I.C.21.c.17 for additional information regarding coding social determinants of health.

15. Syndromes

Follow the Alphabetic Index guidance when coding syndromes. In the absence of Alphabetic Index guidance, assign codes for the documented manifestations of the syndrome. Additional codes for manifestations that are not an integral part of the disease process may also be assigned when the condition does not have a unique code.

16. Documentation of Complications of Care

Code assignment is based on the provider's documentation of the relationship between the condition and the care or procedure, unless otherwise instructed by the classification. The guideline extends to any complications of care, regardless of the chapter the code is located in. It is important to note that not all conditions that occur during or following medical care or surgery are classified as complications. There must be a cause-and-effect relationship between the care provided and the condition, and the documentation must support that the condition is clinically significant. It is not necessary for the provider to explicitly document the term "complication." For example, if the condition alters the course of the surgery as documented in the operative report, then it would be appropriate to report a complication code. Query the provider for clarification if the documentation is not clear as to the relationship between the condition and the care or procedure.

17. Borderline Diagnosis

If the provider documents a "borderline" diagnosis at the time of discharge, the diagnosis is coded as confirmed, unless the classification provides a specific entry (eg, borderline diabetes). If a borderline condition has a specific index entry in *ICD-10-CM*, it should be coded as such. Since borderline conditions are not uncertain diagnoses, no distinction is made between the care setting (inpatient versus outpatient). Whenever the documentation is unclear regarding a borderline condition, coders are encouraged to query for clarification.

18. Use of Sign/Symptom/Unspecified Codes

Sign/symptom and "unspecified" codes have acceptable, even necessary, uses. While specific diagnosis codes should be reported when they are supported by the available medical record documentation and clinical knowledge of the patient's health condition, there are instances when signs/ symptoms or unspecified codes are the best choices for accurately reflecting the healthcare encounter. Each health care encounter should be coded to the level of certainty known for that encounter.

As stated in the introductory section of these official coding guidelines, a joint effort between the healthcare provider and the coder is essential to achieve complete and accurate documentation, code assignment, and reporting of diagnoses and procedures. The importance of consistent, complete documentation in the medical record cannot be overemphasized. Without such documentation accurate coding cannot be achieved. The entire record should be reviewed to determine the specific reason for the encounter and the conditions treated.

If a definitive diagnosis has not been established by the end of the encounter, it is appropriate to report codes for sign(s) and/or symptom(s) in lieu of a definitive diagnosis. When sufficient clinical information isn't known or available about a particular health condition to assign a more specific code, it is acceptable to report the appropriate "unspecified" code (eg, a diagnosis of pneumonia has been determined, but not the specific type). Unspecified codes should be reported when they are the codes that most accurately reflect what is known about the patient's condition

at the time of that particular encounter. It would be inappropriate to select a specific code that is not supported by the medical record documentation or conduct medically unnecessary diagnostic testing in order to determine a more specific code.

19. Coding for Healthcare Encounters in Hurricane Aftermath

a. Use of External Cause of Morbidity Codes

An external cause of morbidity code should be assigned to identify the cause of the injury(ies) incurred as a result of the hurricane. The use of external cause of morbidity codes is supplemental to the application of *ICD-10-CM* codes. External cause of morbidity codes are never to be recorded as a principal diagnosis (first-listed in non-inpatient settings). The appropriate injury code should be sequenced before any external cause codes. The external cause of morbidity codes capture how the injury or health condition happened (cause), the intent (unintentional or accidental; or intentional, such as suicide or assault), the place where the event occurred, the activity of the patient at the time of the event, and the person's status (e.g., civilian, military). They should not be assigned for encounters to treat hurricane victims' medical conditions when no injury, adverse effect or poisoning is involved. External cause of morbidity codes should be assigned for each encounter for care and treatment of the injury. External cause of morbidity codes may be assigned in all health care settings. For the purpose of capturing complete and accurate *ICD-10-CM* data in the aftermath of the hurricane, a healthcare setting should be considered as any location where medical care is provided by licensed healthcare professionals.

b. Sequencing of External Causes of Morbidity Codes

Codes for cataclysmic events, such as a hurricane, take priority over all other external cause codes except child and adult abuse and terrorism and should be sequenced before other external cause of injury codes. Assign as many external cause of morbidity codes as necessary to fully explain each cause. For example, if an injury occurs as a result of a building collapse during the hurricane, external cause codes for both the hurricane and the building collapse should be assigned, with the external causes code for hurricane being sequenced as the first external cause code. For injuries incurred as a direct result of the hurricane, assign the appropriate code(s) for the injuries, followed by the code X37.0-, Hurricane (with the appropriate 7th character), and any other applicable external cause of injury codes. Code X37.0- also should be assigned when an injury is incurred as a result of flooding caused by a levee breaking related to the hurricane. Code X38.-, Flood (with the appropriate 7th character), should be assigned when an injury is from flooding resulting directly from the storm. Code X36.0-, Collapse of dam or man-made structure, should not be assigned when the cause of the collapse is due to the hurricane. Use of code X36.0- is limited to collapses of man-made structures due to earth surface movements, not due to storm surges directly from a hurricane.

c. Other External Causes of Morbidity Code Issues

For injuries that are not a direct result of the hurricane, such as an evacuee that has incurred an injury as a result of a motor vehicle accident, assign the appropriate external cause of morbidity code(s) to describe the cause of the injury, but do not assign code X37.0-, Hurricane. If it is not clear whether the injury was a direct result of the hurricane, assume the injury is due to the hurricane and assign code X37.0-, Hurricane, as well as any other applicable external cause of morbidity codes. In addition to code X37.0-, Hurricane, other possible applicable external cause of morbidity codes include:

X30-, Exposure to excessive natural heat
X31-, Exposure to excessive natural cold
X38-, Flood

d. Use of Z Codes

Z codes (other reasons for healthcare encounters) may be assigned as appropriate to further explain the reasons for presenting for healthcare services, including transfers between healthcare facilities, or provide additional information relevant to a patient encounter. The *ICD-10-CM Official Guidelines for Coding and Reporting* identify which codes may be assigned as principal or first-listed diagnosis only, secondary diagnosis only, or principal/first-listed or secondary (depending on the circumstances). Possible applicable Z codes include:

Z59.0-, Homelessness
Z59.1, Inadequate housing
Z59.5, Extreme poverty
Z75.1, Person awaiting admission to adequate facility elsewhere
Z75.3, Unavailability and inaccessibility of health-care facilities

Z75.4, Unavailability and inaccessibility of other helping agencies
Z76.2, Encounter for health supervision and care of other healthy infant and child
Z99.12, Encounter for respirator [ventilator] dependence during power failure

The external cause of morbidity codes and the Z codes listed above are not an all-inclusive list. Other codes may be applicable to the encounter based upon the documentation. Assign as many codes as necessary to fully explain each healthcare encounter. Since patient history information may be very limited, use any available documentation to assign the appropriate external cause of morbidity and Z codes.

C. Chapter-Specific Coding Guidelines

See each chapter for specific guidelines.

Section II. Selection of Principal Diagnosis

Excluded as not relevant to provider-based coding. Refer to the full *ICD-10-CM* manual if needed.

Section III. Reporting Additional Diagnoses

Excluded as not relevant to provider-based coding. Refer to the full *ICD-10-CM* manual if needed.

Section IV. Diagnostic Coding and Reporting Guidelines for Outpatient Services

These coding guidelines for outpatient diagnoses have been approved for use by hospitals/providers in coding and reporting hospital-based outpatient services and provider-based office visits.

Guidelines in Section I, Conventions, general coding guidelines and chapter-specific guidelines, should also be applied for outpatient services and office visits.

Information about the use of certain abbreviations, punctuation, symbols, and other conventions used in the *ICD-10-CM* Tabular List (code numbers and titles), can be found in Section IA of these guidelines, under "Conventions Used in the Tabular List." Section I.B. contains general guidelines that apply to the entire classification. Section I.C. contains chapter-specific guidelines that correspond to the chapters as they are arranged in the classification. Information about the correct sequence to use in finding a code is also described in Section I.

The terms encounter and visit are often used interchangeably in describing outpatient service contacts and, therefore, appear together in these guidelines without distinguishing one from the other.

Though the conventions and general guidelines apply to all settings, coding guidelines for outpatient and provider reporting of diagnoses will vary in a number of instances from those for inpatient diagnoses, recognizing that:

The Uniform Hospital Discharge Data Set (UHDDS) definition of principal diagnosis does not apply to hospital-based outpatient services and provider-based office visits.

Coding guidelines for inconclusive diagnoses (probable, suspected, rule out, etc.) were developed for inpatient reporting and do not apply to outpatients.

A. Selection of first-listed condition

In the outpatient setting, the term first-listed diagnosis is used in lieu of principal diagnosis.

In determining the first-listed diagnosis the coding conventions of *ICD-10-CM*, as well as the general and disease specific guidelines, take precedence over the outpatient guidelines.

Diagnoses often are not established at the time of the initial encounter/visit. It may take two or more visits before the diagnosis is confirmed.

The most critical rule involves beginning the search for the correct code assignment through the Alphabetic Index. Never search initially in the Tabular List as this will lead to coding errors.

1. Outpatient Surgery

When a patient presents for outpatient surgery (same day surgery), code the reason for the surgery as the first-listed diagnosis (reason for the encounter), even if the surgery is not performed due to a contraindication.

2. Observation Stay

When a patient is admitted for observation for a medical condition, assign a code for the medical condition as the first-listed diagnosis.

When a patient presents for outpatient surgery and develops complications requiring admission to observation, code the reason for the surgery as the first reported diagnosis (reason for the encounter), followed by codes for the complications as secondary diagnoses.

B. Codes from A00.0 through T88.9, Z00 – Z99, *U00–U85*

The appropriate code(s) from A00.0 through T88.9, Z00–Z99 and U00–U85 must be used to identify diagnoses, symptoms, conditions, problems, complaints, or other reason(s) for the encounter/visit.

C. Accurate reporting of *ICD-10-CM* diagnosis codes

For accurate reporting of *ICD-10-CM* diagnosis codes, the documentation should describe the patient's condition, using terminology which includes specific diagnoses as well as symptoms, problems, or reasons for the encounter. There are *ICD-10-CM* codes to describe all of these.

D. Codes that describe symptoms and signs

Codes that describe symptoms and signs, as opposed to diagnoses, are acceptable for reporting purposes when a diagnosis has not been established (confirmed) by the provider. Chapter 18 of *ICD-10-CM*, Symptoms, Signs, and Abnormal Clinical and Laboratory Findings Not Elsewhere Classified (codes R00 – R99) contains many, but not all codes for symptoms.

E. Encounters for circumstances other than a disease or injury

ICD-10-CM provides codes to deal with encounters for circumstances other than a disease or injury. The Factors Influencing Health Status and Contact with Health Services codes (Z00 – Z99) are provided to deal with occasions when circumstances other than a disease or injury are recorded as diagnosis or problems.

See Chapter 21, "Factors influencing health status and contact with health services."

F. Level of Detail in Coding

1. *ICD-10-CM* codes with 3, 4, 5, 6, or 7 characters

ICD-10-CM is composed of codes with 3, 4, 5, 6, or 7 characters. Codes with three characters are included in *ICD-10-CM* as the heading of a category of codes that may be further subdivided by the use of fourth, fifth, sixth, or seventh characters to provide greater specificity.

2. Use of full number of characters required for a code

A three-character code is to be used only if it is not further subdivided. A code is invalid if it has not been coded to the full number of characters required for that code, including the 7th character, if applicable.

3. Highest level of specificity

Code to the highest level of specificity when supported by the medical record documentation.

G. *ICD-10-CM* code for the diagnosis, condition, problem, or other reason for encounter/visit

List first the *ICD-10-CM* code for the diagnosis, condition, problem, or other reason for encounter/visit shown in the medical record to be chiefly responsible for the services provided. List additional codes that describe any coexisting conditions. In some cases, the first-listed diagnosis may be a symptom when a diagnosis has not been established (confirmed) by the provider.

H. Uncertain diagnosis

Do not code diagnoses documented as "probable," "suspected," "questionable," "rule out," "compatible with," "consistent with," or "working diagnosis" or other similar terms indicating uncertainty. Rather, code the condition(s) to the highest degree of certainty for that encounter/visit, such as symptoms, signs, abnormal test results, or other reason for the visit.

Please note: This differs from the coding practices used by short-term, acute care, long-term care and psychiatric hospitals.

I. Chronic diseases

Chronic diseases treated on an ongoing basis may be coded and reported as many times as the patient receives treatment and care for the condition(s)

J. Code all documented conditions that coexist

Code all documented conditions that coexist at the time of the encounter/visit and that require or affect patient care, treatment or management. Do not code conditions that were previously treated and no longer exist. However, history codes (categories Z80–Z87) may be used as secondary codes if the historical condition or family history has an impact on current care or influences treatment.

K. Patients receiving diagnostic services only

For patients receiving diagnostic services only during an encounter/visit, sequence first the diagnosis, condition, problem, or other reason for encounter/visit shown in the medical record to be chiefly responsible for the outpatient services provided during the encounter/visit. Codes for other diagnoses (eg, chronic conditions) may be sequenced as additional diagnoses.

For encounters for routine laboratory/radiology testing in the absence of any signs, symptoms, or associated diagnosis, assign Z01.89, Encounter for other specified special examinations. If routine testing is performed during the same encounter as a test to evaluate a sign, symptom, or diagnosis, it is appropriate to assign both the Z code and the code describing the reason for the non-routine test.

For outpatient encounters for diagnostic tests that have been interpreted by a physician, and the final report is available at the time of coding, code any confirmed or definitive diagnosis(es) documented in the interpretation. Do not code related signs and symptoms as additional diagnoses.

Please note: This differs from the coding practice in the hospital inpatient setting regarding abnormal findings on test results.

L. Patients receiving therapeutic services only

For patients receiving therapeutic services only during an encounter/visit, sequence first the diagnosis, condition, problem, or other reason for encounter/visit shown in the medical record to be chiefly responsible for the outpatient services provided during the encounter/visit. Codes for other diagnoses (eg, chronic conditions) may be sequenced as additional diagnoses.

The only exception to this rule is that when the primary reason for the admission/encounter is chemotherapy or radiation therapy, the appropriate Z code for the service is listed first, and the diagnosis or problem for which the service is being performed is listed second.

M. Patients receiving preoperative evaluations only

For patients receiving preoperative evaluations only, sequence first a code from subcategory Z01.81, Encounter for pre-procedural examinations, to describe the pre-op consultations. Assign a code for the condition to describe the reason for the surgery as an additional diagnosis. Code also any findings related to the pre-op evaluation.

N. Ambulatory surgery

For ambulatory surgery, code the diagnosis for which the surgery was performed. If the postoperative diagnosis is known to be different from the preoperative diagnosis at the time the diagnosis is confirmed, select the postoperative diagnosis for coding, since it is the most definitive.

O. Routine outpatient prenatal visits

See Chapter 15, Pregnancy, childbirth and the puerperium.

P. Encounters for general medical examinations with abnormal findings

The subcategories for encounters for general medical examinations, Z00.0- and encounter for routine child health examination, Z00.12-, provide codes for with and without abnormal findings. Should a general medical examination result in an abnormal finding, the code for general medical examination with abnormal finding should be assigned as the first-listed diagnosis. An examination with abnormal findings refers to a condition/diagnosis that is newly identified or a change in severity of a chronic condition (such as uncontrolled hypertension, or an acute exacerbation of chronic obstructive pulmonary disease) during a routine physical examination. A secondary code for the abnormal finding should also be coded.

Q. Encounters for routine health screenings

See Chapter 21, Factors influencing health status and contact with health services, Screening

Alphabetic Index

Instructions are listed in *italic font*. The "*see*" instruction indicates it is necessary to reference another term while "*see also*" instruction indicates another main term may provide additional entries. It is not necessary to follow a "*see also*" instruction when the current entry directs to a code for the condition. "*Code*" or "*Code to*" directs to the appropriate reference for a condition.

Punctuation

[ ]—used to identify manifestation codes

( )—enclose nonessential words that do not affect code assignment

:—the colon identifies that a term is incomplete and requires additional modifying terms

- - -the hyphen indicates additional characters are found in the tabular list

A

Aarskog's syndrome Q87.19

Abandonment—*see* Maltreatment

Abasia (-astasia) (hysterical) F44.4

Abderhalden-Kaufmann-Lignac syndrome (cystinosis) E72.04

Abdomen, abdominal—*see also* Disease, diseased

- acute R10.0
- angina K55.1
- muscle deficiency syndrome Q79.4

Abdominalgia—*see* Pain(s), abdominal

Abduction contracture, hip or other joint—*see* Contraction, joint

Aberrant (congenital)—*see also* Malposition, congenital

- artery (peripheral) Q27.8
  - eye Q15.8
  - pulmonary Q25.79
  - retina Q14.1
- endocrine gland NEC Q89.2
- hepatic duct Q44.5
- parathyroid gland Q89.2
- pituitary gland Q89.2
- thymus (gland) Q89.2
- thyroid gland Q89.2

Abiotropy R68.89

Ablepharia, ablepharon Q10.3

Abnormal, abnormality, abnormalities—*see also* Anomaly

- auditory perception H93.29-
- autosomes Q99.9
- basal metabolic rate R94.8
- bleeding time R79.1
- blood amino-acid level R79.83
- blood gas level R79.81
- blood pressure
  - elevated R03.0
- brain scan R94.02
- caloric test R94.138
- chemistry, blood R79.9
  - C-reactive protein R79.82
  - drugs—*see* Findings, abnormal, in blood
  - gas level R79.81
  - pancytopenia D61.818
  - PTT R79.1
- chest sounds (friction) (rales) R09.89
- chromosome, chromosomal Q99.9
  - sex Q99.8
    - female phenotype Q97.9
    - male phenotype Q98.9
- clinical findings NEC R68.89
- coagulation D68.9
  - newborn, transient P61.6
  - profile R79.1
  - time R79.1
- cortisol-binding globulin E27.8
- creatinine clearance R94.4
- development, developmental Q89.9
  - central nervous system Q07.9
- diagnostic imaging
  - abdomen, abdominal region NEC R93.5
  - bladder R93.41
  - coronary circulation R93.1
  - head R93.0

Abnormal, abnormality, abnormalities, *continued*

- heart R93.1
- kidney R93.42-
- lung (field) R91.8
- musculoskeletal system NEC R93.7
- renal pelvis R93.41
- retroperitoneum R93.5
- site specified NEC R93.89
- skull R93.0
- testis R93.81-
- ureter R93.41
- urinary organs, specified R93.49
- echocardiogram R93.1
- electrocardiogram [ECG] [EKG] R94.31
- electroencephalogram [EEG] R94.01
- electrolyte—*see* Imbalance, electrolyte
- electromyogram [EMG] R94.131
- electro-oculogram [EOG] R94.110
- electrophysiological intracardiac studies R94.39
- electroretinogram [ERG] R94.111
- feces (color) (contents) (mucus) R19.5
- function studies
  - auditory R94.120
  - bladder R94.8
  - brain R94.09
  - cardiovascular R94.30
  - ear R94.128
  - endocrine NEC R94.7
  - eye NEC R94.118
  - kidney R94.4
  - liver function test R79.89
  - nervous system
    - central NEC R94.09
    - peripheral NEC R94.138
  - pancreas R94.8
  - placenta R94.8
  - pulmonary R94.2
  - special senses NEC R94.128
  - spleen R94.8
  - thyroid R94.6
  - vestibular R94.121
- gait—*see* Gait abnormality
  - hysterical F44.4
- globulin R77.1
  - cortisol-binding E27.8
- heart
  - rate R00.9
    - specified NEC R00.8
  - shadow R93.1
- hemoglobin (disease) (*see also* Disease, hemoglobin) D58.2
  - trait—*see* Trait, hemoglobin, abnormal
- kidney function test R94.4
- loss of
  - weight R63.4
- Mantoux test R76.11
- movement (disorder)—*see also* Disorder, movement
  - involuntary R25.9
    - spasm R25.2
    - tremor R25.1
- neonatal screening P09.9
  - congenital adrenal hyperplasia P09.2
  - congenital endocrine disease P09.2
  - congenital hematologic disorders P09.3
  - critical congenital heart disease P09.5
  - cystic fibrosis P09.4
  - hemoglobinothies P09.3
  - hypothyroidism P09.2
  - inborn errors of metabolism P09.1
  - neonatal hearing loss P09.6
  - red cell membrane defects P09.3
  - sickle cell P09.3
  - specified NEC P09.8
- oculomotor study R94.113
- palmar creases Q82.8
- partial thromboplastin time (PTT) R79.1
- percussion, chest (tympany) R09.89
- phonocardiogram R94.39
- plasma
  - protein R77.9
    - specified NEC R77.8
  - viscosity R70.1
- posture R29.3

Abnormal, abnormality, abnormalities, *continued*

- prothrombin time (PT) R79.1
- pulmonary
  - artery, congenital Q25.79
  - function, newborn P28.89
  - test results R94.2
- pulsations in neck R00.2
- red blood cell(s) (morphology) (volume) R71.8
- renal function test R94.4
- response to nerve stimulation R94.130
- retinal correspondence H53.31
- retinal function study R94.111
- rhythm, heart—*see also* Arrhythmia
- saliva—*see* Abnormal, specimen
- scan
  - kidney R94.4
  - liver R93.2
  - thyroid R94.6
- serum level (of)
  - acid phosphatase R74.8
  - alkaline phosphatase R74.8
  - amylase R74.8
  - enzymes R74.9
    - specified NEC R74.8
  - lipase R74.8
  - triacylglycerol lipase R74.8
- sinus venosus Q21.1
- specimen
  - specified organ, system and tissue NOS R89.9
- sputum (amount) (color) (odor) R09.3
- stool (color) (contents) (mucus) R19.5
  - bloody K92.1
  - guaiac positive R19.5
- transport protein E88.09
- tumor marker NEC R97.8
- urination NEC R39.198
- urine (constituents) R82.90
  - cytological and histological examination R82.89
  - glucose R81
  - hemoglobin R82.3
  - microbiological examination (positive culture) R82.79
  - pyuria R82.81
  - specified substance NEC R82.998
- vectorcardiogram R94.39
- visually evoked potential (VEP) R94.112
- white blood cells D72.9
  - specified NEC D72.89
- X-ray examination—*see* Abnormal, diagnostic imaging

Abnormity (any organ or part)—*see* Anomaly

Abocclusion M26.29

- hemolytic disease (newborn) P55.1

Abortion (complete) (spontaneous) O03.9

- incomplete (spontaneous) O03.4
- missed O02.1
- spontaneous—*see* Abortion (complete) (spontaneous)
  - threatened O20.0
- threatened (spontaneous) O20.0
- tubal O00.10-
  - with intrauterine pregnancy O00.11

Abramov-Fiedler myocarditis (acute isolated myocarditis) I40.1

Abrasion T14.8

- abdomen, abdominal (wall) S30.811
- alveolar process S00.512
- ankle S90.51-
- antecubital space—*see* Abrasion, elbow
- anus S30.817
- arm (upper) S40.81-
- auditory canal—*see* Abrasion, ear
- auricle—*see* Abrasion, ear
- axilla—*see* Abrasion, arm
- back, lower S30.810
- breast S20.11-
- brow S00.81
- buttock S30.810
- calf—*see* Abrasion, leg
- canthus—*see* Abrasion, eyelid
- cheek S00.81
  - internal S00.512
- chest wall—*see* Abrasion, thorax
- chin S00.81

ALPHABETIC INDEX

Abrasion, *continued*

- clitoris S30.814
- cornea S05.0-
- costal region—*see* Abrasion, thorax
- dental K03.1
- digit(s)
  - foot—*see* Abrasion, toe
  - hand—*see* Abrasion, finger
- ear S00.41-
- elbow S50.31-
- epididymis S30.813
- epigastric region S30.811
- epiglottis S10.11
- esophagus (thoracic)
  - cervical S10.11
- eyebrow—*see* Abrasion, eyelid
- eyelid S00.21-
- face S00.81
- finger(s) S60.41-
  - index S60.41-
  - little S60.41-
  - middle S60.41-
  - ring S60.41-
- flank S30.811
- foot (except toe(s) alone) S90.81
  - toe—*see* Abrasion, toe
- forearm S50.81-
  - elbow only—*see* Abrasion, elbow
- forehead S00.81
- genital organs, external
  - male S30.815
- groin S30.811
- gum S00.512
- hand S60.51-
- head S00.91
  - ear—*see* Abrasion, ear
  - eyelid—*see* Abrasion, eyelid
  - lip S00.511
  - nose S00.31
  - oral cavity S00.512
  - scalp S00.01
  - specified site NEC S00.81
- heel—*see* Abrasion, foot
- hip S70.21-
- inguinal region S30.811
- interscapular region S20.419
- jaw S00.81
- knee S80.21-
- labium (majus) (minus) S30.814
- larynx S10.11
- leg (lower) S80.81-
  - knee—*see* Abrasion, knee
  - upper—*see* Abrasion, thigh
- lip S00.511
- lower back S30.810
- lumbar region S30.810
- malar region S00.81
- mammary—*see* Abrasion, breast
- mastoid region S00.81
- mouth S00.512
- nail
  - finger—*see* Abrasion, finger
  - toe—*see* Abrasion, toe
- nape S10.81
- nasal S00.31
- neck S10.91
  - specified site NEC S10.81
  - throat S10.11
- nose S00.31
- occipital region S00.01
- oral cavity S00.512
- orbital region—*see* Abrasion, eyelid
- palate S00.512
- palm—*see* Abrasion, hand
- parietal region S00.01
- pelvis S30.810
- penis S30.812
- perineum
  - female S30.814
  - male S30.810
- periocular area—*see* Abrasion, eyelid

Abrasion, *continued*

- phalanges
  - finger—*see* Abrasion, finger
  - toe—*see* Abrasion, toe
- pharynx S10.11
- pinna—*see* Abrasion, ear
- popliteal space—*see* Abrasion, knee
- prepuce S30.812
- pubic region S30.810
- pudendum
  - female S30.816
  - male S30.815
- sacral region S30.810
- scalp S00.01
- scapular region—*see* Abrasion, shoulder
- scrotum S30.813
- shin—*see* Abrasion, leg
- shoulder S40.21
- skin NEC T14.8
- sternal region S20.319
- submaxillary region S00.81
- submental region S00.81
- subungual
  - finger(s)—*see* Abrasion, finger
  - toe(s)—*see* Abrasion, toe
- supraclavicular fossa S10.81
- supraorbital S00.81
- temple S00.81
- temporal region S00.81
- testis S30.813
- thigh S70.31-
- thorax, thoracic (wall) S20.91
  - back S20.41-
  - front S20.31-
- throat S10.11
- thumb S60.31-
- toe(s) (lesser) S90.41-
  - great S90.41-
- tongue S00.512
- tooth, teeth (dentifrice) (habitual) (hard tissues) (occupational) (ritual) (traditional) K03.1
- trachea S10.11
- tunica vaginalis S30.813
- tympanum, tympanic membrane—*see* Abrasion, ear
- uvula S00.512
- vagina S30.814
- vocal cords S10.11
- vulva S30.814
- wrist S60.81-

Abscess (connective tissue) (embolic) (fistulous) (metastatic) (multiple) (pernicious) (pyogenic) (septic) L02.91

- abdomen, abdominal
  - cavity K65.1
  - wall L02.211
- abdominopelvic K65.1
- accessory sinus—*see* Sinusitis
- adrenal (capsule) (gland) E27.8
- alveolar K04.7
- anorectal K61.2
- anus K61.0
- apical (tooth) K04.7
- appendix K35.33
- areola (acute) (chronic) (nonpuerperal) N61.1
- axilla (region) L02.41
  - lymph gland or node L04.2
- back (any part, except buttock) L02.212
- Bartholin's gland N75.1
- brain (any part) (cystic) (otogenic) G06.0
- breast (acute) (chronic) (nonpuerperal) N61.1
  - newborn P39.0
- buccal cavity K12.2
- buttock L02.31
- cecum K35.33
- cerebellum, cerebellar G06.0
  - sequelae G09
- cerebral (embolic) G06.0
  - sequelae G09
- cervical (meaning neck) L02.11
  - lymph gland or node L04.0
- cheek (external) L02.01
  - inner K12.2

Abscess, *continued*

- chest J86.9
  - with fistula J86.0
  - wall L02.213
- chin L02.01
- circumtonsillar J36
- colostomy K94.02
- cranium G06.0
- dental K04.7
- dentoalveolar K04.7
- ear (middle)—*see also* Otitis, media
  - acute—see Otitis, media
  - external H60.0-
- epididymis N45.4
- epidural G06.2
  - brain G06.0
  - spinal cord G06.1
- erysipelatous—*see* Erysipelas
- esophagus K20.80
- ethmoid (bone) (chronic) (sinus) J32.2
- extradural G06.2
  - brain G06.0
    - sequelae G09
  - spinal cord G06.1
- eyelid H00.03-
- face (any part, except ear, eye and nose) L02.01
- foot L02.61-
- forehead L02.01
- frontal sinus (chronic) J32.1
- gallbladder K81.0
- gluteal (region) L02.31
- groin L02.214
- hand L02.51-
  - head NEC L02.811 part, except ear, eye and nose) L02.01
- horseshoe K61.31
- heel—*see* Abscess, foot
- ileocecal K35.33
- iliac (region) L02.214
  - fossa K35.33
- inguinal (region) L02.214
  - lymph gland or node L04.1
- intersphincterIc K61.4
- intracranial G06.0
- intratonsillar J36
- knee—*see also* Abscess, lower limb
  - joint M00.9
- lateral (alveolar) K04.7
- lingual K14.0
  - tonsil J36
- lip K13.0
- loin (region) L02.211
- lower limb L02.41
- lumbar (tuberculous) A18.01
  - nontuberculous L02.212
- lymph, lymphatic, gland or node (acute)—*see also* Lymphadenitis, acute
  - mesentery I88.0
- marginal, anus K61.0
- maxilla, maxillary M27.2
  - molar (tooth) K04.7
  - premolar K04.7
  - sinus (chronic) J32.0
- mons pubis L02.215
- mouth (floor) K12.2
- myocardium I40.0
- nasal J32.9
- navel L02.216
  - newborn P38.9
    - with mild hemorrhage P38.1
    - without hemorrhage P38.9
- neck (region) L02.11
  - lymph gland or node L04.0
- nipple N61.1
- nose (external) (fossa) (septum) J34.0
  - sinus (chronic)—*see* Sinusitis
- operative wound T81.43
- otogenic G06.0
- palate (soft) K12.2
  - hard M27.2
- parapharyngeal J39.0
- pararectal K61.1
- parietal region (scalp) L02.811

ALPHABETIC INDEX

Abscess, *continued*

- parotid (duct) (gland) K11.3
  - region K12.2
- pectoral (region) L02.213
- perianal K61.0
- periapical K04.7
- periappendicular K35.33
- pericardial I30.1
- pericecal K35.33
- perineum, perineal (superficial) L02.215
  - urethra N34.0
- periodontal (parietal)
  - apical K04.7
- peripharyngeal J39.0
- peripleuritic J86.9
  - with fistula J86.0
- perirectal K61.1
- peritoneum, peritoneal (perforated) (ruptured) K65.1
  - with appendicitis K35.33
  - postoperative T81.43
- peritonsillar J36
- perityphlic K35.33
- phagedenic NOS L02.91
  - pituitary (gland) E23.6
- pleura J86.9
  - with fistula J86.0
- pilonidal L05.01
- postcecal K35.33
  - postoperative (any site) T81.43
- postnasal J34.0
- postpharyngeal J39.0
- posttonsillar J36
- presacral K68.19
- rectum K61.1
- retropharyngeal J39.0
- root, tooth K04.7
- rupture (spontaneous) NOS L02.91
- scalp (any part) L02.811
- scrofulous (tuberculous) A18.2
- septal, dental K04.7
- sinus (accessory) (chronic) (nasal)—*see also* Sinusitis
  - intracranial venous (any) G06.0
- specified site NEC L02.818
- sphenoidal (sinus) (chronic) J32.3
- stitch T81.41
- subarachnoid G06.2
  - brain G06.0
  - spinal cord G06.1
- subcecal K35.33
- subcutaneous—*see also* Abscess, by site
- subdural G06.2
  - brain G06.0
  - sequelae G09
  - spinal cord G06.1
- subgaleal L02.811
- sublingual K12.2
  - gland K11.3
- submandibular (region) (space) (triangle) K12.2
  - gland K11.3
- submaxillary (region) L02.01
  - gland K11.3
- submental L02.01
  - gland K11.3
- supralevator K61.5
- suprarenal (capsule) (gland) E27.8
- temple L02.01
- temporal region L02.01
- temporosphenoidal G06.0
- testes N45.4
- thorax J86.9
  - with fistula J86.0
- thyroid (gland) E06.0
- tongue (staphylococcal) K14.0
- tonsil(s) (lingual) J36
- tonsillopharyngeal J36
- tooth, teeth (root) K04.7
- trunk L02.219
  - abdominal wall L02.211
  - back L02.212
  - chest wall L02.213
  - groin L02.214
  - perineum L02.215
  - umbilicus L02.216

Abscess, *continued*

- umbilicus L02.216
- upper
  - limb L02.41-
- uvula K12.2
- vermiform appendix K35.33
- vulvovaginal gland N75.1
- wound T81.49

Absence (of) (organ or part) (complete or partial)

- albumin in blood E88.09
- alimentary tract (congenital) Q45.8
  - upper Q40.8
- anus (congenital) Q42.3
  - with fistula Q42.2
- aorta (congenital) Q25.41
- appendix, congenital Q42.8
- artery (congenital) (peripheral) Q27.8
  - pulmonary Q25.79
  - umbilical Q27.0
- atrial septum (congenital) Q21.1
- auditory canal (congenital) (external) Q16.1
- auricle (ear), congenital Q16.0
- bile, biliary duct, congenital Q44.5
- canaliculus lacrimalis, congenital Q10.4
- cervix (with uterus) congenital Q51.5
- cilia (congenital) Q10.3
- corpus callosum Q04.0
- digestive organ(s) or tract, congenital Q45.8
  - acquired NEC Z90.49
  - upper Q40.8
- ear, congenital Q16.9
  - acquired H93.8-
  - auricle Q16.0
  - external Q16.0
  - inner Q16.5
  - lobe, lobule Q17.8
  - middle, except ossicles Q16.4
    - ossicles Q16.3
- endocrine gland (congenital) NEC Q89.2
  - acquired E89.89
- eustachian tube (congenital) Q16.2
- eye (acquired)
  - congenital Q11.1
  - muscle (congenital) Q10.3
- eyelid (fold) (congenital) Q10.3
- family member (causing problem in home) NEC *see also* Disruption, family) Z63.32
- fibrinogen (congenital) D68.2
  - acquired D65
- gallbladder (acquired) Z90.49
  - congenital Q44.0
- gamma globulin in blood D80.1
  - hereditary D80.0
- genital organs
  - acquired (female) (male) Z90.79
  - female, congenital Q52.8
    - external Q52.71
    - internal NEC Q52.8
  - male, congenital Q55.8
- genitourinary organs, congenital NEC
  - female Q52.8
  - male Q55.8
- ileum (acquired) Z90.49
  - congenital Q41.2
- incus (acquired)
  - congenital Q16.3
- inner ear, congenital Q16.5
- intestine (acquired) (small) Z90.49
  - congenital Q41.9
    - specified NEC Q41.8
  - large Z90.49
    - congenital Q42.9
    - specified NEC Q42.8
- iris, congenital Q13.1
- jejunum (acquired) Z90.49
  - congenital Q41.1
- kidney(s) (acquired) Z90.5
  - congenital
    - bilateral Q60.1
    - unilateral Q60.0
- labyrinth, membranous Q16.5

Absence, *continued*

- lens (acquired)—*see also* Aphakia
  - congenital Q12.3
- liver (congenital) Q44.79
- muscle (congenital) (pectoral) Q79.8
  - ocular Q10.3
- organ
  - or site, congenital NEC Q89.8
    - acquired NEC Z90.89
- osseous meatus (ear) Q16.4
- parathyroid gland (acquired) E89.2
  - congenital Q89.2
- pituitary gland (congenital) Q89.2
  - acquired E89.3
- punctum lacrimale (congenital) Q10.4
- rectum (congenital) Q42.1
  - with fistula Q42.0
  - acquired Z90.49
- respiratory organ NOS Q34.9
- scrotum, congenital Q55.29
- septum
  - atrial (congenital) Q21.1
- skull bone (congenital) Q75.8
  - with
    - anencephaly Q00.0
    - encephalocele—*see* Encephalocele
    - hydrocephalus Q03.9
      - with spina bifida—*see* Spina bifida, by site, with hydrocephalus
    - microcephaly Q02
- teeth, tooth (congenital) K00.0
  - acquired (complete) K08.109
    - class I K08.101
    - class II K08.102
    - class III K08.103
    - class IV K08.104
  - due to
    - caries K08.139
      - class I K08.131
      - class II K08.132
      - class III K08.133
      - class IV K08.134
    - periodontal disease K08.129
      - class I K08.121
      - class II K08.122
      - class III K08.123
      - class IV K08.124
    - specified NEC K08.199
      - class I K08.191
      - class II K08.192
      - class III K08.193
      - class IV K08.194
    - trauma K08.119
      - class I K08.111
      - class II K08.112
      - class III K08.113
      - class IV K08.114
  - partial K08.409
    - class I K08.401
    - class II K08.402
    - class III K08.403
    - class IV K08.404
    - due to
      - caries K08.439
        - class I K08.431
        - class II K08.432
        - class III K08.433
        - class IV K08.434
      - periodontal disease K08.429
        - class I K08.421
        - class II K08.422
        - class III K08.423
        - class IV K08.424
      - specified NEC K08.499
        - class I K08.491
        - class II K08.492
        - class III K08.493
        - class IV K08.494
      - trauma K08.419
        - class I K08.411
        - class II K08.412
        - class III K08.413
        - class IV K08.414

ALPHABETIC INDEX

Absence, *continued*

- testes (congenital) Q55.0
  - acquired Z90.79
- thymus gland Q89.2
- thyroid (gland) (acquired) E89.0
  - cartilage, congenital Q31.8
  - congenital E03.1
  - tricuspid valve Q22.4
- transverse aortic arch, congenital Q25.49
- umbilical artery, congenital Q27.0
- uterus congenital Q51.0

Absorption

- carbohydrate, disturbance K90.49
- chemical—*see* Table of Drugs and Chemicals
  - through placenta (newborn) P04.9
    - environmental substance P04.6
    - nutritional substance P04.5
    - obstetric anesthetic or analgesic drug P04.0
- drug NEC—*see* Table of Drugs and Chemicals
  - addictive
    - through placenta (newborn) (*see also* newborn, affected by, maternal use of) P04.40
    - cocaine P04.41
    - hallucinogens P04.42
    - specified drug NEC P04.49
  - medicinal
    - through placenta (newborn) P04.19
    - through placenta (newborn) P04.19
    - obstetric anesthetic or analgesic drug P04.0
- fat, disturbance K90.49
  - pancreatic K90.3
- noxious substance—*see* Table of Drugs and Chemicals
- protein, disturbance K90.49
- starch, disturbance K90.49
- toxic substance—*see* Table of Drugs and Chemicals

Abstinence symptoms, syndrome

- alcohol F10.239
- cocaine F14.23
- neonatal P96.1
- nicotine—*see* Dependence, drug, nicotine
- stimulant NEC F15.93
  - with dependence F15.23

Abuse

- alcohol (nondependent) F10.10
  - in remission (early) (sustained) F10.11
  - with
    - intoxication F10.129
      - with delirium F10.121
      - uncomplicated F10.120
    - withdrawal F10.139
      - with
        - ◊ perceptual disturbance F10.132
      - delirium F10.131
    - uncomplicated F10.130
  - counseling and surveillance Z71.41
- amphetamine (or related substance)—*see also* Abuse, drug, stimulant NEC
  - stimulant NEC F15.10
    - with
      - intoxication F15.129
      - ◊ with
        - ◊ delirium F15.121
        - ◊ perceptual disturbance F15.122
- analgesics (non-prescribed) (over the counter) F55.8
- antacids F55.0
- anxiolytic—*see* Abuse, drug, sedative
- barbiturates—*see* Abuse, drug, sedative
- caffeine—*see* Abuse, drug, stimulant NEC
- cannabis, cannabinoids—*see* Abuse, drug, cannabis
- child—*see* Maltreatment, child
- cocaine—*see* Abuse, drug, cocaine
- drug NEC (nondependent) F19.10
  - amphetamine type—*see* Abuse, drug, stimulant NEC
  - anxiolytics—*see* Abuse, drug, sedative
  - barbiturates—*see* Abuse, drug, sedative
  - caffeine—*see* Abuse, drug, stimulant NEC
  - cannabis F12.10
    - in remission (early) (sustained) F12.11
  - cocaine F14.10
    - in remission (early) (sustained) F14.11

Abuse, *continued*

- with
  - intoxication F14.129
  - ◊ uncomplicated F14.120
- counseling and surveillance Z71.51
- herbal or folk remedies F55.1
- hormones F55.3
- hashish—*see* Abuse, drug, cannabis
- inhalant F18.10
  - in remission (early) (sustained) F18.11
- laxatives F55.2
- opioid F11.10
- opioid, unspecified F11.91
  - in remission (early) (sustained) F11.11
- PCP (phencyclidine) (or related substance)—*see* Abuse, drug, hallucinogen
- psychoactive NEC F19.10
- sedative, hypnotic, or anxiolytic F13.10
- sedative, hypnotic, or anxiolytic, unspecified F13.91
  - in remission (early) (sustained) F13.11
- solvent—*see* Abuse, drug, inhalant
- steroids F55.3
- stimulant NEC F15.10
  - in remission (early) (sustained) F15.11
  - with
    - intoxication F15.129
    - ◊ uncomplicated F15.120
  - ◊ vitamins F55.4
- hallucinogens F16.1-
  - unspecified F16.91
- hashish—*see* Abuse, drug, cannabis
- herbal or folk remedies F55.1
- hormones F55.3
- inhalant F18.1-
- laxatives F55.2
- marijuana—*see* Abuse, drug, cannabis
- PCP (phencyclidine) (or related substance) F16.1-
- physical (adult) (child)—*see* Maltreatment
- psychoactive substance F19.1-
- psychological (adult) (child)—*see* Maltreatment
- sexual—*see* Maltreatment
- solvent—*see* Abuse, drug, inhalant

Acalculia R48.8

- developmental F81.2

Acanthamebiasis (with) B60.10

- conjunctiva B60.12
- keratoconjunctivitis B60.13
- meningoencephalitis B60.11
- other specified B60.19

Acanthosis (acquired) (nigricans) L83

- benign Q82.8
- congenital Q82.8
- seborrheic L82.1
  - inflamed L82.0
- tongue K14.3

Acardia, acardius Q89.8

Acardiacus amorphus Q89.8

Acariasis B88.0

- scabies B86

Acarodermatitis (urticarioides) B88.0

Acathisia (drug induced) G25.71

Accelerated atrioventricular conduction I45.6

Accessory (congenital)

- atrioventricular conduction I45.6
- auditory ossicles Q16.3
- biliary duct or passage Q44.5
- carpal bones Q74.0
- cusp
  - pulmonary Q22.3
- cystic duct Q44.5
- endocrine gland NEC Q89.2
- eye muscle Q10.3
- eyelid Q10.3
- face bone(s) Q75.8
- finger(s) Q69.0
- foreskin N47.8
- frontonasal process Q75.8
- gallbladder Q44.1
- genital organ(s)

Accessory, *continued*

- female Q52.8
  - external Q52.79
  - internal NEC Q52.8
- male Q55.8
- genitourinary organs NEC Q89.8
  - female Q52.8
  - male Q55.8
- hallux Q69.2
- heart Q24.8
  - valve, NEC Q24.8
    - pulmonary Q22.3
- hepatic ducts Q44.5
- lacrimal canal Q10.6
- liver Q44.79
  - duct Q44.5
- navicular of carpus Q74.0
- nipple Q83.3
- parathyroid gland Q89.2
- pituitary gland Q89.2
- prepuce N47.8
- sesamoid bones Q74.8
  - foot Q74.2
  - hand Q74.0
- skin tags Q82.8
- tarsal bones Q74.2
- thumb Q69.1
- thymus gland Q89.2
- thyroid gland Q89.2
- toes Q69.2
- uterus Q51.28
- valve, heart
  - pulmonary Q22.3

Accident

See also the ICD-10-CM External Cause of Injuries Table for codes describing accident details.

- birth—*see* Birth, injury
- cerebrovascular (embolic) (ischemic) (thrombotic) I63.9
  - old (without sequelae) Z86.73

Accretio cordis (nonrheumatic) I31.0

Acculturation difficulty Z60.3

Acephalobrachia monster Q89.8

Acephalochirus monster Q89.8

Acephalogaster Q89.8

Acephalostomus monster Q89.8

Acephalothorax Q89.8

Acetonemia R79.89

- in Type 1 diabetes E10.10
  - with coma E10.11

Achalasia (cardia) (esophagus) K22.0

- congenital Q39.5
- pylorus Q40.0

Achlorhydria, achlorhydric (neurogenic) K31.83

- anemia D50.8
- psychogenic F45.8

Achroma, cutis L80

Achromia parasitica B36.0

Achondrogenesis Q77.0

Achondroplasia (osteosclerosis congenita) Q77.4

Achylia gastrica K31.89

- psychogenic F45.8

Acid

- peptic disease K30
- stomach K30
  - psychogenic F45.8

Acidemia E87.2

- metabolic (newborn) P19.9
  - first noted before onset of labor P19.0
  - first noted during labor P19.1
  - noted at birth P19.2

Acidity, gastric (high) K30

- psychogenic F45.8

Acidocytopenia—*see* Agranulocytosis

Acidocytosis D72.10

ALPHABETIC INDEX

Acidosis (lactic) (respiratory) E87.2
- in Type 1 diabetes E10.10
  - with coma E10.11
- metabolic NEC E87.2
  - hyperchlormic, of newborn P74.421
  - mixed metabolic and respiratory, newborn P84
- newborn P84
  - acute metabolic E87.21
  - chronic metabolic E87.22
  - other E87.29
  - unspecified E87.20

Aciduria
- 4-hydroxybutyric E72.81
- gamma-hydroxybutyric E72.81
- glutaric (type I)
  - type II E71.313
  - type III E71.5-

Acladiosis (skin) B36.0

Acleistocardia Q21.1

Acne L70.9
- artificialis L70.8
- atrophica L70.2
- cachecticorum (Hebra) L70.8
- conglobata L70.1
- cystic L70.0
- excoriée des jeunes filles L70.5
- frontalis L70.2
- indurata L70.0
- infantile L70.4
- lupoid L70.2
- necrotic, necrotica (miliaris) L70.2
- neonatal L70.4
- nodular L70.0
- occupational L70.8
- picker's L70.5
- pustular L70.0
- rodens L70.2
- specified NEC L70.8
- tropica L70.3
- varioliformis L70.2
- vulgaris L70.0

Acquired—*see also* Disease, diseased
- immunodeficiency syndrome (AIDS) B20

Acroasphyxia, chronic I73.89

Acrocephalopolysyndactyly Q87.0

Acrocephalosyndactyly Q87.0

Acrocephaly Q75.009

Acrochondrohyperplasia—*see* Syndrome, Marfans

Acrocyanosis I73.89
- newborn P28.2
  - meaning transient blue hands and feet—omit code

Acrodermatitis
- infantile papular L44.4

Acromegaly, acromegalia E22.0

Acronyx L60.0

Acroparesthesia (simple) (vasomotor) I73.89

Action, heart
- disorder I49.9
- irregular I49.9
  - psychogenic F45.8

Activation
- mast cell (disorder) (syndrome) D89.40
  - idiopathic D89.42
  - monoclonal D89.41
  - secondary D89.43
  - specified type NEC D89.49

Active—*see* Disease, diseased

Acute—*see also* Disease, diseased
- abdomen R10.0
- gallbladder—*see* Cholecystitis, acute

Acyanotic heart disease (congenital) Q24.9

Adair-Dighton syndrome (brittle bones and blue sclera, deafness) Q78.0

Adamantinoma
- long bones C40.9-
  - lower limb C40.2-
  - upper limb C40.0-

Adamantinoma, *continued*
- malignant C41.1
  - jaw (bone) (lower) C41.1
    - upper C41.0
- tibial C40.2-

Adams-Stokes (-Morgagni) disease or syndrome I45.9

Adaption reaction—*see* Disorder, adjustment

Addiction (*see also* Dependence) F19.20
- alcohol, alcoholic (ethyl) (methyl) (wood) (without remission) F10.20
  - with remission F10.21
- drug—*see* Dependence, drug
- ethyl alcohol (without remission) F10.20
  - with remission F10.21
- ethyl alcohol (without remission) F10.20
  - with remission F10.21
- methylated spirit (without remission) F10.20
  - with remission F10.21
- tobacco—*see* Dependence, drug, nicotine

Addisonian crisis E27.2

Addison's
- anemia (pernicious) D51.0
- disease (bronze) or syndrome E27.1

Addison-Schilder complex E71.528

Additional—*see also* Accessory
- chromosome(s) Q99.8
  - sex—*see* Abnormal, chromosome, sex
  - 21—*see* Trisomy, 21

Adduction contracture, hip or other joint—*see* Contraction, joint

Adenitis—*see also* lymphadenitis
- acute, unspecified site L04.9
- axillary I88.9
  - acute L04.2
  - chronic or subacute I88.1
- cervical I88.9
  - acute L04.0
  - chronic or subacute I88.1
- chronic, unspecified site I88.1
- due to Pasteurella multocida (p. septica) A28.0
- gangrenous L04.9
- groin I88.9
  - acute L04.1
  - chronic or subacute I88.1
- inguinal I88.9
  - acute L04.1
  - chronic or subacute I88.1
- lymph gland or node, except mesenteric I88.9
  - acute—*see* Lymphadenitis, acute
  - chronic or subacute I88.1
- mesenteric (acute) (chronic) (nonspecific) (subacute) I88.0
- scrofulous (tuberculous) A18.2
- strumous, tuberculous A18.2
- subacute, unspecified site I88.1

Adenocarcinoma—*see also* Neoplasm, malignant, by site in Table of Neoplasms in the complete *ICD-10-CM* manual
- renal cell C64-

Adenoiditis (chronic) J35.02
- with tonsillitis J35.03
- acute J03.90
  - recurrent J03.91
  - specified organism NEC J03.80
    - recurrent J03.81
  - staphylococcal J03.80
    - recurrent J03.81
  - streptococcal J03.00
    - recurrent J03.01

Adenoma—*see also* Neoplasm, benign, by site in Table of Neoplasms in the complete *ICD-10-CM* manual
- apocrine
  - breast D24-
  - specified site NEC—*see* Neoplasm, skin, benign, by site in Table of Neoplasms in the complete *ICD-10-CM* manual
  - unspecified site D23.9
- ceruminous D23.2-

Adenomatosis
- endocrine (multiple) E31.20
  - single specified site—*see* Neoplasm, uncertain behavior, by site in Table of Neoplasms in the complete *ICD-10-CM* manual
- specified site—*see* Neoplasm, benign, by site in Table of Neoplasms in the complete *ICD-10-CM* manual
  - unspecified site D12.6

Adenomatous
- goiter (nontoxic) E04.9
  - with hyperthyroidism—*see* Hyperthyroidism, with, goiter
  - toxic—*see* Hyperthyroidism, with, goiter

Adenopathy (lymph gland) R59.9
- generalized R59.1

Adenosclerosis I88.8

Adenovirus, as cause of disease classified elsewhere B97.0

Adherent—*see also* Adhesions
- labia (minora) N90.89
- pericardium (nonrheumatic) I31.0
  - rheumatic I09.2
- scar (skin) L90.5
- tendon in scar L90.5

Adhesions, adhesive (postinfective)
- cardiac I31.0
  - rheumatic I09.2
- cervicovaginal N88.1
  - congenital Q52.8
- conjunctiva congenital Q15.8
- joint—*see* Ankylosis
  - temporomandibular M26.61-
- labium (majus) (minus), congenital Q52.5
- meninges (cerebral) (spinal) G96.12
  - congenital Q07.8
  - tuberculous (cerebral) (spinal) A17.0
- nasal (septum) (to turbinates) J34.89
- pericardium (nonrheumatic) I31.0
  - focal I31.8
  - rheumatic I09.2
- preputial, prepuce N47.5
- temporomandibular M26.61-
- vagina (chronic) N89.5

Adiponecrosis neonatorum P83.88

Adiposis—*see also* Obesity
- cerebralis E23.6
- adiposogenital dystrophy E23.6

Admission (for)—*see also* Encounter (for)
- aftercare (*see also* Aftercare) Z51.89
  - radiation therapy (antineoplastic) Z51.0
  - sepsis Z51.A
- attention to artificial opening (of) Z43.9
  - artificial vagina Z43.7
  - colostomy Z43.3
  - cystostomy Z43.5
  - enterostomy Z43.4
  - gastrostomy Z43.1
  - ileostomy Z43.2
  - jejunostomy Z43.4
  - nephrostomy Z43.6
  - specified site NEC Z43.8
  - intestinal tract Z43.4
  - urinary tract Z43.6
  - tracheostomy Z43.0
  - ureterostomy Z43.6
  - urethrostomy Z43.6
- change of
  - dressing (nonsurgical) Z48.00
  - surgical dressing Z48.01
- circumcision, ritual or routine (in absence of diagnosis) Z41.2
- counseling—*see also* Counseling
  - dietary Z71.3
  - HIV Z71.7
  - human immunodeficiency virus Z71.7
  - non-attending third party Z71.0
  - procreative management NEC Z31.69
  - travel Z71.84
- desensitization to allergens Z51.6
- dietary surveillance and counseling Z71.3

ALPHABETIC INDEX

Admission (for), *continued*

- ear piercing Z41.3
- examination at health care facility (adult) (*see also* Examination) Z00.00
  - with abnormal findings Z00.01
  - ear Z01.10
    - with abnormal findings NEC Z01.118
  - eye Z01.00
    - with abnormal findings Z01.01
    - after failed exam Z01.02-
  - hearing Z01.10
    - infant or child (over 28 days old) Z00.129
      - with abnormal findings Z00.121
      - with abnormal findings NEC Z01.118
  - vision Z01.00
    - infant or child (over 28 days old) Z00.129
      - with abnormal findings Z00.121
      - with abnormal findings Z01.01
      - after failed exam Z01.02-
- followup examination Z09
- intrauterine device management Z30.431
  - initial prescription Z30.014
- prophylactic (measure)—*see also* Encounter, prophylactic measure
  - vaccination Z23
- radiation therapy (antineoplastic) Z51.0
- removal of
  - dressing (nonsurgical) Z48.00
  - implantable subdermal contraceptive Z30.46
  - intrauterine contraceptive device Z30.432
  - staples Z48.02
  - surgical dressing Z48.01
  - sutures Z48.02
- sensitivity test—*see also* Test, skin
  - allergy NEC Z01.82
  - Mantoux Z11.1
- vision examination Z01.00
  - with abnormal findings Z01.01
  - after failed exam Z01.02-

Adolescent X-linked adrenoleukodystrophy E71.521

Adrenal (gland)—*see* Disease, diseased

Adrenalitis, adrenitis E27.8

- autoimmune E27.1

Adrenogenital syndrome E25.9

- congenital E25.0
- salt loss E25.0

Adrenogenitalism, congenital E25.0

Adrenoleukodystrophy E71.529

- neonatal E71.511
- Xlinked E71.529
  - Addison only phenotype E71.528
  - Addison-Schilder E71.528
  - adolescent E71.521
  - adrenomyeloneuropathy E71.522
  - childhood cerebral E71.520
  - other specified E71.528

Adrenomyeloneuropathy E71.522

Adverse effect—*see* Table of Drugs and Chemicals, categories T36 – T50, with 6th character 5

Aerodermectasia

- subcutaneous (traumatic) T79.7

Aerophagy, aerophagia (psychogenic) F45.8

Afibrinogenemia (*see also* Defect, coagulation) D68.8

- acquired D65
- congenital D68.2

Aftercare (*see also* Care) Z51.89

- following surgery (for) (on)
  - attention to
    - dressings (nonsurgical) Z48.00
      - surgical Z48.01
      - sutures Z48.02
  - circulatory system Z48.812
  - digestive system Z48.815
  - genitourinary system Z48.816
  - nervous system Z48.811
  - oral cavity Z48.814—respiratory system Z48.813
  - sense organs Z48.810
  - skin and subcutaneous tissue Z48.817

Aftercare, *continued*

- specified body system
  - circulatory Z48.812
  - digestive Z48.815
  - genitourinary Z48.816
  - nervous Z48.811
  - oral cavity Z48.814
  - respiratory Z48.813
  - sense organs Z48.810
  - skin and subcutaneous tissue Z48.817
  - teeth Z48.814
- spinal Z47.89
  - teeth Z48.814
- fracture code *to* fracture with seventh character D
- involving
  - removal of
    - dressings (nonsurgical) Z48.00
    - staples Z48.02
    - surgical dressings Z48.01
    - sutures Z48.02

Agammaglobulinemia (acquired) (secondary) (nonfamilial) D80.1

- with
  - immunoglobulin-bearing B-lymphocytes D80.1
  - lymphopenia D81.9
- common variable (CVAgamma) D80.1
- lymphopenic D81.9

Aganglionosis (bowel) (colon) Q43.1

Agenesis

- alimentary tract (complete) (partial) NEC Q45.8
  - upper Q40.8
- anus, anal (canal) Q42.3
  - with fistula Q42.2
- aorta Q25.41
- appendix Q42.8
- artery (peripheral) Q27.9
  - pulmonary Q25.79
  - umbilical Q27.0
- auditory (canal) (external) Q16.1
- auricle (ear) Q16.0
- bile duct or passage Q44.5
- bone Q79.9
- breast (with nipple present) Q83.8
  - with absent nipple Q83.0
- canaliculus lacrimalis Q10.4
- cartilage Q79.9
- cecum Q42.8
- cervix Q51.5
- cilia Q10.3
- clavicle Q74.0
- colon Q42.9
  - specified NEC Q42.8
- corpus callosum Q04.0
- digestive organ(s) or tract (complete) (partial) NEC Q45.8
  - upper Q40.8
- ear Q16.9
  - auricle Q16.0
  - lobe Q17.8
- endocrine (gland) NEC Q89.2
- eustachian tube Q16.2
- eye Q11.1
  - adnexa Q15.8
- eyelid (fold) Q10.3
- face
  - bones NEC Q75.8
- gallbladder Q44.0
- heart Q24.8
  - valve, NEC Q24.8
  - pulmonary Q22.0
- intestine (small) Q41.9
  - large Q42.9
  - specified NEC Q42.8
- iris (dilator fibers) Q13.1
- genitalia, genital (organ(s))
  - female Q52.8
    - external Q52.71
    - internal NEC Q52.8
  - male Q55.8
- incus Q16.3
- labyrinth, membranous Q16.5
- lacrimal apparatus Q10.4
- lens Q12.3

Agenesis, *continued*

- liver Q44.79
- muscle Q79.8
  - eyelid Q10.3
  - ocular Q15.8
- parathyroid (gland) Q89.2
- pelvic girdle (complete) (partial) Q74.2
- pituitary (gland) Q89.2
- punctum lacrimale Q10.4
- rectum Q42.1
  - with fistula Q42.0
- roof of orbit Q75.8
- round ligament Q52.8
- scapula Q74.0
- scrotum Q55.29
- septum
  - atrial Q21.1
- shoulder girdle (complete) (partial) Q74.0
- skull (bone) Q75.8
  - with
    - anencephaly Q00.0
    - encephalocele—*see* Encephalocele
    - hydrocephalus Q03.9
      - with spina bifida—*see* Spina bifida, by site, with hydrocephalus
    - microcephaly Q02
- spinal cord Q06.0
- testicle Q55.0
- thymus (gland) Q89.2
- thyroid (gland) E03.1
  - cartilage Q31.8
  - uterus Q51.0

Aglossia-adactylia syndrome Q87.0

Agnosia (body image) (other senses) (tactile) R48.1

- developmental F88
- verbal R48.1
- auditory R48.1
  - developmental F80.2
  - developmental F80.2

Agranulocytosis (chronic) (cyclical) (genetic) (infantile) (periodic) (pernicious) (*see also* Neutropenia) D70.9

- congenital D70.0
- cytoreductive cancer chemotherapy sequela D70.1
- drug-induced D70.2
  - due to cytoreductive cancer chemotherapy D70.1
- due to infection D70.3
- secondary D70.4
  - drug-induced D70.2
    - due to cytoreductive cancer chemotherapy D70.1

Agraphia (absolute) R48.8

- with alexia R48.0
- developmental F81.81

Ague (dumb)—*see* Malaria

Ahumada-del Castillo syndrome E23.0

AIDS (related complex) B20

AIPH (acute idiopathic pulmonary hemorrhage in infants (over 28 days old)) R04.81

Air

- anterior mediastinum J98.2
- hunger, psychogenic F45.8
- sickness T75.3

Airplane sickness T75.3

Akathisia (drug-induced) (treatment-induced) G25.71

- neuroleptic induced (acute) G25.71

Alactasia, congenital E73.0

Albuminuria, albuminuric (acute) (chronic) (subacute) (*see also* Proteinuria) R80.9

- orthostatic R80.2
- postural R80.2
- scarlatinal A38.8

Alcohol, alcoholic, alcohol-induced

- addiction (without remission) F10.20
  - with remission F10.21
- counseling and surveillance Z71.41
  - family member Z71.42
- intoxication (acute) (without dependence) F10.129
  - with
    - delirium F10.121

ALPHABETIC INDEX

Alcohol, alcoholic, alcohol-induced, *continued*
- ■ dependence F10.229
  - – with delirium F10.221
  - – uncomplicated F10.220
  - – uncomplicated F10.120

Alcohol use
- • unspecified, uncomplicated F10.90
- • unspecified, in remission F10.90

Alcoholism (chronic) (without remission) F10.20
- • with
  - – psychosis—*see* Psychosis
  - – remission F10.21

Alder (-Reilly) anomaly or syndrome (leukocyte granulation) D72.0

Aldrich (-Wiskott) syndrome (eczema-thrombocytopenia) D82.0

Aleukia
- • congenital D70.0
- • hemorrhagica D61.9
  - – congenital D61.09

Alexia R48.0
- • developmental F81.0
- • secondary to organic lesion R48.0

Alkalosis E87.3
- • metabolic E87.3
- • of newborn P74.41

Allergy, allergic (reaction) (to) T78.40
- • air-borne substance NEC (rhinitis) J30.89
- • anaphylactic reaction or shock T78.2
- • angioneurotic edema T78.3
- • animal (dander) (epidermal) (hair) (rhinitis) J30.81
- • bee sting (anaphylactic shock) T63.44-
- • biological—*see* Allergy, drug
- • colitis K52.29
  - – food protein-induced K52.22
- • dander (animal) (rhinitis) J30.81
- • dandruff (rhinitis) J30.81
- • desensitization to allergens, encounter for Z51.6
- • drug, medicament & biological (any) (external) (internal) T78.40
  - – correct substance properly administered—*see* Table of Drugs and Chemicals, by drug, adverse effect
  - – wrong substance given or taken NEC (by accident)—see Table of Drugs and Chemicals, by drug, poisoning
- • due to pollen J30.1
- • dust (house) (stock) (rhinitis) J30.89
  - – with asthma—*see* Asthma, allergic extrinsic
- • eczema—*see* Dermatitis, contact, allergic
- • epidermal (animal) (rhinitis) J30.81
- • feathers (rhinitis) J30.89
- • food (any) (ingested) NEC T78.1
  - – anaphylactic shock—*see* Shock, anaphylactic, due to food
  - – dermatitis—*see* Dermatitis, due to, food
  - – dietary counseling and surveillance Z71.3
  - – in contact with skin L23.6
  - – rhinitis J30.5
  - – status (without reaction) Z91.018
    - ■ beef Z91.014
    - ■ eggs Z91.012
    - ■ lamb Z91.014
    - ■ mammalian meats Z91.014
    - ■ milk products Z91.011
    - ■ peanuts Z91.010
    - ■ pork Z91.014
    - ■ red meats Z91.014
    - ■ seafood Z91.013
    - ■ specified NEC Z91.018
- • gastrointestinal K52.29
  - – food protein-induced K52.22
  - – meaning colitis or gastroenteritis K52.59
  - – meaning other adverse food reaction NEC T78.1
- • grain J30.1
- • grass (hay fever) (pollen) J30.1
  - – asthma—*see* Asthma, allergic extrinsic
- • hair (animal) (rhinitis) J30.81
- • history (of)—*see* History, family of, allergy
- • horse serum—*see* Allergy, serum
- • inhalant (rhinitis) J30.89
  - – pollen J30.1
- • kapok (rhinitis) J30.89

Allergy, allergic, *continued*
- • medicine—*see* Allergy, drug
- • milk protein Z91.011
  - – anaphylactic reaction T78.07
  - – dermatitis L27.2
  - – enterocolitis syndrome K52.21
  - – enteropathy K52.22
  - – gastroenteritis K52.29
  - – gastroesophageal reflux (*see also* Reaction, adverse, food) K21.9
    - ■ with esophagitis K21.0-
  - – proctocolitis K52.29
  - – nasal, seasonal due to pollen J30.1
- • pollen (any) (hay fever) J30.1
  - – asthma—*see* Asthma, allergic extrinsic
- • primrose J30.1
- • primula J30.1
- • purpura D69.0
- • ragweed (hay fever) (pollen) J30.1
  - – asthma—*see* Asthma, allergic extrinsic
- • rose (pollen) J30.1
- • seasonal NEC J30.2
- • Senecio jacobae (pollen) J30.1
- • serum (*see also* Reaction, serum) T80.69
  - – anaphylactic shock T80.59
- • shock (anaphylactic) T78.2
  - – due to
    - ■ administration of blood and blood products T80.51
    - ■ immunization T80.52
    - ■ serum NEC T80.59
    - ■ vaccination T80.52
- • specific NEC T78.49
- • tree (any) (hay fever) (pollen) J30.1
  - – asthma—*see* Asthma, allergic extrinsic
- • upper respiratory J30.9
- • urticaria L50.0
- • vaccine—*see* Allergy, serum
- • wheat—*see* Allergy, food

Alopecia (hereditaria) (seborrheica) L65.9
- • due to cytotoxic drugs NEC L65.8
- • postinfective NEC L65.8
  - – specified NEC L66.89

Alport syndrome Q87.81

ALTE (apparent life threatening event) **in newborn and infant** R68.13

Alteration (of), Altered
- • mental status R41.82
- • pattern of family relationships affecting child Z62.898

Alymphocytosis D72.810
- • thymic (with immunodeficiency) D82.1

Alymphoplasia, thymic D82.1

Amastia (with nipple present) Q83.8
- • with absent nipple Q83.0

Amaurosis (acquired) (congenital)—*see also* Blindness
- • hysterical F44.6
- • Leber's congenital H35.50

Ambiguous genitalia Q56.4

Amblyopia (congenital) (ex anopsia) (partial) (suppression) H53.00-
- • anisometropic—*see* Amblyopia
- • hysterical F44.6
- • suspect H53.04-

Amebiasis
- • acute A06.0
- • intestine A06.0

Ameloblastoma—*see also* Cyst
- • long bones C40.9-
  - – lower limb C40.2-
  - – upper limb C40.0-
- • malignant C41.1
  - – jaw (bone) (lower) C41.1
    - ■ upper C41.0
- • tibial C40.2-

Amenorrhea N91.2

Amsterdam dwarfism Q87.19

Amyelia Q06.0

Amygdalitis—*see* Tonsillitis

Amygdalolith J35.8

Amyotonia M62.89
- • congenita G70.2

Anacidity, gastric K31.83
- • psychogenic F45.8

Anaerosis of newborn P28.89

Analbuminemia E88.09

Anaphylactic
- • purpura D69.0
- • shock or reaction—*see* Shock, anaphylactic

Anaphylactoid shock or reaction—*see* Shock, anaphylactic

Anaphylaxis—*see* Shock, anaphylactic

Anaplasmosis [*A. phagocytophilum*] (transfusion transmitted) A79.82
- • human A77.49

Anarthria R47.1

Anasarca R60.1
- • renal N04.9

Anastomosis
- • arteriovenous ruptured brain I60.8-
  - – intracerebral I61.8
  - – intraparenchymal I61.8
  - – intraventricular I61.5
  - – subarachnoid I60.8-

Android pelvis Q74.2

Anemia (essential) (general) (hemoglobin deficiency) (infantile) (primary) (profound) D64.9
- • achlorhydric D50.8
- • aplastic D61.9
  - – congenital D61.09
  - – drug-induced D61.1
  - – due to
    - ■ drugs D61.1
    - ■ external agents NEC D61.2
    - ■ infection D61.2
    - ■ radiation D61.2
  - – red cell (pure) D60.9
    - ■ chronic D60.0
    - – specified type NEC D60.8
    - – transient D60.1
  - – idiopathic D61.3
  - – red cell (pure) D60.9
    - ■ chronic D60.0
    - ■ congenital D61.01
    - ■ specified type NEC D61.89
  - – toxic D61.2
- • aregenerative
  - – congenital D61.09
- • atypical D64.9
- • Baghdad spring D55.0
- • blood loss (chronic) D50.0
  - – acute D62
- • chlorotic D50.8
- • chronic
  - – hemolytic D58.9
    - ■ idiopathic D59.9
- • chronica congenita aregenerativa D61.09
- • congenital P61.4
  - – aplastic D61.09
  - – Heinz body D58.2
  - – spherocytic D58.0
- • Cooley's (erythroblastic) D56.1
- • deficiency D53.9
  - – 2, 3 diphosphoglycurate mutase D55.29
  - – 2, 3 PG D55.29
  - – enzyme D55.9
    - ■ drug-induced (hemolytic) D59.2
    - ■ glucose-6-phosphate dehydrogenase (G6PD) with anemia D55.0
    - ■ glycolytic D55.29
  - – folate D52.9
    - ■ dietary D52.0
    - ■ drug-induced D52.1
  - – folic acid D52.9
    - ■ dietary D52.0
    - ■ drug-induced D52.1
  - – glucose-6-phosphate dehydrogenase
    - ■ with anemia D55.0
  - – glyceraldehyde phosphate dehydrogenase D55.29
  - – G6PD with anemia D55.0
  - – hexokinase D55.29

ALPHABETIC INDEX

Anemia, *continued*

- nutritional D53.9
  - with
    - poor iron absorption D50.8
  - phosphoglycerate kinase D55.29
  - PK D55.21
  - pyruvate kinase D55.21
  - triose-phosphate isomerase D55.29
- Diamond-Blackfan (congenital hypoplastic) D61.01
- due to (in) (with)
  - antineoplastic chemotherapy D64.81
  - blood loss (chronic) D50.0
    - acute D62
  - chemotherapy, antineoplastic D64.81
  - chronic disease classified elsewhere NEC D63.8
  - chronic kidney disease D63.1
  - end stage renal disease D63.1
  - hemorrhage (chronic) D50.0
    - acute D62
  - loss of blood (chronic) D50.0
    - acute D62
  - myxedema E03.9 [D63.8]
  - prematurity P61.2
- Dyke-Young type (secondary) (symptomatic) D59.19
- enzyme-deficiency, drug-induced D59.2
- erythroblastic
  - familial D56.1
  - newborn (*see also* Disease, hemolytic) P55.9
  - of childhood D56.1
- erythropoietin-resistant anemia (EPO resistant anemia) D63.1
- familial erythroblastic D56.1
- Fanconi('s) D61.03
- favism D55.0
- glucose-6-phosphate dehydrogenase (G6PD) deficiency D55.0
  - with anemia D55.0
  - without anemia D75.A
- Heinz body, congenital D58.2
- hemolytic D58.9
  - acquired D59.9
    - autoimmune NEC D59.19
      - acute D59.9
      - Lederer's D59.19
    - autoimmune D59.10
      - cold D59.12
      - mixed D59.13
      - warm D59.11
  - cold type (primary) (secondary) (symptomatic) D59.12
  - mixed type (primary) (secondary) (symptomatic) D59.13
  - nonspherocytic
    - congenital or hereditary NEC D55.8
      - glucose-6-phosphate dehydrogenase deficiency with anemia D55.0
      - glucose-6-phosphate dehydrogenase deficiency without anemia D75.A
      - pyruvate kinase deficiency D55.21
      - type
        - 0 II D55.29
  - primary
    - autoimmune
      - cold type D59.12
      - mixed type D59.13
      - warm type D59.11
  - secondary D59.4
    - autoimmune D59.1
    - autoimmune
    - cold type D59.12
    - mixed type D59.13
    - warm type D59.11
    - autoimmune
      - cold D59.12
      - mixed D59.13
      - warm D59.11
  - warm type (primary) (secondary) (symptomatic) D59.11
- hemorrhagic (chronic) D50.0
  - acute D62
- Herrick's D57.1
- hookworm B76.9 [D63.8]

Anemia, *continued*

- hypochromic (idiopathic) (microcytic) (normoblastic) D50.9
  - due to blood loss (chronic) D50.0
    - acute D62
- hypoplasia, red blood cells D61.9
  - congenital or familial D61.01
- hypoplastic (idiopathic) D61.9
  - congenital or familial (of childhood) D61.01
- hypoproliferative (refractive) D61.9
  - idiopathic D64.9
- iron deficiency D50.9
  - secondary to blood loss (chronic) D50.0
    - acute D62
  - specified type NEC D50.8
- Joseph-Diamond-Blackfan (congenital hypoplastic) D61.01
- leukoerythroblastic D61.82
- malarial (*see also* Malaria) B54 [D63.8]
- marsh (*see also* Malaria) B54 [D63.8]
- Mediterranean (with other hemoglobinopathy) D56.9
- microcytic (hypochromic) D50.9
  - due to blood loss (chronic) D50.0
    - acute D62
    - familial D56.8
- microdrepanocytosis D57.40
- microelliptopolkilocytic (RiettiGreppi Micheli) D56.9
- myelofibrosis D75.81
- myelophthisic D61.82
- myeloproliferative D47.Z9
- newborn P61.4
  - due to
    - ABO (antibodies, isoimmunization, maternal/fetal incompatibility) P55.1
    - Rh (antibodies, isoimmunization, maternal/fetal incompatibility) P55.0
  - following fetal blood loss P61.3
  - posthemorrhagic (fetal) P61.3
- normocytic (infectional) D64.9
  - due to blood loss (chronic) D50.0
    - acute D62
  - myelophthisic D61.82
- nutritional (deficiency) D53.9
  - with
    - poor iron absorption D50.8
  - of prematurity P61.2
- paludal (*see also* Malaria) B54 [D63.8]
- posthemorrhagic (chronic) D50.0
  - acute D62
  - newborn P61.3
- postoperative (postprocedural)
  - due to (acute) blood loss D62
    - chronic blood loss D50.0
  - specified NEC D64.9
- progressive D64.9
  - malignant D51.0
  - pernicious D51.0
- pure red cell D60.9
  - congenital D61.01
- pyruvate kinase deficiency D55.21
- Rietti-Greppi-Micheli D56.9
- secondary to
  - blood loss (chronic) D50.0
    - acute D62
  - hemorrhage (chronic) D50.0
    - acute D62
- semiplastic D61.89
- sickle-cell—*see* Disease, sickle-cell
- siderogenic (refractory) D50.9
  - due to blood loss (chronic) D50.0
    - acute D62
- syphilitic (acquired) (late) A52.79 [D63.8]
- thalassemia D56.9
- thrombocytopenic—*see* Thrombocytopenia
- toxic D61.2
- tuberculous A18.89 [D63.8]
- Witts' (achlorhydric anemia) D50.8

Anesthesia, anesthetic R20.0

- dissociative F44.6
- functional (hysterical) F44.6
- hysterical F44.6
- testicular N50.9

Aneurysm (anastomotic) (artery) (cirsoid) (diffuse) (false) (fusiform) (multiple) (saccular)

- abdominal (aorta) I71.40
  - infrarenal I71.43
    - ruptured I71.33
  - juxtarenal I71.42
    - ruptured I71.32
  - pararenal I71.41
    - ruptured I71.31
- aorta, aortic (nonsyphilitic) I71.9
  - abdominal I71.40
    - dissecting—*see* Dissection, aorta
    - ruptured I71.30
  - arch I71.22
    - ruptured I71.12
  - arteriosclerotic I71.9
    - ruptured I71.8
  - ascending I71.21
    - ruptured I71.11
  - congenital Q25.43
  - descending I71.9
    - abdominal I71.40
      - ruptured I71.30
    - ruptured I71.8
    - thoracic I71.23
      - ruptured I71.13
  - dissecting—*see* Dissection, aorta
  - root Q25.43
    - ruptured I71.8
  - sinus, congenital Q25.43
  - thoracic I71.20
    - ruptured I71.10
  - thoracoabdominal I71.60
    - paravisceral I71.62
      - ruptured I71.52
    - ruptured I71.50
    - supraceliac I71.61
      - ruptured I71.51
  - thorax, thoracic I71.20
    - arch I71.22
      - ruptured I71.12
    - ascending I71.21
      - ruptured I71.11
    - descending I71.23
      - ruptured I71.13
    - ruptured I71.10
    - arch I71.12
      - ascending I71.11
      - descending I71.13
  - transverse I71.22
  - valve (heart) (*see also* Endocarditis, aortic) I35.8
- arteriovenous (congenital)—*see also* Malformation, arteriovenous
  - brain Q28.2
    - ruptured I60.8-
      - intracerebral I61.8
      - intraparenchymal I61.8
      - intraventricular I61.5
      - subarachnoid I60.8-
  - berry (congenital) (nonruptured) I67.1
    - ruptured I60.7
  - brain I67.1
    - arteriovenous (congenital) (nonruptured) Q28.2
      - acquired I67.1
        - ruptured I60.8-
      - ruptured I60.8-
    - berry (congenital) (nonruptured) I67.1
      - ruptured (*see also* Hemorrhage, intracranial, subarachnoid) I60.7
    - congenital Q28.3
      - ruptured I60.7
    - meninges I67.1
      - ruptured I60.8-
    - miliary (congenital) (nonruptured) I67.1
      - ruptured (*see also* Hemorrhage, intracranial, subarachnoid) I60.7
    - mycotic I33.0ruptured into brain I60.0-
  - cavernous sinus I67.1
    - arteriovenous (congenital) (nonruptured) Q28.3
      - ruptured I60.8-

ALPHABETIC INDEX

Aneurysm, *continued*
- circle of Willis I67.1
  - congenital Q28.3
    - ruptured I60.6
  - ruptured I60.6
- congenital (peripheral) Q27.8
  - brain Q28.3
    - ruptured I60.7
  - pulmonary Q25.79
- ductus arteriosus Q25.0
- endocardial, infective (any valve) I33.0
- infective
  - endocardial (any valve) I33.0
- mycotic
  - endocardial (any valve) I33.0
  - ruptured, brain—*see* Hemorrhage, intracerebral, subarachnoid
- patent ductus arteriosus Q25.0
- pulmonary I28.1
  - arteriovenous Q25.72
  - tricuspid (heart) (valve) I07.8

Angelman syndrome Q93.51

Anger R45.4

Angina (attack) (cardiac) (chest) (heart) (pectoris) (syndrome) (vasomotor) I20.9
- aphthous B08.5
- croupous J05.0
- exudative, chronic J37.0
- Ludovici K12.2
- Ludwig's K12.2
- membranous J05.0
- monocytic—*see* Mononucleosis, infectious
- phlegmonous J36
- refractory, pectoris I20.2
- tonsil J36
- trachealis J05.0

Angioedema (allergic) (any site) (with urticaria) T78.3
- episodic, with eosinophilia D72.118

Angioendothelioma—*see* Neoplasm, uncertain behavior, by site in Table of Neoplasms in the complete *ICD-10-CM* manual
- benign D18.00
  - skin D18.01
  - specified site NEC D18.09
- bone—*see* Neoplasm, bone, malignant in Table of Neoplasms in the complete *ICD-10-CM* manual
- Ewing's—*see* Neoplasm, bone, malignant in Table of Neoplasms in the complete *ICD-10-CM* manual

Angiohemophilia (A) (B) D68.0

Angioma—*see also* Hemangioma, by site
- capillary I78.1
- hemorrhagicum hereditaria I78.0
- malignant—*see* Neoplasm, connective tissue, malignant in Table of Neoplasms in the complete *ICD-10-CM* manual
- plexiform D18.00
  - skin D18.01
  - specified site NEC D18.09
- senile I78.1
- skin D18.01
- specified site NEC D18.09
- spider I78.1
- stellate I78.1

Angiomatosis Q82.8
- encephalotrigeminal Q85.8
- hemorrhagic familial I78.0
- hereditary familial I78.0

Angioneurosis F45.8

Angioneurotic edema (allergic) (any site) (with urticaria) T78.3

Angiopathia, angiopathy I99.9
- peripheral I73.9
  - specified type NEC I73.89

Angiospasm (peripheral) (traumatic) (vessel) I73.9
- cerebral G45.9

Angulation
- femur (acquired)—*see also* Deformity, limb, specified type NEC, thigh
  - congenital Q74.2

Angulation, *continued*
- tibia (acquired)—*see also* Deformity, limb, specified type NEC, lower leg
  - congenital Q74.2
- wrist (acquired)—*see also* Deformity, limb, specified type NEC, forearm
  - congenital Q74.0

Angulus infectiosus (lips) K13.0

Anhydration, anhydremia E86.0
- with
  - hypernatremia E87.0
  - hyponatremia E87.1

Anhydremia E86.0
- with
  - hypernatremia E87.0
  - hyponatremia E87.1

Aniridia (congenital) Q13.1

Anisocoria (pupil) H57.02
- congenital Q13.2

Ankyloblepharon (eyelid) (acquired)
- filiforme (adnatum) (congenital) Q10.3
- total Q10.3

Ankyloglossia Q38.1

Ankylosis (fibrous) (osseous) (joint) M24.60
- jaw (temporomandibular) M26.61-
  - specified site NEC M24.69
  - temporomandibular M26.61-

Anodontia (complete) (partial) (vera) K00.0
- acquired K08.10

Anomaly, anomalous (congenital) (unspecified type) Q89.9
- Alder (-Reilly) (leukocyte granulation) D72.0
- alimentary tract Q45.9
  - upper Q40.9
- ankle (joint) Q74.2
- aorta (arch) NEC Q25.40
  - absence and aplasia Q25.41
  - aneurysm (congenital) Q25.43
  - coarctation (preductal) (postductal) Q25.1
  - dilation (congenital) Q25.44
  - double arch Q25.45
  - hypoplasia Q25.42
  - right aortic arch Q25.47
  - tortuous arch Q25.46
- aqueduct of Sylvius Q03.0
  - with spina bifida—*see* Spina bifida, with hydrocephalus
- arm Q74.0
- artery (peripheral) Q27.9
  - eye Q15.8
  - pulmonary NEC Q25.79
  - retina Q14.1
  - subclavian Q27.8
    - origin Q25.48
  - umbilical Q27.0
- atrial
  - septa Q21.1
- atrioventricular
  - excitation I45.6
  - septum Q21.0
- Axenfeld's Q15.0
- biliary duct or passage Q44.5
- bladder Q64.70
  - absence Q64.5
  - diverticulum Q64.6
  - exstrophy Q64.10
    - cloacal Q64.12
    - extroversion Q64.19
    - specified type NEC Q64.19
    - supravesical fissure Q64.11
  - neck obstruction Q64.31
  - specified type NEC Q64.79
- bone Q79.9
  - arm Q74.0
  - leg Q74.2
  - pelvic girdle Q74.2
  - shoulder girdle Q74.0
  - skull Q75.9
    - with
      - anencephaly Q00.0
      - encephalocele—*see* Encephalocele

Anomaly, *continued*
- hydrocephalus Q03.9
  - ◊ with spina bifida—*see* Spina bifida, by site, with hydrocephalus
- microcephaly Q02
- broad ligament Q50.6
- bursa Q79.9
- anthus Q10.3
- cardiac Q24.9
- carpus Q74.0
- caruncle, lacrimal Q10.6
- cervix Q51.9
- cheek Q18.9
- chin Q18.9
- chromosomes, chromosomal Q99.9
  - D (1)—*see* condition, chromosome 13
  - E (3)—*see* condition, chromosome 18
  - G—*see* condition, chromosome 21
  - sex
    - female phenotype Q97.8
    - gonadal dysgenesis (pure) Q99.1
    - Klinefelter's Q98.4
    - male phenotype Q98.9
    - Turner's Q96.9
    - specified NEC Q99.8
- cilia Q10.3
- clavicle Q74.0
- common duct Q44.5
- communication
  - left ventricle with right atrium Q21.0
- connection
  - pulmonary venous Q26.4
    - partial Q26.3
    - total Q26.2
  - cystic duct Q44.5
- dental
  - arch relationship M26.20
    - specified NEC M26.29
  - dentofacial M26.9
    - dental arch relationship M26.20
      - specified NEC M26.29
    - jaw size M26.00
    - mandibular
      - hypoplasia M26.04
    - malocclusion M26.4
      - dental arch relationship NEC M26.29
    - specified type NEC M26.89
    - temporomandibular joint M26.60-
      - adhesions M26.61-
      - ankylosis M26.61-
      - arthralgia M26.62-
      - articular disc M26.63-
        - specified type NEC M26.69
- dermatoglyphic Q82.8
- digestive organ(s) or tract Q45.9
  - lower Q43.9
  - upper Q40.9
- ductus
  - arteriosus Q25.0
  - botalli Q25.0
- ear (external) Q17.9
- elbow Q74.0
- endocrine gland NEC Q89.2
- eye Q15.9
  - anterior segment Q13.9
    - specified NEC Q13.89
  - posterior segment Q14.9
    - specified NEC Q14.8
  - ptosis (eyelid) Q10.0
    - specified NEC Q15.8
- eyelid Q10.3
  - ptosis Q10.0
- face Q18.9
- fallopian tube Q50.6
- fascia Q79.9
- femur NEC Q74.2
- fibula NEC Q74.2
- finger Q74.0
- flexion (joint) NOS Q74.9
  - hip or thigh Q65.89
- foot NEC Q74.2
  - varus (congenital) Q66.3-

Anomaly, *continued*

- foramen
  - Botalli Q21.1
  - ovale Q21.1
- forearm Q74.0
- forehead Q75.8
- gastrointestinal tract Q45.9
- gallbladder (position) (shape) (size) Q44.1
- genitalia, genital organ(s) or system
  - female Q52.9
    - external Q52.70
    - internal Q52.9
  - male Q55.9
    - hydrocele P83.5
    - specified NEC Q55.8
- genitourinary NEC
  - female Q52.9
  - male Q55.9
- Gerbode Q21.0
- granulation or granulocyte, genetic (constitutional) (leukocyte) D72.0
- gyri Q07.9
- hand Q74.0
- heart Q24.9
  - patent ductus arteriosus (Botalli) Q25.0
  - septum Q21.9
    - auricular Q21.1
    - interatrial Q21.1
    - interventricular Q21.0
      - with pulmonary stenosis or atresia, dextraposition of aorta and hypertrophy of right ventricle Q21.3
    - specified NEC Q21.8
    - ventricular Q21.0
      - with pulmonary stenosis or atresia, dextraposition of aorta and hypertrophy of right ventricle Q21.3
  - tetralogy of Fallot Q21.3
  - valve NEC Q24.8
    - aortic
      - bicuspid valve Q23.81
      - stenosis Q23.0
    - pulmonary Q22.3
      - stenosis Q22.1
- heel NEC Q74.2
- Hegglin's D72.0
- hepatic duct Q44.5
- hip NEC Q74.2
- humerus Q74.0
- hydatid of Morgagni
  - female Q50.5
  - male (epididymal) Q55.4
    - testicular Q55.29
- hypersegmentation of neutrophils, hereditary D72.0
- hypophyseal Q89.2
- ilium NEC Q74.2
- integument Q84.9
- ischium NEC Q74.2
- joint Q74.9
- Jordan's D72.0
- lens Q12.9
- leukocytes, genetic D72.0
  - granulation (constitutional) D72.0
- ligament Q79.9
  - broad Q50.6
  - round Q52.8
- limb Q74.9
  - lower NEC Q74.2
    - reduction deformity—*see* Defect, reduction, limb, lower
  - upper Q74.0
- liver Q44.70
  - duct Q44.5
- lower limb NEC Q74.2
- May (-Hegglin) D72.0
- meningeal bands or folds Q07.9
  - constriction of Q07.8
  - spinal Q06.9
- meninges Q07.9
  - cerebral Q04.8
  - spinal Q06.9
- meningocele Q05.9

Anomaly, *continued*

- mesentery Q45.9
- metacarpus Q74.0
- metatarsus NEC Q74.2
- mitral (leaflets) (valve) Q23.9
  - specified NEC Q23.88
- multiple NEC Q89.7
- muscle Q79.9
- musculoskeletal system, except limbs Q79.9
- neck (any part) Q18.9
- nerve Q07.9
  - acoustic Q07.8
  - optic Q07.8
- nervous system (central) Q07.9
- omphalomesenteric duct Q43.0
- origin
  - artery
    - pulmonary Q25.79
- ovary Q50.39
- oviduct Q50.6
- parathyroid gland Q89.2
- Pelger-Huët (hereditary hyposegmentation) D72.0
- pelvic girdle NEC Q74.2
- pelvis (bony) NEC Q74.2
- penis (glans) Q55.69
- pigmentation L81.9
  - congenital Q82.8
- pituitary (gland) Q89.2
- prepuce Q55.69
- pulmonary Q33.9
  - artery NEC Q25.79
  - valve Q22.3
    - stenosis Q22.1
  - venous connection Q26.4
    - partial Q26.3
    - total Q26.2
- radius Q74.0
- respiratory system Q34.9
  - specified NEC Q34.8
- Rieger O13.81
- rotation
  - hip or thigh Q65.89
- round ligament Q52.8
- sacroiliac (joint) NEC Q74.2
- scapula Q74.0
- sex chromosomes NEC—*see also* Anomaly, chromosomes
  - female phenotype Q97.8
  - male phenotype Q98.9
- shoulder Q74.0
- simian crease Q82.8
- sinus of Valsalva Q25.49
- skull Q75.9
  - with
    - anencephaly Q00.0
    - encephalocele—*see* Encephalocele
    - hydrocephalus Q03.9
      - with spina bifida—*see* Spina bifida, by site, with hydrocephalus
    - microcephaly Q02
- specified organ or site NEC Q89.8
- tarsus NEC Q74.2
- tendon Q79.9
- thigh NEC Q74.2
- thumb Q74.0
- thymus gland Q89.2
- thyroid (gland) Q89.2
  - cartilage Q31.8
- tibia NEC Q74.2
- toe NEC Q74.2
- tooth, teeth K00.9
  - eruption K00.6
- tragus Q17.9
- ulna Q74.0
- umbilical artery Q27.0
- upper limb Q74.0
- ureter Q62.8
  - obstructive NEC Q62.39
    - orthotopic ureterocele Q62.31
- urinary tract Q64.9
- uterus Q51.9
- ventricular
  - septa Q21.0

Anomaly, *continued*

- vitelline duct Q43.0
- wrist Q74.0

Anonychia (congenital) Q84.3

- acquired L60.8

Anorchia, anorchism, anorchidism Q55.0

Anorexia R63.0

- nervosa F50.00
  - atypical F50.9
  - binge-eating type F50.2-
    - with purging F50.02-
  - restricting type F50.01-

Anosmia R43.0

- hysterical F44.6

Anosognosia R41.85

Anovulatory cycle N97.0

Anoxemia R09.02

- newborn P84

Anoxia (pathological) R09.02

- cerebral G93.1
  - newborn P84
- due to
  - drowning T75.1
  - high altitude T70.29
- intrauterine P84
- newborn P84

Anteversion

- femur (neck), congenital Q65.89

Anthrax

- with pneumonia A22.1
- cutaneous A22.0
- colitis A22.2
- gastrointestinal A22.2
- inhalation A22.1
- intestinal A22.2
- pulmonary A22.1
- respiratory A22.1

Anthropoid pelvis Q74.2

Antibody

- antiphospholipid R76.0
  - with
    - hemorrhagic disorder D68.312
    - hypercoagulable state D68.61

Anticardiolipin syndrome D68.61

Anticoagulant, circulating (intrinsic)—*see also* Disorder, hemorrhagic D68.318

- drug-induced (extrinsic)—*see also* Disorder, hemorrhagic D68.32
- iatrogenic D68.32

Antidiuretic hormone syndrome E22.2

Antiphospholipid

- antibody
  - with hemorrhagic disorder D68.312
- syndrome D68.61

Antisocial personality F60.2

Antritis J32.0

- maxilla J32.0
  - acute J01.00
    - recurrent J01.01

Anuria R34

- postrenal N13.8

Anusitis K62.89

Anxiety F41.9

- depression F41.8
- episodic paroxysmal F41.0
- hysteria F41.8
- panic type F41.0
- separation, abnormal (of childhood) F93.0
- social F40.1-
- specified NEC F41.8

Aorta (aortic arch) anomaly Q25.4-

Apepsia K30

- psychogenic F45.8

Apertognathia M26.09

Apert's syndrome Q87.0

ALPHABETIC INDEX

Aphagia R13.0
- psychogenic F50.9

Aphakia (acquired) (postoperative) H27.0-
- congenital Q12.3

Aphasia (amnestic) (global) (nominal) (semantic) (syntactic)
- developmental (receptive type) F80.2
  - expressive type F80.1
  - Wernicke's F80.2
- sensory F80.2
- Wernicke's F80.2

Aphonia (organic) R49.1
- hysterical F44.4
- psychogenic F44.4

Aphthae, aphthous—*see also* Disease, diseased
- Bednar's K12.0
- cachectic K14.0
- oral (recurrent) K12.0
- stomatitis (major) (minor) K12.0
- thrush B37.0
- ulcer (oral) (recurrent) K12.0

Aplasia—*see also* Agenesis
- abdominal muscle syndrome Q79.4
- aorta (congenital) Q25.41
- bone marrow (myeloid) D61.9
  - congenital D61.01
- cervix (congenital) Q51.5
- congenital pure red cell D61.01
- corpus callosum Q04.0
- erythrocyte congenital D61.01
- gallbladder, congenital Q44.0
- parathyroid-thymic D82.1
- Pelizaeus-Merzbacher E75.27
- red cell (with thymoma) D60.9
  - acquired D60.9
    - due to drugs D60.9
  - chronic D60.0
  - congenital D61.01
  - constitutional D61.01
  - due to drugs D60.9
  - hereditary D61.01
  - of infants D61.01
  - primary D61.01
  - pure D61.01
    - due to drugs D60.9
  - transient D60.1
- round ligament Q52.8
- testicle Q55.0
- thymic, with immunodeficiency D82.1
- thyroid (congenital) (with myxedema) E03.1
- uterus Q51.0

Apnea, apneic (of) (spells) R06.81
- newborn NEC P28.4
  - central apnea P28.41
  - mixed neonatal apnea P28.43
  - obstructive apnea P28.42
  - sleep (primary), unspecified P28.30
  - sleep, other P28.39
  - sleep, primary mixed P28.33
  - obstructive P28.4
  - other apnea P28.49
  - sleep (central) (obstructive) (primary) P28.3
  - sleep, primary central P28.31
  - sleep, primary obstructive P28.32
- prematurity P28.4
- sleep G47.30
  - central (primary) G47.31
    - idiopathic G47.31
    - in conditions classified elsewhere G47.37
  - obstructive (adult) (pediatric) G47.33
    - hypopnea G47.33
  - primary central G47.31
  - specified NEC G47.39

Apneumatosis, newborn P28.0

Apophysitis (bone)—*see also* Osteochondropathy
- calcaneus M92.6
- juvenile M92.9

Apoplexia, apoplexy, apoplectic
- heat T67.01

Appendage
- testicular (organ of Morgagni) Q55.29

Appendicitis (pneumococcal) (retrocecal) K37
- with
  - gangrene K35.891
    - with localized peritonitis K35.31
  - perforation NOS K35.32
  - peritoneal abscess K35.33
  - peritonitis NEC K35.33
    - generalized K35.209
  - with
    - ◊ abscess K35.219
      - » with perforation or rupture K35.211
      - » following rupture or perforation of appendix NOS K35.211
      - » without perforation or rupture K35.210
    - ◊ perforation or rupture K35.201
      - following rupture or perforation of appendix NOS K35.201
    - without rupture or perforation of appendix K35.200
  - localized K35.30
    - with
      - ◊ gangrene K35.31
      - ◊ perforation K35.32
      - » and abscess K35.33
    - rupture K35.32
- acute (catarrhal) (fulminating) (gangrenous) (obstructive) (retrocecal) (suppurative) K35.80
  - with
    - gangrene K35.891
    - peritoneal abscess K35.33
    - peritonitis NEC K35.33
      - generalized (with perforation or rupture) K35.209
      - ◊ with
        - » abscess K35.219
        - ❖ with perforation or rupture K35.211
        - ❖ following rupture or perforation of appendix NOS K35.211
        - ❖ without perforation or rupture K35.210
      - » perforation or rupture K35.201
      - ◊ following rupture or perforation of appendix NOS K35.201
      - ◊ without rupture or perforation of appendix K35.200
    - localized K35.30
      - ◊ with
        - » gangrene K35.31
        - » perforation K35.32
        - ❖ and abscess K35.33
  - specified NEC K35.890
    - with gangrene K35.891
- ruptured NOS (with local peritonitis) K35.32

Appendicopathia oxyurica B80

Appendix, appendicular—*see also* Disease, diseased
- Morgagni
  - female Q50.5
  - male (epididymal) Q55.4
    - testicular Q55.29
  - testis Q55.29

Appetite
- depraved—*see* Pica
- excessive R63.2
- lack or loss (*see also* Anorexia) R63.0
  - nonorganic origin F50.89
  - psychogenic F50.89
- perverted (hysterical)—*see* Pica

Apprehensiveness, abnormal F41.9

ARC (AIDS-related complex) B20

Arch
- aortic Q25.49
- bovine Q25.49

Arcuate uterus Q51.810

Arcuatus uterus Q51.810

Argentaffinoma—*see also* Neoplasm, uncertain behavior, by site
- syndrome E34.09

Arnold-Chiari disease, obstruction or syndrome (type II) Q07.00
- with
  - hydrocephalus Q07.02
    - with spina bifida Q07.03
  - spina bifida Q07.01
    - with hydrocephalus Q07.03
- type III—*see* Encephalocele
- type IV Q04.8

Arousals, confusional G47.51

Arrest, arrested
- cardiac I46.9
  - due to
    - cardiac condition I46.2
    - specified condition NEC I46.8
  - newborn P29.81
  - postprocedural I97.12-
- development or growth
  - child R62.50
- epiphyseal
  - complete
    - femur M89.15-
    - humerus M89.12-
    - tibia M89.16-
    - ulna M89.13-
  - forearm M89.13-
    - specified NEC M89.13-
  - ulna—*see* Arrest, epiphyseal, by type, ulna
  - lower leg M89.16-
    - specified NEC M89.168
    - tibia—*see* Arrest, epiphyseal, by type, tibia
  - partial
    - femur M89.15-
    - humerus M89.12-
    - tibia M89.16-
    - ulna M89.13-
  - specified NEC M89.18
- growth plate—*see* Arrest, epiphyseal
- physeal—*see* Arrest, epiphyseal
- respiratory R09.2
  - newborn P28.81

Arrhythmia (auricle) (cardiac) (juvenile) (nodal) (reflex) (supraventricular) (transitory) (ventricle) I49.9
- block I45.9
- newborn
  - bradycardia P29.12
  - occurring before birth P03.819
    - before onset of labor P03.810
    - during labor P03.811
  - tachycardia P29.11
- psychogenic F45.8
- sinus I49.8
- vagal R55

Arrillaga-Ayerza syndrome (pulmonary sclerosis with pulmonary hypertension) I27.0

Arsenical pigmentation L81.8
- from drug or medicament—*see* Table of Drugs and Chemicals

Arteriosclerosis, arteriosclerotic (diffuse) (obliterans) (of) (senile) (with calcification) I70.90
- pulmonary (idiopathic) I27.0

Arteritis I77.6
- cerebral I67.7
  - in
    - systemic lupus erythematosus M32.19
- coronary (artery) I25.89
  - rheumatic I01.8
    - chronic I09.89

Artery, arterial—*see also* Disease, diseased
- single umbilical Q27.0

Arthralgia (allergic)—*see also* Pain, joint
- temporomandibular M26.62-

Arthritis, arthritic (acute) (chronic) (nonpyogenic) (subacute) M19.9-
- due to or associated with
  - acromegaly (*see also* subcategory M14.8-) E22.0
  - bacterial disease (*see also* subcategory M01) A49.9
  - erysipelas (*see also* category M01) A46
  - erythema
    - nodosum L52

ALPHABETIC INDEX

Arthritis, arthritic, *continued*

- hemophilia D66 [M36.2]
- Henoch- (Schönlein) purpura D69.0 [M36.4]
- human parvovirus (*see also* category M01) B97.6
- Lyme disease A69.23
- rat bite fever (*see also* M01) A25.1
- serum sickness (*see also* Reaction, serum) T80.69
- in (due to)
  - acromegaly (*see also* subcategory M14.8-) E22.0
  - endocrine disorder NEC (*see also* subcategory M14.8-) E34.9
  - enteritis, infectious NEC (*see also* category M01) A09
  - erythema
    - multiforme (*see also* subcategory M14.8-) L51.9
    - nodosum (*see also* subcategory M14.8-) L52
  - hemochromatosis (*see also* subcategory M14.8-) E83.118
  - hemoglobinopathy NEC D58.2 [M36.3]
  - hemophilia NEC D66 [M36.2]
  - *Hemophilus influenzae* M00.8- [B96.3]
  - Henoch (-Schönlein)purpura D69.0 [M36.4]
  - hypogammaglobulinemia (*see also* subcategory M14.8-) D80.1
  - hypothyroidism NEC (*see also* subcategory M14.8-) E03.9
  - infection—*see* Arthritis, pyogenic or pyemic
  - infectious disease NEC—*see* category M01
  - Lyme disease A69.23
  - metabolic disorder NEC (*see also* subcategory M14.8-) E88.9
  - respiratory disorder NEC (*see also* subcategory M14.8-) J98.9
  - *Salmonella* (arizonae) (choleraesuis) (typhimurium) A02.23
    - specified organism NEC (*see also* category M01) A08.8
  - sarcoidosis D86.86
  - thalassemia NEC D56.9 [M36.3]
- juvenile M08.90
  - with systemic onset—see Still's disease
  - ankle M08.97-
  - elbow M08.92-
  - foot joint M08.97-
  - hand joint M08.94-
  - hip M08.95-
  - knee M08.96-
  - multiple site M08.99
  - pauciarticular M08.40
    - ankle M08.47-
    - elbow M08.42-
    - foot joint M08.47-
    - hand joint M08.44-
    - hip M08.45-
    - knee M08.46-
    - shoulder M08.41-
    - specified site NEC M08.4A
    - vertebrae M08.48
    - wrist M08.43-
  - rheumatoid—*see* Arthritis, rheumatoid, juvenile
  - shoulder M08.91-
  - specified site NEC M08.9A
  - vertebra M08.98
  - specified type NEC M08.8-
    - ankle M08.87-
    - elbow M08.82-
    - foot joint M08.87-
    - hand joint M08.84-
    - hip M08.85-
    - knee M08.86-
    - multiple site M08.89
    - shoulder M08.81-
    - specified joint NEC M08.88
    - vertebrae M08.88
    - wrist M08.83-
    - wrist M08.93-
- pneumococcal M00.10
  - ankle M00.17-
  - elbow M00.12-
  - foot joint M00.17-
  - hand joint M00.14-
  - hip M00.15-
  - knee M00.16-
  - multiple site M00.19

Arthritis, arthritic, *continued*

  - shoulder M00.11-
  - vertebra M00.18
  - wrist M00.13-
- pyogenic or pyemic (any site except spine) M00.9
  - bacterial NEC M00.80
    - ankle M00.87-
    - elbow M00.82-
    - foot joint M00.87-
    - hand joint M00.84-
    - hip M00.85-
    - knee M00.86-
    - multiple site M00.89
    - shoulder M00.81-
    - vertebra M00.88
    - wrist M00.83-
  - pneumococcal—*see* Arthritis, pneumococcal
  - spine—*see* Spondylopathy, infective
  - staphylococcal—*see* Arthritis, staphylococcal
  - streptococcal—*see* Arthritis, streptococcal NEC
    - pneumococcal—*see* Arthritis, pneumococcal
- rheumatoid M06.9
  - juvenile (with or without rheumatoid factor) M08.00
    - ankle M08.07-
    - elbow M08.02-
    - foot joint M08.07-
    - hand joint M08.04-
    - hip M08.05-
    - knee M08.06-
    - multiple site M08.09
    - shoulder M08.01-
    - vertebra M08.08
    - wrist M08.03-
- septic (any site except spine)—*see* Arthritis, pyogenic or pyemic
- staphylococcal M00.00
  - ankle M00.07-
  - elbow M00.02-
  - foot joint M00.07-
  - hand joint M00.04-
  - hip M00.05-
  - knee M00.06-
  - multiple site M00.09
  - shoulder M00.01-
  - vertebra M00.08
  - wrist M00.03-
- streptococcal NEC M00.20
  - ankle M00.27-
  - elbow M00.22-
  - foot joint M00.07-
  - hand joint M00.24-
  - hip M00.25-
  - knee M00.26-
  - multiple site M00.29
  - shoulder M00.21-
  - vertebra M00.28
  - wrist M00.23-
- suppurative—*see* Arthritis, pyogenic or pyemic
- temporomandibular M26.64-

Arthrodysplasia Q74.9

Arthrogryposis (congenital) Q68.8

- multiplex congenita Q74.3

Arthropathy (*see also* Arthritis) M12.9

- hemophilic NEC D66 [M36.2]
- in (due to)
  - acromegaly E22.0 [M14.8-]
  - *blood disorder NOS D75.9 [M36.3]*
  - endocrine disease NOS E34.9 [M14.8-]
  - erythema
    - multiforme L51.9 [M14.8-]
    - nodosum L52 [M14.8-]
  - hemochromatosis E83.118 [M14.8-]
  - hemoglobinopathy NEC D58.2 [M36.3]
  - hemophilia NEC D66 [M36.2]
  - Henoch-Schönlein purpura D69.0 [M36.4]
  - hypothyroidism E03.9 [M14.8-]
  - infective endocarditis I33.0 [M12.8-]
  - metabolic disease NOS E88.9 [M14.8-]
  - neoplastic disease NOS (*see also* Table of Neoplasms in the complete *ICD-10-CM manual*) D49.9 [M36.1]
  - nutritional deficiency (*see also* subcategory M14.8-) E63.9

Arthropathy, *continued*

  - sarcoidosis D86.86
  - thyrotoxicosis (*see also* subcategory M14.8-) E05.90
  - ulcerative colitis K51.90 [M07.6-]
  - viral hepatitis (postinfectious) NEC B19.9 [M12.8-]
  - Whipple's disease (*see also* subcategory M14.8-) K90.81
- postinfectious NEC B99 [M12.8-]
  - in (due to)
    - viral hepatitis NEC B19.9 [M12.8-]
- temporomandibular joint M26.65-
- traumatic M12.50
  - ankle M12.57-
  - elbow M12.52-
  - foot joint M12.57-
  - hand joint M12.54-
  - hip M12.55-
  - knee M12.56-
  - multiple site M12.59
  - shoulder M12.51-
  - specified joint NEC M12.58
  - vertebrae M12.58
  - wrist M12.53-

Artificial

- opening status (functioning) (without complication) Z93.9
  - gastrostomy Z93.1
  - ileostomy (ileal pouch) (Kock pouch) Z93.2

Asadollahi-Rauch syndrome Q87.85

Ascariasis B77.9

- with
  - complications NEC B77.89
  - intestinal complications B77.0
  - pneumonia, pneumonitis B77.81

Ascites (abdominal) R18.8

- cardiac I50.9
- heart I50.9
- malignant R18.0
- pseudochylous R18.8

Asocial personality F60.2

Aspartylglucosaminuria E77.1

Asperger's disease or syndrome F84.5

Asphyxia, asphyxiation (by) R09.01

- antenatal P84
- birth P84
- bunny bag—*see* Asphyxia, due to, mechanical threat to breathing, trapped in bed clothes
- drowning T75.1
- gas, fumes, or vapor—*see* Table of Drugs and Chemicals
- inhalation—*see* Inhalation
- intrauterine P84
- newborn P84
- pathological R09.01
- postnatal P84
  - mechanical—*see* Asphyxia, due to, mechanical threat to breathing
- prenatal P84
- reticularis R23.1
- strangulation—*see* Asphyxia, due to, mechanical threat to breathing
- submersion T75.1
- traumatic T71.9
  - due to
    - foreign body (in)—*see* Foreign body, respiratory tract, causing, asphyxia
    - low oxygen content of ambient air T71.2-
      - due to
        - ◊ being trapped in
          - ▸ low oxygen environment T71.29
            - ◆ in car trunk T71.221
              - ◇ circumstances undetermined T71.224
              - ◇ done with intent to harm by
                - ✓ another person T71.223
                - ✓ self T71.222
            - ◆ in refrigerator T71.231
              - ◇ circumstances undetermined T71.234
              - ◇ done with intent to harm by
                - ✓ another person T71.233
                - ✓ self T71.232
        - ◊ cave-in T71.21

ALPHABETIC INDEX

Asphyxia, asphyxiation, *continued*

- mechanical threat to breathing (accidental) T71.191
  - circumstances undetermined T71.194
  - done with intent to harm by
    - ◊ another person T71.193
    - ◊ self T71.192
  - hanging T71.161
    - ◊ circumstances undetermined T71.164
    - ◊ done with intent to harm by
      - » another person T71.163
      - » self T71.162
  - plastic bag T71.121
    - ◊ circumstances undetermined T71.124
    - ◊ done with intent to harm by
      - » another person T71.123
      - » self T71.122
  - smothering
    - ◊ in furniture T71.151
      - » circumstances undetermined T71.154
      - » done with intent to harm by
        - ✦ another person T71.153
        - ✦ self T71.152
    - ◊ under
      - » another person's body T71.141
        - ✦ circumstances undetermined T71.144
        - ✦ done with intent to harm T71.143
      - » pillow T71.111
        - ✦ circumstances undetermined T71.114
        - ✦ done with intent to harm by
          - ✱ another person T71.113
          - ✱ self T71.112
  - trapped in bed clothes T71.131
    - ◊ circumstances undetermined T71.134
    - ◊ done with intent to harm by
      - » another person T71.133
      - » self T71.132
- vomiting, vomitus—*see* Foreign body, respiratory tract, causing, asphyxia

Aspiration

- amniotic (clear) fluid (newborn) P24.10
  - with
    - pneumonia (pneumonitis) P24.11
    - respiratory symptoms P24.11
- blood
  - newborn (without respiratory symptoms) P24.20
    - with
      - pneumonia (pneumonitis) P24.21
      - respiratory symptoms P24.21
  - specified age NEC—*see* Foreign body, respiratory tract
- bronchitis J69.0
- food or foreign body (with asphyxiation)—*see* Asphyxia
- liquor (amnii) (newborn) P24.10
  - with
    - pneumonia (pneumonitis) P24.11
    - respiratory symptoms P24.11
- meconium (newborn) (without respiratory symptoms) P24.00
  - with
    - pneumonitis (pneumonitis) P24.01
    - respiratory symptoms P24.01
- milk (newborn) (without respiratory symptoms) P24.30
  - with
    - pneumonia (pneumonitis) P24.31
    - respiratory symptoms P24.31
  - specified age NEC—*see* Foreign body, respiratory tract
- mucus—*see also* Foreign body, by site
  - newborn P24.10
    - with
      - pneumonia (pneumonitis) P24.11
      - respiratory symptoms P24.11
  - neonatal P24.9
  - specific NEC (without respiratory symptoms) P24.80
    - with
      - pneumonia (pneumonitis) P24.81
      - respiratory symptoms P24.81
  - newborn P24.9
    - specific NEC (without respiratory symptoms) P24.80

Aspiration, *continued*

- with
  - pneumonia (pneumonitis) P24.81
  - respiratory symptoms P24.81
- pneumonia J69.0
- pneumonitis J69.0
- syndrome of newborn—*see* Aspiration, by substance, with pneumonia
- vernix caseosa (newborn) P24.80
  - with
    - pneumonia (pneumonitis) P24.81
    - respiratory symptoms P24.81
- vomitus—*see also* Foreign body, respiratory tract
  - newborn (without respiratory symptoms) P24.30
    - with
      - pneumonia (pneumonitis) P24.31
      - respiratory symptoms P24.31

Asplenia (congenital) Q89.01

- functional D73.0

Astasia (-abasia) (hysterical) F44.4

Asthenia, asthenic R53.1

- cardiac (*see also* Failure, heart) I50.9
  - psychogenic F45.8
- cardiovascular (*see also* Failure, heart) I50.9
  - psychogenic F45.8
- heart (*see also* Failure, heart) I50.9
  - psychogenic F45.8
- hysterical F44.4
- myocardial (*see also* Failure, heart) I50.9
  - psychogenic F45.8
- nervous F48.8
- neurocirculatory F45.8

Asthenopia

- hysterical F44.6
- psychogenic F44.6

Asthma, asthmatic (bronchial) (catarrh) (spasmodic) J45.909

- with
  - chronic obstructive bronchitis J44.89
  - chronic obstructive pulmonary disease J44.89
  - exacerbation (acute) J45.901
  - hay fever—*see* Asthma, allergic extrinsic
  - rhinitis, allergic—*see* Asthma, allergic extrinsic
  - status asthmaticus J45.902
- allergic extrinsic J45.909
  - with
    - exacerbation (acute) J45.901
    - status asthmaticus J45.902
- atopic—*see* Asthma, allergic extrinsic
- childhood J45.909
  - with
    - exacerbation (acute) J45.901
    - status asthmaticus J45.902
- cough variant J45.991
- chronic obstructive J44.89
- detergent J69.8
- due to
  - detergent J69.8
- extrinsic, allergic—*see* Asthma, allergic extrinsic
- hay—*see* Asthma, allergic extrinsic
- idiosyncratic—*see* Asthma, nonallergic
- intermittent (mild) J45.20
  - with
    - exacerbation (acute) J45.21
    - status asthmaticus J45.22
- intrinsic, nonallergic—*see* Asthma, nonallergic
- late onset J45.909
  - with
    - exacerbation (acute) J45.901
    - status asthmaticus J45.902
- mild intermittent J45.20
  - with
    - exacerbation (acute) J45.21
    - status asthmaticus J45.22
- mild persistent J45.30
  - with
    - exacerbation (acute) J45.31
    - status asthmaticus J45.32
- mixed J45.909
  - with
    - exacerbation (acute) J45.901
    - status asthmaticus J45.902

Asthma, asthmatic, *continued*

- moderate persistent J45.40
  - with
    - exacerbation (acute) J45.41
    - status asthmaticus J45.42
- nervous—*see* Asthma, nonallergic
- nonallergic (intrinsic) J45.909
  - with
    - exacerbation (acute) J45.901
    - status asthmaticus J45.902
- persistent
  - mild J45.30
    - with
      - exacerbation (acute) J45.31
      - status asthmaticus J45.32
  - moderate J45.40
    - with
      - exacerbation (acute) J45.41
      - status asthmaticus J45.42
  - severe J45.50
    - with
      - exacerbation (acute) J45.51
      - status asthmaticus J45.52
- predominantly allergic J45.909
- severe persistent J45.50
  - with
    - exacerbation (acute) J45.51
    - status asthmaticus J45.52
- specified NEC J45.998

Astroblastoma

- specified site—*see* Neoplasm, malignant, by site in Table of Neoplasms in the complete *ICD-10-CM* manual
- unspecified site C71.9

Astrocytoma (cystic)

- anaplastic
  - specified site—*see* Neoplasm, malignant, by site in Table of Neoplasms in the complete *ICD-10-CM* manual
  - unspecified site C71.9
- fibrillary
  - specified site—*see* Neoplasm, malignant, by site in Table of Neoplasms in the complete *ICD-10-CM* manual
  - unspecified site C71.9
- fibrous
  - specified site—*see* Neoplasm, malignant, by site in Table of Neoplasms in the complete *ICD-10-CM* manual
  - unspecified site C71.9
- gemistocytic
  - specified site—*see* Neoplasm, malignant, by site in Table of Neoplasms in the complete *ICD-10-CM* manual
  - unspecified site C71.9
- juvenile
  - specified site—*see* Neoplasm, malignant, by site in Table of Neoplasms in the complete *ICD-10-CM* manual
  - unspecified site C71.9
- pilocytic
  - specified site—*see* Neoplasm, malignant, by site in Table of Neoplasms in the complete *ICD-10-CM* manual
  - unspecified site C71.9
- piloid
  - specified site—*see* Neoplasm, malignant, by site in Table of Neoplasms in the complete *ICD-10-CM* manual
  - unspecified site C71.9
- protoplasmic
  - specified site—*see* Neoplasm, malignant, by site in Table of Neoplasms in the complete *ICD-10-CM* manual
  - unspecified site C71.9

Astroglioma

- specified site—*see* Neoplasm, malignant, by site in Table of Neoplasms in the complete *ICD-10-CM* manual
- unspecified site C71.9

Asymmetrical face Q67.0

ALPHABETIC INDEX

At risk
- for
  - dental caries Z91.849
    - high Z91.843
    - low Z91.841
    - moderate Z91.842
  - falling Z91.81

Ataxia, ataxy, ataxic R27.0
- autosomal recessive Friedreich G11.11
- cerebellar (hereditary) G11.9
  - with defective DNA repair G11.3
  - early-onset G11.10
  - in
    - myxedema E03.9 [G13.2]
    - neoplastic disease (*see also* Table of Neoplasms in the complete *ICD-10-CM* manual) D49.9 [G32.81]
      - specified disease NEC G32.81
    - late-onset (Marie's) G11.2
  - with
    - essential tremor G11.19
    - myoclonus [Hunt's ataxia] G11.19
    - retained tendon reflexes G11.19
- Friedreich's (heredofamilial) (cerebellar) (spinal) G11.11
- gait R26.0
  - hysterical F44.4
- gluten M35.9 [G32.81]
  - with celiac disease K90.0 [G32.81]
- hereditary G11.9
  - cerebellar—*see* Ataxia, cerebellar
  - spinal (Friedreich's) G11.11
- heredofamilial—*see* Ataxia, hereditary
- Hunt's G11.19
- hysterical F44.4
- Marie's (cerebellar) (heredofamilial) (late- onset) G11.2
- nonorganic origin F44.4
- nonprogressive, congenital G11.0
- psychogenic F44.4
- SangerBrown's (hereditary) G11.2
- spinal
  - hereditary (Friedreich's) G11.11
- spinocerebellar, Xlinked recessive G11.11
- telangiectasia (LouisBar) G11.3

Ataxia-telangiectasia (Louis-Bar) G11.3

Atelectasis (massive) (partial) (pressure) (pulmonary) J98.11
- newborn P28.10
  - due to resorption P28.11
  - partial P28.19
  - primary P28.0
  - secondary P28.19
    - primary (newborn) P28.0

Atelocardia Q24.9

Atheroma, atheromatous (*see also* Arteriosclerosis) I70.90
- aorta, aortic I70.0
  - valve (*see also* Endocarditis, aortic) I35.8
- pulmonary valve (heart) (*see also* Endocarditis, pulmonary) I37.8
- tricuspid (heart) (valve) I36.8
- valve, valvular—*see* Endocarditis

Athlete's
- foot B35.3
- heart I51.7

Athyrea (acquired)—*see also* Hypothyroidism
- congenital E03.1

Atonia, atony, atonic
- capillary I78.8
- congenital P94.2
- esophagus K22.89
- intestine K59.89
  - psychogenic F45.8
- stomach K31.89
  - neurotic or psychogenic F45.8
- uterus (during labor)
  - without hemorrhage O75.89

Atransferrinemia, congenital E88.09

Atresia, atretic
- alimentary organ or tract NEC Q45.8
  - upper Q40.8
- ani, anus, anal (canal) Q42.3
  - with fistula Q42.2

Atresia, atretic, *continued*
- aortic (orifice) (valve) Q23.0
  - congenital with hypoplasia of ascending aorta and defective development of left ventricle (with mitral stenosis) Q23.4
  - in hypoplastic left heart syndrome Q23.4
- aqueduct of Sylvius Q03.0
  - with spina bifida—*see* Spina bifida, with hydrocephalus
- artery NEC Q27.8
  - umbilical Q27.0
- bile duct (common) (congenital) (hepatic) Q44.2
  - acquired—*see* Obstruction, bile duct
- cecum Q42.8
- cervix (acquired) N88.2
  - congenital Q51.828
- choana Q30.0
- colon Q42.9
  - specified NEC Q42.8
- common duct Q44.2
- cystic duct Q44.2
  - acquired K82.8
  - with obstruction K82.0
- digestive organs NEC Q45.8
- esophagus Q39.0
  - with tracheoesophageal fistula Q39.1
- fallopian tube (congenital) Q50.6
  - acquired N97.1
- follicular cyst N83.0-
- foramen of
  - Luschka Q03.1
    - with spina bifida—*see* Spina bifida, with hydrocephalus
  - Magendie Q03.1
    - with spina bifida—*see* Spina bifida, with hydrocephalus
- gallbladder Q44.1
- genital organ
  - external
    - female Q52.79
    - male Q55.8
  - internal
    - female Q52.8
    - male Q55.8
- gullet Q39.0
  - with tracheoesophageal fistula Q39.1
- hymen Q52.3
  - acquired (postinfective) N89.6
- intestine (small) Q41.9
  - large Q42.9
    - specified NEC Q42.8
- iris, filtration angle Q15.0
- mitral valve Q23.2
  - in hypoplastic left heart syndrome Q23.4
- nares (anterior) (posterior) Q30.0
- nose, nostril Q30.0
  - acquired J34.89
- organ or site NEC Q89.8
- oviduct (congenital) Q50.6
  - acquired N97.1
- rectum Q42.1
  - with fistula Q42.0
- ureter Q62.10
  - pelvic junction Q62.11
  - vesical orifice Q62.12
- ureteropelvic junction Q62.11
- ureterovesical orifice Q62.12
- uterus Q51.818
  - acquired N85.8
- vagina (congenital) Q52.4
  - acquired (postinfectional) (senile) N89.5
- vein NEC Q27.8
  - pulmonary Q26.4
    - partial Q26.3
    - total Q26.2

Atrial septal defect
- coronary sinus Q21.13
- inferior sinus venosus Q21.15
- other specified Q21.19
- patent foramen ovale Q21.12
- secundum Q21.11
- sinus venosus, unspecified Q21.16

Atrial septal defect, *continued*
- superior sinus venosus Q21.14
- unspecified Q21.10

Atrioventricular septal defect
- complete Q21.23
- partial Q21.21
- transitional Q21.22
- unspecified as to partial or complete Q21.20

Atrophy, atrophic (of)
- adrenal (capsule) (gland) E27.49
  - primary (autoimmune) E27.1
- buccal cavity K13.79
- facioscapulohumeral (Landouzy-Déjérine) G71.02
- hemifacial Q67.4
  - Romberg G51.8
  - Landouzy-Déjérine G71.02
- laryngitis, infective J37.0
- lip K13.0
- muscle, muscular (diffuse) (general) (idiopathic) (primary)
  - infantile spinal G12.0
  - progressive (bulbar) G12.21
    - infantile (spinal) G12.0
    - spinal G12
      - infantile G12.0
  - pseudohypertrophic G71.02
  - spinal G12.9
    - infantile, type I (Werdnig-Hoffmann) G12.0
- nail L60.3
- pseudohypertrophic (muscle) G71.0
- rhinitis J31.0
- scar L90.5
- suprarenal (capsule) (gland) E27.49
  - primary E27.1
- systemic affecting central nervous system
  - in
    - myxedema E03.9 [G13.2]
    - neoplastic disease (*see also* Table of Neoplasms in the complete *ICD-10-CM* manual) D49.9 [G13.1]
      - specified disease NEC G13.8
- testes N50.0
- thyroid (gland) (acquired) E03.4
  - with cretinism E03.1
  - congenital (with myxedema) E03.1
- turbinate J34.89
- WerdnigHoffmann G12.0

Attack, attacks
- AdamsStokes I45.9
- benign shuddering G25.83
- cyanotic, newborn P28.2
- drop NEC R55
- epileptic—*see* Epilepsy
- hysterical F44.9
- panic F41.0
- shuddering, benign G25.83
- StokesAdams I45.9
- syncope R55
- transient ischemic (TIA) G45.9
  - specified NEC G45.8
- unconsciousness R55
  - hysterical F44.89
- vasomotor R55
- vasovagal (paroxysmal) (idiopathic) R55
- without alteration of consciousness—*see* Epilepsy, syndromes, localization-related, symptomatic, with simple partial seizure

Attention (to)
- artificial
  - opening (of) Z43.9
    - digestive tract NEC Z43.4
      - stomach Z43.1
    - specified NEC Z43.8
    - trachea Z43.0
    - urinary tract NEC Z43.6
      - cystostomy Z43.5
      - nephrostomy Z43.6
      - ureterostomy Z43.6
      - urethrostomy Z43.6
- colostomy Z43.3
- cystostomy Z43.5

ALPHABETIC INDEX

Attention, *continued*

- deficit disorder or syndrome F98.8
  - with hyperactivity—*see* Disorder, attention-deficit hyperactivity
- gastrostomy Z43.1
- ileostomy Z43.2
- jejunostomy Z43.4
- nephrostomy Z43.6
- surgical dressings Z48.01
- sutures Z48.02
- tracheostomy Z43.0
- ureterostomy Z43.6
- uretrhostomy Z43.6

Austin Flint murmur (aortic insufficiency) I35.1

Autism, autistic (childhood) (infantile) F84.0

- atypical F84.9
- spectrum disorder F84.0

Autoantibodies, multiple confirmed islet, with normoglycemia E10.A1

Autoerythrocyte sensitization (syndrome) D69.2

Autographism L50.3

Autoimmune

- disease (systemic) M35.9
- lymphoproliferative syndrome /ALPS/ D89.82
- thyroiditis E06.3

Autoimmunity, confirmed islet, with dysglycemia E10.A2

Automatism G93.89

- with temporal sclerosis G93.81
- epileptic—*see* Epilepsy, localization-related, symptomatic, with complex partial seizures
- paroxysmal, idiopathic—*see* Epilepsy, localization-related, symptomatic, with complex partial seizures

Autosensitivity, erythrocyte D69.2

Aversion

- oral R63.39
  - newborn P92.-
  - nonorganic origin F98.2

Avitaminosis (multiple) (*see also* Deficiency, vitamin) E56.9

- D E55.9
  - with rickets E55.0

AVNRT (atrioventricular nodal re-entrant tachycardia) I47.19

AVRT (atrioventricular nodal re-entrant tachycardia) I47.19

Avulsion (traumatic)

- spleen S36.032

Awareness of heart beat R00.2

Axenfeld's

- anomaly or syndrome Q15.0

Ayerza's disease or syndrome (pulmonary artery sclerosis with pulmonary hypertension) I27.0

Azotemia R79.89

- meaning uremia N19

B

Babesiosis B60.00

- due to
  - Babesia
    - divergens B60.03
    - duncani B60.02
    - KO-1 B60.09
    - microti B60.01
    - MO-1 B60.03
    - species
      - unspecified B60.00
    - venatorum B60.09
  - specified NEC B60.09

Babington's disease (familial hemorrhagic telangiectasia) I78.0

Baby

- crying constantly R68.11
- floppy (syndrome) P94.2

Bacteriuria, bacteruria (asymptomatic) R82.71

Bacillus

- coli infection (*see also* Escherichia coli) B96.20
- Shiga's A03.0
- suipestifer infection—*see* Infection, salmonella

Backache (postural) M54.9

- sacroiliac M53.3

Backward reading (dyslexia) F81.0

Bacteremia R78.81

- with sepsis—*see* Sepsis

Bacterium, bacteria, bacterial

- agent NEC, as cause of disease classified elsewhere B96.89
- in blood—*see* Bacteremia
- in urine R82.71

Bacteriuria, bacteruria R82.71

- urinary tract infection N39.0

Baelz's disease (cheilitis glandularis apostematosa) K13.0

Baerensprung's disease (eczema marginatum) B35.6

Balanitis (circinata) (erosiva) (gangrenosa) (phagedenic) (vulgaris) N48.1

- candidal B37.42

Balanoposthitis N47.6

Band(s)

- gallbladder (congenital) Q44.1
- vagina N89.5

Bandemia D72.825

Bankruptcy, anxiety concerning Z59.89

Bannister's disease T78.3

Bartonellosis A44.9

- cutaneous A44.1
- mucocutaneous A44.1
- specified NEC A44.8
- systemic A44.0

Barton's fracture S52.56-

Basophilia D72.824

Basophilism (cortico-adrenal) (Cushing's) (pituitary) E24.0

Bateman's

- disease B08.1
- purpura (senile) D69.2

Bathing cramp T75.1

Battle exhaustion F43.0

Beach ear—*see* Swimmer's, ear

Beat(s)

- atrial, premature I49.1
- premature I49.40
  - atrial I49.1
  - auricular I49.1
  - supraventricular I49.1

Becker's

- disease
  - myotonia congenita, recessive form G71.12
  - dystrophy G71.01

Beckwith-Wiedemann syndrome Q87.3

Bedbug bite(s)—*see* Bite(s), by site, superficial, insect

Bedclothes, asphyxiation or suffocation by—*see* Asphyxia, traumatic

Bednar's

- aphthae K12.0

Bedwetting—*see* Enuresis

Bee sting (with allergic or anaphylactic shock) T63.44-

Behavior

- drug *seeking* Z76.5
- self-damaging (lifestyle) Z72.89

Bell's

- palsy, paralysis G51.0
  - infant or newborn P11.3

Bence Jones albuminuria or proteinuria NEC R80.3

Bennett's fracture (displaced) S62.21-

Bent

- back (hysterical) F44.4
- nose M95.0
  - congenital Q67.4

Bereavement (uncomplicated) Z63.4

Bergeron's disease (hysterical chorea) F44.4

Besnier's

- lupus pernio D86.3
- prurigo L20.0

Best's disease H35.50

Betalipoproteinemia, broad or floating E78.2

Betting and gambling Z72.6

Bicornate or bicornis uterus Q51.3

Bicuspid aortic valve (at birth) (congenital) Q23.81

- functional, with stenosis—*see* Stenosis, aortic (valve)

Biedl-Bardet syndrome Q87.83

Bifid (congenital)

- scrotum Q55.29
- toe NEC Q74.2
- uterus Q51.3
- uvula Q35.7

Bifurcation (congenital)

- gallbladder Q44.1

Bigorexia F45.22

Bilharziasis—*see also* Schistosomiasis

- cutaneous B65.3

Bilirubin metabolism disorder E80.7

- specified NEC E80.6

Biparta, bipartite

- carpal scaphoid Q74.0

Bird

- face Q75.8

Birth

- injury NOS P15.9
  - brachial plexus NEC P14.3
  - cerebral hemorrhage P10.1
  - eye P15.3
  - fracture
    - clavicle P13.4
    - skull P13.0
  - laceration
    - brain P10.1
    - by scalpel P15.8
  - nerve
    - brachial plexus P14.3
    - facial P11.3
  - paralysis
    - facial nerve P11.3
  - scalp P12.9
  - scalpel wound P15.8
  - specified type NEC P15.8
  - skull NEC P13.1
    - fracture P13.0
- shock, newborn P96.89
- weight
  - low (2499 grams or less)—*see* Low, birthweight
    - extremely (999 grams or less)—*see* Low, birthweight, extreme
  - 4000 grams to 4499 grams P08.1
  - 4500 grams or more P08.0

Birthmark Q82.5

Bisalbuminemia E88.09

Bite(s) (animal) (human)

- abdomen, abdominal
  - wall S31.159
    - epigastric region S31.152
    - left
      - lower quadrant S31.154
      - upper quadrant S31.151
    - periumbillic region S31.155
    - right
      - lower quadrant S31.153
      - upper quadrant S31.150
    - superficial NEC S30.871
      - insect S30.861
- amphibian (venomous)—*see* Table of Drugs and Chemicals, by animal or substance, poisoning
- animal—*see also* Bite
  - venomous—*see* Table of Drugs and Chemicals, by animal or substance, poisoning
- ankle S91.05-
  - superficial NEC S90.57-
    - insect S90.56-
- antecubital space—*see* Bite, elbow
- anus S31.835
  - superficial NEC S30.877
    - insect S30.867

ALPHABETIC INDEX

Bite(s), *continued*

- arm (upper) S41.15-
  - lower—*see* Bite, forearm
  - superficial NEC S40.87-
    - insect S40.86-
- arthropod NEC—*see* Table of Drugs and Chemicals, by animal or substance
- auditory canal (external) (meatus)—*see* Bite, ear
- auricle, ear—*see* Bite, ear
- axilla—*see* Bite, arm
- back—*see also* Bite, thorax, superficial, back
  - lower S31.050
    - superficial NEC S30.870
      - insect S30.860
- bedbug—*see* Bite(s), by site, superficial, insect
- breast
  - superficial NEC S20.17-
    - insect S20.16-
- brow—*see* Bite, head, specified site NEC
- buttock S31.8-
  - left S31.825
  - right S31.815
  - superficial NEC S30.870
    - insect S30.860
- calf—*see* Bite, leg
- canaliculus lacrimalis—*see* Bite, eyelid
- canthus, eye—*see* Bite, eyelid
- centipede—*see* Table of Drugs and Chemicals, by animal or substance, poisoning
- cheek (external) S01.45-
  - internal—*see* Bite, oral cavity
  - superficial NEC S00.87
    - insect S00.86
- chest wall—*see* Bite, thorax
- chigger B88.0
- chin—*see* Bite, head, specified site NEC
- clitoris—*see* Bite, vulva
- costal region—*see* Bite, thorax
- digit(s)
  - hand—*see* Bite, finger
  - toe—*see* Bite, toe
- ear (canal) (external) S01.35-
  - superficial NEC S00.47-
    - insect S00.46-
- elbow S51.05-
  - superficial NEC S50.37-
    - insect S50.36-
- epididymis—*see* Bite, testis
- epigastric region—*see* Bite, abdomen
- epiglottis—*see* Bite, neck, specified site NEC
- esophagus, cervical
  - superficial NEC S10.17
    - insect S10.16
- eyebrow—*see* Bite, eyelid
- eyelid S01.15-
  - superficial NEC S00.27-
    - insect S00.26-
- face NEC—*see* Bite, head, specified site NEC
- finger(s) S61.25-
  - with
    - damage to nail S61.35-
  - index S61.25-
    - with
      - damage to nail S61.35-
    - left S61.251
      - with
        - ◊ damage to nail S61.351
    - right S61.250
      - with
        - ◊ damage to nail S61.350
    - superficial NEC S60.47-
      - insect S60.46-
  - little S61.25-
    - with
      - damage to nail S61.35-
    - superficial NEC S60.47-
      - insect S60.46-
  - middle S61.25-
    - with
      - damage to nail S61.35-
    - superficial NEC S60.47-
      - insect S60.46-

Bite(s), *continued*

  - ring S61.25-
    - with
      - damage to nail S61.35-
    - superficial NEC S60.47-
      - insect S60.46-
  - superficial NEC S60.47-
    - insect S60.46-
  - thumb—*see* Bite, thumb
- flank—*see* Bite, abdomen, wall
- flea—*see* Bite, superficial, insect
- foot (except toe(s) alone) S91.35-
  - superficial NEC S90.87-
    - insect S90.86-
  - toe—*see* Bite, toe
- forearm S51.85-
  - elbow only—*see* Bite, elbow
  - superficial NEC S50.87-
    - insect S50.86-
- forehead—*see* Bite, head, specified site NEC
- genital organs, external
  - female
    - superficial NEC S30.876
      - insect S30.866
    - vagina and vulva—*see* Bite, vulva
  - male
    - penis—*see* Bite, penis
    - scrotum—*see* Bite, scrotum
    - superficial NEC S30.875
      - insect S30.865
    - testes—*see* Bite, testis
- groin—*see* Bite, abdomen, wall
- gum—*see* Bite, oral cavity
- hand S61.45-
  - finger—*see* Bite, finger
  - superficial NEC S60.57-
    - insect S60.56-
  - thumb—*see* Bite, thumb
- head (code *to* Bite *of specific site for* cheek, ear, eyelid, lip, nose, oral cavity, or scalp) S01.95
  - specified site NEC S01.85
    - superficial NEC S00.87
      - insect S00.86
  - superficial NEC S00.97
    - insect S00.96
  - temporomandibular area—*see* Bite, cheek
- heel—*see* Bite, foot
- hip S71.05-
  - superficial NEC S70.27-
    - insect S70.26-
- hymen S31.45
- hypochondrium—*see* Bite, abdomen, wall
- hypogastric region—*see* Bite, abdomen, wall
- inguinal region—*see* Bite, abdomen, wall
- insect—*see* Bite, by site, superficial, insect
- instep—*see* Bite, foot
- interscapular region—*see* Bite, thorax, superficial, back
- jaw—*see* Bite, head, specified site NEC
- knee S81.05-
  - superficial NEC S80.27-
    - insect S80.26-
- labium (majus) (minus)—*see* Bite, vulva
- lacrimal duct—*see* Bite, eyelid
- larynx
  - superficial NEC S10.17
    - insect S10.16
- leg (lower) (code *to* Bite *of specific site for* ankle, foot, knee, upper leg/thigh, or toe) S81.85-
  - superficial NEC S80.87-
    - insect S80.86-
- lip S01.551
  - superficial NEC S00.571
    - insect S00.561
- lizard (venomous)—*see* Table of Drugs and Chemicals, by animal or substance, poisoning
- loin—*see* Bite, abdomen, wall
- lower back—*see* Bite, back, lower
- lumbar region—*see* Bite, back, lower
- malar region—*see* Bite, head, specified site NEC
- mammary—*see* Bite, breast
- marine animals (venomous)—*see* Table of Drugs and Chemicals, by animal or substance, poisoning

Bite(s), *continued*

- mastoid region—*see* Bite, head, specified site NEC
- mouth—*see* Bite, oral cavity
- nail
  - finger—*see* Bite, finger
  - toe—*see* Bite, toe
- nape—*see* Bite, neck, specified site NEC
- nasal (septum) (sinus)—*see* Bite, nose
- nasopharynx—*see* Bite, head, specified site NEC
- neck (code *to* Bite *by specific site for* esophagus, larynx, pharynx, or trachea) S11.95
  - involving
    - specified site NEC S11.85
      - superficial NEC S10.87
        - insect S10.86
    - superficial NEC S10.97
      - insect S10.96
  - throat S11.85
    - superficial NEC S10.17
      - insect S10.16
- nose (septum) (sinus) S01.25
  - superficial NEC S00.37
    - insect S00.36
- occipital region—*see* Bite, scalp
- oral cavity S01.552
  - superficial NEC S00.572
    - insect S00.562
- orbital region—*see* Bite, eyelid
- palate—*see* Bite, oral cavity
- palm—*see* Bite, hand
- parietal region—*see* Bite, scalp
- pelvis S31.050
  - superficial NEC S30.870
    - insect S30.860
- penis S31.25
  - superficial NEC S30.872
    - insect S30.862
- perineum
  - female—*see* Bite, vulva
  - male—*see* Bite, pelvis
- periocular area (with or without lacrimal passages)—*see* Bite, eyelid
- phalanges
  - finger—*see* Bite, finger
  - toe—*see* Bite, toe
- pharynx
  - superficial NEC S10.17
    - insect S10.16
- pinna—*see* Bite, ear
- poisonous—*see* Table of Drugs and Chemicals, by animal or substance, poisoning
- popliteal space—*see* Bite, knee
- prepuce—*see* Bite, penis
- pubic region—*see* Bite, abdomen, wall
- rectovaginal septum—*see* Bite, vulva
- red bug B88.0
- reptile NEC—*see* Table of Drugs and Chemicals, by animal or substance, poisoning
  - nonvenomous—*see* Bite, by site
  - snake—*see* Table of Drugs and Chemicals, by animal or substance, poisoning
- sacral region—*see* Bite, back, lower
- sacroiliac region—*see* Bite, back, lower
- salivary gland—*see* Bite, oral cavity
- scalp S01.05
  - superficial NEC S00.07
    - insect S00.06
- scapular region—*see* Bite, shoulder
- scrotum S31.35
  - superficial NEC S30.873
    - insect S30.863
- sea-snake (venomous)—*see* Table of Drugs and Chemicals, by animal or substance, poisoning
- shin—*see* Bite, leg
- shoulder S41.05-
  - superficial NEC S40.27-
    - insect S40.26-
- snake—*see* Table of Drugs and Chemicals, by animal or substance, poisoning
  - nonvenomous—*see* Bite, by site
- spermatic cord—*see* Bite, testis

ALPHABETIC INDEX

Bite(s), *continued*

- spider (venomous)—*see* Table of Drugs and Chemicals, by animal or substance, poisoning
  - nonvenomous—*see* Bite, by site, superficial, insect
- sternal region—*see* Bite, thorax, superficial, front
- submaxillary region—*see* Bite, head, specified site NEC
- submental region—*see* Bite, head, specified site NEC
- subungual
  - finger(s)—*see* Bite, finger
  - toe—*see* Bite, toe
- superficial—*see* Bite, by site, superficial
- supraclavicular fossa S11.85
- supraorbital—*see* Bite, head, specified site NEC
- temple, temporal region—*see* Bite, head, specified site NEC
- temporomandibular area—*see* Bite, cheek
- testis S31.35
  - superficial NEC S30.873
    - insect S30.863
- thigh S71.15-
  - superficial NEC S70.37-
    - insect S70.36-
- thorax, thoracic (wall) S21.95
  - breast—*see* Bite, breast
  - superficial NEC S20.97
    - back S20.47-
    - front S20.37-
    - insect S20.96
      - back S20.46-
      - front S20.36-
- throat—*see* Bite, neck, throat
- thumb S61.05-
  - with
    - damage to nail S61.15-
  - superficial NEC S60.37-
    - insect S60.36-
- thyroid
  - superficial NEC S10.87
    - insect S10.86
- toe(s) S91.15-
  - with
    - damage to nail S91.25-
  - great S91.15-
    - with
      - damage to nail S91.25-
  - lesser S91.15-
    - with
      - damage to nail S91.25-
  - superficial NEC S90.47-
    - great S90.47-
    - insect S90.46-
      - great S90.46-
- tongue S01.552
- trachea
  - superficial NEC S10.17
    - insect S10.16
- tunica vaginalis—*see* Bite, testis
- tympanum, tympanic membrane—*see* Bite, ear
- umbilical region S31.155
- uvula—*see* Bite, oral cavity
- vagina—*see* Bite, vulva
- venomous—*see* Table of Drugs and Chemicals, by animal or substance, poisoning
- vulva S31.45
  - superficial NEC S30.874
    - insect S30.864
- wrist S61.55-
  - superficial NEC S60.87-
    - insect S60.86-

Biting, cheek or lip K13.1

Biventricular failure (heart) I50.9

Bjorck (-Thorson) syndrome (malignant carcinoid) E34.09

Blackfan-Diamond anemia or syndrome (congenital hypoplastic anemia) D61.01

Blackhead L70.0

Blackout R55

Blastomycosis, blastomycotic B40.9

- cutaneous B40.3
- disseminated B40.7
- generalized B40.7
- North American B40.9

Blastomycosis, blastomycotic, *continued*

- primary pulmonary B40.0
- pulmonary
  - acute B40.0
  - chronic B40.1
  - skin B40.3
  - specified NEC B40.89

Bleeding—*see also* Hemorrhage

- anal K62.5
- anovulatory N97.0
- gastrointestinal K92.2
- intermenstrual (regular) N92.3
  - irregular N92.1
  - irregular N92.6
- nipple N64.59
- nose R04.0
- ovulation N92.3
- pre-pubertal vaginal N93.1
- puberty (excessive, with onset of menstrual periods) N92.2
- rectum, rectal K62.5
  - newborn P54.2
- tendencies—*see* Defect, coagulation
- uterus, uterine NEC N93.9
  - dysfunctional or functional N93.8
- vagina, vaginal (abnormal) N93.9
  - dysfunctional or functional N93.8
  - newborn P54.6
  - pre-pubertal N93.1
- vicarious N94.89

Blennorrhea (acute) (chronic)—*see also* Gonorrhea

- inclusion (neonatal) (newborn) P39.1
- lower genitourinary tract (gonococcal) A54.00
- neonatorum (gonococcal ophthalmia) A54.31

Blepharitis (angularis) (ciliaris) (eyelid) (marginal) (nonulcerative) H01.00-

- left H01.006
  - lower H01.005
  - upper H01.004
  - upper and lower H01.00B
- right H01.003
  - lower H01.002
  - upper H01.001
  - upper and lower H01.00A

Blepharochalasis H02.3-

- congenital Q10.0

Blepharoconjunctivitis H10.50-

Blepharoptosis H02.40-

- congenital Q10.0

Blindness (acquired) (congenital) (both eyes) H54.0X

- emotional (hysterical) F44.6
- hysterical F44.6
- one eye (other eye normal) H54.4-
  - left (normal vision on right) H54.42-
    - low vision on right H54.12-
  - right (normal vision on left) H54.41-
    - low vision on left H54.11-
- sac, fallopian tube (congenital) Q50.6
- word (developmental) F81.0
  - acquired R48.0
  - secondary to organic lesion R48.0

Blister (nonthermal)

- abdominal wall S30.821
- alveolar process S00.522
- ankle S90.52-
- antecubital space—*see* Blister, elbow
- anus S30.827
- arm (upper) S40.82-
- auditory canal—*see* Blister, ear
- auricle—*see* Blister, ear
- axilla—*see* Blister, arm
- back, lower S30.820
- beetle dermatitis L24.89
- breast S20.12-
- brow S00.82
- calf—*see* Blister, leg
- canthus—*see* Blister, eyelid
- cheek S00.82
  - internal S00.522
- chest wall—*see* Blister, thorax
- chin S00.82

Blister, *continued*

- costal region—*see* Blister, thorax
- digit(s)
  - foot—*see* Blister, toe
  - hand—*see* Blister, finger
- due to burn—*see* Burn, by site, second degree
- ear S00.42-
- elbow S50.32-
- epiglottis S10.12
- esophagus, cervical S10.12
- eyebrow—*see* Blister, eyelid
- eyelid S00.22-
- face S00.82
- fever B00.1
- finger(s) S60.42-
  - index S60.42-
  - little S60.42-
  - middle S60.42-
  - ring S60.42-
- foot (except toe(s) alone) S90.82-
  - toe—*see* Blister, toe
- forearm S50.82-
  - elbow only—*see* Blister, elbow
- forehead S00.82
- fracture omit code
- genital organ
  - female S30.826
  - male S30.825
- gum S00.522
- hand S60.52-
- head S00.92
  - ear—*see* Blister, ear
  - eyelid—*see* Blister, eyelid
  - lip S00.521
  - nose S00.32
  - oral cavity S00.522
  - scalp S00.02
  - specified site NEC S00.82
- heel—*see* Blister, foot
- hip S70.22-
- interscapular region S20.429
- jaw S00.82
- knee S80.22-
- larynx S10.12
- leg (lower) S80.82-
  - knee—*see* Blister, knee
  - upper—*see* Blister, thigh
- lip S00.521
- malar region S00.82
- mammary—*see* Blister, breast
- mastoid region S00.82
- mouth S00.522
- multiple, skin, nontraumatic R23.8
- nail
  - finger—*see* Blister, finger
  - toe—*see* Blister, toe
- nasal S00.32
- neck S10.92
  - specified site NEC S10.82
  - throat S10.12
- nose S00.32
- occipital region S00.02
- oral cavity S00.522
- orbital region—*see* Blister, eyelid
- palate S00.522
- palm—*see* Blister, hand
- parietal region S00.02
- pelvis S30.820
- penis S30.822
- periocular area—*see* Blister, eyelid
- phalanges
  - finger—*see* Blister, finger
  - toe—*see* Blister, toe
- pharynx S10.12
- pinna—*see* Blister, ear
- popliteal space—*see* Blister, knee
- scalp S00.02
- scapular region—*see* Blister, shoulder
- scrotum S30.823
- shin—*see* Blister, leg
- shoulder S40.22-
- sternal region S20.32-
- submaxillary region S00.82

Blister, *continued*

- submental region S00.82
- subungual
  - finger(s)—*see* Blister, finger
  - toe(s)—*see* Blister, toe
- supraclavicular fossa S10.82
- supraorbital S00.82
- temple S00.82
- temporal region S00.82
- testis S30.823
- thermal—*see* Burn, second degree, by site
- thigh S70.32-
- thorax, thoracic (wall) S20.92
  - back S20.42-
  - front S20.32-
- throat S10.12
- thumb S60.32-
- toe(s) S90.42-
  - great S90.42-
- tongue S00.522
- trachea S10.12
- tympanum, tympanic membrane—*see* Blister, ear
- upper arm—*see* Blister, arm (upper)
- uvula S00.522
- vagina S30.824
- vocal cords S10.12
- vulva S30.824
- wrist S60.82-

Bloating R14.0

Block, blocked

- arrhythmic I45.9
- atrioventricular (incomplete) (partial) I44.30
  - with atrioventricular dissociation I44.2
  - complete I44.2
    - congenital Q24.6
  - congenital Q24.6
  - first degree I44.0
  - second degree (types I and II) I44.1
  - specified NEC I44.39
  - third degree I44.2
  - types I and II I44.1
- cardiac I45.9
- conduction I45.9
  - complete I44.2
- foramen Magendie (acquired) G91.1
  - congenital Q03.1
    - with spina bifida—*see* Spina bifida, with hydrocephalus
- heart I45.9
  - complete (atrioventricular) I44.2
  - congenital Q24.6
  - first degree (atrioventricular) I44.0
  - second degree (atrioventricular) I44.1
  - third degree (atrioventricular) I44.2
- Mobitz (types I and II) I44.1
- portal (vein) I81
- second degree (types I and II) I44.1
- third degree I44.2
- Wenckebach (types I and II) I44.1

Blocq's disease F44.4

Blood

- constituents, abnormal R78.9
- disease D75.9
- in
  - feces K92.1
    - occult R19.5
  - urine—*see* Hematuria
- occult in feces R19.5
- pressure
  - decreased, due to shock following injury T79.4
  - examination only Z01.30
  - high—*see* Hypertension
    - borderline R03.0
    - incidental reading, without diagnosis of hypertension R03.0
- transfusion
  - reaction or complication—*see* Complications, transfusion
- type Z67-

Blood-forming organs, disease D75.9

Bloom (-Machacek) (-Torre) syndrome Q82.8

Blount disease or osteochondrosis M92.51-

Blue

- baby Q24.9
- dot cataract Q12.0
  - sclera Q13.5

Blurring, visual H53.8

Blushing (abnormal) (excessive) R23.2

BMI—*see* Body, mass index

Boarder, hospital NEC Z76.4

- healthy infant or child Z76.2
  - foundling Z76.1

Blue

- baby Q24.9
- dot cataract Q12.0
- sclera Q13.5
  - with fragility of bone and deafness Q78.0

Boder-Sedgwick syndrome (ataxia-telangiectasia) G11.3

Body, bodies

- mass index (BMI)
  - adult Z68-
  - pediatric
    - 5th percentile to less than 85th percentile for age Z68.52
    - 85th percentile to less than 95th percentile for age Z68.53
    - greater than or equal to ninety-fifth percentile for age Z68.54
    - 95th percentile for age to less than 120% of the 95th percentile for age Z68.54
    - 120% of the 95th percentile for age to less than 140% of the 95th percentile for age Z68.55
    - greater than or equal to 140% of the 95th percentile for age Z68.56
    - less than fifth percentile for age Z68.51
  - rocking F98.4

Boeck's

- disease or sarcoid—*see* Sarcoidosis
- lupoid (miliary) D86.3

Bonnevie-Ullrich syndrome Q87.19

Borderline

- diabetes mellitus (prediabetes) R73.03
- hypertension R03.0
- personality F60.3

Botalli, ductus (patent) (persistent) Q25.0

Botulism (foodborne intoxication) A05.1

- infant A48.51
- non-foodborne A48.52
- wound A48.52

Bouillaud's disease or syndrome (rheumatic heart disease) I01.9

Bourneville's disease Q85.1

Bowleg(s) (acquired) M21.16-

- congenital Q68.5

Brachycardia R00.1

Brachycephaly, non-deformational Q75.022

Bradycardia (sinoatrial) (sinus) (vagal) R00.1

- neonatal P29.12
- tachycardia syndrome I49.5

Bradypnea R06.89

Bradytachycardia I49.5

Brailsford's disease or osteochondrosis—*see* Osteochondrosis, juvenile, radius

Brain—*see also* Disease, diseased

- death G93.82
- syndrome—*see* Syndrome, brain

Brash (water) R12

BRBPR K62.5

Breast—*see also* Disease, diseased

- buds E30.1
  - in newborn P96.89
- nodule N63.0

Breath

- foul R19.6
- holder, child R06.89
- holding spell R06.89
- shortness R06.02

Breathing

- labored—*see* Hyperventilation
- mouth R06.5
- periodic R06.3
  - high altitude G47.32

Breathlessness R06.81

Brennemann's syndrome I88.0

Bright red blood per rectum (BRBPR) K62.5

Briquet's disorder or syndrome F45.0

Brissaud's

- infantilism or dwarfism E23.0
- motor-verbal tic F95.2

Brittle

- bones disease Q78.0
- nails L60.3

Broad—*see also* Disease, diseased

- beta disease E78.2

Broad- or floating-betalipoproteinemia E78.2

Broken

- arm (meaning upper limb)—*see* Fracture, arm
- bone—*see* Fracture
- leg (meaning lower limb)—*see* Fracture, leg
- nose S02.2-
- tooth, teeth—*see* Fracture, tooth

Bromidism, bromism G92.8

- due to
  - correct substance properly administered—*see* Table of Drugs and Chemicals, by drug, adverse effect
  - overdose or wrong substance given or taken—*see* Table of Drugs and Chemicals, by drug, poisoning

Bronchiolitis (acute) (infective) (subacute) J21.9

- with
  - bronchospasm or obstruction J21.9
  - influenza, flu or grippe—*see* Influenza, with, respiratory manifestations NEC
- chronic (fibrosing) (obliterative) J44.89
  - obliterative J44.81
- due to
  - external agent—*see* Bronchitis, acute, due to
  - human metapneumovirus J21.1
  - respiratory syncytial virus (RSV) J21.0
  - specified organism NEC J21.8
- fibrosa obliterans J44.81
- influenzal—*see* Influenza, with, respiratory manifestations NEC
- obliterans—*see also* Bronchiolitis, obliterative J44.81
  - syndrome J44.81
- obliterative (chronic) (subacute)—*see also* Bronchiolitis, obliterans J44.81
  - due to chemicals, gases, fumes or vapors (inhalation)—*see also* Disease, respiratory, chronic, due to chemicals, gases, fumes or vapors J44.81
  - due to fumes or vapors—*see also* Disease, respiratory, chronic, due to chemicals, gases, fumes or vapors J44.81

Bronchitis (diffuse) (fibrinous) (hypostatic) (infective) (membranous) J40

- with
  - influenza, flu or grippe—*see* Influenza, with, respiratory manifestations NEC
  - obstruction (airway) (lung) J44.89
  - tracheitis (15 years of age and above) J40
    - acute or subacute J20.9
    - under 15 years of age J20.9
  - acute or subacute (with bronchospasm or obstruction) J20.9
    - due to
      - Haemophilus influenzae J20.1
      - Mycoplasma pneumoniae J20.0
      - specified organism NEC J20.8
      - Streptococcus J20.2
      - virus
        - coxsackie J20.3
        - echovirus J20.7
        - parainfluenza J20.4
        - respiratory syncytial (RSV) J20.5
        - rhinovirus J20.6
        - viral NEC J20.8

ALPHABETIC INDEX

Bronchitis, *continued*

- allergic (acute) J45.909
  - with
    - exacerbation (acute) J45.901
    - status asthmaticus J45.902
- asthmatic J45.9
  - chronic J44.89
- catarrhal (15 years of age and above) J40
  - acute—see Bronchitis, acute
  - under 15 years of age J20.9
- chronic J42
  - with
    - airways obstruction J44.89
    - asthmatic (obstructive) J44.89
    - emphysematous J44.89
    - obstructive J44.89
  - emphysematous (obstructive) J44.89
  - obstructive (chronic) (diffuse) J44.89
  - mucopurulent
    - acute or subacute J20.9
    - pneumococcal, acute or subacute J20.2
  - viral NEC, acute or subacute (see also Bronchitis, acute) J20.8

Bronchoalveolitis J18.0

Bronchocele meaning goiter E04.0

Bronchomycosis NOS B49 [J99]

- candidal B37.1

Bronchorrhea J98.09

- acute J20.9

Bronchospasm (acute) J98.01

- with
  - bronchiolitis, acute J21.9
  - bronchitis, acute (conditions in J20)—see Bronchitis, acute
- due to external agent—see Disease, diseased, respiratory, acute, due to
- exercise induced J45.990

Bronze baby syndrome P83.88

Bruck-de Lange disease Q87.19

BRUE (brief resolved unexplained event) R68.13

Brugsch's syndrome Q82.8

Bruise (skin surface intact)—see also Contusion

- with
  - open wound—see Wound, open
  - internal organ—see Injury, by site
- newborn P54.5
- scalp, due to birth injury, newborn P12.3

Bruit (arterial) R09.89

- cardiac R01.1

Bruxism

- psychogenic F45.8

Bubo I88.8

- indolent (nonspecific) I88.8
- inguinal (nonspecific) I88.8
  - infective I88.8
- scrofulous (tuberculous) A18.2
- syphilitic (primary) A51.0

Buds

- breast E30.1
  - in newborn P96.89

Bulimia (nervosa) F50.2-

- atypical F50.9
- normal weight F50.9

Bulky

- stools R19.5

Bunion M21.61-

- tailor's M21.62-

Bunionette M21.62-

Buphthalmia, buphthalmos (congenital) Q15.0

Buried

- penis (congenital) Q55.64

Burkitt

- cell leukemia C91.0-
- lymphoma (malignant) C83.7-
  - small noncleaved, diffuse C83.7-
  - spleen C83.77
  - undifferentiated C83.7-

Burkitt, *continued*

- tumor C83.7-
- type
  - acute lymphoblastic leukemia C91.0-
  - undifferentiated C83.7-

Burn (electricity) (flame) (hot gas, liquid or hot object) (radiation) (steam) (thermal) T30.0

- abdomen, abdominal (muscle) (wall) T21.02
  - first degree T21.12
  - second degree T21.22
  - third degree T21.32
- above elbow T22.03-
  - first degree T22.13-
  - left T22.032
    - first degree T22.132
    - second degree T22.232
    - third degree T22.332
  - right T22.031
    - first degree T22.131
    - second degree T22.231
    - third degree T22.331
  - second degree T22.23-
  - third degree T22.33-
- acid (caustic) (external) (internal)—see Corrosion, by site
- alimentary tract
  - esophagus T28.1
  - mouth T28.0
  - pharynx T28.0
- alkaline (caustic) (external) (internal)—see Corrosion, by site
- ankle T25.01-
  - first degree T25.11-
  - left T25.012
    - first degree T25.112
    - second degree T25.212
    - third degree T25.312
  - multiple with foot—see Burn, lower, limb, multiple sites, ankle and foot
  - right T25.011
    - first degree T25.111
    - second degree T25.211
    - third degree T25.311
  - second degree T25.21-
  - third degree T25.31-
- anus—see Burn, buttock
- arm (lower) (upper)—see Burn, upper limb
- axilla T22.04-
  - first degree T22.14-
  - left T22.042
    - first degree T22.142
    - second degree T22.242
    - third degree T22.342
  - right T22.041
    - first degree T22.141
    - second degree T22.241
    - third degree T22.341
  - second degree T22.24-
  - third degree T22.34-
- back (lower) T21.04
  - first degree T21.14
  - second degree T21.24
  - third degree T21.34
  - upper T21.03
    - first degree T21.13
    - second degree T21.23
    - third degree T21.33
- blisters *code as* Burn, second degree, by site
- breast(s)—*see* Burn, chest wall
- buttock(s) T21.05
  - first degree T21.15
  - second degree T21.25
  - third degree T21.35
- calf T24.03-
  - first degree T24.13-
  - left T24.032
    - first degree T24.132
    - second degree T24.232
    - third degree T24.332
  - right T24.031
    - first degree T24.131
    - second degree T24.231

Burn, *continued*

- - third degree T24.331
  - second degree T24.23-
  - third degree T24.33-
- canthus (eye)—see Burn, eyelid
- caustic acid or alkaline—see Corrosion, by site
- cheek T20.06
  - first degree T20.16
  - second degree T20.26
  - third degree T20.36
- chemical (acids) (alkalines) (caustics) (external) (internal)—see Corrosion, by site
- chest wall T21.01
  - first degree T21.11
  - second degree T21.21
  - third degree T21.31
- chin T20.03
  - first degree T20.13
  - second degree T20.23
  - third degree T20.33
- conjunctiva (and cornea)—see Burn, cornea
- cornea (and conjunctiva) T26.1- (see complete *ICD-10-CM* Manual)
- corrosion (external) (internal)—see Corrosion, by site
- deep necrosis of underlying tissue *code as* Burn, third degree, by site
- dorsum of hand T23.069
  - first degree T23.16-
  - left T23.062
    - first degree T23.162
    - second degree T23.262
    - third degree T23.362
  - right T23.061
    - first degree T23.161
    - second degree T23.261
    - third degree T23.361
  - second degree T23.26-
  - third degree T23.36-
- due to ingested chemical agent—see Corrosion, by site
- ear (auricle) (external) (canal) T20.01
  - first degree T20.11
  - second degree T20.21
  - third degree T20.31
- elbow T22.02-
  - first degree T22.12-
  - left T22.022
    - first degree T22.122
    - second degree T22.222
    - third degree T22.322
  - right T22.021
    - first degree T22.121
    - second degree T22.221
    - third degree T22.321
  - second degree T22.22-
  - third degree T22.32-
- epidermal loss *code as* Burn, second degree, by site
- erythema, erythematous *code as* Burn, first degree, by site
- esophagus T28.1
- extent (percentage of body surface)
  - less than 10 percent T31.0
  - 10–19 percent T31.10
    - with 0–9 percent third degree burns T31.10
    - with 10–19 percent third degree burns T31.11
- extremity—see Burn, limb
- eye(s) and adnexa T26.4- (see complete *ICD-10-CM* Manual)
- eyelid(s) T26.0- (See complete *ICD-10-CM* Manual for codes)
- face—see Burn, head
- finger T23.029
  - first degree T23.12-
  - left T23.022
    - first degree T23.122
    - second degree T23.222
    - third degree T23.322
  - multiple sites (without thumb) T23.03-
    - with thumb T23.04-
      - first degree T23.14-
      - left T23.042
        - ◊ first degree T23.142
        - ◊ second degree T23.242
        - ◊ third degree T23.342

Burn, *continued*

- right T23.041
  - ◊ first degree T23.141
  - ◊ second degree T23.241
  - ◊ third degree T23.341
  - ~ second degree T23.24-
  - ~ third degree T23.34-
- ■ first degree T23.13-
- ■ left T23.032
  - ~ first degree T23.132
  - ~ second degree T23.232
  - ~ third degree T23.332
- ■ right T23.031
  - ~ first degree T23.131
  - ~ second degree T23.231
  - ~ third degree T23.331
  - ■ second degree T23.23-
  - ■ third degree T23.33-
- right T23.021
  - ■ first degree T23.121
  - ■ second degree T23.221
  - ■ third degree T23.321
  - ~ second degree T23.22-
  - ~ third degree T23.32-
- flank—*see* Burn, abdomen, abdominal (muscle) (wall)
- foot T25.02-
  - first degree T25.12-
  - left T25.022
    - ■ first degree T25.122
    - ■ second degree T25.222
    - ■ third degree T25.322
  - multiple with ankle—*see* Burn, lower, limb, multiple sites
  - right T25.021
    - ■ first degree T25.121
    - ■ second degree T25.221
    - ■ third degree T25.321
  - second degree T25.22-
  - third degree T25.32-
- forearm T22.01-
  - first degree T22.11-
  - left T22.012
    - ■ first degree T22.112
    - ■ second degree T22.212
    - ■ third degree T22.312
  - right T22.011
    - ■ first degree T22.111
    - ■ second degree T22.211
    - ■ third degree T22.311
  - second degree T22.219
  - third degree T22.319
- forehead T20.06
  - first degree T20.16
  - second degree T20.26
  - third degree T20.36
- fourth degree *code as* Burn, third degree, by site
- friction—*see* Burn, by site
- from swallowing caustic or corrosive substance NEC—*see* Corrosion, by site
- full thickness skin loss *code as* Burn, third degree, by site
- genital organs
  - external
    - ■ female T21.07
      - ~ first degree T21.17
      - ~ second degree T21.27
      - ~ third degree T21.37
    - ■ male T21.06
      - ~ first degree T21.16
      - ~ second degree T21.26
      - ~ third degree T21.36
- groin—*see* Burn, abdomen, abdominal (muscle) (wall)
- hand(s) T23.009
  - back—*see* Burn, dorsum of hand
  - finger—*see* Burn, finger
  - first degree T23.10-
  - left T23.002
    - ■ first degree T23.102
    - ■ second degree T23.202
    - ■ third degree T23.302
  - multiple sites with wrist T23.09-
    - ■ first degree T23.19-

Burn, *continued*

- ■ left T23.092
  - ~ first degree T23.192
  - ~ second degree T23.292
  - ~ third degree T23.392
- ■ right T23.091
  - ~ first degree T23.191
  - ~ second degree T23.291
  - ~ third degree T23.391
  - ■ second degree T23.29-
  - ■ third degree T23.39-
- palm—*see* Burn, palm
- right T23.001
  - ■ first degree T23.101
  - ■ second degree T23.201
  - ■ third degree T23.301
  - ~ second degree T23.20-
  - ~ third degree T23.30-
- thumb—*see* Burn, thumb
- head (and face) (and neck) (*Code by* Burn to specific site for cheek, chin, ear, eye, forehead, lip, neck, nose, or scalp) T20.00
  - first degree T20.10
  - multiple sites T20.09
    - ■ first degree T20.19
    - ■ second degree T20.29
    - ■ third degree T20.39
  - second degree T20.20
  - third degree T20.30
- hip(s)—*see* Burn, thigh
- inhalation—*see* Burn, respiratory tract
  - caustic or corrosive substance (fumes)—*see* Corrosion
- internal organ(s)
  - esophagus T28.1
  - from caustic or corrosive substance (swallowing) NEC—*see* Corrosion, by site
  - mouth T28.0
  - pharynx T28.0
- interscapular region—*see* Burn, back, upper
- knee T24.02-
  - first degree T24.12-
  - left T24.022
    - ■ first degree T24.122
    - ■ second degree T24.222
    - ■ third degree T24.322
  - right T24.021
    - ■ first degree T24.121
    - ■ second degree T24.221
    - ■ third degree T24.321
  - second degree T24.22-
  - third degree T24.32-
- labium (majus) (minus)—*see* Burn, genital organs, external, female
- lacrimal apparatus, duct, gland or sac—*see* Burn, eye, specified site NEC
- larynx T27.0- (*See complete ICD-10-CM* Manual for codes)
  - with lung T27.1-
- leg(s) (lower) (upper)—*see* Burn, lower, limb
- lightning—*see* Burn, by site
- limb(s)
  - lower (except ankle or foot alone)—*see* Burn, lower, limb
  - upper—*see* Burn, upper limb
- lip(s) T20.02
  - first degree T20.12
  - second degree T20.22
  - third degree T20.32
- lower
  - back—*see* Burn, back
  - limb T24.00- (*Code to Burn by specific site for ankle, calf, foot, thigh, knee*)
    - ■ first degree T24.109
    - ■ left T24.002
      - ~ first degree T24.102
      - ~ second degree T24.202
      - ~ third degree T24.302
    - ■ multiple sites, except ankle and foot T24.099
      - ~ ankle and foot T25.09-
        - ◊ first degree T25.19-
        - ◊ left T25.092

Burn, *continued*

- » first degree T25.192
- » second degree T25.292
- » third degree T25.392
- ◊ right T25.091
  - » first degree T25.191
  - » second degree T25.291
  - » third degree T25.391
- ◊ second degree T25.29-
- ◊ third degree T25.39-
- ~ first degree T24.19-
  - ◊ left T24.092
    - ◊ first degree T24.192
    - ◊ second degree T24.292
    - ◊ third degree T24.392
  - ~ right T24.091
    - ◊ first degree T24.191
    - ◊ second degree T24.291
    - ◊ third degree T24.391
  - ~ second degree T24.29-
  - ~ third degree T24.39-
- ■ right T24.001
  - ~ first degree T24.101
  - ~ second degree T24.201
  - ~ third degree T24.301
  - ■ second degree T24.20-
  - ■ thigh—*see* Burn, thigh
  - ■ third degree T24.30-
- toe—*see* Burn, toe
- mouth T28.0
- neck T20.07
  - first degree T20.17
  - second degree T20.27
  - third degree T20.37
- nose (septum) T20.04
  - first degree T20.14
  - second degree T20.24
  - third degree T20.34
- ocular adnexa—*see* Burn, eye
- orbit region—*see* Burn, eyelid
- palm T23.059
  - first degree T23.15-
  - left T23.052
    - ■ first degree T23.152
    - ■ second degree T23.252
    - ■ third degree T23.352
  - right T23.051
    - ■ first degree T23.151
    - ■ second degree T23.251
    - ■ third degree T23.351
  - second degree T23.25-
  - third degree T23.35-
- partial thickness *code as* Burn, unspecified degree, by site
- pelvis—*see* Burn, trunk
- penis—*see* Burn, genital organs, external, male
- perineum
  - female—*see* Burn, genital organs, external, female
  - male—*see* Burn, genital organs, external, male
- periocular area—*see* Burn, eyelid
- pharynx T28.0
- respiratory tract T27.- (*See complete ICD-10-CM* Manual for codes)
- scalp T20.05
  - first degree T20.15
  - second degree T20.25
  - third degree T20.35
- scapular region T22.06-
  - first degree T22.16-
  - left T22.062
    - ■ first degree T22.162
    - ■ second degree T22.262
    - ■ third degree T22.362
  - right T22.061
    - ■ first degree T22.161
    - ■ second degree T22.261
    - ■ third degree T22.361
  - second degree T22.26-
  - third degree T22.36-
- scrotum—*see* Burn, genital organs, external, male
- shoulder T22.05-
  - first degree T22.15-

ALPHABETIC INDEX

Burn, *continued*

- left T22.052
  - first degree T22.152
  - second degree T22.252
  - third degree T22.352
- right T22.051
  - first degree T22.151
  - second degree T22.251
  - third degree T23.351
  - second degree T22.25-
  - third degree T22.35-
- temple—*see* Burn, head
- testis—*see* Burn, genital organs, external, male
- thigh T24.01-
  - first degree T24.11-
  - left T24.012
    - first degree T24.112
    - second degree T24.212
    - third degree T24.312
  - right T24.011
    - first degree T24.111
    - second degree T24.211
    - third degree T24.311
    - second degree T24.21-
    - third degree T24.31-
- thorax (external)—*see* Burn, trunk
- throat (meaning pharynx) T28.0
- thumb(s) T23.01-
  - first degree T23.11-
  - left T23.012
    - first degree T23.112
    - second degree T23.212
    - third degree T23.312
  - multiple sites with fingers T23.04-
    - first degree T23.14-
    - left T23.042
      - first degree T23.142
      - second degree T23.242
      - third degree T23.342
    - right T23.041
      - first degree T23.141
      - second degree T23.241
      - third degree T23.341
    - second degree T23.24-
    - third degree T23.34-
  - right T23.011
    - first degree T23.111
    - second degree T23.211
    - third degree T23.311
    - second degree T23.21-
    - third degree T23.31-
- toe T25.039
  - first degree T25.139
  - left T25.032
    - first degree T25.132
    - second degree T25.232
    - third degree T25.332
  - right T25.031
    - first degree T25.131
    - second degree T25.231
    - third degree T25.331
  - second degree T25.23-
  - third degree T25.33-
- tongue T28.0
- tonsil(s) T28.0
- trachea T27.- (*See* complete *ICD-10-CM* Manual for codes)
- trunk T21.00 (*Code to Burn by specific site for abdominal wall, buttock, upper limb, back, chest wall, genital organs, or scapular region*)
  - first degree T21.10
  - second degree T21.20
  - specified site NEC T21.09
    - first degree T21.19
    - second degree T21.29
    - third degree T21.39
  - third degree T21.30
- unspecified site with extent of body surface involved specified
  - less than 10 percent T31.0
  - 10 –19 percent (0 – 9 percent third degree) T31.10
    - with 10 –19 percent third degree T31.11

Burn, *continued*

- upper limb (*Code to Burn by specific site for above elbow, axilla, elbow, forearm, hand, scapular region, shoulder, upper back, or wrist*) T22.00
  - first degree T22.10
  - multiple sites T22.09-
    - first degree T22.19-
    - left T22.092
      - first degree T22.192
      - second degree T22.292
      - third degree T22.392
    - right T22.091
      - first degree T22.191
      - second degree T22.291
      - third degree T22.391
    - second degree T22.29-
    - third degree T22.39-
  - second degree T22.20
  - third degree T22.3-
- vulva—*see* Burn, genital organs, external, female
- wrist T23.07-
  - first degree T23.17-
  - left T23.072
    - first degree T23.172
    - second degree T23.272
    - third degree T23.372
  - multiple sites with hand T23.09-
    - first degree T23.19-
    - left T23.092
      - first degree T23.192
      - second degree T23.292
      - third degree T23.392
    - right T23.091
      - first degree T23.191
      - second degree T23.291
      - third degree T23.391
    - second degree T23.29-
    - third degree T23.39-
  - right T23.071
    - first degree T23.171
    - second degree T23.271
    - third degree T23.371
  - second degree T23.27-
  - third degree T23.37-

Burnett's syndrome E83.52

Bursitis M71.9

- hip NEC M70.7-
  - trochanteric M70.6-
- radiohumeral M70.3-
- specified NEC M71.50
  - ankle M71.57-
  - due to use, overuse or pressure—*see* Disorder
  - elbow M71.52-
  - foot M71.57-
  - hand M71.54-
  - hip M71.55-
  - knee M71.56-
  - specified site NEC M71.58
  - tibial collateral M76.4-
  - wrist M71.53-

C

Cachexia R64

- dehydration E86.0
- due to
  - underlying condition E88.A
  - with
    - hypernatremia E87.0
    - hyponatremia E87.1
    - hypophyseal E23.0
    - hypopituitary E23.0
    - pituitary E23.0
    - Simmonds' E23.0
- pulmonary R64

CADASIL (cerebral autosomal dominate arteriopathy with subcortical infarcts and leukocephalopathy) I67.850

Café au lait spots L81.3

Caked breast (puerperal, postpartum) O92.79

Calcaneo-apophysitis M92.6

Calciferol (vitamin D) deficiency E55.9

- with rickets E55.0

Calcification

- adrenal (capsule) (gland) E27.49
- cerebral (cortex) G93.89
- choroid plexus G93.89
- kidney N28.89
  - tuberculous B90.9
- lymph gland or node (postinfectional) I89.8
  - tuberculous B90.8
- pericardium (*see also* Pericarditis) I31.1
- pleura
  - tuberculous NEC B90.9
- subcutaneous L94.2
- suprarenal (capsule) (gland) E27.49

Calcinosis (interstitial) (tumoral) (universalis) E83.59

- circumscripta (skin) L94.2
- cutis L94.2

Calciuria 82.994

Calculus, calculi, calculous

- biliary—*see also* Calculus, gallbladder
  - specified NEC K80.80
    - with obstruction K80.81
- bilirubin, multiple—*see* Calculus, gallbladder
- bladder (encysted) (impacted) (urinary) (diverticulum) N21.0
- gallbladder K80.20
  - with
    - bile duct calculus—*see* Calculus, gallbladder, with, bile duct calculus
    - cholecystitis K80.10
      - with obstruction K80.11
      - acute K80.00
        - ◊ with
          - » chronic cholecystitis K80.12
            - ❖ with obstruction K80.13
          - » obstruction K80.01
      - chronic K80.10
        - ◊ with
          - » acute cholecystitis K80.12
            - ❖ with obstruction K80.13
          - » obstruction K80.11
    - specified NEC K80.18
      - ◊ with obstruction K80.19
    - obstruction K80.21
- intestinal (impaction) (obstruction) K56.49
- kidney (impacted) (multiple) (pelvis) (recurrent) (staghorn) N20.0
  - with calculus, ureter N20.2
  - congenital Q63.8
- nose J34.89
- pyelitis (impacted) (recurrent) N20.0
  - with hydronephrosis N13.6
- pyelonephritis (impacted) (recurrent)—*see* category N20
  - with hydronephrosis N13.2
- tonsil J35.8
- ureter (impacted) (recurrent) N20.1
  - with calculus, kidney N20.2
    - with hydronephrosis N13.6
    - with infection N13.6
    - ureteropelvic junction N20.1
- urethra (impacted) N21.1
- urinary (duct) (impacted) (passage) (tract) N20.9
  - with hydronephrosis N13.2
    - with infection N13.6
- vagina N89.8
- xanthine E79.8 [N22]

California

- encephalitis A83.5

Callositas, callosity (infected) L84

Callus (infected) L84

CALME (Childhood asymmetric labium majus enlargement) N90.61

Calorie deficiency or malnutrition (*see also* Malnutrition) E46

Calvé-Perthes disease M91.1-

Camptocormia (hysterical) F44.4

Canal—*see also* Disease, diseased

- atrioventricular common Q21.2

Canavan disease E75.28

ALPHABETIC INDEX

Candidiasis, candidal B37.9
- balanitis B37.42
- bronchitis B37.1
- cheilitis B37.83
- congenital P37.5
- cystitis B37.41
- disseminated B37.7
- endocarditis B37.6
- enteritis B37.82
- esophagitis B37.81
- intertrigo B37.2
- lung B37.1
- meningitis B37.5
- mouth B37.0
- nails B37.2
- neonatal P37.5
- onychia B37.2
- oral B37.0
- osteomyelitis B37.89
- otitis externa B37.84
- paronychia B37.2
- perionyxis B37.2
- pneumonia B37.1
- proctitis B37.82
- pulmonary B37.1
- pyelonephritis B37.49
- sepsis B37.7
- skin B37.2
- specified site NEC B37.89
- stomatitis B37.0
- systemic B37.7
- urethritis B37.41
- urogenital site NEC B37.49
- vagina B37.3
- vulva B37.3
- vulvovaginitis B37.3

Canker (mouth) (sore) K12.0
- rash A38.9

Caput
- crepitus Q75.8

Carbuncle L02.93
- abdominal wall L02.231
- anus K61.0
- axilla L02.43-
- back (any part) L02.232
- breast N61.1
- buttock L02.33
- cheek (external) L02.03
- chest wall L02.233
- chin L02.03
- face NEC L02.03
- finger L02.53-
- flank L02.231
- foot L02.63-
- forehead L02.03
- gluteal (region) L02.33
- groin L02.234
- hand L02.53-
- head NEC L02.831
- heel L02.63-
- hip L02.43-
- knee L02.43-
- lower limb L02.43-
- navel L02.236
- neck L02.13
- nose (external) (septum) J34.0
- partes posteriores L02.33
- pectoral region L02.233
- perineum L02.235
- pinna—*see* Abscess, ear, external
- scalp L02.831
- specified site NEC L02.838
- temple (region) L02.03
- thumb L02.53-
- toe L02.63-
- trunk L02.239
  - abdominal wall L02.231
  - back L02.232
  - chest wall L02.233
  - groin L02.234
  - perineum L02.235
  - umbilicus L02.236

Carbuncle, *continued*
- umbilicus L02.236
- upper limb L02.43-
- urethra N34.0
- vulva N76.4

Carcinoma (malignant)—*see also* Neoplasm, by site, malignant in the Table of Neoplasms in the complete *ICD-10-CM* manual.
- carcinoid D3A.00
  - benign D3A.00
    - appendix D3A.020
    - ascending colon D3A.022
    - bronchus (lung) D3A.090
    - cecum D3A.021
    - colon D3A.029
    - descending colon D3A.024
    - duodenum D3A.010
    - foregut NOS D3A.094
    - hindgut NOS D3A.096
    - ileum D3A.012
    - jejunum D3A.011
    - kidney D3A.093
    - large intestine D3A.029
    - lung (bronchus) D3A.090
    - midgut NOS D3A.095
    - rectum D3A.026
    - sigmoid colon D3A.025
    - small intestine D3A.019
    - specified NEC D3A.098
    - stomach D3A.092
    - thymus D3A.091
    - transverse colon D3A.023
- Merkel cell C4A.-
  - neuroendocrine—*see also* Tumor, neuroendocrine
- renal cell C64-

Cardiac—*see also* Disease, diseased
- death, sudden—*see* Arrest, cardiac
- pacemaker
  - in situ Z95.0
  - management or adjustment Z45.018
- tamponade I31.4

Cardiochalasia K21.9

Cardiomegaly—*see also* Hypertrophy, cardiac
- congenital Q24.8
- idiopathic I51.7

Cardiomyopathy (familial) (idiopathic) I42.9
- constrictive NOS I42.5
- due to
  - Friedreich's ataxia G11.11
  - progressive muscular dystrophy G71.0
- hypertrophic (nonobstructive) I42.2
  - obstructive I42.1
    - congenital Q24.8
- in
  - sarcoidosis D86.85
  - metabolic E88.9 [I43]
  - thyrotoxic E05.90 [I43]
    - with thyroid storm E05.91 [I43]
  - nutritional E63.9 [I43]
- restrictive NEC I42.5
- secondary I42.9
- specified NEC I42.8
- thyrotoxic E05.90 [I43]
  - with thyroid storm E05.91 [I43]

Cardiopathia nigra I27.0

Cardiopathy
- idiopathic I42.9
- mucopolysaccharidosis E76.3 [I52]

Cardiosymphysis I31.0

Care (of) (for) (following)
- family member (handicapped) (sick)
  - unavailable, due to
    - absence (person rendering care) (sufferer) Z74.2
    - inability (any reason) of person rendering care Z74.2
- foundling Z76.1
- palliative Z51.5
- unavailable, due to
  - absence of person rendering care Z74.2
  - inability (any reason) of person rendering care Z74.2
- well baby Z76.2

Caries
- dental K02.9

Carnitine insufficiency E71.40

Carpenter's syndrome Q87.0

Carrier (suspected) of
- bacterial disease NEC Z22.39
  - diphtheria Z22.2
  - intestinal infectious NEC Z22.1
    - typhoid Z22.0
  - meningococcal Z22.31
  - sexually transmitted Z22.4
  - specified NEC Z22.39
  - staphylococcal (Methicillin susceptible) Z22.321
    - Methicillin resistant Z22.322
  - streptococcal Z22.338
    - group B Z22.330
- genetic Z14.8
  - cystic fibrosis Z14.1
  - hemophilia A (asymptomatic) Z14.01
    - symptomatic Z14.02
- gonorrhea Z22.4
- HAA (hepatitis Australian-antigen) Z22.5
- HB (c)(s)-AG Z22.5
- hepatitis (viral) Z22.5
  - Australia-antigen (HAA) Z22.5
  - B surface antigen (HBsAg) Z22.5
  - C Z22.5
  - specified NEC Z22.5
- infectious organism Z22.9
  - specified NEC Z22.8
- meningococci Z22.31
- serum hepatitis—*see* Carrier, hepatitis
- staphylococci (Methicillin susceptible) Z22.321
  - Methicillin resistant Z22.322
- streptococci Z22.338
  - group B Z22.330
- syphilis Z22.4
- venereal disease Z22.4

Car sickness T75.3

Caruncle (inflamed)
- myrtiform N89.8

Caseation lymphatic gland (tuberculous) A18.2

Cassidy (-Scholte) syndrome (malignant carcinoid) E34.09

Casts in urine R82.998

Cat
- cry syndrome Q93.4

Cataract (cortical) (immature) (incipient) H26.9
- anterior
  - and posterior axial embryonal Q12.0
  - pyramidal Q12.0
- blue Q12.0
- central Q12.0
- cerulean Q12.0
- congenital Q12.0
- coralliform Q12.0
- coronary Q12.0
- crystalline Q12.0
- in
  - hypoparathyroidism E20.9 [H28]
  - nutritional disease E63.9 [H28]
- infantile—*see* Cataract, presenile
- juvenile—*see* Cataract, presenile
- nuclear
  - embryonal Q12.0
  - presenile H26.00-
  - zonular (perinuclear) Q12.0

Cataracta—*see also* Cataract
- centralis pulverulenta Q12.0
- cerulea Q12.0
- congenita Q12.0
- coralliformis Q12.0
- coronaria Q12.0
- membranacea
  - congenita Q12.0

Catarrh, catarrhal (acute) (febrile) (infectious) (inflammation) (*see also* Disease, diseased) J00
- chronic J31.0
- gingivitis K05.00
  - plaque induced K05.00
- larynx, chronic J37.0

ALPHABETIC INDEX

Catarrh, catarrhal, *continued*
- liver B15.9
- middle ear, chronic H65.2-
- mouth K12.1
- nasal (chronic)—*see* Rhinitis
- nasopharyngeal (chronic) J31.1
  - acute J00
- pulmonary—*see* Bronchitis
- spring (eye) (vernal)—*see* Conjunctivitis, acute, atopic
- summer (hay)—*see* Fever, hay
- throat J31.2
- tubotympanal—*see also* Otitis, media, acute, subacture, nonsuppurative NEC
  - chronic H65.2-

Catatonic
- stupor R40.1

Cat-scratch disease or fever A28.1

Cavovarus foot, congenital Q66.1-

Cavus foot (congenital) Q66.7-

CDKL5 (Cyclin-Dependent Kinase-Like 5 Deficiency Disorder) G40.42

Cecitis K52.9
- with perforation, peritonitis, or rupture K65.8

Cecoureterocele Q62.32

Celiac
- disease (with steatorrhea) K90.0
- infantilism K90.0

Cells (see Disease, diseased)
- in urine R82.998

Cellulitis (diffuse) (phlegmonous) (septic) (suppurative) L03.90
- abdominal wall L03.311
- ankle L03.11-
- anus K61.0
- axilla L03.11-
- back (any part) L03.312
- breast (acute) (nonpuerperal) N61.0
  - nipple N61.0
- buttock L03.317
- cervical (meaning neck) L03.221
- cheek (external) L03.211
  - internal K12.2
- chest wall L03.313
- chronic L03.90
- drainage site (following operation) T81.49
- ear (external) H60.1-
- erysipelatous—*see* Erysipelas
- face NEC L03.211
- finger (intrathecal) (periosteal) (subcutaneous) (subcuticular) L03.01-
- foot L03.11-
- gangrenous—*see* Gangrene
- gluteal (region) L03.317
- groin L03.314
- head NEC L03.811
  - face (any part, except ear, eye and nose) L03.211
- jaw (region) L03.211
- knee L03.11-
- lip K13.0
- lower limb L03.11-
  - toe—*see* Cellulitis, toe
- mouth (floor) K12.2
- multiple sites, so stated L03.90
- navel L03.316
  - newborn P38.9
    - with mild hemorrhage P38.1
    - without hemorrhage P38.9
- neck (region) L03.221
- nose (septum) (external) J34.0
- orbit, orbital H05.01-
  - periorbital L03.213
- palate (soft) K12.2
- pectoral (region) L03.313
- pelvis, pelvic (chronic)
  - female (*see also* Disease, pelvis, inflammatory) N73.2
    - acute N73.0
  - male K65.0
- perineal, perineum L03.315
- periorbital L03.213

Cellulitis,, *continued*
- perirectal K61.1peritonsillar J36
- preseptal L03.213
- rectum K61.1
- scalp (any part) L03.811
- specified site NEC L03.818
- submandibular (region) (space) (triangle) K12.2
  - gland K11.3
- submaxillary (region) K12.2
  - gland K11.3
- toe (intrathecal) (periosteal) (subcutaneous) (subcuticular) L03.03
- tonsil J36
- trunk L03.319
  - abdominal wall L03.311
  - back (any part) L03.312
  - buttock L03.317
  - chest wall L03.313
  - groin L03.314
  - perineal, perineum L03.315
  - umbilicus L03.316
- upper limb L03.11-
  - axilla L03.11-
  - finger L03.01-
  - thumb L03.01-
- vaccinal T88.0

Central auditory processing disorder H93.25

Cephalematoma, cephalhematoma (calcified)
- newborn (birth injury) P12.0

Cephalgia, cephalalgia—*see also* Headache
- histamine G44.009
  - intractable G44.001
  - not intractable G44.009

Cerumen (accumulation) (impacted) H61.2-

Cervicalgia M54.2

Cervicitis (acute) (chronic) (nonvenereal) (senile (atrophic)) (subacute) (with ulceration) N72
- chlamydial A56.09
- gonococcal A54.03
- trichomonal A59.09

Cervicocolpitis (emphysematosa) (*see also* Cervicitis) N72

Cestode infestation B71.9
- specified type NEC B71.8

Cestodiasis B71.9

Chafing L30.4

Chalasia (cardiac sphincter) K21.9

Chalazion H00.10
- left H00.16
  - lower H00.15
  - upper H00.14
- right H00.13
  - lower H00.12
  - upper H00.11

Chancre (any genital site) (hard) (hunterian) (mixed) (primary) (seronegative) (seropositive) (syphilitic) A51.0
- conjunctiva NEC A51.2
- extragenital A51.2
- eyelid A51.2
- lip A51.2
- nipple A51.2
- palate, soft A51.2
- soft
  - palate A51.2
  - urethra A51.0

Change(s) (in) (of)—*see also* Removal
- circulatory I99.9
- contraceptive device Z30.433
- dressing (nonsurgical) Z48.00
  - surgical Z48.01
- hypertrophic
  - nasal sinus J34.89
  - turbinate, nasal J34.3
  - upper respiratory tract J39.8
- mental status R41.82
- sacroiliac joint M53.3

Change(s), *continued*
- skin R23.9
  - acute, due to ultraviolet radiation L56.9
    - specified NEC L56.8
  - cyanosis R23.0
  - flushing R23.2
  - pallor R23.1
  - petechiae R23.3
  - specified change NEC R23.8
  - swelling—*see* Mass, localized
- vascular I99.9
- voice R49.9
  - psychogenic F44.4

CHARGE association Q89.8

Charley-horse (quadriceps) M62.831
- traumatic (quadriceps) S76.11-

Checking (of)
- implantable subdermal contraceptive Z30.46
- intrauterine contraceptive device Z30.431

Cheese itch B88.0

Cheilitis (acute) (angular) (catarrhal) (chronic) (exfoliative) (gangrenous) (glandular) (infectional) (suppurative) (ulcerative) (vesicular) K13.0
- actinic (due to sun) L56.8
  - other than from sun L56.9
- candidal B37.83

Cheilodynia K13.0

Cheiloschisis—*see* Cleft, lip

Cheilosis (angular) K13.0

Cheiropompholyx L30.1

Chemotherapy (session) (for)
- cancer Z51.11
- neoplasm Z51.11

Cheyne-Stokes breathing (respiration) R06.3

Chickenpox—*see* Varicella

Chigger (infestation) B88.0

Child—*see also* Problem, child
- custody dispute Z65.3

Childhood
- cerebral X-linked adrenoleukodystrophy E71.520
- period of rapid growth Z00.2

Chill(s) R68.83
- with fever R50.9
- congestive in malarial regions B54
- without fever R68.83

Chinese dysentery A03.9

Chlamydia, chlamydial A74.9
- cervicitis A56.09
- conjunctivitis A74.0
- cystitis A56.01
- endometritis A56.11
- epididymitis A56.19
- female
  - pelvic inflammatory disease A56.11
  - pelviperitonitis A56.11
- orchitis A56.19
- peritonitis A74.81
- pharyngitis A56.4
- proctitis A56.3
- salpingitis A56.11
- sexually-transmitted infection NEC A56.8
- specified NEC A74.89
- urethritis A56.01
- vulvovaginitis A56.02

Chlamydiosis—*see* Chlamydia

Chlorotic anemia D50.8

Cholecystitis K81.9
- with
  - gangrene of gallbladder K82.A1
  - perforation of gallbladder K82.A2
- acute (emphysematous) (gangrenous) (suppurative) K81.0
  - with
    - calculus, stones in
    - cystic duct—*see* Calculus, gallbladder, with, cholecystitis, acute
    - gallbladder—*see* Calculus, gallbladder, with, cholecystitis, acute

Cholecystitis, *continued*
- choledocholithiasis—*see* Calculus, gallbladder, with, cholecystitis, acute
- cholelithiasis—*see* Calculus, gallbladder, with, cholecystitis, acute
- chronic cholecystitis K81.2
  - with gallbladder calculus K80.12
    - ◊ with obstruction K80.13
- chronic K81.1
  - with acute cholecystitis K81.2
    - with gallbladder calculus K80.12
      - with obstruction K80.13
- emphysematous (acute)—*see* Cholecystitis, acute
- gangrenous—*see* Cholecystitis, acute
- suppurative—*see* Cholecystitis, acute

Choking sensation R09.89

Cholesteremia E78.0

Cholesterol
- elevated (high) E78.00
  - with elevated (high) triglycerides E78.2
  - screening for Z13.220

Cholesterolemia (essential) (pure) E78.00
- familial E78.01
- hereditary E78.01

Chondritis M94.8X-
- costal (Tietze's) M94.0
- patella, posttraumatic M22.4-

Chondrodysplasia Q78.9
- with hemangioma Q78.4
- calcificans congenita Q77.3
- fetalis Q77.4
- metaphyseal (Jansen's) (McKusick's) (Schmid's) Q78.8
- punctata Q77.3

Chondrodystrophy, chondrodystrophia (familial) (fetalis) (hypoplastic) Q78.9
- calcificans congenita Q77.3
- myotonic (congenital) G71.13
- punctata Q77.3

Chondroectodermal dysplasia Q77.6

Chondrogenesis imperfecta Q77.4

Chondromalacia (systemic) M94.2-
- knee M94.26-
  - patella M22.4-

Chondro-osteodysplasia (Morquio-Brailsford type) E76.219

Chondro-osteodystrophy E76.29

Chondropathia tuberosa M94.0

Chordee (nonvenereal) N48.89
- congenital Q54.4

Chorea (chronic) (gravis) (posthemiplegic) (senile) (spasmodic) G25.5
- drug-induced G25.4
- hysterical F44.4
- progressive G25.5
- with
  - heart involvement I02.0
    - active or acute (conditions in I01-) I02.0
    - rheumatic I02.9
      - with valvular disorder I02.0
    - rheumatic heart disease (chronic) (inactive) (quiescent)—*code to* rheumatic heart condition involved

Choreoathetosis (paroxysmal) G25.5

Chorioretinitis
- in (due to)
  - toxoplasmosis (acquired) B58.01
    - congenital (active) P37.1 *[H32]*

Chromophytosis B36.0

Chylopericardium I31.3
- acute I30.9

Cicatricial (deformity)—*see* Cicatrix

Cicatrix (adherent) (contracted) (painful) (vicious) (*see also* Scar) L90.5
- adenoid (and tonsil) J35.8
- anus K62.89
- brain G93.89
- mouth K13.79
- muscle M62.89

Cicatrix, *continued*
- with contracture—*see* Contraction, muscle NEC
- palate (soft) K13.79
- rectum K62.89
- skin L90.5
  - postinfective L90.5
  - specified site NEC L90.5
  - tuberculous B90.8
- tonsil (and adenoid) J35.8
- tuberculous NEC B90.9
- vagina N89.8
  - postoperative N99.2
- wrist, constricting (annular) L90.5

CINCA (chronic infantile neurological, cutaneous and articular syndrome) M04.2

Circulation
- failure (peripheral) R57.9
  - newborn P29.89
- fetal, persistent P29.38

Circumcision (in absence of medical indication) (ritual) (routine) Z41.2

Cirrhosis, cirrhotic (hepatic) (liver) K74.60
- due to
  - xanthomatosis E78.2
- fatty K76.0
- liver K74.60
  - congenital P78.81
  - pigmentary E83.110
- xanthomatous (biliary) K74.5
  - due to xanthomatosis (familial) (metabolic) (primary) E78.2

Clam digger's itch B65.3

Clammy skin R23.1

Clark's paralysis G80.9

Claudication, intermittent I73.9
- cerebral (artery) G45.9

Clavus (infected) L84

Clawfoot (congenital) Q66.89
- acquired M21.53-

Clawtoe (congenital) Q66.89
- acquired M20.5X-

Cleft (congenital)—*see also* Imperfect, closure
- foot Q72.7
- hand Q71.6
- lip (unilateral) Q36.9
  - with cleft palate Q37.9
    - hard Q37.1
      - with soft Q37.5
    - soft Q37.3
      - with hard Q37.5
  - bilateral Q36.0
    - with cleft palate Q37.8
      - hard Q37.0
        - ◊ with soft Q37.4
      - soft Q37.2
        - ◊ with hard Q37.4
    - median Q36.1
  - palate Q35.9
    - with cleft lip (unilateral) Q37.9
      - bilateral Q37.8
      - hard Q35.1
      - with
        - cleft lip (unilateral) Q37.1
          - ◊ bilateral Q37.0
        - soft Q35.5
          - ◊ with cleft lip (unilateral) Q37.5
            - bilateral Q37.4
    - medial Q35.5
    - soft Q35.3
      - with
        - cleft lip (unilateral) Q37.3
          - ◊ bilateral Q37.2
        - hard Q35.5
          - ◊ with cleft lip (unilateral) Q37.5
            - bilateral Q37.4
- penis Q55.69
- scrotum Q55.29
- uvula Q35.7

Cleidocranial dysostosis Q74.0

Clicking hip (newborn) R29.4

Closed bite M26.29

Closure
- congenital, nose Q30.0
- cranial sutures, premature Q75.009
- foramen ovale, imperfect Q21.1
- hymen N89.6
- interauricular septum, defective Q21.1
- interventricular septum, defective Q21.0
- lacrimal duct—*see also* Stenosis, lacrimal, duct
  - congenital Q10.5
- nose (congenital) Q30.0
  - acquired M95.0
- vagina N89.5

Clot (blood)—*see also* Embolism
- artery (obstruction) (occlusion)—*see* Embolism
- circulation I74.9

Clouded state R40.1
- epileptic—*see* Epilepsy, specified NEC
- paroxysmal—*see* Epilepsy, specified NEC

Cloudy antrum, antra J32.0

Cloverleaf skull Q75.051

Clubfoot (congenital) Q66.89
- acquired M21.54-
- equinovarus Q66.0-
- paralytic M21.54-

Clubhand (congenital) (radial) Q71.4-
- acquired M21.51-

Clumsiness, clumsy child syndrome F82

Cluttering F80.81

Coagulopathy—*see also* Defect, coagulation
- consumption D65
- intravascular D65
  - newborn P60

Coalition
- calcaneo-scaphoid Q66.89
- tarsal Q66.89

Coarctation
- aorta (preductal) (postductal) Q25.1
- pulmonary artery Q25.71

Coccydynia, coccygodynia M53.3

Cockayne's syndrome Q87.19

Cock's peculiar tumor L72.3

Cold J00
- with influenza, flu, or grippe—*see* Influenza, with, respiratory manifestations NEC
- agglutinin disease or hemoglobinuria (chronic) D59.12
- bronchial—*see* Bronchitis
- chest—*see* Bronchitis
- common (head) J00
- head J00
- on lung—*see* Bronchitis
- rose J30.1
- virus J00
- sensitivity, auto-immune D59.12
- symptoms J00

Colibacillosis A49.8
- as the cause of other disease (*see also* Escherichia coli) B96.20
- generalized A41.50

Colic (bilious) (infantile) (intestinal) (recurrent) (spasmodic) R10.83
- abdomen R10.83
  - psychogenic F45.8
- hysterical F45.8
- kidney N23
- mucous K58.9
  - with constipation K58.1
  - with diarrhea K58.0
  - mixed K58.2
  - other K58.8
  - psychogenic F54
- nephritic N23
- psychogenic F45.8
- renal N23
- ureter N23
- uterus NEC N94.89
  - menstrual—*see* Dysmenorrhea

ALPHABETIC INDEX

Colitis (acute) (catarrhal) (chronic) (noninfective) (hemorrhagic) (*see also* Enteritis) K52.9
- allergic K52.29
  - with
    - food protein-induced enterocolitis syndrome K52.21
    - proctocolitis K52.29
- amebic (acute) (*see also* Amebiasis) A06.0
- anthrax A22.2
- C. difficile
  - not specified as recurrent A04.72
  - recurrent A04.71
  - toxic NEC K52.1
    - due to
      - Clostridioides difficile
        - not specified as recurrent A04.72
        - recurrent A04.71
      - Clostridium difficile
        - not specified as recurrent A04.72
        - recurrent A04.71
- Clostridioides difficile
  - not specified as recurrent A04.72
  - recurrent A04.71
- collagenous K52.831
- cystica superficialis K52.89
- dietary counseling and surveillance (for) Z71.3
- dietetic K52.29
- eosinophilic K52.82
- food hypersensitivity K52.29
- giardial A07.1
- granulomatous—*see* Enteritis, regional, large intestine
- infectious—*see* Enteritis, infectious
- indeterminate, so stated K52.3
- left sided K51.50
  - with
    - abscess K51.514
    - complication K51.519
      - specified NEC K51.518
    - fistula K51.513
    - obstruction K51.512
    - rectal bleeding K51.511
- lymphocytic K52.832
- microscopic, other K52.838
  - unspecified K52.839
- noninfective K52.9
  - specified NEC K52.89
- septic—*see* Enteritis, infectious
- spastic K58.9
  - with constipation K58.1
  - with diarrhea K58.0
  - mixed K58.2
  - other K58.8
  - psychogenic F54
- staphylococcal A04.8
  - foodborne A05.0
- ulcerative (chronic) K51.90
  - with
    - complication K51.919
      - abscess K51.914
      - fistula K51.913
      - obstruction K51.912
      - rectal bleeding K51.911
      - specified complication NEC K51.918
  - enterocolitis—*see* Pancolitis, ulcerative
  - ileocolitis—*see* Ileocolitis, ulcerative
  - mucosal proctocolitis—*see* Rectosigmoiditis, ulcerative
  - proctitis—*see* Proctitis, ulcerative
  - pseudopolyposis—*see* Polyp, colon, inflammatory
  - psychogenic F54
  - rectosigmoiditis—*see* Rectosigmoiditis, ulcerative
  - specified type NEC K51.80
    - with
      - complication K51.819
        - abscess K51.814
        - fistula K51.813
        - obstruction K51.812
        - rectal bleeding K51.811
        - specified complication NEC K51.818

Collagenosis, collagen disease (nonvascular) (vascular) M35.9
- specified NEC M35.8

Collapse R55
- adrenal E27.2
- cardiorespiratory R57.0
- cardiovascular R57.0
  - newborn P29.89
- circulatory (peripheral) R57.9
- during or
  - resulting from a procedure, not elsewhere classified T81.10
- general R55
- nasal valve J34.829
  - external J34.8210
    - dynamic J34.8212
    - static J34.8211
  - internal J34.8200
    - dynamic J34.8202
    - static J34.8201
- neurocirculatory F45.8
- nose M95.0
  - lower sidewall or nostril, on inspiration J34.8212
  - upper, middle sidewall, on inspiration J34.8202
- postoperative T81.10
- valvular—*see* Endocarditis
- vascular (peripheral) R57.9
  - newborn P29.89

Colles' fracture S52.53-

Collet (-Sicard) syndrome G52.7

Collodion baby Q80.2

Coloboma (iris) Q13.0
- eyelid Q10.3
- fundus Q14.8
- lens Q12.2
- optic disc (congenital) Q14.2

Colonization
- MRSA (Methicillin resistant Staphylococcus aureus) Z22.322
- MSSA (Methicillin susceptible Staphylococcus aureus) Z22.321
- status—*see* Carrier (suspected) of

Colostomy
- attention to Z43.3
- fitting or adjustment Z46.89
- malfunctioning K94.03
- status Z93.3

Coma R40.20
- with
  - motor response (none) R40.231
    - abnormal R40.233
    - extension R40.232
    - flexion withdrawal R40.234
    - localizes pain R40.235
    - obeys commands R40.236
  - score of
    - 1 R40.231
    - 2 R40.232
    - 3 R40.233
    - 4 R40.234
    - 5 R40.235
    - 6 R40.236
  - opening of eyes (never) R40.211
    - in response to
      - pain R40.212
      - sound R40.213
    - score of
      - 1 R40.211
      - 2 R40.212
      - 3 R40.213
      - 4 R40.214
    - spontaneous R40.214
  - verbal response (none) R40.221
    - confused conversation R40.224
    - inappropriate words R40.223
    - incomprehensible words R40.222
    - oriented R40.225
    - score of
      - 1 R40.221
      - 2 R40.222
      - 3 R40.223
      - 4 R40.224
      - 5 R40.225

Coma, *continued*
- hyperosmolar (diabetic)—*see* Diabetes
- hypoglycemic (diabetic)—*see* Diabetes
  - nondiabetic E15
  - in diabetes—*see* Diabetes
- insulin-induced—*see* Diabetes, coma
- newborn P91.5
- nontraumatic, due to underlying condition R40.2A
- persistent vegetative state R40.3
- secondary R40.2A
- specified NEC, without documented Glasgow coma scale score, or with partial Glasgow coma scale score reported R40.244

Comatose—*see* Coma

Comedo, comedones (giant) L70.0

Common
- arterial trunk Q20.0
- atrioventricular canal Q21.2
- atrium Q21.1
- cold (head) J00
- truncus (arteriosus) Q20.0

Communication
- between
  - pulmonary artery and pulmonary vein, congenital Q25.72
- congenital between uterus and digestive or urinary tract Q51.7
- disorder
  - social pragmatic F80.82

Complaint—*see also* Disease
- bowel, functional K59.9
  - psychogenic F45.8
- intestine, functional K59.9
  - psychogenic F45.8
- kidney—*see* Disease, renal

Complex
- Addison-Schilder E71.528
- Costen's M26.69
- Eisenmenger's (ventricular septal defect) I27.83
- Schilder-Addison E71.528

Complication(s) (from) (of)
- arteriovenous
  - fistula, surgically created T82.9
    - infection or inflammation T82.7
  - shunt, surgically created T82.9
    - infection or inflammation T82.7
  - vascular (counterpulsation) T82.9
    - infection or inflammation T82.7
- cardiac—*see also* Disease, heart
  - device, implant or graft T82.9
    - infection or inflammation T82.7
  - cardiovascular device, graft or implant T82.9
    - infection or inflammation T82.7
  - catheter (device) NEC—*see also* Complications, prosthetic device or implant
    - cystostomy T83.9
      - infection and inflammation T83.510
    - mechanical
      - obstruction T83.090
      - perforation T83.090
      - protrusion T83.090
      - specified NEC T83.090
    - dialysis (vascular) T82.9
      - infection and inflammation T82.7
    - intravenous infusion T82.9
      - infection or inflammation T82.7
    - urethral T83.9
      - indwelling
        - infection and inflammation T83.511
        - specified complication NEC T83.091
          - infection and inflammation T83.511
        - obstruction (mechanical)
        - perforation T83.091
        - protrusion T83.091
        - specified type NEC T83.091
    - urinary NEC
      - infection and inflammation T83.518
      - specified complication NEC T83.098
- chimeric antigen receptor (CAR-T) cell therapy T80.82

Complication(s), *continued*

- circulatory system I99.8
  - postprocedural I97.89
    - following cardiac surgery I97.19-
      - postcardiotomy syndrome I97.0
    - postcardiotomy syndrome I97.0
  - delivery (*see also* Complications, obstetric) O75.9
    - specified NEC O75.89
  - extracorporeal circulation T80.90
  - gastrointestinal K92.9
    - postoperative
      - malabsorption NEC K91.2
  - gastrostomy (stoma) K94.20
    - hemorrhage K94.21
    - infection K94.22
    - malfunction K94.23
    - mechanical K94.23
    - specified complication NEC K94.29
  - genitourinary
    - device or implant T83.9
      - urinary system T83.9
    - infection or inflammation T83.598
      - ◊ indwelling urethral catheter T83.511
  - graft (bypass) (patch)—*see also* Complications, prosthetic device or implant
    - urinary organ
      - infection and inflammation T83.598
      - indwelling urethral catheter T83.511
  - IEC (immune effector cellular) therapy T80.82
  - immune effector cellular (IEC) therapy T80.82
  - infusion (procedure) T80.90
    - infection T80.29
    - sepsis T80.29
    - serum reaction (*see also* Reaction, serum) T80.69
      - anaphylactic shock (*see also* Shock, anaphylactic) T80.59
  - injection (procedure) T80.90
    - drug reaction—*see* Reaction, drug
    - infection T80.29
    - sepsis T80.29
  - labor O75.9
    - specified NEC O75.89
  - metabolic E88.9
    - postoperative E89.89
      - specified NEC E89.89
  - obstetric O75.9
    - specified NEC O75.89
  - perfusion NEC T80.90
  - postprocedural—*see also* Complications, surgical procedure
    - cardiac arrest
      - following cardiac surgery I97.120
      - following other surgery I97.121
    - cardiac functional disturbance NEC
      - following cardiac surgery I97.190
      - following other surgery I97.191
    - cardiac insufficiency
      - following cardiac surgery I97.110
      - following other surgery I97.111
    - heart failure
      - following cardiac surgery I97.130
      - following other surgery I97.131
    - hemorrhage (hematoma) (of)
      - genitourinary organ or structure
        - following procedure on genitourinary organ or structure N99.820
    - specified NEC
      - respiratory system J95.89
  - prosthetic device or implant T85
    - mechanical NEC T85.698
      - ventricular shunt
        - breakdown T85.01
        - displacement T85.02
        - leakage T85.03
        - malposition T85.02
        - obstruction T85.09
        - perforation T85.09
        - protrusion T85.09
        - specified NEC T85.09
  - respiratory system J98.9
    - postoperative J95.89
      - air leak J95.812
      - specified NEC J95.89

Complication(s), *continued*

- surgical procedure (on) T81.9
  - malabsorption (postsurgical) NEC K91.2
    - postcardiotomy syndrome I97.0
    - postcommissurotomy syndrome I97.0
    - postvalvulotomy syndrome I97.0
  - shock (hypovolemic) T81.19
  - stitch abscess T81.41
  - wound infection T81.49
- transfusion (blood) (lymphocytes) (plasma) T80.92
  - circulatory overload E87.71
  - febrile nonhemolytic transfusion reaction R50.84
  - hemochromatosis E83.111
  - hemolytic reaction (antigen unspecified) T80.919
  - incompatibility reaction (antigen unspecified) T80.919
    - acute (antigen unspecified) T80.910
    - delayed (antigen unspecified) T80.911
    - delayed serologic (DSTR) T80.89
  - infection T80.29
    - acute T80.22
  - reaction NEC T80.89
    - sepsis T80.29
    - shock T80.89
- transplant T86.90
  - bone marrow T86.00
    - failure T86.02
    - rejection T86.01
    - failure T86.-
  - heart T86.2-
    - with lung T86.30
    - cardiac allograft vasculopathy T86.290
      - failure T86.32
      - rejection T86.31
    - failure T86.22
    - rejection T86.21
  - infection T86.-
  - kidney T86.10
    - failure T86.12
    - rejection T86.11
  - liver T86.4-
    - failure T86.42
    - rejection T86.41
  - lung T86.81-
    - with heart T86.30
      - failure T86.32
      - rejection T86.31
    - failure T86.811
    - rejection T86.810
  - malignant neoplasm C80.2
  - peripheral blood stem cells T86.5
  - post-transplant lymphoproliferative disorder (PTLD) D47.Z1
  - rejection T86. -
  - specified
    - type NEC T86.-
  - stem cell (from peripheral blood) (from umbilical cord) T86.5
  - umbilical cord stem cells T86.5
- vaccination T88.1-
  - anaphylaxis NEC T80.52-
  - cellulitis T88.0-
  - encephalitis or encephalomyelitis G04.02
  - infection (general) (local) NEC T88.0-
    - meningitis G03.8
  - myelitis G04.89
  - protein sickness T80.62-
  - rash T88.1-
  - reaction (allergic) T88.1-
    - serum T80.62-
  - sepsis T88.0-
  - serum intoxication, sickness, rash, or other serum reaction NEC T80.62-
    - anaphylactic shock T80.52-
  - shock (allergic) (anaphylactic) T80.52-
  - vaccinia (generalized) (localized) T88.1-
- vascular I99.9
  - device or implant T82.9
    - infection or inflammation T82.7
- ventricular (communicating) shunt (device) T85-
  - mechanical
    - breakdown T85.01
    - displacement T85.02

Complication(s), *continued*

- leakage T85.03
- malposition T85.02
- obstruction T85.09
- perforation T85.09
- protrusion T85.09
- specified NEC T85.09

Compression

- brain (stem) G93.5
  - due to
    - contusion (diffuse) (*see also* Injury, intracranial, diffuse) S06.A0
      - with herniation S06.A1
    - focal (*see also* Injury, intracranial, focal) S06.A0
      - with herniation S06.A1
    - injury NEC (*see also* Injury, intracranial, diffuse) S06.A0
      - nontraumatic G93.5
    - traumatic (*see also* Injury, intracranial, diffuse) S06.A0
      - with herniation S06.A1
- facies Q67.1
- with injury *code by* Nature of injury
- laryngeal nerve, recurrent G52.2
  - with paralysis of vocal cords and larynx J38.00
    - bilateral J38.02
    - unilateral J38.01
- nerve (*see also* Disorder, nerve) G58.9
  - root or plexus NOS (in) G54.9
    - neoplastic disease (*see also* Table of Neoplasms in the complete *ICD-10-CM manual*) D49.9 [G55]

Compulsion, compulsive

- neurosis F42.8
- personality F60.5
- states F42.9
- swearing F42.8
  - in Gilles de la Tourette's syndrome F95.2
- tics and spasms F95.9

Concato's disease (pericardial polyserositis) A19.9

- nontubercular I31.1
- pleural—*see* Pleurisy, with, effusion

Concealed penis Q55.64

Concretio cordis I31.1

- rheumatic I09.2

Concretion—*see also* Calculus

- prepuce (male) N47.8
- tonsil J35.8

Concussion (brain) (cerebral) (current) S06.0X-

- syndrome F07.81
- with
  - loss of consciousness of 30 minutes or less S06.0X1
  - loss of consciousness of unspecified duration S06.0X9
  - loss of consciousness status unknown S06.0XA-
- without loss of consciousness S06.0X0

Condition—*see also* Disease

- post COVID-19 U09.9

Conditions arising in the perinatal period—*see* Newborn, affected by

Conduct disorder—*see* Disorder, conduct

Condyloma A63.0

- acuminatum A63.0
- gonorrheal A54.09
- latum A51.31
- syphilitic A51.31
  - congenital A50.07
- venereal, syphilitic A51.31

Conflagration—*see also* Burn

- asphyxia (by inhalation of gases, fumes or vapors) *see* Table of Drugs and Chemicals

Conflict (with)—*see also* Discord

- family Z73.9
- grandparent-child Z62.831
- group home care staff-child Z62.833
- kinship-care child Z62.831
- marital Z63.0
  - involving divorce or estrangement Z63.5
- non-parental relative legal guardian-child Z62.831
- non-parental relative-child Z62.831

ALPHABETIC INDEX

Conflict, *continued*

- non-relative guardian-child Z62.832
- other relative-child Z62.831
- parent-child Z62.820
  - parent-adopted child Z62.821
  - parent-biological child Z62.820
  - parent-foster child Z62.822
  - parent-step child Z62.823

Confusional arousals G47.51

Congestion, congestive

- brain G93.89
- breast N64.59
- catarrhal J31.0
- chest R09.89
- glottis J37.0
- larynx J37.0
- lung R09.89
  - active or acute—*see* Pneumonia

Conjunctivitis (staphylococcal) (streptococcal) NOS H10.9

- acute H10.3-
  - atopic H10.1-
  - chemical H10.21-
  - mucopurulent H10.02-
    - viral—*see* Conjunctivitis, viral
  - toxic H10.21-
- blennorrhagic (gonococcal) (neonatorum) A54.31
- chemical (acute) H10.21-
- chlamydial A74.0
  - neonatal P39.1
- epidemic (viral) B30.9
- gonococcal (neonatorum) A54.31
- in (due to)
  - Chlamydia A74.0
  - gonococci A54.31
  - rosacea H10.82-
- inclusion A74.0
- infantile P39.1
  - gonococcal A54.31
- neonatal P39.1
  - gonococcal A54.31
- viral B30.9

Conradi (-Hunermann) disease Q77.3

Conscious simulation (of illness) Z76.5

Consecutive—*see* Disease, diseased

Consolidation lung (base)—*see* Pneumonia, lobar

Constipation (atonic) (neurogenic) (simple) (spastic) K59.00

- chronic K59.09
  - idiopathic K59.04
- drug-induced K59.03
- functional K59.04
- outlet dysfunction K59.02
- psychogenic F45.8
- slow transit K59.01
- specified NEC K59.09

Constriction—*see also* Stricture

- external
  - abdomen, abdominal (wall) S30.841
  - alveolar process S00.542
  - ankle S90.54-
  - antecubital space S50.84-
  - arm (upper) S40.84-
  - auricle S00.44-
  - axilla S40.84-
  - back, lower S30.840
  - breast S20.14-
  - brow S00.84
  - buttock S30.840
  - calf S80.84-
  - canthus S00.24-
  - cheek S00.84
    - internal S00.542
  - chest wall—*see* Constriction, external, thorax
  - chin S00.84
  - clitoris S30.844
  - costal region—*see* Constriction, external, thorax
  - digit(s)
    - foot—*see* Constriction, external, toe
    - hand—*see* Constriction, external, finger
  - ear S00.44-
  - elbow S50.34-
  - epididymis S30.843

Constriction, *continued*

- epigastric region S30.841
- esophagus, cervical S10.14
- eyebrow S00.24-
- eyelid S00.24-
- face S00.84
- finger(s) S60.44-
  - index S60.44-
  - little S60.44-
  - middle S60.44-
  - ring S60.44-
- flank S30.841
- foot (except toe(s) alone) S90.84-
  - toe—*see* Constriction, external, toe
- forearm S50.84-
  - elbow only S50.34-
- forehead S00.84
- genital organs, external
  - female S30.846
  - male S30.845
- groin S30.841
- gum S00.542
- hand S60.54-
- head S00.94
  - ear S00.44-
  - eyelid S00.24-
  - lip S00.541
  - nose S00.34
  - oral cavity S00.542
  - scalp S00.04
  - specified site NEC S00.84
- heel S90.84-
- hip S70.24-
- inguinal region S30.841
- interscapular region S20.449
- jaw S00.84
- knee S80.24-
- labium (majus) (minus) S30.844
- larynx S10.14
- leg (lower) S80.84-
  - knee S80.24-
  - upper S70.34-
- lip S00.541
- lower back S30.840
- lumbar region S30.840
- malar region S00.84
- mammary S20.14-
- mastoid region S00.84
- mouth S00.542
- nail
  - finger—*see* Constriction, external, finger
  - toe—*see* Constriction, external, toe
- nasal S00.34
- neck S10.94
  - specified site NEC S10.84
  - throat S10.14
- nose S00.34
- occipital region S00.04
- oral cavity S00.542
- orbital region S00.24-
- palate S00.542
- palm S60.54-
- parietal region S00.04
- pelvis S30.840
- penis S30.842
- perineum
  - female S30.844
  - male S30.840
- periocular area S00.24-
- phalanges
  - finger—*see* Constriction, external, finger
  - toe—*see* Constriction, external, toe
- pharynx S10.14
- pinna S00.44-
- popliteal space S80.24-
- prepuce S30.842
- pubic region S30.840
- pudendum
  - female S30.846
  - male S30.845
- sacral region S30.840
- scalp S00.04
- scapular region S40.24-

Constriction, *continued*

- scrotum S30.843
- shin S80.84-
- shoulder S40.24-
- sternal region S20.349
- submaxillary region S00.84
- submental region S00.84
- subungual
  - finger(s)—*see* Constriction, external, finger
  - toe(s)—*see* Constriction, external, toe
- supraclavicular fossa S10.84
- supraorbital S00.84
- temple S00.84
- temporal region S00.84
- testis S30.843
- thigh S70.34-
- thorax, thoracic (wall) S20.94
  - back S20.44-
  - front S20.34-
  - throat S10.14
- thumb S60.34-
- toe(s) (lesser) S90.44-
  - great S90.44-
- tongue S00.542
- trachea S10.14
- tunica vaginalis S30.843
- uvula S00.542
- vagina S30.844
- vulva S30.844
- wrist S60.84-
- prepuce (acquired) (congenital) N47.1
- pylorus (adult hypertrophic) K31.1
  - congenital or infantile Q40.0
  - newborn Q40.0

Constrictive—*see* Disease, diseased

Consultation

- medical—*see* Counseling
- specified reason NEC Z71.89
- without complaint or sickness Z71.9
  - specified reason NEC Z71.89

Consumption—*see* Tuberculosis

Contact (with)—*see also* Exposure (to)

- AIDS virus Z20.6
- anthrax Z20.810
- aromatic amines Z77.020
- arsenic Z77.010
- asbestos Z77.090
- bacterial disease NEC Z20.818
- body fluids (potentially hazardous) Z77.21
- benzene Z77.021
- chemicals (chiefly nonmedicinal) (hazardous) NEC Z77.098
- chromium compounds Z77.018
- communicable disease Z20.9
  - bacterial NEC Z20.818
  - specified NEC Z20.89
  - viral NEC Z20.828
  - Zika virus Z20.821
- coronavirus (disease) (novel) 2019 Z20.822
- dyes Z77.098
- Escherichia coli (E. coli) Z20.01
- German measles Z20.4
- gonorrhea Z20.2
- hazardous metals NEC Z77.018
- hazardous substances NEC Z77.29
- hazards in the physical environment NEC Z77.128
- hazards to health NEC Z77.9
- HIV Z20.6
- HTLV-III/LAV Z20.6
- human immunodeficiency virus Z20.6
- infection Z20.9
  - specified NEC Z20.89
- intestinal infectious disease NEC Z20.09
  - Escherichia Coli (E. coli) Z20.01
- lead Z77.011
- meningococcus Z20.811
- mold (toxic) Z77.120
- nickel dust Z77.018
- poliomyelitis Z20.89
- positive maternal group B streptococcus P00.82
- rabies Z20.3
- rubella Z20.4

ALPHABETIC INDEX

Contact, *continued*
- sexually-transmitted disease Z20.2
- smallpox (laboratory) Z20.89
- syphilis Z20.2
- tuberculosis Z20.1
- varicella Z20.820
- venereal disease Z20.2
- viral disease NEC Z20.828
- viral hepatitis Z20.5
- Zika virus Z20.821

Contamination, food—*see* Intoxication, foodborne

Contraception, contraceptive
- advice Z30.09
- counseling Z30.09
- device (intrauterine) (in situ) Z97.5
  - checking Z30.431
  - in place Z97.5
  - initial prescription Z30.014
    - barrier Z30.018
    - diaphragm Z30.018
    - subdermal implantable Z30.017
    - transdermal patch hormonal Z30.016
    - vaginal ring hormonal Z30.015
  - maintenance Z30.40
    - barrier Z30.49
    - diaphragm Z30.49
    - subdermal implantable Z30.46
    - transdermal patch hormonal Z30.45
    - vaginal ring hormonal Z30.44
  - reinsertion Z30.433
  - removal Z30.432
  - replacement Z30.433
- emergency (postcoital) Z30.012
- initial prescription Z30.019
  - injectable Z30.013
  - intrauterine device Z30.014
  - pills Z30.011
  - postcoital (emergency) Z30.012
  - specified type NEC Z30.018
  - subdermal implantable Z30.019
- maintenance Z30.40
  - examination Z30.8
  - injectable Z30.42
  - intrauterine device Z30.431
  - pills Z30.41
  - specified type NEC Z30.49
  - subdermal implantable Z30.46
  - transdermal patch Z30.45
  - vaginal ring Z30.44
- management Z30.9
  - specified NEC Z30.8
- postcoital (emergency) Z30.012
- prescription Z30.019
  - repeat Z30.40
- surveillance (drug)—*see* Contraception, maintenance

Contraction(s), contracture, contracted
- Achilles tendon—*see also* Short, tendon, Achilles
  - congenital Q66.89
- bladder N32.89
  - neck or sphincter N32.0
- congenital Q65.89
  - hysterical F44.4
  - knee M24.56-
  - shoulder M24.51-
  - wrist M24.53-
- hip Q65.89
  - elbow M24.52-
  - foot joint M24.57-
  - hand joint M24.54-
  - hip M24.55-
- hourglass
  - bladder N32.89
    - congenital Q64.79
  - gallbladder K82.0
    - congenital Q44.1
  - stomach K31.89
    - congenital Q40.2
    - psychogenic F45.8
- hysterical F44.4

Contraction(s), contracture, contracted, *continued*
- joint (abduction) (acquired) (adduction) (flexion) (rotation) M24.5-
  - ankle M24.57-
  - congenital NEC Q68.8
- muscle (postinfective) (postural) NEC M62.40
  - with contracture of joint—*see* Contraction, joint
  - congenital Q79.8
    - sternocleidomastoid Q68.0
  - hysterical F44.4
  - posttraumatic—*see* Strabismus, paralytic
  - psychogenic F45.8
    - conversion reaction F44.4
  - psychogenic F45.8
    - conversion reaction F44.4
- premature
  - atrium I49.1
  - supraventricular I49.1
- pylorus NEC—*see also* Pylorospasm
  - psychogenic F45.8
- sternocleidomastoid (muscle), congenital Q68.0
- stomach K31.89
  - hourglass K31.89
    - congenital Q40.2
    - psychogenic F45.8
  - psychogenic F45.8
- tendon (sheath) M62.40
  - ankle M62.47-
  - foot M62.47-
  - forearm M62.43-
  - hand M62.44-
  - lower leg M62.46-
  - multiple sites M62.49
  - neck M62.48
  - pelvic region M62.45-
  - shoulder region M62.41-
  - specified site NEC M62.48
  - thigh M62.45-
  - thorax M62.48
  - trunk M62.48
  - upper arm M62.42-
- urethra—*see also* Stricture, urethra
  - orifice N32.0
- vagina (outlet) N89.5
- vesical N32.89
  - neck or urethral orifice N32.0

Contusion (skin surface intact) T14.8
- abdomen, abdominal (muscle) (wall) S30.1
- adnexa, eye NEC S05.8X-
- alveolar process S00.532
- ankle S90.0-
- antecubital space S50.1-
- anus S30.3
- arm (upper) S40.02-
  - lower (with elbow) S50.1-
- auditory canal S00.43-
- auricle S00.43-
- axilla S40.02-
- back S20.22-
  - lower S30.0
- bone NEC T14.8
- brainstem S06.38-
- breast S20.0-
- brow S00.83
- buttock S30.0
- canthus, eye S00.1-
- cauda equina S34.3
- cerebellar, traumatic S06.37-
- cerebral S06.33-
  - left side S06.32-
  - right side S06.31-
- cheek S00.83
  - internal S00.532
- chest (wall)—*see* Contusion, thorax
- chin S00.83
- clitoris S30.23
- conus medullaris (spine) S34.139
- corpus cavernosum S30.21
- costal region—*see* Contusion, thorax
- ear S00.43-
- elbow S50.0-
  - with forearm S50.1-

Contusion, *continued*
- epididymis S30.22
- epigastric region S30.1
- epiglottis S10.0
- esophagus (thoracic)
  - cervical S10.0
- eyebrow S00.1-
- eyelid (and periocular area) S00.1-
- face NEC S00.83
- femoral triangle S30.1
- finger(s) S60.00
  - with damage to nail (matrix) S60.1-
  - index S60.02-
    - with damage to nail S60.12-
  - little S60.05-
    - with damage to nail S60.15-
  - middle S60.03-
    - with damage to nail S60.13-
  - ring S60.04-
    - with damage to nail S60.14-
  - thumb—*see* Contusion, thumb
- flank S30.1
- foot (except toe(s) alone) S90.3-
  - toe—*see* Contusion, toe
- forearm S50.1-
  - elbow only S50.0-
- forehead S00.83
- genital organs, external
  - female S30.202
  - male S30.201
- groin S30.1
- gum S00.532
- hand S60.22-
  - finger(s)—*see* Contusion, finger
  - wrist S60.21-
- head S00.93
  - ear S00.43-
  - eyelid S00.1-
  - lip S00.531
  - nose S00.33
  - oral cavity S00.532
  - scalp S00.03
  - specified part NEC S00.83
- heel S90.3-
- hip S70.0-
- iliac region S30.1
- inguinal region S30.1
- interscapular region S20.229
- intra-abdominal organ S36.92
  - refer to specific organ under contusion
- jaw S00.83
- kidney S37.01-
  - major (greater than 2 cm) S37.02-
  - minor (less than 2 cm) S37.01-
- knee S80.0-
- labium (majus) (minus) S30.23
- lacrimal apparatus, gland or sac S05.8X-
- larynx S10.0
- leg (lower) S80.1-
  - knee S80.0-
- lip S00.531
- lower back S30.0
- lumbar region S30.0
- lung S27.329
  - bilateral S27.322
  - unilateral S27.321
- malar region S00.83
- mastoid region S00.83
- mouth S00.532
- muscle—*see* Contusion, by site
- nail
  - finger—*see* Contusion, finger, with damage to nail
  - toe—*see* Contusion, toe, with damage to nail
- nasal S00.33
- neck S10.93
  - specified site NEC S10.83
  - throat S10.0
- nerve—*see* Injury, nerve
- newborn P54.5
- nose S00.33
- occipital
  - region (scalp) S00.03
- palate S00.532

ALPHABETIC INDEX

Contusion, *continued*

- parietal
  - region (scalp) S00.03
  - kidney—see Contusion, kidney
- pelvis S30.0
- penis S30.21
- perineum
  - female S30.23
  - male S30.0
- periocular area S00.1-
- pharynx S10.0
- pinna S00.43-
- popliteal space S80.0-
- prepuce S30.21
- pubic region S30.1
- pudendum
  - female S30.202
  - male S30.201
- quadriceps femoris S70.1-
- rectum S36.62
- sacral region S30.0
- scalp S00.03
  - due to birth injury P12.3
- scapular region S40.01-
- scrotum S30.22
- shoulder S40.01-
- skin NEC T14.8
- spermatic cord S30.22
- spinal cord—see Injury, spinal cord, by region
  - cauda equina S34.3
  - conus medullaris S34.139
- spleen S36.02-
  - major S36.021
  - minor S36.020
- sternal region S20.219
- stomach S36.32
- subcutaneous NEC T14.8
- submaxillary region S00.83
- submental region S00.83
- subperiosteal NEC T14.8
- subungual
  - finger—see Contusion, finger, with damage to nail
  - toe—see Contusion, toe, with damage to nail
- supraclavicular fossa S10.83
- supraorbital S00.83
- temple (region) S00.83
- testis S30.22
- thigh S70.1-
- thorax (wall) S20.20
  - back S20.22-
  - front S20.21-
- throat S10.0
- thumb S60.01-
  - with damage to nail S60.11-
- toe(s) (lesser) S90.12-
  - with damage to nail S90.22-
  - great S90.11-
    - with damage to nail S90.21-
    - specified type NEC S90.221
- tongue S00.532
- trachea (cervical) S10.0
- tunica vaginalis S30.22
- tympanum, tympanic membrane S00.43-
- uvula S00.532
- vagina S30.23
- vocal cord(s) S10.0
- vulva S30.23
- wrist S60.21-

Conversion hysteria, neurosis or reaction F44.9

Converter, tuberculosis (test reaction) R76.11

Convulsions (idiopathic) (*see also* Seizure(s)) R56.9

- febrile R56.00
  - with status epilepticus G40.901
  - complex R56.01
    - with status epilepticus G40.901
  - simple R56.00
- infantile P90
  - epilepsy—see Epilepsy
- myoclonic G25.3
- neonatal, benign (familial)—see Epilepsy, generalized, idiopathic
- newborn P90

Convulsions, *continued*

- post traumatic R56.1
- recurrent R56.9
- scarlatinal A38.8

Convulsive—*see also* Convulsions

Cooley's anemia D56.1

Copra itch B88.0

Coprophagy F50.89

Cor

- pulmonale (chronic) I27.81
- triloculare Q20.8
  - biventriculare Q21.1

Corbus' disease (gangrenous balanitis) N48.1

Corn (infected) L84

Cornelia de Lange syndrome Q87.19

Cornual gestation or pregnancy O00.8-

Coronavirus (Infection)

- as cause of diseases classified elsewhere B97.29
- coronavirus-19 U07.1
- COVID-19 U07.1
- SARS-associated B97.21

Corrosion (injury) (acid) (caustic) (chemical) (lime) (external) (internal) T30.4

- extent (percentage of body surface)
  - less than 10 percent T32.0

Coryza (acute) J00

- with grippe or influenza—see Influenza, with, respiratory manifestations NEC

Costen's syndrome or complex M26.69

Costochondritis M94.0

Cot death R99

Cough (affected) (chronic) (epidemic) (nervous) R05.9

- with hemorrhage—see Hemoptysis
- acute R05.1
- bronchial R05
  - with grippe or influenza—see Influenza, with, respiratory manifestations NEC
- chronic R05.3
- functional F45.8
- hysterical F45.8
- laryngeal, spasmodic R05
- paroxysmal, due to Bordetella pertussis (without pneumonia) A37.00
  - with pneumonia A37.01
- persistent R05.3
- psychogenic F45.8
- refractory R05.3
- specified NEC R05.8
- subacute R05.2
- syncope R05.4
- unexplained R05.3

Counseling (for) Z71.9

- abuse NEC
  - perpetrator Z69.82
  - victim Z69.81
- alcohol abuser Z71.41
  - family Z71.42
- child abuse
  - non-parental
    - perpetrator Z69.021
    - victim Z69.020
  - parental
    - perpetrator Z69.011
    - victim Z69.010
- contraceptive Z30.09
- dietary Z71.3
- drug abuser Z71.51
  - family member Z71.52
- exercise Z71.82
- family Z71.89
- for non-attending third party Z71.0
  - related to sexual behavior or orientation Z70.2
- genetic
  - nonprocreative Z71.83
  - procreative NEC Z31.5
- health (advice) (education) (instruction)—*see* Counseling
- human immunodeficiency virus (HIV) Z71.7
- immunization safety Z71.85
- insulin pump use Z46.81

Counseling, *continued*

- medical (for) Z71.9
  - human immunodeficiency virus (HIV) Z71.7
  - on behalf of another Z71.0
  - specified reason NEC Z71.89
- natural family planning
  - to avoid pregnancy Z30.02
- pediatric to adult transitioning Z71.87
- perpetrator (of)
  - abuse NEC Z69.82
  - child abuse
    - non-parental Z69.021
    - parental Z69.011
  - rape NEC Z69.82
  - spousal abuse Z69.12
- procreative NEC Z31.69
- rape victim Z69.81
- safety for (international) travel Z71.84
- socioeconomic factors Z71.88
- specified reason NEC Z71.89
- spousal abuse (perpetrator) Z69.12
  - victim Z69.11
- substance abuse Z71.89
  - alcohol Z71.41
  - drug Z71.51
  - tobacco Z71.6
- tobacco use Z71.6
- travel (international) Z71.84
- use (of)
  - insulin pump Z46.81
- vaccine product safety Z71.85
- victim (of)
  - abuse Z69.81
  - child abuse
    - by parent Z69.010
    - non-parental Z69.020
  - rape NEC Z69.81

COVID-19 U07.1

- condition post U09.9
- contact (with) Z20.822
- exposure (to) Z20.822
- history of (personal) Z86.16
- long (haul) U09.9
  - sequelae (post acute) U09.9

Cowden syndrome, other Q85.82

Coxsackie (virus) (infection) B34.1

- as cause of disease classified elsewhere B97.11
- enteritis A08.3
- meningitis (aseptic) A87.0
- pharyngitis B08.5

Crabs, meaning pubic lice B85.3

Crack baby P04.41

Cracked tooth K03.81

Cradle cap L21.0

Cramp(s) R25.2

- abdominal—*see* Pain, abdominal
- bathing T75.1
- colic R10.83
  - psychogenic F45.8
- due to immersion T75.1
- fireman T67.2
- heat T67.2
- immersion T75.1
- intestinal—*see* Pain, abdominal
  - psychogenic F45.8
- limb (lower) (upper) NEC R25.2
  - sleep related G47.62
- muscle (limb) (general) R25.2
  - due to immersion T75.1
  - psychogenic F45.8
- salt-depletion E87.1
- stoker's T67.2
- swimmer's T75.1

Craniocleidodysostosis Q74.0

Craniofenestria (skull) Q75.8

Craniolacunia (skull) Q75.8

Cranioschisis Q75.8

Craniostenosis Q75.009

ALPHABETIC INDEX

Craniosynostosis Q75.009
- bilateral Q75.002
- coronal Q75.029
  - bilateral Q75.022
  - unilateral Q75.021
- lambdoid Q75.049
  - bilateral Q75.042
  - unilateral Q75.041
- metopic Q75.03
- multi-suture, specified NEC Q75.058
- sagittal Q75.01
- single-suture, specified NEC Q75.08
- unilateral Q75.001

Crepitus
- caput Q75.8
- joint—*see* Derangement, joint, specified type NEC

Crib death R99

Cribriform hymen Q52.3

Cri-du-chat syndrome Q93.4

Crigler-Najjar disease or syndrome E80.5

Crisis
- abdomen R10.0
- acute reaction F43.0
- addisonian E27.2
- adrenal (cortical) E27.2
- celiac K90.0
- Dietl's N13.8
- emotional—*see also* Disorder, adjustment
  - acute reaction to stress F43.0
  - other reactions to severe stress F43.89
  - specific to childhood and adolescence F93.8
- oculogyric H51.8
  - psychogenic F45.8
- psychosexual identity F64.2
- sickle-cell D57.00
  - with
    - acute chest syndrome D57.01
    - cerebral vascular involvement D57.03
    - crisis (painful) D57.00
      - with complication specified NEC D57.09
    - splenic sequestration D57.02
    - vasoocclusive pain D57.00
- state (acute reaction) F43.0

Crocq's disease (acrocyanosis) I73.89

Crohn's disease—*see* Enteritis, regional

Crooked septum, nasal J34.2

Croup, croupous (catarrhal) (infectious) (inflammatory) (nondiphtheritic) J05.0
- bronchial J20.9

Crush, crushed, crushing T14.8
- ankle S97.0-
- arm (upper) (and shoulder) S47.- (See complete *ICD-10-CM* Manual for codes)
- finger(s) S67.1-
  - with hand (and wrist) S67.2-
  - index S67.19-
  - little S67.19-
  - middle S67.19-
  - ring S67.19-
  - thumb—*see* Crush, thumb
- foot S97.8-
  - toe—*see* Crush, toe
- hand (except fingers alone) S67.2-
  - with wrist S67.4-
- thumb S67.0-
  - with hand (and wrist) S00.44-
- toe(s) S97.10-
  - great S97.11-
  - lesser S97.12-
- wrist S67.3-
  - with hand S67.4-

Crusta lactea L21.0

Crying (constant) (continuous) (excessive)
- child, adolescent, or adult R45.83
- infant (baby) (newborn) R68.11

Cryptitis (anal) (rectal) K62.89

Cryptopapillitis (anus) K62.89

Cryptophthalmos Q11.2
- syndrome Q87.0

Cryptorchid, cryptorchism, cryptorchidism Q53.9
- bilateral Q53.20
  - abdominal Q53.211
  - perineal Q53.22
- unilateral Q53.10
  - abdominal Q53.111
  - perineal Q53.12

Cryptosporidiosis A07.2
- hepatobiliary B88.8
- respiratory B88.8

Crystalluria R82.998

Cubitus
- congenital Q68.8
- valgus (acquired) M21.0-
  - congenital Q68.8
- varus (acquired) M21.1-
  - congenital Q68.8

Cultural deprivation or shock Z60.3

Curvature
- organ or site, congenital NEC—*see* Distortion
- penis (lateral) Q55.61
- Pott's (spinal) A18.01
- radius, idiopathic, progressive (congenital) Q74.0
- spine (acquired) (angular) (idiopathic) (incorrect) (postural)
  - congenital Q67.5
  - due to or associated with
    - osteitis
    - deformans M88.88
    - tuberculosis (Pott's curvature) A18.01
  - tuberculous A18.01

Cushingoid due to steroid therapy E24.2
- correct substance properly administered—*see* Table of Drugs and Chemicals, by drug, adverse effect
- overdose or wrong substance given or taken—*see* Table of Drugs and Chemicals, by drug, poisoning

Cushing's
- syndrome or disease E24.9
  - drug-induced E24.2
  - iatrogenic E24.2
  - pituitary-dependent E24.0
  - specified NEC E24.8
- ulcer—*see* Ulcer, peptic, acute

Cutaneous—*see also* Disease, diseased
- hemorrhage R23.3

Cutis—*see also* Disease, diseased
- hyperelastica Q82.8
- osteosis L94.2
- verticis gyrata Q82.8
  - acquired L91.8

Cyanosis R23.0
- due to
  - patent foramen botalli Q21.1
  - persistent foramen ovale Q21.1
- enterogenous D74.8

Cyanotic heart disease I24.9
- congenital Q24.9

Cycle
- anovulatory N97.0
- menstrual, irregular N92.6

Cyclical vomiting, in migraine (*see also* Vomiting, cyclical) G43.A0
- psychogenic F50.89

Cyclical vomiting syndrome unrelated to migraine R11.15

Cycloid personality F34.0

Cyclopia, cyclops Q87.0

Cyclopism Q87.0

Cyclothymia F34.0

Cyclothymic personality F34.0

Cylindruria R82.998

Cynanche
- tonsillaris J36

Cyst (colloid) (mucous) (simple) (retention)
- adenoid (infected) J35.8
- antrum J34.1
- anus K62.89

Cyst, *continued*
- arachnoid, brain (acquired) G93.0
  - congenital Q04.6
- Baker's M71.2-
  - choroid plexus Q04.6
- Bartholin's gland N75.0
- bone (local) NEC M85.60
  - specified type NEC M85.60
    - ankle M85.67-
    - foot M85.67-
    - forearm M85.63-
    - hand M85.64-
    - jaw M27.40
      - developmental (nonodontogenic) K09.1
      ◊ odontogenic K09.0
    - lower leg M85.66-
    - multiple site M85.69
    - neck M85.68
    - rib M85.68
    - shoulder M85.61-
    - skull M85.68
    - specified site NEC M85.68
    - thigh M85.65-
    - toe M85.67-
    - upper arm M85.62-
    - vertebra M85.68
- brain (acquired) G93.0
  - congenital Q04.6
  - third ventricle (colloid), congenital Q04.6
- breast (benign) (blue dome) (pedunculated) (solitary) N60.0-
  - canal of Nuck (female) N94.89
    - congenital Q52.4
  - choledochus, congenital Q44.4
  - common (bile) duct
    - congenital NEC Q89.8
  - fallopian tube Q50.4
  - kidney Q61.00
    - more than one (multiple) Q61.02
    - specified as polycystic Q61.3
      - infantile type NEC Q61.19
  - ovary Q50.1
  - oviduct Q50.4
  - congenital NEC Q89.8
  - kidney Q61.00
    - more than one (multiple) Q61.02
    - specified as polycystic Q61.3
      ◊ infantile type NEC Q61.19
        - collecting duct dilation Q61.11
    - solitary Q61.01
  - prepuce Q55.69
  - thymus (gland) Q89.2
- corpus
  - albicans N83.29-
  - luteum (hemorrhagic) (ruptured) N83.1-
- craniobuccal pouch E23.6
- craniopharyngeal pouch E23.6
- Dandy-Walker Q03.1
  - with spina bifida—*see* Spina bifida
- dental (root) K04.8
  - developmental K09.0
  - eruption K09.0
  - primordial K09.0
- dentigerous (mandible) (maxilla) K09.0
- dermoid—*see* Neoplasm, benign, by site in Table of Neoplasms in the complete *ICD-10-CM* manual
  - implantation
    - vagina N89.8
  - developmental K09.1
    - odontogenic K09.0
  - dura (cerebral) G93.0
    - spinal G96.198
  - epoophoron Q50.5
  - eruption K09.0
  - esophagus K22.89
  - ethmoid sinus J34.1
  - eye NEC H57.89
  - eyelid (sebaceous) H02.82-
    - infected—*see* Hordeolum
    - left H02.826
      - lower H02.825
      - upper H02.824

ALPHABETIC INDEX

Cyst, *continued*

- right H02.823
  - ■ lower H02.822
  - ■ upper H02.821
- fallopian tube N83.8
  - congenital Q50.4
- follicle (graafian) (hemorrhagic) N83.0-
- follicular (atretic) (hemorrhagic) (ovarian) N83.0-
  - dentigerous K09.0
  - odontogenic K09.0
  - skin L72.9
    - ■ specified NEC L72.8
- frontal sinus J34.1
- gingiva K09.0
- graafian follicle N83.0-
- granulosal lutein (hemorrhagic) N83.1-
- hemangiomatous D18.00
  - skin D18.01
  - specified site NEC D18.09
- hydatid (*see also* Echinococcus)
  - Morgagni
    - ■ male (epididymal) Q55.4
    - ■ testicular Q55.29
- hymen N89.8
  - embryonic Q52.4
- hypophysis, hypophyseal (duct) (recurrent) E23.6
  - cerebri E23.6
- implantation (dermoid)
  - vagina N89.8
- intrasellar E23.6
- jaw (bone) M27.40
  - developmental (odontogenic) K09.0
- kidney (acquired) N28.1
  - congenital Q61.00
  - more than one (multiple) Q61.02
    - ■ specified as polycystic Q61.3
    - infantile type (autosomal recessive) NEC Q61.19
      - ◊ collecting duct dilation Q61.11
  - simple N28.1
  - solitary (single) Q61.01
    - ■ acquired N28.1
- lateral periodontal K09.0
- lens H27.8
  - congenital Q12.8
- lip (gland) K13.0
- lutein N83.1-
- mandible M27.40
  - dentigerous K09.0
- maxilla M27.40
  - dentigerous K09.0
- meninges (cerebral) G93.0
  - spinal G96.19-
- Morgagni (hydatid)
  - male (epididymal) Q55.4
    - ■ testicular Q55.29
- Müllerian duct Q50.4
  - appendix testis Q55.29
  - cervix Q51.6
  - fallopian tube Q50.4
  - female Q50.4
  - male Q55.29
- nerve root
  - cervical G96.191
  - lumbar G96.191
  - sacral G96.191
  - thoracic G96.191
- nervous system NEC G96.89
- nose (turbinates) J34.1
  - sinus J34.1
- odontogenic, developmental K09.0
- omentum (lesser) congenital Q45.8
- ovary, ovarian (twisted) N83.20-
  - adherent N83.20-
  - corpus
    - ■ albicans N83.29-
    - ■ luteum (hemorrhagic) N83.1-
  - developmental Q50.1
  - due to failure of involution NEC N83.20-
  - follicular (graafian) (hemorrhagic) N83.0-
  - hemorrhagic N83.20-
  - retention N83.29-
  - serous N83.20-

Cyst, *continued*

- specified NEC N83.29-
  - theca lutein (hemorrhagic) N83.1-
- paramesonephric duct Q50.4
  - female Q50.4
  - male Q55.29
- paranephric N28.1
- paraphysis, cerebri, congenital Q04.6
- paraoophoron Q50.5
- parovarian Q50.5
- pericardial (congenital) Q24.8
  - acquired (secondary) I31.8
- pericoronal K09.0
- periodontal K04.8
  - lateral K09.0
- perineural G96.191
- peripelvic (lymphatic) N28.1
- periventricular, acquired, newborn P91.1
- pilar L72.11
- pilonidal (infected) (rectum) L05.91
  - with abscess L05.01
- pituitary (duct) (gland) E23.6
- porencephalic Q04.6
  - acquired G93.0
- prepuce N47.4
  - congenital Q55.69
- primordial (jaw) K09.0
- Rathke's pouch E23.6
- rectum (epithelium) (mucous) K62.89
- renal—*see* Cyst, kidney
- retention (ovary) N83.29-
- sebaceous (duct) (gland) L72.3
  - eyelid—*see* Cyst, eyelid
  - genital organ NEC
    - ■ female N94.89
    - ■ male N50.89
  - scrotum L72.3
- serous (ovary) N83.20-
- sinus (accessory) (nasal) J34.1
- skin L72.9
  - sebaceous L72.3
- solitary
  - bone—*see* Cyst, bone
  - jaw M27.40
  - kidney N28.1
- sphenoid sinus J34.1
- spinal meninges G96.198
- subdural (cerebral) G93.0
  - spinal cord G96.198
- Tarlov G96.191
- testis N44.2
  - tunica albuginea N44.1
- theca lutein (ovary) N83.1-
- thyroglossal duct (infected) (persistent) Q89.2
- thyrolingual duct (infected) (persistent) Q89.2
- tonsil J35.8
- trichilemmal (proliferating) L72.12
- trichodermal L72.12
- turbinate (nose) J34.1
- vagina, vaginal (implantation) (inclusion) (squamous cell) (wall) N89.8
  - embryonic Q52.4
- wolffian
  - female Q50.5
  - male Q55.4

Cystic—*see also* Disease, diseased

- corpora lutea (hemorrhagic) N83.1-
- kidney (congenital) Q61.9
  - infantile type NEC Q61.19
    - ■ collecting duct dilatation Q61.11
  - medullary Q61.5
- ovary N83.20-

Cysticerosis, cysticerciasis B69.9

- with
  - epileptiform fits B69.0
- brain B69.0
- central nervous system B69.0
  - cerebral B69.0
  - specified NEC B69.89

Cystinosis (malignant) E72.04

Cystitis (exudative) (hemorrhagic) (septic) (suppurative) N30.90

- acute N30.00
  - with hematuria N30.01
- of trigone N30.00
  - ■ with hematuria N30.31
- blennorrhagic (gonococcal) A54.01
- chlamydial A56.01
- gonococcal A54.01
- trichomonal A59.03

Cystoma—*see also* Neoplasm, benign, by site in Table of Neoplasms in the complete *ICD-10-CM* manual

- simple (ovary) N83.29-

Cytomegalic inclusion disease

- congenital P35.1

Cytomegalovirus infection B25.9

Cytopenia D75.9

D

Da Costa's syndrome F45.8

Dacryocystitis

- neonatal P39.1

Dacryostenosis—*see also* Stenosis, lacrimal

- congenital Q10.5

Dactylitis

- bone—see Osteomyelitis
- sickle-cell D57.00
  - Hb C D57.219
  - Hb SS D57.00
  - specified NEC D57.819
- skin L08.9
- tuberculous A18.03

Dactylosymphysis Q70.9

- fingers—*see* Syndactylism, complex, fingers
- toes—*see* Syndactylism, complex, toes

Damage

- brain (nontraumatic) G93.9
  - anoxic, hypoxic G93.1
  - child NEC G80.9
  - due to birth injury P11.2
- cerebral NEC—*see* Damage, brain
- eye, birth injury P15.3
- lung
  - dabbing (related) U07.0
  - electronic cigarette (related) U07.0
  - vaping (associated) (device) (product) (use) U07.0
- organ
  - dabbing (related) U07.0
  - electronic cigarette (related) U07.0
  - vaping (device) (product) (use) (associated) U07.0
- vascular I99.9

Dandruff L21.0

Dandy-Walker syndrome Q03.1

- with spina bifida—*see* Spina bifida

Danlos' syndrome Q79.60

- classical Ehlers-Danlos syndrome Q79.61
- hypermobile Ehlers-Danlos syndrome Q79.62
- other Ehlers-Danlos syndromes Q79.69
- vascular Ehlers-Danlos syndrome Q79.63

Darier (-White) disease (congenital) Q82.8

- meaning erythema annulare centrifugum L53.1

Darier-Roussy sarcoid D86.3

De la Tourette's syndrome F95.2

De Lange's syndrome Q87.19

De Morgan's spots (senile angiomas) I78.1

De Toni-Fanconi (-Debré) syndrome E72.09

- with cystinosis E72.04

Dead

- fetus, retained (mother) O36.4
  - early pregnancy O02.1

Deaf-mutism (acquired) (congenital) NEC H91.3

- hysterical F44.6

Deafness (acquired) (complete) (hereditary) (partial) H91.9-

- with blue sclera and fragility of bone Q78.0
- central—*see* Deafness, sensorineural

ALPHABETIC INDEX

Deafness, *continued*
- conductive H90.2
  - and sensorineural, mixed H90.8
    - bilateral H90.6
  - bilateral H90.0
  - unilateral H90.1-
    - with restrictive hearing on contralateral side H90.A-
- congenital H90.5
  - with blue sclera and fragility of bone Q78.0
- emotional (hysterical) F44.6
- functional (hysterical) F44.6
- high frequency H91.9-
- hysterical F44.6
- low frequency H91.9-
- mixed conductive and sensorineural H90.8
  - bilateral H90.6
  - unilateral H90.7-
- nerve—*see* Deafness, sensorineural
- neural—*see* Deafness, sensorineural
- noise-induced—*see also* subcategory H83.3
- psychogenic (hysterical) F44.6
- sensorineural H90.5
  - and conductive, mixed H90.8
    - bilateral H90.6
  - bilateral H90.3
  - unilateral H90.4-
- sensory—*see* Deafness, sensorineural
- word (developmental) H93.25

Death (cause unknown) (of) (unexplained) (unspecified cause) R99
- brain G93.82
- cardiac (sudden) (with successful resuscitation)—*code to underlying disease*
  - family history of Z82.41
  - personal history of Z86.74
  - family member (assumed) Z63.4

Debility (chronic) (general) (nervous) R53.81
- congenital or neonatal NOS P96.9
- nervous R53.81

Débove's disease (splenomegaly) R16.1

Decalcification
- teeth K03.89

Decrease(d)
- absolute neutrophil count—*see* Neutropenia
- blood
  - glucose
    - level 1 E16.A1
    - level 2 E16.A2
    - level 3 E16.A3
  - platelets—*see* Thrombocytopenia
  - pressure R03.1
    - due to shock following
      - injury T79.4
      - operation T81.19
- function
  - ovary in hypopituitarism E23.0
  - pituitary (gland) (anterior) (lobe) E23.0
    - posterior (lobe) E23.0
- hematocrit R71.0
- hemoglobin R71.0
- leukocytes D72.819
  - specified NEC D72.818
- lymphocytes D72.810
- respiration, due to shock following injury T79.4
- tolerance
  - fat K90.49
  - glucose R73.09
  - salt and water E87.8
- vision NEC H54.7
- white blood cell count D72.819
  - specified NEC D72.818

Defect, defective Q89.9
- 3-beta-hydroxysteroid dehydrogenase E25.0
- 11-hydroxylase E25.0
- 21-hydroxylase E25.0
- atrial septal (ostium secundum type) Q21.1
  - ostium primum type Q21.2
- atrioventricular
  - canal Q21.2
  - septum Q21.2

Defect, defective, *continued*
- auricular septal Q21.1
- bilirubin excretion NEC E80.6
- bulbar septum Q21.0
- cell membrane receptor complex (CR3) D71
- circulation I99.9
  - congenital Q28.9
  - newborn Q28.9
- coagulation (factor) (*see also* Deficiency) D68.9
  - newborn, transient P61.6
- conduction (heart) I45.9
  - bone—*see* Deafness, conductive
- coronary sinus Q21.1
- cushion, endocardial Q21.2
- degradation, glycoprotein E77.1
- diaphragm
  - with elevation, eventration or hernia—*see* Hernia, diaphragm
  - congenital Q79.1
    - with hernia Q79.0
    - gross (with hernia) Q79.0
- extensor retinaculum M62.89
- filling
  - bladder R93.41
  - kidney R93.42-
  - renal pelvis R93.41
  - ureter R93.41
  - urinary organs, specified NEC R93.49
- GABA (gamma aminobutyric acid) metabolic E72.81
- Gerbode Q21.0
- glucose transport, blood-brain barrier E74.810
- glycoprotein degradation E77.1
- home, technical, preventing adequate care Z59.19
- interatrial septal Q21.1
- interauricular septal Q21.1
- interventricular septal Q21.0
  - with dextroposition of aorta, pulmonary stenosis and hypertrophy of right ventricle Q21.3
  - in tetralogy of Fallot Q21.3
- learning (specific)—*see* Disorder, learning
- lymphocyte function antigen-1 (LFA-1) D84.0
- lysosomal enzyme, post-translational modification E77.0
- modification, lysosomal enzymes, post-translational E77.0
- obstructive, congenital
  - ureter Q62.39
    - orthotopic ureterocele Q62.31
- osteochondral NEC—*see also* Deformity M95.8
- ostium
  - primum Q21.2
  - secundum Q21.1
- platelets, qualitative D69.1
  - constitutional D68.0
- reduction
  - limb
    - lower Q72.9-
      - longitudinal
        ◊ femur Q72.4-
        ◊ fibula Q72.6-
        ◊ tibia Q72.5-
      - specified type NEC Q72.89-
    - upper Q71.9-
      - longitudinal
        ◊ radius Q71.4-
        ◊ ulna Q71.5-
      - specified type NEC Q71.89-
- respiratory system, congenital Q34.9
- septal (heart) NOS Q21.9
  - atrial Q21.1
  - ventricular (*see also* Defect, ventricular septal) Q21.0
- sinus venosus Q21.1
- speech R47.9
  - developmental F80.9
  - specified NEC R47.89
- vascular (local) I99.9
  - congenital Q27.9
- ventricular septal Q21.0
  - in tetralogy of Fallot Q21.3
- vision NEC H54.7

Defibrination (syndrome) D65
- newborn P60

Deficiency, deficient
- 3-beta-hydroxysteroid dehydrogenase E25.0
- 11-hydroxylase E25.0
- 21-hydroxylase E25.0
- AADC (aromatic L-amino acid decarboxylase) E70.81
- abdominal muscle syndrome Q79.4
- acid sphingomyelinase (ASMD) E75.249
  - type
    - A E75.240
    - A/B E75.244
    - B E75.241
- adenosine deaminase (ADA) D81.30
  - deaminase 2 D81.32
  - other adenosine deaminase D81.39
  - severe combined immunodeficiency due to adenosine deaminase deficiency D81.31
    - type 1 (without SCID) (without severe combined immunodeficiency) D81.39
    - type 2 D81.32
- anti-hemophilic
  - factor (A) D66
    - B D67
    - C D68.1
  - globulin (AHG) NEC D66
- antidiuretic hormone E23.2
- aromatic L-amino acid decarboxylase (AADC) E70.81
- attention (disorder) (syndrome) F98.8
  - with hyperactivity—*see* Disorder, attention-deficit hyperactivity
- beta-glucuronidase E76.29
- calcium (dietary) E58
- carnitine E71.40
  - due to
    - hemodialysis E71.43
    - inborn errors of metabolism E71.42
    - Valproic acid therapy E71.43
  - iatrogenic E71.43
  - muscle palmityltransferase E71.314
  - primary E71.41
  - secondary E71.448
- cell membrane receptor complex (CR3) D71
- central nervous system G96.89
- clotting (blood) (*see also* Deficiency) D68.9
- coagulation NOS D68.9
- combined glucocorticoid and mineralocorticoid E27.49
- corticoadrenal E27.40
- craniofacial axis Q75.009
  - primary E27.1
- dehydrogenase
  - long chain/very long chain acyl CoA E71.310
  - medium chain acyl CoA E71.311
  - short chain acyl CoA E71.312
- diet E63.9
- disaccharidase E73.9
- enzymes, circulating NEC E88.09
- essential fatty acid (EFA) E63.0
- factor—*see also* Deficiency
  - IX (congenital) (functional) (hereditary) (with functional defect) D67
  - VIII (congenital) (functional) (hereditary) (with functional defect) D66
    - with vascular defect D68.0
  - XI (congenital) (hereditary) D68.1
- fibrinogen (congenital) (hereditary) D68.2
  - acquired D65
- GABA (gamma aminobutyric acid) metabolic E72.81
- GABA-T (gamma aminobutyric acid) metabolic E72.81
- gammaglobulin in blood D80.1
  - hereditary D80.0
- glucocorticoid E27.49
  - mineralocorticoid E27.49
- glucose-6-phosphate dehydrogenase (G6PD) with anemia D55.0
- glucose-6-phosphate dehydrogenase (G6PD) without anemia D75.A
- glucose transporter protein type 1 E74.810
- glucuronyl transferase E80.5
- Glut1 E74.810
- gonadotropin (isolated) E23.0
- growth hormone (idiopathic) (isolated) E23.0
- hearing—*see* Deafness
- high grade F70
- hemoglobin D64.9

ALPHABETIC INDEX

Deficiency, deficient, *continued*

- hormone
  - anterior pituitary (partial) NEC E23.0
    - growth E23.0
  - growth (isolated) E23.0
  - pituitary E23.0
- hypoxanthine-(guanine)-phosphoribosyltransferase (HG-PRT) (total H-PRT) E79.1
- immunity D84.9
  - cell-mediated D84.89
    - with thrombocytopenia and eczema D82.0
  - combined D81.9
- infantile neurovisceral acid sphingomyelinase E75.240
- kappa-light chain D80.8
- lacrimal fluid (acquired)—*see also* Syndrome
  - congenital Q10.6
- lactase
  - congenital E73.0
  - secondary E73.1
- lysosome-associated membrane protein 2 [LAMP2] E74.05
- menadione (vitamin K) E56.1
  - newborn P53
- mineralocorticoid E27.49
  - with glucocorticoid E27.49
- moral F60.2
- multiple sulfatase (MSD) E75.26
  - *Add-* succinic semialdehyde dehydrogenase E72.81
  - *Revise from-* sulfatase E75.29
  - *Revise to-* sulfatase E75.26
- muscle
  - carnitine (palmityltransferase) E71.314
- NADH diaphorase or reductase (congenital) D74.0
- NADH-methemoglobin reductase (congenital) D74.0
- natrium E87.1
- parathyroid (gland) E20.9
- phosphoenolpyruvate carboxykinase E74.4
- phosphomannomutase E74.818
- phosphomannose isomerase E74.818
- phosphomannosyl mutase E74.818
- pituitary hormone (isolated) E23.0
- plasma thromboplastin
  - antecedent (PTA) D68.1
  - component (PTC) D67
- plasminogen (type 1) (type 2) E88.02
- platelet NEC D69.1
  - constitutional D68.0
- protein (*see also* Malnutrition) E46
- pseudocholinesterase E88.09
- PTA (plasma thromboplastin antecedent) D68.1
- pyruvate
  - carboxylase E74.4
  - dehydrogenase E74.4
- salt E87.1
- secretion
  - urine R34
- short stature homeobox gene (SHOX)
  - with
    - dyschondrosteosis Q78.8
    - short stature (idiopathic) E34.3
    - Turner's syndrome Q96.9
- sodium (Na) E87.1
- thrombokinase D68.2
  - newborn P53
- vascular I99.9
- vasopressin E23.2
- vitamin (multiple) NOS E56.9
  - K E56.1
    - of newborn P53

Deficit—*see also* Deficiency

- attention and concentration R41.840
  - disorder—*see* Attention, deficit
- concentration R41.840
- oxygen R09.02

Deflection

- radius M21.83-
- septum (acquired) (nasal) (nose) J34.2
- spine—*see* Curvature, spine
- turbinate (nose) J34.2

Defluvium

- capillorum—*see* Alopecia
- unguium L60.8

Deformity Q89.9

- abdominal wall
  - acquired M95.8
  - congenital Q79.59
- alimentary tract, congenital Q45.9
  - upper Q40.9
- anus (acquired) K62.89
  - congenital Q43.9
- aorta (arch) (congenital) Q25.40
- aortic
  - cusp or valve (congenital) Q23.88
    - acquired (*see also* Endocarditis, aortic) I35.8
- artery (congenital) (peripheral) NOS Q27.9
  - umbilical Q27.0
- atrial septal Q21.1
- bile duct (common) (congenital) (hepatic) Q44.5
  - acquired K83.8
- biliary duct or passage (congenital) Q44.5
  - acquired K83.8
- bladder (neck) (trigone) (sphincter) (acquired) N32.89
  - congenital Q64.79
- bone (acquired) NOS M95.9
  - congenital Q79.9
- brain (congenital) Q04.9
  - acquired G93.89
- bursa, congenital Q79.9
- cerebral, acquired G93.89
  - congenital Q04.9
- cheek (acquired) M95.2
  - congenital Q18.9
- chin (acquired) M95.2
  - congenital Q18.9
- choroid (congenital) Q14.3
  - plexus Q07.8
    - acquired G96.198
- clavicle (acquired) M95.8
  - congenital Q68.8
- cystic duct (congenital) Q44.5
  - acquired K82.8
- Dandy-Walker Q03.1
  - with spina bifida—*see* Spina bifida
- diaphragm (congenital) Q79.1
  - acquired J98.6
- digestive organ NOS Q45.9
- ductus arteriosus Q25.0
- ear (acquired) H61.1-
  - congenital (external) Q17.9
- ectodermal (congenital) NEC Q84.9
- endocrine gland NEC Q89.2
- eye, congenital Q15.9
- face (acquired) M95.2
  - congenital Q18.9
- flexion (joint) (acquired) (*see also* Deformity, limb, flexion) M21.20
  - congenital NOS Q74.9
    - hip Q65.89
- foot (acquired)—*see also* Deformity, limb, lower leg
  - cavovarus (congenital) Q66.1-
  - congenital NOS Q66.9-
    - specified type NEC Q66.89
    - specified type NEC M21.6X-
  - valgus (congenital) Q66.6
    - acquired M21.07-
  - varus (congenital) NEC Q66.3-
    - acquired M21.17-
- forehead (acquired) M95.2
  - congenital Q75.8
- frontal bone (acquired) M95.2
  - congenital Q75.8
- gallbladder (congenital) Q44.1
  - acquired K82.8
- gastrointestinal tract (congenital) NOS Q45.9
  - acquired K63.89
- genitalia, genital organ(s) or system NEC
  - female (congenital) Q52.9
    - acquired N94.89
    - external Q52.70
  - male (congenital) Q55.9
    - acquired N50.89
- head (acquired) M95.2
  - congenital Q75.8

Deformity, *continued*

- heart (congenital) Q24.9
  - septum Q21.9
    - auricular Q21.1
      - ventricular Q21.0
- hepatic duct (congenital) Q44.5
  - acquired K83.8
- humerus (acquired) M21.82-
  - congenital Q74.0
- hypophyseal (congenital) Q89.2
- ilium (acquired) M95.5
  - congenital Q74.2
- integument (congenital) Q84.9
- ischium (acquired) M95.5
  - congenital Q74.2
- ligament (acquired)—*see* Disorder
  - congenital Q79.9
- limb (acquired) M21.90
  - congenital Q38.0
  - congenital, except reduction deformity Q74.9
  - flat foot M21.4-
  - flexion M21.20
    - ankle M21.27-
    - elbow M21.22-
    - finger M21.24-
    - hip M21.25-
    - knee M21.26-
    - shoulder M21.21-
    - toe M21.27-
    - wrist M21.23-
  - foot
    - drop M21.37-
    - flat—*see* Deformity, limb, flat foot
    - specified NEC M21.6X-
  - forearm M21.93-
  - hand M21.94-
  - lower leg M21.96-
    - specified type NEC M21.80
      - forearm M21.83-
      - lower leg M21.86-
      - thigh M21.85-
        - unequal length M21.70
      - thigh M21.95-
      - upper arm M21.82-
- lip (acquired) NEC K13.0
- liver (congenital) Q44.0
  - acquired K76.89
- Madelung's (radius) Q74.0
- meninges or membrane (congenital) Q07.9
  - cerebral Q04.8
    - acquired G96.198
  - spinal cord (congenital) Q06.-
    - acquired G96.198
- metacarpus (acquired)—*see* Deformity, limb, forearm
  - congenital Q74.0
- mitral (leaflets) (valve) I05.8
  - parachute Q23.2
  - stenosis, congenital Q23.2
- mouth (acquired) K13.79
  - congenital Q38.6
  - multiple, congenital NEC Q89.7
- muscle (acquired) M62.89
  - congenital Q79.9
    - sternocleidomastoid Q68.0
- musculoskeletal system (acquired) M95.9
  - congenital Q79.9
  - specified NEC M95.8
- nail (acquired) L60.8
  - congenital Q84.6
- nasal—*see* Deformity, nose
- neck (acquired) M95.3
  - congenital Q18.9
    - sternocleidomastoid Q68.0
- nervous system (congenital) Q07.9
- nose (acquired) (cartilage) M95.0
  - bone (turbinate) M95.0
  - congenital Q30.9
    - bent or squashed Q67.4
    - septum (acquired) J34.2
      - congenital Q30.8
- ovary (congenital) Q50.39
- parathyroid (gland) Q89.2

Deformity, *continued*

- pelvis, pelvic (acquired) (bony) M95.5
  - congenital Q74.2
- penis (glans) (congenital) Q55.69
  - acquired N48.89
- pinna, acquired H61.1-
  - congenital Q17.9
- pituitary (congenital) Q89.2
  - posture—*see* Dorsopathy
- prepuce (congenital) Q55.69
  - acquired N47.8
- rectum (congenital) Q43.9
  - acquired K62.89
- respiratory system (congenital) Q34.9
- rotation (joint) (acquired)—*see* Deformity, limb, specified site NEC
  - congenital Q74.9
  - hip M21.85-
    - congenital Q65.89
- sacroiliac joint (congenital) Q74.2
- septum, nasal (acquired) J34.2
- scapula (acquired) M95.8
  - congenital Q68.8
- shoulder (joint) (acquired) M21.92-
  - congenital Q74.0
- skull (acquired) M95.2
  - congenital Q75.8
    - with
      - anencephaly Q00.0
      - encephalocele—*see* Encephalocele
      - hydrocephalus Q03.9
        - ◊ with spina bifida—*see* Spina bifida, by site, with hydrocephalus
      - microcephaly Q02
- spinal
  - nerve root (congenital) Q07.9
- Sprengel's (congenital) Q74.0
- sternocleidomastoid (muscle), congenital Q68.0
- thymus (tissue) (congenital) Q89.2
- thyroid (gland) (congenital) Q89.2
- toe (acquired) M20.6-
  - congenital Q66.9-
  - hallux valgus M20.1-
- tricuspid (leaflets) (valve) I07.8
  - atresia or stenosis Q22.4
  - Ebstein's Q22.5
- trunk (acquired) M95.8
  - congenital Q89.9
- urachus (congenital) Q64.4
- urinary tract (congenital) Q64.9
  - urachus Q64.4
- vagina (acquired) N89.8
  - congenital Q52.4
- valgus NEC M21.00
  - knee M21.06-
- varus NEC M21.10
  - knee M21.16-
- vesicourethral orifice (acquired) N32.89
  - congenital NEC Q64.79
  - wrist drop M21.33-

Degeneration, degenerative

- brain (cortical) (progressive) G31.9
  - childhood G31.9
    - specified NEC G31.89
  - cystic G31.89
    - congenital Q04.6
  - in
    - congenital hydrocephalus Q03.9
      - with spina bifida—*see also* Spina bifida
    - Hunter's syndrome E76.1
- cerebrovascular I67.9
  - due to hypertension I67.4
- cortical (cerebellar) (parenchymatous) G31.89
- cutis L98.8
- extrapyramidal G25.9
- fatty
  - liver NEC K76.0
- intervertebral disc
  - sacrococcygeal region M53.3
- kidney N28.89
  - cystic, congenital Q61.9
  - fatty N28.89
  - polycystic Q61.3

Degeneration, degenerative, *continued*

- infantile type (autosomal recessive) NEC Q61.19
  - collecting duct dilatation Q61.11
- muscle (fatty) (fibrous) (hyaline) (progressive) M62.89
  - heart—*see* Degeneration, myocardial
- myocardial, myocardium (fatty) (hyaline) (senile) I51.5
  - with rheumatic fever (conditions in I00) I09.0
    - active, acute or subacute I01.2
      - with chorea I02.0
    - inactive or quiescent (with chorea) I09.0
- nasal sinus (mucosa) J32.9
  - frontal J32.1
  - maxillary J32.0
- nervous system G31.9
  - fatty G31.89
  - specified NEC G31.89
- ovary N83.8
  - cystic N83.20-
  - microcystic N83.20-
- pituitary (gland) E23.6
- pulmonary valve (heart) I37.8
- sinus (cystic)—*see also* Sinusitis
- skin L98.8
  - colloid L98.8
- spinal (cord) G31.89
  - familial NEC G31.89
  - fatty G31.89
- tricuspid (heart) (valve) I07.9
- turbinate J34.89

Deglutition

- paralysis R13.0
  - hysterical F44.4
- pneumonia J69.0

Dehiscence (*of*)

- closure
  - laceration (internal) (external) T81.33
  - traumatic laceration (external) (internal) T81.33
- traumatic injury wound repair T81.33
- wound T81.30
  - traumatic repair T81.33

Dehydration E86.0

- hypertonic E87.0
- hypotonic E87.1
- newborn P74.1

Delay, delayed

- closure, ductus arteriosus (Botalli) P29.38
- conduction (cardiac) (ventricular) I45.9
- development R62.50
  - intellectual (specific) F81.9
  - language F80.9
    - due to hearing loss F80.4
  - learning F81.9
  - pervasive F84.9
  - physiological R62.50
    - specified stage NEC R62.0
  - reading F81.0
  - sexual E30.0
  - speech F80.9
    - due to hearing loss F80.4
  - spelling F81.81
- gastric emptying K30
- menarche E30.0
- milestone R62.0
- passage of meconium (newborn) P76.0
- primary respiration P28.9
- puberty (constitutional) E30.0
- separation of umbilical cord P96.82
- sexual maturation, female E30.0
- sleep phase syndrome G47.21
- vaccination Z28.9

Deletion(s)

- autosome Q93.9
  - identified by fluorescence in situ hybridization (FISH) Q93.89
  - identified by in situ hybridization (ISH) Q93.89
- chromosome
  - seen only at prometaphase Q93.89
  - part of NEC Q93.59
  - short arm
    - 5p Q93.4
    - 22q11.2 Q93.81
  - specified NEC Q93.89

Deletion(s), *continued*

- microdeletions NEC Q93.88

Delinquency (juvenile) (neurotic) F91.8

- group Z72.810

Delinquent immunization status Z28.3

Delirium, delirious (acute or subacute) (not alcohol- or drug-induced) R41.0

- exhaustion F43.0

Delivery (childbirth) (labor)

- cesarean (for)
  - fetal-maternal hemorrhage O43.01-
  - placental insufficiency O36.51-
  - placental transfusion syndromes
    - fetomaternal O43.01-
    - fetus to fetus O43.02-
    - maternofetal O43.01-
  - pre-eclampsiaO14.9-
    - mild O14.0-
    - moderate O14.0-
    - severe
      - with hemolysis, elevated liver enzymes and low platelet count (HELLP) O14.2-
  - complicated O75.9
    - by
      - premature rupture, membranes (*see also* Pregnancy, complicated by, premature rupture of membranes) O42.90
  - missed (at or near term) O36.4

Dementia (degenerative (primary)) (persisting) (unspecified severity) (without behavioral disturbance, psychotic disturbance, mood disturbance, and anxiety) F03.90

- in (due to)
  - hypercalcemia E83.52 [*F02.80*]
    - with behavioral disturbance E83.52 [*F02.81*]
  - hypothyroidism, acquired E03.9 [*F02.80*]
    - with behavioral disturbance E03.9 [*F02.81*]
  - due to iodine deficiency E01.8 [*F02.80*]
    - with behavioral disturbance E01.8 [*F02.81*]

Demodex folliculorum (infestation) B88.0

Demyelination, demyelinization

- central nervous system G37.9
  - specified NEC G37.89
- corpus callosum (central) G37.1
- disseminated, acute G36.9
  - specified NEC G36.8
- global G35
- in optic neuritis G36.0

Dentia praecox K00.6

Dentigerous cyst K09.0

Dentin

- sensitive K03.89

Dentition (syndrome) K00.7

- delayed K00.6
- difficult K00.7
- precocious K00.6
- premature K00.6
- retarded K00.6

Dependence (on) (syndrome) F19.20

- with remission F19.21
- alcohol (ethyl) (methyl) (without remission) F10.20
  - with
    - anxiety disorder F10.280
    - intoxication F10.229
      - with delirium F10.221
      - uncomplicated F10.220
    - counseling and surveillance Z71.41
    - in remission F10.21
- amphetamine(s) (type)—*see* Dependence, drug, stimulant NEC
- benzedrine—*see* Dependence, drug, stimulant NEC
- bhang—*see* Dependence, drug, cannabis
- caffeine—*see* Dependence, drug, stimulant NEC
- cannabis (sativa) (indica) (resin) (derivatives) (type)— F12.20
  - withdrawal F12.23
- coca (leaf) (derivatives)—*see* Dependence, drug, cocaine
- cocaine—*see* Dependence, drug, cocaine
- combinations of drugs F19.20
- dagga—*see* Dependence, drug, cannabis

ALPHABETIC INDEX

Dependence, *continued*

- dexamphetamine—*see* Dependence, drug, stimulant NEC
- dexedrine—*see* Dependence, drug, stimulant NEC
- dextro-nor-pseudo-ephedrine—*see* Dependence, drug, stimulant NEC
- diazepam—*see* Dependence, drug
- drug NEC F19.20
  - cannabis F12.20
    - with
      - intoxication F12.229
        - ◊ uncomplicated F12.220
      - in remission F12.21
      - in remission, unspecified F12.91
  - cocaine F14.20
    - with
      - intoxication F14.229
        - ◊ uncomplicated F14.220
      - withdrawal F14.23
      - in remission F14.21
      - in remission, unspecified F14.91
      - withdrawal symptoms in newborn P96.1
  - counseling and surveillance Z71.51
  - inhalant F18.20
    - with
      - intoxication F18.229
        - ◊ uncomplicated F18.220
      - in remission F18.21
  - nicotine F17.200
    - with disorder F17.209
      - in remission F17.201
      - ~ specified disorder NEC F17.208
      - ~ withdrawal F17.203
    - chewing tobacco F17.220
      - ~ with disorder F17.229
        - ◊ in remission F17.221
        - ◊ specified disorder NEC F17.228
        - ◊ withdrawal F17.223
    - cigarettes F17.210
      - ~ with disorder F17.219
        - ◊ in remission F17.211
        - ◊ specified disorder NEC F17.218
    - specified product F17.290
      - ~ with disorder F17.299
        - ◊ in remission F17.291
        - ◊ specified disorder NEC F17.298
        - ◊ withdrawal F17.293
  - psychoactive NEC F19.20
  - sedative, anxiolytic or hypnotic F13.-
  - sedative, anxiolytic or hypnotic, unspecified, in remission F13.91
  - stimulant NEC F15.20
    - with
      - ~ intoxication F15.229
        - ◊ uncomplicated F15.220
      - ~ withdrawal F15.23
      - in remission F15.21
- ethyl
  - alcohol (without remission) F10.20
    - with remission F10.21
- ganja—*see* Dependence, drug, cannabis
- glue (airplane) (sniffing)—*see* Dependence, drug, inhalant
- hashish—*see* Dependence, drug, cannabis
- hemp—*see* Dependence, drug, cannabis
- Indian hemp—*see* Dependence, drug, cannabis
- inhalants—*see* Dependence, drug, inhalant
- maconha—*see* Dependence, drug, cannabis
- marijuana—*see* Dependence, drug, cannabis
- methyl
  - alcohol (without remission) F10.20
    - with remission F10.21
- nicotine—*see* Dependence, drug, nicotine
- on
  - assistance with personal care Z74.1
  - care provider (because of) Z74.9
    - no other household member able to render care Z74.2
  - machine Z99.89
    - enabling NEC Z99.89
    - specified type NEC Z99.89
  - renal dialysis (hemodialysis) (peritoneal) Z99.2

Dependence, *continued*

- respirator Z99.11
- ventilator Z99.11
- wheelchair Z99.3
- oxygen (long-term) (supplemental) Z99.81
- PCP (phencyclidine) (*see also* Abuse, drug) F16.20
- phencyclidine (PCP) (and related substances) (*see also* Abuse, drug) F16.20
- phenmetrazine—*see* Dependence, drug, stimulant NEC
- polysubstance F19.20
- psychostimulant NEC—*see* Dependence, drug, stimulant NEC
- sedative, anxiolytic or hypnotic F13.-
- specified drug NEC—*see* Dependence, drug
- stimulant NEC—*see* Dependence, drug, stimulant NEC
- substance NEC—*see* Dependence, drug
- supplemental oxygen Z99.81
- tobacco—*see* Dependence, drug, nicotine
  - counseling and surveillance Z71.6
- volatile solvents—*see* Dependence, drug, inhalant

Depletion

- extracellular fluid E86.9
- plasma E86.1
- salt or sodium E87.1
  - causing heat exhaustion or prostration T67.4
  - nephropathy N28.9
- volume NOS E86.9

Depolarization, premature I49.40

- atrial I49.1
- specified NEC I49.49

Deposit

- bone in Boeck's sarcoid D86.89

Depression (acute) (mental) F32.A

- anaclitic—*see* Disorder, adjustment
- anxiety F41.8
  - persistent F34.1
- atypical (single episode) F32.89
- basal metabolic rate R94.8
- bone marrow D75.89
- central nervous system R09.2
- cerebral R29.818
  - newborn P91.4
- major F32.9
- medullary G93.89
- nervous F34.1
- neurotic F34.1
- psychogenic (reactive) (single episode) F32.9
- psychoneurotic F34.1
- reactive (psychogenic) (single episode) F32.9
  - psychotic (single episode) F32.3
- recurrent—*see* Disorder, depressive, recurrent
- respiratory center G93.89
- situational F43.21
- skull Q67.4
- specified NEC (single episode) F32.89

Deprivation

- cultural Z60.3
- emotional NEC Z65.8
  - affecting infant or child—*see* Maltreatment, child, psychological
- material due to limited financial resources, specified NEC Z59.87
- social Z60.4
  - affecting infant or child—*see* Maltreatment, child, psychological abuse

De Quervain's

- syndrome E34.51
- thyroiditis (subacute granulomatous thyroiditis) E06.1

Derangement

- joint (internal) M24.9
  - ankylosis—*see* Ankylosis
  - specified type NEC M24.8-
    - ankle M24.87-
    - elbow M24.82-
    - foot joint M24.87-
    - hand joint M24.84-
    - hip M24.85-
    - shoulder M24.81-
  - temporomandibular M26.69

Dermatitis (eczematous) L30.9

- acarine B88.0
- ammonia L22
- arsenical (ingested) L27.8
- artefacta L98.1
  - psychogenic F54
- atopic L20.9
  - psychogenic F54
  - specified NEC L20.89
- cercarial B65.3
- contact (occupational) L25.9
  - allergic L23.9
    - due to
      - adhesives L23.1
      - cement L24.5
      - chemical products NEC L23.5
      - chromium L23.0
      - cosmetics L23.2
      - dander (cat) (dog) L23.81
      - drugs in contact with skin L23.3
      - dyes L23.4
      - food in contact with skin L23.6
      - hair (cat) (dog) L23.81
      - insecticide L23.5
      - metals L23.0
      - nickel L23.0
      - plants, non-food L23.7
      - plastic L23.5
      - rubber L23.5
      - specified agent NEC L23.89
    - due to
      - dander (cat) (dog) L23.81
      - hair (cat) (dog) L23.81
    - irritant L24.9
      - due to
        - body fluids L24.A0
        - digestive L24.B1
        - fecal or urinary L24.B3
        - incontinence (dual) (fecal) (urinary) L24.A2
        - saliva L24.A1
        - specified NEC L24.A9
      - related to
        - colostomy L24.B3
        - endotracheal tube L24.A9
        - enterocutaneous fistula L24.B3
        - gastrostomy L24.B1
        - ileostomy L24.B3
        - jejunostomy L24.B1
        - respiratory L24.B2
        - saliva or spit fistula L24.B1
        - stoma or fistula L24.B0
        - tracheostomy L24.B2
- contusiformis L52
- desquamative L30.8
- diabetic—*see* E08-E13 with .620
- diaper L22
- due to
  - adhesive(s) (allergic) (contact) (plaster) L23.1
  - alcohol (irritant) (skin contact) L24.2
    - taken internally L27.8
  - alkalis (contact) (irritant) L24.5
  - arsenic (ingested) L27.8
  - cereal (ingested) L27.2
  - chemical(s) NEC L25.3
    - taken internally L27.8
  - coffee (ingested) L27.2
  - cosmetics (contact) L25.0
    - allergic L23.2
  - dander (cat) (dog) L23.81
  - Demodex species B88.0
  - Dermanyssus gallinae B88.0
  - drugs and medicaments (generalized) (internal use) L27.0
    - in contact with skin L25.1
      - allergic L23.3
    - localized skin eruption L27.1
    - specified substance—*see* Table of Drugs and Chemicals
  - dyes (contact) L25.2
    - allergic L23.4
  - fish (ingested) L27.2
  - flour (ingested) L27.2

ALPHABETIC INDEX

Dermatitis, *continued*

- food (ingested) L27.2
  - in contact with skin L25.4
- fruit (ingested) L27.2
- furs (allergic) (contact) L23.81
- hair (cat) (dog) L23.81
- infrared rays
- ingestion, ingested substance L27.9
  - chemical NEC L27.8
  - drugs and medicaments—*see* Dermatitis, due to, drugs and medicaments
  - food L27.2
  - specified NEC L27.8
- insecticide in contact with skin L24.5
- internal agent L27.9
  - drugs and medicaments (generalized)—*see* Dermatitis, due to, drugs and medicaments
  - food L27.2
- irradiation—*see* Dermatitis, due to, radiation
- lacquer tree (allergic) (contact) L23.7
- light (sun) NEC
  - acute L56.8
- Lyponyssoides sanguineus B88.0
- milk (ingested) L27.2
- petroleum products (contact) (irritant) (substances in T52.0) L24.2
- plants NEC (contact) L25.5
  - allergic L23.7
- plasters (adhesive) (any) (allergic) (contact) L23.1
- primrose (allergic) (contact) L23.7
- primula (allergic) (contact) L23.7
- radiation
  - nonionizing (chronic exposure)
  - sun NEC
    - acute L56.8
- ragweed (allergic) (contact) L23.7
- Rhus (allergic) (contact) (diversiloba) (radicans) (toxicodendron) (venenata) (verniciflua) L23.7
- Senecio jacobaea (allergic) (contact) L23.7
- solvents (contact) (irritant) (substances in categories T52) L24.2
- specified agent NEC (contact) L25.8
  - allergic L23.89
- sunshine NEC
  - acute L56.8
- ultraviolet rays (sun NEC) (chronic exposure)
  - acute L56.8
- vaccine or vaccination L27.0
  - specified substance—*see* Table of Drugs and Chemicals
- dyshydrotic L30.1
- dysmenorrheica N94.6
- exfoliative, exfoliativa (generalized) L26
  - neonatorum L00
- eyelid H01.9
  - allergic H01.11-
    - left H01.116
      - lower H01.115
      - upper H01.114
    - right H01.113
      - lower H01.112
      - upper H01.111
  - due to
    - Demodex species B88.0
- facta, factitia, factitial L98.1
  - psychogenic F54
- flexural NEC L20.82
- friction L30.4
- gangrenosa, gangrenous infantum L08.0
- harvest mite B88.0
- infectious eczematoid L30.3
- infective L30.3
- irritant—*see* Dermatitis, contact
- Jacquet's (diaper dermatitis) L22
- Leptus B88.0
- mite B88.0
- napkin L22
- purulent L08.0
- pyococcal L08.0
- pyogenica L08.0
- Ritter's (exfoliativa) L00
- schistosome B65.3

Dermatitis, *continued*

- seborrheic L21.9
  - infantile L21.1
  - specified NEC L21.8
- sensitization NOS L23.9
- septic L08.0
- suppurative L08.0
- traumatic NEC L30.4
- ultraviolet (sun) (chronic exposure)
  - acute L56.8

Dermatographia L50.3

Dermatolysis (exfoliativa) (congenital) Q82.8

Dermatomegaly NEC Q82.8

Dermatomycosis B36.9

- furfuracea B36.0
- specified type NEC B36.8

Dermatomyositis (acute) (chronic)—*see also*

Dermatopolymyositis

- in (due to) neoplastic disease (*see also* Table of Neoplasms in the complete *ICD-10-CM* manual) D49.9 [M36.0]
- juvenile M33.00
  - with
    - myopathy M33.02
    - respiratory involvement M33.01
    - specified organ involvement NEC M33.09
  - without myopathy M33.03
- specified NEC M33.10
  - with
    - myopathy M33.12
    - respiratory involvement M33.11
    - specified organ involvement NEC M33.19
  - without myopathy M33.13

Dermatoneuritis of children *see* Poisoning

Dermatophytosis (epidermophyton) (infection) (Microsporum) (tinea) (Trichophyton) B35.9

- beard B35.0
- body B35.4
- capitis B35.0
- corporis B35.4
- deep-seated B35.8
- disseminated B35.8
- foot B35.3
- granulomatous B35.8
- groin B35.6
- hand B35.2
- nail B35.1
- perianal (area) B35.6
- scalp B35.0
- specified NEC B35.8

Dermatophytosis M33.90

- with
  - myopathy M33.92
  - respiratory involvement M33.91
  - specified organ involvement NEC M33.99
- juvenile M33.00
  - with
    - myopathy M33.02
    - respiratory involvement M33.01
    - specified organ involvement NEC M33.09
  - without myopathy M33.93

Dermatopolyneuritis—*see* Poisoning

Dermatorrhexis (Ehlers-Danos) Q79.60

Dermatosis L98.9

- eyelid (noninfectious) H01.9
  - factitial L98.1
  - menstrual NEC L98.8

Dermophytosis—*see* Dermatophytosis

Despondency F32.A

Destruction, destructive—*see also* Damage

- joint—*see also* Derangement, joint, specified type NEC
  - sacroiliac M53.3
- rectal sphincter K62.89
- septum (nasal) J34.89

Detergent asthma J69.8

Deterioration

- general physical R53.81

Development

- abnormal, bone Q79.9
- arrested R62.50
  - bone—*see* Arrest, development or growth, bone
  - child R62.50
    - due to malnutrition E45
- defective, congenital—*see also* Anomaly, by site
  - left ventricle Q24.8
    - in hypoplastic left heart syndrome Q23.4
- delayed (*see also* Delay, development) R62.50
  - arithmetical skills F81.2
  - language (skills) (expressive) F80.1
  - learning skill F81.9
  - mixed skills F88
  - motor coordination F82
  - reading F81.0
  - specified learning skill NEC F81.89
  - speech F80.9
  - spelling F81.81
  - written expression F81.81
- imperfect, congenital—*see also* Anomaly, by site
  - heart Q24.9
  - lungs Q33.6
- incomplete
  - bronchial tree Q32.4
  - organ or site not listed—*see* Hypoplasia, by site
  - respiratory system Q34.9
- sexual, precocious NEC E30.1
- tardy, mental (*see also* Disability, intellectual) F79

Developmental—*see* Disease, diseased

- testing, infant or child—*see* Examination, child

Deviation (in)

- midline (jaw) (teeth) (dental arch) M26.29
  - specified site NEC—*see* Malposition
- nasal septum J34.2
  - congenital Q67.4
- septum (nasal) (acquired) J34.2
  - congenital Q67.4
- sexual transvestism F64.1
- teeth, midline M26.29

Device

- cerebral ventricle (communicating) in situ Z98.2
- drainage, cerebrospinal fluid, in situ Z98.2

Devil's

- pinches (purpura simplex) D69.2

Dextaposition, aorta Q20.3

- in tetralogy of Fallot Q21.3

Dextrocardia (true) Q24.0

- with
  - complete transposition of viscera Q89.3
  - situs inversus Q89.3

Dextrotransposition, aorta Q20.3

Dhobi itch B35.6

Di George's syndrome D82.1

Diabetes, diabetic (mellitus) (sugar) E11.9

- with
  - coma due to
    - hyperosmolarity E11.01
    - hypoglycemia E11.641
    - ketoacidosis E11.11
  - bronzed E83.110
  - dietary counseling and surveillance Z71.3
  - due to drug or chemical E09.9
    - with
      - amyotrophy E09.44
      - arthropathy NEC E09.618
      - autonomic (poly)neuropathy E09.43
      - cataract E09.36
      - Charcot's joints E09.610
      - chronic kidney disease E09.22
      - circulatory complication NEC E09.59
      - complication E09.8
        - specified NEC E09.69
      - dermatitis E09.620
      - foot ulcer E09.621
      - gangrene E09.52
      - gastroparesis E09.43
      - glomerulonephrosis, intracapillary E09.21
      - glomerulosclerosis, intercapillary E09.21
      - hyperglycemia E09.65

ALPHABETIC INDEX

Diabetes, diabetic (mellitus) (sugar), *continued*

- ■ hyperosmolarity E09.00
  - ~ with coma E09.01
- ■ hypoglycemia E09.649
  - ~ with coma E09.641
- ■ ketoacidosis E09.10
  - ~ with coma E09.11
- ■ kidney complications NEC E09.29
- ■ Kimmelsteil-Wilson disease E09.21
- ■ mononeuropathy E09.41
- ■ myasthenia E09.44
- ■ necrobiosis lipoidica E09.620
- ■ nephropathy E09.21
- ■ neuralgia E09.42
- ■ neurologic complication NEC E09.49
- ■ neuropathic arthropathy E09.610
- ■ neuropathy E09.40
- ■ ophthalmic complication NEC E09.39
- ■ oral complication NEC E09.638
- ■ periodontal disease E09.630
- ■ peripheral angiopathy E09.51
  - ~ with gangrene E09.52
- ■ polyneuropathy E09.42
- ■ renal complication NEC E09.29
- ■ renal tubular degeneration E09.29
- ■ retinopathy E09.319
  - ~ with macular edema E09.311
  - ~ nonproliferative E09.329
    - ◊ with macular edema E09.321
    - ◊ mild E09.329
      - » with macular edema E09.321
    - ◊ moderate E09.339
      - » with macular edema E09.331
    - ◊ severe E09.349
      - » with macular edema E09.341
  - ~ proliferative E09.359
    - ◊ with macular edema E09.351
- ■ skin complication NEC E09.628
- ■ skin ulcer NEC E09.622
- due to underlying condition E08.9
  - ~ with
    - ■ amyotrophy E08.44
    - ■ arthropathy NEC E08.618
    - ■ autonomic (poly)neuropathy E08.43
    - ■ cataract E08.36
    - ■ Charcot's joints E08.610
    - ■ chronic kidney disease E08.22
    - ■ circulatory complication NEC E08.59
    - ■ complication E08.8
      - ~ specified NEC E08.69
    - ■ dermatitis E08.620
    - ■ foot ulcer E08.621
    - ■ gangrene E08.52
    - ■ gastroparesis E08.43
    - ■ glomerulonephrosis, intracapillary E08.21
    - ■ glomerulosclerosis, intercapillary E08.21
    - ■ hyperglycemia E08.65
    - ■ hyperosmolarity E08.00
      - ~ with coma E08.01
    - ■ hypoglycemia E08.649
      - ~ with coma E08.641
    - ■ ketoacidosis E08.10
      - ~ with coma E08.11
    - ■ kidney complications NEC E08.29
    - ■ Kimmelsteil-Wilson disease E08.21
    - ■ mononeuropathy E08.41
    - ■ myasthenia E08.44
    - ■ necrobiosis lipoidica E08.620
    - ■ nephropathy E08.21
    - ■ neuralgia E08.42
    - ■ neurologic complication NEC E08.49
    - ■ neuropathic arthropathy E08.610
    - ■ neuropathy E08.40
    - ■ ophthalmic complication NEC E08.39
    - ■ oral complication NEC E08.638
    - ■ periodontal disease E08.630
    - ■ peripheral angiopathy E08.51
      - ~ with gangrene E08.52
    - ■ polyneuropathy E08.42
    - ■ renal complication NEC E08.29
    - ■ renal tubular degeneration E08.29

Diabetes, diabetic (mellitus) (sugar), *continued*

- ■ retinopathy E08.319
  - ~ with macular edema E08.311
  - ~ nonproliferative E08.329
    - ◊ with macular edema E08.321
    - ◊ mild E08.329
      - » with macular edema E08.321
    - ◊ moderate E08.339
      - » with macular edema E08.331
    - ◊ severe E08.349
      - » with macular edema E08.341
  - ~ proliferative E08.359
    - ◊ with macular edema E08.351
- ■ skin complication NEC E08.628
- ■ skin ulcer NEC E08.622
- gestational (in pregnancy)
  - ~ affecting newborn P70.0
  - ~ diet controlled O24.410
  - ~ insulin (and diet) controlled O24.414
  - ~ oral hypoglycemic drug controlled O24.415
- inadequately controlled—*code to* Diabetes, by type, with hyperglycemia
- insipidus E23.2
  - ~ nephrogenic N25.1
  - ~ pituitary E23.2
- insulin dependent—*code to* type of diabetes
- juvenile-onset—*see* Diabetes, type 1
- ketosis-prone—*see* Diabetes, type 1
- latent R73.09
- neonatal (transient) P70.2
- non-insulin dependent—*code to* type of diabetes
- out of control—*code to* Diabetes, by type, with hyperglycemia
- poorly controlled—*code to* Diabetes, by type, with hyperglycemia
- postpancreatectomy—*see* Diabetes
- postprocedural—*see* Diabetes
- prediabetes R73.03
- secondary diabetes mellitus NEC—*see* Diabetes
- steroid-induced—*see* Diabetes, due to drug or chemical
- type 1 E10.9
  - ~ early-stage E10.A-
  - ~ presymptomatic E10.A0
    - ■ Stage 1 E10.A1
    - ■ Stage 2 E10.A2
  - ~ with
    - ■ amyotrophy E10.44
    - ■ arthropathy NEC E10.618
    - ■ autonomic (poly)neuropathy E10.43
    - ■ cataract E10.36
    - ■ Charcot's joints E10.610
    - ■ chronic kidney disease E10.22
    - ■ circulatory complication NEC E10.59
    - ■ complication E10.8
      - ~ specified NEC E10.69
    - ■ dermatitis E10.620
    - ■ foot ulcer E10.621
    - ■ gangrene E10.52
    - ■ gastroparesis E10.43
    - ■ glomerulonephrosis, intracapillary E10.21
    - ■ glomerulosclerosis, intercapillary E10.21
    - ■ hyperglycemia E10.65
    - ■ hypoglycemia E10.649
      - ~ with coma E10.641
    - ■ ketoacidosis E10.10
      - ~ with coma E10.11
    - ■ kidney complications NEC E10.29
    - ■ Kimmelsteil-Wilson disease E10.21
    - ■ mononeuropathy E10.41
    - ■ myasthenia E10.44
    - ■ necrobiosis lipoidica E10.620
    - ■ nephropathy E10.21
    - ■ neuralgia E10.42
    - ■ neurologic complication NEC E10.49
    - ■ neuropathic arthropathy E10.610
    - ■ neuropathy E10.40
    - ■ ophthalmic complication NEC E10.39
    - ■ oral complication NEC E10.638
    - ■ periodontal disease E10.630
    - ■ peripheral angiopathy E10.51
      - ~ with gangrene E10.52
    - ■ polyneuropathy E10.42
    - ■ renal complication NEC E10.29

Diabetes, diabetic (mellitus) (sugar), *continued*

- ■ renal tubular degeneration E10.29
- ■ retinopathy E10.319
  - ~ with macular edema E10.311
  - ~ nonproliferative E10.329
    - ◊ with macular edema E10.321
    - ◊ mild E10.329
      - » with macular edema E10.321
    - ◊ moderate E10.339
      - » with macular edema E10.331
    - ◊ severe E10.349
      - » with macular edema E10.341
  - ~ proliferative E10.359
    - ◊ with macular edema E10.351
- ■ skin complication NEC E10.628
- ■ skin ulcer NEC E10.622
- type 2 E11.9
  - ~ with
    - ■ amyotrophy E11.44
    - ■ arthropathy E11.618
    - ■ autonomic (poly)neuropathy E11.43
    - ■ cataract E11.36
    - ■ Charcot's joints E11.610
    - ■ chronic kidney disease E11.22
    - ■ circulatory complication NEC E11.59
    - ■ complication E11.8
      - ~ specified NEC E11.69
    - ■ dermatitis E11.620
    - ■ foot ulcer E11.621
    - ■ gangrene E11.52
    - ■ gastroparesis E11.43
    - ■ glomerulonephrosis, intracapillary E11.21
    - ■ glomerulosclerosis, intercapillary E11.21
    - ■ hyperglycemia E11.65
    - ■ hyperosmolarity E11.00
      - ~ with coma E11.01
    - ■ hypoglycemia E11.649
      - ~ with coma E11.641
    - ■ ketoacidosis E11.10
      - ~ with coma E11.11
    - ■ kidney complications NEC E11.29
    - ■ Kimmelsteil-Wilson disease E11.21
    - ■ mononeuropathy E11.41
    - ■ myasthenia E11.44
    - ■ necrobiosis lipoidica E11.620
    - ■ nephropathy E11.21
    - ■ neuralgia E11.42
    - ■ neurologic complication NEC E11.49
    - ■ neuropathic arthropathy E11.610
    - ■ neuropathy E11.40
    - ■ ophthalmic complication NEC E11.39
    - ■ oral complication NEC E11.638
    - ■ periodontal disease E11.630
    - ■ peripheral angiopathy E11.51
      - ~ with gangrene E11.52
    - ■ polyneuropathy E11.42
    - ■ renal complication NEC E11.29
    - ■ renal tubular degeneration E11.29
    - ■ retinopathy E11.319
      - ~ with macular edema E11.311
      - ~ nonproliferative E11.329
        - ◊ with macular edema E11.321
        - ◊ mild E11.329
          - » with macular edema E11.321
        - ◊ moderate E11.339
          - » with macular edema E11.331
        - ◊ severe E11.349
          - » with macular edema E11.341
      - ~ proliferative E11.359
        - ◊ with macular edema E11.351
    - ■ skin complication NEC E11.628
    - ■ skin ulcer NEC E11.622

Diagnosis deferred R69

Dialysis (intermittent) (treatment)

- noncompliance (with) Z91.158
  - ~ due to financial hardship Z91.151
- renal (hemodialysis) (peritoneal), status Z99.2

Diamond-Blackfan anemia (congenital hypoplastic) D61.01

Diamond-Gardener syndrome (autoerythrocyte sensitization) D69.2

Diaper rash L22

Diaphoresis (excessive) R61

Diaphragmatitis, diaphragmitis J98.6

Diarrhea, diarrheal (disease) (infantile) (inflammatory) R19.7
- allergic K52.29
- amebic (*see also* Amebiasis) A06.0
  - acute A06.0
- cachectic NEC K52.89
- chronic (noninfectious) K52.9
- dietetic K52.29
- due to
  - Campylobacter A04.5
  - C. difficile A04.7-
  - Escherichia coli A04.4
    - enteroaggregative A04.4
    - enterohemorrhagic A04.3
    - enteropathogenic A04.0
    - enterotoxigenic A04.1
    - specified NEC A04.4
  - food hypersensitivity K52.29
  - specified organism NEC A08.8
    - bacterial A04.8
    - viral A08.39
- dysenteric A09
- endemic A09
- epidemic A09
- functional K59.1
  - following gastrointestinal surgery K91.89
  - psychogenic F45.8
- Giardia lamblia A07.1
- giardial A07.1
- infectious A09
- mite B88.0
- neonatal (noninfectious) P78.3
- nervous F45.8
- noninfectious K52.9
- psychogenic F45.8
- specified
  - bacterial A04.8
  - virus NEC A08.39

Diastasis
- cranial bones M84.88
  - congenital NEC Q75.8
- joint (traumatic)—*see* Dislocation

Diathesis
- hemorrhagic (familial) D69.9
  - newborn NEC P53

Didymytis N45.1
- with orchitis N45.3

Dietary
- surveillance and counseling Z71.3

Dietl's crisis N13.8

Difficult, difficulty (in)
- acculturation Z60.3
- feeding R63.30
  - newborn P92.9
    - breast P92.5
    - specified NEC P92.8
  - nonorganic (infant or child) F98.29
- reading (developmental) F81.0
  - secondary to emotional disorders F93.9
- spelling (specific) F81.81
  - with reading disorder F81.89
  - due to inadequate teaching Z55.8
- swallowing—*see* Dysphagia
- walking R26.2

DiGeorge's syndrome (thymic hypoplasia) D82.1

Dilatation
- aorta (congenital) Q25.44
- bladder (sphincter) N32.89
  - congenital Q64.79
- colon K59.39
  - congenital Q43.1
  - psychogenic F45.8
  - toxic K59.31
- common duct (acquired) K83.8
  - congenital Q44.5
- cystic duct (acquired) K82.8
  - congenital Q44.5

Dilatation, *continued*
- ileum K59.89
  - psychogenic F45.8
- jejunum K59.89
  - psychogenic F45.8
- Meckel's diverticulum (congenital) Q43.0
- rectum K59.39
- sphincter ani K62.89
- stomach K31.89
  - acute K31.0
  - psychogenic F45.8
- vesical orifice N32.89

Dilated, dilation—*see* Dilatation

Diminished, diminution
- hearing (acuity)—*see* Deafness
- sense or sensation (cold) (heat) (tactile) (vibratory) R20.8
- vision NEC H54.7

Dimitri-Sturge-Weber disease Q85.8

Dimple
- congenital, sacral Q82.6
  - parasacral Q82.6
  - parasacral, pilonidal or postanal—*see* Cyst, pilonidal

Diphallus Q55.69

Diphtheria, diphtheritic (gangrenous) (hemorrhagic) A36.9
- carrier Z22.2

Diplegia (upper limbs) G83.0
- lower limbs G82.20

Dipsomania F10.20
- with
  - remission F10.21

Dirt-eating child F98.3

Disability, disabilities
- intellectual F79
  - with
    - autistic features F84.9
    - pathogenic CHAMP1 (genetic) (variant) F78.A9
    - pathogenic HNRNPH2 (genetic) (variant) F78.A9
    - pathogenic SATB2 (genetic) (variant) F78.A9
    - pathogenic SETBP1 (genetic) (variant) F78.A9
    - pathogenic STXBP1 (genetic) (variant) F78.A9
    - pathogenic SYNGAP1 (genetic) (variant) F78.A1
    - autosomal dominant F78.A9
    - autosomal recessive F78.A9
    - genetic related F78.A9
  - with
    - pathogenic CHAMP1 (variant) F78.A9
    - pathogenic HNRNPH2 (variant) F78.A9
    - pathogenic SATB2 (variant) F78.A9
    - pathogenic SETBP1 (variant) F78.A9
    - pathogenic STXBP1 (variant) F78.A9
    - pathogenic SYNGAP1 (variant) F78.A1
    - specified NEC F78.A9
  - SYNGAP1-related F78.A1
    - in
      - ◊ autosomal dominant mental retardation F78.A9
      - ◊ autosomal recessive mental retardation F78.A9
      - ◊ SATB2-associated syndrome F78.A9
      - ◊ SETBP1 disorder F78.A9
      - ◊ STXBP1 encephalopathy with epilepsy (*see also* Encephalopathy; and *see also* Epilepsy) F78.A9
      - ◊ X-linked mental retardation (syndromic) (Bain type) F78.A9
    - mild (I.Q.50 – 69) F70
    - moderate (I.Q.35 – 49) F71
    - profound (I.Q. under 20) F73
    - severe (I.Q.20 – 34) F72
    - specified level NEC F78
- knowledge acquisition F81.9
- learning F81.9
- limiting activities Z73.6
- spelling, specific F81.81

Disappearance of family member Z63.4

Discharge (from)
- abnormal finding in—*see* Abnormal, specimen
- breast (female) (male) N64.52
- diencephalic autonomic idiopathic—*see* Epilepsy, specified NEC

Discharge, *continued*
- ear—*see also* Otorrhea
- excessive urine R35.89
- nipple N64.52
- penile R36.9
- postnasal R09.82
- urethral R36.9
  - without blood R36.0
- vaginal N89.8

Discoloration
- nails L60.8

Discord (with)
- family Z63.8

Discordant connection
- ventriculoarterial Q20.3

Discrepancy
- leg length (acquired)—*see* Deformity, limb, unequal length
  - congenital—*see* Defect, reduction, limb, lower

Disease, diseased—*see also* Syndrome
- acid-peptic K30
- Adams-Stokes (-Morgagni) (syncope with heart block) I45.9
- adenoids (and tonsils) J35.9
- airway
  - reactive—*see* Asthma
- Alexander G31.86
- alligator-skin Q80.9
- angiospastic I73.9
  - cerebral G45.9
- Antopol E74.05
- anus K62.9
  - specified NEC K62.89
- aortic (heart) (valve) I35.9
  - rheumatic I06.9
- autoimmune (systemic) NOS M35.9
  - hemolytic D59.1
    - cold type (primary) (secondary) (symptomatic) D59.12
    - drug-induced D59.0
    - mixed type (primary) (secondary) (symptomatic) D59.13
    - warm type (primary) (secondary) (symptomatic) D59.11
  - thyroid E06.3
- autoinflammatory M04.9
  - NOD2-associated M04.8
- Ayerza's (pulmonary artery sclerosis with pulmonary hypertension) I27.0
- Babington's (familial hemorrhagic telangiectasia) I78.0
- Baelz's (cheilitis glandularis apostematosa) K13.0
- Bannister's T78.3
- basal ganglia G25.9
  - specified NEC G25.89
- Bateman's B08.1
- Becker
  - myotonia congenita G71.12
- bladder N32.9
  - specified NEC N32.89
- bleeder's D66
- blood D75.9
  - vessel I99.9
- Blount M92.51-
- Bouillaud's (rheumatic heart disease) I01.9
- Bourneville (-Brissaud) (tuberous sclerosis) Q85.1
- bowel K63.9
  - functional K59.9
    - psychogenic F45.8
- brain G93.9
  - parasitic NEC B71.9 [G94]
  - specified NEC G93.89
- broad
  - beta E78.2
- bronze Addison's E27.1
- Canavan E75.28
  - carcinoid E34.00
    - heart E34.01
    - specified NEC E34.09
- cardiopulmonary, chronic I27.9
- cardiovascular (atherosclerotic) I25.10
- celiac (adult) (infantile) K90.0

ALPHABETIC INDEX

Disease, diseased, *continued*

- cerebrovascular I67.9
  - acute I67.89
  - hereditary NEC I67.858
  - specified NEC I67.89
- chigo, chigoe B88.1
- childhood granulomatous D71
- chlamydial A74.9
  - specified NEC A74.89
- cold
  - agglutinin or hemoglobinuria D59.12
  - hemagglutinin (chronic) D59.12
- collagen NOS (nonvascular) (vascular) M35.9
  - specified NEC M35.8
- colon K63.9
  - functional K59.9
    - congenital Q43.2
- Concato's (pericardial polyserositis) A19.9
  - nontubercular I31.1
  - pleural—*see* Pleurisy, with, effusion
- congenital Q07.9
  - nonautoimmune hemolytic D59.4
- conjunctiva H11.9
  - chlamydial A74.0
  - viral B30.9
- connective tissue, systemic (diffuse) M35.9
  - in (due to)
    - hypogammaglobulinemia D80.1 [M36.8]
  - specified NEC M35.8
  - COVID-19 U07.1
- Crocq's (acrocyanosis) I73.89
- cystic
  - kidney, congenital Q61.9
- cytomegalic inclusion (generalized) B25.9
  - congenital P35.1
- cytomegaloviral B25.9
- Danon E74.05
- Dèbove's (splenomegaly) R16.1
- demyelinating, demyelinizating (nervous system) G37.9
  - multiple sclerosis G35
  - specified NEC G37.89
- de Quervain's (tendon sheath) M65.4
  - thyroid (subacute granulomatous thyroiditis) E06.1
- diaphorase deficiency D74.0
- diaphragm J98.6
- diarrheal, infectious NEC A09
- disruptive F91.9
  - mood dysregulation F34.81
  - specified NEC F91.8
- disruptive behavior F91.9
- Duchenne-Griesinger G71.01
- Duchenne's
  - muscular dystrophy G71.01
  - pseudohypertrophy, muscles G71.01
- Dupré's (meningism) R29.1
- dysmorphic body F45.22
- Eddowes' (brittle bones and blue sclera) Q78.0
- Edsall's T67.2
- Eichstedt's (pityriasis versicolor) B36.0
- Eisenmenger's (irreversible) I27.83
- Ellis-van Creveld (chondroectodermal dysplasia) Q77.6
- end stage renal (ESRD) N18.6
- English (rickets) E55.0
- Erb (-Landouzy) G71.02
- esophagus K22.9
  - functional K22.4
  - psychogenic F45.8
- eustachian tube—*see* Disorder, eustachian tube
- facial nerve (seventh) G51.9
  - newborn (birth injury) P11.3
- Fanconi('s) D61.03
- fascia NEC—*see also* Disorder, muscle
  - inflammatory—*see* Myositis
  - specified NEC M62.89
- Fede's K14.0
- female pelvic inflammatory (*see also* Disease, pelvis, inflammatory) N73.9
- fifth B08.3
- Fothergill's
  - scarlatina anginosa A38.9
- Friedreich's
  - combined systemic or ataxia G11.11
  - myoclonia G25.3

Disease, diseased, *continued*

- frontal sinus—*see* Sinusitis, frontal
- fungus NEC B49
- Gaisböck's (polycythemia hypertonica) D75.1
- gastroesophageal reflux (GERD) K21.9
  - with esophagitis K21.0-
- gastrointestinal (tract) K92.9
  - functional K59.9
    - psychogenic F45.8
  - specified NEC K92.89
- Gee (-Herter) (-Heubner) (-Thaysen) (nontropical sprue) K90.0
- genital organs
  - female N94.9
  - male N50.9
- Gibert's (pityriasis rosea) L42
- Gilles de la Tourette's (motor-verbal tic) F95.2
- glycogen storage
  - lysosomal E74.02
    - with acid maltase deficiency E74.02
    - without acid maltase deficiency E74.05
  - type IIB E74.05
- Goldstein's (familial hemorrhagic telangiectasia) I78.0
- graft-versus-host (GVH) D89.813
  - acute D89.810
  - acute on chronic D89.812
  - chronic D89.811
- granulomatous (childhood) (chronic) D71
- Grisel's M43.6
- Gruby's (tinea tonsurans) B35.0
- Guinon's (motor-verbal tic) F95.2
  - follicles L73.9
    - specified NEC L73.8
- Hamman's (spontaneous mediastinal emphysema) J98.2
- hand, foot, and mouth B08.4
- heart (organic) I51.9
  - with
    - pulmonary edema (acute) (*see also* Failure, ventricular, left) I50.1
    - rheumatic fever (conditions in I00)
      - active I01.9
        - ◊ with chorea I02.0
        - ◊ specified NEC I01.8
      - inactive or quiescent (with chorea) I09.9
        - ◊ specified NEC I09.89
  - aortic (valve) I35.9
  - black I27.0
  - congenital Q24.9
    - cyanotic Q24.9
    - specified NEC Q24.8
  - fibroid—*see* Myocarditis
  - functional I51.89
    - psychogenic F45.8
  - hyperthyroid (*see also* Hyperthyroidism) E05.90 [I43]
    - with thyroid storm E05.91 [I43]
  - kyphoscoliotic I27.1
  - mitral I05.9
    - specified NEC I0
  - psychogenic (functional) F45.8
  - pulmonary (chronic) I27.9
    - in schistosomiasis B65.9 [I52]
    - specified NEC I27.89
  - rheumatic (chronic) (inactive) (old) (quiescent) (with chorea) I09.9
    - active or acute I01.9
    - with chorea (acute) (rheumatic) (Sydenham's) I02.0
  - thyrotoxic (*see also* Thyrotoxicosis) E05.90 [I43]
    - with thyroid storm E05.91 [I43]
- heavy chain NEC C88.2-
  - alpha C88.3-
  - gamma C88.2-
  - mu C88.2-
- Hebra's
  - pityriasis
    - maculata et circinata L42
- hemoglobin or Hb
  - abnormal (mixed) NEC D58.2
    - with thalassemia D56.9
  - AS genotype D57.3
  - Bart's D56.0
  - C (Hb-C) D58.2
    - with other abnormal hemoglobin NEC D58.2

Disease, diseased, *continued*

- elliptocytosis D58.1
- Hb-S D57.2-
  - sickle-cell D57.2-
    - thalassemia D56.8
- Constant Spring D58.2
- D (Hb-D) D58.2
- E (Hb-E) D58.2
- E-beta thalassemia D56.5
- elliptocytosis D58.1
- H (Hb-H) (thalassemia) D56.0
  - with other abnormal hemoglobin NEC D56.9
  - Constant Spring D56.0
- I thalassemia D56.9
- M D74.0
- S or SS D57.1
  - with
    - acute chest syndrome D57.01
    - cerebral vascular involvement D57.03
    - crisis (painful) D57.00
      - ◊ with complication specified NEC D57.09
      - splenic sequestration D57.02
      - vasoocclusive pain D57.00
    - beta plus D57.44
      - with
        - ◊ acute chest syndrome D57.451
        - ◊ cerebral vascular involvement D57.453
        - ◊ crisis D57.459
          - » with specified complication NEC D57.458
          - ◊ splenic sequestration D57.452
          - » vasoocclusive pain D57.459
      - without crisis D57.44
    - beta zero D57.42
      - with
        - ◊ acute chest syndrome D57.431
          - » with dactylitis D57.434
        - ◊ cerebral vascular involvement D57.433
        - ◊ crisis D57.439
          - » with specified complication NEC D57.438
        - ◊ dactylitis D57.434
        - ◊ splenic sequestration D57.432
        - ◊ vasoocclusive pain D57.439
      - without crisis D57.42
  - SC D57.2-
  - SD D57.8-
  - SE D57.8-
  - spherocytosis D58.0
  - unstable, hemolytic D58.2
- hemolytic (newborn) P55.9
  - autoimmune D59.10
    - cold type (primary) (secondary) (symptomatic) D59.12
    - mixed type (primary) (secondary) (symptomatic) D59.13
    - warm type (primary) (secondary) (symptomatic) D59.11
  - drug-induced D59.0
  - due to or with
    - incompatibility
      - ABO (blood group) P55.1
      - blood (group) (Duffy) (K) (Kell) (Kidd) (Lewis) (M) (S) NEC P55.8
  - hemorrhagic D69.9
    - newborn P53
- Henoch (-Schönlein) (purpura nervosa) D69.0
- hepatic—*see* Disease, liver
- Herter (-Gee) (-Heubner) (nontropical sprue) K90.0
- Heubner-Herter (nontropical sprue) K90.0
- high fetal gene or hemoglobin thalassemia D56.9
- hip (joint) M25.9
  - congenital Q65.89
  - suppurative M00.9
- host-versus-graft D89.813
  - acute D89.810
  - acute on chronic D89.812
  - chronic D89.811
- human immunodeficiency virus (HIV) B20
- hyaline (diffuse) (generalized)
  - membrane (lung) (newborn) P22.0
- hypophysis E23.7
- I-cell E77.0
- IgG4-related D89.84

ALPHABETIC INDEX

Disease, diseased, *continued*

- immune D89.9
- immunoglobulin G4-related D89.84
- inclusion B25.9
  - salivary gland B25.9
- infectious, infective B99.9
  - congenital P37.9
    - specified NEC P37.8
  - viral P35.9
    - specified type NEC P35.8
  - specified NEC B99.8
- inflammatory
  - prepuce
    - balanoposthitis N47.6
  - intestine K63.9
    - functional K59.9
    - psychogenic F45.8
    - specified NEC K59.89
  - jigger B88.1
  - joint—*see also* Disorder, joint
    - sacroiliac M53.3
  - Jourdain's (acute gingivitis) K05.00
    - plaque induced K05.00
  - kidney (functional) (pelvis) N28.9
    - chronic N18.9
      - hypertensive—*see* Hypertension, kidney
      - stage 1 N18.1
      - stage 2 (mild) N18.2
      - stage 3 (moderate) N18.30
      - stage 3a N18.31
      - stage 3b N18.32
      - stage 4 (severe) N18.4
      - stage 5 N18.5
    - cystic (congenital) Q61.9
    - in (due to)
    - multicystic Q61.4
    - polycystic Q61.3
      - childhood type NEC Q61.19
        - collecting duct dilatation Q61.11
- Kimmelstiel (-Wilson) (intercapillary polycystic (congenital) glomerulosclerosis)—*see* E08-E13 with .21
- kissing—*see* Mononucleosis, infectious
- Kok Q89.8
- Kostmann's (infantile genetic agranulocytosis) D70.0
- Lafora body—*see also* Epilepsy, progressive, Lafora G40.C09
- Lenegre's I44.2
- Lev's (acquired complete heart block) I44.2
- lip K13.0
- liver (chronic) (organic) K76.9
  - fatty, nonalcoholic (NAFLD) K76.0
    - gestational alloimmune (GALD) P78.84
- Lobstein's (brittle bones and blue sclera) Q78.0
- Ludwig's (submaxillary cellulitis) K12.2
- lung J98.4
  - dabbing (related) U07.0
  - electronic cigarette (related) U07.0
  - in
  - obstructive (chronic) J44.9
    - with
      - asthma J44.89
      - bronchitis J44.89
    - sarcoidosis D86.0
    - systemic
      - lupus erythematosus M32.13
  - interstitial J84.9
    - of childhood, specified NEC J84.848
    - specified NEC J84.89
  - vaping (device) (product) (use) (associated) U07.0
- Lutembacher's (atrial septal defect with mitral stenosis) Q21.1
- Lyme A69.20
- lymphoproliferative D47.9
  - specified NEC D47.29
  - T-gamma D47.29
  - X-linked D82.3
- maple-syrup-urine E71.0
- Marion's (bladder neck obstruction) N32.0
- medullary center (idiopathic) (respiratory) G93.89
- metabolic, metabolism E88.9
  - bilirubin E80.7
  - glycoprotein E77.9

Disease, diseased, *continued*

- specified NEC E77.8
- minicore G71.29
- Minot's (hemorrhagic disease, newborn) P53
- Minot-von Willebrand-Jürgens (angiohemophilia) D68.0
- mitral (valve) I05.9
- MOG antibody G37.81
- Morgagni-Adams-Stokes (syncope with heart block) I45.9
- Morvan's G60.8
- multicore G71.29
- muscle M62.9
  - specified type NEC M62.89
  - tone, newborn P94.9
    - specified NEC P94.8
- myelin oligodendrocyte glycoprotein antibody G37.81
- myocardium, myocardial (*see also* Degeneration, myocardial) I51.5
  - primary (idiopathic) I42.9
- myoneural G70.9
- nails L60.9
  - specified NEC L60.8
- nasal J34.9
- nemaline body G71.21
- neuromuscular system G70.9
- neutropenic D70.9
- nerve—*see* Disorder, nerve
  - nervous system G98.8 central G96.9
    - specified NEC G96.89
- nose J34.9
- organ
  - dabbing (related) U07.0
  - electronic cigarette (related) U07.0
  - vaping (device) (product) (use) (associated) U07.0
- Osler-Rendu (familial hemorrhagic telangiectasia) I78.0
- ovary (noninflammatory) N83.9
  - cystic N83.20-
  - inflammatory—*see* Salpingo-oophoritis
    - polycystic E28.2
  - specified NEC N83.8
- pancreas K86.9
  - cystic K86.2
  - fibrocystic E84.9
  - specified NEC K86.89
- parasitic B89
  - cerebral NEC B71.9 /G94/
  - intestinal NOS B82.9
  - mouth B37.0
  - skin NOS B88.9
  - *specified type—see* Infestation
  - tongue B37.0
- pelvis, pelvic
  - gonococcal (acute) (chronic) A54.24
  - inflammatory (female) N73.9
    - acute N73.0
    - chronic N73.1
    - specified NEC N73.8
- Pick's I31.1
- pinworm B80
- pituitary (gland) E23.7
- Pollitzer's (hidradenitis suppurativa) L73.2
- polycystic
  - kidney or renal Q61.3
    - childhood type NEC Q61.19
      - collecting duct dilatation Q61.11
  - ovary, ovaries E28.2
- prepuce N47.8
  - inflammatory N47.7
    - balanoposthitis N47.6
- Pringle's (tuberous sclerosis) Q85.1
- Puente's (simple glandular cheilitis) K13.0
- pulmonary—*see also* Disease, lung
  - heart I27.9
    - specified NEC I27.89
  - hypertensive (vascular) I27.20
    - primary (idiopathic) I27.0
  - valve I37.9
    - rheumatic I09.89
- rag picker's or rag sorter's A22.1
- rectum K62.9
  - specified NEC K62.89
- renal (functional) (pelvis) (*see also* Disease, kidney)

Disease, diseased, *continued*

N28.9

- with
  - edema—*see* Nephrosis
  - glomerular lesion—*see* Glomerulonephritis
    - with edema—*see* Nephrosis
  - interstitial nephritis N12
- acute N28.9
- chronic (*see also* Disease, kidney, chronic) N18.9
- cystic, congenital Q61.9
- diabetic—*see* E08-E13 with .22
- end-stage (failure) N18.6
- fibrocystic (congenital) Q61.8
- lupus M32.14
- polycystic (congenital) Q61.3
  - childhood type NEC Q61.19
    - collecting duct dilatation Q61.11
- Rendu-Osler-Weber (familial hemorrhagic telangiectasia) I78.0
- respiratory (tract) J98.9
  - acute or subacute NOS J06.9
    - due to
      - smoke inhalation J70.5
  - newborn P28.9
    - specified type NEC P28.89
  - upper J39.9
    - acute or subacute J06.9
    - streptococcal J06.9
- rickettsial NOS A79.9
  - specified type NEC A79.89
- Riga (-Fede) (cachectic aphthae) K14.0
- Ritter's L00
- Roger's (congenital interventricular septal defect) Q21.0
- Rosenthal's (factor XI deficiency) D68.1
- Rossbach's (hyperchlorhydria) K30
- sacroiliac NEC M53.3
- salivary gland or duct K11.9
  - inclusion B25.9
  - *specified NEC K11.8*
  - virus B25.9
- Schönlein (-Henoch) (purpura rheumatica) D69.0
- scrofulous (tuberculous) A18.2
- scrotum N50.9
- serum NEC (*see also* Reaction, serum) T80.69
- sexually transmitted A64
  - anogenital
    - herpesviral infection—*see* Herpes, anogenital
    - warts A63.0
  - chlamydial infection—*see* Chlamydia
  - gonorrhea—*see* Gonorrhea
  - specified organism NEC A63.8
  - syphilis—*see* Syphilis
  - trichomoniasis—*see* Trichomoniasis
- sickle-cell D57.1
  - with crisis (painful) D57.00
  - with
    - acute chest syndrome D57.01
    - cerebral vascular involvement D57.03
    - crisis (painful) D57.00
      - with complication specified NEC D57.09
      - dactylitis D57.04
    - dactylitis D57.04
    - pain (vaso-occlusive) D57.00
    - splenic sequestration D57.02
  - Hb-C D57.20
    - with
      - acute chest syndrome D57.211
      - cerebral vascular involvement D57.213
      - crisis D57.219
        - ◊ with dactylitis D57.214
        - ◊ with specified complication NEC D57.218
      - dactylitis D57.214
      - pain (vaso-occlusive) D57.219
      - splenic sequestration D57.212
  - Hb-SD D57.80
    - with
      - acute chest syndrome D57.811
      - cerebral vascular involvement D57.813
      - crisis D57.819
        - ◊ with complication specified NEC D57.818
        - ◊ with dactylitis D57.814
      - ◊ dactylitis D57.814
      - pain (vaso-occlusive) D57.819

ALPHABETIC INDEX

Disease, diseased, *continued*

~ splenic sequestration D57.812
- ■ without crisis D57.80
- Hb-SE D57.80
- ■ with crisis D57.819
- ■ with
- ~ acute chest syndrome D57.811
- ~ cerebral vascular involvement D57.813
- ~ crisis D57.819
- ◊ with complication specified NEC D57.818
- ~ splenic sequestration D57.812
- ~ vasoocclusive pain D57.819
- ■ without crisis D57.80
- specified D57.80
- ■ with
- ~ acute chest syndrome D57.811
- ~ cerebral vascular involvement D57.813
- ~ crisis D57.819
- ◊ with complication specified NEC D57.818
- ~ splenic sequestration D57.812
- ~ vasoocclusive pain D57.819
- ■ without crisis D57.80
- spherocytosis D57.80
- ■ with
- ~ acute chest syndrome D57.811
- ~ cerebral vascular involvement D57.813
- ~ crisis D57.819
- ◊ with complication specified NEC D57.818
- ~ splenic sequestration D57.812
- ~ vasoocclusive pain D57.819
- ■ without crisis D57.80
- thalassemia D57.40
- ■ with
- ~ acute chest syndrome D57.411
- ~ with dactylitis D57.414
- ~ cerebral vascular involvement D57.413
- ~ crisis (painful) D57.419
- ◊ with specified complication NEC D57.418
- ~ splenic sequestration D57.412
- ~ vasoocclusive pain D57.419
- ■ beta plus D57.44
- ~ with
- ◊ acute chest syndrome D57.451
- » with dactylitis D57.454
- ◊ cerebral vascular involvement D57.453
- ◊ crisis D57.459
- » with specified complication NEC D57.458
- ◊ dactylitis D57.454
- ◊ pain (vaso-occlusive) D57.459
- ◊ splenic sequestration D57.452
- ~ without crisis D57.44
- ■ beta zero D57.42
- ~ with
- ◊ acute chest syndrome D57.431
- ◊ cerebral vascular involvement D57.433
- ◊ crisis D57.439
- » with specified complication NEC D57.438
- ◊ splenic sequestration D57.432
- ◊ vasoocclusive pain D57.439
- ~ without crisis D57.42
- elliptocytosis D57.8-
- sixth B08.20
- due to human herpesvirus 6 B08.21
- due to human herpesvirus 7 B08.22
- skin L98.9
- due to metabolic disorder NEC E88.9 [L99]
- specified NEC L98.8
- slim (HIV) B20
- South African creeping B88.0
- Startle Q89.8
- Sticker's (erythema infectiosum) B08.3
- Stokes-Adams (syncope with heart block) I45.9
- stomach K31.9
- functional, psychogenic F45.8
- specified NEC K31.89
- striatopallidal system NEC G25.89
- testes N50.9
- thalassemia Hb-S—*see* Disease, sickle-cell, thalassemia
- Thaysen-Gee (nontropical sprue) K90.0
- Thomsen G71.12
- throat J39.2

Disease, diseased, *continued*

- septic J02.0
- thyroid (gland) E07.9
- heart (*see also* Hyperthyroidism) E05.90 [I43]
- ■ with thyroid storm E05.91 [I43]
- specified NEC E07.89
- Tietze's M94.0
- tonsils, tonsillar (and adenoids) J35.9
- tooth, teeth K08.9
- hard tissues K03.9
- ■ specified NEC K03.89
- Tourette's F95.2
- tricuspid I07.9
- nonrheumatic I36.9
- Underwood's (sclerema neonatorum) P83.0
- urinary (tract) N39.9
- bladder N32.9
- ■ specified NEC N32.89
- specified NEC N39.8
- vagabond's B85.1
- vagina, vaginal (noninflammatory) N89.9
- inflammatory NEC N76.89
- specified NEC N89.8
- vascular I99.9
- venereal (*see also* Disease, sexually transmitted) A64
- chlamydial NEC A56.8
- ■ anus A56.3
- ■ genitourinary NOS A56.2
- ■ pharynx A56.4
- ■ rectum A56.3
- viral, virus (*see also* Disease, by type of virus) B34.9
- human immunodeficiency (HIV) B20
- Powassan A84.81
- von Willebrand (-Jürgens) (angiohemophilia) D68.0
- Vrolik's (osteogenesis imperfecta) Q78.0
- wasting NEC E88.A
- due to
- ■ underlying condition E88.A
- Werdnig-Hoffmann G12.0
- Werner-Schultz (neutropenic splenomegaly) D73.81
- white blood cells D72.9
- specified NEC D72.89
- wool sorter's A22.1

Disfigurement (due to scar) L90.5

Dislocation (articular)

- finger S63.2-
- index S63.2-
- interphalangeal S63.27-
- ■ distal S63.29-
- ~ index S63.29-
- ~ little S63.29-
- ~ middle S63.29-
- ~ ring S63.29-
- ■ index S63.2-
- ■ little S63.2-
- ■ middle S63.2-
- ■ proximal S63.28-
- ~ index S63.28-
- ~ little S63.28-
- ~ middle S63.28-
- ~ ring S63.28-
- ■ ring S63.2-
- little S63.2-
- metacarpophalangeal S63.26-
- ■ index S63.26-
- ■ little S63.26-
- ■ middle S63.26-
- ■ ring S63.26-
- middle S63.2-
- ring S63.2-
- thumb—*see* Dislocation
- hip S73.0-
- congenital (total) Q65.2
- ■ bilateral Q65.1
- ■ partial Q65.5
- ~ bilateral Q65.4
- ~ unilateral Q65.3-
- ■ unilateral Q65.0-
- interphalangeal (joint(s))
- finger S63.2-
- ■ distal S63.29-
- ~ index S63.29-

Dislocation, *continued*

- ~ little S63.29-
- ~ middle S63.29-
- ~ ring S63.29-
- ■ index S63.2-
- ■ little S63.2-
- ■ middle S63.2-
- ■ proximal S63.28-
- ~ index S63.28-
- ~ little S63.28-
- ~ middle S63.28-
- ~ ring S63.28-
- ■ ring S63.2-
- ~ thumb S63.12-
- jaw (cartilage) (meniscus) S03.0-
- knee S83.10-
- cap—*see* Dislocation, patella
- congenital Q68.2
- old M23.8X-
- patella—*see* Dislocation, patella
- proximal tibia
- ■ anteriorly S83.11-
- ■ laterally S83.14-
- ■ medially S83.13-
- ■ posteriorly S83.12-
- specified type NEC S83.19-
- lens (complete) H27.10
- anterior H27.12-
- congenital Q12.1
- partial H27.11-
- posterior H27.13-
- traumatic S05.8X-
- mandible S03.0-
- metacarpophalangeal (joint)
- finger S63.26-
- ■ index S63.26-
- ■ little S63.26-
- ■ middle S63.26-
- ■ ring S63.26-
- ■ thumb S63.11-
- partial—*see* Subluxation, by site
- patella S83.00-
- congenital Q74.1
- lateral S83.01-
- recurrent (nontraumatic) M22.0-
- ■ incomplete M22.1-
- specified type NEC S83.09-
- sacroiliac (joint) (ligament) S33.2
- congenital Q74.2
- septum (nasal) (old) J34.2
- temporomandibular S03.0-
- thumb S63.10-

Disorder (of)—*see also* Disease

- acute
- psychotic—*see* Psychosis, acute
- stress F43.0
- adjustment (grief) F43.20
- with
- ■ anxiety F43.22
- ~ with depressed mood F43.23
- ■ conduct disturbance F43.24
- ~ with emotional disturbance F43.25
- ■ depressed mood F43.21
- ~ with anxiety F43.23
- ■ other specified symptom F43.29
- prolonged grief F43.81
- adrenogenital E25.9
- aggressive, unsocialized F91.1
- alcohol-related
- with
- ■ intoxication F10.929
- ~ uncomplicated F10.920
- allergic—*see* Allergy
- alveolar NEC J84.09
- amino-acid
- metabolism—*see* Disturbance, metabolism, amino-acid
- ■ specified NEC E72.89
- neonatal, transitory P74.8
- anaerobic glycolysis with anemia D55.29
- anxiety F41.9
- illness F45.21
- mixed

ALPHABETIC INDEX

Disorder, *continued*

- ■ with depression (mild) F41.8
- – phobic F40.9
  - ■ of childhood F40.8
  - – social F40.1-
  - – specified NEC F41.8
- aromatic amino-acid metabolism E70.9
  - – specified NEC E70.89
- attention-deficit hyperactivity (adolescent) (adult) (child) F90.9
  - – combined type F90.2
  - – hyperactive type F90.1
  - – inattentive type F90.0
  - – specified type NEC F90.8
- attention-deficit without hyperactivity (adolescent) (adult) (child) F90.0
- auditory processing (central) H93.25
- autistic F84.0
- autoimmune D89.89
- autonomic nervous system G90.9
  - – specified NEC G90.89
- avoidant
  - – restrictive food intake F50.82
- balance
  - – acid-base E87.8
    - ■ mixed E87.4
  - – electrolyte E87.8
  - – fluid NEC E87.8
- beta-amino-acid metabolism E72.89
- bilirubin excretion E80.6
- binge-eating F50.81-
- bipolar (I) (type1) F31.9
  - – current (or most recent) episode
    - ■ depressed F31.9
      - – without psychotic features F31.30
        - ◊ mild F31.31
        - ◊ moderate F31.32
        - ◊ severe (without psychotic features) F31.4
    - ■ hypomanic F31.0
    - ■ manic F31.9
      - – without psychotic features F31.10
        - ◊ mild F31.11
        - ◊ moderate F31.12
        - ◊ severe (without psychotic features) F31.13
    - ■ mixed F31.60
      - – mild F31.61
      - – moderate F31.62
- bladder N32.9
  - – specified NEC N32.89
- bleeding D68.9
- body dysmorphic F45.22
- breast
  - – associated with
    - ■ cracked nipple 092.1-
    - ■ galactorrhea O92.6
    - ■ hypogalactia O92.4
    - ■ lactation O92.70
      - – specified NEC O92.79
    - ■ lactation disorder NEC O92.79
    - ■ pregnancy O92.20
      - – specified NEC O92.29
    - ■ puerperium O92.20
      - – specified NEC O92.29
- Briquet's F45.0
- cannabis use
  - – due to drug abuse—*see* Abuse, drug, cannabis
  - – due to drug dependence—*see* Dependence, drug, cannabis
- carbohydrate
  - – metabolism (congenital) E74.9
    - ■ specified NEC E74.89
- carnitine metabolism E71.40
- central auditory processing H93.25
- character NOS F60.9
- citrate metabolism NEC E74.829
- citrate transporter, SLC13A5 E74.820
- coagulation (factor) *(see also* Defect, coagulation) D68.9
  - – newborn, transient P61.6
- coccyx NEC M53.3
- conduct (childhood) F91.9
  - – adjustment reaction—*see* Disorder, adjustment
  - – adolescent onset type F91.2

Disorder, *continued*

- – childhood onset type F91.1
- – depressive F91.8
- – group type F91.2
- – hyperkinetic—*see* Disorder, attention-deficit hyperactivity
- – oppositional defiance F91.3
- – socialized F91.2
- – solitary aggressive type F91.1
- – specified NEC F91.8
- – unsocialized (aggressive) F91.1
- conduction, heart I45.9
- congenital glycosylation (CDG) E74.89
- cornea H18.9
  - – due to contact lens H18.82-
  - – Cyclin-Dependent Kinase-Like 5 Deficiency (CDKL5) G40.42
- cyclothymic F34.0
- defiant oppositional F91.3
- depressive F32.A
  - – major F32.9
    - ■ with psychotic symptoms F32.3
    - ■ in remission (full) F32.5
      - – partial F32.4
    - ■ recurrent F33.9
    - ■ single episode F32.9
      - – mild F32.0
      - – moderate F32.1
      - – severe (without psychotic symptoms) F32.2
        - ◊ with psychotic symptoms F32.3
- developmental F89
  - – arithmetical skills F81.2
  - – coordination (motor) F82
  - – expressive writing F81.81
  - – language F80.9
    - ■ expressive F80.1
    - ■ mixed receptive and expressive F80.2
    - ■ receptive type F80.2
    - ■ specified NEC F80.89
  - – learning F81.9
    - ■ arithmetical F81.2
    - ■ reading F81.0
  - – mixed F88
  - – motor coordination or function F82
  - – pervasive F84.9
    - ■ specified NEC F84.8
  - – phonological F80.0
  - – reading F81.0
  - – scholastic skills—*see also* Disorder, learning
    - ■ mixed F81.89
  - – specified NEC F88
  - – speech F80.9
    - ■ articulation F80.0
    - ■ specified NEC F80.89
  - – written expression F81.81
- diaphragm J98.6
- digestive (system) K92.9
  - – newborn P78.9
    - ■ specified NEC P78.89
  - – postprocedural—*see* Complication, gastrointestinal
  - – psychogenic F45.8
- disc (intervertebral)
  - – with
    - ■ myelopathy
      - – sacroiliac region M53.3
      - – sacrococcygeal region M53.3
  - – specified NEC
    - ■ sacrococcygeal region M53.3
- disruptive F91.9
  - – mood dysregulation F34.81
  - – specified NEC F91.8
- dissocial personality F60.2
- dissociative F44.9
  - – affecting
    - ■ motor function F44.4
      - – and sensation F44.7
    - ■ sensation F44.6
      - – and motor function F44.7
  - – brief reactive F43.0
  - – drug induced hemorrhagic D68.32
- drug related
  - – abuse—*see* Abuse, drug

Disorder, *continued*

- – dependence—*see* Dependence, drug
- dysthymic F34.1
- eating (adult) (psychogenic) F50.9
  - – anorexia—*see* Anorexia
  - – binge F50.81-
  - – bulimia F50.2-
  - – child F98.29
    - ■ pica (in remission) F98.3
    - ■ rumination disorder (in remission) F98.21
  - – other F50.89
  - – pica F50.89
    - ■ childhood (in remission) F98.3
  - – rumination (see also Rumination) R11.10
    - ■ infancy or childhood (in remission) F98.21
- electrolyte (balance) NEC E87.8
  - – acidosis (metabolic) (respiratory) E87.2
  - – alkalosis (metabolic) (respiratory) E87.3
  - – emotional (persistent) F34.9
  - – of childhood F93.9
    - ■ specified NEC F93.8
- esophagus K22.9
  - – functional K22.4
  - – psychogenic F45.8
- eustachian tube H69.9-
  - – specified NEC H69.8-
- factor, coagulation—*see* Defect, coagulation
- fatty acid
  - – metabolism E71.30
    - ■ specified NEC E71.39
  - – oxidation
    - ■ LCAD E71.310
    - ■ MCAD E71.311
    - ■ SCAD E71.312
    - ■ specified deficiency NEC E71.318
- feeding (infant or child) *(see also* Disorder, eating) R63.30
  - – or eating disorder F50.9
  - – pediatric
    - ■ acute R63.31
    - ■ chronic R63.32
  - – specified NEC F50.9
- feigned (with obvious motivation) Z76.5
- fibroblastic M72.9
- fluency
  - – childhood onset F80.81
  - – in conditions classified elsewhere R47.82
- fluid balance E87.8
- follicular (skin) L73.9
  - – specified NEC L73.8
- functional polymorphonuclear neutrophils D71
- gamma-glutamyl cycle E72.89
- gastric (functional) K31.9
  - – motility K30
  - – psychogenic F45.8
  - – secretion K30
- gastrointestinal (functional) NOS K92.9
  - – newborn P78.9
  - – psychogenic F45.8
- gender-identity or -role F64.9
  - – childhood F64.2
  - – effect on relationship F66
  - – of adolescence or adulthood (nontranssexual) F64.0
  - – specified NEC F64.8
  - – uncertainty F66
- genitourinary system
  - – female N94.9
  - – male N50.9
  - – psychogenic F45.8
- glomerular (in) N05.9
  - – disseminated intravascular coagulation D65 *[N08]*
  - – hemolytic-uremic syndrome D59.3
  - – Henoch (-Schönlein) purpura D69.0 *[N08]*
  - – sepsis NEC A41.- *[N08]*
  - – subacute bacterial endocarditis I33.0 *[N08]*
  - – systemic lupus erythematosus M32.14
  - – Waldenström macroglobulinemia C88.0- *[N08]*
- gluconeogenesis E74.4
- glucose transport E74.819
  - – specified NEC E74.818
- glycine metabolism E72.50
  - – hyperoxaluria R82.992

ALPHABETIC INDEX

Disorder, *continued*

- ■ primary E72.53
- glycoprotein E77.9
  - specified NEC E77.8
- habit (and impulse) F63.9
  - specified NEC F63.89
- heart action I49.9
- hemorrhagic NEC D69.9
  - drug-induced D68.32
  - due to
    - ■ extrinsic circulating anticoagulants D68.32
    - ■ increase in
      - anti-IIa D68.32
      - anti-Xa D68.32
- hoarding F42.3
- hypochondriacal F45.20
  - body dysmorphic F45.22
- identity
  - dissociative F44.81
  - of childhood F93.8
- immune mechanism (immunity) D89.9
  - specified type NEC D89.89
- integument, newborn P83.9
  - specified NEC P83.88
- intestine, intestinal
  - carbohydrate absorption NEC E74.39
    - ■ postoperative K91.2
  - functional NEC K59.9
  - psychogenic F45.8
- joint M25.9
  - psychogenic F45.8
- lacrimal system H04.9
- lactation NEC O92.79
- language (developmental) F80.9
  - expressive F80.1
  - mixed receptive and expressive F80.2
  - receptive F80.2
- learning (specific) F81.9
  - acalculia R48.8
  - alexia R48.0
  - mathematics F81.2
  - reading F81.0
  - specified NEC F81.89
    - ■ with impairment in
      - ~ mathematics F81.2
      - ~ reading F81.0
      - ~ written expression F81.81
  - spelling F81.81
  - written expression F81.81
- liver K76.9
  - malarial B54 [K77]
- lung, interstitial, drug-induced J70.4
  - dabbing (related) U07.0
  - e-cigarette (related) U07.0
  - electronic cigarette (related) U07.0
  - vaping (device) (product) (use) (associated) (related) U07.0
- lymphoproliferative, post-transplant (PTLD) D47.Z1
- meninges, specified type NEC G96.198
- menstrual N92.6
  - psychogenic F45.8
  - specified NEC N92.5
- mental (or behavioral) (nonpsychotic) F99
  - following organic brain damage F07.9
    - ■ postconcussional syndrome F07.81
    - ■ specified NEC F07.89
  - infancy, childhood or adolescence F98.9
  - neurotic—*see* Neurosis
- metabolic, amino acid, transitory, newborn P74.8
- metabolism NOS E88.9
  - amino-acid E72.9
    - ■ aromatic
      - ~ hyperphenylalaninemia E70.1
      - ◊ classical phenylketonuria E70.0
    - other specified E70.89
    - ■ branched chain E71.2
      - ~ maple syrup urine disease E71.0
      - ~ propionate NEC E71.128
      - ~ propionic acidemia E71.121
    - ■ glycine E72.50
      - ~ hyperoxaluria R82.992

Disorder, *continued*

- ◊ primary E72.53
- ■ other specified E72.8
  - beta-amino acid E72.8
  - gamma-glutamyl cycle E72.8
- ■ straight-chain E72.8
- bilirubin E80.7
  - ■ specified NEC E80.6
- calcium E83.50
  - ■ hypercalcemia E83.52
  - ■ hypocalcemia E83.51
  - ■ other specified E83.59
- carbohydrate E74.9
  - ■ specified NEC E74.89
- citrate NEC E74.829
- congenital E88.9
- glutamine E72.89
- glycoprotein E77.9
  - ■ specified NEC E77.8
- mitochondrial E88.40
  - ■ MELAS syndrome E88.41
  - ■ MERRF syndrome (myoclonic epilepsy associated with ragged-red fibers) E88.42
  - ■ other specified E88.49
    - ~ beta-amino acid E72.89
    - ~ gamma-glutamyl cycle E72.89
- plasma protein NEC E88.09
- purine E79.9
- pyrimidine E79.9
- pyruvate E74.4
- serine E72.8
- sodium E87.8
- straight chain E72.89
- threonine E72.89
- micturition NEC R39.198
  - feeling of incomplete emptying R39.14
  - hesitancy R39.11
  - need to immediately re-void R39.191
  - poor stream R39.12
  - position dependent R39.192
  - psychogenic F45.8
  - split stream R39.13
  - straining R39.16
  - urgency R39.15
- mitochondrial metabolism E88.40
- mixed
  - anxiety and depressive F41.8
  - of scholastic skills (developmental) F81.89
  - receptive expressive language F80.2
- mood (affective), unspecified F39
- movement G25.9
  - drug-induced G25.70
    - ■ akathisia G25.71
    - ■ specified NEC G25.79
  - treatment-induced G25.9
  - hysterical F44.4
  - stereotyped F98.4
- muscle M62.9
  - psychogenic F45.8
  - specified type NEC M62.89
  - tone, newborn P94.9
    - ■ specified NEC P94.8
- musculoskeletal system, soft tissue
  - psychogenic F45.8
- myoneural G70.9
  - due to lead G70.1
  - specified NEC G70.89
  - toxic G70.1
- nerve G58.9
  - cranial G52.9
    - ■ multiple G52.7
    - ■ seventh NEC G51.8
    - ■ sixth NEC—*see* Strabismus, paralytic, sixth nerve
  - facial G51.9
    - ■ specified NEC G51.8
- nervous system G98.8
  - autonomic (peripheral) G90.9
    - ■ specified NEC G90.89
- neurocognitive
  - mild disorder due to known physiological condition without behavioral disturbance F06.70
  - mild disorder due to known physiological condition

Disorder, *continued*

- with behavioral disturbance F06.71
- neurodevelopmental F89
  - specified NEC F88
- neurohypophysis NEC E23.3
- neuromuscular G70.9
  - hereditary NEC G71.9
  - specified NEC G70.89
  - toxic G70.1
- neurotic F48.9
  - specified NEC F48.8
- neutrophil, polymorphonuclear D71
- non-rapid eye movement sleep arousal
  - sleep terror type F51.4
  - sleepwalking type F51.3
- nose J34.9
  - specified NEC J34.89
- obsessive-compulsive F42.9
  - excoriation (skin picking) disorder F42.4
  - hoarding disorder F42.3
  - mixed obsessional thoughts and acts F42.2
  - other F42.8
- oppositional defiant F91.3
- overanxious F41.1
  - of childhood F93.8
- pain
  - with related psychological factors F45.42
  - exclusively related to psychological factors F45.41
- panic F41.0
- parietoalveolar NEC J84.09
- paroxysmal, mixed R56.9
- peroxisomal E71.50
  - biogenesis
    - ■ neonatal adrenoleukodystrophy E71.511
    - ■ specified disorder NEC E71.518
    - ■ Zellweger syndrome E71.510
  - rhizomelic chondrodysplasia punctata E71.540
  - specified form NEC E71.548
    - ■ group 1 E71.518
    - ■ group 2 E71.53
    - ■ group 3 E71.542
  - X-linked adrenoleukodystrophy E71.529
    - ■ adolescent E71.521
    - ■ adrenomyeloneuropathy E71.522
    - ■ childhood E71.520
    - ■ specified form NEC E71.528
  - Zellweger-like syndrome E71.54
- persistent
  - (somatoform) pain F45.41
  - affective (mood) F34.9
- personality *(see also* Personality) F60.9
  - affective F34.0
  - aggressive F60.3
  - amoral F60.2
  - anankastic F60.5
  - antisocial F60.2
  - anxious F60.6
  - asocial F60.2
  - avoidant F60.6
  - borderline F60.3
  - compulsive F60.5
  - cyclothymic F34.0
  - dissocial F60.2
  - emotional instability F60.3
  - expansive paranoid F60.0
  - explosive F60.3
  - histrionic F60.4
  - hysterical F60.4
  - labile F60.3
  - moral deficiency F60.2
  - obsessional F60.5
  - obsessive (-compulsive) F60.5
  - paranoid F60.0
  - pseudosocial F60.2
  - psychopathic F60.2
  - schizoid F60.1
  - type A F60.5
  - unstable (emotional) F60.3
- pervasive, developmental F84.9
- pigmentation L81.9
  - choroid, congenital Q14.3
  - diminished melanin formation L81.6
  - iron L81.8

Disorder, *continued*
- specified NEC L81.8
- pituitary gland E23.7
  - specified NEC E23.6
- polymorphonuclear neutrophils D71
- postconcussional F07.81
- postprocedural (postoperative)—*see* Complications, postprocedural
- post-traumatic stress (PTSD) F43.10
  - acute F43.11
  - chronic F43.12
- premenstrual dysphoric (PMDD) F32.81
- prepuce N47.8
- psychogenic NOS (*see also* Disease, diseased) F45.9
  - anxiety F41.8
  - appetite F50.9
  - asthenic F48.8
  - cardiovascular (system) F45.8
  - compulsive F42.8
  - cutaneous F54
  - depressive F32.9
  - digestive (system) F45.8
  - dysmenorrheic F45.8
  - dyspneic F45.8
  - endocrine (system) F54
  - eye NEC F45.8
  - feeding—*see* Disorder, eating
  - functional NEC F45.8
  - gastric F45.8
  - gastrointestinal (system) F45.8
  - genitourinary (system) F45.8
  - heart (function) (rhythm) F45.8
  - hyperventilatory F45.8
  - hypochondriacal—*see* Disorder, hypochondriacal
  - intestinal F45.8
  - joint F45.8
  - learning F81.9
  - limb F45.8
  - lymphatic (system) F45.8
  - menstrual F45.8
  - micturition F45.8
  - monoplegic NEC F44.4
  - motor F44.4
  - muscle F45.8
  - musculoskeletal F45.8
  - neurocirculatory F45.8
  - obsessive F42.8
  - organ or part of body NEC F45.8
  - paralytic NEC F44.4
  - phobic F40.9
  - physical NEC F45.8
  - rectal F45.8
  - respiratory (system) F45.8
  - rheumatic F45.8
  - specified part of body NEC F45.8
  - stomach F45.8
- psychomotor NEC F44.4
  - hysterical F44.4
- psychoneurotic—*see also* Neurosis
  - mixed NEC F48.8
- psychophysiologic—*see* Disorder, somatoform
- psychosexual development F66
  - identity of childhood F64.2
- psychosomatic NOS—*see* Disorder, somatoform
  - multiple F45.0
  - undifferentiated F45.1
- psychotic—*see* Psychosis
  - puberty E30.9
  - specified NEC E30.8
- pulmonary (valve)—*see* Endocarditis, pulmonary
- pyruvate metabolism E74.4
- reading R48.0
  - developmental (specific) F81.0
- REM sleep behavior G47.52
- receptive language F80.2
- refraction H52.7
- respiratory function, impaired—*see also* Failure, respiration
  - postprocedural—*see* Complication
  - psychogenic F45.8
- rumination (infant or child) (in remission) F98.21
- sacrum, sacrococcygeal NEC M53.3

Disorder, *continued*
- schizoid of childhood F84.5
- seizure (*see also* Epilepsy) G40.909
- semantic pragmatic F80.89
  - with autism F84.0
- sense of smell R43.1
  - psychogenic F45.8
- separation anxiety, of childhood F93.0
- shyness, of childhood and adolescence F40.10
- sibling rivalry F93.8
- sickle-cell (sickling) (homozygous)—*see* Disease, sickle-cell
  - heterozygous D57.3
  - specified type NEC D57.8-
  - trait D57.3
- sinus (nasal) J34.9
  - specified NEC J34.89
- skin L98.9
  - hypertrophic L91.9
    - specified NEC L91.8
  - newborn P83.9
    - specified NEC P83.88
  - picking F42.4
- SLC13A5 Citrate Transporter Disorder E74.820
- sleep G47.9
  - circadian rhythm G47.20
    - advanced sleep phase type G47.22
    - delayed sleep phase type G47.21
    - free running type G47.24
    - in conditions classified elsewhere G47.27
    - irregular sleep wake type G47.23
    - jet lag type G47.25
    - non-24 hour sleep-wake type G47.24
    - specified NEC G47.29
  - terrors F51.4
  - walking F51.3
- sleep-wake pattern or schedule—*see* Disorder, sleep, circadian rhythm G47.9
- social
  - anxiety (of childhood) F40.10
    - generalized F40.11
  - functioning in childhood F94.9
    - specified NEC F94.8
  - pragmatic F80.82
- somatization F45.0
- somatoform F45.9
  - pain (persistent) F45.41
  - somatization (multiple) (long-lasting) F45.0
  - specified NEC F45.8
  - undifferentiated F45.1
- specific
  - arithmetical F81.2
  - developmental, of motor F82
  - reading F81.0
  - speech and language F80.9
  - spelling F81.81
  - written expression F81.81
- speech R47.9
  - articulation (functional) (specific) F80.0
  - developmental F80.9
  - specified NEC R47.89
- spelling (specific) F81.81
- stereotyped, habit or movement F98.4
- stomach (functional)—*see* Disorder, gastric
- stress F43.9
  - acute F43.0
  - post-traumatic F43.10
    - acute F43.11
    - chronic F43.12
- temperature regulation, newborn P81.9
- thyroid (gland) E07.9
  - function NEC, neonatal, transitory P72.2
  - iodine-deficiency related E01.8
    - specified NEC E07.89
- tic—*see* Tic
- tobacco use
  - mild F17.200
  - moderate or severe F17.200
- tooth K08.9
  - eruption K00.6
- Tourette's F95.2

Disorder, *continued*
- trauma and stressor related F43.9
- tubulo-interstitial (in)
  - lymphoma NEC C85.9- *[N16]*
  - Salmonella infection A02.25
  - sarcoidosis D86.84
  - sepsis A41.9 *[N16]*
    - streptococcal A40.9 *[N16]*
  - systemic lupus erythematosus M32.15
  - toxoplasmosis B58.83
  - transplant rejection T86.-- *[N16]*
  - unsocialized aggressive F91.1
- vision, binocular H53.30
  - abnormal retinal correspondence H53.31
  - diplopia H53.2
- white blood cells D72.9
  - specified NEC D72.89

Disorientation R41.0

Displacement, displaced
- acquired traumatic of bone, cartilage, joint, tendon NEC—*see* Dislocation
- bladder (acquired) N32.89
  - congenital Q64.19
- canaliculus (lacrimalis), congenital Q10.6
- device, implant or graft (*see also* Complications, by site and type, mechanical) T85.628
- fallopian tube (acquired) N83.4-
  - congenital Q50.6
  - opening (congenital) Q50.6
- gallbladder (congenital) Q44.1
- intervertebral disc NEC
  - sacrococcygeal region M53.3
- lachrymal, lacrimal apparatus or duct (congenital) Q10.6
- lens, congenital Q12.1
- macula (congenital) Q14.1
- Meckel's diverticulum Q43.0
- nail (congenital) Q84.6
  - acquired L60.8
- ovary (acquired) N83.4-
  - congenital Q50.39
- oviduct (acquired) N83.4-
  - congenital Q50.6
- sacro-iliac (joint) (congenital) Q74.2
  - current injury S33.2
- uterine opening of oviducts or fallopian tubes Q50.6
- ventricular septum Q21.0

Disproportion
- fiber-type G71.20
  - congenital G71.29

Disruption (of)
- closure of
  - laceration (external) (internal) T81.33
  - traumatic laceration (external) (internal) T81.33
- family Z63.8
  - due to
    - absence of family member due to military deployment Z63.31
    - absence of family member NEC Z63.32
    - alcoholism and drug addiction in family Z63.72
    - bereavement Z63.4
    - death (assumed) or disappearance of family member Z63.4
    - divorce or separation Z63.5
    - drug addiction in family Z63.72
    - stressful life events NEC Z63.79
- wound T81.30
  - operation T81.31
  - traumatic injury repair T81.33
- traumatic injury wound repair T81.33

Dissection
- aorta
  - thoracic I71.019
    - aortic arch I71.011
    - ascending aorta I71.010
    - descending thoracic aorta I71.012

Dissociation
- auriculoventricular or atrioventricular (AV) (any degree) (isorhythmic) I45.89
  - with heart block I44.2

Dissociative reaction, state F44.9

ALPHABETIC INDEX

Distension, distention

- abdomen R14.0
- bladder N32.89
- stomach K31.89
  - acute K31.0
  - psychogenic F45.8

Distortion(s) (congenital)

- bile duct or passage Q44.5
- cervix (uteri) Q51.9
- clavicle Q74.0
- common duct Q44.5
- cystic duct Q44.5
- ear (auricle) (external) Q17.3
  - inner Q16.5
  - middle Q16.4
  - ossicles Q16.3
- endocrine NEC Q89.2
- eustachian tube Q17.8
- eye (adnexa) Q15.8
- face bone(s) NEC Q75.8
- fallopian tube Q50.6
- foot Q66.9-
- genitalia, genital organ(s)
  - female Q52.8
    - external Q52.79
    - internal NEC Q52.8
- hepatic duct Q44.5
- intrafamilial communications Z63.8
- lens Q12.8
- liver Q44.79
- oviduct Q50.6
- parathyroid (gland) Q89.2
- pituitary (gland) Q89.2
- sacroiliac joint Q74.2
- scapula Q74.0
- shoulder girdle Q74.0
- skull bone(s) NEC Q75.8
  - with
    - anencephalus Q00.0
    - encephalocele—*see* Encephalocele
    - hydrocephalus Q03.9
      - with spina bifida—*see* Spina bifida, with hydrocephalus
    - microcephaly Q02
- thymus (gland) Q89.2
- thyroid (gland) Q89.2
- toe(s) Q66.9-

Distress

- abdomen—*see* Pain, abdominal
- acute respiratory R06.03
  - syndrome (adult) (child) J80
- epigastric R10.13
- fetal P84
- gastrointestinal (functional) K30
  - psychogenic F45.8
- intestinal (functional) NOS K59.9
  - psychogenic F45.8
- relationship, with spouse or intimate partner Z63.0
- respiratory R06.03
  - distress syndrome, child J80
  - newborn P22.9
    - specified NEC P22.8
  - orthopnea R06.01
  - psychogenic F45.8
  - shortness of breath R06.02

Disturbance(s)—*see also* Disease

- absorption K90.9
  - calcium E58
  - carbohydrate K90.49
  - fat K90.49
    - pancreatic K90.3
  - protein K90.49
  - starch K90.49
  - vitamin—*see* Deficiency
- acid-base equilibrium E87.8
  - mixed E87.4
- activity and attention (with hyperkinesis)—*see* Disorder, attention-deficit hyperactivity
- assimilation, food K90.9
- blood clotting (mechanism) (*see also* Defect, coagulation) D68.9

Disturbance(s), *continued*

- cerebral
  - status, newborn P91.9
    - specified NEC P91.88
- circulatory I99.9
- conduct (*see also* Disorder, conduct) F91.9
  - adjustment reaction—*see* Disorder, adjustment
  - disruptive F91.9
  - hyperkinetic—*see* Disorder, attention-deficit hyperactivity
  - socialized F91.2
  - specified NEC F91.8
  - unsocialized F91.1
- digestive K30
  - psychogenic F45.8
- electrolyte—*see also* Imbalance, electrolyte
  - newborn, transitory P74.49
    - hyperchloremia P74.421
    - hyperchloremic metabolic acidosis P74.421
    - hypochloremia P74.422
  - potassium balance
    - hyperkalemia P74.31
    - hypokalemia P74.32
  - sodium balance
    - hypernatremia P74.21
    - hyponatremia P74.22
    - specified type NEC P74.49
- emotions specific to childhood and adolescence F93.9
  - endocrine (gland)
  - involving relationship problems F93.8
  - mixed F93.8
  - neonatal, transitory specified P72.8
  - specified NEC F93.8
  - with
    - anxiety and fearfulness NEC F93.8
    - oppositional disorder F91.3
    - sensitivity (withdrawal) F40.10
    - shyness F40.10
    - social withdrawal F40.10
- equilibrium R42
- gait—*see* Gait abnormality
  - hysterical F44.4
  - psychogenic F44.4
- gastrointestinal (functional) K30
  - psychogenic F45.8
- heart, functional (conditions in I44-I50)
  - due to presence of (cardiac) prosthesis I97.19-
  - postoperative I97.89
    - cardiac surgery I97.19-
- keratinization NEC
  - lip K13.0
- metabolism E88.9
  - amino-acid E72.9
    - straight-chain E72.89
  - general E88.9
  - glutamine E72.89
  - neonatal, transitory P74.9
    - calcium and magnesium P71.9
    - specified type NEC P71.8
  - carbohydrate metabolism P70.9
    - specified type NEC P70.8
    - specified NEC P74.8
  - threonine E72.8
- nervous, functional R45.0
- nutritional E63.9
  - nail L60.3
- ocular motion H51.9
  - psychogenic F45.8
- oculogyric H51.8
  - psychogenic F45.8
- oculomotor H51.9
  - psychogenic F45.8
- personality (pattern) (trait) (*see also* Disorder, personality) F60.9
- potassium balance, newborn
  - hyperkalemia P74.31
  - hypokalemia P74.32
- psychomotor F44.4
- rhythm, heart I49.9
- sensation (cold) (heat) (localization) (tactile discrimination) (texture) (vibratory) NEC R20.9
  - hysterical F44.6

Disturbance(s), *continued*

- sensory—*see* Disturbance
- situational (transient)—*see also* Disorder, adjustment
  - acute F43.0
- sleep G47.9
  - nonorganic origin F51.9
- smell R43.9
  - and taste (mixed) R43.8
  - anosmia R43.0
  - parosmia R43.1
  - specified NEC R43.8
- sodium balance, newborn
  - hypernatremia P74.21
  - hyponatremia P74.22
- speech R47.9
  - developmental F80.9
  - specified NEC R47.89
- taste R43.9
  - and smell (mixed) R43.8
  - parageusia R43.2
  - specified NEC R43.8
- temperature
  - regulation, newborn P81.9
    - specified NEC P81.8
  - sense R20.8
    - hysterical F44.6
- tooth
  - eruption K00.6
- vascular I99.9
- vision, visual H53.9
  - specified NEC H53.8
- voice R49.9
  - psychogenic F44.4
  - specified NEC R49.8

Diuresis R35.89

Diverticulum, diverticula (multiple)

- Meckel's (displaced) (hypertrophic) Q43.0
- pericardium (congenital) (cyst) Q24.8
  - acquired I31.8

Division

- glans penis Q55.69

Divorce, causing family disruption Z63.5

Dizziness R42

- hysterical F44.89
- psychogenic F45.8

DNR (do not resuscitate) Z66

Dohle body panmyelopathic syndrome D72.0

Dolichocephaly Q67.2

- non-deformational Q75.01

Dorsalgia M54.9

- psychogenic F45.41

Dorsopathy M53.9

Double

- albumin E88.09
- aortic arch Q25.45
- uterus Q51.2-

Doubled up Z59.01

Down syndrome Q90.9

Drinking (alcohol)

- excessive, to excess NEC (without dependence) F10.10
  - habitual (continual) (without remission) F10.20
    - with remission F10.21

Drip, postnasal (chronic) R09.82

- due to
  - allergic rhinitis—*see* Rhinitis, allergic
  - common cold J00
  - nasopharyngitis—*see* Nasopharyngitis
  - other known condition—*code* to condition
  - sinusitis—*see* Sinusitis

Drop (in)

- attack NEC R55
- hematocrit (precipitous) R71.0
- hemoglobin R71.0

Dropped heart beats I45.9

Dropsy, dropsical—*see also* Hydrops

- abdomen R18.8
- brain—*see* Hydrocephalus
- newborn due to isoimmunization P56.0

ALPHABETIC INDEX

Drowned, drowning (near) T75.1

Drowsiness R40.0

Drug
- abuse counseling and surveillance Z71.51
- addiction—*see* Dependence
- dependence—*see* Dependence
- habit—*see* Dependence
- harmful use—*see* Abuse, drug
- induced fever R50.2
- overdose—*see* Table of Drugs and Chemicals, by drug, poisoning
- poisoning—*see* Table of Drugs and Chemicals, by drug, poisoning
- resistant organism infection (*see also* Resistant, organism, to, drug) Z16.30
- therapy
  - long term (current) (prophylactic)—*see* Therapy, drug long-term (current) (prophylactic)
  - short term—omit code
- wrong substance given or taken in error—*see* Table of Drugs and Chemicals, by drug, poisoning

Drunkenness (without dependence) F10.129
- acute in alcoholism F10.229
- chronic (without remission) F10.20
  - with remission F10.21
- pathological (without dependence) F10.129
  - with dependence F10.229

Dry, dryness—*see also* Disease, diseased
- mouth R68.2
  - due to dehydration E86.0
- nose J34.89

Dubin-Johnson disease or syndrome E80.6

Dubowitz' syndrome Q87.19

Duchenne-Griesinger disease G71.01

Duchenne's
- disease or syndrome
  - muscular dystrophy G71.01
- paralysis
  - birth injury P14.0
  - due to or associated with
    - muscular dystrophy G71.01

Duffy phenotype—*see* Phenotype, Duffy

Duodenitis (nonspecific) (peptic) K29.80
- with bleeding K29.81

Duplication, duplex—*see also* Accessory
- alimentary tract Q45.8
- biliary duct (any) Q44.5
- cystic duct Q44.5
- digestive organs Q45.8
- frontonasal process Q75.8
- liver Q44.79

Dupré's disease (meningism) R29.1

Dwarfism E34.3
- achondroplastic Q77.4
- congenital E34.3
- constitutional E34.3
- hypochondroplastic Q77.4
- hypophyseal E23.0
- infantile E34.3
- Laron-type E34.3
- Lorain (-Levi) type E23.0
- metatropic Q77.8
- nephrotic-glycosuric (with hypophosphatemic rickets) E72.09
- nutritional E45
- penis Q55.69
- pituitary E23.0
- renal N25.0
- thanatophoric Q77.1

Dysarthria R47.1

Dysbasia R26.2
- hysterical F44.4
- nonorganic origin F44.4
- psychogenic F44.4

Dysbetalipoproteinemia (familial) E78.2

Dyscalculia R48.8
- developmental F81.2

Dyschezia K59.00

Dyscranio-pygo-phalangy Q87.0
- stomach K31.89
  - psychogenic F45.8

Dysentery, dysenteric (catarrhal) (diarrhea) (epidemic) (hemorrhagic) (infectious) (sporadic) (tropical) A09
- amebic (*see also* Amebiasis) A06.0
  - acute A06.0
- arthritis (*see also* category M01) A09
  - bacillary (*see also* category M01) A03.9
- bacillary A03.9
  - arthritis (*see also* category M01)
  - Shigella A03.9
    - boydii A03.2
    - dysenteriae A03.0
    - flexneri A03.1
    - group A A03.0
    - group B A03.1
    - group C A03.2
    - group D A03.3
    - sonnei A03.3
    - specified type NEC A03.8
- candidal B37.82
- Chinese A03.9
- Giardia lamblia A07.1
- Lamblia A07.1
- monilial B37.82
- Salmonella A02.0
- viral (*see also* Enteritis, viral) A08.4

Dysequilibrium R42

Dysesthesia R20.8
- hysterical F44.6

Dysfunction
- autonomic
  - somatoform F45.8
- bladder N31.9
  - neuromuscular NOS N31.9
- bleeding, uterus N93.8
- cerebral G93.89
- colon K59.9
  - psychogenic F45.8
- feeding, pediatric
  - acute R63.31
  - chronic R63.32
- hypophysis E23.7
- hypothalamic NEC E23.3
- meibomian gland, of eyelid H02.88-
  - left H02.886
    - lower H02.885
    - upper H02.884
    - upper and lower eyelids H02.88B
  - right H02.883
    - lower H02.882
    - upper H02.881
    - upper and lower eyelids H02.88A
- multifidus muscles, lumbar region M62.85
- physiological NEC R68.89
  - psychogenic F59
- pituitary (gland) E23.3
- rectum K59.9
  - psychogenic F45.8
- sexual (due to) R37
- sinoatrial node I49.5
- somatoform autonomic F45.8
- temporomandibular (joint) M26.69
  - joint-pain syndrome M26.62-
- ventricular I51.9
  - with congestive heart failure I50.9

Dysgenesis
- gonadal (due to chromosomal anomaly) Q96.9
- renal
  - bilateral Q60.4
  - unilateral Q60.3
- reticular D72.0
- tidal platelet D69.3

Dyshidrosis, dysidrosis L30.1

Dyskeratosis L85.8
- congenital Q82.8

Dyskinesia G24.9
- hysterical F44.4
- nonorganic origin F44.4
- psychogenic F44.4

Dyslalia (developmental) F80.0

Dyslexia R48.0
- developmental F81.0

Dyslipidemia E78.5

Dysmenorrhea (essential) (exfoliative) N94.6
- congestive (syndrome) N94.6
- primary N94.4
- psychogenic F45.8
- secondary N94.5

Dysmetabolic syndrome X E88.810

Dysmorphia
- muscle F45.22

Dysmorphism (due to)
- alcohol Q86.0

Dysmorphophobia (non-delusional) F45.22

Dysorexia R63.0
- psychogenic F50.89

Dysostosis
- cleidocranial, cleidocranialis Q74.0
- multiplex E76.01

Dyspareunia N94.10
- deep N94.12
- other specified N94.19
- superficial (introital) N94.11

Dyspepsia R10.13
- atonic K30
- functional (allergic) (congenital) (gastrointestinal) (occupational) (reflex) K30
- nervous F45.8
- neurotic F45.8
- psychogenic F45.8

Dysphagia R13.10
- cervical R13.19
- functional (hysterical) F45.8
- hysterical F45.8
- nervous (hysterical) F45.8
- neurogenic R13.19
- oral phase R13.11
- oropharyngeal phase R13.12
- pharyngeal phase R13.13
- pharyngoesophageal phase R13.14
- psychogenic F45.8
- specified NEC R13.19

Dysphagocytosis, congenital D71

Dysphasia
- developmental
  - expressive type F80.1
  - receptive type F80.2

Dysphonia R49.0
- functional F44.4
- hysterical F44.4
- psychogenic F44.4

Dyspituitarism E23.3

Dysplasia—*see also* Anomaly
- acetabular, congenital Q65.89
- alveolar capillary, with vein misalignment J84.843
- anus (histologically confirmed) (mild) (moderate) K62.82
- asphyxiating thoracic (congenital) Q77.2
- brain Q07.9
- bronchopulmonary, perinatal P27.1
- chondroectodermal Q77.6
- colon D12.6
- dystrophic Q77.5
- ectodermal (anhidrotic) (congenital) (hereditary) Q82.4
  - hydrotic Q82.8
- high grade, focal D12.6
- hip, congenital Q65.89
- joint, congenital Q74.8
- kidney Q61.4
  - multicystic Q61.4
- leg Q74.2
- lung, congenital (not associated with short gestation) Q33.6
- oculodentodigital Q87.0
- renal Q61.4
  - multicystic Q61.4
- skin L98.8
- spondyloepiphyseal Q77.7
- thymic, with immunodeficiency D82.1

ALPHABETIC INDEX

Dysplasminogenemia E88.02

Dyspnea (nocturnal) (paroxysmal) R06.00
- asthmatic (bronchial) J45.909
  - with
    - exacerbation (acute) J45.901
  - bronchitis J45.909
    - with
      - θ exacerbation (acute) J45.901
      - θ status asthmaticus J45.902
    - status asthmaticus J45.902
- functional F45.8
- hyperventilation R06.4
- hysterical F45.8
- newborn P28.89
- orthopnea R06.01
- psychogenic F45.8
- shortness of breath R06.02
- transfusion-associated dyspnea (TAD) J95.87

Dyspraxia R27.8
- developmental (syndrome) F82

Dysproteinemia E88.09

Dysrhythmia
- cardiac I49.9
  - newborn
    - bradycardia P29.12
    - occurring before birth P03.819
      - before onset of labor P03.810
      - during labor P03.811
    - tachycardia P29.11
  - postoperative I97.89
- cerebral or cortical—*see* Epilepsy

Dyssomnia—*see* Disorder, sleep

Dyssynergia
- cerebellaris myoclonica (Hunt's ataxia) G11.19

Dystocia
- affecting newborn P03.1

Dystonia G24.9
- cervical G24.3
- deformans progressiva G24.1
- drug induced NEC G24.09
  - acute G24.02
  - specified NEC G24.09
- familial G24.1
- idiopathic G24.1
  - familial G24.1
  - nonfamilial G24.2
  - orofacial G24.4
- lenticularis G24.8
- musculorum deformans G24.1
- neuroleptic induced (acute) G24.02
- orofacial (idiopathic) G24.4
- oromandibular G24.4
  - due to drug G24.01
- specified NEC G24.8
- torsion (familial) (idiopathic) G24.1
  - acquired G24.8
  - genetic G24.1
  - symptomatic (nonfamilial) G24.2

Dystonic movements R25.8

Dystrophy, dystrophia
- adiposogenital E23.6
- autosomal recessive, childhood type, muscular dystrophy resembling Duchenne or Becker G71.01
- Becker's type G71.01
- cornea (hereditary) H18.50-
  - endothelial H18.51-
  - epithelial H18.52-
  - granular H18.53-
  - lattice H18.54-
  - macular H18.55-
  - specified type NEC H18.59-
- Duchenne's type G71.01
- Erb's G71.02
- Fuchs' H18.51-
- Gower's muscular G71.01
- infantile neuraxonal G31.89
- Landouzy-Déjérine G71.02
- Leyden-Möbius G71.09

Dystrophy, dystrophia, *continued*
- muscular G71.00
  - autosomal recessive, childhood type, muscular dystrophy resembling Duchenne or Becker G71.01
  - benign (Becker type) G71.01
    - capuloperoneal with early contractures [Emery-Dreifuss] G71.09
  - congenital (hereditary) (progressive) (with specific morphological abnormalities of the muscle fiber) G71.09
  - distal G71.09
  - Duchenne type G71.01
  - Emery-Dreifuss G71.09
  - Erb type G71.02
  - facioscapulohumeral G71.02
  - Gower's G71.01
  - hereditary (progressive) G71.09
  - Landouzy-Déjérine type G71.02
  - limb-girdle G71.09
  - progressive (hereditary) G71.09
  - pseudohypertrophic (infantile) G71.01
  - scapulohumeral G71.02
  - scapuloperoneal G71.09
  - severe (Duchenne type) G71.01
  - specified type NEC G71.09
- nail L60.3
- ocular G71.09
- oculocerebrorenal E72.03
- oculopharyngeal G71.09
- retinal (hereditary) H35.50
  - involving
    - sensory area H35.53
- scapuloperoneal G71.09
- skin NEC L98.8
- thoracic, asphyxiating Q77.2
- ungulum L60.3

Dysuria R30.0
- psychogenic F45.8

E

Ear—*see also* Disease, diseased
- piercing Z41.3
- wax (impacted) H61.2-

Earache—*see* subcategory H92.0

Ebola virus disease A98.4

Eccentro-osteochondrodysplasia E76.29

Ecchymosis R58
- newborn P54.5
- spontaneous R23.3
- traumatic—*see* Contusion

Echovirus, as cause of disease classified elsewhere B97.12

Ectasia, ectasis
- annuloaortic I35.8

Ecthyma L08.0
- gangrenosum L08.0

Ectodermosis erosiva pluriorificialis L51.1

Ectopic, ectopia (congenital)
- abdominal viscera Q45.8
  - due to defect in anterior abdominal wall Q79.59
- atrial beats I49.1
- beats I49.49
  - atrial I49.1
- bladder Q64.10
- lens, lentis Q12.1
- testis Q53.00
  - bilateral Q53.02
  - unilateral Q53.01
- thyroid Q89.2
- vesicae Q64.10

Ectropion H02.10-
- cervix N86
  - with cervicitis N72
- congenital Q10.1
- lip (acquired) K13.0
  - congenital Q38.0

Eczema (acute) (chronic) (erythematous) (fissum) (rubrum) (squamous) (see also Dermatitis) L30.9
- contact—*see* Dermatitis, contact

Eczema, *continued*
- dyshydrotic L30.1
- flexural L20.82
- infantile L20.83
  - intertriginous L21.1
  - seborrheic L21.1
- intertriginous NEC L30.4
  - infantile L21.1
- intrinsic (allergic) L20.84
- marginatum (hebrae) B35.6
- pustular L30.3
- vaccination, vaccinatum T88.1

Eddowes (-Spurway) syndrome Q78.0

Edema, edematous (infectious) (pitting) (toxic) R60.9
- with nephritis—*see* Nephrosis
- allergic T78.3
- angioneurotic (allergic) (any site) (with urticaria) T78.3
- brain (cytotoxic) (vasogenic) G93.6
  - due to birth injury P11.0
  - newborn (anoxia or hypoxia) P52.4
    - birth injury P11.0
- circumscribed, acute T78.3
- conjunctiva H11.42-
- due to
  - salt retention E87.0
- epiglottis—*see* Edema, glottis
- essential, acute T78.3
- eyelid NEC H02.84-
  - left H02.846
    - lower H02.845
    - upper H02.844
  - right H02.843
    - lower H02.842
    - upper H02.841
- generalized R60.1
- glottis, glottic, glottidis (obstructive) (passive) J38.4
  - allergic T78.3
- intracranial G93.6
- legs R60.0
- localized R60.0
- lower limbs R60.0
- lung J81.1
  - acute J81.0
  - due to
    - high altitude T70.29
    - near drowning T75.1
- newborn P83.30
  - hydrops fetalis—*see* Hydrops, fetalis
  - specified NEC P83.39
- penis N48.89
- periodic T78.3
- Quincke's T78.3
- salt E87.0

Edentulism—*see* Absence, teeth, acquired

Edsall's disease T67.2

Educational handicap Z55.9
- less than a high school diploma or GED Z55.5
- specified NEC Z55.8

Edward's syndrome—*see* Trisomy, 18

Effect, adverse
- abuse—*see* Maltreatment
- altitude (high)—*see* Effect, adverse, high altitude
- biological, correct substance properly administered—*see* Effect, adverse, drugs and medicaments
- blood (derivatives) (serum) (transfusion)—*see* Complications, transfusion
- chemical substance—*see* Table of Drugs and Chemicals
- cold (temperature) (weather)
  - frostbite—*see* Frostbite
- drugs and medicaments T88.7
  - specified drug—*see* Table of Drugs and Chemicals, by drug, adverse effect
  - specified effect—*code to* condition
- electric current, electricity (shock) T75.4
  - burn—*see* Burn
- exposure—*see* Exposure
- external cause NEC T75.89
- foodstuffs T78.1
  - allergic reaction—*see* Allergy, food
    - causing anaphylaxis—*see* Shock, anaphylactic, due to food

DYSPLASMINOGENEMIA–EFFECT, ADVERSE

Effect, adverse, *continued*

- noxious—*see* Poisoning, food, noxious
- gases, fumes, or vapors
  - specified agent—*see* Table of Drugs and Chemicals
- glue (airplane) sniffing
  - due to drug abuse—*see* Abuse, drug, inhalant
  - due to drug dependence—*see* Dependence, drug, inhalant
- heat—*see* Heat
- high altitude NEC T70.29
  - anoxia T70.29
  - on
    - ears T70.0
    - sinuses T70.1
  - polycythemia D75.1
- hot weather—*see* Heat
- hunger T73.0
- immersion, foot—*see* Immersion
- immunization—*see* Complications, vaccination
- immunological agents—*see* Complications, vaccination
- infusion—*see* Complications, infusion
- lack of care of infants—*see* Maltreatment, child
- medical care T88.9
  - specified NEC T88.8
- medicinal substance, correct, properly administered—*see* Effect, adverse, drugs and medicaments
- motion T75.3
- serum NEC (*see also* Reaction, serum) T80.69
- specified NEC T78.8
- strangulation—*see* Asphyxia, traumatic
- submersion T75.1
- toxic—*see* Table of Drugs and Chemicals, by animal or substance, poisoning
- transfusion—*see* Complications, transfusion
- ultraviolet (radiation) (rays) NOS
  - burn—*see* Burn
  - dermatitis or eczema—*see* Dermatitis, due to, ultraviolet rays
    - acute L56.8
- vaccine (any)—*see* Complications, vaccination
- whole blood—*see* Complications, transfusion

Effect(s) (of) (from)—*see* Effect, adverse

Effects, late—*see* Sequelae

Effort syndrome (psychogenic) F45.8

Effusion

- brain (serous) G93.6
- bronchial—*see* Bronchitis
- cerebral G93.6
- cerebrospinal—*see also* Meningitis
  - vessel G93.6
- chest—*see* Effusion, pleura
- intracranial G93.6
- joint M25.40
  - ankle M25.47-
  - elbow M25.42-
  - foot joint M25.47-
  - hand joint M25.44-
  - hip M25.45-
  - knee M25.46-
  - shoulder M25.41-
  - specified joint NEC M25.48
  - wrist M25.43-
- malignant pleural J91.0
- pericardium, pericardial (noninflammatory) I31.3
  - acute—*see* Pericarditis, acute
- peritoneal (chronic) R18.8
- pleura, pleurisy, pleuritic, pleuropericardial J90
  - due to systemic lupus erythematosus M32.13
  - in conditions classified elsewhere J91.8
  - malignant J91.0
  - newborn P28.89
- spinal—*see* Meningitis
- thorax, thoracic—*see* Effusion, pleura

Ehlers-Danlos syndrome Q79.60

- classical Ehlers-Danlos syndrome Q79.61
- hypermobile Ehlers-Danlos syndrome Q79.62
- other Ehlers-Danlos syndromes Q79.69
- vascular Ehlers-Danlos syndrome Q79.63

Ehrlichiosis A77.40

- due to
- E. chaffeensis A77.41

Eichstedt's disease B36.0

Eisenmenger's

- complex or syndrome I27.83
- defect Q21.8

Ekbom's syndrome (restless legs) G25.81

Ekman's syndrome (brittle bones and blue sclera) Q78.0

Elastic skin Q82.8

Elastoma (juvenile) Q82.8

Electric current, electricity, effects (concussion) (fatal) (nonfatal) (shock) T75.4

- burn—*see* Burn

Electrocution T75.4

- from electroshock gun (taser) T75.4

Electrolyte imbalance E87.8

Elevated, elevation

- alanine transaminase (ALT) R74.01
- ALT (alanine transaminase) R74.01
- aspartate transaminase (AST) R74.01
- AST (aspartate transaminase) R74.01
- basal metabolic rate R94.8
- blood pressure—*see also* Hypertension
  - reading (incidental) (isolated) (nonspecific), no diagnosis of hypertension R03.0
- blood sugar R73.9
- body temperature (of unknown origin) R50.9
- C-reactive protein (CRP) R79.82
- cancer antigen 125 [CA 125] R97.1
- carcinoembryonic antigen [CEA] R97.0
- cholesterol E78.00
  - with high triglycerides E78.2
- erythrocyte sedimentation rate R70.0
- fasting glucose R73.01
- finding on laboratory examination—*see* Findings, abnormal, inconclusive, without diagnosis
- glucose tolerance (oral) R73.02
- lactic acid dehydrogenase (LDH) level R74.02
- leukocytes D72.829
- lipoprotein a (Lp(a)) level E78.41
- liver function
  - study R94.5
  - test R79.89
    - alkaline phosphatase R74.8
    - aminotransferase R74.01
    - bilirubin R17
    - hepatic enzyme R74.8
    - lactate dehydrogenase R74.02
- lymphocytes D72.820
- scapula, congenital Q74.0
- sedimentation rate R70.0
- SGOT R74.0
- SGPT R74.0
- transaminase level R74.0
- triglycerides E78.1
  - with high cholesterol E78.2
- troponin R77.8
- tumor associated antigens [TAA] NEC R97.8
- tumor specific antigens [TSA] NEC R97.8
- white blood cell count D72.829
  - specified NEC D72.828

Elliptocytosis (congenital) (hereditary) D58.1

- Hb C (disease) D58.1
- hemoglobin disease D58.1
- sickle-cell (disease) D57.8-
  - trait D57.3

Elongated, elongation (congenital)—*see also* Distortion

- bone Q79.9
- cystic duct Q44.5
- frenulum, penis Q55.69
- labia minora (acquired) N90.69

Embolism (multiple) (paradoxical) I74.9

- artery I74.9
- cavernous sinus (venous—*see* Embolism, intracranial, venous sinus
  - pituitary E23.6
- portal (vein) I81
- pulmonary (acute) (artery) (vein) I26.99
  - chronic I27.82
- pyemic (multiple) I76
  - following
    - Hemophilus influenzae A41.3

Embolism, *continued*

- pneumococcal A40.3
  - with pneumonia J13
- specified organism NEC A41.89
- staphylococcal A41.2
- streptococcal A40.9
- renal (artery) N28.0
  - vein I82.3
- vein (acute) I82.90
  - renal I82.3

Embryoma—*see also* Neoplasm, uncertain behavior, by site in Table of Neoplasms in the complete *ICD-10-CM* manual

- kidney C64.-
- malignant—*see also* Neoplasm, malignant, by site in Table of Neoplasms in the complete *ICD-10-CM* manual
  - kidney C64.-

Emesis—*see* Vomiting

Emotional lability R45.86

Emotionality, pathological F60.3

Emphysema

- cellular tissue (traumatic) T79.7
- connective tissue (traumatic) T79.7
- eyelid(s) H02.89
  - traumatic T79.7
- interstitial J98.2
  - congenital P25.0
  - perinatal period P25.0
- laminated tissue T79.7
- mediastinal J98.2
  - newborn P25.2
- subcutaneous (traumatic) T79.7
  - nontraumatic J98.2
- traumatic T79.7

Empyema (acute) (chest) (double) (pleura) (supradiaphragmatic) (thorax) J86.9

- with fistula J86.0
- gallbladder K81.0

Enanthema, viral B09

Encephalitis (chronic) (hemorrhagic) (idiopathic) (nonepidemic) (spurious) (subacute) G04.90

- acute A86
  - disseminated G04.00
    - infectious G04.01
    - noninfectious G04.81
    - postimmunization (postvaccination) G04.02
    - postinfectious G04.01
  - inclusion body A85.8
  - necrotizing hemorrhagic G04.30
    - postimmunization G04.32
    - postinfectious G04.31
    - specified NEC G04.39
  - toxic NEC G92.8
- **Encephalomyelitis** (*see also* Encephalitis) G04.90
  - acute disseminated G04.00
    - infectious G04.01
    - noninfectious G04.81
    - postimmunization G04.02
    - postinfectious G04.01
  - acute necrotizing hemorrhagic G04.30
    - postimmunization G04.32
    - postinfectious G04.31
    - specified NEC G04.39
  - equine A83.9
    - Eastern A83.2
  - in diseases classified elsewhere G05.3
  - postchickenpox B01.11
  - postinfectious NEC G04.01
  - postmeasles B05.0
  - postvaccinal G04.02
  - postvaricella B01.11

Encephalopathy (acute) G93.40

- acute necrotizing hemorrhagic G04.30
  - postimmunization G04.32
  - postinfectious G04.31
  - specified NEC G04.39
- congenital Q07.9
- developmental and epileptic G93.45
- due to
  - drugs (*see also* Table of Drugs and Chemicals) G92.-
- early infantile epileptic G93.45

ALPHABETIC INDEX

Encephalopathy, *continued*

- hepatic K76.82
- hyperbilirubinemic, newborn P57.9
  - due to isoimmunization (conditions in P55) P57.0
- hypertensive I67.4
- hypoglycemic E16.2
- hypoxic—*see* Damage, brain, anoxic
- hypoxic ischemic P91.60
  - mild P91.61
  - moderate P91.62
  - severe P91.63
- in (due to) (with)
  - birth injury P11.1
  - hyperinsulinism E16.1 [G94]
  - influenza—*see* Influenza, with, encephalopathy
  - lack of vitamin (*see also* Deficiency, vitamin) E56.9 [G32.89]
  - neoplastic disease (*see also* Neoplasm) D49.9 [G13.1]
  - serum (*see also* Reaction, serum) T80.69
  - trauma (postconcussional) F07.81
    - current injury—*see* Injury, intracranial
  - vaccination G04.02
- lead—*see* Poisoning, lead
- metabolic G93.41
  - drug induced G92.8
  - toxic G92.9
- neonatal P91.819
  - in diseases classified elsewhere P91.811
- postcontusional F07.81
  - current injury—*see* Injury, intracranial, diffuse
- postradiation G93.89
- toxic G92.9
  - metabolic G92.8
- traumatic (postconcussional) F07.81
  - current injury—*see* Injury, intracranial

Encephalocele Q01.9

- frontal Q01.0
- nasofrontal Q01.1
- occipital Q01.2
- specified NEC Q01.8

Encephalomalacia (brain) (cerebellar) (cerebral)—*see* Softening, brain

Encephalomyelitis (*see also* Encephalitis) G04.90

- acute disseminated G04.00
  - infectious G04.01
  - noninfectious G04.81
  - postimmunization G04.02
  - postinfectious G04.01
- acute necrotizing hemorrhagic G04.30
  - postimmunization G04.32
  - postinfectious G04.31
  - specified NEC G04.39
- congenital Q07.9
- due to
  - drugs (*see also* Table of Drugs and Chemicals) G92
- equine A83.9
  - Eastern A83.2
- hyperbilirubinemic, newborn P57.9
  - due to isoimmunization (conditions in P55) P57.0
- hypertensive I67.4
- hypoglycemic E16.2
- hypoxic—*see* Damage, brain, anoxic
- hypoxic ischemic P91.60
  - mild P91.61
  - moderate P91.62
  - severe P91.63
- in diseases classified elsewhere G05.3
- in (due to) (with)
  - birth injury P11.1
  - hyperinsulinism E16.1 [G94]
  - influenza—*see* Influenza, with, encephalopathy
  - lack of vitamin (*see also* Deficiency, vitamin) E56.9 [G32.89]
  - neoplastic disease (*see also* Table of Neoplasms in the complete *ICD-10-CM* manual) D49.9 [G13.1]
  - serum (*see also* Reaction, serum) T80.69
  - trauma (postconcussional) F07.81
    - current injury—*see* Injury, intracranial
  - vaccination G04.02
- lead—*see* Poisoning, lead

Encephalomyelitis, *continued*

- metabolic G93.41
  - drug induced G92.8
  - toxic G92.9
- neonatal P91.819
  - in diseases classified elsewhere P91.811
- postchickenpox B01.11
- postcontusional F07.81
  - current injury—*see* Injury, intracranial, diffuse
- postinfectious NEC G04.01
- postmeasles B05.0
- postradiation G93.89
- postvaccinal G04.02
- postvaricella B01.11
  - specified NEC G04.39
- toxic G92.9
  - metabolic G92.8
- traumatic (postconcussional) F07.81
  - current injury—*see* Injury, intracranial

Encephalorrhagia—*see* Hemorrhage, intracranial, intracerebral

Encephalosis, posttraumatic F07.81

Encopresis R15.9

- functional F98.1
- nonorganic origin F98.1
- psychogenic F98.1

Encounter (with health service) (for) Z76.89

- administrative purpose only Z02.9
  - examination for
    - adoption Z02.82
    - armed forces Z02.3
    - child welfare Z02.84
    - disability determination Z02.71
    - driving license Z02.4
    - employment Z02.1
    - insurance Z02.6
    - medical certificate NEC Z02.79
    - residential institution admission Z02.2
    - school admission Z02.0
    - sports Z02.5
  - specified reason NEC Z02.89
- aftercare—*see* Aftercare
- check-up—*see* Examination
- child welfare screening exam
- chemotherapy for neoplasm Z51.11
- counseling—*see* Counseling
- desensitization to allergens Z51.6
- ear piercing Z41.3
- examination—*see* Examination
- expectant parent(s) (adoptive) pre-birth pediatrician visit Z76.81
- fluoride varnish application Z29.3
- genetic
  - nonprocreative Z71.83
  - procreative counseling Z31.5
  - testing—*see* Test
- hearing conservation and treatment Z01.12
- HIV
  - pre-exposure prophylaxis Z29.81
  - PrEP Z29.81
- instruction (in)
  - child care (postpartal) (prenatal) Z32.3
  - natural family planning
    - to avoid pregnancy Z30.02
- laboratory (as part of a general medical examination) Z00.00
  - with abnormal findings Z00.01
- mental health services (for)
  - abuse NEC
    - perpetrator Z69.82
    - victim Z69.81
  - child abuse/neglect (psychological) (sexual)
    - non-parental
      - perpetrator Z69.021
      - victim Z69.020
    - parental
      - perpetrator Z69.011
      - victim Z69.010
  - spousal or partner abuse (psychological)
    - perpetrator Z69.12
    - victim Z69.11

Encounter, *continued*

- observation (for) (ruled out)
  - condition suspected related to home physiologic monitoring device Z03.83
    - newborn Z05.81
      - apnea alarm Z05.81
      - bradycardia alarm Z05.81
      - malfunction of home cardiorespiratory monitor Z05.81
    - non-specific findings home physiologic monitoring device Z05.81
    - pulse oximeter alarm without findings Z05.81
  - exposure to (suspected)
    - anthrax Z03.810
    - biological agent NEC Z03.818
  - conditions related to home physiologic monitoring device Z03.83
- palliative care Z51.5
- pediatrician visit, by expectant parent(s) (adoptive) Z76.81
- pregnancy
  - supervision of—*see* Pregnancy, supervision of
  - test Z32.00
    - result negative Z32.02
    - result positive Z32.01
- prophylactic measures
  - antivenin Z29.12
  - ear piercing Z41.3
  - fluoride administration Z29.3
  - HIV pre-exposure Z29.81
  - other specified Z29.8
  - rabies immune globulin Z29.14
  - respiratory syncytial virus (RSV) immune globulin Z29.11
  - Rho(D) immune globulin Z29.13
  - specified NEC Z29.89
  - unspecified Z29.9
- radiation therapy (antineoplastic) Z51.0
- radiological (as part of a general medical examination) Z00.00
  - with abnormal findings Z00.01
- repeat cervical smear to confirm findings of recent normal smear following initial abnormal smear Z01.42
- respiratory syncytial (RSV) virus immune globulin administration Z29.11
- suspected condition, ruled out
  - fetal anomaly Z03.73
  - fetal growth Z03.74
- suspected exposure (to), ruled out
  - anthrax Z03.810
  - biological agents NEC Z03.818
- therapeutic drug level monitoring Z51.81
- to determine fetal viability of pregnancy O36.80
- training
  - insulin pump Z46.81
- X-ray of chest (as part of a general medical examination) Z00.00
  - with abnormal findings Z00.01

Endocarditis (chronic) (marantic) (nonbacterial) (thrombotic) (valvular) I38

- with rheumatic fever (conditions in I00)
  - active—*see* Endocarditis, acute, rheumatic
  - inactive or quiescent (with chorea) I09.1
- acute or subacute I33.9
  - infective I33.0
  - rheumatic (aortic) (mitral) (pulmonary) (tricuspid) I01.1
    - with chorea (acute) (rheumatic) (Sydenham's) I02.0
- aortic (heart) (nonrheumatic) (valve) I35.8
  - with
    - mitral disease I08.0
      - with tricuspid (valve) disease I08.3
      - active or acute I01.1
        - ◊ with chorea (acute) (rheumatic) (Sydenham's) I02.0
  - rheumatic fever (conditions in I00)
    - active—*see* Endocarditis, acute, rheumatic
    - inactive or quiescent (with chorea) I06.9
  - tricuspid (valve) disease I08.2
    - with mitral (valve) disease I08.3
  - acute or subacute I33.9

ALPHABETIC INDEX

Endocarditis, *continued*

- arteriosclerotic I35.8
- rheumatic I06.9
  - with mitral disease I08.0
    - with tricuspid (valve) disease I08.3
    - active or acute I01.1
      - ◊ with chorea (acute) (rheumatic) (Sydenham's) I02.0
  - active or acute I01.1
    - with chorea (acute) (rheumatic) (Sydenham's) I02.0
  - specified NEC I06.8
- specified cause NEC I35.8
- atypical verrucous (Libman-Sacks) M32.11
- bacterial (acute) (any valve) (subacute) I33.0
- candidal B37.6
- constrictive I33.0
- due to
  - Serratia marcescens I33.0
- infectious or infective (acute) (any valve) (subacute) I33.0
- lenta (acute) (any valve) (subacute) I33.0
- Libman-Sacks M32.11
- malignant (acute) (any valve) (subacute) I33.0
- mitral (chronic) (double) (fibroid) (heart) (inactive) (valve) (with chorea) I05.9
  - with
    - aortic (valve) disease I08.0
      - with tricuspid (valve) disease I08.3
    - active or acute I01.1
      - ◊ with chorea (acute) (rheumatic) (Sydenham's) I02.0
    - rheumatic fever (conditions in I00)
      - active—*see* Endocarditis, acute, rheumatic
      - inactive or quiescent (with chorea) I05.9
  - active or acute I01.1
    - with chorea (acute) (rheumatic) (Sydenham's) I02.0
    - bacterial I33.0
  - nonrheumatic I34.8
    - acute or subacute I33.9
  - specified NEC I05.8
- monilial B37.6
- mycotic (acute) (any valve) (subacute) I33.0
- pneumococcal (acute) (any valve) (subacute) I33.0
- pulmonary (chronic) (heart) (valve) I37.8
  - with rheumatic fever (conditions in I00)
    - active—*see* Endocarditis, acute, rheumatic
    - inactive or quiescent (with chorea) I09.89
    - with aortic, mitral or tricuspid disease I08.8
  - acute or subacute I33.9
  - rheumatic I01.1
    - with chorea (acute) (rheumatic) (Sydenham's) I02.0
  - arteriosclerotic I37.8
  - congenital Q22.2
- purulent (acute) (any valve) (subacute) I33.0
- rheumatic (chronic) (inactive) (with chorea) I09.1
  - active or acute (aortic) (mitral) (pulmonary) (tricuspid) I01.1
    - with chorea (acute) (rheumatic) (Sydenham's) I02.0
- septic (acute) (any valve) (subacute) I33.0
- streptococcal (acute) (any valve) (subacute) I33.0
- subacute—*see* Endocarditis, acute
- suppurative (acute) (any valve) (subacute) I33.0
- toxic I33.9
- tricuspid (chronic) (heart) (inactive) (rheumatic) (valve) (with chorea) I07.9
  - with
    - aortic (valve) disease I08.2
      - mitral (valve) disease I08.3
    - mitral (valve) disease I08.1
      - aortic (valve) disease I08.3
    - rheumatic fever (conditions in I00)
      - active—*see* Endocarditis, acute, rheumatic
      - inactive or quiescent (with chorea) I07.8
  - active or acute I01.1
    - with chorea (acute) (rheumatic) (Sydenham's) I02.0
  - arteriosclerotic I36.8
  - nonrheumatic I36.8
    - acute or subacute I33.9

Endocarditis, *continued*

- specified cause, except rheumatic I36.8
- ulcerative (acute) (any valve) (subacute) I33.0
- vegetative (acute) (any valve) (subacute) I33.0
- verrucous (atypical) (nonbacterial) (nonrheumatic) M32.11

Endocardium, endocardial—*see also* Disease, diseased

- cushion defect Q21.2

Endocervicitis—*see also* Cervicitis

- hyperplastic N72

Endometritis (decidual) (nonspecific) (purulent) (senile) (atrophic) (suppurative) N71.9

- acute N71.0
- blennorrhagic (gonococcal) (acute) (chronic) A54.24
- cervix, cervical (with erosion or ectropion)—*see also* Cervicitis
  - hyperplastic N72
- chlamydial A56.11
- gonococcal, gonorrheal (acute) (chronic) A54.24
- hyperplastic N85.00-
  - cervix N72

Engman's disease L30.3

Engorgement

- breast N64.59
  - newborn P83.4
  - puerperal, postpartum O92.79

Enlargement, enlarged—*see also* Hypertrophy

- adenoids J35.2
  - with tonsils J35.3
- gingival K06.1
- labium majus (childhood asymmetric) CALME N90.61
- lymph gland or node R59.9
  - generalized R59.1
  - localized R59.0
- tonsils J35.1
  - with adenoids J35.3
- vestibular aqueduct Q16.5

Enteritis (acute) (diarrheal) (hemorrhagic) (noninfective) K52.9

- aertrycke infection A02.0
- allergic K52.29
  - with
    - eosinophilic gastritis or gastroenteritis K52.81
    - food protein-induced enterocolitis syndrome (FPIES) K52.21
    - food protein-induced enteropathy K52.22
- amebic (acute) A06.0
- bacillary NOS A03.9
- candidal B37.82
- chronic (noninfectious) K52.9
  - ulcerative—*see* Colitis, ulcerative
- Clostridioides difficile
  - not specified as recurrent A04.72
  - recurrent A04.71
- Clostridium
  - botulinum (food poisoning) A05.1
  - difficile
    - not specified as recurrent A04.72
    - recurrent A04.71
- coxsackie virus A08.39
- dietetic K52.29
- due to
  - Clostridium difficile A04.7-
  - coxsackie virus A08.39
  - echovirus A08.39
  - enterovirus NEC A08.39
  - food hypersensitivity K52.29
  - torovirus A08.39
- echovirus A08.39
- enterovirus NEC A08.39
- eosinophilic K52.81
- epidemic (infectious) A09
- fulminant (*see also* Ischemia, intestine) K55.019
  - ischemic K55.9
    - acute (*see also* Ischemia, intestine) K55.019
- giardial A07.1
- infectious NOS A09
  - due to
    - Arizona (bacillus) A02.0
    - Campylobacter A04.5

Enteritis, *continued*

- Clostridioides difficile
  - not specified as recurrent A04.72
  - recurrent A04.71
- Escherichia coli A04.4
  - enteroaggregative A04.4
  - enterohemorrhagic A04.3
  - enteropathogenic A04.0
  - enterotoxigenic A04.1
  - specified NEC A04.4
- enterovirus A08.39
  - specified
    - bacteria NEC A04.8
    - virus A08.39
  - virus NEC A08.39
- toxic NEC K52.1
  - due to
    - ◊ Clostridioides difficile
      - ▸ not specified as recurrent A04.72
      - ▸ recurrent A04.71
    - ◊ Clostridium difficile
      - ▸ not specified as recurrent A04.72
      - ▸ recurrent A04.71
- virus NEC A08.4
  - specified type NEC A08.39
- necroticans A05.2
- noninfectious K52.9
- parasitic NEC B82.9
- regional (of) K50.90
  - with
    - complication K50.919
      - abscess K50.914
      - fistula K50.913
      - intestinal obstruction K50.912
      - rectal bleeding K50.911
      - specified complication NEC K50.918
  - large intestine (colon) (rectum) K50.10
    - with
      - complication K50.119
        - ◊ abscess K50.114
        - ◊ fistula K50.113
        - ◊ intestinal obstruction K50.112
        - ◊ rectal bleeding K50.111
        - ◊ small intestine (duodenum) (ileum) (jejunum) involvement K50.80
          - ▸ with
            - ❖ complication K50.819
              - ✦ abscess K50.814
              - ✦ fistula K50.813
              - ✦ intestinal obstruction K50.812
              - ✦ rectal bleeding K50.811
              - ✦ specified complication NEC K50.818
        - ◊ specified complication NEC K50.118
  - rectum—*see* Enteritis, regional, large intestine
  - small intestine (duodenum) (ileum) (jejunum) K50.00
    - with
      - complication K50.019
        - ◊ abscess K50.014
        - ◊ fistula K50.013
        - ◊ intestinal obstruction K50.012
        - ◊ large intestine (colon) (rectum) involvement K50.80
          - ▸ with
            - ❖ complication K50.819
              - ✦ abscess K50.814
              - ✦ fistula K50.813
              - ✦ intestinal obstruction K50.812
              - ✦ rectal bleeding K50.811
              - ✦ specified complication NEC K50.818
        - ◊ rectal bleeding K50.011
        - ◊ specified complication NEC K50.018
- rotaviral A08.0
- Salmonella, salmonellosis (arizonae) (choleraesuis) (enteritidis) (typhimurium) A02.0
- septic A09
- staphylococcal A04.8
  - due to food A05.0
- torovirus A08.39
- toxic NEC K52.1
  - due to
    - Clostridioides difficile
      - not specified as recurrent A04.72
      - recurrent A04.71

ALPHABETIC INDEX

Enteritis, *continued*
- ■ Clostridium difficile
  - ~ not specified as recurrent A04.72
  - ~ recurrent A04.71
- viral A08.4
  - enterovirus A08.39
  - Rotavirus A08.0
  - specified NEC A08.39
  - virus specified NEC A08.39

Enterobiasis B80

Enterobius vermicularis (infection) (infestation) B80

Enterocolitis (*see also* Enteritis) K52.9
- due to
  - Clostridioides difficile
    - ■ not specified as recurrent A04.72
    - ■ recurrent A04.71
  - Clostridium difficile
    - ■ not specified as recurrent A04.72
    - ■ recurrent A04.71
- fulminant ischemic (*see also* Ischemia, intestine) K55.059
- hemorrhagic (acute) (*see also* Ischemia, intestine) K55.059
- infectious NEC A09
- necrotizing
  - due to
    - ■ Clostridioides difficile
      - not specified as recurrent A04.72
      - recurrent A04.71
    - ■ Clostridium difficile
      - not specified as recurrent A04.72
      - recurrent A04.71
  - in newborn P77.9
    - ■ stage 1 (without pneumatosis, without perforation) P77.1
    - ■ stage 2 (with pneumatosis, without perforation) P77.2
    - ■ stage 3 (with pneumatosis, with perforation) P77.3
  - stage 1 (excluding newborns) K55.31
  - stage 2 (excluding newborns) K55.32
  - stage 3 (excluding newborns) K55.33
  - unspecified K55.30
- noninfectious K52.9
  - newborn—*see* Enterocolitis, necrotizing
- protein-induced syndrome K52.21
- pseudomembranous (newborn) A04.7-

Enteropathy K63.9
- food protein-induced enterocolitis K52.22
- gluten-sensitive
  - celiac K90.0
  - non-celiac K90.41
- protein-losing K90.49

Enterorrhagia K92.2

Enterospasm—*see also* Syndrome, irritable, bowel
- psychogenic F45.8

Enterovirus, as cause of disease classified elsewhere B97.10
- coxsackievirus B97.11
- echovirus B97.12
- other specified B97.19

Enthesopathy (peripheral) M77.9
- ankle and tarsus M77.5
  - specified type NEC—*see* Enthesopathy, foot, specified type NEC
- elbow region M77.8
  - lateral epicondylitis—*see* Epicondylitis, lateral
  - medial epicondylitis—*see* Epicondylitis, medial
- foot NEC M77.9
  - specified type NEC M77.5-
- forearm M77.9
- hand M77.9
- hip —*see* Enthesopathy, lower limb, specified type NEC
- iliac crest spur—*see* Spur, bone, iliac crest
- lateral epicondylitis—*see* Epicondylitis, lateral
- lower limb (excluding foot) M76.9
  - Achilles tendinitis—*see* Tendinitis, Achilles
  - anterior tibial syndrome M76.81-
  - iliac crest spur—*see* Spur, bone, iliac crest
  - iliotibial band syndrome—*see* Syndrome, iliotibial band

Enthesopathy (peripheral), *continued*
- pelvic region—*see* Enthesopathy, lower limb, specified type NEC
  - posterior tibial syndrome M76.82-
  - specified type NEC M76.89-
  - tibial collateral bursitis—*see* Bursitis, tibial collateral
- medial epicondylitis—*see* Epicondylitis, medial
- metatarsalgia—*see* Metatarsalgia
- multiple sites M77.9
- pelvis M77.9
- posterior tibial syndrome M76.82-
- psoas tendinitis—*see* Tendinitis
- shoulder M77.9
- specified site NEC M77.9
- specified type NEC M77.8
- upper arm M77.9
- wrist and carpus NEC M77.8

Entropion (eyelid) (paralytic)
- congenital Q10.2

Enuresis R32
- functional F98.0
- habit disturbance F98.0
- nocturnal N39.44
  - psychogenic F98.0
- nonorganic origin F98.0
- psychogenic F98.0

Eosinophilia (allergic) (hereditary) (idiopathic) (secondary) D72.10
- familial D72.19
- hereditary D72.19
- in disease classified elsewhere D72.18
- with
  - angiolymphoid hyperplasia (ALHE) D18.01

Eosinophilia-myalgia syndrome M35.8

Ependymoblastoma
- specified site—*see* Neoplasm, malignant, by site in Table of Neoplasms in the complete *ICD-10-CM* manual
- unspecified site C71.9

Ependymoma (epithelial) (malignant)
- anaplastic
  - specified site—*see* Neoplasm, malignant, by site in Table of Neoplasms in the complete *ICD-10-CM* manual
  - unspecified site C71.9
- benign specified site—*see* Neoplasm, benign, by site in Table of Neoplasms in the complete *ICD-10-CM* manual
- specified site—*see* Neoplasm, malignant, by site in Table of Neoplasms in the complete *ICD-10-CM* manual
- unspecified site C71.9

Ependymopathy G93.89

Epiblepharon (congenital) Q10.3

Epicanthus, epicanthic fold (eyelid) (congenital) Q10.3

Epicondylitis (elbow)
- lateral M77.1-
- medial M77.0-

Epidermodysplasia verruciformis B07.8

Epidermolysis
- bullosa (congenital) Q81.9
  - dystrophica Q81.2
  - letalis Q81.1
  - simplex Q81.0
  - specified NEC Q81.8
- necroticans combustiformis L51.2
  - due to drug—*see* Table of Drugs and Chemicals, by drug

Epididymitis (acute) (nonvenereal) (recurrent) (residual) N45.1
- with orchitis N45.3
- blennorrhagic (gonococcal) A54.23
- chlamydial A56.19
- gonococcal A54.23
- syphilitic A52.76

Epididymo-orchitis (*see also* Epididymitis) N45.3

Epiglottitis, epiglottiditis (acute) J05.10
- with obstruction J05.11
- chronic J37.0

Epilepsia partialis continua (*see also* Kozhevnikof's epilepsy) G40.1-

Epilepsy, epileptic, epilepsia (attack) (cerebral) (convulsion) (fit) (seizure) G40.909
- *Note:* the following terms are to be considered equivalent to intractable: pharmacoresistant (pharmacologically resistant), treatment resistant, refractory (medically) and poorly controlled
- benign childhood with centrotemporal EEG spikes—*see* Epilepsy, localization-related, idiopathic
- benign myoclonic in infancy G40.80-
- childhood
  - with occipital EEG paroxysms—*see* Epilepsy, localization-related, idiopathic
- generalized
  - specified NEC G40.409
    - ■ intractable G40.419
      - with status epilepticus G40.411
      - without status epilepticus G40.419
    - ■ not intractable G40.409
      - with status epilepticus G40.401
      - without status epilepticus G40.409
- impulsive petit mal—*see* Epilepsy, juvenile myoclonic
- KCNQ2-related G40.842
  - intractable G40.844
    - ■ with status epilepticus G40.843
    - ■ without status epilepticus G40.844
  - not intractable G40.842
    - ■ with status epilepticus G40.841
    - ■ without status epilepticus G40.842
- Lafora progressive myoclonus (*see also* Epilepsy, progressive, Lafora) G40.C09
- myoclonus, myoclonic—*see also* Epilepsy, generalized, specified NEC
  - progressive—*see also* Epilepsy, generalized, idiopathic
    - ■ Lafora G40.C09
      - not intractable G40.C09
      - ◊ with status epilepticus G40.C01
      - ◊ without status epilepticus G40.C09
- localization-related (focal) (partial)
- myoclonus, myoclonic—*see also* Epilepsy, generalized, specified NEC
  - progressive—*see also* Epilepsy, generalized, idiopathic
    - ■ Lafora G40.C09
      - intractable G40.C19
      - ◊ with status epilepticus G40.C11
      - ◊ without status epilepticus G40.C19
    - not intractable G40.C09
      - ◊ with status epilepticus G40.C01
      - ◊ without status epilepticus G40.C09
- not intractable G40.909
  - with status epilepticus G40.901
  - without status epilepticus G40.909
- on awakening—*see* Epilepsy, generalized, specified NEC
- parasitic NOS B71.9 [G94]
- progressive (familial) myoclonic—*see* Epilepsy, myoclonus, progressive
  - Lafora—*see also* Epilepsy, progressive, Lafora G40.C09
- spasms G40.822
  - intractable G40.824
    - ■ with status epilepticus G40.823
    - ■ without status epilepticus G40.824
  - not intractable G40.822
    - ■ with status epilepticus G40.821
    - ■ without status epilepticus G40.822
- specified NEC G40.802
  - intractable G40.804
    - ■ with status epilepticus G40.803
    - ■ without status epilepticus G40.804
  - not intractable G40.802
    - ■ with status epilepticus G40.801
    - ■ without status epilepticus G40.802
- syndromes
  - generalized
  - localization-related (focal) (partial)
    - ■ idiopathic
      - with seizures of localized onset
      - ◊ intractable G40.019
        - » without status epilepticus G40.019
  - specified NEC G40.802

ALPHABETIC INDEX

Epilepsy, epileptic, epilepsia, *continued*
- ■ intractable G40.804
  - – with status epilepticus G40.803
  - – without status epilepticus G40.804
- ■ not intractable G40.802
  - – with status epilepticus G40.801
  - – without status epilepticus G40.802
- tonic (-clonic)—*see* Epilepsy, generalized, specified NEC

Epiloia Q85.1

Epimenorrhea N92.0

Epipharyngitis—*see* Nasopharyngitis

Epiphysitis—*see also* Osteochondropathy
- juvenile M92.9

Episode
- depressive F32.A
  - – major F32.9
    - ■ mild F32.0
    - ■ moderate F32.1
    - ■ severe (without psychotic symptoms) F32.2
    - – with psychotic symptoms F32.3
  - – recurrent F33.9
    - ■ brief F33.8
    - – specified NEC F32.89

Epispadias (female) (male) Q64.0

Epistaxis (multiple) R04.0
- hereditary I78.0

Equinovarus (congenital) (talipes) Q66.0-

Equivalent
- convulsive (abdominal)—*see* Epilepsy, specified NEC
- epileptic (psychic)—*see* Epilepsy, localization-related, symptomatic, with complex partial seizures

Erb (-Duchenne) paralysis (birth injury) (newborn) P14.0

Erb-Goldflam disease or syndrome G70.00
- with exacerbation (acute) G70.01
- in crisis G70.01

Erb's
- disease G71.02
- palsy, paralysis (brachial) (birth) (newborn) P14.0
- pseudohypertrophic muscular dystrophy G71.02

Erdheim's syndrome (acromegalic macrospondylitis) E22.0

Erosio interdigitalis blastomycetica B37.2

Erosion
- cervix (uteri) (acquired) (chronic) (congenital) N86
  - – with cervicitis N72

Eructation R14.2
- nervous or psychogenic F45.8

Eruption
- drug (generalized) (taken internally) L27.0
  - – fixed L27.1
  - – in contact with skin—*see* Dermatitis, due to drugs and medicaments
  - – localized L27.1
- napkin L22
- skin (nonspecific) R21
  - – due to inoculation/vaccination (generalized) (*see also* Dermatitis, due to, vaccine) L27.0
    - ■ localized L27.1
  - – feigned L98.1
- tooth, teeth, abnormal (incomplete) (late) (premature) (sequence) K00.6

Erysipelas (gangrenous) (infantile) (newborn) (phlegmonous) (suppurative) A46
- external ear A46 *[H62.4-]*

Erythema, erythematous (infectional) (inflammation) L53.9
- arthriticum epidemicum A25.1
- chronicum migrans (Borrelia burgdorferi) A69.20
- diaper L22
- gluteal L22
- ichthyosiforme congenitum bullous Q80.3
- induratum (nontuberculous) L52
- infectiosum B08.3
- intertrigo L30.4
- marginatum L53.2
  - – in (due to) acute rheumatic fever I00
- migrans A26.0
  - – chronicum A69.20
  - – tongue K14.1

Erythema, erythematous, *continued*
- multiforme (major) (minor) L51.9
  - – bullous, bullosum L51.1
  - – conjunctiva L51.1
  - – specified NEC L51.8
- napkin L22
- neonatorum P83.88
  - – toxic P83.1
- nodosum L52
- rash, newborn P83.88
- solare L55.0
- toxic, toxicum NEC L53.0
  - – newborn P83.1

Erythremia (acute) C94.0-
- secondary D75.1

Erythroblastopenia (*see also* Aplasia, red cell) D60.9
- congenital D61.01

Erythroblastophthisis D61.09

Erythroblastosis (fetalis) (newborn) P55.9
- due to
  - – ABO (antibodies) (incompatibility) (isoimmunization) P55.1

Erythrocyanosis (crurum) I73.89

Erythrocytosis (megalosplenic) (secondary) D75.1
- familial D75.0
- oval, hereditary—*see* Elliptocytosis
- secondary D75.1
- stress D75.1

Erythroderma (secondary) (*see also* Erythema) L53.9
- bullous ichthyosiform, congenital Q80.3
- desquamativum L21.1
- ichthyosiform, congenital (bullous) Q80.3
- neonatorum P83.88
- psoriaticum L40.8

Erythrodysesthesia, palmar plantar (PPE) L27.1

Erythrogenesis imperfecta D61.09

Erythrophagocytosis D75.89

Escherichia coli (E. coli), as cause of disease classified elsewhere B96.20
- non-0157 Shiga toxin-producing (with known O group) B96.22
- non-Shiga toxin-producing B96.29
- 0157 with confirmation of Shiga toxin when H antigen is unknown, or is not H7 B96.21
- 0157:H- (nonmotile)with confirmation of Shiga toxin B96.21
- 0157:H7 with or without confirmation of Shiga toxin-production B96.21
- Shiga toxin-producing (with unspecified O group) (STEC) B96.23
  - 0157 B96.21
- 0157:H7 with or without confirmation of Shiga toxin-production B96.21
  - – specified NEC B96.22
- specified NEC B96.29

Esophagitis (acute) (alkaline) (chemical) (chronic) (infectional) (necrotic) (peptic) (postoperative) K20.9-
- candidal B37.81
- due to gastrointestinal reflux disease K21.0-
- eosinophilic K20.0
- reflux K21.0-
- specified NEC K20.80

Estrangement (marital) Z63.5
- parent-child NEC Z62.890

Ethmoiditis (chronic) (nonpurulent) (purulent)—*see also* Sinusitis, ethmoidal
- influenzal—*see* Influenza manifestations NEC

Evaluation (for) (of)
- development state
  - – adolescent Z00.3
  - – period of
    - ■ delayed growth in childhood Z00.70
    - – with abnormal findings Z00.71
    - ■ rapid growth in childhood Z00.2
  - – puberty Z00.3
- growth and developmental state (period of rapid growth) Z00.2

Evaluation, *continued*
- period of
  - – delayed growth in childhood Z00.70
    - ■ with abnormal findings Z00.71
  - – rapid growth in childhood Z00.2
- suspected condition—*see* Observation

Evans syndrome D69.41

Event
- apparent life threatening in newborn and infant (ALTE) R68.13
- brief resolved unexplained event (BRUE) R68.13

Eversion
- cervix (uteri) N86
  - – with cervicitis N72

Evisceration
- birth injury P15.8

Examination (for) (following) (general) (of) (routine) Z00.00
- with abnormal findings Z00.01
- abuse, physical (alleged), ruled out
  - – child Z04.72
- adolescent (development state) Z00.3
- alleged rape or sexual assault (victim), ruled out
  - – child Z04.42
- annual (adult) (periodic) (physical) Z00.00
  - – with abnormal findings Z00.01
  - – gynecological Z01.419
    - ■ with abnormal findings Z01.411
- blood—*see* Examination, laboratory
- blood pressure Z01.30
  - – with abnormal findings Z01.31
- cervical Papanicolaou smear Z12.4
  - – as part of routine gynecological examination Z01.419
    - ■ with abnormal findings Z01.411
- child (over 28 days old) Z00.129
  - – with abnormal findings Z00.121
  - – under 28 days old—*see* Newborn, examination
- contraceptive (drug) maintenance (routine) Z30.8
  - – device (intrauterine) Z30.431
- developmental—*see* Examination, child
- ear Z01.10
  - – with abnormal findings NEC Z01.118
- eye Z01.00
  - – with abnormal findings Z01.01
  - – after failed exam Z01.02
- following
  - – accident NEC Z04.3
    - ■ transport Z04.1
    - ■ work Z04.2
  - – assault, alleged, ruled out
    - ■ child Z04.72
  - – motor vehicle accident Z04.1
  - – treatment (for) Z09
    - ■ combined NEC Z09
    - – fracture Z09
      - – malignant neoplasm Z08
      - ■ malignant neoplasm Z08
    - ■ mental disorder Z09
    - ■ specified condition NEC Z09
- follow-up (routine) (following) Z09
  - – chemotherapy NEC Z09
    - ■ malignant neoplasm Z08
  - – fracture Z09
    - – malignant neoplasm Z08
  - – radiotherapy NEC Z09
    - ■ malignant neoplasm Z08
  - – surgery NEC Z09
    - ■ malignant neoplasm Z08
- forced labor exploitation Z04.82
- forced sexual exploitation Z04.81
- gynecological Z01.419
  - – with abnormal findings Z01.411
  - – for contraceptive maintenance Z30.8
- health—*see* Examination, medical
- hearing Z01.10
  - – with abnormal findings Z01.118
  - – following failed hearing screening Z01.110
- infant or child (28 days and older) Z00.129
  - ■ with abnormal findings Z00.121
- immunity status testing Z01.84
- laboratory (as part of a general medical examination) Z00.00

ALPHABETIC INDEX

Examination, *continued*
- with abnormal findings Z00.01
- preprocedural Z01.812
- lactating mother Z39.1
- medical (adult) (for) (of) Z00.00
  - with abnormal findings Z00.01
  - administrative purpose only Z02.9
    - specified NEC Z02.89
  - admission to
    - school Z02.0
      - following illness or medical treatment Z02.0
    - summer camp Z02.89
  - adoption Z02.82
  - blood alcohol or drug level Z02.83
  - camp (summer) Z02.89
  - general (adult) Z00.00
    - with abnormal findings Z00.01
  - medicolegal reasons NEC Z04.89
  - participation in sport Z02.5
  - pre-operative—*see* Examination, pre-procedural
  - pre-procedural
    - cardiovascular Z01.810
    - respiratory Z01.811
    - specified NEC Z01.818
  - preschool children
    - for admission to school Z02.0
  - sport competition Z02.5
- medicolegal reason NEC Z04.89
  - following
    - forced labor exploitation Z04.82
    - forced sexual exploitation Z04.81
- newborn—*see* Newborn, examination
- pelvic (annual) (periodic) Z01.419
  - with abnormal findings Z01.411
- period of rapid growth in childhood Z00.2
- periodic (adult) (annual) (routine) Z00.00
  - with abnormal findings Z00.01
- physical (adult)—*see also* Examination, medical Z00.00
  - sports Z02.5
- pre-chemotherapy (antineoplastic) Z01.818
- pre-procedural (pre-operative)
  - cardiovascular Z01.810
  - laboratory Z01.812
  - respiratory Z01.811
  - specified NEC Z01.818
- prior to chemotherapy (antineoplastic) Z01.818
- radiological (as part of a general medical examination) Z00.00
  - with abnormal findings Z00.01
- repeat cervical smear to confirm findings of recent normal smear following initial abnormal smear Z01.42
- skin (hypersensitivity) Z01.82
- special (*see also* Examination) Z01.89
  - specified type NEC Z01.89
- specified type or reason NEC Z04.89
- urine—*see* Examination, laboratory
- vision Z01.00
  - following failed vision screening Z01.020
    - with abnormal findings Z01.021
  - infant or child (over 28 days old) Z00.129
    - with abnormal findings Z00.121
  - with abnormal findings Z01.01

Exanthem, exanthema—*see also* Rash
- with enteroviral vesicular stomatitis B08.4
- subitum B08.20
  - due to human herpesvirus 6 B08.21
  - due to human herpesvirus 7 B08.22
- viral, virus B09
  - specified type NEC B08.8

Excess, excessive, excessively
- alcohol level in blood R78.0
- crying
  - in child, adolescent, or adult R45.83
  - in infant R68.11
- development, breast N62
- drinking (alcohol) NEC (without dependence) F10.10
  - habitual (continual) (without remission) F10.20
- eating R63.2
- foreskin N47.8
- gas R14.0

Excess, excessive, excessively, *continued*
- large
  - colon K59.39
    - congenital Q43.8
    - toxic K59.31
  - infant P08.0
  - organ or site, congenital NEC—*see* Anomaly, by site
- long
  - organ or site, congenital NEC—*see* Anomaly, by site
- menstruation (with regular cycle) N92.0
  - with irregular cycle N92.1
- napping Z72.821
- natrium E87.0
- secretion—*see also* Hypersecretion
  - sweat R61
- skin and subcutaneous tissue L98.7
  - eyelid (acquired)—*see* Blepharochalasis
    - congenital Q10.3
- sodium (Na) E87.0
- sweating R61
- thirst R63.1
  - due to deprivation of water T73.1
- weight
  - gain R63.5
  - loss R63.4

Excitability, abnormal, under minor stress (personality disorder) F60.3

Excitation
- anomalous atrioventricular I45.6

Excoriation (traumatic)—*see also* Abrasion
- neurotic L98.1
- skin picking disorder F42.4

Exhaustion, exhaustive (physical NEC) R53.83
- battle F43.0
- cardiac—*see* Failure, heart
- delirium F43.0
- heat (*see also* Heat, exhaustion) T67.5
  - due to
    - salt depletion T67.4
    - water depletion T67.3
- psychosis F43.0

Exomphalos Q79.2
- meaning hernia—*see* Hernia, umbilicus

Exotropia—*see* Strabismus, divergent concomitant

Explanation of
- investigation finding Z71.2
- medication Z71.89

Exploitation
- labor
  - confirmed
    - adult forced T74.61
    - child forced T74.62
  - suspected
    - adult forced T76.61
    - child forced T76.62
- sexual
  - confirmed
    - adult forced T74.51
    - child T74.52
  - suspected
    - adult forced T76.51
    - child T76.52

Exposure (to) (*see also* Contact) T75.89
- AIDS virus Z20.6
- anthrax Z20.810
- aromatic amines Z77.020
- aromatic (hazardous) compounds NEC Z77.028
- aromatic dyes NOS Z77.028
- arsenic Z77.010
- asbestos Z77.090
- bacterial disease NEC Z20.818
- benzene Z77.021
- body fluids (potentially hazardous) Z77.21
- chemicals (chiefly nonmedicinal) (hazardous) NEC Z77.098
- chromium compounds Z77.018
- communicable disease Z20.9
  - bacterial NEC Z20.818
  - specified NEC Z20.89
  - viral NEC Z20.828
- coronavirus (disease) (novel) 2019 Z20.822

Exposure, *continued*
- dyes Z77.098
- environmental tobacco smoke (acute) (chronic) Z77.22
- Escherichia coli (E. coli) Z20.01
- German measles Z20.4
- gonorrhea Z20.2
- hazardous metals NEC Z77.018
- hazardous substances NEC Z77.29
- hazards in the physical environment NEC Z77.128
- hazards to health NEC Z77.9
- human immunodeficiency virus (HIV) Z20.6
- human T-lymphotropic virus type-1 (HTLV-1) Z20.89
- infestation (parasitic) NEC Z20.7
- intestinal infectious disease NEC Z20.09
  - Escherichia coli (E. coli) Z20.01
- lead Z77.011
- meningococcus Z20.811
- mold (toxic) Z77.120
- nickel dust Z77.018
- poliomyelitis Z20.89
- polycyclic aromatic hydrocarbons Z77.028
- prenatal (drugs) (toxic chemicals)—*see* Newborn, noxious substances transmitted via placenta or breast milk
- rabies Z20.3
- rubella Z20.4
- second hand tobacco smoke (acute) (chronic) Z77.22
  - in the perinatal period P96.81
- sexually-transmitted disease Z20.2
- smallpox (laboratory) Z20.89
- syphilis Z20.2
- tuberculosis Z20.1
- varicella Z20.820
- venereal disease Z20.2
- viral disease NEC Z20.828
- Zika virus Z20.821

Exstrophy
- abdominal contents Q45.8
- bladder Q64.10
  - cloacal Q64.12
  - specified type NEC Q64.19
  - supravesical fissure Q64.11

Extrasystoles (supraventricular) I49.49
- atrial I49.1
- auricular I49.1

Extravasation
- pelvicalyceal N13.8
- pyelosinus N13.8
- vesicant agent
  - antineoplastic chemotherapy T80.810
  - other agent NEC T80.818

F

Failure, failed
- aortic (valve) I35.8
  - rheumatic I06.8
- biventricular I50.82
- cardiorenal (chronic) I50.9
- cardiorespiratory (*see also* Failure, heart) R09.2
- circulation, circulatory (peripheral) R57.9
  - newborn P29.89
- compensation—*see* Disease, heart
- compliance with medical treatment or regimen—*see* Noncompliance
- expansion terminal respiratory units (newborn) (primary) P28.0
- gain weight (child over 28 days old) R62.51
  - newborn P92.6
- heart (acute) (senile) (sudden) I50.9
  - biventricular I50.82
  - combined left-right sided I50.82
  - compensated I50.9
  - congestive (compensated) (decompensated) I50.9
    - with rheumatic fever (conditions in I00)
      - active I01.8
      - inactive or quiescent (with chorea) I09.81
    - newborn P29.0
    - rheumatic (chronic) (inactive) (with chorea) I09.81
      - active or acute I01.8
      - ◊ with chorea I02.0

ALPHABETIC INDEX

Failure, failed, *continued*

- decompensated I50.9
  - ■ newborn P29.0
- diastolic (congestive) (left ventricular) I50.3-
  - ■ combined with systolic (congestive) I50.40
    - ~ acute (congestive) I50.41
      - ◊ and (on) chronic (congestive) I50.43
    - ~ chronic (congestive) I50.42
      - ◊ and (on) acute (congestive) I50.43
- due to presence of cardiac prosthesis I97.13-
- following cardiac surgery I97.13-
- high output NOS I50.83
- low output (syndrome) NOS I50.9
- postprocedural I97.13-
- specified NEC I50.89
- Note: heart failure stages A, B, C, and D are based on the American College of Cardiology and American Heart Association stages of heart failure, which complement and should not be confused with the New York Heart Association Classification of Heart Failure, into Class I, Class II, Class III, and Class IV
- stage A Z91.89
- stage B—*see also* Failure, heart, by type as diastolic or systolic I50.9
- stage C—*see also* Failure, heart, by type as diastolic or systolic I50.9
- stage D—*see also* Failure, heart, by type as diastolic or systolic, chronic I50.84
- systolic (congestive) (left ventricular) I50.2-
  - ■ combined with diastolic (congestive) I50.40
    - ~ acute (congestive) I50.41
    - ~ chronic (congestive) I50.42
      - ◊ and (on) acute (congestive) I50.43
- intestinal failure K90.83
- kidney (*see also* Disease, kidney, chronic) N19
  - acute (*see also* Failure, renal, acute) N17.9-
  - diabetic—*see* E08-E13 with .22
- lactation (complete) O92.3
  - partial O92.4
- mitral I05.9
- myocardial, myocardium (*see also* Failure, heart) I50.9
  - chronic (*see also* Failure, heart, congestive) I50.9
  - congestive (*see also* Failure, heart, congestive) I50.9
- newborn screening P09.-
- ovulation causing infertility N97.0
- renal N19
  - with
    - ■ tubular necrosis (acute) N17.0
  - acute N17.9
    - ■ with
      - ~ cortical necrosis N17.1
      - ~ medullary necrosis N17.2
      - ~ tubular necrosis N17.0
      - ■ specified NEC N17.8
  - chronic N18.9
  - congenital P96.0
  - end stage N18.6
    - ■ due to hypertension I12.0
- respiration, respiratory J96.90
  - with
    - ■ hypercapnia J96.92
    - ■ hypercarbia J96.92
    - ■ hypoxia J96.91
  - acute J96.00
    - ■ with
      - ~ hypercapnia J96.02
      - ~ hypercarbia J96.02
      - ~ hypoxia J96.01
  - center G93.89
  - chronic J96.10
    - ■ with
      - ~ hypercapnia J96.12
      - ~ hypercarbia J96.12
      - ~ hypoxia J96.11
  - newborn P28.5
  - postprocedural (acute) J95.821
    - ■ acute and chronic J95.822
- to thrive (child over 28 days old) R62.51
  - newborn P92.6
- transplant T86.-
  - bone
    - ■ marrow T86.02

Failure, failed, *continued*

- heart T86.22
  - ■ with lung(s) T86.32
- kidney T86.12
- liver T86.42
- lung(s) T86.811
  - ■ with heart T86.32
- stem cell (peripheral blood) (umbilical cord) T86.5
- ventricular (*see also* Failure, heart) I50.9
  - left I50.1
    - ■ with rheumatic fever (conditions in I00)
      - ~ active I01.8
        - ◊ with chorea I02.0
      - ~ inactive or quiescent (with chorea) I09.81
    - ■ rheumatic (chronic) (inactive) (with chorea) I09.81
      - ~ active or acute I01.8
        - ◊ with chorea I02.0
  - right (*see also* Failure, heart, congestive) I50.9
- vital centers, newborn P91.88

Fainting (fit) R55

Fallot's

- tetrad or tetralogy Q21.3

Family, familial—*see also* Disease, diseased

- disruption Z63.8
  - involving divorce or separation Z63.5
- planning advice Z30.09
- problem Z63.9
  - specified NEC Z63.8
- retinoblastoma C69.2-

Fanconi('s) anemia D61.03

Fanconi hypoplastic anemia D61.03

Fanconi panmyelopathy D61.03

Fasciitis M72.9

- infective M72.8
- necrotizing M72.6
- necrotizing M72.6

Fascioscapulohumeral myopathy G71.02

Fast pulse R00.0

Fat

- in stool R19.5

Fatigue R53.83

- auditory deafness—*see* Deafness
- chronic R53.82
- combat F43.0
- general R53.83
- muscle M62.89

Fatigue syndrome

- myalgic encephalomyelitis/chronic fatigue syndrome G93.32
- other postinfection and related fatigue syndromes G93.39
- postviral fatigue syndrome G93.31

Fatty—*see also* Disease, diseased

- liver NEC K76.0
  - nonalcoholic K76.0

Faucitis J02.9

Favism (anemia) D55.0

Favus—*see* Dermatophytosis

Fear complex or reaction F40.9

Fear of—*see* Phobia

Febris, febrile—*see also* Fever

- rubra A38.9

Fecal

- incontinence R15.9
- smearing R15.1
- soiling R15.1
- urgency R15.2

Fecalith (impaction) K56.41

Fede's disease K14.0

Feeble rapid pulse due to shock following injury T79.4

Feeble-minded F70

Feeding

- difficulties R63.30
- problem R63.39
  - newborn P92.9
    - ■ specified NEC P92.8
  - nonorganic (adult)—*see* Disorder, eating

Feeling (of)

- foreign body in throat R09.89

Feet—*see* Disease, diseased

Feigned illness Z76.5

Fetid

- breath R19.6

Fetus, fetal—*see also* Disease, diseased

- alcohol (syndrome) (dysmorphic) Q86.0
- lung tissue P28.0

Fever (inanition) (of unknown origin) (persistent) (with chills) (with rigor) R50.9

- African tick bite A77.8
- American
  - mountain (tick) A93.2
  - spotted A77.0
- Bullis A77.0
- catarrhal (acute) J00
  - chronic J31.0
- cerebrospinal meningococcal A39.0
- Colorado tick (virus) A93.2
- due to
  - conditions classified elsewhere R50.81
  - heat T67.0-
- ephemeral (of unknown origin) R50.9
- epidemic hemorrhagic A98.5
- erysipelatous—*see* Erysipelas
- glandular—*see* Mononucleosis, infectious
- Haverhill A25.1
- hay (allergic) J30.1
  - with asthma (bronchial) J45.909
    - ■ with
      - ~ exacerbation (acute) J45.901
      - ~ status asthmaticus J45.902
  - due to
    - ■ allergen other than pollen J30.89
    - ■ pollen, any plant or tree J30.1
- heat (effects) T67.0-
- hemorrhagic (arthropod-borne) NOS A94
  - arenaviral A96.9
- intermittent (bilious)—*see also* Malaria
  - of unknown origin R50.9
- Lone Star A77.0
- mountain
  - meaning Rocky Mountain spotted fever A77.0
  - tick (American) (Colorado) (viral) A93.2
- newborn P81.9
  - environmental P81.0
- non-exanthematous tick A93.2
- persistent (of unknown origin) R50.9
- petechial A39.0
- postimmunization R50.83
- postoperative R50.82
  - due to infection T81.40
- posttransfusion R50.84
- postvaccination R50.83
- presenting with conditions classified elsewhere R50.81
- rat-bite A25.9
  - due to
    - ■ Spirillum A25.0
    - ■ Streptobacillus moniliformis A25.1
- relapsing (Borrelia) A68.9
  - louse borne A68.0
  - Novy's
    - ■ louse-borne A68.0
    - ■ tick-bourne A68.1
  - tick borne A68.1
- rheumatic (active) (acute) (chronic) (subacute) I00
  - with central nervous system involvement I02.9
  - active with heart involvement (*see* category) I01
  - inactive or quiescent with
    - ■ cardiac hypertrophy I09.89
    - ■ carditis I09.9
    - ■ endocarditis I09.1
      - ~ aortic (valve) I06.9
        - ◊ with mitral (valve) disease I08.0
      - ~ mitral (valve) I05.9
        - ◊ with aortic (valve) disease I08.0
      - ~ pulmonary (valve) I09.89
      - ~ tricuspid (valve) I07.8
    - ■ heart disease NEC I09.89
    - ■ heart failure (congestive) (conditions in I50) I09.81

Fever, *continued*
- left ventricular failure (conditions in I50.1–I50.4-) I09.81
- myocarditis, myocardial degeneration (conditions in I51.4) I09.0
  - pancarditis I09.9
    - pericarditis I09.2
- Rocky Mountain spotted A77.0
- rose J30.1
- Sao Paulo A77.0
- scarlet A38.9
- specified NEC A96.8
  - viral A99
    - specified NEC A98.8
- spirillary A25.0
- spotted A77.9
  - American A77.0
  - Brazilian A77.0
  - cerebrospinal meningitis A39.0
  - Columbian A77.0
  - due to Rickettsia
    - rickettsii A77.0
  - Ehrlichiosis A77.40
    - due to
      - E. chaffeensis A77.41
  - Rocky Mountain spotted A77.0
- streptobacillary A25.1
- swine A02.8
- thermic T67.0-
- unknown origin R50.9
- uveoparotid D86.69
- West Nile (viral) A92.30
  - with
    - complications NEC A92.39
    - cranial nerve disorders A92.32
    - encephalitis A92.31
    - encephalomyelitis A92.31
    - neurologic manifestation NEC A92.32
    - optic neuritis A92.32
    - polyradiculitis A92.32
- yellow A95.9
  - jungle A95.0
  - sylvatic A95.0
  - urban A95.1
- Zika virus A92.5

Fibrillation
- atrial or auricular (established) I48.91
  - cardiac I49.8
  - chronic I48.20
    - persistent I48.19
  - paroxysmal I48.0
  - permanent I48.21
  - persistent (chronic) (NOS) (other) I48.19
    - longstanding I48.11
- heart I49.8
  - muscular M62.89
  - ventricular I49.01

Fibrinogenopenia D68.8
- acquired D65
- congenital D68.2

Fibrinolysis (hemorrhagic) (acquired) D65
- newborn, transient P60

Fibrocystic
- disease—*see also* Fibrosis, cystic
  - pancreas E84.9

Fibromatosis M72.9
- gingival K06.1

Fibromyxolipoma D17.9

Fibroplasia, retrolental H35.17-

Fibrosis, fibrotic
- anal papillae K62.89
- cystic (of pancreas) E84.9
  - with
    - distal intestinal obstruction syndrome E84.19
    - fecal impaction E84.19
    - intestinal manifestations NEC E84.19
    - pulmonary manifestations E84.0
    - specified manifestations NEC E84.8
- meninges G96.198
- pericardium I31.0

Fibrosis, fibrotic, *continued*
- rectal sphincter K62.89
- retroperitoneal K68.2
- skin L90.5

Fiedler's
- myocarditis (acute) I40.1

Fifth disease B08.3

Filatov's disease—*see* Mononucleosis, infectious

Fimbrial cyst Q50.4

Financial problem affecting care NOS Z59.-
- financial insecurity Z59.86

Findings, abnormal, inconclusive, without diagnosis—*see also* Abnormal
- alcohol in blood R78.0
- antenatal screening of mother O28.9
  - biochemical O28.1
  - chromosomal O28.5
  - cytological O28.2
  - genetic O28.5
  - hematological O28.0
  - radiological O28.4
  - specified NEC O28.8
  - ultrasonic O28.3
- bacteriuria R82.71
- bicarbonate E87.8
- blood sugar R73.09
  - high R73.9
  - low (transient) E16.2
- casts or cells, urine R82.998
- chloride E87.8
- cholesterol E78.9
  - high E78.00
    - with high triglycerides E78.2
- creatinine clearance R94.4
- crystals, urine R82.998
- culture
  - blood R78.81
  - positive—*see* Positive, culture
- echocardiogram R93.1
- electrolyte level, urinary R82.998
- function study NEC R94.8
  - bladder R94.8
  - endocrine NEC R94.7
    - kidney R94.4
    - liver R94.5
    - pancreas R94.8
    - placenta R94.8
    - pulmonary R94.2
    - spleen R94.8
    - thyroid R94.6
- glycosuria R81
- heart
  - shadow R93.1
  - sounds R01.2
- hematinuria R82.3
- hemoglobinuria R82.3
- in blood (of substance not normally found in blood) R78.9
  - alcohol (excessive level) R78.0
  - lead R78.71
- lactic acid dehydrogenase (LDH) R74.02
- liver function test (*see also* Elevated, liver function, test) R79.89
- neonatal screening/newborn state mandated P09.-
- PPD R76.11
- radiologic (X-ray) R93.89
  - abdomen R93.5
  - intrathoracic organs NEC R93.1
  - musculoskeletal
    - limbs R93.6
    - other than limb R93.7
  - retroperitoneum R93.5
  - testis R93.81-
- scan NEC R94.8
  - bladder R94.8
  - bone R94.8
  - kidney R94.4
  - liver R93.2
  - lung R94.2
  - pancreas R94.8
  - placental R94.8

Findings, abnormal, inconclusive, without diagnosis, *continued*
- spleen R94.8
- thyroid R94.6
- sedimentation rate, elevated R70.0
- SGOT R74.01
- SGPT R74.01
- sodium (deficiency) E87.1
  - excess E87.0
- stress test R94.39
- thyroid (function) (metabolic rate) (scan) (uptake) R94.6
- transaminase (level) R74.01
- triglycerides E78.9
  - high E78.1
    - with high cholesterol E78.2
- tuberculin skin test (without active tuberculosis) R76.11
- urine
  - bacteriuria R82.71
  - casts or cells R82.998
  - culture positive R82.79
  - glucose R81
  - hemoglobin R82.3
  - sugar R81
- vectorcardiogram (VCG) R94.39

Fire, Saint Anthony's—*see* Erysipelas

Fissure, fissured
- anus, anal K60.2
  - acute K60.0
  - chronic K60.1
  - congenital Q43.8
- lip K13.0
  - congenital—see Cleft, lip
- nipple N64.0
  - associated with
    - lactation O92.13
    - puerperium O92.12

Fistula (cutaneous) L98.8
- abdominothoracic J86.0
- accessory sinuses—*see* Sinusitis
- anorectal (infectional) K60.50
  - complex K60.529
  - chronic K60.522
    - initial K60.521
    - new K60.521
    - occurring following complete healing K60.523
    - persistent K60.522
    - recurrent K60.523
    - extrasphincteríc K60.52-
  - high intersphincteric K60.52-
  - low intersphincteric K60.51-
    - simple K60.519
    - chronic K60.512
      - initial K60.511
      - new K60.511
      - occurring following complete healing K60.513
      - persistent K60.512
      - recurrent K60.513
    - superficial K60.51-
  - suprasphincteríc K60.52-
  - transsphincteric K60.52-
- anus, anal (recurrent) (infectional) K60.30
  - complex K60.329
    - chronic K60.322
      - initial K60.321
      - new K60.321
      - occurring following complete healing K60.323
      - persistent K60.322
      - recurrent K60.323
  - congenital Q43.6
    - with absence, atresia and stenosis Q42.2
  - extrasphincteríc K60.42-
  - high intersphincteric K60.32-
  - low intersphincteric K60.31-
    - simple K60.319
      - chronic K60.312
        - initial K60.311
        - new K60.311
        - occurring following complete healing K60.313
        - persistent K60.312
    - superficial K60.31-
  - suprasphincteríc K60.32-
  - transsphincteric K60.32-

Fistula, *continued*

- arteriovenous (acquired) (nonruptured) I77.0
  - brain I67.1
    - congenital Q28.2
      - ruptured—*see* Fistula, arteriovenous, brain, ruptured
    - ruptured I60.8-
      - intracerebral I61.8
      - intraparenchymal I61.8
      - intraventricular I61.5
      - subarachnoid I60.8-
  - cerebral—*see* Fistula, arteriovenous, brain
  - congenital (peripheral)—*see also* Malformation, arteriovenous
    - brain Q28.2
      - ruptured I60.8-
        - pulmonary Q25.72
    - pulmonary I28.0
      - congenital Q25.72
  - surgically created (for dialysis) Z99.2
- brain G93.89
- breast N61.0
- bronchial J86.0
- bronchocutaneous, bronchomediastinal, bronchopleural, bronchopleuro-mediastinal (infective) J86.0
- bronchoesophageal J86.0
  - congenital Q39.2
    - with atresia of esophagus Q39.1
- bronchovisceral J86.0
- buccal cavity (infective) K12.2
- cerebrospinal (fluid) G96.08
- chest (wall) J86.0
- colovesical N32.1
- costal region J86.0
- cystic duct
  - congenital Q44.5
- diaphragm J86.0
- esophagobronchial J86.0
  - congenital Q39.2
    - with atresia of esophagus Q39.1
- esophagocutaneous K22.89
- esophagopleural-cutaneous J86.0
- esophagotracheal J86.0
  - congenital Q39.2
    - with atresia of esophagus Q39.1
- esophagus K22.89
  - congenital Q39.2
    - with atresia of esophagus Q39.1
- ethmoid—*see* Sinusitis, ethmoidal
- hepatopleural J86.0
- hepatopulmonary J86.0
- in ano K60.30
- ischiorectal (fossa) K61.39
- lip K13.0
  - congenital Q38.0
- lung J86.0
- mammary (gland) N61.0
- maxillary J32.0
- mediastinal J86.0
- mediastinobronchial J86.0
- mediastinocutaneous J86.0
- mouth K12.2
- nasal J34.89
  - sinus—*see* Sinusitis
- nose J34.89
- oral (cutaneous) K12.2
  - maxillary J32.0
- oroantral J32.0
- parotid (gland) K11.4
  - region K12.2
- perianal K60.30
- perineo rectal K60.40
- perirectal K60.40
- pleura, pleural, pleurocutaneous, pleuroperitoneal J86.0
- pleuropericardial I31.8
- pulmonary J86.0
  - arteriovenous I28.0
    - congenital Q25.72
- pulmonoperitoneal J86.0
- rectal (infectional) K60.40
  - complex K60.429
    - chronic K60.422
    - initial K60.421

Fistula, *continued*

- new K60.421
- occurring following complete healing K60.423
- persistent K60.422
- recurrent K60.423
- rectum (to skin) K60.40
  - congenital Q43.6
    - with absence, atresia and stenosis Q42.0
- skin L98.8
- submaxillary (gland) K11.4
  - region K12.2
- thoracic J86.0
- thoracoabdominal J86.0
- thoracogastric J86.0
- thoracointestinal J86.0
- thorax J86.0
- thyroglossal duct Q89.2
- tracheoesophageal J86.0
  - congenital Q39.2
    - with atresia of esophagus Q39.1

Fit R56.9

- epileptic—*see* Epilepsy
- fainting R55
- newborn P90

Flail

- chest S22.5
  - chest compression and cardiopulmonary resuscitation M96.A4
  - newborn (birth injury) P13.8
- joint (paralytic) M25.2-
  - ankle M25.27-
  - elbow M25.22-
  - foot joint M25.27-
  - hand joint M25.24-
  - hip M25.25-
  - knee M25.26-
  - shoulder M25.21-
  - specified joint NEC M25.28
  - wrist M25.23-

Flat

- foot (acquired) (fixed type) (painful) (postural)—*see also* Deformity, limb, flat foot
  - congenital (rigid) (spastic) (everted) Q66.5-
- pelvis M95.5
  - congenital Q74.2

Flattening

- nose (congenital) Q67.4
  - acquired M95.0

Flatulence R14.3

- psychogenic F45.8

Flexion

- deformity, joint (*see also* Deformity, limb, flexion) M21.20
  - hip, congenital Q65.89

Flint murmur (aortic insufficiency) I35.1

Floating

- gallbladder, congenital Q44.1

Flooding N92.0

Floppy

- baby syndrome (nonspecific) P94.2

Flu—*see also* Influenza

- avian (*see also* Influenza, due to, identified novel influenza A virus) J09.X2
- bird (*see also* Influenza, due to, identified novel influenza A virus) J09.X2
- intestinal NEC A08.4
- swine (viruses that normally cause infections in pigs) (*see also* Influenza, due to, identified novel influenza A virus) J09.X2

Fluid

- abdomen R18.8
- loss (acute) E86.9
- peritoneal cavity R18.8
- retention R60.9

Fluoride varnish application Z29.3

Fluorosis

- dental K00.3

Flutter

- atrial or auricular I48.92
  - atypical I48.4
  - type I I48.3
  - type II I48.4
  - typical I48.3
- heart I49.8
  - atrial or auricular I48.92
  - atypical I48.4
  - type I I48.3
  - type II I48.4
  - typical I48.3
  - ventricular I49.02
- ventricular I49.02

FNHTR (febrile nonhemolytic transfusion reaction) R50.84

Follicle

- graafian, ruptured, with hemorrhage N83.0-

Folliculitis (superficial) L73.9

- cyst N83.0-
- gonococcal (acute) (chronic) A54.01

Folling's disease E70.0

Follow-up—*see* Examination, follow-up

Food

- allergy L27.2
- asphyxia (from aspiration or inhalation)—*see* Foreign body, by site
- choked on—*see* Foreign body, by site
- cyst N83.0-
- deprivation T73.0
  - specified kind of food NEC E63.8
- insecurity Z59.41
- intoxication—*see* Poisoning, food
- lack of T73.0
- poisoning—*see* Poisoning, food
- rejection NEC—*see* Disorder, eating
- strangulation or suffocation—*see* Foreign body, by site
- toxemia—*see* Poisoning, food

Foramen ovale (nonclosure) (patent) (persistent) Q21.1

Foreign body

- alimentary tract T18.9
  - esophagus—*see* Foreign body, esophagus
  - mouth T18.0
  - multiple sites T18.8
  - specified site NEC T18.8
- auditory canal—*see* Foreign body, entering through orifice, ear
- bronchus T17.50 (*See complete ICD-10-CM Manual for codes*)
- canthus—*see* Foreign body, conjunctival sac
- conjunctival sac T15.1-
- cornea T15.0-
- entering through orifice
  - accessory sinus T17.0
  - alimentary canal T18.9
    - multiple parts T18.8
    - specified part NEC T18.8
  - alveolar process T18.0
  - antrum (Highmore's) T17.0
  - anus T18.5
  - appendix T18.4
  - auditory canal T16.-
  - auricle T16.-
  - bronchioles—*see* Foreign body, respiratory tract
  - bronchus (main)—*see* Foreign body, bronchus
  - buccal cavity T18.0
  - canthus (inner) T15.1-
  - conjunctival sac T15.1-
  - digestive organ or tract NOS T18.9
    - multiple parts T18.8
    - specified part NEC T18.8
  - ear (external) T16.-
  - esophagus—*see* Foreign body, esophagus
  - eye (external) NOS T15.-
    - conjunctival sac T15.1-
    - cornea T15.0-
    - specified part NEC T15. -
  - eyeball T15. -
  - eyelid T15.1-
    - with
      - laceration—*see* Laceration, eyelid, with foreign body

ALPHABETIC INDEX

Foreign body, *continued*

- puncture—*see* Puncture, eyelid, with foreign body
- superficial injury—*see* Foreign body, superficial, eyelid
- gastrointestinal tract T18.9
  - multiple parts T18.8
  - specified part NEC T18.8
- genitourinary tract T19.9
  - multiple parts T19.8
  - specified part NEC T19.8
- Highmore's antrum T17.0
- hypopharynx—*see* Foreign body, pharynx
- lacrimal apparatus (punctum) T15.-
- larynx—*see* Foreign body, larynx
- lung—*see* Foreign body, respiratory tract
- maxillary sinus T17.0
- mouth T18.0
- nasal sinus T17.0
- nasopharynx—*see* Foreign body, pharynx
- nose (passage) T17.1
- nostril T17.1
- pharynx—*see* Foreign body, pharynx
- piriform sinus—*see* Foreign body, pharynx
- respiratory tract—*see* Foreign body, respiratory tract
- sinus (accessory) (frontal) (maxillary) (nasal) T17.0
  - piriform—*see* Foreign body, pharynx
- suffocation by—*see* Foreign body, by site
- tear ducts or glands—*see* Foreign body, entering through orifice, eye, specified part NEC
- throat—*see* Foreign body, pharynx
- tongue T18.0
- tonsil, tonsillar (fossa)—*see* Foreign body, pharynx
- trachea—*see* Foreign body, trachea
- vagina T19.2
- vulva T19.2
- esophagus T18.108
  - causing
    - injury NEC T18.108
      - food (bone) (seed) T18.128
      - gastric contents (vomitus) T18.118
      - specified type NEC T18.19-
    - tracheal compression T18.100
      - food (bone) (seed) T18.120
      - gastric contents (vomitus) T18.110
      - specified type NEC T18.190
- feeling of, in throat R09.89
- fragment—*see* Retained, foreign body fragments (type of)
- genitourinary tract T19.9
  - vagina T19.2
  - vulva T19.2
- granuloma (old) (soft tissue)—*see also* Granuloma, foreign body
  - skin L92.3
- in
  - laceration—*see* Laceration, by site, with foreign body
  - puncture wound—*see* Puncture, by site, with foreign body
  - soft tissue (residual) M79.5
- ingestion, ingested NOS T18.9
- inhalation or inspiration—*see* Foreign body, by site
- larynx T17.308
  - causing
    - asphyxiation T17.300
      - food (bone) (seed) T17.320
      - gastric contents (vomitus) T17.310
      - specified type NEC T17.390
    - injury NEC T17.308
      - food (bone) (seed) T17.328
      - gastric contents (vomitus) T17.318
      - specified type NEC T17.398
- old or residual
  - soft tissue (residual) M79.5
- pharynx T17.208
  - causing
    - asphyxiation T17.200
      - food (bone) (seed) T17.220
      - gastric contents (vomitus) T17.210
      - specified type NEC T17.290
    - injury NEC T17.208
      - food (bone) (seed) T17.228

Foreign body, *continued*

- gastric contents (vomitus) T17.218
- specified type NEC T17.298
- respiratory tract T17.908
  - bronchioles—*see* Foreign body, respiratory tract, specified site NEC
  - bronchus—*see* Foreign body, bronchus
  - causing
    - asphyxiation T17.900
      - food (bone) (seed) T17.920
      - gastric contents (vomitus) T17.910
      - specified type NEC T17.990
    - injury NEC T17.908
      - food (bone) (seed) T17.928
      - gastric contents (vomitus) T17.918
      - specified type NEC T17.998
  - larynx—*see* Foreign body, larynx
  - multiple parts—*see* Foreign body, respiratory tract
  - nasal sinus T17.0
  - nasopharynx—*see* Foreign body, pharynx
  - nose T17.1
  - nostril T17.1
  - pharynx—*see* Foreign body, pharynx
  - specified site NEC T17.80- (*See complete ICD-10-CM Manual for codes*)
    - fragments—*see* Retained, foreign body fragments (type of)
    - soft tissue M79.5
    - throat—*see* Foreign body, pharynx
    - trachea—*see* Foreign body, trachea
- superficial, without open wound
  - abdomen, abdominal (wall) S30.851
  - alveolar process S00.552
  - ankle S90.55-
  - antecubital space S40.85-
  - anus S30.857
  - arm (upper) S40.85-
  - auditory canal S00.45-
  - axilla S40.85-
  - back, lower S30.850
  - breast S20.15-
  - brow S00.85
  - buttock S30.850
  - calf S80.85-
  - canthus S00.25-
  - cheek S00.85
    - internal S00.552
  - chest wall S20.95
  - chin S00.85
  - clitoris S30.854
  - costal region S20.95
  - digit(s)
    - hand—*see* Foreign body, superficial, without open wound, finger
    - foot—*see* Foreign body, superficial, without open wound, toe
  - ear S00.45-
  - elbow S50.35-
  - epididymis S30.853
  - epigastric region S30.851
  - epiglottis S10.15
  - esophagus, cervical S10.15
  - eyebrow S00.25-
  - eyelid S00.25-
  - face S00.85
  - finger(s) S60.45-
    - index S60.45-
    - little S60.45-
    - middle S60.45-
    - ring S60.45-
  - flank S30.851
  - foot (except toe(s) alone) S90.85-
    - toe—*see* Foreign body, superficial, without open wound, toe
  - forearm S50.85-
    - elbow only S50.35-
  - forehead S00.85
  - genital organs, external
    - female S30.856
    - male S30.855
  - groin S30.851
  - gum S00.552
  - hand S60.55-

Foreign body, *continued*

- head S00.95
  - ear S00.45-
  - eyelid S00.25-
  - lip S00.551
  - nose S00.35
  - oral cavity S00.552
  - scalp S00.05
  - specified site NEC S00.85
- heel—*see* Foreign body, superficial, without open wound, foot
- hip S70.25-
- inguinal region S30.851
- interscapular region S20.459
- jaw S00.85
- knee S80.25-
- labium (majus) (minus) S30.854
- larynx S10.15
- leg (lower) S80.85-
  - knee S80.25-
  - upper—*see* Foreign body, superficial, without open wound, thigh
- lip S00.551
- lower back S30.850
- lumbar region S30.850
- malar region S00.85
- mammary—*see* Foreign body, superficial, without open wound, breast
- mastoid region S00.85
- mouth S00.552
- nail
  - finger—*see* Foreign body, superficial, without open wound, finger
  - toe—*see* Foreign body, superficial, without open wound, toe
- nape S10.85
- nasal S00.35
- neck S10.95
  - specified site NEC S10.85
  - throat S10.15
- nose S00.35
- occipital region S00.05
- oral cavity S00.552
- orbital region—*see* Foreign body, superficial, without open wound, eyelid
- palate S00.552
- palm—*see* Foreign body, superficial, without open wound, hand
- parietal region S00.05
- pelvis S30.850
- penis S30.852
- perineum
  - female S30.854
  - male S30.850
- periocular area S00.25-
- phalanges
  - finger—*see* Foreign body, superficial, without open wound, finger
  - toe—*see* Foreign body, superficial, without open wound, toe
- pharynx S10.15
- pinna S00.45-
- popliteal space S80.25-
- prepuce S30.852
- pubic region S30.850
- pudendum
  - female S30.856
  - male S30.855
- sacral region S30.850
- scalp S00.05
- scapular region S40.25-
- scrotum S30.853
- shin S80.85-
- shoulder S40.25-
- sternal region S20.359
- submaxillary region S00.85
- submental region S00.85
- subungual
  - finger(s)—*see* Foreign body, superficial, without open wound, finger
  - toe(s)—*see* Foreign body, superficial, without open wound, toe
- supraclavicular fossa S10.85

ALPHABETIC INDEX

Foreign body, *continued*
- supraorbital S00.85
- temple S00.85
- temporal region S00.85
- testis S30.853
- thigh S70.35-
- thorax, thoracic (wall) S20.95
  - ■ back S20.45-
  - ■ front S20.35-
- throat S10.15
- thumb S60.35-
- toe(s) (lesser) S90.45-
  - ■ great S90.45-
- tongue S00.552
- trachea S10.15
- tunica vaginalis S30.853
- tympanum, tympanic membrane S00.45-
- uvula S00.552
- vagina S30.854
- vocal cords S10.15
- vulva S30.854
- wrist S60.85-
- swallowed T18.9
- trachea T17.40- *(See complete ICD-10-CM Manual for codes)*
- type of fragment—*see* Retained, foreign body fragments (type of)

Fothergill's
- disease (trigeminal neuralgia)—*see also* Neuralgia
  - scarlatina anginosa A38.9

Foul breath R19.6

Foundling Z76.1

FPIES (food protein-induced enterocolitis syndrome) K52.21

Fracture (abduction) (adduction) (separation) T14.8
- acetabulum S32.40-
  - column
    - ■ anterior (displaced) (iliopubic) S32.43-
      - ~ nondisplaced S32.43-
    - ■ posterior (displaced) (ilioischial) S32.44-
      - ~ nondisplaced S32.44-
  - dome (displaced) S32.48-
    - ■ nondisplaced S32.48
  - specified NEC S32.49-
  - transverse (displaced) S32.45-
    - ■ with associated posterior wall fracture (displaced) S32.46-
      - ~ nondisplaced S32.46-
    - ■ nondisplaced S32.45-
  - wall
    - ■ anterior (displaced) S32.41-
      - ~ nondisplaced S32.41-
    - ■ medial (displaced) S32.47-
      - ~ nondisplaced S32.47-
    - ■ posterior (displaced) S32.42-
      - ~ with associated transverse fracture (displaced) S32.46-
        - ◊ nondisplaced S32.46-
      - ~ nondisplaced S32.42-
- ankle S82.89-
  - bimalleolar (displaced) S82.84-
    - ■ nondisplaced S82.84-
  - lateral malleolus only (displaced) S82.6-
    - ■ nondisplaced S82.6-
  - medial malleolus (displaced) S82.5-
    - ■ associated with Maisonneuve's fracture—*see* Fracture, Maisonneuve's
    - ■ nondisplaced S82.5-
  - talus—*see* Fracture
  - trimalleolar (displaced) S82.85-
    - ■ nondisplaced S82.85-
- arm (upper)—*see also* Fracture, humerus, shaft
  - humerus—*see* Fracture, humerus
  - radius—*see* Fracture, radius
  - ulna—*see* Fracture, ulna
- astragalus—*see* Fracture
- Barton's—*see* Barton's fracture
- base of skull—*see* Fracture, skull, base
- basicervical (basal) (femoral) S72.0
- Bennett's—*see* Bennett's fracture
- bimalleolar—*see* Fracture, ankle, bimalleolar
- blowout S02.3-

Fracture, *continued*
- bone NEC T14.8
  - birth injury P13.9
  - following insertion of orthopedic implant, joint prosthesis or bone plate—*see* Fracture
- burst—*see* Fracture, traumatic, by site
- calcaneus—*see* Fracture, tarsal, calcaneus
- carpal bone(s) S62.10-
  - capitate (displaced) S62.13-
    - ■ nondisplaced S62.13-
  - cuneiform—*see* Fracture, carpal bone, triquetrum
  - hamate (body) (displaced) S62.14-
    - ■ hook process (displaced) S62.15-
      - ~ nondisplaced S62.15-
    - ■ nondisplaced S62.14-
  - larger multangular—*see* Fracture, carpal bones, trapezium
  - lunate (displaced) S62.12-
    - ■ nondisplaced S62.12-
  - navicular S62.00-
    - ■ distal pole (displaced) S62.01-
      - ~ nondisplaced S62.01-
    - ■ middle third (displaced) S62.02-
      - ~ nondisplaced S62.02-
    - ■ proximal third (displaced) S62.03-
      - ~ nondisplaced S62.03-
    - ■ volar tuberosity—*see* Fracture, carpal bones, navicular, distal pole
  - os magnum—*see* Fracture, carpal bones, capitate
  - pisiform (displaced) S62.16-
    - ■ nondisplaced S62.16-
  - semilunar—*see* Fracture, carpal bones, lunate
  - smaller multangular—*see* Fracture, carpal bones, trapezoid
  - trapezium (displaced) S62.17-
    - ■ nondisplaced S62.17-
  - trapezoid (displaced) S62.18-
    - ■ nondisplaced S62.18-
  - triquetrum (displaced) S62.11-
    - ■ nondisplaced S62.11-
  - unciform—*see* Fracture, carpal bones, hamate
- clavicle S42.00-
  - acromial end (displaced) S42.03-
    - ■ nondisplaced S42.03-
  - birth injury P13.4
  - lateral end—*see* Fracture, clavicle, acromial end
  - shaft (displaced) S42.02-
    - ■ nondisplaced S42.02-
  - sternal end (anterior) (displaced) S42.01-
    - ■ nondisplaced S42.01-
    - ■ posterior S42.01-
- coccyx S32.2
- collar bone—*see* Fracture, clavicle
- Colles'—*see* Colles' fracture
- coronoid process—*see* Fracture, ulna, upper end, coronoid process
- costochondral, costosternal junction—*see* Fracture, rib
- cranium—*see* Fracture, skull
- cricoid cartilage S12.8
- cuboid (ankle)—*see* Fracture, tarsal, cuboid
- cuneiform
  - foot—*see* Fracture, tarsal, cuneiform
  - wrist—*see* Fracture, carpal, triquetrum
- delayed union—*see* Delay
- due to
  - birth injury—*see* Birth, injury, fracture
- Dupuytren's—*see* Fracture, ankle, lateral malleolus only
- elbow S42.40-
- ethmoid (bone) (sinus)—*see* Fracture, skull, base
- face bone S02.92-
- fatigue—*see also* Fracture, stress
- femur, femoral S72.9-
  - basicervical (basal) S72.0
  - birth injury P13.2
  - capital epiphyseal S79.01-
  - condyles, epicondyles—*see* Fracture, femur, lower end
  - distal end—*see* Fracture, femur, lower end
  - epiphysis
    - ■ head—*see* Fracture, femur, upper end, epiphysis
    - ■ lower—*see* Fracture, femur, lower end, epiphysis
    - ■ upper—*see* Fracture, femur, upper end, epiphysis

Fracture, *continued*
  - head—*see* Fracture, femur, upper end, head
  - intertrochanteric—*see* Fracture, femur
  - intratrochanteric—*see* Fracture, femur
  - lower end S72.40-
    - ■ condyle (displaced) S72.41-
      - ~ lateral (displaced) S72.42-
        - ◊ nondisplaced S72.42-
      - ~ medial (displaced) S72.43-
        - ◊ nondisplaced S72.43-
      - ~ nondisplaced S72.41-
    - ■ epiphysis (displaced) S72.44-
      - ~ nondisplaced S72.44-
    - ■ physeal S79.10-
      - ~ Salter-Harris
        - ◊ Type I S79.11-
        - ◊ Type II S79.12-
        - ◊ Type III S79.13-
        - ◊ Type IV S79.14-
      - ~ specified NEC S79.19-
    - ■ specified NEC S72.49-
    - ■ supracondylar (displaced) S72.45-
      - ~ with intracondylar extension (displaced) S72.46-
        - ◊ nondisplaced S72.46-
      - ~ nondisplaced S72.45-
    - ■ torus S72.47-
  - neck—*see* Fracture, femur, upper end, neck
  - pertrochanteric—*see* Fracture, femur
  - shaft (lower third) (middle third) (upper third) S72.30-
    - ■ comminuted (displaced) S72.35-
      - ~ nondisplaced S72.35-
    - ■ oblique (displaced) S72.33-
      - ~ nondisplaced S72.33-
    - ■ segmental (displaced) S72.36-
      - ~ nondisplaced S72.36-
    - ■ specified NEC S72.39-
    - ■ spiral (displaced) S72.34-
      - ~ nondisplaced S72.34-
    - ■ transverse (displaced) S72.32-
      - ~ nondisplaced S72.32-
  - specified site NEC—*see* subcategory S72.8
  - transcervical—*see* Fracture, femur, upper end, neck
  - transtrochanteric—*see* Fracture, femur, trochanteric
  - upper end S72.00-
    - ■ cervicotrochanteric—*see* Fracture, femur, upper end, neck, base
    - ■ epiphysis (displaced) S72.02-
      - ~ nondisplaced S72.02-
    - ■ midcervical (displaced) S72.03-
      - ~ nondisplaced S72.03-
    - ■ neck S72.00-
      - ~ base (displaced) S72.04-
        - ◊ nondisplaced S72.04-
    - ■ pertrochanteric—*see* Fracture, femur, upper end
    - ■ physeal S79.00-
      - ~ Salter-Harris type I S79.01-
      - ~ specified NEC S79.09-
    - ■ transcervical—*see* Fracture, femur, upper end, midcervical
- fibula (shaft) (styloid) S82.40-
  - comminuted (displaced or nondisplaced) S82.45- *(See complete ICD-10-CM Manual for codes)*
    - ■ involving ankle or malleolus—*see* Fracture, fibula
    - ■ lateral malleolus (displaced) S82.6-
      - ~ nondisplaced S82.6-
    - ■ lower end
      - ~ physeal S89.30-
        - ◊ Salter-Harris
          - » Type I S89.31-
          - » Type II S89.32-
        - ◊ specified NEC S89.39-
      - ~ specified NEC S82.83-
      - ~ torus S82.82-
  - oblique (displaced or nondisplaced) S82.43- *(See complete ICD-10-CM Manual for codes)*
  - segmental (displaced or nondisplaced) S82.46- *(See complete ICD-10-CM Manual for codes)*
  - spiral (displaced or nondisplaced) S82.44- *(See complete ICD-10-CM Manual for codes)*

ALPHABETIC INDEX

Fracture, *continued*

– transverse (displaced or nondisplaced) S82.42- (*See complete ICD-10-CM Manual for codes*)
  - ■ upper end
    - ~ physeal S89.20-
    - ◊ Salter-Harris
      - » Type I S89.21-
      - » Type II S89.22-
    - ◊ specified NEC S89.29-
    - ~ specified NEC S82.83-
    - ~ torus S82.81-
- finger (except thumb) S62.6-
  - – distal phalanx (displaced) S62.63-
    - ■ nondisplaced S62.66-
  - – index S62.6-
    - ■ distal phalanx (displaced) S62.63-
      - ~ nondisplaced S62.66-
    - ■ medial phalanx (displaced) S62.62-
      - ~ nondisplaced S62.65-
    - ■ proximal phalanx (displaced) S62.61-
      - ~ nondisplaced S62.64-
  - – little S62.6-
    - ■ distal phalanx (displaced) S62.63-
      - ~ nondisplaced S62.66-
    - ■ medial phalanx (displaced) S62.62-
      - ~ nondisplaced S62.65-
    - ■ proximal phalanx (displaced) S62.61-
      - ~ nondisplaced S62.64-
  - – medial phalanx (displaced) S62.62-
    - ■ nondisplaced S62.65-
  - – middle S62.6-
    - ■ distal phalanx (displaced) S62.63-
      - ~ nondisplaced S62.66-
    - ■ medial phalanx (displaced) S62.62-
      - ~ nondisplaced S62.65-
    - ■ proximal phalanx (displaced) S62.61-
      - ~ nondisplaced S62.64-
  - – proximal phalanx (displaced) S62.61-
    - ■ nondisplaced S62.64-
  - – ring S62.6-
    - ■ distal phalanx (displaced) S62.63-
      - ~ nondisplaced S62.66-
    - ■ medial phalanx (displaced) S62.62-
      - ~ nondisplaced S62.65-
    - ■ proximal phalanx (displaced) S62.61-
      - ~ nondisplaced S62.64-
  - – thumb—*see* Fracture, thumb
- foot S92.90-
  - – astragalus—*see* Fracture, tarsal, talus
  - – calcaneus—*see* Fracture, tarsal, calcaneus
  - – cuboid—*see* Fracture, tarsal, cuboid
  - – cuneiform—*see* Fracture, tarsal, cuneiform
  - – metatarsal—*see* Fracture, metatarsal bone
  - – navicular—*see* Fracture, tarsal, navicular
  - – sesamoid S92.81-
  - – talus—*see* Fracture, tarsal, talus
  - – tarsal—*see* Fracture, tarsal
  - – toe—*see* Fracture, toe
- forearm S52.9-
  - – radius—*see* Fracture, radius
  - – ulna—*see* Fracture, ulna
- fossa (anterior) (middle) (posterior) S02.19-
- frontal (bone) (skull) S02.0-
  - – sinus S02.19-
- greenstick—*see* Fracture, by site
- hallux—*see* Fracture, toe, great
- hand
  - – carpal—*see* Fracture, carpal bone
  - – finger (except thumb)—*see* Fracture, finger
  - – metacarpal—*see* Fracture, metacarpal
  - – navicular (scaphoid) (hand)—*see* Fracture, carpal bone, navicular
  - – thumb—*see* Fracture, thumb
- healed or old
  - – with complications—*code by* Nature of the complication
- heel bone—*see* Fracture, tarsal, calcaneus
- Hill-Sachs S42.29-
- hip—*see* Fracture, femur, neck
- humerus S42.30-
  - – anatomical neck—*see* Fracture, humerus, upper end
  - – articular process—*see* Fracture, humerus, lower end

Fracture, *continued*

  - – capitellum—*see* Fracture, humerus, lower end, condyle, lateral
  - – distal end—*see* Fracture, humerus, lower end
  - – epiphysis
    - ■ lower—*see* Fracture, humerus, lower end, physeal
    - ■ upper—*see* Fracture, humerus, upper end, physeal
  - – external condyle—*see* Fracture, humerus, lower end, condyle, lateral
  - – great tuberosity—*see* Fracture, humerus, upper end, greater tuberosity
  - – intercondylar—*see* Fracture, humerus, lower end
  - – internal epicondyle—*see* Fracture, humerus, lower end, epicondyle, medial
  - – lesser tuberosity—*see* Fracture, humerus, upper end, lesser tuberosity
  - – lower end S42.40-
    - ■ condyle
      - ~ lateral (displaced) S42.45-
        - ◊ nondisplaced S42.45-
      - ~ medial (displaced) S42.46-
        - ◊ nondisplaced S42.46-
    - ■ epicondyle
      - ~ lateral (displaced) S42.43-
        - ◊ nondisplaced S42.43-
      - ~ medial (displaced) S42.44-
        - ◊ incarcerated S42.44-
        - ◊ nondisplaced S42.44-
    - ■ physeal S49.10-
      - ~ Salter-Harris
        - ◊ Type I S49.11-
        - ◊ Type II S49.12-
        - ◊ Type III S49.13-
        - ◊ Type IV S49.14-
      - ~ specified NEC S49.19-
    - ■ specified NEC (displaced) S42.49-
      - ~ nondisplaced S42.49-
    - ■ supracondylar (simple) (displaced) S42.41-
      - ~ comminuted (displaced) S42.42-
        - ◊ nondisplaced S42.42-
      - ~ nondisplaced S42.41-
    - ■ torus S42.48-
    - ■ transcondylar (displaced) S42.47-
      - ~ nondisplaced S42.47-
  - – proximal end—*see* Fracture, humerus, upper end
  - – shaft S42.30-
    - ■ comminuted (displaced) S42.35-
      - ~ nondisplaced S42.35-
    - ■ greenstick S42.31-
    - ■ oblique (displaced) S42.33
      - ~ nondisplaced S42.33-
    - ■ segmental (displaced) S42.36-
      - ~ nondisplaced S42.36-
    - ■ specified NEC S42.39-
    - ■ spiral (displaced) S42.34-
      - ~ nondisplaced S42.34-
    - ■ transverse (displaced) S42.32-
      - ~ nondisplaced S42.32-
  - – supracondylar—*see* Fracture, humerus, lower end
  - – surgical neck—*see* Fracture, humerus, upper end, surgical neck
  - – trochlea—*see* Fracture, humerus, lower end, condyle, medial
  - – tuberosity—*see* Fracture, humerus, upper end
  - – upper end S42.20-
    - ■ anatomical neck—*see* Fracture, humerus, upper end, specified NEC
    - ■ articular head—*see* Fracture, humerus, upper end, specified NEC
    - ■ epiphysis—*see* Fracture, humerus, upper end, physeal
    - ■ greater tuberosity (displaced) S42.25-
      - ~ nondisplaced S42.25-
    - ■ lesser tuberosity (displaced) S42.26-
      - ~ nondisplaced S42.26-
    - ■ physeal S49.00-
      - ~ Salter-Harris
        - ◊ Type I S49.01-
        - ◊ Type II S49.02-
        - ◊ Type III S49.03-
        - ◊ Type IV S49.04-
      - ~ specified NEC S49.09-

Fracture, *continued*

    - ■ specified NEC (displaced) S42.29-
      - ~ nondisplaced S42.29-
    - ■ surgical neck (displaced) S42.21-
      - ~ four-part S42.24-
        - ◊ nondisplaced S42.21-
      - ~ three-part S42.23-
      - ~ two-part (displaced) S42.22-
        - ◊ nondisplaced S42.22-
    - ■ torus S42.27-
    - ■ transepiphyseal—*see* Fracture, humerus, upper end, physeal
- hyoid bone S12.8
- ilium S32.30-
  - – avulsion (displaced) S32.31-
    - ■ nondisplaced S32.31-
  - – specified NEC S32.39-
- impaction, impacted—*code as* Fracture, by site
- innominate bone—*see* Fracture, ilium
- instep—*see* Fracture, foot
- ischium S32.60-
  - – avulsion (displaced) S32.61-
    - ■ nondisplaced S32.61-
  - – specified NEC S32.69-
- jaw (bone) (lower)—*see* Fracture, mandible
- knee cap—*see* Fracture, patella
- larynx S12.8
- late effects—*see* Sequelae
- leg (lower)
  - – ankle—*see* Fracture, ankle
  - – femur—*see* Fracture, femur
  - – fibula—*see* Fracture, fibula
  - – malleolus—*see* Fracture, ankle
  - – patella—*see* Fracture, patella
  - – specified site NEC S82.89-
  - – tibia—*see* Fracture, tibia
- lumbosacral spine S32.9
- Maisonneuve's (displaced) S82.86-
  - – nondisplaced S82.86-
- malar bone (see also Fracture) S02.40-
- malleolus—*see* Fracture, ankle
- malunion—*see* Fracture, by site
- mandible (lower jaw (bone)) S02.609-
  - – alveolus S02.67-
  - – angle (of jaw) S02.65-
  - – body, unspecified S02.60-
  - – condylar process S02.61-
  - – coronoid process S02.63-
  - – ramus, unspecified S02.64-
  - – specified site NEC S02.69-
  - – subcondylar process S02.62-
  - – symphysis S02.66-
- march—*see* Fracture
- metacarpal S62.30-
  - – base (displaced) S62.31-
    - ■ nondisplaced S62.34-
  - – fifth S62.30-
    - ■ base (displaced) S62.31-
      - ~ nondisplaced S62.34-
    - ■ neck (displaced) S62.33-
      - ~ nondisplaced S62.36-
    - ■ shaft (displaced) S62.32-
      - ~ nondisplaced S62.35-
    - ■ specified NEC S62.39-
  - – first S62.20-
    - ■ base NEC (displaced) S62.23-
      - ~ nondisplaced S62.23-
    - ■ Bennett's—*see* Bennett's fracture
    - ■ neck (displaced) S62.25-
      - ~ nondisplaced S62.25-
    - ■ shaft (displaced) S62.24-
      - ~ nondisplaced S62.24-
    - ■ specified NEC S62.29-
  - – fourth S62.30-
    - ■ base (displaced) S62.31-
      - ~ nondisplaced S62.34-
    - ■ neck (displaced) S62.33-
      - ~ nondisplaced S62.36-
    - ■ shaft (displaced) S62.32-
      - ~ nondisplaced S62.35-
    - ■ specified NEC S62.39-
  - – neck (displaced) S62.33-
    - ■ nondisplaced S62.36-

ALPHABETIC INDEX

Fracture, *continued*

- Rolando's—*see* Rolando's fracture
- second S62.30-
  - ■ base (displaced) S62.31-
    - ~ nondisplaced S62.34-
  - ■ neck (displaced) S62.33-
    - ~ nondisplaced S62.36-
  - ■ shaft (displaced) S62.32-
    - ~ nondisplaced S62.35-
  - ■ specified NEC S62.39-
  - shaft (displaced) S62.32-
    - ■ nondisplaced S62.35-
  - third S62.30-
    - ■ base (displaced) S62.31-
      - ~ nondisplaced S62.34-
    - ■ neck (displaced) S62.33-
      - ~ nondisplaced S62.36-
    - ■ shaft (displaced) S62.32-
      - ~ nondisplaced S62.35-
    - ■ specified NEC S62.39-
  - specified NEC S62.39-
- metatarsal bone S92.30-
  - fifth (displaced) S92.35-
    - ■ nondisplaced S92.35-
  - first (displaced) S92.31-
    - ■ nondisplaced S92.31-
  - fourth (displaced) S92.34-
    - ■ nondisplaced S92.34-
  - physeal S99.10-
    - ■ Salter-Harris
      - ~ Type I S99.11-
      - ~ Type II S99.12-
      - ~ Type III S99.13-
      - ~ Type IV S99.14-
  - second (displaced) S92.32-
    - ■ nondisplaced S92.32-
  - third (displaced) S92.33-
    - ■ nondisplaced S92.33-
    - ■ specified NEC S99.19-
- Monteggia's—*see* Monteggia's fracture
- multiple
  - hand (and wrist) NEC—*see* Fracture, by site
  - ribs—*see* Fracture, rib, multiple
- nasal (bone(s)) S02.2-
- navicular (scaphoid) (foot)—*see also* Fracture, tarsal bone(s), navicular
  - hand—*see* Fracture, carpal bone(s), navicular
- neck S12.9
  - cervical vertebra S12.9
    - ■ fifth (displaced) S12.400
      - ~ nondisplaced S12.401
    - ■ first (displaced) S12.000
      - ~ burst (stable) S12.0-
        - ◊ unstable S12.0-
      - ~ nondisplaced S12.001
      - ~ posterior arch (displaced) S12.030
        - ◊ nondisplaced S12.031
    - ■ fourth (displaced) S12.300
      - ~ nondisplaced S12.301
    - ■ second (displaced) S12.100
      - ~ nondisplaced S12.101
    - ■ seventh (displaced) S12.600
      - ~ nondisplaced S12.601–
    - ■ sixth (displaced) S12.500
      - ~ nondisplaced S12.501
    - ■ third (displaced) S12.200
      - ~ nondisplaced S12.201
  - hyoid bone S12.8
  - larynx S12.8
  - specified site NEC S12.8
  - thyroid cartilage S12.8
  - trachea S12.8
- newborn—*see* Birth, injury, fracture
- nonunion—*see* Nonunion, fracture
- nose, nasal (bone) (septum) S02.2-
- occiput—*see* Fracture, skull, base, occiput
- olecranon (process) (ulna)—*see* Fracture, ulna, upper end, olecranon process
- orbit, orbital (bone) (region) S02.85
  - calcis—*see* Fracture, tarsal bone(s), calcaneus
  - floor (blow-out) S02.3-
  - magnum—*see* Fracture, carpal bone(s), capitate

Fracture, *continued*

- pubis—*see* Fracture, pubis
- roof S02.12-
- wall
  - ■ lateral S02.83-
  - ■ medial S02.84-
- other, chest compression and cardiopulmonary resuscitation M96.A9
- palate S02.8-
- parietal bone (skull) S02.0-
- patella S82.00-
  - comminuted (displaced or nondisplaced) S82.04- (*See complete ICD-10-CM Manual for codes*)
  - longitudinal (displaced or nondisplaced) S82.02- (*See complete ICD-10-CM Manual for codes*)
  - osteochondral (displaced or nondisplaced) S82.01- (*See complete ICD-10-CM Manual*)
  - transverse (displaced or nondisplaced) S82.03- (*See complete ICD-10-CM Manual for codes*)
- pedicle (of vertebral arch)—*see* Fracture, vertebra
- pelvis, pelvic (bone) S32.9
  - acetabulum—*see* Fracture, acetabulum
  - ilium—*see* Fracture, ilium
  - ischium—*see* Fracture, ischium
  - multiple
    - ■ without disruption of pelvic ring (circle) S32.82
  - pubis—*see* Fracture, pubis
  - specified site NEC S32.89
  - sacrum—*see* Fracture, sacrum
- phalanx
  - foot—*see* Fracture, toe
  - hand—*see* Fracture, finger
- pisiform—*see* Fracture, carpal bone(s), pisiform
- pond—*see* Fracture, skull
- prosthetic device, internal—*see* Complications, prosthetic device, by site, mechanical
- pubis S32.50-
  - with disruption of pelvic ring—*see* Disruption
  - specified site NEC S32.59-
  - superior rim S32.51-
- radius S52.9-
  - distal end—*see* Fracture, radius, lower end
  - head—*see* Fracture, radius, upper end, head
  - lower end S52.50-
    - ■ Barton's—*see* Barton's fracture
    - ■ Colles'—*see* Colles' fracture
    - ■ extraarticular NEC S52.55-
    - ■ intraarticular NEC S52.57-
    - ■ physeal S59.20-
      - ~ Salter-Harris
        - ◊ Type I S59.21-
        - ◊ Type II S59.22-
        - ◊ Type III S59.23-
        - ◊ Type IV S59.24-
      - ~ specified NEC S59.29-
    - ■ Smith's—*see* Smith's fracture
    - ■ specified NEC S52.59-
    - ■ styloid process (displaced) S52.51-
      - ~ nondisplaced S52.51-
    - ■ torus S52.52-
  - neck—*see* Fracture, radius, upper end
  - proximal end—*see* Fracture, radius, upper end
  - shaft S52.30-
    - ■ bent bone S52.38-
    - ■ comminuted (displaced) S52.35-
      - ~ nondisplaced S52.35-
    - ■ Galeazzi's—*see* Galeazzi's fracture
    - ■ greenstick S52.31-
    - ■ oblique (displaced) S52.33-
      - ~ nondisplaced S52.33-
    - ■ segmental (displaced) S52.36-
      - ~ nondisplaced S52.36-
    - ■ specified NEC S52.39-
    - ■ spiral (displaced) S52.34-
      - ~ nondisplaced S52.34-
    - ■ transverse (displaced) S52.32-
      - ~ nondisplaced S52.32-
  - upper end S52.10-
    - ■ head (displaced) S52.12-
      - ~ nondisplaced S52.12-
    - ■ neck (displaced) S52.13-
      - ~ nondisplaced S52.13-
    - ■ specified NEC S52.18-

Fracture, *continued*

- ■ physeal S59.10-
  - ~ Salter-Harris
    - ◊ Type I S59.11-
    - ◊ Type II S59.12-
    - ◊ Type III S59.13-
    - ◊ Type IV S59.14-
  - ~ specified NEC S59.19-
- ■ torus S52.11-
- ramus
  - inferior or superior, pubis—*see* Fracture, pubis
  - mandible—*see* Fracture, mandible
- rib S22.3-
  - multiple S22.4-
    - ■ with flail chest—*see* Flail, chest
  - multiple fractures, chest compression and cardiopulmonary resuscitation M96.A3
  - one rib, chest compression and cardiopulmonary resuscitation M96.A2
  - with flail chest—*see* Flail, chest
- root, tooth—*see* Fracture, tooth
- sacrum S32.10
  - specified NEC S32.19
  - Type
    - ■ 1 S32.14
    - ■ 2 S32.15
    - ■ 3 S32.16
    - ■ 4 S32.17
  - Zone
    - ■ I S32.119
      - ~ displaced (minimally) S32.111
        - ◊ severely S32.112
      - ~ nondisplaced S32.110
    - ■ II S32.129
      - ~ displaced (minimally) S32.121
        - ◊ severely S32.122
      - ~ nondisplaced S32.120
    - ■ III S32.139
      - ~ displaced (minimally) S32.131
        - ◊ severely S32.132
      - ~ nondisplaced S32.130
- scaphoid (hand)—*see also* Fracture, carpal bone(s), navicular
  - foot—*see* Fracture, tarsal, navicular
- semilunar bone, wrist—*see* Fracture, carpal, lunate
- sequelae—*see* Sequelae
- sesamoid bone
  - foot S92.81-
  - hand—*see* Fracture, carpal bone(s)
  - other—*code by site* under Fracture
- shepherd's—*see* Fracture, tarsal bone(s), talus
- shoulder (girdle) S42.9-
- sinus (ethmoid) (frontal) S02.19-
- skull S02.91-
  - base S02.10-
    - ■ occiput S02.119
      - ~ condyle S02.11-
        - ◊ type I S02.11-
        - ◊ type II S02.11-
        - ◊ type III S02.11
      - ~ specified NEC S02.118-
    - ■ specified NEC S02.19-
  - birth injury P13.0
  - frontal bone S02.0-
  - parietal bone S02.0-
  - specified site NEC S02.8-
  - temporal bone S02.19-
  - vault S02.0-
- Smith's—*see* Smith's fracture
- sphenoid (bone) (sinus) S02.19-
- stave (of thumb)—*see* Fracture, metacarpal, first
- sternum S22.20-
  - chest compression and cardiopulmonary resuscitation M96.A1
  - with flail chest—*see* Flail, chest
  - body S22.22
  - manubrium S22.21
  - xiphoid (process) S22.24
- stress M84.30-
  - ankle M84.37-
  - carpus M84.34-
  - clavicle M84.31-
  - femoral neck M84.359

ALPHABETIC INDEX

Fracture, *continued*

- femur M84.35-
- fibula M84.36-
- finger M84.34-
- hip M84.359
- humerus M84.32-
- ilium M84.350
- ischium M84.350
- metacarpus M84.34-
- metatarsus M84.37-
- pelvis M84.350
- radius M84.33-
- rib M84.38
- scapula M84.31-
- skull M84.38
- tarsus M84.37-
- tibia M84.36-
- toe M84.37-
- ulna M84.33-
- supracondylar, elbow—*see* Fracture, humerus, lower end, supracondylar
- symphysis pubis—*see* Fracture, pubis
- talus (ankle bone)—*see* Fracture, tarsal bone(s), talus
- tarsal bone(s) S92.20-
  - astragalus—*see* Fracture, tarsal bone(s), talus
  - calcaneus S92.00-
    - anterior process (displaced) S92.02-
      - nondisplaced S92.02-
    - body (displaced) S92.01-
      - nondisplaced S92.01-
    - extraarticular NEC (displaced) S92.05-
      - nondisplaced S92.05-
    - intraarticular (displaced) S92.06-
      - nondisplaced S92.06-
    - physeal S99.00-
      - Salter-Harris
      ◊ Type I S99.01-
      ◊ Type II S99.02-
      ◊ Type III S99.03-
      ◊ Type IV S99.04-
      - specified NEC S99.09-
    - tuberosity (displaced) S92.04-
      - avulsion (displaced) S92.03-
      ◊ nondisplaced S92.03-
      - nondisplaced S92.04-
  - cuboid (displaced) S92.21-
    - nondisplaced S92.21-
  - cuneiform
    - intermediate (displaced) S92.23-
      - nondisplaced S92.23-
    - lateral (displaced) S92.22-
      - nondisplaced S92.22-
    - medial (displaced) S92.24-
      - nondisplaced S92.24-
  - navicular (displaced) S92.25-
    - nondisplaced S92.25-
  - scaphoid—*see* Fracture, tarsal bone(s), navicular
  - talus S92.10-
    - avulsion (displaced) S92.15-
      - nondisplaced S92.15-
    - body (displaced) S92.12-
      - nondisplaced S92.12-
    - dome (displaced) S92.14-
      - nondisplaced S92.14-
    - head (displaced) S92.12-
      - nondisplaced S92.12-
    - lateral process (displaced) S92.14-
      - nondisplaced S92.14-
    - neck (displaced) S92.11-
      - nondisplaced S92.11-
    - posterior process (displaced) S92.13-
      - nondisplaced S92.13-
    - specified NEC S92.19-
- temporal bone (styloid) S02.19-
- thorax (bony) S22.9
  - with flail chest—*see* Flail, chest
  - rib S22.3-
    - multiple S22.4-
      - with flail chest—*see* Flail, chest
- thumb S62.50-
  - distal phalanx (displaced) S62.52-
    - nondisplaced S62.52-

Fracture, *continued*

- proximal phalanx (displaced) S62.51-
  - nondisplaced S62.51-
- thyroid cartilage S12.8
- tibia (shaft) S82.20-
  - comminuted (displaced or nondisplaced) S82.25- *(See complete ICD-10-CM Manual)*
  - condyles—*see* Fracture, tibia
  - distal end—*see* Fracture, tibia
  - epiphysis
    - lower—*see* Fracture, tibia
    - upper—*see* Fracture, tibia
  - head (involving knee joint)—*see* Fracture, tibia
  - intercondyloid eminence—*see* Fracture, tibia
  - involving ankle or malleolus—*see* Fracture, ankle, medial malleolus
  - lower end S82.30-
    - physeal S89.10-
      - Salter-Harris
      ◊ Type I S89.11-
      ◊ Type II S89.12-
      ◊ Type III S89.13-
      ◊ Type IV S89.14-
      - specified NEC S89.19-
    - pilon (displaced) S82.87-
      - nondisplaced S82.87-
      - specified NEC S82.39-
    - torus S82.31-
  - malleolus—*see* Fracture, ankle, medial malleolus
  - oblique (displaced or nondisplaced) S82.23- - *(See complete ICD-10-CM Manual)*
  - pilon—*see* Fracture, tibia
  - proximal end—*see* Fracture, tibia
  - segmental (displaced or nondisplaced) S82.26- - *(See complete ICD-10-CM Manual)*
  - spiral (displaced) S82.24-
    - nondisplaced S82.24-
  - transverse (displaced or nondisplaced) S82.22- - *(See complete ICD-10-CM Manual)*
  - tuberosity—*see* Fracture, tibia
  - upper end S82.10-
    - bicondylar (displaced) or nondisplaced) S82.14— *(See complete ICD-10-CM Manual)*
    - lateral condyle (displaced) or nondisplaced) S82.12—*(See complete ICD-10-CM Manual)*
    - medial condyle (displaced) or nondisplaced) S82.13—*(See complete ICD-10-CM Manual)*
    - physeal S89.00-
      - Salter-Harris
      ◊ Type I S89.01-
      ◊ Type II S89.02-
      ◊ Type III S89.03-
      ◊ Type IV S89.04-
      - specified NEC S89.09-
    - plateau—*see* Fracture, tibiar
    - spine (displaced or nondisplaced) S82.11- *(See complete ICD-10-CM Manual)*
    - torus S82.16-
    - specified NEC S82.19-
    - tuberosity (displaced or nondisplaced) S82.15- *(See complete ICD-10-CM Manual)*
- toe S92.91-
  - great (displaced) S92.4-
    - distal phalanx (displaced) S92.42-
      - nondisplaced S92.42-
      - nondisplaced S92.4-
    - proximal phalanx (displaced) S92.41-
      - nondisplaced S92.41-
      - specified NEC S92.49-
  - lesser (displaced) S92.5-
    - distal phalanx (displaced) S92.53-
      - nondisplaced S92.53-
    - middle phalanx (displaced) S92.52-
      - nondisplaced S92.52-
      - nondisplaced S92.5-
    - proximal phalanx (displaced) S92.51-
      - nondisplaced S92.51-
    - specified NEC S92.59-
- tooth (root) S02.5-
- trachea (cartilage) S12.8
- trapezium or trapezoid bone—*see* Fracture, carpal bone(s)
- trimalleolar—*see* Fracture, ankle, trimalleolar

Fracture, *continued*

- triquetrum (cuneiform of carpus)—*see* Fracture, carpal bone(s), triquetrum
- trochanter—*see* Fracture, femur
- tuberosity (external)—*code by* site under Fracture
- ulna (shaft) S52.20-
  - bent bone S52.28-
  - coronoid process—*see* Fracture, ulna, upper end, coronoid process
  - distal end—*see* Fracture, ulna, lower end
  - head S52.60-
  - lower end S52.60-
    - physeal S59.00-
      - Salter-Harris
      ◊ Type I S59.01-
      ◊ Type II S59.02-
      ◊ Type III S59.03-
      ◊ Type IV S59.04-
      - specified NEC S59.09-
    - specified NEC S52.69-
    - styloid process (displaced) S52.61-
      - nondisplaced S52.61-
    - torus S52.62-
  - proximal end—*see* Fracture, ulna, upper end
  - shaft S52.20-
    - comminuted (displaced) S52.25-
      - nondisplaced S52.25-
    - greenstick S52.21-
    - Monteggia's—*see* Monteggia's fracture
    - oblique (displaced) S52.23-
      - nondisplaced S52.23-
    - segmental (displaced) S52.26-
      - nondisplaced S52.26-
    - specified NEC S52.29-
    - spiral (displaced) S52.24-
      - nondisplaced S52.24-
    - transverse (displaced) S52.22-
      - nondisplaced S52.22-
  - upper end S52.00-
    - coronoid process (displaced) S52.04-
      - nondisplaced S52.04-
    - olecranon process (displaced) S52.02-
      - with intraarticular extension S52.03-
      - nondisplaced S52.02-
      ◊ with intraarticular extension S52.03-
    - specified NEC S52.09-
    - torus S52.01-
- unciform—*see* Fracture, carpal bone(s), hamate
- vault of skull S02.0-
- vertebra, vertebral (arch) (body) (column) (neural arch) (pedicle) (spinous process) (transverse process)
  - atlas—*see* Fracture, neck, cervical vertebra, first
  - axis—*see* Fracture, neck, cervical vertebra, second
  - cervical (teardrop) S12.9
    - axis—*see* Fracture, neck, cervical vertebra, second
    - first (atlas)—*see* Fracture, neck, cervical vertebra, first
    - second (axis)—*see* Fracture, neck, cervical vertebra, second
- vertex S02.0-
- vomer (bone) S02.2-
- wrist S62.10-
  - carpal—*see* Fracture, carpal bone
  - navicular (scaphoid) (hand)—*see* Fracture, carpal bone(s), navicular
- zygoma S02.402
  - left side S02.40F
  - right side S02.40E

Fragile, fragility

- bone, congenital (with blue sclera) Q78.0
- X chromosome Q99.2

Fragilitas

- ossium (with blue sclerae) (hereditary) Q78.0

Frank's essential thrombocytopenia D69.3

Fraser's syndrome Q87.0

Freckle(s) L81.2

Frederickson's hyperlipoproteinemia, type

- IIA E78.0
- IIB and III E78.2

Freeman Sheldon syndrome Q87.0

ALPHABETIC INDEX

Frenum, frenulum
- tongue (shortening) (congenital) Q38.1

Frequency micturition (nocturnal) R35.0
- psychogenic F45.8

Friction
- burn—*see* Burn, by site
- sounds, chest R09.89

Friedreich's
- ataxia G11.11
- combined systemic disease G11.11
- facial hemihypertrophy Q67.4
- sclerosis (cerebellum) (spinal cord) G11.11

Fröhlich's syndrome E23.6

Fucosidosis E77.1

Fugue R68.89
- reaction to exceptional stress (transient) F43.0

Fulminant, fulminating—*see* Disease, diseased

Functional—*see also* Disease, diseased
- bleeding (uterus) N93.8

Fungus, fungous
- cerebral G93.89
- disease NOS B49
- infection—*see* Infection, fungus

Funnel
- breast (acquired) M95.4
  – congenital Q67.6
- chest (acquired) M95.4
  – congenital Q67.6
- pelvis (acquired) M95.5
  – congenital Q74.2

FUO (fever of unknown origin) R50.9

Furfur L21.0
- microsporon B36.0

Furuncle L02.92
- abdominal wall L02.221
- ankle L02.42-
- anus K61.0
- axilla (region) L02.42-
- back (any part) L02.222
- breast N61.1
- buttock L02.32
- cheek (external) L02.02
- chest wall L02.223
- chin L02.02
- face L02.02
- flank L02.221
- foot L02.62-
- forehead L02.02
- gluteal (region) L02.32
- groin L02.224
- hand L02.52-
- head L02.821
  – face L02.02
- hip L02.42-
- knee L02.42-
- leg (any part) L02.42-
- lower limb L02.42-
- malignant A22.0
- mouth K12.2
- navel L02.226
- neck L02.12
- nose J34.0
- partes posteriores L02.32
- pectoral region L02.223
- perineum L02.225
- scalp L02.821
- specified site NEC L02.828
- submandibular K12.2
- temple (region) L02.02
- thumb L02.52-
- toe L02.62-
- trunk L02.229
  – abdominal wall L02.221
  – back L02.222
  – chest wall L02.223
  – groin L02.224
  – perineum L02.225
  – umbilicus L02.226
- umbilicus L02.226

Furuncle, *continued*
- upper limb L02.42-
- vulva N76.4

Fusion, fused (congenital)
- astragaloscaphoid Q74.2
- atria Q21.1
- auricles, heart Q21.1
- choanal Q30.0
- cusps, heart valve NEC Q24.8
  – pulmonary Q22.1
- fingers Q70.0-
- hymen Q52.3
- limb, congenital Q74.8
  – lower Q74.2
  – upper Q74.0
- nares, nose, nasal, nostril(s) Q30.0
- ossicles Q79.9
  – auditory Q16.3
- pulmonic cusps Q22.1
- sacroiliac (joint) (acquired) M43.28
  – congenital Q74.2
- toes Q70.2
- ventricles, heart Q21.0

Fussy baby R68.12

G

Gain in weight (abnormal) (excessive)—*see also* Weight, gain

Gaisböck's disease (polycythemia hypertonica) D75.1

Gait abnormality R26.9
- ataxic R26.0
- hysterical (ataxic) (staggering) F44.4
- paralytic R26.1
- spastic R26.1
- specified type NEC R26.89
- staggering R26.0
- unsteadiness R26.81
- walking difficulty NEC R26.2

Galactocele (breast)
- puerperal, postpartum O92.79

Galactophoritis N61.0

Galactorrhea O92.6
- not associated with childbirth N64.3

GALD (gestational alloimmune liver disease) P78.84

Galeazzi's fracture S52.37-

Gallbladder—*see also* Disease, diseased
- acute K81.0

Gambling Z72.6
- gamma heavy chain C88.2-

Ganglion (compound) (diffuse) (joint) (tendon (sheath)) M67.40
- ankle M67.47-
- foot M67.47-
- forearm M67.43-
- hand M67.44-
- lower leg M67.46-
- multiple sites M67.49
- pelvic region M67.45-
- shoulder region M67.41-
- specified site NEC M67.48
- thigh region M67.45-
- upper arm M67.42-
- wrist M67.43-

Ganglionitis
- newborn (birth injury) P11.3

Gangliosidosis E75.10
- GM2 E75.00
  – Sandhoff disease E75.01
  – Tay-Sachs disease E75.02

Gangrene, gangrenous (connective tissue) (dropsical) (dry) (moist) (skin) (ulcer) (*see also* Necrosis)
- appendix K35.80
  – with
    - peritonitis, localized (*see also* Appendicitis) K35.31
- epididymis (infectional) N45.1
- erysipelas—*see* Erysipelas
- glossitis K14.0
- laryngitis J04.0

Gangrene, gangrenous, *continued*
- pancreas
  – idiopathic
    - infected K85.02
      - uninfected K85.01
  – infected K85.82
  – uninfected K85.81
- quinsy J36
- testis (infectional) N45.2
  – noninfective N44.8
- uvulitis K12.2

Gardner-Diamond syndrome (autoerythrocyte sensitization) D69.2

Gargoylism E76.01

Gartner's duct
- cyst Q52.4
- persistent Q50.6

Gas R14.3
- excessive R14.0
- on stomach R14.0
- pains R14.1

Gastrectasis K31.0
- psychogenic F45.8

Gastric—*see* Disease, diseased

Gastritis (simple) K29.70
- with bleeding K29.71
- acute (erosive) K29.00
  – with bleeding K29.01
  – dietary counseling and surveillance Z71.3
- eosinophilic K52.81
- viral NEC A08.4

Gastroduodenitis K29.90
- with bleeding K29.91
- virus, viral A08.4
  – specified type NEC A08.39

Gastroenteritis (acute) (chronic) (noninfectious) (*see also* Enteritis) K52.9
- allergic K52.29
  – with
    - eosinophilic gastritis or gastroenteritis K52.81
    - food protein-induced enterocolitis syndrome K52.21
    - food protein-induced enteropathy K52.22
- dietetic K52.29
- eosinophilic K52.81
- epidemic (infectious) A09
- food hypersensitivity K52.29
- infectious—*see* Enteritis, infectious
- noninfectious K52.9
  – specified NEC K52.89
- rotaviral A08.0
- Salmonella A02.0
- viral NEC A08.4
  – acute infectious A08.39
  – infantile (acute) A08.39
  – rotaviral A08.0
  – severe of infants A08.39
  – specified type NEC A08.39

Gastroenteropathy (*see also* Gastroenteritis) K52.9
- infectious A09

Gastrojejunitis (*see also* Enteritis) K52.9

Gastropathy K31.9
- erythematous K29.70
- exudative K90.89

Gastrorrhagia K92.2
- psychogenic F45.8

Gastroschisis (congenital) Q79.3

Gastrospasm (neurogenic) (reflex) K31.89
- neurotic F45.8
- psychogenic F45.8

Gastrostomy
- attention to Z43.1
- status Z93.1

Gee (-Herter) (-Thaysen) disease (nontropical sprue) K90.0

Gemistocytoma
- specified site—*see* Neoplasm, malignant, by site in Table of Neoplasms in the complete *ICD-10-CM* manual
- unspecified site C71.9

ALPHABETIC INDEX

General, generalized—*see* Disease, diseased

Genetic

- carrier (status)
  - cystic fibrosis Z14.1
  - hemophilia A (asymptomatic) Z14.01
    - symptomatic Z14.02
  - specified NEC Z14.8
- susceptibility to disease NEC Z15.89
  - epilepsy Z15.1
  - neurodevelopmental disorders Z15.1
  - obesity Z15.2

Genu

- congenital Q74.1
- extrorsum (acquired) M21.16-
  - congenital Q74.1
- introrsum (acquired) M21.06-
  - congenital Q74.1
- recurvatum (acquired) M21.86-
  - congenital Q68.2
- valgum (acquired) (knock-knee) M21.06-
  - congenital Q74.1
- varum (acquired) (bowleg) M21.16-
  - congenital Q74.1

Geographic tongue K14.1

Geophagia—*see* Pica

Gerbode defect Q21.0

GERD (gastroesophageal reflux disease) K21.9

Gerhardt's

- syndrome (vocal cord paralysis) J38.00
  - bilateral J38.02
  - unilateral J38.01

German measles—*see also* Rubella

- exposure to Z20.4

Germinoblastoma (diffuse) C85.9-

- follicular C82.9-

Gerstmann's syndrome R48.8

- developmental F81.2

Gianotti-Crosti disease L44.4

Giant

- urticaria T78.3

Giardiasis A07.1

Gibert's disease or pityriasis L42

Giddiness R42

- hysterical F44.89
- psychogenic F45.8

Gigantism (cerebral) (hypophyseal) (pituitary) E22.0

- constitutional E34.4

Gilbert's disease or syndrome E80.4

Gilles de la Tourette's disease or syndrome (motor-verbal tic) F95.2

Gingivitis

- acute (catarrhal) K05.00
  - plaque induced K05.00

Gingivoglossitis K14.0

Gingivostomatitis

- herpesviral B00.2

Glaucoma

- childhood Q15.0
- congenital Q15.0
- in (due to)
  - endocrine disease NOS E34.9 *[H42]*
  - Lowe's syndrome E72.03 *[H42]*
  - metabolic disease NOS E88.9 *[H42]*
  - Rieger anomaly Q13.81 *[H42]*
- infantile Q15.0
- newborn Q15.0
- secondary (to)
  - trauma H40.3-
  - traumatic—*see also* Glaucoma, secondary, trauma
  - newborn (birth injury) P15.3

Gleet (gonococcal) A54.01

Glioblastoma (multiforme)

- with sarcomatous component
  - specified site—see Neoplasm, malignant, by site in Table of Neoplasms in the complete *ICD-10-CM* manual
  - unspecified site C71.9

Glioblastoma, *continued*

- giant cell
  - specified site—see Neoplasm, malignant, by site in Table of Neoplasms in the complete *ICD-10-CM* manual
  - unspecified site C71.9
- specified site—see Neoplasm, malignant, by site in Table of Neoplasms in the complete *ICD-10-CM* manual
  - unspecified site C71.9

Glioma (malignant)

- astrocytic
  - specified site—see Neoplasm, malignant, by site in Table of Neoplasms in the complete *ICD-10-CM* manual
  - unspecified site C71.9
- mixed
  - specified site—see Neoplasm, malignant, by site in Table of Neoplasms in the complete *ICD-10-CM* manual
  - unspecified site C71.9
- nose Q30.8
- specified site NEC—see Neoplasm, malignant, by site in Table of Neoplasms in the complete *ICD-10-CM* manual
  - specified site—see Neoplasm, uncertain behavior, by site in Table of Neoplasms in the complete *ICD-10-CM* manual
- unspecified site C71.9

Gliosarcoma

- specified site—see Neoplasm, malignant, by site in Table of Neoplasms in the complete *ICD-10-CM* manual
- unspecified site C71.9

Gliosis (cerebral) G93.89

Globinuria R82.3

Globus (hystericus) F45.8

Glomangioma D18.00

- skin D18.01
- specified site NEC D18.09

Glomangiomyoma D18.00

- intra-abdominal D18.03
- intracranial D18.02
- skin D18.01
- specified site NEC D18.09

Glomerulonephritis (*see also* Nephritis) N05.9

- with
  - C3
    - glomerulonephritis N05.A
    - glomerulopathy N05.A
    - with dense deposit disease N05.6
  - edema—*see* Nephrosis
  - minimal change N05.0
  - minor glomerular abnormality N05.0
- acute N00.9
- chronic N03.9
- in (due to)
  - defibrination syndrome D65 *[N08]*
  - disseminated intravascular coagulation D65 *[N08]*
  - *hemolytic-uremic syndrome* D59.3
  - Henoch (-Schönlein) purpura D69.0 *[N08]*
  - sepsis A41.9 *[N08]*
    - streptococcal A40- *[N08]*
  - subacute bacterial endocarditis I33.0 *[N08]*
  - systemic lupus erythematosus M32.14
  - Waldenstrom macroglobulinemia C88.0- *[N08]*
- poststreptococcal NEC N05.9
  - acute N00.9
  - chronic N03.9
- proliferative NEC (*see also* N00-N07 with fourth character .8) N05.8
  - diffuse (lupus) M32.14

Glossitis (chronic superficial) (gangrenous) (Moeller's) K14.0

- areata exfoliativa K14.1
- benign migratory K14.1
- cortical superficial, sclerotic K14.0
- interstitial, sclerous K14.0
- superficial, chronic K14.0

Glottitis (*see also* Laryngitis) J04.0

Glue

- ear H65.3-
- sniffing (airplane)—*see* Abuse, drug
  - dependence—*see* Dependence, drug

Glue, *continued*

- GLUT1 deficiency syndrome 1, infantile onset E74.810
- GLUT1 deficiency syndrome 2, childhood onset E74.810

Glycogenosis (diffuse) (generalized)

- pulmonary interstitial J84.842

Glycopenia E16.2

Glycosuria R81

- renal E74.818

Goiter (plunging) (substernal) E04.9

- with
  - hyperthyroidism (recurrent)—*see* Hyperthyroidism, with, goiter
  - thyrotoxicosis—*see* Hyperthyroidism, with, goiter
- adenomatous—*see* Goiter, nodular
- congenital
  - transitory, with normal functioning P72.0
- due to
  - iodine-deficiency (endemic) E01.2
- endemic (iodine-deficiency) E01.2
  - diffuse E01.0
  - multinodular E01.1
- iodine-deficiency (endemic) E01.2
  - diffuse E01.0
  - multinodular E01.1
  - nodular E01.1
- lingual Q89.2
- lymphadenoid E06.3
- neonatal NEC P72.0
- nodular (nontoxic) (due to) E04.9
  - endemic E01.1
  - iodine-deficiency E01.1
  - sporadic E04.9
- nontoxic E04.9
  - diffuse (colloid) E04.0
  - multinodular E04.2
  - simple E04.0
  - specified NEC E04.8
  - uninodular E04.1
- simple E04.0

Goldberg syndrome Q89.8

Goldberg-Maxwell syndrome E34.51

Goldenhar (-Gorlin) syndrome Q87.0

Goldflam-Erb disease or syndrome G70.00

- with exacerbation (acute) G70.01
- in crisis G70.01

Goldscheider's disease Q81.8

Goldstein's disease (familial hemorrhagic telangiectasia) I78.0

Gonococcus, gonococcal (disease) (infection) (*see also* Disease, diseased) A54.9

- conjunctiva, conjunctivitis (neonatorum) A54.31
- eye A54.30
  - conjunctivitis A54.31
  - newborn A54.31
- fallopian tubes (acute) (chronic) A54.24
- genitourinary (organ) (system) (tract) (acute)
  - lower A54.00
- pelviperitonitis A54.24
- pelvis (acute) (chronic) A54.24
- pyosalpinx (acute) (chronic) A54.24
- urethra (acute) (chronic) A54.01
  - with abscess (accessory gland) (periurethral) A54.1
- vulva (acute) (chronic) A54.02

Gonorrhea (acute) (chronic) A54.9

- Bartholin's gland (acute) (chronic) (purulent) A54.02
  - with abscess (accessory gland) (periurethral) A54.1
- bladder A54.01
- cervix A54.03
- conjunctiva, conjunctivitis (neonatorum) A54.31
- contact Z20.2
- exposure to Z20.2
- fallopian tube A54.24
- lower genitourinary tract A54.00
- ovary (acute) (chronic) A54.24
- pelvis (acute) (chronic) A54.24
  - female pelvic inflammatory disease A54.24
- urethra A54.01
- vagina A54.02
- vulva A54.02

ALPHABETIC INDEX

Gorlin-Chaudry-Moss syndrome Q87.0

Gougerot-Carteaud disease or syndrome (confluent reticulate papillomatosis) L83

Gouley's syndrome (constrictive pericarditis) I31.1

Gout, gouty (acute) (attack) (flare)—*see also* Gout M10.9
- idiopathic M10.0-
  - ankle M10.07-
  - elbow M10.02-
  - foot joint M10.07-
  - hand joint M10.04-
  - hip M10.05-
  - knee M10.06-
  - multiple site M10.09
  - shoulder M10.01-
  - vertebrae M10.08

Gower's
- muscular dystrophy G71.01
- syndrome (vasovagal attack) R55

Graft-versus-host disease D89.813
- acute D89.810
- acute on chronic D89.812
- chronic D89.811

Grain mite (itch) B88.0

Granular—*see also* Disease, diseased
- inflammation, pharynx J31.2

Granuloma L92.9
- abdomen
  - from residual foreign body L92.3
  - pyogenicum L98.0
- annulare (perforating) L92.0
- beryllium (skin) L92.3
- brain (any site) G06.0
- candidal (cutaneous) B37.2
- cerebral (any site) G06.0
- foreign body (in soft tissue) NEC M60.2-
  - ankle M60.27-
  - foot M60.27-
  - forearm M60.23-
  - hand M60.24-
  - lower leg M60.26-
  - pelvic region M60.25-
  - shoulder region M60.21-
  - skin L92.3
  - specified site NEC M60.28
  - subcutaneous tissue L92.3
  - thigh M60.25-
  - upper arm M60.22-
- gland (lymph) I88.8
- hepatic NEC K75.3
  - in (due to)
    - sarcoidosis D86.89
- Hodgkin C81.9-
- intracranial (any site) G06.0
- monilial (cutaneous) B37.2
- operation wound T81.89
  - foreign body—*see* Foreign body
  - stitch T81.89
- orbit, orbital H05.11-
- pyogenic, pyogenicum (of) (skin) L98.0
- rectum K62.89
- reticulohistiocytic D76.3
- septic (skin) L98.0
- silica (skin) L92.3
- skin L92.9
  - from residual foreign body L92.3
  - pyogenicum L98.0
- stitch (postoperative) T81.89
- suppurative (skin) L98.0
- telangiectacticum (skin) L98.0
- umbilical (umbilicus) P83.81

Granulomatosis L92.9
- with polyangiitis M31.3
- eosinophilic, with polyangiitis [EGPA] M30.1
- progressive septic D71

Grawitz tumor C64.-

Green sickness D50.8

Grief F43.21
- prolonged F43.29
- reaction (*see also* Disorder, adjustment) F43.20

Grinding, teeth
- psychogenic F45.8
- sleep related G47.63

Grisel's disease M43.6

Growing pains, children R29.898

Growth (fungoid) (neoplastic) (new)—*see also* Table of Neoplasms in the complete *ICD-10-CM* manual
- adenoid (vegetative) J35.8
- benign—*see* Neoplasm, benign, by site in Table of Neoplasms in the complete *ICD-10-CM* manual
- malignant—*see* Neoplasm, malignant, by site in Table of Neoplasms in the complete *ICD-10-CM* manual
- rapid, childhood Z00.2
- secondary—*see* Neoplasm, secondary, by site in Table of Neoplasms in the complete *ICD-10-CM* manual

Gruby's disease B35.0

Guerin-Stern syndrome Q74.3

Guinon's disease (motor-verbal tic) F95.2

Gumboil K04.7

Gynecological examination (periodic) (routine) Z01.419
- with abnormal findings Z01.411

Gynecomastia N62

Gyrate scalp Q82.8

H

H-ABC (hypomyelination with atrophy of the basal ganglia and cerebellum) G23.3

Haemophilus (H.) influenzae, as cause of disease classified elsewhere B96.3

Hailey-Hailey disease Q82.8

Hair—*see also* Disease, diseased
- plucking F63.3
  - in stereotyped movement disorder F98.4
- tourniquet syndrome—*see also* Constriction, external, by site
  - finger S60.44-
  - penis S30.842
  - thumb S60.34-
  - toe S90.44-

Hairball in stomach T18.2

Hair-pulling, pathological (compulsive) F63.3

Halitosis R19.6

Hallerman-Streiff syndrome Q87.0

Hallucination R44.3
- auditory R44.0
- gustatory R44.2
- olfactory R44.2
- specified NEC R44.2
- tactile R44.2
- visual R44.1

Hallux
- deformity (acquired) NEC M20.5X-
- limitus M20.5X-
- rigidus congenital Q74.2
- valgus (acquired) M20.1-
  - congenital Q66.6
- varus congenital Q66.3-

Hamartoma, hamartoblastoma Q85.9

Hamartosis Q85.9

Hammer toe (acquired) NEC—*see also* Deformity, toe, hammer toe
- congenital Q66.89

Hand-foot syndrome L27.1

Handicap, handicapped
- educational Z55.9
  - specified NEC Z55.8

Hangover (alcohol) F10.129

Hanhart's syndrome Q87.0

Hardening
- brain G93.89

Hardship, material, due to limited financial resources, specified NEC Z59.87

Harelip (complete) (incomplete)—*see* Cleft, lip

Harlequin (newborn) Q80.4

Harmful use (of)
- alcohol F10.10
- cannabinoids—*see* Abuse, drug, cannabis
- cocaine—*see* Abuse, drug, cocaine
- drug—*see* Abuse, drug
- hallucinogens—*see* Abuse, drug
- PCP (phencyclidine)—*see* Abuse, drug

Hashimoto's (struma lymphomatosa) E06.3

Hashitoxicosis (transient) E06.3

Haverhill fever A25.1

Hay fever (*see also* Fever, hay) J30.1

Hb (abnormal)
- Bart's disease D56.0
- disease—*see* Disease, hemoglobin
- trait—*see* Trait

Head—*see* Disease, diseased

Headache R51.9
- with
  - orthostatic component NEC R51.0
  - positional component NEC R51.0
- cervicogenic G44.86
- chronic daily R51.9
- cluster G44.009
  - intractable G44.001
  - not intractable G44.009
- daily chronic R51.9
- histamine G44.009
  - intractable G44.001
  - not intractable G44.009
- migraine (type)—*see also* Migraine G43.909
- nasal septum R51.9
- periodic syndromes in adults and children G43.C0
  - with refractory migraine G43.C1
  - intractable G43.C1
  - not intractable G43.C0
  - without refractory migraine G43.C0
- tension (-type) G44.209
  - chronic G44.229
    - intractable G44.221
    - not intractable G44.229
  - episodic G44.219
    - intractable G44.211
    - not intractable G44.219
  - intractable G44.201
  - not intractable G44.209

Hearing examination Z01.10
- abnormal findings NEC Z01.118
- following failed hearing screening Z01.110
- for hearing conservation and treatment Z01.12
- infant or child (over 28 days old) Z00.12-

Heart—*see* condition

Heart beat
- abnormality R00.9
  - specified NEC R00.8
- awareness R00.2
- rapid R00.0
- slow R00.1

Heartburn R12
- psychogenic F45.8

Heat (effects) T67.9
- apoplexy T67.01
- burn (*see also* Burn) L55.9
- cramps T67.2
- exertional T67.02
- exhaustion T67.5
  - anhydrotic T67.3
  - due to
    - salt (and water) depletion T67.4
    - water depletion T67.3
      - with salt depletion T67.4
- fatigue (transient) T67.6
- fever T67.01
- hyperpyrexia T67.01
- prickly L74.0
- pyrexia T67.01
- rash L74.0
- stroke T67.01
  - exertional T67.02
  - specified NEC T67.09
- syncope T67.1

ALPHABETIC INDEX

Heavy-for-dates NEC (infant) (4000g to 4499g) P08.1
- exceptionally (4500g or more) P08.0

Heerfordt's disease D86.89

Hegglin's anomaly or syndrome D72.0

Heinz body anemia, congenital D58.2

Heloma L84

Hemangioendothelioma—*see also* Neoplasm, uncertain behavior, by site in Table of Neoplasms in the complete *ICD-10-CM* manual
- benign D18.00
  - skin D18.01
  - specified site NEC D18.09
- bone (diffuse)—*see* Neoplasm, bone, malignant in Table of Neoplasms in the complete *ICD-10-CM* manual
- epithelioid—*see also* Neoplasm, uncertain behavior, by site in Table of Neoplasms in the complete *ICD-10-CM* manual
  - malignant—*see* Neoplasm, malignant, by site in Table of Neoplasms in the complete *ICD-10-CM* manual
- malignant—*see* Neoplasm, connective tissue, malignant in Table of Neoplasms in the complete *ICD-10-CM* manual

Hemangiofibroma—*see* Neoplasm, benign, by site in Table of Neoplasms in the complete *ICD-10-CM* manual

Hemangiolipoma—*see* Lipoma

Hemangioma D18.00
- arteriovenous D18.00
  - skin D18.01
  - specified site NEC D18.09
- capillary I78.1
  - skin D18.01
  - specified site NEC D18.09
- cavernous D18.00
  - skin D18.01
  - specified site NEC D18.09
- epithelioid D18.00
  - skin D18.01
  - specified site NEC D18.09
- histiocytoid D18.00
  - skin D18.01
  - specified site NEC D18.09
- infantile D18.00
  - skin D18.01
  - specified site NEC D18.09
- intramuscular D18.00
  - skin D18.01
  - specified site NEC D18.09
- juvenile D18.00
- malignant—*see* Neoplasm, connective tissue, malignant in Table of Neoplasms in the complete *ICD-10-CM* manual
- plexiform D18.00
  - skin D18.01
  - specified site NEC D18.09
- racemose D18.00
  - skin D18.01
  - specified site NEC D18.09
- sclerosing—*see* Neoplasm, skin, benign in Table of Neoplasms in the complete *ICD-10-CM* manual
- simplex D18.00
  - skin D18.01
  - specified site NEC D18.09
- skin D18.01
- specified site NEC D18.09
- venous D18.00
  - skin D18.01
  - specified site NEC D18.09
- verrucous keratotic D18.00
  - skin D18.01
  - specified site NEC D18.09

Hemangiomatosis (systemic) I78.8
- involving single site—see Hemangioma

Hemarthrosis (nontraumatic) M25.00
- ankle M25.07-
- elbow M25.02-
- foot joint M25.07-
- hand joint M25.04-
- hip M25.05-
- in hemophilic arthropathy—*see* Arthropathy, hemophilic

Hemarthrosis, *continued*
- knee M25.06-
- shoulder M25.01-
- specified joint NEC M25.08
- traumatic—*see* Sprain, by site
- vertebrae M25.08
- wrist M25.03

Hematemesis K92.0
- with ulcer—*code by site under* Ulcer, with hemorrhage K27.4
- newborn, neonatal P54.0
  - due to swallowed maternal blood P78.2

Hematocele
- female NEC N94.89
  - with ectopic pregnancy O00.90
    - ■ with uterine pregnancy O00.91

Hematochezia (*see also* Melena) K92.1

Hematoma (traumatic) (skin surface intact)—*see also* Contusion
- with
  - injury of internal organs—*see* Injury, by site
  - open wound—*see* Wound, open
- auricle—*see* Contusion, ear
  - nontraumatic—*see* Disorder
- birth injury NEC P15.8
- brain (traumatic)
  - with
    - ■ cerebral laceration or contusion (diffuse)—*see* Injury, intracranial, diffuse
  - cerebellar, traumatic S06.37-
    - newborn NEC P52.4
    - ■ birth injury P10.1
  - intracerebral, traumatic—*see* Injury, intracranial, intracerebral hemorrhage
  - nontraumatic—*see* Hemorrhage, intracranial
  - subarachnoid, arachnoid, traumatic—*see* Injury, intracranial, subarachnoid hemorrhage
  - subdural, traumatic—*see* Injury, intracranial, subdural hemorrhage
- breast (nontraumatic) N64.89
- cerebral—*see* Hematoma, brain
- cerebrum
  - left S06.35-
  - right S06.34-
- face, birth injury P15.4
- genital organ NEC (nontraumatic)
  - female (nonobstetric) N94.89
  - ■ traumatic S30.202
- internal organs—*see* Injury, by site
- intracerebral, traumatic—*see* Injury, intracranial, intracerebral hemorrhage
- intraoperative—*see* Complications
- labia (nontraumatic) (nonobstetric) N90.89
- pelvis (female) (nontraumatic) (nonobstetric) N94.89
  - traumatic—*see* Injury, by site
- perianal (nontraumatic) K64.5
- pinna H61.12-
- retroperitoneal K68.3
- superficial, newborn P54.5
- vagina (ruptured) (nontraumatic) N89.8

Hematomyelitis G04.90

Hematopneumothorax (*see* Hemothorax)

Hematopoiesis, cyclic D70.4

Hematuria R31.9
- benign (familial) (of childhood)
  - essential microscopic R31.1
- gross R31.0
- microscopic NEC (with symptoms) R31.29
  - asymptomatic R31.21
  - benign essential R31.1

Hemiatrophy R68.89
- face, facial, progressive (Romberg) G51.8

Hemichorea G25.5

Hemiplegia G81.9-
- ascending NEC G81.9-
  - spinal G95.89
- flaccid G81.0-
- hysterical F44.4
- newborn NEC P91.88
  - birth injury P11.9

Hemiplegia, *continued*
- spastic G81.1-
  - congenital G80.2

Hemispasm (facial) R25.2

Hemitremor R25.1

Hemochromatosis E83.119
- due to repeated red blood cell transfusion E83.111
- hereditary (primary) E83.110
- neonatal P78.84
- primary E83.110
- specified NEC E83.118

Hemoglobin—*see also* Disease, diseased
- abnormal (disease)—*see* Disease, hemoglobin
- AS genotype D57.3
- Constant Spring D58.2
- E-beta thalassemia D56.5
- fetal, hereditary persistence (HPFH) D56.4
- H Constant Spring D56.0
- low NOS D64.9
- S (Hb S), heterozygous D57.3

Hemoglobinemia D59.9
- paroxysmal D59.6
  - nocturnal D59.5

Hemoglobinopathy (mixed) D58.2
- with thalassemia D56.8
- sickle-cell D57.1
  - with thalassemia D57.40
    - ■ with
      - acute chest syndrome D57.411
      - cerebral vascular involvement D57.413
      - crisis (painful) D57.419
      - with specified complication NEC D57.418
        - ◊ splenic sequestration D57.412
        - ◊ vasoocclusive pain D57.419
    - ■ without crisis D57.40

Hemoglobinuria R82.3
- with anemia, hemolytic, acquired (chronic) NEC D59.6
- cold (paroxysmal) (with Raynaud's syndrome) D59.6
  - agglutinin D59.12
- due to exertion or hemolysis NEC D59.6
- intermittent D59.6
- march D59.6
- nocturnal (paroxysmal) D59.5
- paroxysmal (cold) D59.6
  - nocturnal D59.5

Hemopericardium I31.2
- newborn P54.8

Hemophilia (classical) (familial) (hereditary) D66
- A D66
- B D67
- C D68.1
- acquired D68.311
- autoimmune D68.311
- secondary D68.311
- vascular D68.0

Hemoptysis R04.2
- newborn P26.9

Hemorrhage, hemorrhagic (concealed) R58
- acute idiopathic pulmonary, in infants R04.81
- adenoid J35.8
- adrenal (capsule) (gland) E27.49
  - medulla E27.8
  - newborn P54.4
- alveolar
  - lung, newborn P26.8
- anemia (chronic) D50.0
  - acute D62
- antepartum (with)
  - before 20 weeks gestation O20.9
    - ■ specified type NEC O20.8
    - ■ threatened abortion O20.0
  - anus K62.5
- basilar (ganglion) I61.0
- bowel K92.2
  - newborn P54.3
- brain (miliary) (nontraumatic)—*see* Hemorrhage, intracranial, intracerebral
  - due to
    - ■ birth injury P10.1

ALPHABETIC INDEX

Hemorrhage, hemorrhagic, *continued*
- newborn P52.4
  - birth injury P10.1
- brainstem (nontraumatic) I61.3
  - traumatic S06.38-
- breast N64.59
- bulbar I61.5
- cecum K92.2
- cerebellar, cerebellum (nontraumatic) I61.4
  - newborn P52.6
  - traumatic S06.37-
- cerebral, cerebrum—*see also* Hemorrhage, intracranial, intracerebral
  - newborn (anoxic) P52.4
    - birth injury P10.1
  - lobe I61.1
- cerebromeningeal I61.8
- cerebrospinal—*see* Hemorrhage, intracranial, intracerebral
- colon K92.2
- conjunctiva H11.3-
  - newborn P54.8
- corpus luteum (ruptured) cyst N83.1-
- cortical (brain) I61.1
- cranial—*see* Hemorrhage, intracranial
- cutaneous R23.3
  - due to autosensitivity, erythrocyte D69.2
  - newborn P54.5
- disease D69.9
  - newborn P53
- duodenum, duodenal K92.2
  - ulcer—*see* Ulcer, duodenum, with, hemorrhage
- epicranial subaponeurotic (massive), birth injury P12.2
- epidural (traumatic)—*see also* Injury, intracranial
  - nontraumatic I62.1
- esophagus K22.89
  - varix I85.01
- extradural (traumatic)—*see* Injury, intracranial, epidural hemorrhage
  - birth injury P10.8
  - newborn (anoxic) (nontraumatic) P52.8
  - nontraumatic I62.1
- gastric—*see* Hemorrhage, stomach
- gastroenteric K92.2
  - newborn P54.3
- gastrointestinal (tract) K92.2
  - newborn P54.3
- genitourinary (tract) NOS R31.9
- graafian follicle cyst (ruptured) N83.0-
- intermenstrual (regular) N92.3
  - irregular N92.1
- internal (organs) EC R58
  - capsule I61.0
  - newborn P54.8
- intestine K92.2
  - newborn P54.3
- intra-alveolar (lung), newborn P26.8
- intracerebral (nontraumatic)—*see* Hemorrhage, intracranial, intracerebral
- intracranial, intracerebral
- intracranial (nontraumatic) I62.9
  - birth injury P10.9
  - epidural, nontraumatic I62.1
  - extradural, nontraumatic I62.1
  - intracerebral (nontraumatic) (in) I61.9
    - brain stem I61.3
    - cerebellum I61.4
    - hemisphere I61.2
      - cortical (superficial) I61.1
      - subcortical (deep) I61.0
    - intraventricular I61.5
    - multiple localized I61.6
    - newborn P52.4
      - birth injury P10.1
    - specified NEC I61.8
    - superficial I61.1
  - subarachnoid (nontraumatic) (from) I60.9
    - intracranial (cerebral) artery I60.7
      - anterior communicating I60.2-
      - basilar I60.4
      - carotid siphon and bifurcation I60.0-
      - communicating I60.7
        - ◊ anterior I60.2-
        - ◊ posterior I60.3-

Hemorrhage, hemorrhagic, *continued*
  - middle cerebral I60.1-
  - posterior communicating I60.3-
  - specified artery NEC I60.6
  - vertebral I60.5-
- newborn P52.5
  - birth injury P10.3
  - specified NEC I60.8-
  - traumatic S06.6X-
- subdural (nontraumatic) I62.00
  - acute I62.01
  - birth injury P10.0
  - chronic I62.03
  - newborn (anoxic) (hypoxic) P52.8
    - birth injury P10.0
  - spinal G95.19
  - subacute I62.02
  - traumatic—*see* Injury, intracranial, subdural hemorrhage
- intrapontine I61.3
- intraventricular I61.5
  - newborn (nontraumatic) (*see also* Newborn, affected by, hemorrhage) P52.3
    - due to birth injury P10.2
    - grade
      - 1 P52.0
      - 2 P52.1
      - 3 P52.21
      - 4 P52.22
- lenticular striate artery I61.0
- lung R04.89
  - newborn P26.9
    - massive P26.1
    - specified NEC P26.8
- medulla I61.3
- membrane (brain) I60.8-
- meninges, meningeal (brain) (middle) I60.8-
- mouth K13.79
- mucous membrane NEC R58
  - newborn P54.8
- nail (subungual) L60.8
- nasal turbinate R04.0
  - newborn P54.8
- newborn P54.9
  - specified NEC P54.8
- nipple N64.59
- nose R04.0
  - newborn P54.8
- ovary NEC N83.8
- pericardium, pericarditis I31.2
- peritonsillar tissue J35.8
  - due to infection J36
- pituitary (gland) E23.6
- petechial R23.3
  - due to autosensitivity, erythrocyte D69.2
- pons, pontine I61.3
- posterior fossa (nontraumatic) I61.8
  - newborn P52.6
- postnasal R04.0
- pulmonary R04.89
  - newborn P26.9
    - massive P26.1
    - specified NEC P26.8
- purpura (primary) D69.3
- rectum (sphincter) K62.5
  - newborn P54.2
- retroperitoneal K68.3
- skin R23.3
  - newborn P54.5
- slipped umbilical ligature P51.8
- stomach K92.2
  - newborn P54.3
  - ulcer—*see* Ulcer, stomach, with, hemorrhage
- subconjunctival—*see also* Hemorrhage, conjunctiva
  - birth injury P15.3
- subcortical (brain) I61.0
- subcutaneous R23.3
- subependymal
  - newborn P52.0
    - with intraventricular extension P52.1
      - and intracerebral extension P52.22
- subungual L60.8

Hemorrhage, hemorrhagic, *continued*
- suprarenal (capsule) (gland) E27.49
  - newborn P54.4
- tonsil J35.8
- ulcer—*code by site* under Ulcer, with hemorrhage K27.4
- umbilicus, umbilical
  - cord
    - after birth, newborn P51.9
    - newborn P51.9
      - massive P51.0
      - slipped ligature P51.8
      - stump P51.9
- uterus, uterine (abnormal) N93.9
  - dysfunctional or functional N93.8
  - intermenstrual (regular) N92.3
    - irregular N92.1
  - pubertal N92.2
- vagina (abnormal) N93.9
  - newborn P54.6
- ventricular I61.5
- viscera NEC R58
  - newborn P54.8

Hemorrhoids (bleeding) (without mention of degree) K64.9
- 1st degree (grade/stage I) (without prolapse outside of anal canal) K64.0
- 2nd degree (grade/stage II) (that prolapse with straining but retract spontaneously) K64.1
- 3rd degree (grade/stage III) (that prolapse with straining and require manual replacement back inside anal canal) K64.2
- 4th degree (grade/stage IV) (with prolapsed tissue that cannot be manually replaced) K64.3
- external K64.4
  - with
    - thrombosis K64.5
- internal (without mention of degree) K64.8
- prolapsed K64.8
- skin tags
  - anus K64.4
  - residual K64.4
- specified NEC K64.8
- strangulated (*see also* Hemorrhoids, by degree) K64.8
- thrombosed (*see also* Hemorrhoids, by degree) K64.5
- ulcerated (*see also* Hemorrhoids, by degree) K64.8

Hemothorax
- newborn P54.8

Henoch (-Schönlein) disease or syndrome (purpura) D69.0

Hepatitis K75.9
- acute (infectious) (viral) B17.9
- B B19.10
  - acute B16.9
- C (viral) B19.20
  - acute B17.10
  - chronic B18.2
- catarrhal (acute) B15.9
- chronic K73.9
  - active NEC K73.2
- epidemic B15.9
- fulminant NEC K75.3
  - neonatal giant cell P59.29
- history of
  - B Z86.19
  - C Z86.19
- homologous serum—*see* Hepatitis, viral, type B
- in (due to)
  - congenital (active) P37.1 [K77]
- infectious, infective (acute) (chronic) (subacute) B15.9
- neonatal (idiopathic) (toxic) P59.29
- newborn P59.29
- viral, virus B19.9
  - acute B17.9
    - C B18.2
  - in remission, any type—*code to* Hepatitis, chronic, by type
  - type
    - A B15.9
    - B 19.10
      - acute B16.9
    - C B19.20
      - acute B17.10
      - chronic B18.2

ALPHABETIC INDEX

Hepatitis—*see also* Hypertrophy, liver
- congenital Q44.79
- in mononucleosis
  - gammaherpesviral B27.09
  - infectious specified NEC B27.89

Hereditary alpha tryptasemia (syndrome) D89.44

Herlitz' syndrome Q81.1

Hernia, hernial (acquired) (recurrent) K46.9
- with
  - gangrene—*see* Hernia, by site, with, gangrene
  - incarceration—*see* Hernia, by site, with, obstruction
  - irreducible—*see* Hernia, by site, with, obstruction
  - obstruction—*see* Hernia, by site, with, obstruction
  - strangulation—*see* Hernia, by site, with, obstruction
- abdomen, abdominal K46.-
- bladder (mucosa) (sphincter)
  - congenital (female) (male) Q79.51
- diaphragm, diaphragmatic K44.9
  - with
    - gangrene (and obstruction) K44.1
    - obstruction K44.0
  - congenital Q79.0
- direct (inguinal)—*see* Hernia, inguinal
- diverticulum, intestine—*see* Hernia
- double (inguinal)—*see* Hernia, inguinal, bilateral
- epigastric (*see also* Hernia, ventral) K43.9
- esophageal hiatus—*see* Hernia, hiatal
- external (inguinal)—*see* Hernia, inguinal
- foramen magnum G93.5
  - congenital Q01.8
- hiatal (esophageal) (sliding) K44.9
  - with
    - gangrene (and obstruction) K44.1
    - obstruction K44.0
  - congenital Q40.1
- indirect (inguinal)—*see* Hernia, inguinal
- incisional K43.2
  - with
    - gangrene (and obstruction) K43.1
    - obstruction K43.0
- inguinal (direct) (external) (funicular) (indirect) (internal) (oblique) (scrotal) (sliding) K40.90
  - with
    - gangrene (and obstruction) K40.40
      - not specified as recurrent K40.40
      - recurrent K40.41
    - obstruction K40.30
      - not specified as recurrent K40.30
      - recurrent K40.31
  - bilateral K40.20
    - with
      - gangrene (and obstruction) K40.10
        - ◊ not specified as recurrent K40.10
        - ◊ recurrent K40.11
      - obstruction K40.00
        - ◊ not specified as recurrent K40.00
        - ◊ recurrent K40.01
    - not specified as recurrent K40.20
    - recurrent K40.21
  - not specified as recurrent K40.90
  - recurrent K40.91
  - unilateral K40.90
    - with
      - gangrene (and obstruction) K40.40
        - ◊ not specified as recurrent K40.40
        - ◊ recurrent K40.41
      - obstruction K40.30
        - ◊ not specified as recurrent K40.30
        - ◊ recurrent K40.31
    - not specified as recurrent K40.90
    - recurrent K40.91
- irreducible—*see also* Hernia, by site, with obstruction
  - with gangrene—*see* Hernia, by site, with gangrene
- linea (alba) (semilunaris)—*see* Hernia, ventral
- midline—*see* Hernia, ventral
- oblique (inguinal)—*see* Hernia, inguinal
- obstructive—*see also* Hernia, by site, with obstruction
  - with gangrene—*see* Hernia, by site, with gangrene
- scrotum, scrotal—*see* Hernia, inguinal
- sliding (inguinal)—*see also* Hernia, inguinal
  - hiatus—*see* Hernia, hiatal
- spigelian—*see* Hernia, ventral

Hernia, hernial, *continued*
- spinal—*see* Spina bifida
- strangulated—*see also* Hernia, by site, with obstruction
  - with gangrene—*see* Hernia, by site, with gangrene
- subxiphoid—*see* Hernia, ventral
- supra-umbilicus—*see* Hernia, ventral
- tunica vaginalis Q55.29
- umbilicus, umbilical K42.9
  - with
    - gangrene (and obstruction) K42.1
    - obstruction K42.0
  - ventral K43.9
    - recurrent—*see* Hernia, incisional
    - incisional K43.2
      - with
        - gangrene (and obstruction) K43.1
        - obstruction K43.0
      - specified NEC K43.9

Herniation—*see also* **Hernia**
- brain (stem) G93.5
  - nontraumatic G93.5
  - traumatic S06.A1
- cerebral G93.5
  - nontraumatic G93.5
  - traumatic S06.A1

Herpangina B08.5

Herpes, herpesvirus, herpetic B00.9
- anogenital A60.9
  - urogenital tract A60.00
    - cervix A60.03
    - male genital organ NEC A60.02
    - penis A60.01
    - specified site NEC A60.09
    - vagina A60.04
    - vulva A60.04
- circinatus B35.4
- encephalitis B00.4
  - due to herpesvirus 7 B10.09
  - specified NEC B10.09
- genital, genitalis A60.00
  - female A60.09
  - male A60.02
- gingivostomatitis B00.2
- human B00.9
  - 1—*see* Herpes, simplex
  - 2—*see* Herpes, simplex
  - 4—*see* Mononucleosis, Epstein-Barr (virus)
  - 7
    - encephalitis B10.09
- meningitis (simplex) B00.3
- pharyngitis, pharyngotonsillitis B00.2
- simplex B00.9
  - complicated NEC B00.89
  - congenital P35.2
  - specified complication NEC B00.89
  - visceral B00.89
- stomatitis B00.2
- tonsurans B35.0 visceral B00.89
- whitlow B00.89

Herter-Gee Syndrome K90.0

Hesitancy
- of micturition R39.11
- urinary R39.11

Heubner-Herter disease K90.0

Hiccup, hiccough R06.6
- psychogenic F45.8

Hidden penis (congenital) Q55.64

Hidradenitis (axillaris) (suppurative) L73.2

High
- altitude effects T70.20
  - anoxia T70.29
  - on
    - ears T70.0
    - sinuses T70.1
  - polycythemia D75.1
- arch
  - foot Q66.7-
  - palate, congenital Q38.5
- basal metabolic rate R94.8

High, *continued*
- blood pressure—*see also* Hypertension
  - borderline R03.0
  - reading (incidental) (isolated) (nonspecific), without diagnosis of hypertension R03.0
- cholesterol E78.00
  - with high triglycerides E78.2
- expressed emotional level within family Z63.8
- palate, congenital Q38.5
- risk
  - infant NEC Z76.2
  - sexual behavior (heterosexual) Z72.51
    - bisexual Z72.53
    - homosexual Z72.52
- scrotal testis, testes
  - bilateral Q53.23
  - unilateral Q53.13
- temperature (of unknown origin) R50.9
- triglycerides E78.1
  - with high cholesterol E78.2

Hippel's disease Q85.8

Hirschsprung's disease or megacolon Q43.1

Hirsutism, hirsuties L68.0

Hirudiniasis
- external B88.3

Histiocytosis D76.3
- lipid, lipoid D76.3
- mononuclear phagocytes NEC D76.1
- non-Langerhans cell D76.3
- polyostotic sclerosing D76.3
- sinus, with massive lymphadenopathy D76.3
- syndrome NEC D76.3

Histoplasmosis B39.9
- with pneumonia NEC B39.2
  - capsulati B39.4
- disseminated B39.3
- generalized B39.3
- pulmonary B39.2
  - acute B39.0
  - chronic B39.1

History
- family (of)—*see also* History, personal (of)
  - alcohol abuse Z81.1
  - allergy NEC Z84.89
  - anemia Z83.2
  - arthritis Z82.61
  - asthma Z82.5
  - blindness Z82.1
  - cardiac death (sudden) Z82.41
  - carrier of genetic disease Z84.81
  - chromosomal anomaly Z82.79
  - chronic
    - disabling disease NEC Z82.8
      - lower respiratory disease Z82.5
    - colonic polyps Z83.71
  - congenital malformations and deformations Z82.79
    - polycystic kidney Z82.71
  - consanguinity Z84.3
  - deafness Z82.2
  - diabetes mellitus Z83.3
  - disability NEC Z82.8
  - disease or disorder (of)
    - allergic NEC Z84.89
    - behavioral NEC Z81.8
    - blood and blood-forming organs Z83.2
    - cardiovascular NEC Z82.49
    - chronic disabling NEC Z82.8
    - digestive Z83.79
    - ear NEC Z83.52
    - elevated lipoprotein(a) (Lp(a)) Z83.430
    - endocrine NEC Z83.49
    - eye NEC Z83.518
      - glaucoma Z83.511
    - familial hypercholesterolemia Z83.42
    - genitourinary NEC Z84.2
    - glaucoma Z83.511
    - hematological Z83.2
    - immune mechanism Z83.2
    - infectious NEC Z83.1
    - ischemic heart Z82.49
    - kidney Z84.1

ALPHABETIC INDEX

History, *continued*

- ■ lipoprotein metabolism Z83.438
- ■ mental NEC Z81.8
- ■ metabolic Z83.49
- ■ musculoskeletal NEC Z82.69
- ■ neurological NEC Z82.0
- ■ nutritional Z83.49
- ■ parasitic NEC Z83.1
- ■ psychiatric NEC Z81.8
- ■ respiratory NEC Z83.6
- ■ skin and subcutaneous tissue NEC Z84.0
- ■ specified NEC Z84.89
- – drug abuse NEC Z81.3
- – elevated lipoprotein (a) (LP(a)) Z83.430
- – epilepsy Z82.0
- – familial hypercholesterolemia Z83.42
- – genetic disease carrier Z84.81
- – glaucoma Z83.511
- – hearing loss Z82.2
- – human immunodeficiency virus (HIV) infection Z83.0
- – Huntington's chorea Z82.0
- – hypercholesterolemia (familial) Z83.42
- – hyperlipidemia, familial combined Z83.438
- – intellectual disability Z81.0
- – leukemia Z80.6
- – lipidemia NEC Z83.438
- – malignant neoplasm (of) NOS Z80.9
  - ■ bladder Z80.52
  - ■ breast Z80.3
  - ■ bronchus Z80.1
  - ■ digestive organ Z80.0
  - ■ gastrointestinal tract Z80.0
  - ■ genital organ Z80.49
    - – ovary Z80.41
    - – prostate Z80.42
    - – specified organ NEC Z80.49
    - – testis Z80.43
  - ■ hematopoietic NEC Z80.7
  - ■ intrathoracic organ NEC Z80.2
  - ■ kidney Z80.51
  - ■ lung Z80.1
  - ■ lymphatic NEC Z80.7
  - ■ ovary Z80.41
  - ■ prostate Z80.42
  - ■ respiratory organ NEC Z80.2
  - ■ specified site NEC Z80.8
  - ■ testis Z80.43
  - ■ trachea Z80.1
  - ■ urinary organ or tract Z80.59
    - – bladder Z80.52
    - – kidney Z80.51
- – mental
  - ■ disorder NEC Z81.8
- – multiple endocrine neoplasia (MEN) syndrome Z83.41
- – osteoporosis Z82.62
- – personal (of)—*see also* History, family (of)
  - ■ drug therapy
    - – ICI (immune checkpoint inhibitor) drug therapy Z92.26
  - ■ ICI (immune checkpoint inhibitor) drug therapy Z92.26
  - ■ immune checkpoint inhibitor (ICI) therapy Z92.26
- – polycystic kidney Z82.71
- – polyps (colon) Z83.71
- – psychiatric disorder Z81.8
- – psychoactive substance abuse NEC Z81.3
- – respiratory condition NEC Z83.6
  - ■ asthma and other lower respiratory conditions Z82.5
- – self-harmful behavior Z81.8
- – SIDS (sudden infant death syndrome) Z84.82
- – skin condition Z84.0
- – specified condition NEC Z84.89
- – stroke (cerebrovascular) Z82.3
- – substance abuse NEC Z81.4
  - ■ alcohol Z81.1
  - ■ drug NEC Z81.3
  - ■ psychoactive NEC Z81.3
  - ■ tobacco Z81.2
- – sudden cardiac death Z82.41
- – sudden infant death syndrome Z84.82
- – tobacco abuse Z81.2
- – violence, violent behavior Z81.8

History, *continued*

- – visual loss Z82.1
- personal (of)—*see also* History, family (of)
  - – abuse
    - ■ childhood Z62.819
      - – financial Z62.814
    - – forced labor or sexual exploitation in childhood Z62.813
    - – intimate partner Z62.815
    - – physical Z62.810
    - – psychological Z62.811
    - – sexual Z62.810
  - – alcohol dependence F10.21
  - – allergy (to) Z88.9
    - ■ antibiotic agent NEC Z88.1
    - ■ drugs, medicaments and biological substances Z88.9
      - – specified NEC Z88.8
    - ■ food Z91.018
      - – additives Z91.02
      - – beef Z91.014
      - – eggs Z91.012
      - – lamb Z91.014
      - – mammalian meats Z91.014
      - – milk products Z91.011
      - – peanuts Z91.010
      - – pork Z91.014
      - – red meats Z91.014
      - – seafood Z91.013
      - – specified food NEC Z91.018
    - ■ insect Z91.038
      - – bee Z91.030
    - ■ latex Z91.040
    - ■ medicinal agents Z88.9
      - – specified NEC Z88.8
    - ■ narcotic agent Z88.5
    - ■ nonmedicinal agents Z91.048
    - ■ penicillin Z88.0
    - ■ serum Z88.7
    - ■ sulfonamides Z88.2
    - ■ vaccine Z88.7
  - – anaphylactic shock Z87.892
  - – anaphylaxis Z87.892
  - – behavioral disorders Z86.59
  - – brain injury (traumatic) Z87.820
  - – cancer—*see* History, personal (of), malignant neoplasm (of)
  - – cardiac arrest (death), successfully resuscitated Z86.74
  - – CAR-T (Chimeric Antigen Receptor T-cell) therapy Z92.850
  - – cellular therapy Z92.859
    - ■ specified NEC Z92.858
  - – cerebral infarction without residual deficit Z86.73
  - – chemotherapy for neoplastic condition Z92.21
  - – Chimeric Antigen Receptor T-cell (CAR-T) therapy Z92.850
  - – cleft lip (corrected) Z87.730
  - – cleft palate (corrected) Z87.730
  - – congenital malformation (corrected) Z87.798
    - ■ circulatory system (corrected) Z87.74
    - ■ digestive system (corrected) NEC Z87.738
    - ■ ear (corrected) Z87.721
    - ■ eye (corrected) Z87.720
    - ■ face and neck (corrected) Z87.790
    - ■ genitourinary system (corrected) NEC Z87.718
    - ■ heart (corrected) Z87.74
    - ■ integument (corrected) Z87.76
    - ■ limb(s) (corrected) Z87.76
    - ■ musculoskeletal system (corrected) Z87.76
    - ■ neck (corrected) Z87.790
    - ■ nervous system (corrected) NEC Z87.728
    - ■ respiratory system (corrected) Z87.75
    - ■ sense organs (corrected) NEC Z87.728
    - ■ specified NEC Z87.798
  - – coronavirus (disease) (novel) 2019 Z86.16
  - – disease or disorder (of) Z87.898
    - ■ blood and blood-forming organs Z86.2
    - ■ connective tissue NEC Z87.39
    - ■ ear Z86.69
    - ■ endocrine Z86.39
      - – specified type NEC Z86.39
    - ■ eye Z86.69

History, *continued*

- ■ hematological Z86.2
- ■ Hodgkin Z85.71
- ■ immune mechanism Z86.2
- ■ infectious Z86.19
  - – Methicillin resistant Staphylococcus aureus (MRSA) Z86.14
  - – tuberculosis Z86.11
- ■ mental NEC Z86.59
- ■ metabolic Z86.39
  - – specified type NEC Z86.39
- ■ musculoskeletal NEC Z87.39
- ■ nervous system Z86.69
- ■ nutritional Z86.39
- ■ respiratory system NEC Z87.09
- ■ sense organs Z86.69
- ■ specified site or type NEC Z87.898
- ■ urinary system NEC Z87.448
- – drug therapy
  - ■ antineoplastic chemotherapy Z92.21
  - ■ immunosupression Z92.25
  - ■ inhaled steroids Z92.240
  - ■ monoclonal drug Z92.22
  - ■ specified NEC Z92.29
  - ■ steroid Z92.241
  - ■ systemic steroids Z92.241
- – encephalitis Z86.61
- – extracorporeal membrane oxygenation (ECMO) Z92.81
- – fall, falling Z91.81
- – forced labor or sexual exploitation in childhood Z62.813
- – gene therapy Z92.86
- – hepatitis
  - ■ B Z86.19
  - ■ C Z86.19
- – Hodgkin disease Z85.71
- – hypospadias (corrected) Z87.710
- – immunosupression therapy Z92.25
- – infection NEC Z86.19
  - ■ central nervous system Z86.61
  - ■ latent tuberculosis Z86.15
  - ■ Methicillin resistant Staphylococcus aureus (MRSA) Z86.14
- – in situ neoplasm
  - ■ breast Z86.000
  - ■ cervix uteri Z86.001
  - ■ digestive organs, specified NEC Z86.004
  - ■ esophagus Z86.003
  - ■ genital organs, specified NEC Z86.002
  - ■ melanoma Z86.006
  - ■ middle ear Z86.005
  - ■ oral cavity Z86.003
  - ■ respiratory system Z86.005
  - ■ skin Z86.007
  - ■ specified NEC Z86.008
  - ■ stomach Z86.003
- – in utero procedure while a fetus Z98.871
- – latent tuberculosis Z86.15
- – leukemia Z85.6
- – lymphoma (non-Hodgkin) Z85.72
- – malignant melanoma (skin) Z85.820
- – malignant neoplasm (of) Z85.9
  - ■ bone Z85.830
  - ■ brain Z85.841
  - ■ carcinoid—*see* History, personal (of), malignant neoplasm, by site, carcinoid
  - ■ endocrine gland NEC Z85.858
  - ■ eye Z85.840
  - ■ hematopoietic NEC Z85.79
  - ■ kidney NEC Z85.528
    - – carcinoid Z85.520
- – maltreatment Z91.89
- – melanoma Z85.820
- – meningitis Z86.61
- – mental disorder Z86.59
- – Methicillin resistant Staphylococcus aureus (MRSA) Z86.14
- – neglect (in)
  - ■ childhood Z62.812
- – neoplasm
  - ■ in situ—*see* Table of Neoplasms in the complete *ICD-10-CM* manual

ALPHABETIC INDEX

History, *continued*
- ■ malignant—see Table of Neoplasms in the complete *ICD-10-CM* manual
- ■ uncertain behavior Z86.03
- – nephrotic syndrome Z87.441
- – nicotine dependence Z87.891
- – noncompliance with medical treatment or regimen—see Noncompliance
- – nutritional deficiency Z86.39
- – parasuicide (attempt) Z91.51
- – physical trauma NEC Z87.828
  - ■ self-harm or suicide attempt Z91.51
- – pneumonia (recurrent) Z87.01
- – poisoning NEC Z91.89
  - ■ self-harm or suicide attempt Z91.51
- – procedure while a fetus Z98.871
- – prolonged reversible ischemic neurologic deficit (PRIND) Z86.73
- – psychological
  - ■ abuse
    - – child Z62.811
    - ■ trauma, specified NEC Z91.49
  - – respiratory condition NEC Z87.09
  - – retained foreign body fully removed Z87.821
  - – risk factors NEC Z91.89
  - – self-harm
    - ■ nonsuicidal Z91.52
    - ■ suicidal Z91.51
  - – self-inflicted injury without suicidal intent Z91.52
    - ■ self-injury Z91.52
    - ■ nonsuicidal Z91.52
  - – self-mutilation Z91.52
  - – self-poisoning attempt Z91.51
  - – specified NEC Z87.898
  - – steroid therapy (systemic) Z92.241
    - ■ inhaled Z92.240
  - – stroke without residual deficits Z86.73
  - – substance abuse NEC F10-F19
  - – sudden cardiac arrest Z86.74
  - – sudden cardiac death successfully resuscitated Z86.74
  - – suicidal behavior Z91.51
  - – suicide attempt Z91.51
  - – surgery NEC Z98.890
  - – tobacco dependence Z87.891
  - – transient ischemic attack (TIA) without residual deficits Z86.73
  - – trauma (physical) NEC Z87.828
    - ■ psychological NEC Z91.49
    - ■ self-harm Z91.51
  - – traumatic brain injury Z87.820

HIV (*see also* Human, immunodeficiency virus) B20
- ● laboratory evidence (nonconclusive) R75
- ● positive, seropositive Z21
- ● nonconclusive test (in infants) R75

Hives (bold)—*see* Urticaria

Hoarseness R49.0

Hoffmann's syndrome E03.9 *[G73.7]*

Homelessness Z59.00
- ● sheltered Z59.01
- ● unsheltered Z59.02

Homocysteinemia R79.83

Hooded
- ● clitoris Q52.6
- ● penis Q55.69

Hordeolum (eyelid) (externum) (recurrent) H00.01-
- ● internum H00.02-
  - – left H00.026
    - ■ lower H00.025
    - ■ upper H00.024
  - – right H00.023
    - ■ lower H00.022
    - ■ upper H00.021
- ● left H00.016
  - – lower H00.015
  - – upper H00.014
- ● right H00.013
  - – lower H00.012
  - – upper H00.011

Horseshoe kidney (congenital) Q63.1

Hospitalism in children—*see* Disorder, adjustment

Household, housing circumstance affecting care Z59.9
- ● specified NEC Z59.89

HSCT-TMA (hematopoietic stem cell transplantation-associated thrombotic microangiopathy) M31.11

Human
- ● bite (open wound)—*see also* Bite
  - – intact skin surface—*see* Bite
- ● herpesvirus—*see* Herpes
- ● immunodeficiency virus (HIV) disease (infection) B20
  - – asymptomatic status Z21
  - – contact Z20.6
  - – counseling Z71.7
  - – exposure to Z20.6
  - – laboratory evidence R75
- ● papillomavirus (HPV)
  - – screening for Z11.51

Hunger T73.0
- ● air, psychogenic F45.8

Hunter's
- ● syndrome E76.1

Hunt's
- ● dyssynergia cerebellaris myoclonica G11.19

Hutchinson's
- ● disease, meaning
  - – pompholyx (cheiropompholyx) L30.1

Hyaline membrane (disease) (lung) (pulmonary) (newborn) P22.0

Hydatid
- ● Morgagni
  - – female Q50.5
  - – male (epididymal) Q55.4
    - ■ testicular Q55.29

Hydradenitis (axillaris) (suppurative) L73.2

Hydramnios O40.-

Hydrarthrosis—*see also* Effusion, joint
- ● intermittent M12.4-
  - – ankle M12.47-
  - – elbow M12.42-
  - – foot joint M12.47-
  - – hand joint M12.44-
  - – hip M12.45-
  - – knee M12.46-
  - – multiple site M12.49
  - – shoulder M12.41-
  - – specified joint NEC M12.48
  - – wrist M12.43-

Hydroadenitis (axillaris) (suppurative) L73.2

Hydrocele (spermatic cord) (testis) (tunica vaginalis) N43.3
- ● communicating N43.2
  - – congenital P83.5
- ● congenital P83.5
- ● encysted N43.0
- ● female NEC N94.89
- ● infected N43.1
- ● newborn P83.5
- ● round ligament N94.89
- ● specified NEC N43.2
- ● spinalis—*see* Spina bifida
- ● vulva N90.89

Hydrocephalus (acquired) (external) (internal) (malignant) (recurrent) G91.9
- ● aqueduct Sylvius stricture Q03.0
- ● communicating G91.0
- ● congenital (external) (internal) Q03.9
  - – with spina bifida Q05.4
    - ■ cervical Q05.0
    - ■ dorsal Q05.1
    - ■ lumbar Q05.2
    - ■ lumbosacral Q05.2
    - ■ sacral Q05.3
    - ■ thoracic Q05.1
    - ■ thoracolumbar Q05.1
  - – specified NEC Q03.8
- ● due to toxoplasmosis (congenital) P37.1
- ● foramen Magendie block (acquired) G91.1
  - – congenital (*see also* Hydrocephalus, congenital) Q03.1

Hydrocephalus, *continued*
- ● in (due to)
  - – infectious disease NEC B89 [G91.4]
  - – neoplastic disease NEC (*see also* Table of Neoplasms in the complete *ICD-10-CM manual*) G91.4
  - – parasitic disease B89 [G91.4]
- ● newborn Q03.9
  - – with spina bifida—*see* Spina bifida, with hydrocephalus
- ● noncommunicating G91.1
- ● normal pressure G91.2
  - – secondary G91.0
- ● obstructive G91.1
- ● otitic G93.2
- ● post-traumatic NEC G91.3
- ● secondary G91.4
  - – post-traumatic G91.3
- ● specified NEC G91.8

Hydromicrocephaly Q02

Hydromphalos (since birth) Q45.8

Hydronephrosis (atrophic) (early) (functionless) (intermittent) (primary) (secondary) NEC N13.30
- ● with
  - – obstruction (by) (of)
    - ■ renal calculus N13.2
    - ■ ureteral NEC N13.1
      - – calculus N13.2
    - ■ ureteropelvic junction N13.0
      - – congenital Q62.11
      - – with infection N13.6
  - – ureteral stricture NEC N13.1
- ● congenital Q62.0
- ● specified type NEC N13.39

Hydroperitoneum R18.8

Hydrophthalmos Q15.0

Hydrops R60.9
- ● abdominis R18.8
- ● endolymphatic H81.0-
- ● fetalis P83.2
  - – due to
    - ■ ABO isoimmunization P56.0
    - ■ alpha thalassemia D56.0
    - ■ hemolytic disease P56.90
      - – specified NEC P56.99
    - ■ isoimmunization (ABO) (Rh) P56.0
    - ■ other specified nonhemolytic disease NEC P83.2
    - ■ Rh incompatibility P56.0
  - ● newborn (idiopathic) P83.2
    - – due to
      - ■ ABO isoimmunization P56.0
      - ■ alpha thalassemia D56.0
      - ■ hemolytic disease P56.90
        - – specified NEC P56.99
      - ■ isoimmunization (ABO) (Rh) P56.0
      - ■ Rh incompatibility P56.0
- ● pericardium—*see* Pericarditis
- ● spermatic cord—*see* Hydrocele

Hydropyonephrosis N13.6

Hydrorhea (nasal) J34.89

Hydrosadenitis (axillaris) (suppurative) L73.2

Hydroxykynureninuria E70.89

Hyperacidity (gastric) K31.89
- ● psychogenic F45.8

Hyperactive, hyperactivity F90.9
- ● bowel sounds R19.12
- ● child F90.9
  - – attention deficit—*see* Disorder, attention-deficit hyperactivity
- ● detrusor muscle N32.81
- ● gastrointestinal K31.89
  - – psychogenic F45.8
- ● nasal mucous membrane J34.3

Hyperadrenocorticism E24.9
- ● congenital E25.0
- ● iatrogenic E24.2
  - – correct substance properly administered—*see* Table of Drugs and Chemicals, by drug, adverse effect
  - – overdose or wrong substance given or taken—*see* Table of Drugs and Chemicals, by drug, poisoning

HISTORY - HYPERADRENOCORTICISM

ALPHABETIC INDEX

Hyperadrenocorticism, *continued*
- not associated with Cushing's syndrome E27.0
- pituitary-dependent E24.0

Hyperalimentation R63.2

Hyperbetalipoproteinemia (familial) E78.0
- with prebetalipoproteinemia E78.2

Hyperbicarbonatemia P74.41

Hyperbilirubinemia
- constitutional E80.6
- familial conjugated E80.6
- neonatal (transient)—*see* Jaundice, newborn

Hypercalcemia, hypocalciuric, familial E83.52

Hypercalciuria, idiopathic R82.994

Hypercapnia R06.89
- newborn P84

Hyperchloremia E87.8

Hyperchlorhydria K31.89
- neurotic F45.8
- psychogenic F45.8

Hypercholesterolemia (essential) (primary) (pure) E78.00
- with hyperglyceridemia, endogenous E78.2
- dietary counseling and surveillance Z71.3
- familial E78.01
- family history of Z83.42
- hereditary E78.01

Hyperchylia gastrica, psychogenic F45.8

Hypercorticalism, pituitary-dependent E24.0

Hypercorticosolism—*see* Cushing's, syndrome

Hypercorticosteronism E24.2
- correct substance properly administered—*see* Table of Drugs and Chemicals, by drug, adverse effect
- overdose or wrong substance given or taken—*see* Table of Drugs and Chemicals, by drug, poisoning

Hypercortisonism E24.2
- correct substance properly administered—*see* Table of Drugs and Chemicals, by drug, adverse effect
- overdose or wrong substance given or taken—*see* Table of Drugs and Chemicals, by drug, poisoning

Hyperekplexia Q89.8

Hyperelectrolytemia E87.8

Hyperemesis R11.10
- with nausea R11.2
- projectile R11.12
- psychogenic F45.8

Hyperemia (acute) (passive) R68.89
- anal mucosa K62.89
- ear internal, acute—*see* subcategory H83.0
- labyrinth—*see* subcategory H83.0

Hyperexplexia Q89.8

Hyperfunction
- adrenal cortex, not associated with Cushing's syndrome E27.0
  - virilism E25.9
    - congenital E25.0

Hyperglycemia, hyperglycemic (transient) R73.9
- coma—*see* Diabetes, by type, with coma
- postpancreatectomy E89.1

Hyperheparinemia D68.32

Hyperhidrosis, hyperidrosis R61
- generalized R61
- psychogenic F45.8
- secondary R61
  - focal L74.52

Hyperinsulinism (functional) E16.1
- therapeutic misadventure (from administration of insulin)—*see* subcategory T38.3

Hyperkeratosis (*see also* Keratosis) L85.9
- follicularis Q82.8
- universalis congenita Q80.8

Hyperlipemia, hyperlipidemia E78.5
- combined E78.2
  - familial E78.49
- group
  - A E78.00
  - C E78.2

Hyperlipemia, hyperlipidemia, *continued*
- mixed E78.2
  - specified NEC E78.49

Hyperlipoproteinemia E78.5
- Fredrickson's type
  - IIa E78.00
  - IIb E78.2
  - III E78.2
- low-density-lipoprotein-type (LDL) E78.00
- very-low-density-lipoprotein-type (VLDL) E78.1

Hypermagnesemia E83.41
- neonatal P71.8

Hypermenorrhea N92.0

Hypermetropia (congenital) H52.0-

Hypermobility, hypermotility
- colon—*see* Syndrome, irritable bowel
  - psychogenic F45.8
- intestine (*see also* Syndrome, irritable bowel) K58.9
  - psychogenic F45.8
- stomach K31.89
  - psychogenic F45.8
- syndrome M35.7

Hypernatremia E87.0

Hypernephroma C64.-

Hyperopia—*see* Hypermetropia

Hyperorexia nervosa F50.2-

Hyperosmolality E87.0

Hyperostosis (monomelic)—*see also* Disorder
- skull M85.2
  - congenital Q75.8

Hyperperistalsis R19.2
- psychogenic F45.8

Hyperpigmentation—*see also* Pigmentation
- melanin NEC L81.4

Hyperplasia, hyperplastic
- adenoids J35.2
- adrenal (capsule) (cortex) (gland) E27.8
  - with
    - sexual precocity (male) E25.9
      - congenital E25.0
    - virilism, adrenal E25.9
      - congenital E25.0
    - virilization (female) E25.9
      - congenital E25.0
  - congenital E25.0
  - salt-losing E25.0
- angiolymphoid, eosinophilia (ALHE) D18.01
- bone NOS Q79.9
  - face Q75.8
  - skull—*see* Hypoplasia, skull
- cervix (uteri) (basal cell) (endometrium) (polypoid)
  - congenital Q51.828
- endocervicitis N72
- epithelial L85.9
  - nipple N62
  - skin L85.9
- face Q18.8
  - bone(s) Q75.8
- genital
  - female NEC N94.89
  - male N50.89
- gingiva K06.1
- gum K06.1
- liver (congenital) Q44.79
- nose
  - lymphoid J34.89
  - polypoid J33.9
- tonsils (faucial) (infective) (lingual) (lymphoid) J35.1
  - with adenoids J35.3

Hyperpnea—*see* Hyperventilation

Hyperproteinemia E88.09

Hyperpyrexia R50.9
- heat (effects) T67.01
- rheumatic—*see* Fever, rheumatic
- unknown origin R50.9

Hypersecretion
- ACTH (not associated with Cushing's syndrome) E27.0
  - pituitary E24.0

Hypersecretion, *continued*
- corticoadrenal E24.9
- cortisol E24.9
- gastric K31.89
  - psychogenic F45.8
- hormone(s)
  - ACTH (not associated with Cushing's syndrome E27.0
    - pituitary E24.0
  - antidiuretic E22.2
  - growth E22.0

Hypersegmentation, leukocytic, hereditary D72.0

Hypersensitive, hypersensitiveness, hypersensitivity—*see also* Allergy
- gastrointestinal K52.29
  - psychogenic F45.8
- reaction T78.40

Hypertension, hypertensive (accelerated) (benign) (essential) (idiopathic) (malignant) (systemic) I10
- benign, intracranial G93.2
- borderline R03.0
- complicating
  - pregnancy
    - gestational (pregnancy induced) (transient) (without proteinuria)
      - with proteinuria O14.9
        - ◊ mild pre-eclampsia O14.0-
        - ◊ moderate pre-eclampsia O14.0-
        - ◊ severe pre-eclampsia O14.1-
          - with hemolysis, elevated liver enzymes and low platelet count (HELLP) O14.2-
      - pre-existing
        - with
          - ◊ pre-eclampsia O11.-
            - essential O10.01-
            - secondary O10.41-
        - crisis I16.9
        - emergency I16.1
        - encephalopathy I67.4
        - kidney I12.9
          - with
            - stage 5 chronic kidney disease (CKD) or end stage renal disease (ESRD) I12.0
        - lesser circulation I27.0
        - newborn P29.2
          - pulmonary (persistent) P29.30
        - psychogenic F45.8
        - pulmonary I27.20
          - with
            - cor pulmonale (chronic) I27.29
            - right heart ventricular strain/failure I27.29
          - due to
            - hematologic disorders I27.29
            - left heart disease I27.22
            - lung diseases and hypoxia I27.23
            - metabolic disorders I27.29
            - specified systemic disorders NEC I27.29
          - group 1 (associated) (drug-induced) (toxin-induced) I27.21
          - group 2 I27.22
          - group 3 I27.23
          - group 4 I27.24
          - group 5 I27.29
          - of newborn (persistent) P29.3
          - primary (idiopathic) I27.0
            - secondary
              - arterial I27.21
              - specified NEC I27.29
          - resistant (apparent treatment) (treatment) (true) I1A.0
        - urgency I16.0

Hyperthermia (of unknown origin)—*see also* Hyperpyrexia
- newborn P81.9
  - environmental P81.0

Hyperthyroidism (latent) (pre-adult) (recurrent) E05.90
- with
  - goiter (diffuse) E05.00
    - with thyroid storm E05.01
  - storm E05.91
- intracranial (benign) G93.2
- neonatal, transitory P72.1

ALPHABETIC INDEX

Hypertony, hypertonia, hypertonicity
- stomach K31.89
  - psychogenic F45.8

Hypertrophy, hypertrophic
- adenoids (infective) J35.2
  - with tonsils J35.3
- anal papillae K62.89
- bladder (sphincter) (trigone) N32.89
- brain G93.89
- breast N62
  - newborn P83.4
  - pubertal, massive N62
- cardiac (chronic) (idiopathic) I51.7
  - with rheumatic fever (conditions in I00)
    - active I01.8
    - inactive or quiescent (with chorea) I09.89
  - congenital NEC Q24.8
  - rheumatic (with chorea) I09.89
    - active or acute I01.8
      - with chorea I02.0
- foot (congenital) Q74.2
- frenulum, frenum (tongue) K14.8
  - lip K13.0
- gland, glandular R59.9
  - generalized R59.1
  - localized R59.0
- gum (mucous membrane) K06.1
- hemifacial 67.4
- lingual tonsil (infective) J35.1
  - with adenoids J35.3
- lip K13.0
  - congenital Q18.6
- liver R16.0
  - congenital Q44.79
- lymph, lymphatic gland R59.9
  - generalized R59.1
  - localized R59.0
- Meckel's diverticulum (congenital) Q43.0
- mucous membrane
  - gum K06.1
  - nose (turbinate) J34.3
- myocardium—*see also* Hypertrophy, cardiac
  - idiopathic I42.2
- nasal J34.89
  - alae J34.89
  - bone J34.89
  - cartilage J34.89
  - mucous membrane (septum) J34.3
  - sinus J34.89
  - turbinate J34.3
- nasopharynx, lymphoid (infectional) (tissue) (wall) J35.2
- nipple N62
- palate (hard) M27.8
  - soft K13.79
- pharyngeal tonsil J35.2
- pharynx J39.2
  - lymphoid (infectional) (tissue) (wall) J35.2
- pituitary (anterior) (fossa) (gland) E23.6
- prepuce (congenital) N47.8
  - female N90.89
- pseudomuscular G71.09
- pylorus (adult) (muscle) (sphincter) K31.1
  - congenital or infantile Q40.0
- rectal, rectum (sphincter) K62.89
- rhinitis (turbinate) J31.0
- scar L91.0
  - specified NEC L91.8
- skin L91.9
- testis N44.8
  - congenital Q55.29
- toe (congenital) Q74.2
  - acquired—*see also* Deformity, toe
- tonsils (faucial) (infective) (lingual) (lymphoid) J35.1
  - with adenoids J35.3
- uvula K13.79
- ventricle, ventricular (heart)—*see also* Hypertrophy, cardiac
  - congenital Q24.8
  - in tetralogy of Fallot Q21.3
- vulva N90.60
  - childhood asymmetric labium majus enlargement (CALME) N90.61
  - other specified N90.69

Hyperuricemia (asymptomatic) E79.0

Hyperuricosuria R82.993

Hyperventilation (tetany) R06.4
- hysterical F45.8
- psychogenic F45.8
- syndrome F45.8

Hypoacidity, gastric K31.89
- psychogenic F45.8

Hypoadrenalism, hypoadrenia E27.40
- primary E27.1

Hypoadrenocorticism E27.40
- pituitary E23.0
- primary E27.1

Hypoalbuminemia E88.09

Hypoaldosteronism E27.40

Hypocalcemia E83.51
- autosomal dominant E20.810
  - type 1 (ADH1) E20.810
  - type 2 (ADH2) E20.810
- dietary E58
- neonatal P71.1
  - due to cow's milk P71.0
  - phosphate-loading (newborn) P71.1

Hypochloremia E87.8

Hypochlorhydria K31.89
- neurotic F45.8
- psychogenic F45.8

Hypochondria, hypochondriac, hypochondriasis (reaction) F45.21
- sleep F51.03

Hypochondrogenesis Q77.0

Hypochondroplasia Q77.4

Hypochromasia, blood cells D50.8

Hypocitraturia R82.991

Hypoeosinophilia D72.89

Hypofibrinogenemia D68.8
- acquired D65
- congenital (hereditary) D68.2

Hypofunction
- adrenocortical E27.40
  - primary E27.1
- corticoadrenal NEC E27.40
- pituitary (gland) (anterior) E23.0

Hypogalactia O92.4

Hypogammaglobulinemia (*see also* Agammaglobulinemia) D80.1
- hereditary D80.0
- nonfamilial D80.1
- transient, of infancy D80.7

Hypoglycemia (spontaneous) E16.2
- coma E15
  - diabetic—*see* Diabetes
- diabetic—*see* Diabetes
- dietary counseling and surveillance Z71.3
- due to insulin E16.0
  - therapeutic misadventure—*see* subcategory T38.3
- level
  - 1 E16.A1
  - 2 E16.A2
  - 3 E16.A3
- neonatal (transitory) P70.4
- transitory neonatal P70.4

Hypogonadism
- female E28.39
- hypogonadotropic E23.0
- ovarian (primary) E28.39
- pituitary E23.0

Hypometabolism R63.8

Hypomotility
- gastrointestinal (tract) K31.89
  - psychogenic F45.8
- intestine K59.89
  - psychogenic F45.8
- stomach K31.89
  - psychogenic F45.8

Hypomyelination—hypogonadotropic hypogonadism—hypodontia G11.5

Hypomyelination with atrophy of the basal ganglia and cerebellum (H-ABC) G23.3

Hyponatremia E87.1

Hypo-osmolality E87.1

Hypoparathyroidism E20.9
- autoimmune E20.812
- due to impaired parathyroid hormone secretion, unspecified E20.819
- familial E20.89
- idiopathic E20.0
- neonatal, transitory P71.4
- postprocedural E89.2
- secondary, in diseases classified elsewhere E20.811
- specified NEC E20.89
  - due to impaired parathyroid hormone secretion E20.818

Hypoperfusion (in)
- newborn P96.89

Hypophyseal, hypophysis—*see also* Disease, diseased
- gigantism E22.0

Hypopituitarism (juvenile) E23.0
- drug-induced E23.1
- iatrogenic NEC E23.1

Hypoplasia, hypoplastic
- alimentary tract, congenital Q45.8
  - upper Q40.8
- anus, anal (canal) Q42.3
  - with fistula Q42.2
- aorta, aortic Q25.42
  - ascending, in hypoplastic left heart syndrome Q23.4
  - valve Q23.1
    - in hypoplastic left heart syndrome Q23.4
- artery (peripheral) Q27.8
  - pulmonary Q25.79
  - umbilical Q27.0
- biliary duct or passage Q44.5
- bone NOS Q79.9
  - marrow D61.9
    - megakaryocytic D69.49
  - skull—*see* Hypoplasia, skull
- brain Q02
- cecum Q42.8
- cephalic Q02
- clavicle (congenital) Q74.0
- colon Q42.9
  - specified NEC Q42.8
- corpus callosum Q04.0
- digestive organ(s) or tract NEC Q45.8
  - upper (congenital) Q40.8
- ear (auricle) (lobe) Q17.2
  - middle Q16.4
- endocrine (gland) NEC Q89.2
- erythroid, congenital D61.01
- eye Q11.2
- eyelid (congenital) Q10.3
- focal dermal Q82.8
- gallbladder Q44.0
- genitalia, genital organ(s)
  - female, congenital Q52.8
    - external Q52.79
    - internal NEC Q52.8
  - in adiposogenital dystrophy E23.6
- intestine (small) Q41.9
  - large Q42.9
    - specified NEC Q42.8
- jaw M26.09
  - lower M26.04
- kidney(s)
  - bilateral Q60.4
  - unilateral Q60.3
- left heart syndrome Q23.4
- liver Q44.79
- lung (lobe) (not associated with short gestation) Q33.6
  - associated with immaturity, low birth weight, prematurity, or short gestation P28.0
- mandible, mandibular M26.04
- medullary D61.9
- megakaryocytic D69.49
- metacarpus—*see* Defect, reduction, limb, upper, specified type NEC

ALPHABETIC INDEX

Hypoplasia, hypoplastic, *continued*

- metatarsus—*see* Defect, reduction, limb, lower, specified type NEC
- optic nerve H47.03-
- ovary, congenital Q50.39
- parathyroid (gland) Q89.2
- pelvis, pelvic girdle Q74.2
- penis (congenital) Q55.62
- pituitary (gland) (congenital) Q89.2
- pulmonary (not associated with short gestation) Q33.6
  - associated with short gestation P28.0
- rectum Q42.1
  - with fistula Q42.0
- scapula Q74.0
- shoulder girdle Q74.0
- skin Q82.8
- skull (bone) Q75.8
  - with
    - anencephaly Q00.0
    - encephalocele—*see* Encephalocele
    - hydrocephalus Q03.9
      - with spina bifida—*see* Spina bifida, by site, with hydrocephalus
    - microcephaly Q02
- thymic, with immunodeficiency D82.1
- thymus (gland) Q89.2
  - with immunodeficiency D82.1
- thyroid (gland) E03.1
  - cartilage Q31.2
- umbilical artery Q27.0
- zonule (ciliary) Q12.8

Hypoplasminogenemia E88.02

Hypopnea, obstructive sleep apnea G47.33

Hypoproteinemia E77.8

Hypopyrexia R68.0

Hyposecretion

- ACTH E23.0
- antidiuretic hormone E23.2
- ovary E28.39
- vasopressin E23.2

Hyposegmentation, leukocytic, hereditary D72.0

Hypospadias Q54.9

- balanic Q54.0
- coronal Q54.0
- glandular Q54.0
- penile Q54.1
- penoscrotal Q54.2
- perineal Q54.3
- specified NEC Q54.8

Hypotension (arterial) (constitutional) I95.9

- intracranial G96.810
  - following
    - lumbar cerebrospinal fluid shunting G97.83
    - specified procedure NEC G97.84
    - ventricular shunting (ventriculostomy) G97.2
  - specified NEC G96.819
  - spontaneous G96.811
- orthostatic (chronic) I95.1
- postural I95.1

Hypothermia (accidental) T68

- low environmental temperature T68
- neonatal P80.9
  - environmental (mild) NEC P80.8
  - mild P80.8
  - severe (chronic) (cold injury syndrome) P80.0
  - specified NEC P80.8
- not associated with low environmental temperature R68.0

Hypothyroidism (acquired) E03.9

- congenital (without goiter) E03.1
  - with goiter (diffuse) E03.0
- due to
  - iodine-deficiency, acquired E01.8
    - subclinical E02
- iodine-deficiency (acquired) E01.8
  - congenital—*see* Syndrome
  - subclinical E02
- neonatal, transitory P72.2
- specified NEC E03.8

Hypotonia, hypotonicity, hypotony

- congenital (benign) P94.2

Hypoventilation R06.89

Hypovolemia E86.1

- surgical shock T81.19
- traumatic (shock) T79.4

Hypoxemia R09.02

- newborn P84

Hypoxia (*see also* Anoxia) R09.02

- intrauterine P84
- newborn P84

Hysteria, hysterical (conversion) (dissociative state) F44.9

- anxiety F41.8
- psychosis, acute F44.9

I

Ichthyoparasitism due to Vandellia cirrhosa B88.8

Ichthyosis (congenital) Q80.9

- fetalis Q80.4
- hystrix Q80.8
- lamellar Q80.2
- palmaris and plantaris Q82.8
- simplex Q80.0
- vera Q80.8
- vulgaris Q80.0
- X-linked Q80.1

Icterus—*see also* Jaundice

- conjunctiva R17
  - newborn P59.9
- hemorrhagic (acute) (leptospiral) (spirochetal) A27.0
  - newborn P53
- infectious B15.9

Ictus solaris, solis T67.01

Ideation

- homicidal R45.850
- suicidal R45.851

Identity disorder (child) F64.9

- gender role F64.2
- psychosexual F64.2

Idioglossia F80.0

Idiopathic—*see* Disease, diseased

Idiot, idiocy (congenital) F73

- microcephalic Q02

IgE asthma J45.909

IIAC (idiopathic infantile arterial calcification) Q28.8

Ileitis (chronic) (noninfectious) (*see also* Enteritis) K52.9

- infectious A09
- regional (ulcerative)—*see* Enteritis, regional, small intestine
- segmental—*see* Enteritis, regional
- terminal (ulcerative)—*see* Enteritis, regional, small intestine

Ileocolitis (*see also* Enteritis) K52.9

- regional—*see* Enteritis, regional
- infectious A09
- ulcerative K51.0-

Ileus (bowel) (colon) (inhibitory) (intestine) K56.7

- adynamic K56.0
- meconium P76.0
  - in cystic fibrosis E84.11
  - meaning meconium plug (without cystic fibrosis) P76.0
- neurogenic K56.0
  - Hirschsprung's disease or megacolon Q43.1
- newborn
  - due to meconium P76.0
  - in cystic fibrosis E84.11
    - meaning meconium plug (without cystic fibrosis) P76.0
  - transitory P76.1
- obstructive K56.69
- paralytic K56.0

Illness (*see also* Disease) R69

Imbalance R26.89

- constituents of food intake E63.1
- electrolyte E87.8
  - neonatal, transitory NEC P74.49

Imbalance, *continued*

- potassium
  - hyperkalemia P74.31
  - hypokalemia P74.32
- sodium
  - hypernatremia P74.21
  - hyponatremia P74.22
- endocrine E34.9
- eye muscle NOS H50.9
- hysterical F44.4
- posture R29.3
- protein-energy—*see* Malnutrition

Immaturity (less than 37 completed weeks)—*see also* Preterm, newborn

- extreme of newborn (less than 28 completed weeks of gestation) (less than 196 completed days of gestation) (unspecified weeks of gestation) P07.20
  - gestational age
    - 23 completed weeks (23 weeks, 0 days through 23 weeks, 6 days) P07.22
    - 24 completed weeks (24 weeks, 0 days through 24 weeks, 6 days) P07.23
    - 25 completed weeks (25 weeks, 0 days through 25 weeks, 6 days) P07.24
    - 26 completed weeks (26 weeks, 0 days through 26 weeks, 6 days) P07.25
    - 27 completed weeks (27 weeks, 0 days through 27 weeks, 6 days) P07.26
    - less than 23 completed weeks P07.21
- fetus or infant light-for-dates—*see* Light-for-dates
- lung, newborn P28.0
- organ or site NEC—*see* Hypoplasia
- pulmonary, newborn P28.0
- sexual (female) (male), after puberty E30.0

Immersion T75.1

Immunization—*see also* Vaccination

- ABO—*see* Incompatibility, ABO
  - in newborn P55.1
- complication—*see* Complications, vaccination
- encounter for Z23
- not done (not carried out) Z28.9
  - because (of)
    - acute illness of patient Z28.01
    - allergy to vaccine (or component) Z28.04
    - caregiver refusal Z28.82
    - chronic illness of patient Z28.02
    - contraindication NEC Z28.09
    - delay in delivery of vaccine Z28.83
    - group pressure Z28.1
    - guardian refusal Z28.82
    - immune compromised state of patient Z28.03
    - lack of availability of vaccine Z28.83
    - manufacturer delay of vaccine Z28.83
    - parent refusal Z28.82
    - patient's belief Z28.1
    - patient had disease being vaccinated against Z28.81
    - patient refusal Z28.21
    - religious beliefs of patient Z28.1
    - specified reason NEC Z28.89
      - of patient Z28.29
    - unavailability of vaccine Z28.83
    - unspecified patient reason Z28.20
- Rh factor
  - affecting management of pregnancy NEC O36.09-
    - anti-D antibody O36.01-

Immunocompromised NOS D84.9

Immunodeficiency D84.9

- with
  - adenosine-deaminase deficiency D81.30
    - adenosine deaminase 2 D81.32
    - other adenosine deaminase D81.39
    - severe combined immunodeficiency due to adenosine deaminase deficiency D81.31
  - antibody defects D80.9
    - specified type NEC D80.8
  - thrombocytopenia and eczema D82.0
- common variable D83.9
  - with
    - abnormalities of B-cell numbers and function D83.0

ALPHABETIC INDEX

Immunodeficiency, *continued*
- ■ autoantibodies to B- or T-cells D83.2
- ■ immunoregulatory T-cell disorders D83.1
- ■ specified type NEC D83.8
- • due to
  - – conditions classified elsewhere D84.81
  - – drugs D84.821
  - – external causes D84.822
  - – medication (current or past) D84.821
- • combined D81.9
  - – severe D81.9
    - ■ due to adenosine deaminase deficiency D81.31
- • following hereditary defective response to Epstein-Barr virus (EBV) D82.3
- • severe combined (SCID) D81.9
  - – due to adenosine deaminase deficiency D81.31
- • specified type NEC D84.89

Immunodeficient NOS D84.9

Immunosuppressed NOS D84.9

Impaction, impacted
- • bowel, colon, rectum (*see also* Impaction, fecal) K56.49
- • cerumen (ear) (external) H61.2-
- • fecal, feces K56.41
- • intestine (calculous) NEC (*see also* Impaction, fecal) K56.49
- • turbinate J34.89

Impaired, impairment (function)
- • auditory discrimination—*see* Abnormal, auditory perception
- • dual sensory Z73.82
- • fasting glucose R73.01
- • glucose tolerance (oral) R73.02
- • hearing—*see* Deafness
- • heart—*see* Disease, heart
- • rectal sphincter R19.8
- • vision NEC H54.7
  - – both eyes H54.3

Impediment, speech R47.9
- • psychogenic (childhood) F98.8
- • slurring R47.81
- • specified NEC R47.89

Imperception auditory (acquired)—*see also* Deafness
- • congenital H93.25

Imperfect
- • aeration, lung (newborn) NEC—*see* Atelectasis
- • closure (congenital)
  - – alimentary tract NEC Q45.8
    - ■ lower Q43.8
    - ■ upper Q40.8
  - – atrioventricular ostium Q21.2
  - – atrium (secundum) Q21.1
  - – branchial cleft NOS Q18.2
    - ■ cyst Q18.0
    - ■ fistula Q18.0
    - ■ sinus Q18.0
  - – choroid Q14.3
  - – ductus
    - ■ arteriosus Q25.0
    - ■ Botalli Q25.0
  - – ear drum (causing impairment of hearing) Q16.4
  - – esophagus with communication to bronchus or trachea Q39.1
  - – eyelid Q10.3
  - – foramen
    - ■ botalli Q21.1
    - ■ ovale Q21.1
  - – genitalia, genital organ(s)or system
    - ■ female Q52.8
      - – external Q52.79
      - – internal NEC Q52.8
    - ■ male Q55.8
  - – interatrial ostium or septum Q21.1
  - – interauricular ostium or septum Q21.1
  - – interventricular ostium or septum Q21.0
  - – omphalomésenteric duct Q43.0
  - – ostium
    - ■ interatrial Q21.1
    - ■ interauricular Q21.1
    - ■ interventricular Q21.0
  - – roof of orbit Q75.8
  - – septum

Imperfect, *continued*
- ■ atrial (secundum) Q21.1
  - ■ interatrial (secundum) Q21.1
  - ■ interauricular (secundum) Q21.1
  - ■ interventricular Q21.0
    - – in tetralogy of Fallot Q21.3
  - ■ ventricular Q21.0
    - – with pulmonary stenosis or atresia, dextraposition of aorta, and hypertrophy of right ventricle Q21.3
    - – in tetralogy of Fallot Q21.3
- – skull Q75.009
  - ■ with
    - – anencephaly Q00.0
    - – encephalocele—*see* Encephalocele
    - – hydrocephalus Q03.9
      - ◊ with spina bifida—*see* Spina bifida, by site, with hydrocephalus
    - – microcephaly Q02
    - – spine (with meningocele)—*see* Spina bifida
    - – vitelline duct Q43.0
  - • posture R29.3
  - • rotation, intestine Q43.3
  - • septum, ventricular Q21.0

Imperfectly descended testis—*see* Cryptorchid

Imperforate (congenital)—*see also* Atresia
- • anus Q42.3
  - – with fistula Q42.2
- • esophagus Q39.0
  - – with tracheoesophageal fistula Q39.1
- • hymen Q52.3
- • jejunum Q41.1
- • rectum Q42.1
  - – with fistula Q42.0

Impervious (congenital)—*see also* Atresia
- • anus Q42.3
  - – with fistula Q42.2
- • bile duct Q44.2
- • esophagus Q39.0
  - – with tracheoesophageal fistula Q39.1
- • intestine (small) Q41.9
  - – large Q42.9
    - ■ specified NEC Q42.8
- • rectum Q42.1
  - – with fistula Q42.0

Impetigo (any organism) (any site) (circinate) (contagiosa) (simplex) (vulgaris) L01.00
- • external ear L01.00 [H62.4-]
- • furfuracea L30.5

Implantation
- • cyst
  - – vagina N89.8

Impression, basilar Q75.8

Improper care (child) (newborn)—*see* Maltreatment

Improperly tied umbilical cord (causing hemorrhage) P51.8

Impulsiveness (impulsive) R45.87

Inability to swallow—*see* Aphagia

Inadequate, inadequacy
- • development
  - – child R62.50
  - – genitalia
    - ■ after puberty NEC E30.0
    - ■ congenital
      - – female Q52.8
        - ◊ external Q52.79
        - ◊ internal Q52.8
      - – male Q55.8
  - – lungs Q33.6
    - ■ associated with short gestation P28.0
  - – organ or site not listed—*see* Anomaly, by site
- • drinking-water supply Z58.6
- • eating habits Z72.4
- • environment, household Z59.11
- • family support Z63.8
- • food (supply) NEC Z59.48
  - – hunger effects T73.0
- • household care, due to
  - – family member
    - – technical defects in home Z59.19
    - – space Z59.19

Inadequate, inadequacy, *continued*
- – specified NEC Z59.19
  - ■ handicapped or ill Z74.2
  - ■ temporarily away from home Z74.2
- • housing Z59.10
  - – environmental temperature Z59.11
  - – heating Z59.11
  - – utilities Z59.12
- • intrafamilial communication Z63.8
- • material resources due to limited financial resources, specified NEC Z59.87
- • mental—*see* Disability, intellectual
- • pulmonary
  - – function R06.89
    - ■ newborn P28.5
  - – ventilation, newborn P28.5
- • social
  - – insurance Z59.71
  - – skills NEC Z73.4
  - – welfare support Z59.72

Inanition R64
- • fever R50.9

Inappropriate
- • diet or eating habits Z72.4
- • secretion
  - – antidiuretic hormone (ADH) (excessive) E22.2
  - – pituitary (posterior) E22.2
- • sinus tachycardia, so stated (IST) I47.11

Inattention at or after birth—*see* Neglect

Incarceration, incarcerated
- • exomphalos K42.0
  - – gangrenous K42.1
- • hernia—*see also* Hernia, by site, with obstruction
  - – with gangrene—*see* Hernia, by site, with gangrene
- • omphalocele K42.0
- • rupture—*see* Hernia, by site
- • sarcoepiplomphalocele K42.0
  - – with gangrene K42.1

Incision, incisional
- • hernia K43.2
  - – with
    - ■ gangrene (and obstruction) K43.1
    - ■ obstruction K43.0

Inclusion
- • azurophilic leukocytic D72.0
- • blennorrhea (neonatal) (newborn) P39.1
- • gallbladder in liver (congenital) Q44.1

Incompatibility
- • ABO
  - – affecting management of pregnancy O36.11-
    - ■ anti-A sensitization O36.11-
    - ■ anti-B sensitization O36.19-
    - ■ specified NEC O36.19-
  - – infusion or transfusion reaction T80.30-
    - – newborn P55.1
  - – blood (group) (Duffy) (K(ell)) (Kidd) (Lewis) (M) (S) NEC
    - – affecting management of pregnancy O36.11-
      - ■ anti-A sensitization O36.11-
      - ■ anti-B sensitization O36.19-
    - – infusion or transfusion reaction T80.89
      - – newborn P55.8
- • Rh (blood group) (factor)
  - – affecting management of pregnancy NEC O36.09-
    - ■ anti-D antibody O36.01-
  - – infusion or transfusion reaction—*see* Complication(s), transfusion, incompatibility reaction, Rh (factor)
  - – newborn P55.0
- • rhesus—*see* Incompatibility, Rh

Incompetency, incompetent, incompetence
- • annular
  - – aortic (valve)—*see* Insufficiency, aortic
  - – mitral (valve) I34.0
  - – pulmonary valve (heart) I37.1
- • aortic (valve)—*see* Insufficiency, aortic
- • cardiac valve—*see* Endocarditis
- • pulmonary valve (heart) I37.1
  - – congenital Q22.3

ALPHABETIC INDEX

Incomplete—*see also* Disease, diseased
- bladder, emptying R33.9
- defecation R15.0
- expansion lungs (newborn) NEC—*see* Atelectasis
- rotation, intestine Q43.3

Incontinence R32
- anal sphincter R15.9
- feces R15.9
  - nonorganic origin F98.1
- psychogenic F45.8
- rectal R15.9
- urethral sphincter R32
- urine (urinary) R32
  - nocturnal N39.44
  - nonorganic origin F98.0

Increase, increased
- abnormal, in development R63.8
- function
  - adrenal
    - cortex—*see* Cushing's, syndrome
    - pituitary (gland) (anterior) (lobe) E22.9
    - posterior E22.2
  - intracranial pressure (benign) G93.2
  - pressure, intracranial G93.2
  - sphericity, lens Q12.4

Indeterminate sex Q56.4

India rubber skin Q82.8

Indigestion (acid) (bilious) (functional) K30
- due to decomposed food NOS A05.9
- nervous F45.8
- psychogenic F45.8

Induration
- brain G93.89
- breast (fibrous) N64.51
- chancre
  - congenital A50.07
  - extragenital NEC A51.2

Inertia
- stomach K31.89
  - psychogenic F45.8

Infancy, infantile, infantilism—*see also* Disease, diseased
- celiac K90.0
- genitalia, genitals (after puberty) E30.0
- Herter's (nontropical sprue) K90.0
- intestinal K90.0
- Lorain E23.0
- pituitary E23.0
- uterus—*see* Infantile, genitalia

Infant(s)—*see also* Infancy
- excessive crying R68.11
- irritable child R68.12
- lack of care—*see* Neglect
- liveborn (singleton) Z38.2
  - born in hospital Z38.00
    - by cesarean Z38.01
  - born outside hospital Z38.1
  - multiple NEC Z38.8
    - born in hospital Z38.68
      - by cesarean Z38.69
    - born outside hospital Z38.7
  - quadruplet Z38.8
    - born in hospital Z38.63
      - by cesarean Z38.64
    - born outside hospital Z38.7
  - quintuplet Z38.8
    - born in hospital Z38.65
      - by cesarean Z38.66
    - born outside hospital Z38.7
  - triplet Z38.8
    - born in hospital Z38.61
      - by cesarean Z38.62
    - born outside hospital Z38.7
  - twin Z38.5
    - born in hospital Z38.30
      - by cesarean Z38.31
    - born outside hospital Z38.4
- of diabetic mother (syndrome of) P70.1
  - gestational diabetes P70.0

Infantile—*see also* Disease, diseased
- genitalia, genitals E30.0
- os, uterine E30.0
- penis E30.0
- uterus E30.0

Infantilism—*see* Infancy

Infarct, infarction
- adrenal (capsule) (gland) E27.49
- cerebral (acute) (chronic) (*see also* Occlusion, artery) I63.9-
  - neonatal P91.82-
  - perinatal (arterial ischemic) P91.82-
- hypophysis (anterior lobe) E23.6
  - diffuse acute K55.062
  - focal (segmental) K55.061
  - intestine, part unspecified
  - unspecified extent K55.069
- large intestine
  - diffuse acute K55.042
  - focal (segmental) K55.041
  - unspecified extent K55.049
- myocardium, myocardial (acute) (with stated duration of 4 weeks or less)
  - postprocedural
    - following cardiac surgery I97.190
    - following other surgery I97.191
- pituitary (gland) E23.6
- small intestine
  - diffuse acute K55.022
  - focal (segmental) K55.021
  - unspecified extent K55.029
- suprarenal (capsule) (gland) E27.49

Infection
- with
  - drug resistant organism—*see* Resistance, organism(s), to, drug—*see also* specific organism
  - organ dysfunction (acute) R65.20
  - with septic shock R65.21
- acromioclavicular M00.9
- adenoid (and tonsil) J03.90
  - chronic J35.02
- adenovirus NEC
  - as cause of disease classified elsewhere B97.0
  - unspecified nature or site B34.0
- alveolus, alveolar (process) K04.7
- antrum (chronic)—*see* Sinusitis, acute, maxillary
- anus, anal (papillae) (sphincter) K62.89
- axillary gland (lymph) L04.2
- bacterial NOS A49.9
  - as cause of disease classified elsewhere B96.89
    - Enterococcus B95.2
    - Escherichia coli [E. coli] (*see also* Escherichia coli B96.20
    - Helicobacter pylori [H. pylori] B96.81
    - Hemophilus influenzae [H. influenzae] B96.3
    - Mycoplasma pneumoniae [M. pneumoniae] B96.0
    - Proteus (mirabilis) (morganii) B96.4
    - Pseudomonas (aeruginosa) (mallei) (pseudomallei) B96.5
    - Staphylococcus B95.8
      - aureus (methicillin susceptible) (MSSA) B95.61
        - ◊ methicillin resistant (MRSA) B95.62
      - specified NEC B95.7
    - Streptococcus B95.5
      - group A B95.0
      - group B B95.1
      - pneumoniae B95.3
      - specified NEC B95.4
      - specified NEC A48.8
- Blastomyces, blastomycotic—*see also* Blastomycosis
  - North American B40.9
- Borrelia burgdorferi A69.20
- brain (*see also* Encephalitis) G04.90
  - membranes—*see* Meningitis
  - septic G06.0
    - meninges—*see* Meningitis, bacterial
- buttocks (skin) L08.9
- Campylobacter, intestinal A04.5
  - as cause of disease classified elsewhere B96.81
- Candida (albicans) (tropicalis)—*see* Candidiasis
- candiru B88.8

Infection, *continued*
- central line-associated T80.219
  - bloodstream (CLABSI) T80.211
  - specified NEC T80.218
- cervical gland (lymph) L04.0
- Chlamydia, chlamydial A74.9
  - anus A56.3
  - genitourinary tract A56.2
    - lower A56.00
    - specified NEC A56.19
  - pharynx A56.4
  - rectum A56.3
  - sexually transmitted NEC A56.8
- Clostridium NEC
  - botulinum (food poisoning) A05.1
    - infant A48.51
    - wound A48.52
  - difficile
    - foodborne (disease) A04.7-
    - necrotizing enterocolitis A04.7-
    - sepsis A41.4
  - perfringens
    - due to food A05.2
    - foodborne (disease) A05.2
    - necrotizing enterocolitis A05.2
    - sepsis A41.4
  - welchii
    - foodborne (disease) A05.2
    - sepsis A41.4
- congenital P39.9
  - Candida (albicans) P37.5
  - cytomegalovirus P35.1
  - herpes simplex P35.2
  - infectious or parasitic disease P37.9
    - specified NEC P37.8
  - listeriosis (disseminated) P37.2
  - rubella P35.0
  - toxoplasmosis (acute) (subacute) (chronic) P37.1
  - urinary (tract) P39.3
- coronavirus-2019 U07.1
- coronavirus NEC B34.2
  - as cause of disease classified elsewhere B97.29
  - severe acute respiratory syndrome (SARS associated) B97.21
- COVID-19 U07.1
- cytomegalovirus, cytomegaloviral B25.9
  - congenital P35.1
  - maternal, maternal care for (suspected) damage to fetus O35.3
  - mononucleosis B27.10
    - with
      - complication NEC B27.19
      - meningitis B27.12
      - polyneuropathy B27.11
- dental (pulpal origin) K04.7
- due to or resulting from
  - central venous catheter T80.219
    - bloodstream T80.211
    - exit or insertion site T80.212
    - localized T80.212
    - port or reservoir T80.212
    - specified NEC T80.218
    - tunnel T80.212
  - device, implant or graft (*see also* Complications, by site and type, infection or inflammation) T85.79
    - arterial graft NEC T82.7
    - catheter NEC T85.79
      - dialysis (renal) T82.7
      - infusion NEC T82.7
      - urinary T83.518
        - ◊ cystostomy T83.510
        - ◊ Hopkins T83.518
        - ◊ ileostomy T83.518
        - ◊ nephrostomy T83.512
        - ◊ specified NEC T83.518
        - ◊ urethral indwelling T83.511
        - ◊ urostomy T83.518
  - Hickman catheter T80.219
    - bloodstream T80.211
    - localized T80.212
    - specified NEC T80.218
  - immunization or vaccination T88.0

ALPHABETIC INDEX

Infection, *continued*

- infusion, injection or transfusion NEC T80.29
  - ■ acute T80.22
- peripherally inserted central catheter (PICC) T80.219
  - ■ bloodstream T80.211
  - ■ localized T80.212
  - ■ specified NEC T80.218
- portacath (port-a-cath) T80.219
  - ■ bloodstream T80.211
  - ■ localized T80.212
  - ■ specified NEC T80.218
- postoperative (postprocedural) T81.4
  - ■ sepsis T81.49
  - ■ specified surgical site NEC T81.4-
  - ■ superficial incisional surgical site T81.41
- surgery T81.40
- triple lumen catheter T80.219
  - ■ bloodstream T80.211
  - ■ localized T80.212
  - ■ specified NEC T80.218
- umbilical venous catheter T80.219
  - ■ bloodstream T80.211
  - ■ localized T80.212
  - ■ specified NEC T80.218
- ear (middle)—*see also* Otitis, media
  - external—*see* Otitis, externa, infective
  - inner—*see* subcategory H83.0
- echovirus
  - as cause of disease classified elsewhere B97.12
  - unspecified nature or site B34.1
- endocardium I33.0
- Enterobius vermicularis B80
- enterovirus B34.1
  - as cause of disease classified elsewhere B97.10
  - ■ coxsackievirus B97.11
  - ■ echovirus B97.12
  - ■ specified NEC B97.19
- erythema infectiosum B08.3
- Escherichia (E.) coli NEC A49.8
  - as cause of disease classified elsewhere (*see also* Escherichia coli) B96.20
  - congenital P39.8
  - ■ sepsis P36.4
  - generalized A41.51
  - intestinal—*see* Enteritis, infectious, due to, Escherichia coli
- eyelid H01.-
  - abscess—*see* Abscess, eyelid
  - blepharitis—*see* Blepharitis
  - chalazion—*see* Chalazion
  - dermatosis (noninfectious)—*see* Dermatitis, eyelid
  - hordeolum—*see* Hordeolum
  - specified NEC H01.8
- finger (skin) L08.9
  - nail L03.01-
  - ■ fungus B35.1
- focal
  - teeth (pulpal origin) K04.7
  - tonsils J35.01
- foot (skin) L08.9
  - dermatophytic fungus B35.3
- fungus NOS B49
  - beard B35.0
  - dermatophytic—*see* Dermatophytosis
  - foot B35.3
  - groin B35.6
  - hand B35.2
  - nail B35.1
  - perianal (area) B35.6
  - scalp B35.0
  - skin B36.9
    - ■ foot B35.3
    - ■ hand B35.2
    - ■ toenails B35.1
- Giardia lamblia A07.1
- gingiva (chronic)
  - acute K05.00
  - ■ plaque induced K05.00
- gram-negative bacilli NOS A49.9
- gum (chronic)
  - acute K05.00
  - ■ plaque induced K05.00

Infection, *continued*

- Helicobacter pylori A04.8
  - as the cause of disease classified elsewhere B96.81
- Hemophilus
  - influenzae NEC A49.2
  - ■ as cause of disease classified elsewhere B96.3
  - generalized A41.3
- herpes (simplex)—*see also* Herpes
  - congenital P35.2
  - disseminated B00.7
  - herpesvirus, herpesviral—*see* Herpes
- hip (joint) NEC M00.9
  - skin NEC L08.9
- human
  - papilloma virus A63.0
- hydrocele N43.0
- inguinal (lymph) glands L04.1
- joint NEC M00.9
- knee (joint) NEC M00.9
  - joint M00.9
  - skin L08.9
- leg (skin) NOS L08.9
- listeria monocytogenes—*see also* Listeriosis
  - congenital P37.2
- local, skin (staphylococcal) (streptococcal) L08.9
  - abscess—*code by* site under Abscess
  - cellulitis—*code by* site under Cellulitis
  - ulcer—*see* Ulcer
- lung (*see also* Pneumonia) J18.9
  - virus—*see* Pneumonia, viral
- lymph gland—*see also* Lymphadenitis, acute
  - mesenteric I88.0
- lymphoid tissue, base of tongue or posterior pharynx, NEC (chronic) J35.03
- Malassezia furfur B36.0
- mammary gland N61.0
- meningococcal (*see also* Disease, diseased) A39.9
  - cerebrospinal A39.0
  - meninges A39.0
  - meningococcemia A39.4
  - ■ acute A39.2
  - ■ chronic A39.3
- mesenteric lymph nodes or glands NEC I88.0
- metatarsophalangeal M00.9
- mouth, parasitic B37.0
- mu heavy chain disease C88.2-
- Mycoplasma NEC A49.3
  - pneumoniae, as cause of disease classified elsewhere B96.0
- myocardium NEC I40.0
- nail (chronic)
  - with lymphangitis—*see* Lymphangitis, acute
  - finger L03.01-
  - ■ fungus B35.1
  - ingrowing L60.0
  - toe L03.03-
  - ■ fungus B35.1
- newborn P39.9
  - intra-amniotic NEC P39.2
  - skin P39.4
  - specified type NEC P39.8
- nipple N61.0
- Oidium albicans B37.9
- operative wound T81.49
- Oxyuris vermicularis B80
- pancreas (acute) K85.92
  - abscess—*see* Pancreatitis, acute
  - specified NEC K85.82
- parameningococcus A39.9
- paraurethral ducts N34.2
- parvovirus NEC B34.3
  - as the cause of disease classified elsewhere B97.6
- Pasteurella NEC A28.0
  - multocida A28.0
  - pseudotuberculosis A28.0
  - septica (cat bite) (dog bite) A28.0
- perinatal period P39.9
  - specified type NEC P39.8
- perirectal K62.89
- perirenal—*see* Infection, kidney
- peritoneal—*see* Peritonitis

Infection, *continued*

- pharynx—*see also* Pharyngitis
  - coxsackievirus B08.5
  - posterior, lymphoid (chronic) J35.03
- pinworm B80
- pityrosporum furfur B36.0
- pleuro-pneumonia-like organism (PPLO) NEC A49.3
  - as cause of disease classified elsewhere B96.0
- pneumococcus, pneumococcal NEC A49.1
  - as cause of disease classified elsewhere B95.3
  - generalized (purulent) A40.3
  - ■ with pneumonia J13
- port or reservoir T80.212
- postoperative T81.40
  - surgical site
  - ■ deep incisional T81.42
  - ■ organ and space T81.43
  - ■ specified NEC T81.49
  - ■ superficial incisional T81.41
- postprocedural T81.40
- prepuce NEC N47.7
  - with penile inflammation N47.6
- Proteus (mirabilis) (morganii) (vulgaris) NEC A49.8
  - as cause of disease classified elsewhere B96.4
- Pseudomonas NEC A49.8
  - as cause of disease classified elsewhere B96.5
  - pneumonia J15.1
- rectum (sphincter) K62.89
- renal
  - pelvis and ureter (cystic) N28.85
- respiratory (tract) NEC J98.8
  - acute J22
  - chronic J98.8
  - influenzal (upper) (acute)—*see* Influenza, with, respiratory manifestations NEC
  - lower (acute) J22
  - ■ chronic—*see* Bronchitis
  - rhinovirus J00
  - syncytial virus (RSV) J06.9 [B97.4]
  - upper (acute) NOS J06.9
  - ■ streptococcal J06.9
  - ■ viral NOS J06.9
- rhinovirus
  - as cause of disease classified elsewhere B97.89
  - unspecified nature or site B34.8
- rickettsial NOS A79.9
- roundworm (large) NEC B82.0
  - Ascariasis (*see also* Ascariasis) B77.9
- Salmonella (aertrycke) (arizonae) (callinarum) (choleraesuis) (enteritidis) (suipestifer) (typhimurium)
  - with
  - ■ (gastro) enteritis A02.0
  - ■ specified manifestation NEC A02.8
  - due to food (poisoning) A02.9
- scabies B86
- Shigella A03.9
  - boydii A03.2
  - dysenteriae A03.0
  - flexneri A03.1
  - group
  - ■ A A03.0
  - ■ B A03.1
  - ■ C A03.2
  - ■ D A03.3
- shoulder (joint) NEC M00.9
  - skin NEC L08.9
- skin (local) (staphylococcal) (streptococcal) L08.9
  - abscess—*code by* site under Abscess
  - cellulitis—*code by* site under Cellulitis
- spinal cord NOS (*see also* Myelitis) G04.91
  - abscess G06.1
  - meninges—*see* Meningitis
  - streptococcal G04.89
- staphylococcal, unspecified site
  - aureus (methicillin susceptible) (MSSA) A49.01
  - ■ methicillin resistant (MRSA) A49.02
  - as cause of disease classified elsewhere B95.8
  - ■ aureus (methicillin susceptible) (MSSA) B95.61
    - ~ methicillin resistant (MRSA) B95.62
  - ■ specified NEC B95.7
  - food poisoning A05.0
  - generalized (purulent) A41.2
  - pneumonia—*see* Pneumonia, staphylococcal

ALPHABETIC INDEX

Infection, *continued*

- streptobacillus moniliformis A25.1
- streptococcal NEC A49.1
  - as the cause of disease classified elsewhere B95.5
  - congenital
    - sepsis P36.10
      - group B P36.0
    - specified NEC P36.19
  - generalized (purulent) A40.9
- subcutaneous tissue, local L08.9
- threadworm B80
- toe (skin) L08.9
  - cellulitis L03.03-
    - fungus B35.1
  - nail L03.03-
    - fungus B35.1
- tongue NEC K14.0
  - parasitic B37.0
- tooth, teeth K04.7
  - periapical K04.7
- TORCH—*see* Infection, congenital
  - without active infection P00.2
- Trichomonas A59.9
  - cervix A59.09
  - specified site NEC A59.8
  - urethra A59.03
  - urogenitalis A59.00
  - vagina A59.01
  - vulva A59.01
- Trombicula (irritans) B88.0
- tuberculous
  - latent (LTBI) Z22.7
  - NEC—*see* Tuberculosis
- tunnel T80.212
- urinary (tract) N39.0
  - bladder—*see* Cystitis
  - newborn P39.3
  - urethra—*see* Urethritis
- varicella B01.9
- Vibrio
  - parahaemolyticus (food poisoning) A05.3
  - vulnificus
    - foodborne intoxication A05.5
- virus, viral NOS B34.9
  - adenovirus
    - as the cause of disease classified elsewhere B97.0
    - unspecified nature or site B34.0
  - as the cause of disease classified elsewhere B97.89
    - adenovirus B97.0
    - coxsackievirus B97.11
    - echovirus B97.12
    - enterovirus B97.10
      - coxsackievirus B97.11
      - echovirus B97.12
      - specified NEC B97.19
    - parvovirus B97.6
    - specified NEC B97.89
  - central nervous system A89
    - enterovirus NEC A88.8
      - meningitis A87.0
  - coxsackie B34.1
    - as cause of disease classified elsewhere B97.11
  - ECHO
    - as cause of disease classified elsewhere B97.12
    - unspecified nature or site B34.1
  - enterovirus, as cause of disease classified elsewhere B97.10
    - coxsackievirus B97.11
    - echovirus B97.12
    - specified NEC B97.19
  - exanthem NOS B09
  - respiratory syncytial (RSV)
    - as cause of disease classified elsewhere B97.4
    - bronchiolitis J21.0
    - bronchitis J20.5
    - bronchopneumonia J12.1
    - otitis media H65.- [B97.4]
    - pneumonia J12.1
    - upper respiratory infection J06.9 [B97.4]
  - rhinovirus
    - as the cause of disease specified elsewhere B97.89

Infection, *continued*

- specified type NEC B33.8
  - as the cause of disease specified elsewhere B97.89
- yeast (*see also* Candidiasis) B37.9
- Zika virus A92.5
  - congenital P35.4

Infertility

- female N97.9
  - associated with
    - anovulation N97.0
    - Stein-Leventhal syndrome E28.2
  - due to
    - Stein-Leventhal syndrome E28.2

Infestation B88.9

- Acariasis B88.0
  - demodex folliculorum B88.0
  - sarcoptes scabiei B86
  - trombiculae B88.0
- arthropod NEC B88.2
- Ascaris lumbricoides—*see* Ascariasis
- candiru B88.8
- cestodes B71.9
- chigger B88.0
- chigo, chigoe B88.1
- crab-lice B85.3
- Demodex (folliculorum) B88.0
- Dermanyssus gallinae B88.0
- Enterobius vermicularis B80
- eyelid
  - in (due to)
    - phthiriasis B85.3
- fluke B66.9
  - specified type NEC B66.8
- Giardia lamblia A07.1
- helminth
  - intestinal B82.0
    - enterobiasis B80
  - intestinal NEC B82.9
- Linguatula B88.8
- Lyponyssoides sanguineus B88.0
- mites B88.9
  - scabic B86
- Monilia (albicans)—*see* Candidiasis
- mouth B37.0
- nematode NEC (intestinal) B82.0
  - Enterobius vermicularis B80
  - physaloptera B80
  - Oxyuris vermicularis B80
- parasite, parasitic B89
  - eyelid B89
  - intestinal NOS B82.9
  - mouth B37.0
  - skin B88.9
  - tongue B37.0
- Pediculus B85.2
  - body B85.1
  - capitis (humanus) (any site) B85.0
  - corporis (humanus) (any site) B85.1
  - mixed (classifiable to more than one of the titles B85.0-B85.3) B85.4
  - pubis (any site) B85.3
- Pentastoma B88.8
- pest Z59.19
- Phthirus (pubis) (any site) B85.3
  - with any infestation classifiable to B85.0-B85.2 B85.4
- pinworm B80
- pubic louse B85.3
- red bug B88.0
- sand flea B88.1
- Sarcoptes scabiei B86
- scabies B86
- Schistosoma B65.9
  - cercariae B65.3
- skin NOS B88.9
- specified type NEC B88.8
- tapeworm B71.9
- Tetranychus molestissimus B88.0
- threadworm B80
- tongue B37.0
- Trombicula (irritans) B88.0

Infestation, *continued*

- Tunga penetrans B88.1
- Vandella cirrhosa B88.8

Infiltrate, infiltration

- leukemic—*see* Leukemia
- lung R91.8
- lymphatic (*see also* Leukemia) C91.9-
  - gland I88.9
- on chest x-ray R91.8
- pulmonary R91.8
- vesicant agent
  - antineoplastic chemotherapy T80.810
  - other agent NEC T80.818

Inflammation, inflamed, inflammatory (with exudation)

- anal canal, anus K62.89
- areola N61.0
- areolar tissue NOS L08.9
- breast N61.0
- bronchi—*see* Bronchitis
- catarrhal J00
- cerebrospinal
  - meningococcal A39.0
- due to device, implant or graft—*see also* Complications, by site and type, infection or inflammation
  - arterial graft T82.7
  - catheter T85.79
    - cardiac T82.7
    - dialysis (renal) T82.7
    - infusion T82.7
    - urinary T83.518
      - cystostomy T83.510
      - Hopkins T83.518
      - ileostomy T83.518
      - nephrostomy T83.512
      - specified NEC T83.518
      - urethral indwelling T83.511
      - urostomy T83.518
  - electronic (electrode) (pulse generator) (stimulator)
    - vascular NEC T82.7
- duodenum K29.80
  - with bleeding K29.81
- esophagus K20.9-
- follicular, pharynx J31.2
- gland (lymph)—*see* Lymphadenitis
- glottis—*see* Laryngitis
- granular, pharynx J31.2
- leg NOS L08.9
- lip K13.0
- mouth K12.1
- nipple N61.0
- orbit (chronic) H05.10-
  - acute H05.00
    - abscess—*see* Abscess
    - granuloma—*see* Granuloma, orbit
- parotid region L08.9
- perianal K62.89
- pericardium—*see* Pericarditis
- perineum (female) (male) L08.9
- perirectal K62.89
- peritoneum—*see* Peritonitis
- polyp, colon (*see also* Polyp, colon, inflammatory) K51.40
- rectum (*see also* Proctitis) K62.89
- respiratory, upper (*see also* Infection, respiratory, upper) J06.9
- skin L08.9
- subcutaneous tissue L08.9
- tongue K14.0
- tonsil—*see* Tonsillitis
- vein—*see also* Phlebitis
  - intracranial or intraspinal (septic) G08
  - thrombotic I80.9
    - leg—*see* Phlebitis, leg
- lower extremity—*see* Phlebitis, leg

Influenza (bronchial) (epidemic) (respiratory (upper) (unidentified influenza virus) J11.1

- with
  - digestive manifestations J11.2
  - encephalopathy J11.81
  - enteritis J11.2
  - gastroenteritis J11.2
  - gastrointestinal manifestations J11.2

Influenza, *continued*
- laryngitis J11.1
- myocarditis J11.82
- otitis media J11.83
- pharyngitis J11.1
- pneumonia J11.00
  - ■ specified type J11.08
- respiratory manifestations NEC J11.1
- specified manifestation NEC J11.89
- A (non-novel) J10-
- A/H5N1 (*see also* Influenza, due to, identified novel influenza A virus) J09.X2
- avian (*see also* Influenza, due to, identified novel influenza A virus) J09.X2
- B J10-
- bird (*see also* Influenza, due to, identified novel influenza A virus) J09.X2
- C J10-
- novel (2009) H1N1 influenza (*see also* Influenza, due to, identified influenza virus NEC) J10.1
- novel influenza A/H1N1 (*see also* Influenza, due to, identified influenza virus NEC) J10.1
- due to
  - avian (*see also* Influenza, due to, identified novel influenza A virus) J09.X2
  - identified influenza virus NEC J10.1
    - ■ with
      - ~ digestive manifestations J10.2
      - ~ encephalopathy J10.81
      - ~ enteritis J10.2
      - ~ gastroenteritis J10.2
      - ~ gastrointestinal manifestations J10.2
      - ~ laryngitis J10.1
      - ~ myocarditis J10.82
      - ~ otitis media J10.83
      - ~ pharyngitis J10.1
      - ~ pneumonia (unspecified type) J10.00
        - ◊ with same identified influenza virus J10.01
        - ◊ specified type NEC J10.08
      - ~ respiratory manifestations NEC J10.1
      - ~ specified manifestation NEC J10.89
  - identified novel influenza A virus J09.X2
    - ■ with
      - ~ digestive manifestations J09.X3
      - ~ encephalopathy J09.X9
      - ~ enteritis J09.X3
      - ~ gastroenteritis J09.X3
      - ~ gastrointestinal manifestations J09.X3
      - ~ laryngitis J09.X2
      - ~ myocarditis J09.X9
      - ~ otitis media J09.X9
      - ~ pharyngitis J09.X2
      - ~ pneumonia J09.X1
      - ~ respiratory manifestations NEC J09.X2
      - ~ specified manifestation NEC J09.X9
      - ~ upper respiratory symptoms J09.X2
- of other animal origin, not bird or swine (*see also* Influenza, due to, identified novel influenza A virus) J09.X2
- swine (viruses that normally cause infections in pigs) (*see also* Influenza, due to, identified novel influenza A virus) J09.X2

Influenza-like disease—*see* Influenza

Influenzal—*see* Influenza

Ingestion
- chemical—*see* Table of Drugs and Chemicals, by substance, poisoning
- drug or medicament
  - correct substance properly administered—*see* Table of Drugs and Chemicals, by drug, adverse effect
  - overdose or wrong substance given or taken—*see* Table of Drugs and Chemicals, by drug, poisoning
- foreign body—*see* Foreign body, alimentary tract

Ingrowing
- hair (beard) L73.1
- nail (finger) (toe) L60.0

Inguinal—*see also* Disease, diseased
- testicle Q53.9
  - bilateral Q53.212
  - unilateral Q53.112

Inhalation
- anthrax A22.1
- gases, fumes, or vapors
  - specified agent—*see* Table of Drugs and Chemicals, by substance T59.89-
- liquid or vomitus—*see* Asphyxia
- meconium (newborn) P24.00
  - with
    - pneumonia (pneumonitis) P24.01
    - ■ with respiratory symptoms P24.01
- mucus—*see* Asphyxia
- oil or gasoline (causing suffocation)—*see* Foreign body, by site
- smoke T59.81-
  - with respiratory conditions J70.5

Injury (*see also* specified type of injury) T14.90

See also the ICD-10-CM External Cause of Injuries Table for codes describing accident details.

- ankle S99.91-
  - specified type NEC S99.81-
- blood vessel NEC T14.8
  - carotid artery (common) (external) (internal, extracranial)
    - ■ internal, intracranial S06.8-
  - hand (level) S65.9-
    - ■ laceration S65.91-
    - ■ specified
      - ~ type NEC S65.99-
  - neck S15.9
    - ■ specified site NEC S15.8
  - palmar arch (superficial) S65.2-
    - ■ deep S65.30-
      - ~ laceration S65.31-
      - ~ specified type NEC S65.39-
    - ■ laceration S65.21-
    - ■ specified type NEC S65.29-
- brachial plexus S14.3
  - newborn P14.3
- brainstem S06.38-
- cord
  - spermatic (pelvic region)
    - ■ scrotal region S39.848
- eye S05.9-
  - conjunctiva S05.0-
  - cornea
    - ■ abrasion S05.0-
- foot S99.92-
  - specified type NEC S99.82-
- genital organ(s)
  - external S39.94
    - ■ specified NEC S39.848
- head S09.90
  - with loss of consciousness S06.9-
  - specified NEC S09.8
- heart (traumatic)
  - non-traumatic (acute) (chronic) (non-ischemic) I5A
- internal T14.8
  - pelvis, pelvic (organ) S39.9-
    - ~ specified NEC S39.83
  - intra-abdominal S36.90
- intracranial (traumatic) (*see also,* if applicable, Compression, brain, traumatic) S06.9-
  - cerebellar hemorrhage, traumatic—*see* Injury, intracranial
  - cerebral edema, traumatic S06.1X-
    - ■ diffuse S06.1X-
    - ■ focal S06.1X-
      - ~ diffuse (axonal) S06.2X-
  - epidural hemorrhage (traumatic) S06.4X-
  - focal brain injury S06.30-
    - ■ contusion—*see* Contusion, cerebral
  - intracerebral hemorrhage, traumatic S06.36-
    - ■ left side S06.35-
    - ■ right side S06.34-
    - ■ specified NEC S06.89-
  - subarachnoid hemorrhage, traumatic S06.6X-
  - subdural hemorrhage, traumatic S06.5X-
- intrathoracic
  - lung S27.30-
    - ■ aspiration J69.0
    - ■ bilateral S27.302

Injury, *continued*
- ■ contusion S27.329
  - ~ bilateral S27.322
  - ~ unilateral S27.321
- ■ unilateral S27.301
- pneumothorax S27.0-
- kidney S37.0-
  - acute (nontraumatic) N17.9
  - contusion—*see* Contusion, kidney
- lung—*see also* Injury, intrathoracic, lung
  - aspiration J69.0
  - dabbing (related) U07.0
  - electronic cigarette (related) U07.0
  - EVALI- [e-cigarette, or vaping, product use associated] U07.0
  - transfusion-related (TRALI) J95.84
  - vaping (device) (product) (use) (associated) U07.0
- multiple NOS T07
- muscle
  - finger
    - ■ extensor S56.4-
      - ~ hand level S66.3-
        - ◊ strain S66.31-
      - ~ laceration S56.42-
      - ~ strain S56.41-
    - ■ flexor (forearm level) S56.1-
      - ~ hand level S66.1-
        - ◊ laceration S66.12- (See complete *ICD-10-CM Manual*)
      - ~ strain S66.11-
      - ~ laceration S56.12-
      - ~ strain S56.11-
    - ■ intrinsic S66.5-
      - ~ strain S66.51-
  - foot S96.9-
    - ■ intrinsic S96.2-
      - ~ laceration S96.22-
      - ~ strain S96.21-
    - ■ laceration S96.92-
    - ■ specified
      - ~ site NEC S96.8-
        - ◊ strain S96.81-
      - ~ strain S96.91-
  - forearm (level) S56.90-
    - ■ extensor S56.5-
      - ~ laceration S56.52-
      - ~ strain S56.51-
    - ■ flexor
      - ~ laceration S56.22-
      - ~ strain S56.21-
    - ■ laceration S56.92-
    - ■ specified
      - ~ site NEC S56.8-
        - ◊ laceration S56.82-
        - ◊ strain S56.81-
      - ~ strain S56.91-
  - hand (level) S66.9-
    - ■ strain S66.91-
  - thumb
    - ■ abductor (forearm level) S56.3-
      - ~ laceration S56.32-
      - ~ strain S56.31-
    - ■ extensor (forearm level) S56.3-
      - ~ hand level S66.2-
        - ◊ strain S66.21-
      - ~ laceration S56.32-
      - ~ specified type NEC S56.39-
      - ~ strain S56.31-
    - ■ flexor (forearm level) S56.0 -
      - ~ hand level S66.0-
        - ◊ laceration S66.02-
        - ◊ strain S66.01-
      - ~ laceration S56.02-
      - ~ strain S56.01-
    - ■ intrinsic S66.4-
      - ~ strain S66.41-
  - toe—*see also* Injury, muscle, foot
    - ■ extensor, long S96.1-
      - ~ laceration S96.12-
      - ~ strain S96.11-
    - ■ flexor, long S96.0-
      - ~ laceration S96.02-
      - ~ strain S96.01-

ALPHABETIC INDEX

Injury, *continued*

- neck (level) S16.9
  - ■ laceration S16.2
  - ■ specified type NEC S16.8
  - ■ strain S16.1
- nerve NEC T14.8
  - facial S04.5-
    - ■ newborn P11.3
  - lumbar spinal
    - ■ peripheral S34.6
    - ■ root S34.21
    - ■ sympathetic S34.5
  - sacral spinal peripheral S34.6
    - ■ root S34.22
    - ■ sympathetic S34.5
- pelvis, pelvic (floor) S39.93
  - specified NEC S39.83
- postcardiac surgery (syndrome) I97.0
- rectovaginal septum NEC S39.83
- scalp S09.90
  - newborn (birth injury) P12.9
    - ■ due to monitoring (electrode) (sampling incision) P12.4
    - ■ specified NEC P12.89
      - caput succedaneum P12.81
- self-inflicted, without suicidal intent R45.88
- spermatic cord (pelvic region)
  - scrotal region S39.848
- spinal (cord)
  - cervical (neck) S14.109
    - ■ C1 level S14.101
    - ■ C2 level S14.102
    - ■ C3 level S14.103
    - ■ C4 level S14.104
    - ■ C5 level S14.105
    - ■ C6 level S14.106
    - ■ C7 level S14.107
    - ■ C8 level S14.108
  - lumbar S34.109
    - ■ complete lesion S34.11- (*See* complete *ICD-10-CM* Manual)
    - ■ incomplete lesion S34.129
      - L1 level S34.121
      - L2 level S34.122
      - L3 level S34.123
      - L4 level S34.124
      - L5 level S34.125
    - ■ L1 level S34.101
    - ■ L2 level S34.102
    - ■ L3 level S34.103
    - ■ L4 level S34.104
    - ■ L5 level S34.105
  - sacral S34.139
    - ■ complete lesion S34.131
    - ■ incomplete lesion S34.132
  - thoracic S24.109
    - ■ T1 level S24.101
    - ■ T2–T6 level S24.102
    - ■ T7–T10 level S24.103
    - ■ T11–T12 level S24.104
- spleen S36.0-
  - laceration S36.03-
    - ■ superficial (capsular) (minor) S36.030
- toe S99.92-
  - specified type NEC S99.82-
- transfusion-related acute lung (TRALI) J95.84
- vagina S39.93
  - abrasion S30.814
  - bite S31.45
    - ■ insect S30.864
    - ■ superficial NEC S30.874
  - contusion S30.23
  - external constriction S30.844
  - insect bite S30.864
  - laceration S31.41
    - ■ with foreign body S31.42
  - open wound S31.4-
  - puncture S31.43
    - ■ with foreign body S31.44
  - superficial S30.95
    - ■ foreign body S30.854

Injury, *continued*

- vulva S39.94
  - abrasion S30.814
  - bite S31.45
    - ■ insect S30.864
    - ■ superficial NEC S30.874
  - contusion S30.23
  - external constriction S30.844
  - insect bite S30.864
  - laceration S31.41
    - ■ with foreign body S31.42
  - open wound S31.4-
  - puncture S31.43
    - ■ with foreign body S31.44
  - superficial S30.95
    - ■ foreign body S30.854
- whiplash (cervical spine) S13.4

Insecurity

- financial Z59.86
- food Z59.41
- transportation Z59.82

Insensitivity

- adrenocorticotropin hormone (ACTH) E27.49
- androgen E34.50
  - complete E34.51
  - partial E34.52

Insolation (sunstroke) T67.01

Insomnia (organic) G47.00

- adjustment F51.02
  - adjustment disorder F51.02
- behavioral, of childhood Z73.819
  - combined type Z73.812
  - limit setting type Z73.811
  - sleep-onset association type Z73.810
- childhood Z73.819
- chronic F51.04
  - somatized tension F51.04
- conditioned F51.04
- due to
  - anxiety disorder F51.05
  - depression F51.05
  - medical condition G47.01
  - mental disorder NEC F51.05
- idiopathic F51.01
- learned F51.3
- nonorganic origin F51.01
- not due to a substance or known physiological condition F51.01
  - specified NEC F51.09
- paradoxical F51.03
- primary F51.01
- psychiatric F51.05
- psychophysiologic F51.04
- related to psychopathology F51.05
- short-term F51.02
- specified NEC G47.09
- stress-related F51.02
- transient F51.02
- without objective findings F51.02

Inspissated bile syndrome (newborn) P59.1

Instability

- emotional (excessive) F60.3
- housing
  - housed Z59.819
    - ■ with risk of homelessness Z59.811
    - ■ homelessness in past 12 months Z59.812
- joint (post-traumatic) M25.30
  - specified site NEC M25.39
- personality (emotional) F60.3
- vasomotor R55

Insufficiency, insufficient

- adrenal (gland) E27.40
  - primary E27.1
- adrenocortical E27.40
  - primary E27.1
- anus K62.89
- aortic (valve) I35.1
  - with
    - ■ mitral (valve) disease I08.0
      - with tricuspid (valve) disease I08.3

Insufficiency, insufficient, *continued*

- ■ stenosis I35.2
- ■ tricuspid (valve) disease I08.2
  - with mitral (valve) disease I08.3
- congenital Q23.1
- rheumatic I06.1
  - ■ with
    - mitral (valve) disease I08.0
      - ◊ with tricuspid (valve) disease I08.3
    - stenosis I06.2
      - ◊ with mitral (valve) disease I08.0
        - ⁕ with tricuspid (valve) disease I08.3
  - tricuspid (valve) disease I08.2
    - ◊ with mitral (valve) disease I08.3
  - specified cause NEC I35.1
- cardiac—*see also* Insufficiency, myocardial
  - due to presence of (cardiac) prosthesis I97.11-
  - postprocedural I97.11-
- corticoadrenal E27.40
  - primary E27.1
- health insurance coverage Z59.71
- kidney N28.9
  - acute N28.9
  - chronic N18.9
- mitral (valve) I34.0
  - with
    - ■ aortic valve disease I08.0
      - with tricuspid (valve) disease I08.3
    - ■ obstruction or stenosis I05.2
      - with aortic valve disease I08.0
    - ■ tricuspid (valve) disease I08.1
      - with aortic (valve) disease I08.3
  - congenital Q23.3
  - rheumatic I05.1
    - ■ with
      - aortic valve disease I08.0
        - ◊ with tricuspid (valve) disease I08.3
      - obstruction or stenosis I05.2
        - ◊ with aortic valve disease I08.0
          - ⁕ with tricuspid (valve) disease I08.3
    - tricuspid (valve) disease I08.1
      - ◊ with aortic (valve) disease I08.3
  - ■ active or acute I01.1
    - with chorea, rheumatic (Sydenham's) I02.0
  - specified cause, except rheumatic I34.0
- muscle—*see also* Disease, muscle
  - heart—*see* Insufficiency, myocardium, myocardial
  - ocular NEC H50.9
- myocardial, myocardium (with arteriosclerosis) I50.9
  - with
    - ■ rheumatic fever (conditions in I00) I09.0
      - active, acute or subacute I01.2
        - ◊ with chorea I02.0
      - inactive or quiescent (with chorea) I09.0
  - congenital Q24.8
  - newborn P29.0
  - rheumatic I09.0
    - ■ active, acute, or subacute I01.2
  - placental (mother) O36.51
- pulmonary J98.4
  - newborn P28.89
  - valve I37.1
    - ■ with stenosis I37.2
    - ■ congenital Q22.2
    - ■ rheumatic I09.89
      - with aortic, mitral or tricuspid (valve) disease I08.8
- renal (acute) N28.9
  - chronic N18.9
- respiratory R06.89
  - newborn P28.5
- rotation—*see* Malrotation
- suprarenal E27.40
  - primary E27.1
- tarso-orbital fascia, congenital Q10.3
- thyroid (gland) (acquired) E03.9
  - congenital E03.1
- tricuspid (valve) (rheumatic) I07.1
  - with
    - ■ aortic (valve) disease I08.2
      - with mitral (valve) disease I08.3
    - ■ mitral (valve) disease I08.1
      - with aortic (valve) disease I08.3

ALPHABETIC INDEX

Insufficiency, insufficient, *continued*
- ■ obstruction or stenosis I07.2
  - – with aortic (valve) disease I08.2
    - ◊ with mitral (valve) disease I08.3
  - – congenital Q22.8
  - – nonrheumatic I36.1
    - ■ with stenosis I36.2
- • urethral sphincter R32
- • velopharyngeal
  - – acquired K13.79
  - – congenital Q38.8
- • welfare support Z59.72

Intertrigo L30.4
- • labialis K13.0

Intervertebral annulus fibrosus defect
- • large, lumbar region M51.A2
- • large, lumbosacral region M51.A5
- • lumbar region, unspecified size M51.A0
- • small, lumbar region M51.A1
- • small, lumbosacral region M51.A4

Intolerance
- • carbohydrate K90.49
- • disaccharide, hereditary E73.0
- • fat NEC K90.49
  - – pancreatic K90.3
- • food K90.49
  - – dietary counseling and surveillance Z71.3
- • gluten
  - – celiac K90.0
  - – non-celiac K90.41
- • lactose E73.9
  - – specified NEC E73.8
- • milk NEC K90.49
  - – lactose E73.9
- • protein K90.49
- • starch NEC K90.49

Intoxication
- • drug
  - – acute (without dependence)—*see* Abuse, drug, by type, with intoxication
    - ■ with dependence—*see* Dependence, drug, by type with intoxication
  - – addictive
    - ■ via placenta or breast milk—*see* Absorption, drug
  - – newborn P93.8
    - ■ gray baby syndrome P93.0
  - – overdose or wrong substance given or taken—*see* Table of Drugs and Chemicals, by drug, poisoning
- • foodborne A05.9
  - – bacterial A05.9
  - – classical (Clostridium botulinum) A05.1
  - – due to
    - ■ Bacillus cereus A05.4
    - ■ bacterium A05.9
      - – specified NEC A05.8
    - ■ Clostridium
      - – botulinum A05.1
      - – perfringens A05.2
      - – welchii A05.2
    - ■ Salmonella A02.9
      - – with
        - ◊ (gastro) enteritis A02.0
        - ◊ specified manifestation NEC A02.8
    - ■ Staphylococcus A05.0
    - ■ Vibrio
      - – parahaemolyticus A05.3
      - – vulnificus A05.5
  - – enterotoxin, staphylococcal A05.0
  - – noxious—*see* Poisoning, food, noxious
- • meaning
  - – inebriation—*see* category F10
  - – poisoning—*see* Table of Drugs and Chemicals
- • serum (*see also* Reaction, serum) T80.69

Intraabdominal testis, testes
- • bilateral Q53.211
- • unilateral Q53.111

Intrahepatic gallbladder Q44.1

Intrauterine contraceptive device
- • checking Z30.431
- • insertion Z30.430
  - – immediately following removal Z30.433

Intrauterine contraceptive device, *continued*
- • in situ Z97.5
- • management Z30.431
  - – reinsertion Z30.433
  - – removal Z30.432
  - – replacement Z30.433

Intussusception (bowel) (colon) (enteric) (ileocecal) (ileocolic) (intestine) (rectum) K56.1

Invagination (bowel, colon, intestine or rectum) K56.1

Inversion
- • albumin-globulin (A-G) ratio E88.09
- • nipple N64.59
- • testis (congenital) Q55.29

Investigation (*see also* Examination) Z04.9

I. Q.
- • under 20 F73
- • 20–34 F72
- • 35–49 F71
- • 50–69 F70

IRDS (type I) P22.0
- • type II P22.1

Iritis
- • diabetic—*see* E08–E13 with .39

Irradiated enamel (tooth, teeth) K03.89

Irradiation effects, adverse T66

Irregular, irregularity
- • action, heart I49.9
- • bleeding N92.6
- • breathing R06.89
- • menstruation (cause unknown) N92.6
- • periods N92.6
- • respiratory R06.89
- • septum (nasal) J34.2
- • sleep-wake pattern (rhythm) G47.23

Irritable, irritability R45.4
- • bladder N32.89
- • bowel (syndrome) K58.9
  - – with constipation K58.1
  - – with diarrhea K58.0
  - – mixed K58.2
  - – other K58.8
  - – psychogenic F45.8
- • cerebral, in newborn P91.3
- • colon K58.9
  - – with constipation K58.1
  - – with diarrhea K58.0
  - – mixed K58.2
  - – other K58.8
  - – psychogenic F45.8
- • heart (psychogenic) F45.8
- • infant R68.12stomach K31.89
  - – psychogenic F45.8

Irritation
- • anus K62.89
- • bladder N32.89
- • gastric K31.89
  - – psychogenic F45.8
- • nervous R45.0
- • perineum NEC L29.3
- • peripheral autonomic nervous system G90.89
- • sympathetic nerve NEC G90.89
- • stomach K31.89
  - – psychogenic F45.8
- • vaginal N89.8

Ischemia, ischemic I99.8
- • brain—*see* Ischemia, cerebral
- • cerebral (chronic) (generalized) I67.82
  - – intermittent G45.9
  - – newborn P91.0
  - – recurrent focal G45.8
  - – transient G45.9
- • intestine, unspecified part
  - – diffuse acute (reversible) K55.052
  - – focal (segmental) acute (reversible) K55.051
  - – unspecified extent K55.059
- • large intestine
  - – diffuse acute (reversible) K55.032
  - – focal (segmental) acute (reversible) K55.031
  - – unspecified extent K55.039

Ischemia, ischemic, *continued*
- • small intestine
  - – diffuse acute (reversible) K55.012
  - – focal (segmental) acute (reversible) K55.011
  - – unspecified extent K55.019

Ischuria R34

Isoimmunization NEC—*see also* Incompatibility
- • affecting management of pregnancy (ABO) (with hydrops fetalis) O36.11-
  - – anti-A sensitization O36.11-
  - – anti-B sensitization O36.19-
  - – anti-c sensitization O36.09-
  - – anti-C sensitization O36.09-
  - – anti-e sensitization O36.09-
  - – anti-E sensitization O36.09-
  - – Rh NEC O36.09-
    - ■ anti-D antibody O36.01-
  - – specified NEC O36.19-
- • newborn P55.9
  - – with
    - ■ hydrops fetalis P56.0
    - ■ kernicterus P57.0
  - – ABO (blood groups) P55.1
  - – Rhesus (Rh) factor P55.0
  - – specified type NEC P55.8

Isolation, isolated
- • dwelling Z59.89
- • family Z63.79
- • social Z60.4

Issue of
- • medical certificate Z02.79
  - – for disability determination Z02.71
- • repeat prescription (appliance) (glasses) (medicinal substance, medicament, medicine) Z76.0
  - – contraception—*see* Contraception

IST (inappropriate sinus tachycardia, so stated) I47.11

Itch, itching—*see also* Pruritus
- • baker's L23.6
- • barber's B35.0
- • cheese B88.0
- • clam digger's B65.3
- • copra B88.0
- • dhobi B35.6
- • grain B88.0
- • grocer's B88.0
- • harvest B88.0
- • jock B35.6
- • Malabar B35.5
  - – beard B35.0
  - – foot B35.3
  - – scalp B35.0
- • meaning scabies B86
- • Norwegian B86
- • perianal L29.0
- • poultrymen's B88.0
- • sarcoptic B86
- • scabies B86
- • scrub B88.0
- • straw B88.0
- • swimmer's B65.3
- • winter L29.89

Ixodiasis NEC B88.8

J

Jacquet's dermatitis (diaper dermatitis) L22

Jamaican
- • neuropathy G92.8
- • paraplegic tropical ataxic-spastic syndrome G92.8

Jaundice (yellow) R17
- • breast-milk (inhibitor) P59.3
- • catarrhal (acute) B15.9
- • cholestatic (benign) R17
- • due to or associated with
  - – delayed conjugation P59.8
    - ■ associated with (due to) preterm delivery P59.0
  - – preterm delivery P59.0
- • epidemic (catarrhal) B15.9
- • familial nonhemolytic (congenital) (Gilbert) E80.4
  - – Crigler-Najjar E80.5
- • febrile (acute) B15.9

ALPHABETIC INDEX

Jaundice, *continued*

- infectious (acute) (subacute) B15.9
- neonatal—*see* Jaundice, newborn
- newborn P59.9
  - due to or associated with
    - ABO
      - antibodies P55.1
      - incompatibility, maternal/fetal P55.1
      - isoimmunization P55.1
    - breast milk inhibitors to conjugation P59.3
      - associated with preterm delivery P59.0
    - Crigler-Najjar syndrome E80.5
    - delayed conjugation P59.8
      - associated with preterm delivery P59.0
    - Gilbert syndrome E80.4
    - hemolytic disease P55.9
      - ABO isoimmunization P55.1
    - hepatocellular damage P59.20
      - specified NEC P59.29
    - hypothyroidism, congenital E03.1
    - inspissated bile syndrome P59.1
    - mucoviscidosis E84.9
    - preterm delivery P59.0
  - spherocytosis (congenital) D58.0
- nonhemolytic congenital familial (Gilbert) E80.4
- symptomatic R17
  - newborn P59.9

Jealousy

- childhood F93.8
- sibling F93.8

Jejunitis—*see* Enteritis

Jejunostomy status Z93.4

Jejunum, jejunal—*see* Disease, diseased

Jerks, myoclonic G25.3

Jervell-Lange-Nielsen syndrome I45.81

Jeune's disease Q77.2

Jigger disease B88.1

Job's syndrome (chronic granulomatous disease) D71

Joseph-Diamond-Blackfan anemia (congenital hypoplastic) D61.01

K

Kallmann's syndrome E23.0

Kaposi's

- vaccinia T88.1

Kartagener's syndrome or triad (sinusitis, bronchiectasis, situs inversus) Q89.3

Karyotype

- 46,XX Q98.3
  - with streak gonads Q50.32
  - hermaphrodite (true) Q99.1
  - male Q98.3
- 47,XXX Q97.0
- 47,XYY Q98.5

Kawasaki's syndrome M30.3

Kaznelson's syndrome (congenital hypoplastic anemia) D61.01

Kelis L91.0

Keloid, cheloid L91.0

- Hawkin's L91.0
- scar L91.0

Keloma L91.0

Keratitis (nodular) (nonulcerative) (simple) (zonular) H16.9

- dendritic (a) (herpes simplex) B00.52
- disciform (is) (herpes simplex) B00.52
  - varicella B01.81
- gonococcal (congenital or prenatal) A54.33
- herpes, herpetic (simplex) B00.52
- in (due to)
  - exanthema (*see also* Exanthem) B09
  - herpes (simplex) virus B00.52
  - measles B05.81
- postmeasles B05.81

Keratoconjunctivitis H16.20-

- herpes, herpetic (simplex) B00.52
- in exanthema (*see also* Exanthem) B09
- postmeasles B05.81

Keratoderma, keratodermia (congenital) (palmaris et plantaris) (symmetrical) Q82.8

Keratoglobus H18.79

- congenital Q15.8
  - with glaucoma Q15.0

Keratoma

- palmaris and plantaris hereditarium Q82.8

Keratosis

- congenital, specified NEC Q80.8
- female genital NEC N94.89
- follicularis Q82.8
  - congenita Q82.8
  - spinulosa (decalvans) Q82.8
- gonococcal A54.89
- nigricans L83
- palmaris et plantaris (inherited) (symmetrical) Q82.8
  - acquired L85.1
- tonsillaris J35.8
- vegetans Q82.8

Kerion (celsi) B35.0

Kink, kinking

- ureter (pelvic junction) N13.5
  - with
    - hydronephrosis N13.1

Kleeblattschaedel skull Q75.051

Klinefelter's syndrome Q98.4

Klumpke (-Déjerine) palsy, paralysis (birth) (newborn) P14.1

Knee—*see* Disease, diseased

Knock knee (acquired) M21.06-

- congenital Q74.1

Knot(s)

- intestinal, syndrome (volvulus) K56.2

Knotting (of)

- intestine K56.2

Köebner's syndrome Q81.8

Koplik's spots B05.9

Kraft-Weber-Dimitri disease Q85.8

Kraurosis

- ani K62.89

Kreotoxism A05.9

Kwashiokor E40

Kyphoscoliosis, kyphoscoliotic (acquired) (*see also* Scoliosis) M41.9

- congenital Q67.5
- heart (disease) I27.1

Kyphosis, kyphotic (acquired) M40.209

- Morquio-Brailsford type (spinal) E76.219

L

Labile

- blood pressure R09.89

Labium leporinum—*see* Cleft, lip

Labyrinthitis (circumscribed) (destructive) (diffuse) (inner ear) (latent) (purulent) (suppurative) H83.0

Laceration

- abdomen, abdominal
  - wall S31.119
    - with
      - foreign body S31.129
    - epigastric region S31.112
      - with
        - ◊ foreign body S31.122
    - left
      - ~ lower quadrant S31.114
        - ◊ with
          - » foreign body S31.124
      - ~ upper quadrant S31.111
        - ◊ with
          - » foreign body S31.121
    - periumbilic region S31.115
      - ~ with
        - ◊ foreign body S31.125
    - right
      - ~ lower quadrant S31.113
        - ◊ with
          - » foreign body S31.123

Laceration, *continued*

- ~ upper quadrant S31.110
  - ◊ with
    - » foreign body S31.120
- Achilles tendon S86.02-
- ankle S91.01-
  - with
    - foreign body S91.02-
- antecubital space—*see* Laceration
- anus (sphincter) S31.831
  - with
    - foreign body S31.832
  - nontraumatic, nonpuerperal—*see* Fissure, anus
- arm (upper) S41.11-
  - with foreign body S41.12-
  - lower—*see* Laceration, forearm
- auditory canal (external) (meatus)—*see* Laceration, ear
- auricle, ear—*see* Laceration, ear
- axilla—*see* Laceration, arm
- back—*see also* Laceration, thorax, back
  - lower S31.010
    - with
      - foreign body S31.020
- brainstem S06.38-
- buttock S31.8-
  - with foreign body S31.8-
  - left S31.821
    - with foreign body S31.822
  - right S31.811
    - with foreign body S31.812
- calf—*see* Laceration, leg
- canaliculus lacrimalis—*see* Laceration, eyelid
- canthus, eye—*see* Laceration, eyelid
- capsule, joint—*see* Sprain
- cerebellum, traumatic S06.37-
- cerebral
  - left side S06.32-
  - during birth P10.8
    - with hemorrhage P10.1
  - right side S06.31-
- cheek (external) S01.41-
  - with foreign body S01.42-
  - internal—*see* Laceration, oral cavity
- chest wall—*see* Laceration, thorax
- chin—*see* Laceration, head, specified site NEC
- digit(s)
  - hand—*see* Laceration, finger
  - foot—*see* Laceration, toe
- ear (canal) (external) S01.31-
  - with foreign body S01.32-
  - drum S09.2-
- elbow S51.01-
  - with foreign body S51.02-
- epididymis—*see* Laceration, testis
- epigastric region—*see* Laceration, abdomen, wall, epigastric region
- esophagus K22.89
- eyebrow—*see* Laceration, eyelid
- eyelid S01.11-
  - with foreign body S01.12-
- face NEC—*see* Laceration, head, specified site NEC
- finger(s) S61.21-
  - with
    - damage to nail S61.31-
      - with
        - ◊ foreign body S61.32-
    - foreign body S61.22-
  - index S61.21-
    - with
      - damage to nail S61.31-
        - ◊ with
          - » foreign body S61.32-
        - ~ foreign body S61.22-
    - left S61.211
      - ~ with
        - ◊ damage to nail S61.311
          - » with
            - ◊ foreign body S61.221
    - right S61.210
      - ~ with
        - ◊ damage to nail S61.310
          - » with

ALPHABETIC INDEX

Laceration, *continued*
- ◈ foreign body S61.320
- ◊ foreign body S61.220
- little S61.218
  - ■ with
    - ~ damage to nail S61.31-
    - ◊ with
      - ▸ foreign body S61.32-
      - ~ foreign body S61.22-
  - ■ left S61.217
    - ~ with
    - ◊ damage to nail S61.317
      - ▸ with
        - ◈ foreign body S61.327
      - ◊ foreign body S61.227
  - ■ right S61.216
    - ~ with
    - ◊ damage to nail S61.316
      - ▸ with
        - ◈ foreign body S61.326
      - ◊ foreign body S61.226
- middle S61.218
  - ■ with
    - ~ damage to nail S61.31-
    - ◊ with
      - ▸ foreign body S61.32-
      - ~ foreign body S61.22-
  - ■ left S61.213
    - ~ with
    - ◊ damage to nail S61.313
      - ▸ with
        - ◈ foreign body S61.323
      - ◊ foreign body S61.223
  - ■ right S61.212
    - ~ with
    - ◊ damage to nail S61.312
      - ▸ with
        - ◈ foreign body S61.322
      - ◊ foreign body S61.222
- ring S61.218
  - ■ with
    - ~ damage to nail S61.31-
    - ◊ with
      - ▸ foreign body S61.32-
      - ~ foreign body S61.22-
  - ■ left S61.215
    - ~ with
    - ◊ damage to nail S61.315
      - ▸ with
        - ◈ foreign body S61.325
      - ◊ foreign body S61.225
  - ■ right S61.214
    - ~ with
    - ◊ damage to nail S61.314
      - ▸ with
        - ◈ foreign body S61.324
      - ◊ foreign body S61.224
- flank S31.119
  - ~ with foreign body S31.129
- foot (except toe(s) alone) S91.31-
  - ~ with foreign body S91.32-
  - left S91.312
    - ■ with foreign body S91.322
  - right S91.311
    - ■ with foreign body S91.321
  - toe—*see* Laceration, toe
- forearm S51.81-
  - ~ with
    - ■ foreign body S51.82-
  - elbow only—*see* Laceration
  - left S51.812
    - ■ with
      - ~ foreign body S51.822
  - right S51.811
    - ■ with
      - ~ foreign body S51.821
- forehead S01.81
  - ~ with foreign body S01.82
- gum—*see* Laceration, oral cavity
- hand S61.41-
  - ~ with
    - ■ foreign body S61.42-

Laceration, *continued*
- finger—*see* Laceration, finger
- left S61.412
  - ■ with
    - ~ foreign body S61.422
- right S61.411
  - ■ with
    - ~ foreign body S61.421
- thumb—*see* Laceration, thumb
- head S01.91
  - ~ with foreign body S01.92
  - cheek—*see* Laceration, cheek
  - ear—*see* Laceration, ear
  - eyelid—*see* Laceration, eyelid
  - lip—*see* Laceration, lip
  - nose—*see* Laceration, nose
  - oral cavity—*see* Laceration, oral cavity
  - scalp S01.01
    - ■ with foreign body S01.02
  - specified site NEC S01.81
    - ■ with foreign body S01.82
  - temporomandibular area—*see* Laceration, cheek
- heel—*see* Laceration, foot
- hip S71.01-
  - ~ with foreign body S71.02-
  - left S71.012
    - ■ with foreign body S71.022
  - right S71.011
    - ■ with foreign body S71.021
- hypochondrium—*see* Laceration, abdomen, wall
- hypogastric region—*see* Laceration, abdomen, wall
- inguinal region—*see* Laceration, abdomen, wall
- instep—*see* Laceration, foot
- interscapular region—*see* Laceration, thorax, back
- jaw—*see* Laceration, head, specified site NEC
- joint capsule—*see* Sprain, by site
- knee S81.01-
  - ~ with foreign body S81.02-
- labium (majus) (minus)—*see* Laceration, vulva
- lacrimal duct—*see* Laceration, eyelid
- leg (lower) S81.81-
  - ~ with foreign body S81.82-
  - foot—*see* Laceration, foot
  - knee—*see* Laceration, knee
  - left S81.812
    - ■ with foreign body S81.822
  - right S81.811
    - ■ with foreign body S81.821
  - upper—*see* Laceration, thigh
- ligament—*see* Sprain
- lip S01.511
  - ~ with foreign body S01.521
- loin—*see* Laceration, abdomen, wall
- lower back—*see* Laceration, back, lower
- lumbar region—*see* Laceration, back, lower
- malar region—*see* Laceration, head, specified site NEC
- mammary—*see* Laceration
- mastoid region—*see* Laceration, head, specified site NEC
- mouth—*see* Laceration, oral cavity
- muscle—*see* Injury, muscle, by site, laceration
- nail
  - finger—*see* Laceration, finger, with, damage to nail
  - toe—*see* Laceration, toe, with, damage to nail
- nasal (septum) (sinus)—*see* Laceration, nose
- nasopharynx—*see* Laceration, head, specified site NEC
- neck S11.91
  - ~ with foreign body S11.92
- nerve—*see* Injury, nerve
- nose (septum) (sinus) S01.21
  - ~ with foreign body S01.22
- ocular NOS
  - adnexa NOS S01.11-
- oral cavity S01.512
  - ~ with foreign body S01.522
- palate—*see* Laceration, oral cavity
- palm—*see* Laceration, hand
- pelvic S31.010
  - ~ with
    - ■ foreign body S31.020
- penis S31.21
- perineum
  - female S31.41

Laceration, *continued*
- ■ with
  - ~ foreign body S31.42
- male S31.119
  - ■ with foreign body S31.129
- periocular area (with or without lacrimal passages)—*see* Laceration, eyelid
- periumbillic region—*see* Laceration, abdomen, wall, periumbillic
- phalanges
  - finger—*see* Laceration, finger
  - toe—*see* Laceration, toe
- pinna—*see* Laceration, ear
- popliteal space—*see* Laceration, knee
- prepuce—*see* Laceration, penis
- pubic region S31.119
  - ~ with foreign body S31.129
- pudendum—*see* Laceration
- rectovaginal septum—*see* Laceration, vagina
- rectum S36.63
- sacral region—*see* Laceration, back, lower
- sacroiliac region—*see* Laceration, back, lower
- salivary gland—*see* Laceration, oral cavity
- scalp S01.01
  - ~ with foreign body S01.02
- scapular region—*see* Laceration, shoulder
- scrotum S31.31
- shin—*see* Laceration, leg
- shoulder S41.01-
  - ~ with foreign body S41.02-
  - left S41.012
    - ■ with foreign body S41.022
  - right S41.011
    - ■ with foreign body S41.021
- spleen S36.03-
  - superficial (minor) S36.030
- submaxillary region—*see* Laceration, head, specified site NEC
- submental region—*see* Laceration, head, specified site NEC
- subungual
  - finger(s)—*see* Laceration, finger, with, damage to nail
  - toe(s)—*see* Laceration, toe, with, damage to nail
- temple, temporal region—*see* Laceration, head, specified site NEC
- temporomandibular area—*see* Laceration, cheek
- tendon—*see* Injury, muscle, by site, laceration
  - Achilles S86.02-
- testis S31.31
- thigh S71.11-
  - ~ with foreign body S71.12-
- thorax, thoracic (wall) S21.91
  - ~ with foreign body S21.92
  - ■ back S21.22-
    - front S21.12-
  - back S21.21-
    - ■ with
      - ~ foreign body S21.22-
    - front S21.11-
      - ■ with
        - ~ foreign body S21.12-
- thumb S61.01-
  - ~ with
    - ■ damage to nail S61.11-
      - ~ with
        - ◊ foreign body S61.12-
    - ■ foreign body S61.02-
  - left S61.012
    - ■ with
      - ~ damage to nail S61.112
        - ◊ with
          - ▸ foreign body S61.122
        - ~ foreign body S61.022
  - right S61.011
    - ■ with
      - ~ damage to nail S61.111
        - ◊ with
          - ▸ foreign body S61.121
        - ~ foreign body S61.021
- toe(s) S91.11-
  - ~ with

ALPHABETIC INDEX

Laceration, *continued*

- ■ damage to nail S91.21-
  - ~ with
    - ◊ foreign body S91.22-
  - ■ foreign body S91.12-
- great S91.11-
  - ■ with
    - ~ damage to nail S91.21-
    - ◊ with
      - » foreign body S91.22-
    - ~ foreign body S91.12-
  - ■ left S91.112
    - ~ with
    - ◊ damage to nail S91.212
      - » with
        - ✦ foreign body S91.222
      - ◊ foreign body S91.122
  - ■ right S91.111
    - ~ with
    - ◊ damage to nail S91.211
      - » with
        - ✦ foreign body S91.221
      - ◊ foreign body S91.121
- lesser S91.11-
  - ■ with
    - ~ damage to nail S91.21-
    - ◊ with
      - » foreign body S91.22-
    - ~ foreign body S91.12-
  - ■ left S91.115
    - ~ with
    - ◊ damage to nail S91.215
      - » with
        - ✦ foreign body S91.225
      - ◊ foreign body S91.125
  - ■ right S91.114
    - ~ with
    - ◊ damage to nail S91.214
      - » with
        - ✦ foreign body S91.224
      - ◊ foreign body S91.124
- tongue—*see* Laceration, oral cavity
- tunica vaginalis—*see* Laceration, testis
- tympanum, tympanic membrane—*see* Laceration, ear, drum
- umbilical region S31.115
  - with foreign body S31.125
- uvula—*see* Laceration, oral cavity
- vagina S31.41
  - with
    - foreign body S31.42
  - nonpuerperal, nontraumatic N89.8
  - old (postpartal) N89.8
- vulva S31.41
  - with
    - foreign body S31.42
- wrist S61.51-
  - with
    - foreign body S61.52-
  - left S61.512
    - ■ with
      - ~ foreign body S61.522
  - right S61.511
    - ■ with
      - ~ foreign body S61.521

Lack of

- adequate
  - food Z59.48
  - sleep Z72.820
- air conditioning Z59.11
- appetite (*see* Anorexia) R63.0
- basic services in physical environment Z58.81
- care
  - in home Z74.2
  - of infant (at or after birth) T76.02
    - ■ confirmed T74.02
- coordination R27.9
  - ataxia R27.0
  - specified type NEC R27.8
- development (physiological) R62.50
  - failure to thrive (child over 28 days old) R62.51
    - ■ newborn P92.6

Lack of, *continued*

- short stature R62.52
- specified type NEC R62.59
- electricity services Z59.12
- energy R53.83
- food Z59.48
- gas services Z59.12
- growth R62.52
- heating Z59.11
- housing (permanent) (temporary) Z59.00
  - adequate Z59.10
- material resources due to limited financial resources, specified NEC Z59.87
- oil services Z59.12
- ovulation N97.0
- person able to render necessary care Z74.2
- physical exercise Z72.3
- safe drinking water Z58.6
- shelter Z59.02
- water T73.1
  - safe drinking Z58.6
  - services Z59.12

Lactation, lactating (breast) (puerperal, postpartum)

- associated
  - cracked nipple O92.13
  - retracted nipple O92.03
- defective O92.4
- disorder NEC O92.79
- excessive O92.6
- failed (complete) O92.3
  - partial O92.4
- mastitis NEC N61.1
- mother (care and/or examination) Z39.1
- nonpuerperal N64.3

Lafora disease—*see also* Epilepsy, progressive, Lafora G40.C09

Lacunar skull Q75.8

Lalling F80.0

Lambliasis, lambliosis A07.1

Landouzy-Déjerine dystrophy or facioscapulohumeral atrophy G71.02

Lapsed immunization schedule status Z28.3

Large

- baby (regardless of gestational age) (4000g-4499g) P08.1

Large-for-dates (infant) (4000g to 4499g) P08.1

- affecting management of pregnancy O36.6-
- exceptionally (4500g or more) P08.0

Larsen-Johansson disease or osteochondrosis—*see* Osteochondrosis, juvenile, patella

Laryngismus (stridulus) J38.5

- congenital P28.89

Laryngitis (acute) (edematous) (fibrinous) (infective) (infiltrative) (malignant) (membranous) (phlegmonous) (pneumococcal) (pseudomembranous) (septic) (subglottic) (suppurative) (ulcerative) J04.0

- with
  - influenza, flu, or grippe—*see* Influenza, laryngitis
  - tracheitis (acute)—*see* Laryngotracheitis
- atrophic J37.0
- catarrhal J37.0
- chronic J37.0
  - with tracheitis (chronic) J37.1
- Hemophilus influenzae J04.0
- H. influenzae J04.0
- hypertrophic J37.0
- influenzal—*see* Influenza, respiratory manifestations NEC
- obstructive J05.0
- sicca J37.0
- spasmodic J05.0
  - acute J04.0
- streptococcal J04.0
- stridulous J05.0

Laryngomalacia (congenital) Q31.5

Laryngopharyngitis (acute) J06.0

- chronic J37.0

Laryngoplegia J38.00

- bilateral J38.02
- unilateral J38.01

Laryngotracheitis (acute) (infectional) (infective) (viral) J04.2

- atrophic J37.1
- catarrhal J37.1
- chronic J37.1
- Hemophilus influenzae J04.2
- hypertrophic J37.1
- influenzal—*see* Influenza, respiratory manifestations NEC
- sicca J37.1
- spasmodic J38.5
  - acute J05.0
- streptococcal J04.2

Laryngotracheobronchitis—*see* Bronchitis

Late

- talker R62.0
- walker R62.0

Late effects—*see* Sequela

Latent tuberculosis (LTBI) Z22.7

Launois' syndrome (pituitary gigantism) E22.0

Laurence-Moon syndrome Q87.84

Lax, laxity—*see also* Relaxation

- ligament(ous)—*see also* Disorder
  - familial M35.7
- skin congenital Q82.8

Lazy leukocyte syndrome D70.8

Leak, leakage

- air NEC J93.82
  - postprocedural J95.812
- cerebrospinal fluid G96.00
  - cranial
    - postoperative G96.08
      - ■ specified NEC G96.08
      - ■ spontaneous G96.01
      - ■ traumatic G96.08
  - spinal
    - ■ postoperative G96.09
    - ■ post-traumatic G96.09
    - ■ specified NEC G96.09
    - ■ spontaneous G96.02
  - spontaneous
    - ■ from
      - ~ skull base G96.01
      - ~ spine G96.02
- device, implant or graft—*see also* Complications, by site and type, mechanical
  - persistent air J93.82

Leaky heart—*see* Endocarditis

Learning defect (specific) F81.9

Leber's

- congenital amaurosis H35.50

Lederer's anemia D59.19

Legg (-Calvé)-Perthes disease, syndrome or osteochondrosis M91.1-

Leiner's disease L21.1

Lenegre's disease I44.2

Lengthening, leg—*see* Deformity, limb

Lennox-Gastaut syndrome G40.812

- intractable G40.814
  - with status epilepticus G40.813
  - without status epilepticus G40.814
- not intractable G40.812
  - with status epilepticus G40.811
  - without status epilepticus G40.812

Lenticonus (anterior) (posterior) (congenital) Q12.8

Lentiglobus (posterior) (congenital) Q12.8

Lentigo (congenital) L81.4

Leptocytosis, hereditary D56.9

Leptomeningitis (chronic) (circumscribed) (hemorrhagic) (nonsuppurative)—*see* Meningitis

Leptomeningopathy G96.198

Leptus dermatitis B88.0

Leri-Weill syndrome Q77.8

Lesch-Nyhan syndrome E79.1

ALPHABETIC INDEX

Lesion(s) (nontraumatic)
- angiocentric immunoproliferative D47.Z9
- anorectal K62.9
- aortic (valve) I35.9
- basal ganglion G25.9
- brain G93.9
  - congenital Q04.9
    - hypertensive I67.4
- buccal cavity K13.79
- cardiac (*see also* Disease, heart) I51.9
  - congenital Q24.9
- cerebrovascular I67.9
  - degenerative I67.9
  - hypertensive I67.4
- chorda tympani G51.8
- hypothalamic E23.7
- joint—*see* Disorder, joint
  - sacroiliac (old) M53.3
- lip K13.0
- maxillary sinus J32.0
- mitral I05.9
- motor cortex NEC G93.89
- mouth K13.79
- nervous system, congenital Q07.9
- nose (internal) J34.89
- oral mucosa K13.70
- peptic K27.9
- primary (*see also* Syphilis, primary) A51.0
- pulmonary J98.4
  - valve I37.9
- sacroiliac (joint) (old) M53.3
- sinus (accessory) (nasal) J34.89
- skin L98.9
  - suppurative L08.0
- tonsillar fossa J35.9
- tricuspid (valve) I07.9
  - nonrheumatic I36.9
- vascular I99.9
- vagina N89.8
- vulva N90.89

Lethargy R53.83

Leukemia, leukemic C95.9-
- acute lymphoblastic C91.0-
- acute myeloblastic (minimal differentiation) (with maturation) C92.0-
- AML (1/ETO) (M0) (M1) (M2) (without a FAB classification) NOS C92.0-
- chronic myelomonocytic C93.1-
- CMML (-1) (-2) (with eosinophilia) C93.1-
- juvenile myelomonocytic C93.3-
- lymphoid C91.9-
- monocytic (subacute) C93.9-
- myelogenous (*see also* Category C92) C92.9-
- myeloid C92.9-
- subacute lymphocytic C91.9-

Leukemoid reaction (*see also* Reaction, leukemoid) D72.823-

Leukocytopenia D72.819

Leukocytosis D72.829
- eosinophilic D72.19

Leukodystrophy G31.80
- with vanishing white matter disease G11.6
- LMNB1-related autosomal dominant G90.8
- pol III-related G11.5

Leukoencephalitis G04.81
- acute (subacute) hemorrhagic G36.1
  - postimmunization or postvaccinal G04.02
- postinfectious G04.01

Leukoencephalopathy (Encephalopathy) G93.49
- with calcifications and cysts G93.43
- megalencephalic, with subcortical cysts G93.42
- postimmunization and postvaccinal G04.02
- reversible, posterior G93.6

Leukomalacia, cerebral, newborn P91.2

Leukomelanoparthy, hereditary D72.0
- periventricular P91.2

Leukonychia (punctata) (striata) L60.8
- congenital Q84.4

Leukopathia unguium L60.8
- congenital Q84.4

Leukopenia D72.819
- basophilic D72.818
- chemotherapy (cancer) induced D70.1
- congenital D70.0
- cyclic D70.0
- drug induced NEC D70.2
  - due to cytoreductive cancer chemotherapy D70.1
- eosinophilic D72.818
- familial D70.0
- infantile genetic D70.0
- malignant D70.9
- periodic D70.0
- transitory neonatal P61.5

Leukoplakia
- anus K62.89
- rectum K62.89

Leukorrhea N89.8
- due to Trichomonas (vaginalis) A59.00
- trichomonal A59.00

Leukosarcoma C85.9-

Levocardia (isolated) Q24.1
- with situs inversus Q89.3

Lev's disease or syndrome (acquired complete heart block) I44.2

Leyden-Moebius dystrophy G71.09

Liar, pathologic F60.2

Libman-Sacks disease M32.11

Lice (infestation) B85.2
- body (Pediculus corporis) B85.1
- crab B85.3
- head (Pediculus corporis) B85.0
- mixed (classifiable to more than one of the titles B85.0–B85.3) B85.4
- pubic (Phthirus pubis) B85.3

Lichen L28.0
- congenital Q82.8
- pilaris Q82.8
  - acquired L85.8

Light
- for gestational age—*see* Light for dates
- headedness R42

Light-for-dates (infant) P05.00
- with weight of
  - 499 grams or less P05.01
  - 500–749 grams P05.02
  - 750–999 grams P05.03
  - 1000–1249 grams P05.04
  - 1250–1499 grams P05.05
  - 1500–1749 grams P05.06
  - 1750–1999 grams P05.07
  - 2000–2499 grams P05.08
  - 2500 g and over P05.09
- and small-for-dates—*see* Small for dates
- affecting management of pregnancy O36.59-

Ligneous thyroiditis E06.5

Lindau (-von Hippel) disease Q85.8

Line(s)
- Harris'—*see* Arrest, epiphyseal

Lingua
- geographica K14.1

Linguatulosis B88.8

Lipochondrodystrophy E76.01

Lipochrome histiocytosis (familial) D71

Lipodystrophy (progressive) E88.1
- intestinal K90.81

Lipoid—*see also* Disease, diseased
- histiocytosis D76.3
- nephrosis N04.9

Lipoma D17.9
- infiltrating D17.9
- intramuscular D17.9
- pleomorphic D17.9
- site classification
  - arms (skin) (subcutaneous) D17.2-
  - connective tissue D17.30
    - intra-abdominal D17.5
    - intrathoracic D17.4

Lipoma, *continued*
  - peritoneum D17.79
  - retroperitoneum D17.79
  - specified site NEC D17.39
  - spermatic cord D17.6
- face (skin) (subcutaneous) D17.0
- genitourinary organ NEC D17.72
- head (skin) (subcutaneous) D17.0
- intra-abdominal D17.5
- intrathoracic D17.4
- kidney D17.71
- legs (skin) (subcutaneous) D17.2-
- neck (skin) (subcutaneous) D17.0
- peritoneum D17.79
- retroperitoneum D17.79
- skin D17.30
  - specified site NEC D17.39
  - specified site NEC D17.79
- spermatic cord D17.6
- subcutaneous D17.30
  - specified site NEC D17.39
- trunk (skin) (subcutaneous) D17.1
- unspecified D17.9
- spindle cell D17.9

Lipoproteinemia E78.5
- broad-beta E78.2
- floating-beta E78.2

Lisping F80.0

Listeriosis, Listerellosis A32.9
- congenital (disseminated) P37.2
- cutaneous A32.0
- neonatal, newborn (disseminated) P37.2
- oculoglandular A32.81
- specified NEC A32.89

Lithemia E79.0

Little leaguer's elbow—*see* Epicondylitis, medial

Little's disease G80.9

Livedo (annularis) (racemosa) (reticularis) R23.1

Living alone (problems with) Z60.2
- with handicapped person Z74.2

Living in a shelter (motel) (scattered site housing) (temporary or transitional living situation) Z59.01

Lobstein (-Ekman) disease or syndrome Q78.0

Lone Star fever A77.0

Long
- COVID (-19) (*see also* COVID-19) U09.9
- QT syndrome I45.81

Long-term (current) (prophylactic) drug therapy (use of)
- alkylating agent Z79.630
- antibiotics Z79.2
  - short-term use—omit code
- anti-inflammatory, non-steroidal (NSAID) Z79.1
- antimetabolite agent Z79.631
- antitumor antibiotic Z79.632
- aspirin Z79.82
- calcineurin inhibitor Z79.621
- drug, specified NEC Z79.899
- hypoglycemic, oral, drugs Z79.84
- immunomodulators Z79.61
- immunomodulators and immunosuppressants, unspecified Z79.60
- immunosuppressive biologic Z79.620
- inhibitors of nucleotide synthesis Z79.624
- injectable non-insulin antidiabetic drugs Z79.85
- insulin Z79.4
- Janus kinase inhibitor Z79.622
- mammalian target of rapamycin (mTOR) inhibitor Z79.623
- mitotic inhibitor Z79.633
- myelosuppressive agent Z79.64
- non-insulin antidiabetic drug, injectable Z79.899
- non-steroidal anti-inflammatories (NSAID) Z79.1
- other immunomodulators and immunosuppressants Z79.69
- steroids
  - inhaled Z79.51
  - systemic Z79.52
- topoisomerase inhibitorZ79.634

ALPHABETIC INDEX

Longitudinal stripes or grooves, nails L60.8
- congenital Q84.6

Lorain (-Levi) short stature syndrome E23.0

Lordosis M40.50
- acquired—*see* Lordosis, specified type NEC
- congenital Q76.429
  - lumbar region Q76.426
  - lumbosacral region Q76.427
  - sacral region Q76.428
  - sacrococcygeal region Q76.428
  - thoracolumbar region Q76.425
- lumbar region M40.56
- lumbosacral region M40.57
- postural—*see* Lordosis, specified type NEC
- specified type NEC M40.40
  - lumbar region M40.46
  - lumbosacral region M40.47
  - thoracolumbar region M40.45
- thoracolumbar region M40.55

Loss (of)
- appetite (*see* Anorexia) R63.0
  - hysterical F50.89
  - nonorganic origin F50.89
  - psychogenic F50.89
- blood—*see* Hemorrhage
- consciousness, transient R55
  - traumatic—*see* Injury, intracranial
- control, sphincter, rectum R15.9
  - nonorganic origin F98.1
- fluid (acute) E86.9
  - with
    - hypernatremia E87.0
    - hyponatremia E87.1
- hearing—*see also* Deafness
  - central NOS H90.5
  - conductive H90.2
    - bilateral H90.0
    - unilateral
      - with
        - ◊ restricted hearing on the contralateral side H90.A1-
        - ◊ unrestricted hearing on the contralateral side H90.1-
  - mixed conductive and sensorineural hearing loss H90.8
    - bilateral H90.6
    - unilateral
      - with
        - ◊ restricted hearing on the contralateral side H90.A3-
        - ◊ unrestricted hearing on the contralateral side H90.7-
  - neural NOS H90.5
  - perceptive NOS H90.5
  - sensorineural NOS H90.5
    - bilateral H90.3
    - unilateral
      - with
        - ◊ restricted hearing on the contralateral side H90.A2-
        - ◊ unrestricted hearing on the contralateral side H90.4-
  - sensory NOS H90.5
- parent in childhood Z63.4
- self-esteem, in childhood Z62.898
- sense of
  - smell—*see* Disturbance, sensation
  - taste—*see* Disturbance, sensation
  - touch R20.8
- sensory R44.9
  - dissociative F44.6
- vision, visual H54.7
- weight (abnormal) (cause unknown) R63.4

Louis-Bar syndrome (ataxia-telangiectasia) G11.3

Louping ill (encephalitis) A84.89

Louse, lousiness—*see* Lice

Low
- achiever, school Z55.3
- back syndrome M54.50
- basal metabolic rate R94.8

Low, *continued*
- birthweight (2499 grams or less) P07.10
  - with weight of
    - 1000–1249 grams P07.14
    - 1250–1499 grams P07.15
    - 1500–1749 grams P07.16
    - 1750–1999 grams P07.17
    - 2000–2499 grams P07.18
  - extreme (999 grams or less) P07.00
    - with weight of
      - 499 grams or less P07.01
      - 500–749 grams P07.02
      - 750–999 grams P07.03
  - for gestational age—*see* Light for dates
- blood pressure—*see also* Hypotension
  - reading (incidental) (isolated) (nonspecific) R03.1
- cardiac reserve—*see* Disease, heart
- hematocrit D64.9
- hemoglobin D64.9
- salt syndrome E87.1
- self-esteem R45.81
- vision H54.2X-
  - one eye (other eye normal) H54.5-
    - left (normal vision on right) H54.52A-
    - other eye blind—*see* Blindness
    - right (normal vision on left) H54.511-

Low-density-lipoprotein-type (LDL) hyperlipoproteinemia E78.00

Lowe's syndrome E72.03

Lown-Ganong-Levine syndrome I45.6

Ludwig's angina or disease K12.2

Luetscher's syndrome E86.0

Lumbago, lumbalgia M54.50
- with sciatica M54.4-

Lumbermen's itch B88.0

Lump—*see also* Mass
- breast N63.0
  - axillary tail N63.3-
  - left N63.2-
  - right N63.1-
  - subareolar N63.4-

Lupoid (miliary) of Boeck D86.3

Lupus
- anticoagulant D68.62
  - with
    - hemorrhagic disorder D68.312
- erythematosus (discoid) (local)
  - disseminated M32.9
  - systemic M32.9
    - with organ or system involvement M32.10
      - endocarditis M32.11
      - lung M32.13
      - pericarditis M32.12
      - renal (glomerular) M32.14
        - ◊ tubulo-interstitial M32.15
      - specified organ or system NEC M32.19
    - drug-induced M32.0
    - inhibitor (presence of) D68.62
      - with
        - ◊ hemorrhagic disorder D68.312
  - nephritis (chronic) M32.14

Lutembacher's disease or syndrome (atrial septal defect with mitral stenosis) Q21.1

Luxation—*see also* Dislocation
- eyeball (nontraumatic)
  - birth injury P15.3
- lens (old) (partial) (spontaneous)
  - congenital Q12.1

Lyell's syndrome L51.2
- due to drug L51.2
  - correct substance properly administered—*see* Table of Drugs and Chemicals, by drug, adverse effect
  - overdose or wrong substance given or taken—*see* Table of Drugs and Chemicals, by drug, poisoning

Lyme disease A69.20

Lymphadenitis I88.9
- acute L04.9
  - axilla L04.2
  - face L04.0

Lymphadenitis, *continued*
- head L04.0
- hip L04.3
- limb
  - lower L04.3
  - upper L04.2
- neck L04.0
- shoulder L04.2
- specified site NEC L04.8
- trunk L04.1
- any site, except mesenteric I88.9
  - chronic I88.1
  - subacute I88.1
- chronic I88.1
  - mesenteric I88.0
- gonorrheal A54.89
- infective—*see* Lymphadenitis, acute
- mesenteric (acute) (chronic) (nonspecific) (subacute) I88.0
  - tuberculous A18.39
- mycobacterial A31.8
- purulent—*see* Lymphadenitis, acute
- pyogenic—*see* Lymphadenitis, acute
- regional, nonbacterial I88.8
- septic—*see* Lymphadenitis, acute
- subacute, unspecified site I88.1
- suppurative—*see* Lymphadenitis, acute
- syphilitic
  - late A52.79

Lymphadenoid goiter E06.3

Lymphadenopathy (generalized) R59.1
- due to toxoplasmosis (acquired) B58.89
  - congenital (acute) (subacute) (chronic) P37.1

Lymphadenosis R59.1

Lymphangitis I89.1
- with
  - abscess—*code by site under* Abscess
  - cellulitis—*code by site under* Cellulitis
- acute L03.91
  - abdominal wall L03.321
  - auricle (ear)—*see* Lymphangitis, acute
  - axilla L03.12-
  - back (any part) L03.322
  - buttock L03.327
  - cervical (meaning neck) L03.222
  - cheek (external) L03.212
  - chest wall L03.323
- digit
  - finger—*see* Cellulitis, finger
  - toe—*see* Cellulitis, toe
- ear (external) H60.1-
- eyelid—*see* Abscess, eyelid
- face NEC L03.212
- finger (intrathecal) (periosteal) (subcutaneous) (subcuticular) L03.02-
- gluteal (region) L03.327
- groin L03.324
- head NEC L03.891
  - face (any part, except ear, eye and nose) L03.212
- jaw (region) L03.212
- lower limb L03.12-
- navel L03.326
- neck (region) L03.222
- orbit, orbital—*see* Cellulitis, orbit
- pectoral (region) L03.323
- perineal, perineum L03.325
- scalp (any part) L03.891
- specified site NEC L03.898
- strumous tuberculous A18.2
- subacute (any site) I89.1
- toe (intrathecal) (periosteal) (subcutaneous) (subcuticular) L03.04-
- trunk L03.329
  - abdominal wall L03.321
  - back (any part) L03.322
  - buttock L03.327
  - chest wall L03.323
  - groin L03.324
  - perineal, perineum L03.325
  - umbilicus L03.326
- umbilicus L03.326
- upper limb L03.12-

ALPHABETIC INDEX

Lymphocytoma, benign cutis L98.8

Lymphocytopenia D72.810

Lymphocytosis (symptomatic) D72.820
- infectious (acute) B33.8

Lymphogranulomatosis (malignant)—*see also* Lymphoma, Hodgkin
- benign (Boeck's sarcoid) (Schaumann's) D86.1

Lymphohistiocytosis, hemophagocytic (familial) D76.1

Lymphoma (of) (malignant) C85.90
- anaplastic large cell
  - ALK-negative C84.7
  - ALK-positive C84.6
  - CD30-positive C84.6
- B-cell C85.1
- cutaneous follicle center C82.6-
- diffuse follicle center C82.5-
- diffuse large cell C83.3-
  - anaplastic C83.3
  - B-cell C83.3
  - CD30-positive C83.3-
  - centroblastic C83.3-
  - extranodal and solid organ sites NEC C83.398
  - primary central nervous system (brain) (meninges) (PCNSL) (spinal cord) C83.390
  - immunoblastic C83.3-
- follicular C82.9-
  - grade
    - I C82.0-
    - II C82.1-
    - III C82.2-
    - IIIa C82.3-
    - IIIb C82.4-
  - specified NEC C82.8-

Lymphoplasmacytic leukemia—*see* Leukemia, chronic lymphocytic, B-cell type
- follicular C82.9-
  - grade
    - I C82.0-
    - II C82.1-
    - III C82.2-
    - IIIa C82.3-
    - IIIb C82.4-
  - specified NEC C82.8-
- histiocytic C85.9-
  - true C96.A
- Hodgkin C81.9-
  - lymphocyte depleted classical C81.3-
  - mixed cellularity classical C81.2-
  - nodular
    - lymphocyte predominant C81.0
  - Lennert's C84.4-
- lymphoepithelioid C84.4-
- lymphoplasmacytic C83.0-
  - with IgM-production C88.0-
- mature T-cell NEC C84.4-
- mature T/NK-cell C84.9-
  - specified NEC C84.Z-
- non-follicular (diffuse) C83.9-
  - specified NEC C83.8-
  - nodular sclerosis (classical) C81.1-
- non-Hodgkin (*see also* Lymphoma, by type) C85.9-
- peripheral T-cell, not classified C84.4-
  - plasmablastic C83.3-
  - subtype not specified C83.3-
  - T-cell rich C83.3-
- primary central nervous system (brain) (meninges) (PCNSL) (spinal cord) C83.390
  - Burkitt C83. 79
  - diffuse large B-cell C83.390
  - lymphoblastic C83.59

Lymphopenia D72.810

Lymphoproliferation, X-linked disease D82.3

Lymphosarcoma (diffuse) (*see also* Lymphoma) C85.9-

M

Macrocolon (*see also* Megacolon) Q43.1

Macrocornea Q15.8
- with glaucoma Q15.0

Macrocytosis D75.89

Macrodactylia, macrodactylism (fingers) (thumbs) Q74.0
- toes Q74.2

Macrogenitosomia (adrenal) (male) (praecox) E25.9
- congenital E25.0

Macroglobulinemia (idiopathic) (primary) C88.0-
- Waldenstrom C88.0-

Macrophthalmos Q11.3
- in congenital glaucoma Q15.0

Macrosigmoid K59.39
- congenital Q43.2
- toxic K59.31

Macrospondylitis, acromegalic E22.0

Maculae ceruleae B85.1

Madelung's
- deformity (radius) Q74.0
- disease
  - radial deformity Q74.0

Main en griffe (acquired)
- congenital Q74.0

Maintenance (encounter for)
- antineoplastic chemotherapy Z51.11
- antineoplastic radiation therapy Z51.0

Malabsorption K90.9
- calcium K90.89
- carbohydrate K90.49
- disaccharide E73.9
- fat K90.49
- intestinal K90.9
  - specified NEC K90.89
- lactose E73.9
- postgastrectomy K91.2
- postsurgical K91.2
- protein K90.49
- starch K90.49
- syndrome K90.9
  - postsurgical K91.2

Maladaptation—*see* Maladjustment

Maladie de Roger Q21.0

Maladjustment
- educational Z55.4
- family Z63.9
- social Z60.9
  - due to
    - acculturation difficulty Z60.3
    - exclusion and isolation Z60.4
    - rejection Z60.4

Malaise R53.81

Malaria, malarial (fever) B54
- clinically diagnosed (without parasitological confirmation) B54
- congenital NEC P37.4
  - falciparum P37.3
- congestion, congestive B54
- hemorrhagic B54
- recurrent B54
- remittent B54
- specified type NEC (parasitologically confirmed) B53.8
- spleen B54
- typhoid B54

Malassimilation K90.9

Mal de mer T75.3

Maldescent, testis Q53.9
- bilateral Q53.20
  - abdominal Q53.211
  - perineal Q53.22
- unilateral Q53.10
  - abdominal Q53.111
  - perineal Q53.12

Maldevelopment—*see also* Anomaly
- brain Q07.9
- hip Q74.2
  - congenital dislocation Q65.2
    - bilateral Q65.1
    - unilateral Q65.0-
- mastoid process Q75.8
- toe Q74.2

Male type pelvis Q74.2

Malformation (congenital)—*see also* Anomaly
- alimentary tract Q45.9
  - specified type NEC Q45.8
  - upper Q40.9
    - specified type NEC Q40.8
- aorta Q25.40
  - absence Q25.41
  - aneurysm, congenital Q25.43
  - aplasia Q25.41
  - atresia Q25.29
    - aortic arch Q25.21
  - coarctation (preductal) (postductal) Q25.1
  - dilatation, congenital Q25.44
  - hypoplasia Q25.42
  - patent ductus arteriosus Q25.0
  - specified type NEC Q25.49
  - stenosis Q25.1
    - supravalvular Q25.3
- arteriovenous, aneurysmatic (congenital) Q27.3-
  - brain Q28.2
    - ruptured I60.8-
      - intracerebral I61.8
      - intraparenchymal I61.8
      - intraventricular I61.5
      - subarachnoid I60.8-
  - cerebral—*see also* Malformation, arteriovenous, brain Q28.2
  - peripheral Q27.3-
- bile duct Q44.5
- bone Q79.9
  - face Q75.9
    - specified type NEC Q75.8
  - skull Q75.9
    - specified type NEC Q75.8
- broad ligament Q50.6
- bursa Q79.9
- corpus callosum (congenital) Q04.0
- digestive system NEC, specified type NEC Q45.8
- dura Q07.9
  - brain Q04.9
  - spinal Q06.9
- ear Q17.9
  - causing impairment of hearing Q16.9
  - external Q17.9
    - accessory auricle Q17.0
    - absence of
      - auditory canal Q16.1
      - auricle Q16.0
    - macrotia Q17.1
    - microtia Q17.2
    - misplacement Q17.4
    - misshapen NEC Q17.3
    - prominence Q17.5
    - specified type NEC Q17.8
  - inner Q16.5
  - middle Q16.4
    - absence of eustachian tube Q16.2
    - ossicles (fusion) Q16.3
  - ossicles Q16.3
    - external Q17.9
- eye Q15.9
  - lid Q10.3
  - specified NEC Q15.8
- fallopian tube Q50.6
- great
  - vein Q26.9
    - anomalous
      - pulmonary venous connection Q26.4
        - partial Q26.3
        - total Q26.2
- heart Q24.9
  - specified type NEC Q24.8
- integument Q84.9
- joint Q74.9
  - ankle Q74.2
  - sacroiliac Q74.2
- kidney Q63.9
  - accessory Q63.0
  - giant Q63.3
  - horseshoe Q63.1
  - hydronephrosis (congenital) Q62.0
  - malposition Q63.2
  - specified type NEC Q63.8

ALPHABETIC INDEX

Malformation, *continued*

- lacrimal apparatus Q10.6
- liver Q44.70
- meninges or membrane (congenital) Q07.9
  - cerebral Q04.8
  - spinal (cord) Q06.9
- multiple types NEC Q89.7
- musculoskeletal system Q79.9
- nervous system (central) Q07.9
- ovary Q50.39
- parathyroid gland Q89.2
- penis Q55.69
  - aplasia Q55.5
  - curvature (lateral) Q55.61
  - hypoplasia Q55.62
- pulmonary
  - arteriovenous Q25.72
  - artery Q25.9
    - atresia Q25.5
    - specified type NEC Q25.79
- respiratory system Q34.9
- scrotum—*see* Malformation, testis and scrotal transposition
- sense organs NEC Q07.9
- specified NEC Q89.8
- tendon Q79.9
- testis and scrotum Q55.20
  - aplasia Q55.0
  - hypoplasia Q55.1
  - polyorchism Q55.21
  - retractile testis Q55.22
  - scrotal transposition Q55.23
  - specified NEC Q55.29
- thyroid gland Q89.2
- tongue (congenital) Q38.3
  - hypertrophy Q38.2
  - tie Q38.1
- urinary system Q64.9

Malibu disease L98.8

Malignancy—*see also* Neoplasm

- unspecified site (primary) C80.1

Malignant—*see* Disease, diseased

Malingerer, malingering Z76.5

Mallet finger (acquired) M20.01-

- congenital Q74.0

Malnutrition E46

- degree
  - first E44.1
  - mild (protein) E44.1
  - moderate (protein) E44.0
  - second E44.0
- following gastrointestinal surgery K91.2
- lack of care, or neglect (child) (infant) T76.02
  - confirmed T74.02
- protein E46
  - calorie E46
    - mild E44.1
    - moderate E44.0
  - energy E46
    - mild E44.1
    - moderate E44.0

Malocclusion (teeth) M26.4

- temporomandibular (joint) M26.69

Malposition

- arterial trunk Q20.0
- cervix—*see* Malposition
- congenital
  - alimentary tract Q45.8
  - liver Q44.79
    - lower Q43.8
    - upper Q40.8
  - aorta Q25.4
  - artery (peripheral) Q27.8
    - pulmonary Q25.79
  - biliary duct or passage Q44.5
  - clavicle Q74.0
  - digestive organ or tract NEC Q45.8
    - lower Q43.8
    - upper Q40.8
  - endocrine (gland) NEC Q89.2
  - fallopian tube Q50.6

Malposition, *continued*

- finger(s) Q68.1
  - supernumerary Q69.0
- gallbladder Q44.1
- gastrointestinal tract Q45.8
- genitalia, genital organ(s) or tract
  - female Q52.8
    - external Q52.79
    - internal NEC Q52.8
  - male Q55.8
- heart Q24.8
  - dextrocardia Q24.0
  - with complete transposition of viscera Q89.3
- hepatic duct Q44.5
- hip (joint) Q65.89
- ovary Q50.39
- parathyroid (gland) Q89.2
- pituitary (gland) Q89.2
- scapula Q74.0
- shoulder Q74.0
- symphysis pubis Q74.2
- thymus (gland) Q89.2
- thyroid (gland) (tissue) Q89.2
  - cartilage Q31.8
- toe(s) Q66.9-
  - supernumerary Q69.2
- gastrointestinal tract, congenital Q45.8

Malposture R29.3

Malrotation

- cecum Q43.3
- colon Q43.3
- intestine Q43.3
- kidney Q63.2

Maltreatment

- adult
  - financial
    - confirmed T74.A1
    - suspected T76.A1
- child
  - abandonment
    - confirmed T74.02
    - suspected T76.02
  - bullying
    - confirmed T74.32
    - suspected T76.32
  - confirmed T74.92
  - history of—*see* History, personal (of), abuse
  - intimidation (through social media)
  - financial
    - confirmed T74.A2
    - suspected T76.A2
    - confirmed T74.32
    - suspected T76.32
  - neglect
    - confirmed T74.02
    - history of—*see* History, personal (of), abuse
    - suspected T76.02
  - physical abuse
    - confirmed T74.12
    - history of—*see* History, personal (of), abuse
    - suspected T76.12
  - psychological abuse
    - confirmed T74.32
    - history of—*see* History, personal (of), abuse
    - suspected T76.32
  - sexual abuse
    - confirmed T74.22
    - history of—*see* History, personal (of), abuse
    - suspected T76.22
  - suspected T76.92
  - personal history of Z91.89

Mammillitis N61.0

Mammitis—*see* Mastitis

Mammogram (examination) Z12.39

- routine Z12.31

Mammoplasia N62

Manic depression F31.9

Mannosidosis E77.1

Maple-syrup-urine disease E71.0

Marchesani (-Weill) syndrome Q87.0

Marie's

- cerebellar ataxia (late-onset) G11.2
- disease or syndrome (acromegaly) E22.0

Marion's disease (bladder neck obstruction) N32.0

Mark

- port wine Q82.5
- raspberry Q82.5
- strawberry Q82.5
- tattoo L81.8

Maroteaux-Lamy syndrome (mild) (severe) E76.29

Marrow (bone)

- arrest D61.9

Masculinization (female) with adrenal hyperplasia E25.9

- congenital E25.0

Mass

- abdominal R19.00
  - epigastric R19.06
  - generalized R19.07
  - left lower quadrant R19.04
  - left upper quadrant R19.02
  - periumbillic R19.05
  - right lower quadrant R19.03
  - right upper quadrant R19.01
  - specified site NEC R19.09
- breast (*see also* Lump, breast) N63.0
- chest R22.2
- cystic—*see* Cyst
- ear H93.8-
- head R22.0
- intra-abdominal (diffuse) (generalized)—*see* Mass, abdominal
- kidney N28.89
- liver R16.0
- localized (skin) R22.9
  - chest R22.2
  - head R22.0
  - limb
    - lower R22.4-
    - upper R22.3-
  - neck R22.1
  - trunk R22.2
- lung R91.8
- malignant—*see* Neoplasm, malignant, by site in Table of Neoplasms in the complete *ICD-10-CM* manual
- neck R22.1
- pelvic (diffuse) (generalized)—*see* Mass, abdominal
- specified organ NEC—*see* Disease, by site
- splenic R16.1
- substernal thyroid—*see* Goiter
- superficial (localized) R22.9
- umbilical (diffuse) (generalized) R19.09

Mast cell

- disease, systemic tissue D47.02
- leukemia C94.3-
- neoplasm
  - malignant C96.20
    - specified type NEC C96.29
  - of uncertain behavior NEC D47.09
- sarcoma C96.22
- tumor D47.09

Mastalgia N64.4

Mastitis (acute) (diffuse) (nonpuerperal) (subacute) N61.0

- infective N61.0
  - newborn P39.0
- neonatal (noninfective) P83.4
  - infective P39.0

Mastocytosis D47.09

- aggressive systemic C96.21
- cutaneous (diffuse) (maculopapular) D47.01
  - congenital Q82.2
  - of neonatal onset Q82.2
  - of newborn onset Q82.2
- indolent systemic D47.02
- isolated bone marrow D47.02
- malignant C96.29
- systemic (indolent) (smoldering)
  - with an associated hematological non-mast cell lineage disease (SM-AHNMD) D47.02

Mastodynia N64.4

ALPHABETIC INDEX

Mastodalgia—*see* subcategory H92.0

Mastoplasia, mastoplastia N62

Masturbation (excessive) F98.8

Maternal care (suspected) O35.0-
- central nervous system malformation or damage in fetus O35.00X
  - agenesis of the corpus callosum O35.01X-
  - anencephaly O35.02X-
  - choroid plexus cysts O35.03X-
  - encephalocele, not applicable or unspecified O35.04X-
  - holoprosencephaly, not applicable or unspecified O35.05X-
  - hydrocephaly O35.06X-
  - microcephaly O35.07X-
  - other O35.09X-
  - spina bifida O35.08X-
- chromosomal abnormality in fetus
  - fetal cardiac anomalies O35.BXX-
  - fetal facial abnormalities O35.AXX-
  - fetal gastrointestinal anomalies O35.DXX-
  - fetal genitourinary anomalies O35.EXX-
  - fetal lower extremities anomalies O35.HXX-
  - fetal musculoskeletal anomalies of trunk O35.FXX
  - fetal pulmonary anomalies O35.CXX-
  - fetal upper extremities anomalies O35.GXX
  - other chromosomal abnormality O35.19X-
  - sex chromosome abnormality O35.15X-
  - trisomy 13 O35.11X-
  - trisomy 18 O35.12X-
  - trisomy 21 O35.13X-
  - Turner's syndrome O35.14X-
  - unspecified O35.10X-

May (-Hegglin) anomaly or syndrome D72.0

McQuarrie's syndrome (idiopathic familial hypoglycemia) E16.2

Measles (black) (hemorrhagic) (suppressed) B05.9
- with
  - complications NEC B05.89
  - encephalitis B05.0
  - intestinal complications B05.4
  - keratitis (keratoconjunctivitis) B05.81
  - meningitis B05.1
  - otitis media B05.3
  - pneumonia B05.2
- French—*see* Rubella
- German—*see* Rubella
- Liberty—*see* Rubella

Meckel-Gruber syndrome Q61.9

Meckel's diverticulitis, diverticulum (displaced) (hypertrophic) Q43.0

Meconium
- ileus, newborn P76.0
  - in cystic fibrosis E84.11
  - meaning meconium plug (without cystic fibrosis) P76.0
- obstruction, newborn P76.0
  - due to fecaliths P76.0
  - in mucoviscidosis E84.11
- plug syndrome (newborn) NEC P76.0

MED13L (mediator complex subunit 13L) syndrome Q87.85

Mediastinopericarditis—*see also* Pericarditis
- acute I30.9
- adhesive I31.0
- chronic I31.8
  - rheumatic I09.2

Mediator complex subunit 13L (MED13L) syndrome Q87.85

Medulloblastoma
- desmoplastic C71.6
- specified site—*see* Neoplasm, malignant, by site in Table of Neoplasms in the complete *ICD-10-CM* manual
- unspecified site C71.6

Medullomyoblastoma
- specified site—*see* Neoplasm, malignant, by site in Table of Neoplasms in the complete *ICD-10-CM* manual
- unspecified site C71.6

Meekeren-Ehlers-Danlos syndrome Q79.69
- classical Ehlers-Danlos syndrome Q79.61
- hypermobile Ehlers-Danlos syndrome Q79.62
- other Ehlers-Danlos syndromes Q79.69
- vascular Ehlers-Danlos syndrome Q79.63

Megacolon (acquired) (functional) (not Hirschsprung's disease) (in) K59.39
- congenital, congenitum (aganglionic) Q43.1
  - Hirschsprung's (disease) Q43.1
  - toxic K59.31

Megalerythema (epidemic) B08.3

Megalocornea Q15.8
- with glaucoma Q15.0

Megalodactylia (fingers) (thumbs) (congenital) Q74.0
- toes Q74.2

Megarectum K62.89

Megasigmoid K59.39
- congenital Q43.2
- toxic K59.31

Melancholia F32.A
- hypochondriac F45.29
- intermittent (single episode) F32.89
  - recurrent episode F33.9

Melanocytosis, neurocutaneous Q82.8

Melanoderma, melanodermia L81.4

Melanodontia, infantile K03.89

Melanodontoclasia K03.89

Melanoma (malignant) C43.9
- benign—*see* Nevus
- skin C43.-

Melanosis L81.4
- Riehl's L81.4
- tar L81.4
- toxic L81.4

MELAS syndrome E88.41

Melena K92.1
- with ulcer—*code by site under* Ulcer, with hemorrhage K27.4
- due to swallowed maternal blood P78.2
- newborn, neonatal P54.1
  - due to swallowed maternal blood P78.2

Membrane(s), membranous—*see also* Disease, diseased
- over face of newborn P28.9

Menarche
- delayed E30.0
- precocious E30.1

Meningism—*see* Meningismus

Meningismus (infectional) (pneumococcal) R29.1
- due to serum or vaccine R29.1
- influenzal—*see* Influenza

Meningitis (basal) (basic) (brain) (cerebral) (cervical) (congestive) (diffuse) (hemorrhagic) (infantile) (membranous) (metastatic) (nonspecific) (pontine) (progressive) (simple) (spinal) (subacute) (sympathetic) (toxic) G03.9
- abacterial G03.0
- arbovirus A87.8
- aseptic G03.0
- bacterial G00.9
  - Escherichia Coli (E. coli) G00.8
  - gram-negative G00.9
  - H. influenzae G00.0
  - pneumococcal G00.1
  - specified organism NEC G00.8
  - streptococcal (acute) G00.2
- candidal B37.5
- caseous (tuberculous) A17.0
- cerebrospinal A39.0
- clear cerebrospinal fluid NEC G03.0
- coxsackievirus A87.0
- diplococcal (gram positive) A39.0
- echovirus A87.0
- enteroviral A87.0
- epidemic NEC A39.0
- Escherichia Coli (E. coli) G00.8
- fibrinopurulent G00.9
  - specified organism NEC G00.8
- gram-negative cocci G00.9

Meningitis, *continued*
- gram-positive cocci G00.9
- Haemophilus (influenzae) G00.0
- H. influenzae G00.0
- in (due to)
  - bacterial disease NEC A48.8 [G01]
  - chickenpox B01.0
  - Diplococcus pneumoniae G00.1
  - enterovirus A87.0
  - herpes (simplex) virus B00.3
  - infectious mononucleosis B27.92
  - Lyme disease A69.21
  - measles B05.1
  - parasitic disease NEC B89 [G02]
  - Streptococcal pneumoniae G00.1
  - varicella B01.0
  - viral disease NEC A87.8
  - whooping cough A37.90
- infectious G00.9
- influenzal (H. influenzae) G00.0
- meningococcal A39.0
- monilial B37.5
- mycotic NEC B49 [G02]
- Neisseria A39.0
- nonbacterial G03.0
- nonpyogenic G03.0
- ossificans G96.198
- pneumococcal streptococcus pneumoniae G00.1
- postmeasles B05.1
- purulent G00.9
  - specified organism NEC G00.8
- pyogenic G00.9
  - specified organism NEC G00.8
- septic G00.9
  - specified organism NEC G00.8
- serosa circumscripta NEC G03.0
- serous NEC G93.2
- specified organism NEC G00.8
- sterile G03.0
- streptococcal (acute) G00.2
- suppurative G00.9
  - specified organism NEC G00.8
- tuberculous A17.0
- viral NEC A87.9

Meningocele (spinal)— *see also* Spina bifida
- acquired (traumatic) G96.198

Meningococcemia A39.4
- acute A39.2
- chronic A39.3

Meningococcus, meningococcal (*see also* Disease, diseased) A39.9
- carrier (suspected) of Z22.31
- meningitis (cerebrospinal) A39.0

Meningoencephalitis (*see also* Encephalitis) G04.90
- acute NEC (*see also* Encephalitis, viral) A86
  - disseminated G04.00
    - postimmunization or postvaccination G04.02
  - California A83.5
- herpesviral, herpetic B00.4
  - due to herpesvirus 7 B10.09
  - specified NEC B10.09
- in (due to)
  - diseases classified elsewhere G05.3
  - Haemophilus influenzae (H. Influenzae) G00.0
  - herpes B00.4
    - due to herpesvirus 7 B10.09
    - specified NEC B10.09
  - H. influenzae G00.0
  - Lyme disease A69.22
  - toxoplasmosis (acquired) B58.2
    - congenital P37.1
- infectious (acute) (viral) A86
- parasitic NEC B89 [G05.3]
- pneumococcal G04.2
- toxic NEC G92.8
- virus NEC A86

Meningoencephalomyelitis—*see also* Encephalitis
- acute NEC (viral) A86
  - disseminated G04.00
    - postimmunization or postvaccination G04.02
    - postinfectious G04.01

MASTODALGIA-MENINGOENCEPHALOMYELITIS

ALPHABETIC INDEX

Meningoencephalomyelitis, *continued*
- due to
  - Toxoplasma or toxoplasmosis (acquired) B58.2
    - congenital P37.1
  - postimmunization or postvaccination G04.02

Meningomyelitis—*see also* Meningoencephalitis
- in diseases classified elsewhere G05.4

Menkes' disease or syndrome E83.09
- meaning maple-syrup-urine disease E71.0

Menometrorrhagia N92.1

Menorrhagia (primary) N92.0
- pubertal (menses retained) N92.2

Menostaxis N92.0

Menses, retention N94.89

Menstrual—*see* Menstruation

Menstruation
- absent—*see* Amenorrhea
- anovulatory N97.0
- cycle, irregular N92.6
- during pregnancy O20.8
- excessive (with regular cycle) N92.0
  - with irregular cycle N92.1
  - at puberty N92.2
- frequent N92.0
- irregular N92.6
  - specified NEC N92.5
- latent N92.5
- membranous N92.5
- painful (*see also* Dysmenorrhea) N94.6 primary N94.4
  - psychogenic F45.8
  - secondary N94.5
- passage of clots N92.0
- precocious E30.1
- protracted N92.5
- retained N94.89
- retrograde N92.5
- suppression N94.89
- vicarious (nasal) N94.89

Mental—*see also* Disease, diseased
- observation without need for further medical care Z03.89

MERRF syndrome (myoclonic epilepsy associated with ragged-red fiber) E88.42

Metabolic syndrome E88.810

Metal
- pigmentation L81.8

Metaplasia
- gastric intestinal K31.A-

Metatarsus, metatarsal—*see also* Disease, diseased
- valgus (abductus), congenital Q66.6
- varus (adductus) (congenital) Q66.22-
  - primus Q66.21-

Methemoglobinemia D74.9
- congenital D74.0
- enzymatic (congenital) D74.0
- Hb M disease D74.0
- hereditary D74.0
- toxic D74.8

Metropathia hemorrhagica N93.8

Metrorrhagia N92.1
- psychogenic F45.8

Metrostaxis N93.8

Meyer-Schwickerath and Weyers syndrome Q87.0

Mibelli's disease (porokeratosis) Q82.8

Micrencephalon, micrencephaly Q02

Microalbuminuria R80.9

Microangiopathy (peripheral)
- thrombotic M31.10

Microcephalus, microcephalic, microcephaly Q02
- due to toxoplasmosis (congenital) P37.1

Microdeletions NEC Q93.88

Microdrepanocytosis D57.40
- with
  - acute chest syndrome D57.411
  - cerebral vascular involvement D57.413

Microdrepanocytosis, *continued*
- crisis (painful) D57.419
  - with specified complication NEC D57.418
- splenic sequestration D57.412
- vasoocclusive pain D57.419

Microencephalon Q02

Microgenitalia, congenital
- female Q52.8
- male Q55.8

Microlentia (congenital) Q12.8

Microophthalmos, microphthalmia (congenital) Q11.2
- due to toxoplasmosis P37.1

Micropenis Q55.62

Microphakia (congenital) Q12.8

Microsporon furfur infestation B36.0

Micturition
- disorder NEC R39.198
  - psychogenic F45.8
- frequency R35.0
  - psychogenic F45.8
- hesitancy R39.11
- need to immediately re-void R39.191
- painful
  - dysuria R30.0
  - psychogenic F45.8
  - poor stream R39.12
- position dependent R39.192
- urgency R39.15

Migraine (idiopathic) G43.909
- with aura (acute-onset) (prolonged) (typical) (without headache) G43.109
  - with refractory migraine G43.119
    - with status migrainosus G43.111
    - without status migrainosus G43.119
  - not intractable G43.109
  - chronic G43.E09
    - with refractory migraine G43.E19
      - ~ with status migrainosus G43.E11
      - ~ without status migrainosus G43.E19
    - intractable
      - ~ with status migrainosus G43.E11
      - ~ without status migrainosus G43.E19
    - not intractable
      - ~ with status migrainosus G43.E01
      - ~ without status migrainosus G43.E09
    - without refractory migraine G43.E09
      - ~ with status migrainosus G43.E01
      - ~ without status migrainosus G43.E09
    - with status migrainosus G43.101
    - without status migrainosus G43.109
  - without mention of refractory migraine G43.109
    - with status migrainosus G43.101
    - without status migrainosus G43.109
- with refractory migraine G43.919
  - with status migrainosus G43.911
  - without status migrainosus G43.919
- basilar—*see* Migraine, with aura
- classical—*see* Migraine, with aura
- common—*see* Migraine, without aura
- complicated G43.109
- equivalents—*see* Migraine, with aura
- intractable G43.919
  - with status migrainosus G43.911
  - without status migrainosus G43.919
- menstrual G43.829
  - with refractory migraine G43.839
    - with status migrainosus G43.831
    - without status migrainosus G43.839
  - intractable G43.839
    - with status migrainosus G43.831
    - without status migrainosus G43.839
  - not intractable G43.829
    - with status migrainosus G43.821
    - without status migrainosus G43.829
  - without refractory migraine G43.829
    - with status migrainosus G43.821
    - without status migrainosus G43.829
- menstrually related—*see* Migraine, menstrual
- not intractable G43.909
  - with status migrainosus G43.901
  - without status migrainosus G43.919

Migraine, *continued*
- post-traumatic G44.309
  - acute G44.319
    - intractable G44.311
    - not intractable G44.319
  - chronic G44.329
    - intractable G44.321
    - not intractable G44.329
  - intractable G44.301
  - not intractable G44.309
- specified NEC G43.809
  - intractable G43.819
    - with status migrainosus G43.811
    - without status migrainosus G43.819
  - not intractable G43.809
    - with status migrainosus G43.801
    - without status migrainosus G43.809
- triggered seizures—*see* Migraine, with aura
- without aura G43.009
  - with refractory migraine G43.019
    - with status migrainosus G43.011
    - without status migrainosus G43.019
  - not intractable
    - with status migrainosus G43.001
    - without status migrainosus G43.009
  - without mention of refractory migraine G43.009
    - with status migrainosus G43.001
    - without status migrainosus G43.009
- without refractory migraine G43.909
  - with status migrainosus G43.901
  - without status migrainosus G43.919

Migrant, social Z59.00

Migration, anxiety concerning Z60.3

Migratory, migrating—*see also* Disease, diseased
- person Z59.00
- testis Q55.29

Miliaria L74.3
- alba L74.1
- crystallina L74.1
- rubra L74.0

Milk
- crust L21.0
- poisoning—*see* Poisoning, food, noxious
- sickness—*see* Poisoning, food, noxious
- spots I31.0

Milk-alkali disease or syndrome E83.52

Minot's disease (hemorrhagic disease), newborn P53

Mirror writing F81.0

Misadventure (of) (prophylactic) (therapeutic)—*see also* Complications T88.9
- administration of insulin (by accident)—*see* subcategory T38.3

Miscarriage O03.9

Misperception, sleep state F51.02

Missed
- delivery O36.4

Missing—*see* Absence

Mite(s) (infestation) B88.9
- diarrhea B88.0
- grain (itch) B88.0
- hair follicle (itch) B88.0
- in sputum B88.0

Mittelschmerz N94.0

Mixed—*see* Disease, diseased

MNGIE (Mitochondrial Neurogastrointestinal Encephalopathy) syndrome E88.49

Mobile, mobility
- gallbladder, congenital Q44.1

Mobitz heart block (atrioventricular) I44.1

Moebius, Möbius
- syndrome Q87.0
  - congenital oculofacial paralysis (with other anomalies) Q87.0

Moeller's glossitis K14.0

Mohr's syndrome (Types I and II) Q87.0

Molding, head (during birth)—omit code

ALPHABETIC INDEX

Mole (pigmented)—*see also* Nevus
- tubal O00.10
  - with intrauterine pregnancy O00.11

Molimen, molimina (menstrual) N94.3

Molluscum contagiosum (epitheliale) B08.1

Moniliasis (*see also* Candidiasis) B37.9
- neonatal P37.5

Monitoring (encounter for)
- therapeutic drug level Z51.81

Monocytopenia D72.818

Monocytosis (symptomatic) D72.821

Mononeuropathy G58.9

Mononucleosis, infectious B27.90
- with
  - complication NEC B27.99
  - meningitis B27.92
  - polyneuropathy B27.91
- cytomegaloviral B27.10
  - with
    - complication NEC B27.19
    - meningitis B27.12
    - polyneuropathy B27.11
- Epstein-Barr (virus) B27.00
  - with
    - complication NEC B27.09
    - meningitis B27.02
    - polyneuropathy B27.01
- gammaherpesviral B27.00
  - with
    - complication NEC B27.09
    - meningitis B27.02
    - polyneuropathy B27.01
- specified NEC B27.80
  - with
    - complication NEC B27.89
    - meningitis B27.82
    - polyneuropathy B27.81

Monoplegia G83.3-
- hysterical (transient) F44.4
- psychogenic (conversion reaction) F44.4

Monorchism, monorchidism Q55.0

Monosomy (*see also* Deletion, chromosome) Q93.9
- specified NEC Q93.89
- X Q96.9

Monster, monstrosity (single) Q89.7

Monteggia's fracture (-dislocation) S52.27-

Morbidity not stated or unknown R69

Morbilli—*see* Measles

Morbus—*see also* Disease
- angelicus, anglorum E55.0
- celiacus K90.0
- hemorrhagicus neonatorum P53
- maculosus neonatorum P54.5

Morgagni's
- cyst, organ, hydatid, or appendage
  - female Q50.5
  - male (epididymal) Q55.4
  - testicular Q55.29

Morgagni-Stokes-Adams syndrome I45.9

Morgagni-Turner (-Albright) **syndrome** Q96.9

Moron (I.Q.50-69) F70

Morvan's disease or syndrome G60.8

Mosaicism, mosaic (autosomal) (chromosomal)
- 45,X/other cell lines NEC with abnormal sex chromosome Q96.4
- 45,X/46,XX Q96.3
- sex chromosome
  - female Q97.8
  - lines with various numbers of X chromosomes Q97.2
  - male Q98.7
- XY Q96.3

Motion sickness (from travel, any vehicle) (from roundabouts or swings) T75.3

Mountain
- sickness T70.29
  - with polycythemia, acquired (acute) D75.1
- tick fever A93.2

MRSA (Methicillin resistant Staphylococcus aureus)
- infection A49.02
  - as the cause of disease classified elsewhere B95.62
- sepsis A41.02

MSD (multiple sulfatase deficiency) E75.26

MSSA (Methicillin susceptible Staphylococcus aureus)
- infection A49.02
  - as the cause of disease classified elsewhere B95.61
- sepsis A41.01

Mucinosis (cutaneous) (focal) (papular) (reticular erythematous) (skin) L98.5
- oral K13.79

Mucocele
- buccal cavity K13.79
- nasal sinus J34.1
- nose J34.1
- sinus (accessory) (nasal) J34.1
- turbinate (bone) (middle) (nasal) J34.1

Mucolipidosis
- I E77.1
- II, III E77.0

Mucopolysaccharidosis E76.3
- beta-glucuronidase deficiency E76.29
- cardiopathy E76.3 [I52]
- Hunter's syndrome E76.1
- Hurler's syndrome E76.01
- Maroteaux-Lamy syndrome E76.29
- Morquio syndrome E76.219
  - A E76.210
  - B E76.211
  - classic E76.210
- Sanfilippo syndrome E76.22
- specified NEC E76.29
- type
  - I
    - Hurler's syndrome E76.01
    - Hurler-Scheie syndrome E76.02
    - Scheie's syndrome E76.03
  - II E76.1
  - III E76.22
  - IV E76.219
  - IVA E76.210
  - IVB E76.211
  - VI E76.29
  - VII E76.29

Mucositis (ulcerative) K12.30
- nasal J34.81

Mucoviscidosis E84.9
- with meconium obstruction E84.11

Mucus
- asphyxiation or suffocation—*see* Asphyxia
- in stool R19.5
- plug—*see* Asphyxia

Muguet B37.0

Multicystic kidney (development) Q61.4

Multisystem inflammatory syndrome (in adult) (in children) M35.81

Mumps B26.9

Murmur (cardiac) (heart) (organic) R01.1
- aortic (valve)—*see* Endocarditis, aortic
- benign R01.0
- diastolic—*see* Endocarditis
- Flint I35.1
- functional R01.0
- Graham Steell I37.1
- innocent R01.0
- mitral (valve)—*see* Insufficiency, mitral
- nonorganic R01.0
- presystolic, mitral—*see* Insufficiency, mitral
- pulmonic (valve) I37.8
- systolic R01.1
- tricuspid (valve) I07.9
- valvular—*see* Endocarditis

Muscle, muscular—*see also* Disease, diseased
- carnitine (palmityltransferase) deficiency E71.314

Muscle wasting and atrophy, not elsewhere classified, back
- cervical M62.5A0
- thoracic M62.5A1
- lumbosacral M62.5A2

Muscular dystrophy, limb girdle
- autosomal dominant limb girdle G71.031
- autosomal recessive, due to calpain-3 dysfunction G71.032
- due to
  - alpha sarcoglycan dysfunction G71.0341
  - anoctamin-5 dysfunction G71.035
  - beta sarcoglycan dysfunction G71.0342
  - dysferlin dysfunction G71.033
  - other G71.038
  - other sarcoglycan dysfunction G71.0349
  - sarcoglycan dysfunction, unspecified G71.0340
  - unspecified G71.039

Mutation(s)
- surfactant, of lung J84.83

Mutism—*see also* Aphasia
- deaf (acquired) (congenital) NEC H91.3
- elective (adjustment reaction) (childhood) F94.0
- hysterical F44.4
- selective (childhood) F94.0

Myalgia M79.1-
- traumatic NEC T14.8

Myasthenia G70.9
- congenital G70.2
- cordis—*see* Failure, heart
- developmental G70.2
- gravis G70.00
  - with exacerbation (acute) G70.01
  - in crisis G70.01
  - neonatal, transient P94.0
  - pseudoparalytica G70.00
    - with exacerbation (acute) G70.01
    - in crisis G70.01
- stomach, psychogenic F45.8
- syndrome
  - in
    - diabetes mellitus—*see* E08-E13 with .44
    - neoplastic disease (*see also* Table of Neoplasms in the complete *ICD-10-CM manual*) D49.9 [G73.3]
    - thyrotoxicosis E05.90 [G73.3]
      - with thyroid storm E05.91 [G73.3]

Myasthenic M62.81

Mycoplasma (M.) pneumoniae, as cause of disease classified elsewhere B96.0

Mycosis, mycotic B49
- fungoides (extranodal) (solid organ) C84.0-
- mouth B37.0
- nails B35.1
- stomatitis B37.0
- vagina, vaginitis (candidal) B37.3

Myelitis (acute) (ascending) (childhood) (chronic) (descending) (diffuse) (disseminated) (idiopathic) (pressure) (progressive) (spinal cord) (subacute) (*see also* Encephalitis) G04.91
- flaccid G04.82
- in diseases classified elsewhere G05.4
- post-chicken pox B01.12
- postimmunization G04.02
- postinfectious G04.89
- postvaccinal G04.02
- specified NEC G04.89
- toxic G92.9
- varicella B01.12

Myelogenous—*see* Disease, diseased

Myeloid—*see* Disease, diseased

Myelokathexis D70.9

Myelopathy (spinal cord) G95.9
- in (due to)
  - infection—*see* Encephalitis
  - mercury—*see* subcategory T56.1
  - neoplastic disease (*see also* Table of Neoplasms in the complete *ICD-10-CM manual*) D49.9 [G99.2]

Myelophthisis D61.82

ALPHABETIC INDEX

Myelosclerosis D75.89
- disseminated, of nervous system G35

Myelosis
- acute C92.0-
- aleukemic C92.9-
- nonleukemic D72.828
- subacute C92.9-

Myocardiopathy (congestive) (constrictive) (familial) (hypertrophic nonobstructive) (idiopathic) (infiltrative) (obstructive) (primary) (restrictive) (sporadic) (*see also* Cardiomyopathy) I42.9
- hypertrophic obstructive I42.1
- in (due to)
  - Friedreich's ataxia G11.11 [I43]
  - progressive muscular dystrophy G71.09 [I43]
- secondary I42.9
- thyrotoxic E05.90 [I43]
  - with storm E05.91 [I43]

Myocarditis (with arteriosclerosis) (chronic) (fibroid) (interstitial) (old) (progressive) (senile) I51.4
- with
  - rheumatic fever (conditions in I00) I09.0
    - active—*see* Myocarditis, acute, rheumatic
    - inactive or quiescent (with chorea) I09.0
- active I40.9
  - rheumatic I01.2
    - with chorea (acute) (rheumatic) (Sydenham's) I02.0
- acute or subacute (interstitial) I40.9
  - due to
    - streptococcus (beta-hemolytic) I01.2
  - idiopathic I40.1
  - rheumatic I01.2
    - with chorea (acute) (rheumatic) (Sydenham's) I02.0
  - specified NEC I40.8
- bacterial (acute) I40.0
- eosinophilic I40.1
- epidemic of newborn (Coxsackie) B33.22
- Fiedler's (acute) (isolated) I40.1
- giant cell (acute) (subacute) I40.1
- granulomatous (idiopathic) (isolated) (nonspecific) I40.1
- idiopathic (granulomatous) I40.1
- in (due to)
  - Lyme disease A69.29
  - sarcoidosis D86.85
- infective I40.0
- influenzal—*see* Influenza, myocarditis
- isolated (acute) I40.1
- nonrheumatic, active I40.9
- parenchymatous I40.9
- pneumococcal I40.0
- rheumatic (chronic) (inactive) (with chorea) I09.0
  - active or acute I01.2
    - with chorea (acute) (rheumatic) (Sydenham's) I02.0
- septic I40.0
- staphylococcal I40.0
- suppurative I40.0
- toxic I40.8
- virus, viral I40.0
  - of newborn (Coxsackie) B33.22

Myoclonus, myoclonic, myoclonia (familial) (essential) (multifocal) (simplex) G25.3
- drug-induced G25.3
- epilepsy (*see also* Epilepsy, generalized, specified NEC) G40.4-
  - familial (progressive) G25.3
- familial progressive G25.3
- Friedreich's G25.3
- jerks G25.3
- massive G25.3
- palatal G25.3
- pharyngeal G25.3

Myofibromatosis
- infantile Q89.8

Myopathy G72.9
- autosomal (dominant) (recessive) G71.228
  - other specified NEC G71.228
- benign congenital G71.20
- central core G71.29

Myopathy, *continued*
- centronuclear G71.228
- congenital (benign) G71.20
- distal G71.09
- facioscapulohumeral G71.02hyaline body G71.29
- in (due to)
  - Cushing's syndrome E24.9 [G73.7]
  - hyperadrenocorticism E24.9 [G73.7]
  - *hypopituitarism E23.0 [G73.7]*
  - hypothyroidism E03.9 [G73.7]
  - myxedema E03.9 [G73.7]
  - sarcoidosis D86.87
  - scarlet fever A38.1
  - systemic lupus erythematosus M32.19
  - thyrotoxicosis (hyperthyroidism) E05.90 *[G73.7]*
    - with thyroid storm E05.91 *[G73.7]*
- limb-girdle G71.09
- myosin storage G71.29
  - myotubular (centronuclear) G71.220
    - X-linked G71.220
- nemaline G71.21
- ocular G71.09
- oculopharyngeal G71.09
- rod (body) G71.21
- scapulohumeral G71.02

Myopia (axial) (congenital) H52.1-

Myositis M60.9
- in (due to)
  - sarcoidosis D86.87
- infective M60.009
  - arm
    - left M60.001
    - right M60.000
  - leg
    - left M60.004
    - right M60.003
  - lower limb
    - ankle M60.07-
    - foot M60.07-
    - lower leg M60.06-
    - thigh M60.05-
    - toe M60.07-
  - multiple sites M60.09
  - specified site NEC M60.08
  - upper limb
    - finger M60.04-
    - forearm M60.03-
    - hand M60.04-
    - shoulder region M60.01-
    - upper arm M60.02-

Myospasia impulsiva F95.2

Myotonia (acquisita) (intermittens) M62.89
- congenita (acetazolamide responsive) (dominant) (recessive) G71.12
- levior G71.12

Myriapodiasis B88.2

Myringitis H73.2-
- with otitis media—*see* Otitis, media
- acute H73.00-
  - bullous H73.01-
- bullous—*see* Myringitis, acute, bullous
- chronic H73.1-

Myxadenitis labialis K13.0

Myxedema (adult) (idiocy) (infantile) (juvenile) (*see also* Hypothyroidism) E03.9
- circumscribed E05.90
  - with storm E05.91
- congenital E00.1
- cutis L98.5
- localized (pretibial) E05.90
  - with storm E05.91

Myxolipoma D17.9

N

Naegeli's
- disease Q82.8

Nail—*see also* Disease, diseased
- biting F98.8

Nanism, nanosomia—*see* Dwarfism

Napkin rash L22

Narcosis R06.89

Narcotism—*see* Dependence

NARP (Neuropathy, Ataxia and Retinitis pigmentosa) syndrome E88.49

Narrowness, abnormal, eyelid Q10.3

Nasopharyngeal—*see also* Disease, diseased
- pituitary gland Q89.2
- torticollis M43.6

Nasopharyngitis (acute) (infective) (streptococcal) (subacute) J00
- chronic (suppurative) (ulcerative) J31.1

Nasopharynx, nasopharyngeal—*see* Disease, diseased

Natal tooth, teeth K00.6

Nausea (without vomiting) R11.0
- with vomiting R11.2
- marina T75.3
- navalis T75.3

Near drowning T75.1

Nearsightedness—*see* Myopia

Near-syncope R55

Necrolysis, toxic epidermal L51.2
- due to drug
  - correct substance properly administered—*see* Table of Drugs and Chemicals, by drug, adverse effect
  - overdose or wrong substance given or taken—*see* Table of Drugs and Chemicals, by drug, poisoning

Necrosis, necrotic (ischemic)—*see also* Gangrene
- adrenal (capsule) (gland) E27.49
- antrum J32.0
- cortical (acute) (renal) N17.1
- ethmoid (bone) J32.2
- fat, fatty (generalized)—*see also* Disorder, specified type NEC
  - skin (subcutaneous), newborn P83.0
  - subcutaneous due to birth injury P15.6
- kidney (bilateral) N28.0
  - acute N17.9
  - cortical (acute) (bilateral) N17.1
  - medullary (bilateral) (in acute renal failure) (papillary) N17.2
  - papillary (bilateral) (in acute renal failure) N17.2
  - tubular N17.0
    - medullary (acute) (renal) N17.2
- papillary (acute) (renal) N17.2
- pharynx J02.9
  - in granulocytopenia—*see* Neutropenia
- phosphorus—*see* subcategory T54.2
- pituitary (gland) E23.0
- subcutaneous fat, newborn P83.88
- suprarenal (capsule) (gland) E27.49
- tonsil J35.8
- tubular (acute) (anoxic) (renal) (toxic) N17.0
  - postprocedural N99.0

Need (for)
- care provider because (of)
  - assistance with personal care Z74.1
  - continuous supervision required Z74.3
  - impaired mobility Z74.09
  - no other household member able to render care Z74.2
  - specified reason NEC Z74.8
- immunization—*see* Vaccination
- vaccination—*see* Vaccination

Neglect
- child (childhood)
  - confirmed T74.02
  - history of Z62.812
  - suspected T76.02
- emotional, in childhood Z62.898

Nelaton's syndrome G60.8

Neonatal—*see also* Newborn
- acne L70.4
- bradycardia P29.12
- screening, abnormal findings on P09.-
- tachycardia P29.11
- tooth, teeth K00.6

ALPHABETIC INDEX

Neonatorum—*see* Disease, diseased

Neoplasia
- intraepithelial (histologically confirmed)
  - anal (AIN) (histologically confirmed) K62.82
    - grade I K62.82
    - grade II K62.82

Neoplasm, neoplastic—*see also* Table of Neoplasms in the complete *ICD-10-CM* manual.
- lipomatous, benign—*see* Lipoma

Nephralgia N23

Nephritis, nephritic (albuminuric) (azotemic) (congenital) (disseminated) (epithelial) (familial) (focal) (granulomatous) (hemorrhagic) (infantile) (nonsuppurative, excretory) (uremic) N05.9
- with
  - C3
    - glomerulonephritis N05.A
    - glomerulopathy N05.A
    - with dense deposit disease N05.6
  - acute N00.9
    - with
      - C3
        - glomerulonephritis N00.A
        - glomerulopathy N00.A
        - ◊ with dense deposit disease N00.6
        - ◊ dense deposit disease N00.6
      - diffuse
        - crescentic glomerulonephritis N00.7
        - endocapillary proliferative glomerulonephritis N00.4
        - membranous glomerulonephritis N00.2
        - mesangial proliferative glomerulonephritis N00.3
        - mesangiocapillary glomerulonephritis N00.5
      - focal and segmental glomerular lesions N00.1
      - minor glomerular abnormality N00.0
      - specified morphological changes NEC N00.8
  - chronic N03.9
    - with
      - C3
        - glomerulonephritis N03.A
        - glomerulopathy N03.A
        - ◊ with dense deposit disease N03.6
  - croupous N00.9
  - due to
    - diabetes mellitus—*see* E08-E13 with .21
    - subacute bacterial endocarditis I33.0
    - systemic lupus erythematosus (chronic) M32.14
  - in
    - diabetes mellitus—*see* E08-E13 with .21
  - polycystic Q61.3
    - autosomal
      - dominant Q61.2
      - recessive NEC Q61.19
    - childhood type NEC Q61.19
    - infantile type NEC Q61.19
  - poststreptococcal N05.9
    - acute N00.9
    - chronic N03.9
  - rapidly progressive N01.-
    - with
      - C3
        - glomerulonephritis N01.A
        - glomerulopathy N01.A
        - ◊ with dense deposit disease N01.6
  - tubulo-interstitial (in) N12
    - acute (infectious) N10
  - war N00.9

Nephroblastoma (epithelial) (mesenchymal) C64.-

Nephrocystitis, pustular—*see* Nephritis, tubulo-interstitial

Nephroma C64.-

Nephronephritis—*see* Nephrosis

Nephronophthisis Q61.5

Nephropathy (*see also* Nephritis) N28.9
- analgesic N14.0
  - with medullary necrosis, acute N17.2
- diabetic—*see* E08-E13 with .21
- hereditary NEC N07.9
  - with
    - C3

Nephropathy, *continued*
- glomerulonephritis N07.A
- glomerulopathy N07.A
- ◊ with dense deposit disease N07.6
- membranous (diffuse) N06.20
  - with
    - nephrotic syndrome N04.20
      - primary N04.21
      - secondary N04.22
  - idiopathic, with nephrotic syndrome N04.21
    - primary N06.21
      - with nephrotic syndrome N04.21
    - secondary N06.22
      - with nephrotic syndrome N04.22
- obstructive N13.8
- phenacetin N17.2
- vasomotor N17.0
- IgA N02.B-
  - with glomerular lesion N02.B1
    - focal and segmental hyalinosis or sclerosis N02.B2
    - membranoproliferative (diffuse) N02.B3
    - membranous (diffuse) N02.B4
    - mesangial proliferative (diffuse) N02.B5
    - mesangiocapillary (diffuse) N02.B6
    - proliferative NEC N02.B9
    - specified pathology NEC N02.B9

Nephrosis, nephrotic (Epstein's) (syndrome) (congenital) N04.9
- with
  - glomerular lesion N04.1
  - hypocomplementemic N04.5
- acute N04.9
- anoxic—*see* Nephrosis, tubular
- chemical—*see* Nephrosis, tubular
- Finnish type (congenital) Q89.8
- hemoglobin N10
- hemoglobinuric—*see* Nephrosis, tubular
- in
  - diabetes mellitus—*see* E08-E13 with .21
- lipoid N04.9
- minimal change N04.0
- myoglobin N10
- radiation N04.9
- toxic—*see* Nephrosis, tubular
- tubular (acute) N17.0
  - postprocedural N99.0
  - radiation N04.9

Nerves R45.0

Nervous (*see also* Disease, diseased) R45.0
- heart F45.8
- stomach F45.8
- tension R45.0

Nervousness R45.0

Nettleship's syndrome—*see* Urticaria pigmentosa

Neuralgia, neuralgic (acute) M79.2
- ciliary G44.009
  - intractable G44.001
  - not intractable G44.009
- ear—*see* subcategory H92.0
- migrainous G44.009
  - intractable G44.001
  - not intractable G44.009
- perineum R10.2
- pubic region R10.2
- scrotum R10.2
- spermatic cord R10.2

Neurasthenia F48.8
- cardiac F45.8
- gastric F45.8
- heart F45.8

Neuritis (rheumatoid) M79.2
- cranial nerve
  - due to Lyme disease A69.22
  - fifth or trigeminal G51.0
  - seventh or facial G51.8
    - newborn (birth injury) P11.3
  - sixth or abducent—*see* Strabismus, paralytic, sixth nerve
- facial G51.8
  - newborn (birth injury) P11.3
- serum (*see also* Reaction, serum) T80.69

Neuroblastoma
- specified site—*see* Neoplasm, malignant, by site in Table of Neoplasms in the complete *ICD-10-CM* manual
- unspecified site C74.90

Neurocirculatory asthenia F45.8

Neurodermatitis (circumscribed) (circumscripta) (local) L28.0
- atopic L20.81
- diffuse (Brocq) L20.81
- disseminated L20.81

Neurofibromatosis (multiple) (nonmalignant) Q85.00
- acoustic Q85.02
- malignant—*see* Neoplasm, nerve, malignant in Table of Neoplasms in the complete *ICD-10-CM* manual
- specified NEC Q85.09
- type 1 (von Recklinghausen) Q85.01
- type 2 Q85.02

Neurogenic—*see also* Disease, diseased
- bladder (*see also* Dysfunction) N31.9
  - cauda equina syndrome G83.4
- bowel NEC K59.2
- heart F45.8

Neuromyopathy G70.9
- paraneoplastic D49.9 [G13.0]

Neuropathy, neuropathic G62.9
- hereditary G60.9
  - motor and sensory (types I-IV) G60.0
  - sensory G60.8
  - specified NEC G60.8
- idiopathic G60.9
  - progressive G60.3
  - specified NEC G60.8
- peripheral (nerve) (*see also* Polyneuropathy) G62.9
  - autonomic G90.9
    - in (due to)
      - hyperthyroidism E05.90 [G99.0]
        - ◊ with thyroid storm E05.91 [G99.0]

Neurosis, neurotic F48.9
- anankastic F42.8
- anxiety (state) F41.1
  - panic type F41.0
- bladder F45.8
- cardiac (reflex) F45.8
- cardiovascular F45.8
- character F60.9
- colon F45.8
- compulsive, compulsion F42.9
- conversion F44.9
- cutaneous F45.8
- excoriation F42.4
- gastric F45.8
- gastrointestinal F45.8
- heart F45.8
- hysterical F44.9
- incoordination F45.8
  - larynx F45.8
  - vocal cord F45.8
- intestine F45.8
- larynx (sensory) F45.8
  - hysterical F44.4
- mixed NEC F48.8
- musculoskeletal F45.8
- obsessional F42.9
- obsessive-compulsive F42.9
- ocular NEC F45.8
- pharynx F45.8
- phobic F40.9
- posttraumatic (situational) F43.10
  - acute F43.11
  - chronic F43.12
- rectum F45.8
- respiratory F45.8
- rumination F45.8
- state F48.9
- stomach F45.8
- traumatic F43.10
  - acute F43.11
  - chronic F43.12
- vasomotor F45.8
- visceral F45.8

Neurospongioblastosis diffusa Q85.1

Neutropenia, neutropenic (chronic) (genetic) (idiopathic) (immune) (infantile) (malignant) (pernicious) (splenic) D70.9
- congenital (primary) D70.0
- cyclic D70.4
- cytoreductive cancer chemotherapy sequela D70.1
- drug-induced D70.2
  - due to cytoreductive cancer chemotherapy D70.1
- due to infection D70.3
- fever D70.9
- neonatal, transitory (isoimmune) (maternal transfer) P61.5
- periodic D70.4
- secondary (cyclic) (periodic) (splenic) D70.4
  - drug-induced D70.2
    - due to cytoreductive cancer chemotherapy D70.1
- toxic D70.8

Neutrophilia, hereditary giant D72.0

Nevus D22-
- achromic—*see* Neoplasm, skin, benign in Table of Neoplasms in the complete *ICD-10-CM* manual
- amelanotic—*see* Neoplasm, skin, benign in Table of Neoplasms in the complete *ICD-10-CM* manual
- angiomatous D18.00
  - skin D18.01
  - specified site NEC D18.09
- araneus I78.1
- blue—(*see* Neoplasm, skin, benign for blue, cellular, giant, or Jadassohn's or other than malignant in Table of Neoplasms in the complete *ICD-10-CM* manual)
  - malignant—*see* Melanoma
- capillary D18.00
  - skin D18.01
  - specified site NEC D18.09
- cavernous D18.00
  - skin D18.01
  - specified site NEC D18.09
- cellular—*see* Neoplasm, skin, benign in Table of Neoplasms in the complete *ICD-10-CM* manual
  - blue—*see* Neoplasm, skin, benign in Table of Neoplasms in the complete *ICD-10-CM* manual
- comedonicus Q82.5
- dermal—*see* Neoplasm, skin, benign in Table of Neoplasms in the complete *ICD-10-CM* manual
  - with epidermal nevus—*see* Neoplasm, skin, benign in Table of Neoplasms in the complete *ICD-10-CM* manual
- dysplastic—*see* Neoplasm, skin, benign in Table of Neoplasms in the complete *ICD-10-CM* manual
- flammeus Q82.5
- hemangiomatous D18.00
  - skin D18.01
  - specified site NEC D18.09
- lymphatic D18.1
- meaning hemangioma D18.00
  - skin D18.01
  - specified site NEC D18.09
- multiplex Q85.1
- non-neoplastic I78.1
- portwine Q82.5
- sanguineous Q82.5
- skin D22.9
  - abdominal wall D22.5
  - ala nasi D22.39
  - ankle D22.7-
  - anus, anal D22.5
  - arm D22.6-
  - auditory canal (external) D22.2-
  - auricle (ear) D22.2-
  - auricular canal (external) D22.2-
  - axilla, axillary fold D22.5
  - back D22.5
  - breast D22.5
  - brow D22.39
  - buttock D22.5
  - canthus (eye) D22.1-
  - cheek (external) D22.39
  - chest wall D22.5
  - chin D22.39
  - ear (external) D22.2-
    - external meatus (ear) D22.2-
  - eyebrow D22.39
  - eyelid (lower) (upper) D22.1-

Nevus, *continued*
  - face D22.3-
  - finger D22.6-
  - flank D22.5
  - foot D22.7-
  - forearm D22.6-
  - forehead D22.39
  - foreskin D29.0
  - genital organ (external) NEC
    - female D28.0
    - male D29.9
  - gluteal region D22.5
  - groin D22.5
  - hand D22.6-
  - heel D22.7-
  - helix D22.2-
  - hip D22.7-
  - interscapular region D22.5
  - jaw D22.39
  - knee D22.7-
  - leg D22.7-
  - lip (lower) (upper) D22.0
  - lower limb D22.7-
  - nail D22.9
    - finger D22.6-
    - toe D22.7-
  - nasolabial groove D22.39
  - nates D22.5
  - neck D22.4
  - nose (external) D22.39
  - palpebra D22.1-
  - penis D29.0
  - perianal skin D22.5
  - perineum D22.5
  - pinna D22.2-
  - popliteal fossa or space D22.7-
  - scalp D22.4
  - shoulder D22.6-
  - submammary fold D22.5
  - temple D22.39
  - thigh D22.7-
  - toe D22.7-
  - trunk NEC D22.5
  - umbilicus D22.5
  - upper limb D22.6-
  - vulva D28.0
  - specified site NEC -*see* Neoplasm, by site, benign in Table of Neoplasms in the complete *ICD-10-CM* manual
- Sutton's benign D22.9
  - spider I78.1
  - stellar I78.1
- strawberry Q82.5
- unius lateris Q82.5
- Unna's Q82.5
- vascular Q82.5
- verrucous Q82.5

Newborn (infant) (liveborn) (singleton) Z38.2
- abstinence syndrome P96.1
- acne L70.4
- affected by
  - abruptio placenta P02.1
  - amniocentesis (while in utero) P00.6
  - amnionitis P02.78
  - apparent life threatening event (ALTE) R68.13
  - bleeding (into)
    - cerebral cortex P52.22
    - germinal matrix P52.0
    - ventricles P52.1
  - breech delivery P03.0
  - cardiac arrest P29.81
  - cerebral ischemia P91.0
  - Cesarean delivery P03.4
  - chemotherapy agents P04.1
  - chorioamnionitis P02.78
  - cocaine (crack) P04.41
  - complications of labor and delivery P03.9
    - specified NEC P03.89
  - compression of umbilical cord NEC P02.5
  - contracted pelvis P03.1
  - cyanosis P28.2

Newborn, *continued*
  - delivery P03.9
    - Cesarean P03.4
    - forceps P03.2
    - vacuum extractor P03.3
  - drugs of addiction P04.40
    - cocaine P04.41
    - hallucinogens P04.42
    - specified drug NEC P04.49
  - entanglement (knot) in umbilical cord P02.5
  - fetal (intrauterine)
    - growth retardation P05.9
    - inflammatory response syndrome (FIRS) P02.70
    - FIRS (fetal inflammatory response syndrome) P02.70
  - forceps delivery P03.2
  - heart rate abnormalities
    - bradycardia P29.12
    - intrauterine P03.819
      - before onset of labor P03.810
      - during labor P03.811
    - tachycardia P29.11
  - hemorrhage (antepartum) P02.1
    - intraventricular (nontraumatic) P52.3
      - grade 1 P52.0
      - grade 2 P52.1
      - grade 3 P52.21
      - grade 4 P52.22
    - subependymal P52.0
      - with intracerebral extension P52.22
      - with intraventricular extension P52.1
        - 0 with enlargement of ventricles P52.21
      - without intraventricular extension P52.0
  - hypoxic ischemic encephalopathy [HIE] P91.60
    - mild P91.61
    - moderate P91.62
    - severe P91.63
  - induction of labor P03.89
  - intrauterine (fetal) blood loss P50.9
  - intrauterine (fetal) hemorrhage P50.9
  - malpresentation (malposition) NEC P03.1
  - maternal (complication of) (use of)
    - alcohol P04.3
    - amphetamines P04.16
    - analgesia (maternal) P04.0
    - anesthesia (maternal) P04.0
    - anticonvulsants P04.13
    - antidepressants P04.15
    - antineoplastic chemotherapy P04.11
    - anxiolytics P04.1A
    - blood loss P02.1
    - cannabis P04.81
    - circulatory disease P00.3
    - condition P00.9
      - specified NEC P00.89
    - cytotoxic drugs P04.12
    - delivery P03.9
      - Cesarean P03.4
      - forceps P03.2
      - vacuum extractor P03.3
    - diabetes mellitus (pre-existing) P70.1
    - disorder P00.9
      - specified NEC P00.89
    - drugs (addictive) (illegal) NEC P04.49
    - group B streptococcus (GBS) colonization (positive) P00.82
    - hemorrhage P02.1
    - incompetent cervix P01.0
    - infectious disease P00.2
    - malpresentation before labor P01.7
    - medical procedure P00.7
    - medication (legal) (maternal use) (prescribed) P04.19
    - opiates P04.14
      - administered for procedures during pregnancy or labor and delivery P04.0
    - parasitic disease P00.2
    - placenta previa P02.0
    - premature rupture of membranes P01.1
    - respiratory disease P00.3
    - sedative-hypnotics P04.17
      - tranquilizers administered for procedures during pregnancy or labor and delivery P04.0
    - surgical procedure P00.6

ALPHABETIC INDEX

Newborn, *continued*

- ■ medication (legal) (maternal use) (prescribed) P04.19
- ■ specified type NEC P04.18
- membranitis P02.78
- methamphetamine(s) P04.49
- mixed metabolic and respiratory acidosis P84
- neonatal abstinence syndrome P96.1
- noxious substances transmitted via placenta or breast milk P04.9
  - ■ cannabis P04.81
  - ■ specified NEC P04.89
- placenta previa P02.0
- placental
  - ■ abnormality (functional) (morphological) P02.20
    - – specified NEC P02.29
  - ■ dysfunction P02.29
  - ■ infarction P02.29
  - ■ insufficiency P02.29
  - ■ separation NEC P02.1
  - ■ transfusion syndromes P02.3
- placentitis P02.78
- prolapsed cord P02.4
- respiratory arrest P28.81
- slow intrauterine growth P05.9
- tobacco P04.2
- twin to twin transplacental transfusion P02.3
- umbilical cord (tightly) around neck P02.5
- umbilical cord condition P02.60
  - ■ short cord P02.69
  - ■ specified NEC P02.69
- uterine contractions (abnormal) P03.6
- vasa previa P02.69
  - ■ from intrauterine blood loss P50.0
- apnea P28.4
  - primary P28.3
  - obstructive P28.4
  - sleep (central) (obstructive) (primary) P28.3
- born in hospital Z38.00
  - by cesarean Z38.01
- born outside hospital Z38.1
- breast buds P96.89
- breast engorgement P83.4
- check-up—*see* Newborn, examination
- convulsion P90
- dehydration P74.1
- examination
  - 8 to 28 days old Z00.111
  - under 8 days old Z00.110
- fever P81.9
  - environmentally-induced P81.0
- hyperbilirubinemia P59.9
  - of prematurity P59.0
- hypernatremia P74.21
- hyponatremia P74.22
- infection P39.9
  - candidal P37.5
  - specified NEC P39.8
  - urinary tract P39.3
- jaundice P59.9
  - due to
    - ■ breast milk inhibitor P59.3
    - ■ hepatocellular damage P59.20
      - – specified NEC P59.29
    - ■ preterm delivery P59.0
  - of prematurity P59.0
  - specified NEC P59.8
- mastitis P39.0
  - infective P39.0
  - noninfective P83.4
- multiple born NEC Z38.8
  - born in hospital Z38.68
    - ■ by cesarean Z38.69
  - born outside hospital Z38.7
- omphalitis P38.9
  - with mild hemorrhage P38.1
  - without hemorrhage P38.9
- post-term P08.21
- prolonged gestation (over 42 completed weeks) P08.22
- quadruplet Z38.8
  - born in hospital Z38.63
    - ■ by cesarean Z38.64
  - born outside hospital Z38.7

Newborn, *continued*

- quintuplet Z38.8
  - born in hospital Z38.65
    - ■ by cesarean Z38.66
  - born outside hospital Z38.7
- seizure P90
- sepsis (congenital) P36.9
  - due to
    - ■ anaerobes NEC P36.5
    - ■ Escherichia coli P36.4
    - ■ Staphylococcus P36.30
      - – aureus P36.2
      - – specified P36.39
    - ■ Streptococcus P36.10
      - – group B P36.0
      - – specified NEC P36.19
      - – specified NEC P36.8
- triplet Z38.8
  - born in hospital Z38.61
    - ■ by cesarean Z38.62
  - born outside hospital Z38.7
- twin Z38.5
  - born in hospital Z38.30
    - ■ by cesarean Z38.31
  - born outside hospital Z38.4
- vomiting P92.09
  - bilious P92.01
- weight check Z00.111

Niemann-Pick disease or syndrome E75.249

- specified NEC E75.248
- type
  - A E75.240
  - A/B E75.244
  - B E75.241
  - C E75.242
  - D E75.243

Night

- sweats R61
- terrors (child) F51.4

Nightmares (REM sleep type) F51.5

Nipple—*see* Disease, diseased

Nitrosohemoglobinemia D74.8

Nocturia R35.1

- psychogenic F45.8

Nocturnal—*see* Disease, diseased

Node(s)—*see also* Nodule

- Osler's I33.0

Nodule(s), nodular

- breast NEC N63.0
- cutaneous—*see* Swelling, localized
- inflammatory—*see* Inflammation
- lung, solitary (subsegmental branch of the bronchial tree) R91.1
  - multiple R91.8
- retrocardiac R09.89
- solitary, lung (subsegmental branch of the bronchial tree) R91.1
  - multiple R91.8
- subcutaneous—*see* Swelling, localized

Nonclosure—*see also* Imperfect, closure

- ductus arteriosus (Botallo's) Q25.0
- foramen
  - botalli Q21.1
  - ovale Q21.1

Noncompliance Z91.199

- with
  - dietary regimen Z91.119
    - ■ due to
      - – financial hardship Z91.110
      - – specified reason NEC Z91.118
  - dialysis Z91.158
    - ■ due to financial hardship Z91.151
  - medical treatment, specified NEC Z91.199
    - ■ due to
      - – financial hardship Z91.190
      - – specified reason NEC Z91.198
  - medication regimen NEC Z91.148
  - underdosing—*see also* Table of Drugs and Chemicals, categories T36-T50, with final character 6 Z91.148

Noncompliance, *continued*

- ■ intentional NEC Z91.128
  - – by caregiver
    - ◊ due to
      - ◊ financial hardship Z91.A20
      - ◊ specified reason NEC Z91.A28
  - ■ due to financial hardship of patient Z91.120
    - – unintentional NEC Z91.138
      - ◊ by caregiver Z91.A3
      - ◊ due to patient's age related debility Z91.130
  - renal dialysis Z91.158
    - ■ due to financial hardship Z91.151
- caregiver
  - with patient's
    - ■ dietary regimen
      - – due to
        - ◊ financial hardship Z91.A10
        - ◊ specified reason NEC Z91.A18
    - ■ medical treatment and regimen
      - – due to financial hardship Z91.A91
      - – specified reason NEC Z91.A98
    - ■ medication regimen
      - – due to financial hardship Z91.A41
      - – specified reason NEC Z91.A48
    - ■ renal dialysis
      - – due to financial hardship Z91.A51
      - – specified reason NEC Z91.A58

Nondescent (congenital)—*see also* Malposition, congenital

- testicle Q53.9
  - bilateral Q53.20
    - ■ abdominal Q53.211
    - ■ perineal Q53.22
  - unilateral Q53.10
    - ■ abdominal Q53.111
    - ■ perineal Q53.12

Nondevelopment

- brain Q02
  - part of Q04.3
- heart Q24.8
- organ or site, congenital NEC—*see* Hypoplasia

Nonexpansion, lung (newborn) P28.0

Nonovulation N97.0

Non-palpable testicle(s)

- bilateral R39.84
- unilateral R39.83

Nonpneumatization, lung NEC P28.0

Nonrheumatic mitral (valve) disorders

- annulus calcification I34.81
- other I34.89

Nonunion

- fracture—*see* Fracture, by site
- organ or site, congenital NEC—*see* Imperfect, closure
- symphysis pubis, congenital Q74.2

Noonan's syndrome Q87.19

Norcardiosis, nocardiasis A43.9

- cutaneous A43.1
- lung A43.0
- pneumonia A43.0
- pulmonary A43.0
- specified site NEC A43.8

Normocytic anemia (infectional) due to blood loss (chronic) D50.0

- acute D62

Norwegian itch B86

Nose, nasal—*see* Disease, diseased

Nosebleed R04.0

Nose-picking F98.8

Nosophobia F45.22

Nostalgia F43.20

Nothnagel's

- syndrome—*see* Strabismus, paralytic, third nerve
- vasomotor acroparesthesia I73.89

Novy's relapsing fever A68.9

- louse-borne A68.0
- tick-borne A68.1

ALPHABETIC INDEX

Noxious
- foodstuffs, poisoning by—*see* Poisoning, food, noxious, plants NEC
- substances transmitted through placenta or breast milk P04.9

Nursemaid's elbow S53.03-

Nutrition deficient or insufficient (*see also* Malnutrition) E46
- due to
  - insufficient food T73.0
  - lack of
    - care (child) T76.02
    - food T73.0

Nycturia R35.1
- psychogenic F45.8

Nystagmus H55.00
- benign paroxysmal—*see* Vertigo, benign paroxysmal
- central positional H81.4
- congenital H55.01
- dissociated H55.04
- latent H55.02
- miners' H55.09
- positional
  - benign paroxysmal H81.4
    - central H81.4
- specified form NEC H55.09
- visual deprivation H55.03

O

Obesity E66.9
- with alveolar hypoventilation E66.2
- class
  - 1 E66.811
  - 2 E66.812
  - 3 E66.813
- constitutional E66.89
- dietary counseling and surveillance Z71.3
- drug-induced E66.1
- due to
  - drug E66.1
  - excess calories E66.09
    - morbid E66.01
    - severe E66.01
- endocrine E66.89
- endogenous E66.89
- familial E66.89
- glandular E66.89
- hypothyroid—*see* Hypothyroidism
- morbid E66.01
  - with alveolar hypoventilation E66.2
  - due to excess calories E66.01
  - with obesity hypoventilation syndrome (OHS) E66.2
- nutritional E66.09
- pituitary E23.6
- severe E66.01
- specified type NEC E66.89

Observation (following) (for) (without need for further medical care) Z04.9
- accident NEC Z04.3
  - at work Z04.2
  - transport Z04.1
- adverse effect of drug Z03.6
- alleged rape or sexual assault (victim), ruled out
  - child Z04.42
- criminal assault Z04.89
- development state
  - adolescent Z00.3
  - period of rapid growth in childhood Z00.2
  - puberty Z00.3
- disease, specified NEC Z03.89
- following work accident Z04.2
- forced labor exploitation Z04.82
- forced sexual exploitation Z04.81
- newborn (for suspected condition, ruled out)—*see* Newborn, affected by (suspected to be), maternal (complication of) (use of)
  - suspected condition, related to exposure from the mother or birth process—*see* Newborn, affected by, maternal

Observation, *continued*
- ruled out Z05.9
  - specified condition NEC Z05.8
  - specified condition NEC Z05.89
- suicide attempt, alleged NEC Z03.89
  - self-poisoning Z03.6
- suspected, ruled out—*see also* Suspected condition
  - abuse, physical
    - child Z04.72
  - accident at work Z04.2
  - child battering victim Z04.72
  - condition NEC Z03.89
  - drug poisoning or adverse effect Z03.6
  - exposure (to)
    - anthrax Z03.810
    - biological agent NEC Z03.818
  - foreign body
    - aspirated (inhaled) Z03.822
    - ingested Z03.821
    - inserted (injected), in (eye) (orifice) (skin) Z03.823
  - inflicted injury NEC Z04.89
  - newborn, ruled-out
    - cardiac condition Z05.0
    - connective tissue condition Z05.73
    - gastrointestinal condition Z05.5
    - genetic condition Z05.41
    - genitourinary condition Z05.6
    - immunologic condition Z05.43
    - infectious condition Z05.1
    - metabolic condition Z05.42
    - musculoskeletal condition Z05.72
    - neurological condition Z05.2
    - other condition Z05.8
    - respiratory condition Z05.3
    - skin and subcutaneous tissue condition Z05.71
    - unspecified suspected condition Z05.9
  - suicide attempt, alleged Z03.89
    - self-poisoning Z03.6
  - toxic effects from ingested substance (drug) (poison) Z03.6
- toxic effects from ingested substance (drug) (poison) Z03.6

Obsession, obsessional state F42

Obsessive-compulsive neurosis or reaction F42.8
- mixed thoughts and acts F42.2

Obstruction, obstructed, obstructive
- airway J98.8
  - with
    - asthma J45.909
      - with
        - ◊ exacerbation (acute) J45.901
        - ◊ status asthmaticus J45.902
    - bronchitis (chronic) J44.89
- aqueduct of Sylvius G91.1
  - congenital Q03.0
    - with spina bifida—*see* Spina bifida, by site, with hydrocephalus
- artery (*see also* Embolism, artery) I74.9
- bile duct or passage (common) (hepatic) (noncalculous) K83.1
  - with calculus K80.51
  - congenital (causing jaundice) Q44.3
- bladder-neck (acquired) N32.0
  - congenital Q64.31
- cystic duct—*see also* Obstruction, gallbladder
  - with calculus K80.21
- device, implant or graft (*see also* Complications, by site and type, mechanical) T85.698
  - catheter NEC T85.628
    - cystostomy T83.090
    - Hopkins T83.098
    - ileostomy T83.098
    - nephrostomy T83.092
    - urethral indwelling T83.091
    - urinary T83.098
    - urostomy T83.098
  - ventricular intracranial shunt T85.09
- fecal K56.41
  - with hernia—*see* Hernia, by site, with obstruction
- foramen of Monro (congenital) Q03.8
  - with spina bifida—*see* Spina bifida, by site, with hydrocephalus

Obstruction, obstructed, obstructive, *continued*
- foreign body—*see* Foreign body
- gallbladder K82.0
  - with calculus, stones K80.21
  - congenital Q44.1
- intestine K56.609
  - adynamic K56.0
  - complete K56.601
  - congenital (small) Q41.9
    - large Q42.9
      - specified part NEC Q42.8
  - incomplete K56.600
  - neurogenic K56.0
    - Hirschsprung's disease or megacolon Q43.1
  - newborn P76.9
    - due to
      - fecaliths P76.8
      - inspissated milk P76.2
      - meconium (plug) P76.0
        - ◊ in mucoviscidosis E84.11
    - specified NEC P76.8
  - partial K56.600
  - reflex K56.0
  - specified NEC K56.699
    - complete K56.691
    - incomplete K56.690
    - partial K56.690
  - volvulus K56.2
- kidney (calices) (*see also* Hydronephrosis) N28.89
- lacrimal (passages) (duct)
  - by
    - stenosis—*see* Stenosis, lacrimal
    - congenital Q10.5
  - neonatal H04.53-
- lacrimonasal duct—*see* Obstruction, lacrimal
- meconium (plug)
  - newborn P76.0
    - due to fecaliths P76.0
    - in mucoviscidosis E84.11
- nasal J34.89
- nasolacrimal duct—*see also* Obstruction, lacrimal
  - congenital Q10.5
- nose J34.89
- portal (circulation) (vein) I81
- pulmonary valve (heart) I37.0
- pylorus
  - congenital or infantile Q40.0
- rectum K62.4
- renal N28.89
  - outflow N13.8
  - pelvis, congenital Q62.39
- sinus (accessory) (nasal) J34.89
- stomach NEC K31.89
  - congenital Q40.2
  - due to pylorospasm K31.3
- ureter (functional) (pelvic junction) NEC N13.5
  - with
    - hydronephrosis N13.1
    - congenital Q62.39
    - urinary (moderate) N13.9
  - organ or tract (lower) N13.9
    - specified NEC N13.8
  - uropathy N13.9
- vagina N89.5
- vesical NEC N32.0
- vesicourethral orifice N32.0
  - congenital Q64.31

Occlusion, occluded
- anus K62.4
  - congenital Q42.3
    - with fistula Q42.2
- aqueduct of Sylvius G91.1
  - congenital Q03.0
    - with spina bifida—*see* Spina bifida, by site, with hydrocephalus
- artery (*see also* Embolism, artery) I70.9
- choanal Q30.0
- fallopian tube N97.1
  - congenital Q50.6
- gallbladder—*see also* Obstruction, gallbladder
  - congenital (causing jaundice) Q44.1

ALPHABETIC INDEX

Occlusion, occluded, *continued*

- hymen N89.6
  - congenital Q52.3
- nose J34.89
  - congenital Q30.0
- oviduct N97.1
  - congenital Q50.6
- posterior lingual, of mandibular teeth M26.29
- teeth (mandibular) (posterior lingual) M26.29
- ureter (complete) (partial) N13.5
  - congenital Q62.10
  - ureteropelvic junction N13.5
    - congenital Q62.11
  - ureterovesical orifice N13.5
    - congenital Q62.12
- vagina N89.5
- ventricle (brain) NEC G91.1

Occult

- blood in feces (stools) R19.5

Oculogyric crisis or disturbance H51.8

- psychogenic F45.8

Odontoclasia K03.89

Oligoastrocytoma

- specified site—*see* Neoplasm, malignant, by site in Table of Neoplasms in the complete *ICD-10-CM* manual
- unspecified site C71.9

Oligocythemia D64.9

Oligodendroblastoma

- specified site—*see* Neoplasm, malignant in Table of Neoplasms in the complete *ICD-10-CM* manual
- unspecified site C71.9

Oligodendroglioma

- anaplastic type
  - specified site—*see* Neoplasm, malignant, by site in Table of Neoplasms in the complete *ICD-10-CM* manual
  - unspecified site C71.9
- specified site—*see* Neoplasm, malignant, by site in Table of Neoplasms in the complete *ICD-10-CM* manual
- unspecified site C71.9

Oligodontia—*see* Anodontia

Oligoencephalon Q02

Oligohydramnios O41.0-

Oligophrenia—*see also* Disability, intellectual

- phenylpyruvic E70.0

Oliguria R34

- postprocedural N99.0

Omphalitis (congenital) (newborn) P38.9

- with mild hemorrhage P38.1
- without hemorrhage P38.9

Omphalocele Q79.2

Omphalomesenteric duct, persistent Q43.0

Omphalorrhagia, newborn P51.9

Onanism (excessive) F98.8

Onychia—*see also* Cellulitis

- with lymphangitis—*see* Lymphangitis, acute
- candidal B37.2
- dermatophytic B35.1

Onychocryptosis L60.0

Onycholysis L60.1

Onychomadesis L60.8

Onychomycosis (finger) (toe) B35.1

Onychophagia F98.8

Onychophosis L60.8

Onychoptosis L60.8

Onyxis (finger) (toe) L60.0

Oophoritis (cystic) (infectional) (interstitial) N70.92

- with salpingitis N70.93

Ophthalmia (see *also* Conjunctivitis) H10.9

- blennorrhagic (gonococcal) (neonatorum) A54.31
- gonococcal (neonatorum) A54.31
- neonatorum, newborn P39.1
  - gonococcal A54.31

Orchitis (gangrenous) (nonspecific) (septic) (suppurative) N45.2

- blennorrhagic (gonococcal) (acute) (chronic) A54.23
- chlamydial A56.19
- gonococcal (acute) (chronic) A54.23
- mumps B26.0
- syphilitic A52.76

Orotaciduria, oroticaciduria (congenital) (hereditary) (pyrimidine deficiency) E79.8

- anemia D53.0

Orthopnea R06.01

Osgood-Schlatter disease or osteochondrosis M92.52-

Osler (-Weber)-Rendu disease I78.0

Osler's nodes I33.0

Ossification

- diaphragm J98.6
- falx cerebri G96.198
- fontanel, premature Q75.009
- meninges (cerebral) (spinal) G96.198

Osteitis—*see also* Osteomyelitis

- deformans M88.9
- fragilitans Q78.0
  - in (due to)
    - malignant neoplasm of bone C41.9
    - neoplastic disease (*see also* Table of Neoplasms in the complete *ICD-10-CM* manual) D49.9
      - carpus D49.9
      - clavicle D49.9
      - femur D49.9
      - fibula D49.9
      - finger D49.9
      - humerus D49.9
      - ilium D49.9
      - ischium D49.9
      - metacarpus D49.9
      - metatarsus D49.9
      - multiple sites D49.9
      - neck D49.9
      - radius D49.9
      - rib D49.9
      - scapula D49.9
      - skull D49.9
      - tarsus D49.9
      - tibia D49.9
      - toe D49.9
      - ulna D49.9
      - vertebra D49.9
  - skull M88.0
  - specified NEC—*see* Paget's disease, bone, by site
  - vertebra M88.1
- tuberculosa A18.09
  - cystica D86.89
  - multiplex cystoides D86.89

Osteochondritis—*see also* Osteochondropathy

- juvenile M92.9
  - patellar M92.4-

Osteochondrodysplasia Q78.9

- with defects of growth of tubular bones and spine Q77.9
- specified NEC Q78.8

Osteochondropathy M93.9-

- slipped upper femoral epiphysis—*see* Slipped, epiphysis, upper femoral

Osteochondrosis—*see also* Osteochondropathy

- acetabulum (juvenile) M91.0
- astragalus (juvenile) M92.6-
- Blount's M92.51-
- Buchanan's M91.0
- Burns' M92.1-
- calcaneus (juvenile) M92.6-
- capitular epiphysis (femur) (juvenile) M91.1-
- carpal (juvenile) (lunate) (scaphoid) M92.21-
- coxae juvenilis M91.1-
- deformans juvenilis, coxae M91.1-
- Diaz's M92.6-
- femoral capital epiphysis (juvenile) M91.1-
- femur (head), juvenile M91.1-
- fibula (juvenile) M92.5-
- foot NEC (juvenile) M92.8
- Freiberg's M92.7-
- Haas' (juvenile) M92.0-

Osteochondrosis, *continued*

- Haglund's M92.6-
- hip (juvenile) M91.1-
- humerus (capitulum) (head) (juvenile) M92.0-
- ilium, iliac crest (juvenile) M91.0
- ischiopubic synchondrosis M91.0
- Iselin's M92.7-
- juvenile, juvenilis M92.9
  - after congenital dislocation of hip reduction M91.8-
  - arm M92.3-
    - capitular epiphysis (femur) M91.1-
    - clavicle, sternal epiphysis M92.3-
    - coxae M91.1-
    - deformans M92.9
    - fibula M92.50-
    - foot NEC M92.8
    - hand M92.20-
      - carpal lunate M92.21-
      - metacarpal head M92.22-
      - specified site NEC M92.29-
    - head of femur M91.1-
    - hip and pelvis M91.9-
      - femoral head M91.1-
      - pelvis M91.0
        - specified NEC M91.8-
      - humerus M92.0-
    - limb
      - lower NEC M92.8
      - upper NEC M92.3-
    - medial cuneiform bone M92.6-
    - metatarsus M92.7-
    - patella M92.4-
    - radius M92.1-
    - specified site NEC M92.8
    - tarsus M92.6-
    - tibia M92.50-
      - proximal M92.51-
      - tubercle M92.52
    - ulna M92.1-
    - upper limb NEC M92.3-
- Kienbōck's M92.21-
- Köhler's
  - patellar M92.4-
  - tarsal navicular M92.6-
- Legg-Perthes (-Calvé) (-Waldenström) M91.1-
- limb
  - lower NEC (juvenile) M92.8
  - tibia and fibula M92.59-
  - upper NEC (juvenile) M92.3-
- lunate bone carpal (juvenile) M92.21-
- Mauclaire's M92.22-
- metacarpal (head) (juvenile) M92.22-
- metatarsus (fifth) (head) (juvenile) (second) M92.7-
- navicular (juvenile) M92.6-
- os
  - calcis (juvenile) M92.6-
  - tibiale externum (juvenile) M92.6-
- Osgood-Schlatter M92.52-
- Panner's M92.0-
- patellar center (juvenile) (primary) (secondary) M92.4-
- pelvis (juvenile) M91.0
- Pierson's M91.0
- radius (head) (juvenile) M92.1-
- Sever's M92.6-
- Sinding-Larsen M92.4-
- symphysis pubis (juvenile) M91.0
- talus (juvenile) M92.6-
- tarsus (navicular) (juvenile) M92.6-
- tibia (proximal) (tubercle) (juvenile) M92.5-
- ulna (lower) (juvenile) M92.1-
- van Neck's M91.0

Osteogenesis imperfecta Q78.0

Osteomyelitis (general) (infective) (localized) (neonatal) (purulent) (septic) (staphylococcal) (streptococcal) (suppurative) (with periostitis) M86.9

- acute M86.10
  - carpus M86.14-
  - clavicle M86.11-
  - femur M86.15-
  - fibula M86.16-
  - finger M86.14-
  - humerus M86.12-

Osteomyelitis, *continued*
- ilium M86.18
- ischium M86.18
- metacarpus M86.14-
- metatarsus M86.17-
- multiple sites M86.19
- neck M86.18
- radius M86.13-
- rib M86.18
- scapula M86.11-
- skull M86.18
- tarsus M86.17-
- tibia M86.16-
- toe M86.17-
- ulna M86.13-

Osteonecrosis M87.9
- secondary
  - due to
    - hemoglobinopathy NEC D58.2 [M90.50]
      - carpus D58.2 [M90.54-]
      - clavicle D58.2 [M90.51-]
      - femur D58.2 [M90.55-]
      - fibula D58.2 [M90.56-]
      - finger D58.2 [M90.54-]
      - humerus D58.2 [M90.52-]
      - ilium D58.2 [M90.55-]
      - ischium D58.2 [M90.55-]
      - metacarpus D58.2 [M90.54-]
      - metatarsus D58.2 [M90.57-]
      - multiple sites D58.2 [M90.58]
      - neck D58.2 [M90.58]
      - radius D58.2 [M90.53-]
      - rib D58.2 [M90.58]
      - scapula D58.2 [M90.51-]
      - skull D58.2 [M90.58]
      - tarsus D58.2 [M90.57-]
      - tibia D58.2 [M90.56-]
      - toe D58.2 [M90.57-]
      - ulna D58.2 [M90.53-]
      - vertebra D58.2 [M90.58]

Osteophyte M25.70
- ankle M25.77-
- elbow M25.72-
- foot joint M25.77-
- hand joint M25.74-
- hip M25.75-
- knee M25.76-
- shoulder M25.71-
- spine M25.78
- vertebrae M25.78
- wrist M25.73-

Osteopsathyrosis (idiopathica) Q78.0

Osteosclerosis Q78.2
- acquired M85.8-
- congenita Q77.4
- fragilitas (generalisata) Q78.2
- myelofibrosis D75.81

Osteosis
- cutis L94.2

Ostium
- atrioventriculare commune Q21.2
- primum (arteriosum) (defect) (persistent) Q21.2
- secundum (arteriosum) (defect) (patent) (persistent) Q21.1

Ostrum-Furst syndrome Q75.8

Otalgia—*see* subcategory H92.0

Otitis (acute) H66.9-
- with effusion—*see also* Otitis, media, nonsuppurative
  - purulent—*see* Otitis, media
- chronic—*see also* Otitis, media, chronic
  - with effusion—*see also* Otitis, media, nonsuppurative
- externa H60.9-
  - abscess—*see also* Abscess, ear, external
  - acute (noninfective) H60.50-
    - infective—*see* Otitis, externa, infective
  - cellulitis—*see* Cellulitis, ear
  - in (due to)
    - aspergillosis B44.89
    - candidiasis B37.84
    - erysipelas A46 [H62.4-]

Otitis, *continued*
- herpes (simplex) virus infection B00.1
- impetigo L01.00 [H62.4-]
- infectious disease NEC B99 [H62.4-]
- mycosis NEC B36.9 [H62.4-]
- parasitic disease NEC B89 [H62.4-]
- viral disease NEC B34.9 [H62.4-]
- infective NEC H60.39-
  - abscess—*see* Abscess, ear, external
  - cellulitis—*see* Cellulitis, ear
  - swimmer's ear H60.33-
- mycotic NEC B36.9 [H62.4-]
  - in
    - aspergillosis B44.89
    - candidiasis B37.84
    - moniliasis B37.84
- specified NEC—*see* subcategory H60.8-
- tropical NEC B36.8
  - in
    - aspergillosis B44.89
    - candidiasis B37.84
    - moniliasis B37.84
- interna—*see* subcategory H83.0
- media (hemorrhagic) (staphylococcal) (streptococcal) H66.9-
  - with effusion (nonpurulent)—*see* Otitis, media, nonsuppurative
  - acute, subacute H66.9-
    - allergic—*see* Otitis, media, nonsuppurative, acute or subacute NEC allergic
    - exudative—*see* Otitis, media, nonsuppurative, acute or subacute NEC allergic
    - mucoid—*see* Otitis, media, nonsuppurative, acute or subacute NEC allergic
    - necrotizing—*see also* Otitis, media, suppurative, acute
      - in
        - measles B05.3
        - scarlet fever A38.0
    - nonsuppurative NEC—*see* Otitis, media, nonsuppurative, acute or subacute NEC allergic
    - purulent—*see* Otitis, media, suppurative, acute or subacute NEC allergic
    - sanguinous—*see* Otitis, media, nonsuppurative, acute or subacute NEC allergic
    - secretory—*see* Otitis, media, nonsuppurative, acute or subacute NEC allergic, serous
    - seromucinous—*see* Otitis, media, nonsuppurative, acute or subacute NEC allergic
    - serous—*see* Otitis, media, nonsuppurative, acute or subacute NEC allergic, serous
    - suppurative—*see* Otitis, media, suppurative, acute
  - allergic—*see* Otitis, media, nonsuppurative
  - catarrhal—*see* Otitis, media, nonsuppurative
  - chronic H66.9-
    - with effusion (nonpurulent)—*see* Otitis, media, nonsuppurative, chronic
    - allergic—*see* Otitis, media, nonsuppurative, chronic, allergic
    - benign suppurative—*see* Otitis, media, suppurative, chronic
    - catarrhal—*see* Otitis, media, nonsuppurative, chronic, serous
    - exudative—*see* Otitis, media, suppurative, chronic
    - mucinous—*see* Otitis, media, nonsuppurative, chronic, mucoid
    - mucoid—*see* Otitis, media, nonsuppurative, chronic, mucoid
    - nonsuppurative NEC—*see* Otitis, media, nonsuppurative, chronic
    - purulent—*see* Otitis, media, suppurative, chronic
    - secretory—*see* Otitis, media, nonsuppurative, chronic
    - seromucinous—*see* Otitis, media, nonsuppurative, chronic
    - serous—*see* Otitis, media, nonsuppurative, chronic, serous
    - suppurative—*see* Otitis, media, suppurative, chronic
    - transudative—*see* Otitis, media, nonsuppurative, chronic, mucoid
  - exudative—*see* Otitis, media, suppurative

Otitis, *continued*
- in (due to) (with)
  - influenza—*see* Influenza, with, otitis media
  - measles B05.3
  - scarlet fever A38.0
  - tuberculosis A18.6
  - viral disease NEC B34.- [H67.-]
- mucoid—*see* Otitis, media, nonsuppurative
- nonsuppurative H65.9-
  - acute or subacute NEC allergic H65.11- (6th characters 1—3, 9)
    - recurrent H65.11- (6th characters 4—7)
  - secretory—*see* Otitis, media, nonsuppurative, serous
  - serous H65.0- (6th characters 0—3)
    - recurrent H65.0- (6th characters 4—7)
  - chronic H65.49-
    - allergic H65.41-
    - mucoid H65.3-
    - serous H65.2-
- postmeasles B05.3
- purulent—*see* Otitis, media, suppurative
- secretory—*see* Otitis, media, nonsuppurative
- seromucinous—*see* Otitis, media, nonsuppurative
- serous—*see* Otitis, media, nonsuppurative
- suppurative H66.4-
  - acute H66.00- (6th characters 1–3, 9)
    - with rupture of ear drum H66.01- (6th characters 1–3, 9)
  - recurrent H66.00- (6th characters 4–7)
    - with rupture of ear drum H66.01- (6th characters 4–7)
  - chronic (*see also* subcategory) H66.3
    - atticoantral H66.2-
    - tubotympanic (benign) H66.1-
  - transudative—*see* Otitis, media, nonsuppurative
  - tuberculous A18.6

Otomycosis (diffuse) NEC B36.9 [H62.4-]
- in
  - aspergillosis B44.89
  - candidiasis B37.84
  - moniliasis B37.84

Otorrhea H92.1-
- cerebrospinal (fluid) G96.01
  - postoperative G96.08
  - specified NEC G96.08
  - spontaneous G96.01
  - traumatic G96.08

Ovary, ovarian—*see also* Disease, diseased
- vein syndrome N13.8

Overactive—*see also* Hyperfunction
- bladder N32.81
- hypothalamus E23.3

Overactivity R46.3
- child—*see* Disorder, attention-deficit hyperactivity

Overbite (deep) (excessive) (horizontal) (vertical) M26.29

Overconscientious personality F60.5

Overeating R63.2
- nonorganic origin F50.89
- psychogenic F50.89

Overgrowth
- bacterial
  - small intestinal K63.8219
    - fungal K63.822
    - hydrogen-subtype K63.8211
    - hydrogen sulfide-subtype K63.8212
- bone—*see* Hypertrophy, bone
- intestinal methanogen K63.829

Overlapping toe (acquired)—*see also* Deformity, toe
- congenital (fifth toe) Q66.89

Overload
- circulatory, due to transfusion (blood) (blood components) (TACO) E87.71
- fluid E87.70
  - due to transfusion (blood) (blood components) E87.71
  - specified NEC E87.79
- iron, due to repeated red blood cell transfusions E83.111
- potassium (K) E87.5
- sodium (Na) E87.0

Overnutrition—*see* Hyperalimentation

Overproduction—*see also* Hypersecretion
- growth hormone E22.0

Overriding
- toe (acquired)—*see also* Deformity, toe
  - congenital Q66.89

Overstrained R53.83

Overweight E66.3

Overworked R53.83

Ovulation (cycle)
- failure or lack of N97.0
- pain N94.0

Oxycephaly, oxycephalic Q75.009

Oxyuriasis B80

Oxyuris vermicularis (infestation) B80

Ozena J31.0

P

Pachydermatocele (congenital) Q82.8

Paget's disease
- bone M88.9
  - carpus M88.84-
  - clavicle M88.81-
  - femur M88.85-
  - fibula M88.86-
  - finger M88.84-
  - humerus M88.82-
  - ilium M88.85-
  - in neoplastic disease D49.9 *[M90.6-]*
  - ischium M88.85-
  - metacarpus M88.84-
  - metatarsus M88.87-
  - multiple sites M88.89
  - neck M88.88
  - radius M88.83-
  - rib M88.88
  - scapula M88.81-
  - skull M88.0
  - specified NEC M88.88
  - tarsus M88.87-
  - tibia M88.86-
  - toe M88.87-
  - ulna M88.83-
  - vertebra M88.1
- osteitis deformans—*see* Paget's disease, bone

Pain(s) (*see also* Painful) R52
- abdominal R10.9
  - colic R10.83
  - generalized R10.84
    - with acute abdomen R10.0
  - lower R10.30
    - left quadrant R10.32
    - pelvic or perineal R10.2
    - periumbilical R10.33
    - right quadrant R10.31
  - rebound—*see* Tenderness, abdominal, rebound
  - severe with abdominal rigidity R10.0
  - tenderness—*see* Tenderness, abdominal
  - upper R10.10
    - epigastric R10.13
    - left quadrant R10.12
    - right quadrant R10.11
- acute R52
  - due to trauma G89.11
  - neoplasm related G89.3
  - postprocedural NEC G89.18
- adnexa (uteri) R10.2
- anus K62.89
- axillary (axilla) M79.62-
- back (postural) M54.9
- bladder R39.89
  - associated with micturition—*see* Micturition, painful
  - chronic R39.82
- breast N64.4
- broad ligament R10.2
- cancer associated (acute) (chronic) G89.3
- chest (central) R07.9
- chronic G89.29
  - neoplasm related G89.3

Pain(s), *continued*
- coccyx M53.3
- due to cancer G89.3
- due to malignancy (primary) (secondary) G89.3
- ear—*see* subcategory H92.0
- epigastric, epigastrium R10.13
- face, facial R51.9
- female genital organs NEC N94.89
- gastric—*see* Pain, abdominal
- generalized NOS R52
- genital organ
  - female N94.89
  - male
    - scrotal N50.82
    - testicular N50.81-
- groin—*see* Pain, abdominal, lower
- hand M79.64-
  - joints M25.54-
- head—*see* Headache
- intermenstrual N94.0
- jaw R68.84
- joint M25.50
  - ankle M25.57-
  - elbow M25.52-
  - finger M25.54-
  - foot M25.57-
  - hand M79.64-
  - hip M25.55-
  - knee M25.56-
  - shoulder M25.51-
  - specified site NEC M25.59
  - toe M25.57-
  - wrist M25.53-
- kidney N23
- laryngeal R07.0
- limb M79.60-
  - lower M79.60-
    - foot M79.67-
    - lower leg M79.66-
    - thigh M79.65-
    - toe M79.67-
  - upper M79.60-
    - axilla M79.62-
    - finger M79.64-
    - forearm M79.63-
    - hand M79.64-
    - upper arm M79.62-
- loin M54.50
- low back M54.5-
- lumbar region M54.50
- mandibular R68.84
- mastoid—*see* subcategory H92.0
- maxilla R68.84
- menstrual (*see also* Dysmenorrhea) N94.6
- mouth K13.79
- muscle—*see* Myalgia
- musculoskeletal (*see also* Pain, by site) M79.18
- myofascial M79.18
- nasal J34.89
- nasopharynx J39.2
- neck NEC M54.2
- nose J34.89
- ocular H57.1-
- ophthalmic H57.1-
- orbital region H57.1-
- ovary N94.89
- ovulation N94.0
- pelvic (female) R10.2
- perineal, perineum R10.2
- postoperative NOS G89.18
- postprocedural NOS G89.18
- premenstrual F32.81
- psychogenic (persistent) (any site) F45.41
- rectum K62.89
- round ligament (stretch) R10.2
- sacroiliac M53.3
- scrotal N50.82
- shoulder M25.51-
- spine M54.9
  - cervical M54.2
  - low back M54.0
    - with sciatica M54.4-
- temporomandibular (joint) M26.62-

Pain(s), *continued*
- testicular N50.81-
- throat R07.0
- tibia M79.66-
- toe M79.67-
- tumor associated G89.3
- ureter N23
- urinary (organ) (system) N23
- uterus NEC N94.89
- vagina R10.2
- vesical R39.89
  - associated with micturition—*see* Micturition, painful
- vulva R10.2

Painful—*see also* Pain
- menstruation—*see* Dysmenorrhea
  - psychogenic F45.8
- micturition—*see* Micturition, painful
- scar NEC L90.5
- wire sutures T81.89

Painter's colic—*see* subcategory T56.0

Palate—*see* Disease, diseased

Palatoplegia K13.79

Palatoschisis—*see* Cleft, palate

Palliative care Z51.5

Pallor R23.1

Palpitations (heart) R00.2
- psychogenic F45.8

Palsy (*see also* Paralysis) G83.9
- Bell's—*see also* Palsy, facial
  - newborn P11.3
- brachial plexus NEC G54.0
  - newborn (birth injury) P14.3
- cerebral (congenital) G80.9
- cranial nerve—*see also* Disorder, nerve, cranial
  - multiple G52.7
    - in
      - neoplastic disease (*see also* Table of Neoplasms in the complete *ICD-10-CM manual*) D49.9 *[G53]*
      - sarcoidosis D86.82
- Erb's P14.0
- facial G51.0
  - newborn (birth injury) P11.3
- Klumpke (-Déjérine) P14.1
- lead—*see* subcategory T56.0
- seventh nerve—*see also* Palsy, facial
  - newborn P11.3

Pancake heart R93.1
- with cor pulmonale (chronic) I27.81

Pancarditis (acute) (chronic) I51.89
- rheumatic I09.89
  - active or acute I01.8

Pancolitis, ulcerative (chronic) K51.00
- with
  - abscess K51.014
  - complication K51.019
  - fistula K51.013
  - obstruction K51.012
  - rectal bleeding K51.011
  - specified complication NEC K51.018

Pancreatitis (annular) (apoplectic) (calcareous) (edematous) (hemorrhagic) (malignant) (subacute) (suppurative) K85.90
- acute K85.90
  - idiopathic K85.00
    - with infected necrosis K85.02
    - with uninfected necrosis K85.01
    - with infected necrosis K85.92
    - with uninfected necrosis K85.91

Pancytopenia (acquired) D61.818
- with
  - malformations D61.09
  - myelodysplastic syndrome—*see* Syndrome, myelodysplastic, pancytopenia (acquired)
- antineoplastic chemotherapy induced D61.810
- congenital D61.09
- drug-induced NEC D61.811
- Fanconi D61.03

ALPHABETIC INDEX

PANDAS (pediatric autoimmune neuropsychiatric disorders associated with streptococcal infections syndrome) D89.89

Panhematopenia D61.9
- congenital D61.09
- constitutional D61.09

Panhemocytopenia D61.9
- congenital D61.09
- constitutional D61.09

Panhypopituitarism E23.0
- prepubertal E23.0

Panic (attack) (state) F41.0
- reaction to exceptional stress (transient) F43.0

Panmyelopathy, familial, constitutional D61.09

Panmyelophthisis D61.82
- congenital D61.09

Pansinusitis (chronic) (hyperplastic) (nonpurulent) (purulent) J32.4
- acute J01.40
  - recurrent J01.41

Pansynostosis Q75.052

Papanicolaou smear, cervix Z12.4
- as part of routine gynecological examination Z01.419
  - with abnormal findings Z01.411
- for suspected neoplasm Z12.4
- routine Z01.419
  - with abnormal findings Z01.411

Papilledema (choked disc) H47.10
- associated with
  - decreased ocular pressure H47.12
  - increased intracranial pressure H47.11
  - retinal disorder H47.13

Papillitis
- anus K62.89
- necrotizing, kidney N17.2
- renal, necrotizing N17.2
- tongue K14.0

Papilloma—*see also* Neoplasm, benign, by site in Table of Neoplasms in the complete *ICD-10-CM* manual
- acuminatum (female) (male) (anogenital) A63.0
- choroid plexus (lateral ventricle) (third ventricle)
  - anaplastic C71.5
  - malignant C71.5
- rectum K62.89

Papillomatosis—*see also* Neoplasm, benign, by site in Table of Neoplasms in the complete *ICD-10-CM* manual
- confluent and reticulated L83

Papillon-Léage and Psaume syndrome Q87.0

Para-albuminemia E88.09

Paracephalus Q89.7

Parageusia R43.2
- psychogenic F45.8

Paralysis, paralytic (complete) (incomplete) G83.9
- anus (sphincter) K62.89
- asthenic bulbar G70.00
  - with exacerbation (acute) G70.01
  - in crisis G70.01
- Bell's G51.0
  - newborn P11.3
- bowel, colon or intestine K56.0
- brachial plexus G54.0
  - birth injury P14.3
  - newborn (birth injury) P14.3
- brain G83.9
- bulbospinal G70.00
  - with exacerbation (acute) G70.01
  - in crisis G70.01
- cardiac (*see also* Failure, heart) I50.9
- Clark's G80.9
- colon K56.0
- conjugate movement (gaze) (of eye) H51.0
  - cortical (nuclear) (supranuclear) H51.0
- deglutition R13.0
  - hysterical F44.4
- diaphragm (flaccid) J98.6
  - due to accidental dissection of phrenic nerve during procedure—*see* Puncture

Paralysis, paralytic, *continued*
- Duchenne's
  - birth injury P14.0
  - due to or associated with
    - muscular dystrophy G71.01
  - due to intracranial or spinal birth injury—*see* Palsy, cerebral
- Erb (-Duchenne) (birth) (newborn) P14.0
- facial (nerve) G51.0
  - birth injury P11.3
  - congenital P11.3
  - following operation NEC—*see* Puncture, accidental complicating surgery
  - newborn (birth injury) P11.3
- gait R26.1
- glottis J38.00
  - bilateral J38.02
  - unilateral J38.01
- Hoppe-Goldflam G70.00
  - with exacerbation (acute) G70.01
  - in crisis G70.01
- hysterical F44.4
- ileus K56.0
- infantile A80.30
- infective A80.-
- inferior nuclear G83.9
- intestine K56.0
- Klumpke (-Déjérine) (birth) (newborn) P14.1
- laryngeal nerve (recurrent) (superior) (unilateral) J38.00
  - bilateral J38.02
  - unilateral J38.01
- larynx J38.00
  - bilateral J38.02
  - unilateral J38.01
- lead—*see* subcategory T56.0
- left side—*see* Hemiplegia
- leg G83.1-
  - both—*see* Paraplegia
  - hysterical F44.4
  - psychogenic F44.4
- lip K13.0
- monoplegic—*see* Monoplegia
- motor G83.9
- muscle, muscular NEC G72.89
- nerve—*see also* Disorder, nerve
  - facial G51.0
    - birth injury P11.3
    - congenital P11.3
    - newborn (birth injury) P11.3
  - seventh or facial G51.0
    - newborn (birth injury) P11.3
- oculofacial, congenital (Moebius) Q87.0
- palate (soft) K13.79
- progressive, spinal G12.25
- pseudohypertrophic (muscle) G71.09
- psychogenic F44.4
- radicular NEC
  - upper limbs, newborn (birth injury) P14.3
- recurrent isolated sleep G47.53
- respiratory (muscle) (system) (tract) R06.81
  - center NEC G93.89
  - congenital P28.89
  - newborn P28.89
- right side—*see* Hemiplegia
- saturnine—*see* subcategory T56.0
- sleep, recurrent isolated G47.53
- spastic G83.9
  - cerebral G80.-
  - congenital (cerebral) G80.-
- spinal (cord) G83.9
- spinal progressive G12.25
  - pseudohypertrophic G71.02
- syndrome G83.9
- sympathetic G90.89
- uveoparotitic D86.89
- uvula K13.79
- vasomotor NEC G90.89
- velum palate K13.79
- vocal cords J38.00
  - bilateral J38.02
  - unilateral J38.01

Paramenia N92.6

Paramyoclonus multiplex G25.3

Paranoid
- personality F60.0
- traits F60.0
- trends F60.0
- type, psychopathic personality F60.0

Paraphimosis (congenital) N47.2

Paraplegia (lower) G82.20
- complete G82.21
- functional (hysterical) F44.4
- hysterical F44.4
- incomplete G82.22
- psychogenic F44.4

Parasitic—*see also* Disease, diseased
- disease NEC B89
- stomatitis B37.0
- sycosis (beard) (scalp) B35.0

Parasitism B89
- intestinal B82.9
- skin B88.9
- specified—*see* Infestation

Parasomnia G47.50
- in conditions classified elsewhere G47.54
- nonorganic origin F51.8
- organic G47.50
- specified NEC G47.59

Paraspadias Q54.9

Paraspasmus facialis G51.8

Parasuicide (attempt)
- history of (personal) Z91.51
  - in family Z81.8

Paratrachoma A74.0

Parencephalitis—*see also* Encephalitis
- sequelae G09

Parent-child conflict—*see* Conflict, parent-child
- estrangement NEC Z62.890

Paresis—*see also* Paralysis
- bowel, colon or intestine K56.0
- pseudohypertrophic G71.09

Paronychia—*see also* Cellulitis
- with lymphangitis—*see* Lymphangitis, digit
- candidal (chronic) B37.2

Parorexia (psychogenic) F50.89

Parosmia R43.1
- psychogenic F45.8

Parry-Romberg syndrome G51.8

Particolored infant Q82.8

Parulis K04.7

Parvovirus, as the cause of disease classified elsewhere B97.6

Passage
- meconium (newborn) during delivery P03.82
- of sounds or bougies—*see* Attention to, artificial, opening

Passive—*see* Disease, diseased
- smoking Z77.22

Past due on rent or mortgage Z59.81-

Pasteurella septica A28.0

PAT (paroxysmal atrial tachycardia) I47.19

Patent—*see also* Imperfect, closure
- ductus arteriosus or Botallo's Q25.0
- foramen
  - botalli Q21.1
  - ovale Q21.1
- interauricular septum Q21.1
- interventricular septum Q21.0
- omphalomesenteric duct Q43.0
- ostium secundum Q21.1
- vitelline duct Q43.0

Pathologic, pathological—*see also* Disease, diseased
- asphyxia R09.01

Pattern, sleep-wake, irregular G47.23

ALPHABETIC INDEX

Patulous—*see also* Imperfect, closure (congenital)
- alimentary tract Q45.8
  - lower Q43.8
  - upper Q40.8

Pause, sinoatrial I49.5

Pectenosis K62.4

Pectus
- carinatum (congenital) Q67.7
- excavatum (congenital) Q67.6
- recurvatum (congenital) Q67.6

Pediculosis (infestation) B85.2
- capitis (head-louse) (any site) B85.0
- corporis (body-louse) (any site) B85.1
- eyelid B85.0
- mixed (classifiable to more than one of the titles B85.0–B85.3) B85.4
- pubis (pubic louse) (any site) B85.3
- vestimenti B85.1
- vulvae B85.3

Pediculus (infestation)—*see* Pediculosis

Pelger-Huët anomaly or syndrome D72.0

Pelizaeus-Merzbacher disease E75.27

Pelvic—*see also* Disease, diseased
- examination (periodic) (routine) Z01.419
  - with abnormal findings Z01.411
- kidney, congenital Q63.2

Pelviperitonitis—*see also* Peritonitis, pelvic
- gonococcal A54.24

Pemphigus
- benign familial (chronic) Q82.8

Pentosuria (essential) E74.89

Perforation, perforated (nontraumatic) (of)
- accidental during procedure (blood vessel) (nerve) (organ)— see Complication
- antrum—see Sinusitis, maxillary
- appendix K35.32
- atrial septum, multiple Q21.1
- by
  - device, implant or graft (*see also* Complications, by site and type, mechanical) T85.628
    - catheter NEC T85.698
      - cystostomy T83.090
      - urinary—*see also* Complications, catheter, urinary T83.098
    - ventricular intracranial shunt T85.09
  - instrument (any) during a procedure, accidental—see Puncture
- cecum K35.32
- ear drum—see Perforation, tympanum
- nasal
  - septum J34.89
    - congenital Q30.3
  - sinus J34.89
    - congenital Q30.8
  - due to sinusitis—see Sinusitis
- palate (*see also* Cleft, palate) Q35.9
- palatine vault (*see also* Cleft, palate, hard) Q35.1
- sinus (accessory) (chronic) (nasal) J34.89
- sphenoidal sinus—see Sinusitis, sphenoidal
- tympanum, tympanic (membrane) (persistent post-traumatic) (postinflammatory) H72.9-
  - attic H72.1-
    - multiple H72.81-
    - total H72.82-
  - central H72.0-
    - multiple H72.81-
    - total H72.82-
  - marginal NEC—*see* subcategory H72.2
    - multiple H72.81-
    - pars flaccida—*see* Perforation, tympanum, attic
    - total H72.82-
  - traumatic, current episode S09.2-
- uvula K13.79

Periadenitis mucosa necrotica recurrens K12.0

Pericardial effusion
- malignant in diseases classified elsewhere I31.31
- other (noninflammatory) I31.39

Pericarditis (with decompensation) (with effusion) I31.9
- with rheumatic fever (conditions in I00)
  - active—*see* Pericarditis, rheumatic
  - inactive or quiescent I09.2
- acute (hemorrhagic) (nonrheumatic) (Sicca) I30.9
  - with chorea (acute) (rheumatic) (Sydenham's) I02.0
  - benign I30.8
  - nonspecific I30.0
  - rheumatic I01.0
    - with chorea (acute) (Sydenham's) I02.0
- adhesive or adherent (chronic) (external) (internal) I31.0
  - acute—*see* Pericarditis, acute
  - rheumatic I09.2
- bacterial (acute) (subacute) (with serous or seropurulent effusion) I30.1
- calcareous I31.1
- cholesterol (chronic) I31.8
  - acute I30.9
- chronic (nonrheumatic) I31.9
  - rheumatic I09.2
- constrictive (chronic) I31.1
- coxsackie B33.23
- fibrinopurulent I30.1
- fibrinous I30.8
- fibrous I31.0
- idiopathic I30.0
- in systemic lupus erythematosus M32.12
- infective I30.1
- meningococcal A39.53
- neoplastic (chronic) I31.8
  - acute I30.9
- obliterans, obliterating I31.0
- plastic I31.0
- pneumococcal I30.1
- purulent I30.1
- rheumatic (active) (acute) (with effusion) (with pneumonia) I01.0
  - with chorea (acute) (rheumatic) (Sydenham's) I02.0
  - chronic or inactive (with chorea) I09.2
- septic I30.1
- serofibrinous I30.8
- staphylococcal I30.1
- streptococcal I30.1
- suppurative I30.1
- syphilitic A52.06
- tuberculous A18.84
- viral I30.1

Perichondritis
- auricle—*see* Perichondritis, ear
- bronchus J98.09
- ear (external) H61.00-
  - acute H61.01-
  - chronic H61.02-
- nose J34.89

Periepididymitis N45.1

Perilabyrinthitis (acute)—*see* subcategory H83.0

Periods—*see also* Menstruation
- heavy N92.0
- irregular N92.6
- shortened intervals (irregular) N92.1

Periorchitis N45.2

Periproctitis K62.89

Peritonitis (adhesive) (bacterial) (fibrinous) (hemorrhagic) (idiopathic) (localized) (perforative) (primary) (with adhesions) (with effusion) K65.9
- with or following
  - abscess K65.1
  - appendicitis
    - with perforation or rupture K35.32
      - generalized K35.20
      - localized K35.30
  - acute (generalized) K65.0
- chlamydial A74.81
- diaphragmatic K65.0
- diffuse K65.0
- disseminated K65.0
- eosinophilic K65.8
  - acute K65.0
- fibropurulent K65.0
- general (ized) K65.0
- meconium (newborn) P78.0

Peritonitis, *continued*
- neonatal P78.1
  - meconium P78.0
- pancreatic K65.0
- pelvic
  - female N73.5
    - acute N73.3
    - chronic N73.4
      - with adhesions N73.6
  - male K65.0
- purulent K65.0
- septic K65.0
- specified NEC K65.8
- spontaneous bacterial K65.2
- subdiaphragmatic K65.0
- subphrenic K65.0
- suppurative K65.0

Peritonsillitis J36

Perlèche NEC K13.0
- due to
  - candidiasis B37.83
  - moniliasis B37.83

Persistence, persistent (congenital)
- anal membrane Q42.3
  - with fistula Q42.2
- atrioventricular canal Q21.2
- branchial cleft NOS Q18.2
  - cyst Q18.0
  - fistula Q18.0
  - sinus Q18.0
- canal of Cloquet Q14.0
- capsule (opaque) Q12.8
- cilioretinal artery or vein Q14.8
- convolutions
  - aortic arch Q25.46
  - fallopian tube Q50.6
  - oviduct Q50.6
  - uterine tube Q50.6
- fetal
  - circulation P29.38
  - hemoglobin, hereditary (HPFH) D56.4
- foramen
  - Botalli Q21.1
  - ovale Q21.1
- hemoglobin, fetal (hereditary) (HPFH) D56.4
- Meckel's diverticulum Q43.0
- omphalomesenteric duct Q43.0
- ostium
  - atrioventriculare commune Q21.2
  - primum Q21.2
  - secundum Q21.1
- ovarian rests in fallopian tube Q50.6
- primary (deciduous)
  - teeth K00.6
- sinus
  - urogenitalis
    - female Q52.8
    - male Q55.8
- thyroglossal duct Q89.2
- thyrolingual duct Q89.2
- truncus arteriosus or communis Q20.0
- tunica vasculosa lentis Q12.2
- vitelline duct Q43.0

Person (with)
- concern (normal) about sick person in family Z63.6
- consulting on behalf of another Z71.0
- feigning illness Z76.5
- living (in)
  - without
    - adequate housing Z59.10
    - air conditioning Z59.11
    - environmental temperature Z59.11
    - heating Z59.11
    - space Z59.19
    - housing (permanent) (temporary) Z59.00
    - person able to render necessary care Z74.2
    - shelter Z59.02

Personal history of (corrected)
- congenital diaphragmatic hernia or other congenital diaphragm malformations Z87.760
- congenital malformations of integument, limbs and musculoskeletal system Z87.768

PATULOUS–PERSONAL HISTORY OF (CORRECTED)

ALPHABETIC INDEX

Personal history of (corrected), *continued*
- gastroschisis Z87.761
- necrotizing enterocolitis of newborn Z87.61
- other conditions arising in the perinatal period Z87.68
- other congenital abdominal wall malformations Z87.763
- persistent cloaca or cloacal malformations Z87.732
- prune belly malformation Z87.762
- tracheoesophageal fistula or atresia Z87.731

Personality (disorder) F60.9
- affective F34.0
- aggressive F60.3
- amoral F60.2
- anacastlc, anankastic F60.5
- antisocial F60.2
- anxious F60.6
- asocial F60.2
- asthenic F60.7
- avoidant F60.6
- borderline F60.3
- compulsive F60.5
- cycloid F34.0
- cyclothymic F34.0
- depressive F34.1
- dissocial F60.2
- emotionally unstable F60.3
- expansive paranoid F60.0
- explosive F60.3
- fanatic F60.0
- histrionic F60.4
- hyperthymic F34.0
- hypothymic F34.1
- hysterical F60.4
- obsessional F60.5
- obsessive (-compulsive) F60.5
- organic F07.0
- overconscientious F60.5
- paranoid F60.0
- pathologic F60.9
- pattern defect or disturbance F60.9
- psychoinfantile F60.4
- psychopathic F60.2
- querulant F60.0
- schizoid F60.1
- sensitive paranoid F60.0
- sociopathic (amoral) (antisocial) (asocial) (dissocial) F60.2
- specified NEC F60.89

Perthes' disease M91.1-

Pertussis (*see also* Whooping cough) A37.90

Perversion, perverted
- appetite F50.89
  - psychogenic F50.89
- function
  - pituitary gland E23.2
    - posterior lobe E22.2
- sense of smell and taste R43.8
  - psychogenic F45.8
- sexual—*see* Deviation, sexual transvestism

Pervious, congenital—*see also* Imperfect, closure
- ductus arteriosus Q25.0

Pes (congenital)—*see also* Talipes
- adductus Q66.89
- cavus Q66.7-
- valgus Q66.6

Petechia, petechiae R23.3
- newborn P54.5

Petit mal seizure—*see* Epilepsy, generalized, specified NEC

Petit's hernia—*see* Hernia

- Peutz-Jeghers disease or syndrome Q85.8

Pfeiffer's disease—*see* Mononucleosis, infectious

Phagedena (dry) (moist) (sloughing)—*see also* Gangrene
- geometric L88

Phakomatosis Q85.9
- Bourneville's Q85.1
- other phakomatoses, not elsewhere classified Q85.89
- specified NEC Q85.8

Pharyngeal pouch syndrome D82.1

Pharyngitis (acute) (catarrhal) (gangrenous) (infective) (malignant) (membranous) (phlegmonous) (pseudomembranous) (simple) (subacute) (suppurative) (ulcerative) (viral) J02.9
- aphthous B08.5
- atrophic J31.2
- chlamydial A56.4
- chronic (atrophic) (granular) (hypertrophic) J31.2
- coxsackievirus B08.5
- enteroviral vesicular B08.5
- follicular (chronic) J31.2
- granular (chronic) J31.2
- herpesvirai B00.2
- hypertrophic J31.2
- infectional, chronic J31.2
- influenzal—*see* Influenza, with, respiratory manifestations NEC
- pneumococcal J02.8
- purulent J02.9
- putrid J02.9
- septic J02.0
- sicca J31.2
- specified organism NEC J02.8
- staphylococcal J02.8
- streptococcal J02.0
- vesicular, enteroviral B08.5
- viral NEC J02.8

Pharyngolaryngitis (acute) J06.0
- chronic J37.0

Pharyngotonsillitis, herpesviral B00.2

Phenomenon
- vasomotor R55
- vasovagal R55
- Wenckebach's I44.1

Phenotype
- Duffy
  - a positive Z67.A2
  - a and b positive Z67.A4
  - b positive Z67.A3
  - Fy (a+b-) Z67.A2
  - Fy (a-b-) Z67.A1
  - Fy (a-b+) Z67.A3
  - Fy (a+b+) Z67.A4
  - null Z67.A1

Phenylketonuria E70.1
- classical E70.0

Phimosis (congenital) (due to infection) N47.1

Phlebitis (infective) (pyemic) (septic) (suppurative) I80.9
- calf muscular vein (NOS) I80.25-
- femoral vein (superficial) I80.1-
- femoropopliteal vein I80.0-
- gastrocnemial vein I80.25-
- hepatic veins I80.8
- iliac vein (common) (external) (internal) I80.21-
- iliofemoral—*see* Phlebitis, femoral vein
- leg I80.3
  - deep (vessels) NEC I80.20-
    - iliac I80.21-
    - popliteal vein I80.22-
    - specified vessel NEC I80.29-
    - tibial vein I80.23-
  - femoral vein (superficial) I80.1-
  - superficial (vessels) I80.0-
- lower limb—*see* Phlebitis, leg
- peroneal vein I80.24-
- popliteal vein—*see* Phlebitis, leg
- saphenous (accessory) (great) (long) (small)—*see* Phlebitis, leg
- soleal vein I80.25-
- specified site NEC I80.8
- tibial vein—*see* Phlebitis, leg
- ulcerative I80.9
  - leg—*see* Phlebitis, leg
- umbilicus I80.8

Phobia, phobic F40.9
- reaction F40.9
- state F40.9

Photodermatitis (sun) L56.8
- chronic L57.8
- due to drug L56.8

Photosensitivity, photosensitization (sun) skin L56.8

Phthiriasis (pubis) B85.3
- with any infestation classifiable to B85.0–B85.2 B85.4

Physical restraint status Z78.1

Pica F50.89
- in adults F50.89
- infant or child (in remission) F98.3

Picking, nose F98.8

Pickwickian syndrome E66.2

Pierre Robin deformity or syndrome Q87.0

Pig-bel A05.2

Pigeon
- breast or chest (acquired) M95.4
  - congenital Q67.7

Pigmentation (abnormal) (anomaly) L81.9
- iron L81.8
- lids, congenital Q82.8
- metals L81.8
- optic papilla, congenital Q14.2
- retina, congenital (grouped) (nevoid) Q14.1
- scrotum, congenital Q82.8
- tattoo L81.8

Piles (*see also* Hemorrhoids) K64.9

Pinhole meatus (*see also* Stricture, urethra) N35.919

Pink
- eye—*see* Conjunctivitis, acute, mucopurulent

Pinworm (disease) (infection) (infestation) B80

Pithecoid pelvis Q74.2

Pitting (*see also* Edema) R60.9
- lip R60.0
- nail L60.8

Pityriasis (capitis) L21.0
- alba L30.5
- circinata (et maculata) L42
- furfuracea L21.0
- maculata (et circinata) L30.5
- rosea L42
- simplex L30.5
- specified type NEC L30.5
- streptogenes L30.5
- versicolor (scrotal) B36.0

Plagiocephaly Q67.3
- non-deformational
  - anterior Q75.021–
  - posterior Q75.04-

Plaque(s)
- epicardial I31.8

Planning, family
- contraception Z30.9
- procreation Z31.69

Plasmacytopenia D72.818

Plasmacytosis D72.822

Platybasia Q75.8

Platyonychia (congenital) Q84.6
- acquired L60.8

Platypelloid pelvis M95.5
- congenital Q74.2

Plethora R23.2
- newborn P61.1

Pleurisy (acute) (adhesive) (chronic) (costal) (diaphragmatic) (double) (dry) (fibrinous) (fibrous) (interlobar) (latent) (plastic) (primary) (residual) (sicca) (sterile) (subacute) (unresolved) R09.1
- with
  - adherent pleura J86.0
  - effusion J90
- pneumococcal J90
- purulent—*see* Pyothorax
- septic—*see* Pyothorax
- serofibrinous—*see* Pleurisy, with effusion
- seropurulent—*see* Pyothorax
- serous—*see* Pleurisy, with effusion
- staphylococcal J86.9
- streptococcal J90
- suppurative—*see* Pyothorax

Pleuropericarditis—*see also* Pericarditis
- acute I30.9

ALPHABETIC INDEX

Pleuro-pneumonia-like organism (PPLO), as the cause of disease classified elsewhere B96.0

Plica
- polonica B85.0
- tonsil J35.8

Plug
- meconium (newborn) NEC syndrome P76.0
- mucus—*see* Asphyxia

Plumbism—*see* subcategory T56.0

PMEI (polymorphic epilepsy in infancy) G40.83-

Pneumatocele (lung) J98.4
- intracranial G93.89

Pneumaturia R39.89

Pneumocephalus G93.89

Pneumococcemia A40.3

Pneumococcus, pneumococcal—*see* Disease, diseased

Pneumohemopericardium I31.2

Pneumomediastinum J98.2
- congenital or perinatal P25.2

Pneumonia (acute) (double) (migratory) (purulent) (septic) (unresolved) J18.9
- with
  - due to specified organism—*see* Pneumonia, in (due to)
  - influenza—*see* Influenza, with, pneumonia
- 2019 (novel) coronavirus J12.82
- anaerobes J15.8
- anthrax A22.1
- Ascaris B77.81
- aspiration J69.0
  - due to
    - aspiration of microorganisms
      - bacterial J15.9
      - viral J12.9
    - food (regurgitated) J69.0
    - gastric secretions J69.0
    - milk (regurgitated) J69.0
    - oils, essences J69.1
    - solids, liquids NEC J69.8
    - vomitus J69.0
  - newborn P24.81
    - amniotic fluid (clear) P24.11
    - blood P24.21
    - food (regurgitated) P24.31
    - liquor (amnii) P24.11
    - meconium P24.01
    - milk P24.31
    - mucus P24.11
    - specified NEC P24.81
    - stomach contents P24.31
- atypical NEC J18.9
- bacillus J15.9
  - specified NEC J15.8
- bacterial J15.9
  - specified NEC J15.8
- Bacteroides (fragilis) (oralis) (melaninogenicus) J15.8
- broncho-, bronchial (confluent) (croupous) (diffuse) (disseminated) (hemorrhagic) (involving lobes) (lobar) (terminal) J18.0
  - aspiration—*see* Pneumonia, aspiration
    - bacterial J15.9
      - specified NEC J15.8
    - diplococcal J13
    - Eaton's agent J15.7
    - Escherichia coli (E. coli) J15.5
    - Friedländer's bacillus J15.0
    - Hemophilus influenzae J14
    - inhalation—*see also* Pneumonia, aspiration
      - of oils or essences J69.1
    - Klebsiella (pneumoniae) J15.0
    - lipid, lipoid J69.1
    - Mycoplasma (pneumoniae) J15.7
    - pleuro-pneumonia-like-organisms (PPLO) J15.7
    - pneumococcal J13
    - Proteus J15.69
    - Pseudomonas J15.1
    - Serratia marcescens J15.69
    - specified organism NEC J16.8

Pneumonia, *continued*
  - streptococcal NEC J15.4
    - group B J15.3
      - pneumoniae J13
- Butyrivibrio (fibriosolvens) J15.8
- Candida B37.1
- chlamydial J16.0
  - congenital P23.1
- Clostridium (haemolyticum) (novyi) J15.8
- confluent—*see* Pneumonia, broncho
- congenital (infective) P23.9
  - due to
    - bacterium NEC P23.6
    - Chlamydia P23.1
    - Escherichia coli P23.4
    - Haemophilus influenzae P23.6
    - infective organism NEC P23.8
    - Klebsiella pneumoniae P23.6
    - Mycoplasma P23.6
    - Pseudomonas P23.5
    - Staphylococcus P23.2
    - Streptococcus (except group B) P23.6
      - group B P23.3
    - viral agent P23.0
  - specified NEC P23.8
- coronavirus (novel) (disease) 2019 J12.82
- croupous—*see* Pneumonia, lobar
- cytomegalovirus (CMV) B25.0
- diplococcal, diplococcus (broncho-) (lobar) J13
- Eaton's agent J15.7
- Enterobacter J15.69
- Escherichia coli (E. coli) J15.5
- Eubacterium J15.8
- Friedländer's bacillus J15.0
- Fusobacterium (nucleatum) J15.8
- giant cell (measles) B05.2
- gram-negative bacteria NEC J15.69
  - anaerobic J15.8
- Hemophilus influenzae (broncho-) (lobar) J14
- human metapneumovirus (hMPV) J12.3
- in (due to)
  - -Acinetobacter baumannii J15.61
    - actinomycosis A42.0
    - adenovirus J12.0
    - anthrax A22.1
    - ascariasis B77.81
    - aspergillosis B44.9
    - Bacillus anthracis A22.1
    - Bacterium anitratum J15.69
    - candidiasis B37.1
    - chickenpox B01.2
    - Chlamydia J16.0
      - neonatal P23.1
    - cytomegalovirus disease B25.0
    - Diplococcus (pneumoniae) J13
    - Eaton's agent J15.7
    - Enterobacter J15.69
    - Escherichia coli (E. coli) J15.5
    - Friedländer's bacillus J15.0
    - gonorrhea A54.84
    - Hemophilus influenzae (H. influenzae) J14
    - Herелlea J15.69
    - human metapneumovirus (hMPV) J12.3
    - Klebsiella (pneumoniae) J15.0
    - measles B05.2
    - Mycoplasma (pneumoniae) J15.7
    - nocardiosis, nocardiasis A43.0
    - parainfluenza virus J12.2
    - pleuro-pneumonia-like-organism (PPLO) J15.7
    - pneumococcus J13
    - Proteus J15.69
    - Pseudomonas NEC J15.1
    - rheumatic fever I00 [J17]
    - Serratia marcescens J15.69
    - specified
      - bacterium NEC J15.8
      - organism NEC J16.8
    - Staphylococcus J15.20
      - aureus (methicillin susceptible) (MSSA) J15.211
        - methicillin resistant (MRSA) J15.212
      - specified NEC J15.29

Pneumonia, *continued*
  - Streptococcus J15.4
    - group B J15.3
      - pneumoniae J13
    - specified NEC J15.4
  - varicella B01.2
  - whooping cough A37.91
    - due to
      - Bordetella parapertussis A37.11
      - Bordetella pertussis A37.01
      - specified NEC A37.81
- inhalation of food or vomit—*see* Pneumonia, aspiration
- interstitial J84.9
  - pseudomonas J15.1
- Klebsiella (pneumoniae) J15.0
- lipid, lipoid (exogenous) J69.1
- lobar (disseminated) (double) (interstitial) J18.1
  - bacterial J15.9
    - specified NEC J15.8
  - Escherichia coli (E. coli) J15.5
  - Friedländer's bacillus J15.0
  - Hemophilus influenzae J14
  - Klebsiella (pneumoniae) J15.0
  - pneumococcal J13
  - Proteus J15.6
  - Pseudomonas J15.1
  - specified organism NEC J16.8
  - staphylococcal—*see* Pneumonia, staphylococcal
  - streptococcal NEC J15.4
  - Streptococcus pneumoniae J13
  - viral, virus—*see* Pneumonia, viral
- lobular—*see* Pneumonia, broncho
- massive—*see* Pneumonia, lobar
- meconium P24.01
- MRSA (methicillin resistant Staphylococcus aureus) J15.212
- MSSA (methicillin susceptible Staphylococcus aureus) J15.211
- multilobar—*see* Pneumonia, by type
- Mycoplasma (pneumoniae) J15.7
- neonatal P23.9
  - aspiration—*see* Aspiration, by substance, with pneumonia
- parainfluenza virus J12.2
- Peptococcus J15.8
- Peptostreptococcus J15.8
- pleuro-pneumonia-like organism (PPLO) J15.7
- pneumococcal (broncho-) (lobar) J13
- postinfectional NEC B99 [J17]
- postmeasles B05.2
- Proteus J15.6
- Pseudomonas J15.1
- respiratory syncytial virus (RSV) J12.1
- resulting from a procedure J95.89
- rheumatic I00 [J17]
- SARS-associated coronavirus J12.81
- Serratia marcescens J15.6
- specified NEC J18.8
  - bacterium NEC J15.8
  - organism NEC J16.8
  - virus NEC J12.89
- staphylococcal (broncho) (lobar) J15.20
  - aureus (methicillin susceptible) (MSSA) J15.211
    - methicillin resistant (MRSA) J15.212
  - specified NEC J15.29
- streptococcal NEC (broncho) (lobar) J15.4
  - group
    - A J15.4
    - B J15.3
    - specified NEC J15.4
- Streptococcus pneumoniae J13
- varicella B01.2
- Veillonella J15.8
- ventilator associated J95.851
- viral, virus (broncho) (interstitial) (lobar) J12.9
  - congenital P23.0
  - human metapneumovirus (hMPV) J12.3
  - parainfluenza J12.2
  - respiratory syncytial (RSV) J12.1
  - SARS-associated coronavirus J12.81
  - specified NEC J12.89

ALPHABETIC INDEX

Pneumonitis (acute) (primary)—*see also* Pneumonia
- aspiration J69.0
- congenital rubella P35.0
- due to
  - detergent J69.8
  - food, vomit (aspiration) J69.0
  - inhalation
    - ■ blood J69.8
    - ■ essences J69.1
    - ■ food (regurgitated), milk, vomit J69.0
    - ■ oils, essences J69.1
    - ■ saliva J69.0
    - ■ solids, liquids NEC J69.8
    - – oils, essences J69.1
  - solids, liquids NEC J69.8
  - toxoplasmosis (acquired) B58.3
    - ■ congenital P37.1
  - ventilator J95.851
- meconium P24.01
- rubella, congenital P35.0
- ventilator associated J95.851

Pneumopathy NEC J98.4
- alveolar J84.09
- parietoalveolar J84.09

Pneumopericarditis—*see also* Pericarditis
- acute I30.9

Pneumopericardium—*see also* Pericarditis
- congenital P25.3
- newborn P25.3

Pneumophagia (psychogenic) F45.8

Pneumopyopericardium I30.1

Pneumopyothorax—*see* Pyopneumothorax
- with fistula J86.0

Pneumothorax NOS J93.9
- acute J93.83
- chronic J93.81
- congenital P25.1
- perinatal period P25.1
- postprocedural J95.811
- specified NEC J93.83
- spontaneous NOS J93.83
  - newborn P25.1
  - primary J93.11
  - secondary J93.12
  - tension J93.0
- tense valvular, infectional J93.0
- tension (spontaneous) J93.0
- traumatic S27.0

Podencephalus Q01.9

Poikiloderma L81.6
- congenital Q82.8

Pointed ear (congenital) Q17.3

Poison ivy, oak, sumac or other plant dermatitis (allergic) (contact) L23.7

Poisoning (acute)—*see also* Table of Drugs and Chemicals
- algae and toxins T65.82-
- Bacillus B (aertrycke) (cholerae (suis)) (paratyphosus) (suipestifer) A02.9
  - botulinus A05.1
- bacterial toxins A05.9
- berries, noxious—*see* Poisoning, food, noxious, berries
- botulism A05.1
- Clostridium botulinum A05.1
- drug—*see* Table of Drugs and Chemicals, by drug, poisoning
- epidemic, fish (noxious)—*see* Poisoning, food, noxious or naturally toxic, seafood
  - bacterial A05.9
- fava bean D55.0
- food (acute) (diseased) (infected) (noxious) NEC A05.9
  - bacterial—*see* Intoxication, foodborne, by agent
  - due to
    - ■ Bacillus (aertrycke) (choleraesuis) (paratyphosus) (suipestifer) A02.9
    - ~ botulinus A05.1
    - ■ Clostridium (perfringens) (Welchii) A05.2
    - ■ salmonella (aertrycke) (choleraesuis) (enteritidis) (gallinarum) (paratyphi) (suipestifer) A02.9

Poisoning, *continued*
  - ~ with
    - ◊ gastroenteritis A02.0
    - ◊ sepsis A02.1
    - ■ staphylococcus A05.0
    - ■ Vibrio
    - – parahaemolyticus A05.3
    - – vulnificus A05.5
  - noxious or naturally toxic
    - ■ berries—*see* subcategory T62.1-
    - ■ fish—*see* Poisoning, food, noxious or naturally toxic, seafood
    - ■ mushrooms—*see* subcategory T62.0X-
    - ■ plants NEC—*see* subcategory T62.2X-
    - ■ seafood—*see* Poisoning, food, noxious or naturally toxic, seafood
    - ■ specified NEC—*see* subcategory T62.8X-
- kreotoxism, food A05.9
- lead T56.0-
- methamphetamines, underdosing T43.65-
- mushroom—*see* Poisoning, food, noxious, mushroom
- mussels—*see also* Poisoning
  - bacterial—*see* Intoxication, foodborne, by agent
- shellfish (amnesic) (azaspiracid) (diarrheic) (neurotoxic) (noxious) (paralytic) T61.78-
- Staphylococcus, food A05.0

Poliomyelitis (acute) (anterior) (epidemic) A80.9
- congenital P35.8 (if included in tabular list)
- imported A80.1
- indigenous A80.2
  - spinal, acute A80.9
- nonepidemic A80.9
- paralytic
  - specified NEC A80.39
  - wild virus

Pollakiuria R35.0
- psychogenic F45.8

Pollinosis J30.1

Pollitzer's disease L73.2

Polycystic (disease)
- degeneration, kidney Q61.3
  - autosomal recessive (infantile type) NEC Q61.19
- kidney Q61.3
  - autosomal
    - ■ recessive NEC Q61.19
  - autosomal recessive (childhood type) NEC Q61.19
  - infantile type NEC Q61.19
- ovary, ovaries E28.2

Polycythemia (secondary) D75.1
- acquired D75.1
- benign (familial) D75.0
- due to
  - donor twin P61.1
  - erythropoietin D75.1
  - fall in plasma volume D75.1
  - high altitude D75.1
  - maternal-fetal transfusion P61.1
  - stress D75.1
- emotional D75.1
- erythropoietin D75.1
- familial (benign) D75.0
- Gaisböck's (hypertonica) D75.1
- high altitude D75.1
- hypertonica D75.1
- hypoxemic D75.1
- neonatorum P61.1
- nephrogenous D75.1
- relative D75.1
- secondary D75.1
- spurious D75.1
- stress D75.1

Polycytosis cryptogenica D75.1

Polydactylism, polydactyly Q69.9
- toes Q69.2

Polydipsia R63.1

Polydystrophy, pseudo-Hurler E77.0

Polyhydramnios O40.-

Polymenorrhea N92.0

Polyneuritis, polyneuritic—*see also* Polyneuropathy
- cranialis G52.7
- inflammatory G61.9

Polyneuropathy (peripheral) G62.9
- hereditary G60.9
  - specified NEC G60.8
- in (due to)
  - hypoglycemia E16.2 *[G63]*
  - infectious
    - ■ disease NEC B99 *[G63]*
    - ■ mononucleosis B27.91
  - Lyme disease A69.22
  - neoplastic disease (*see also* Table of Neoplasms in the complete *ICD-10-CM* manual) D49.9 *[G63]*
  - sarcoidosis D86.89
  - systemic
    - ■ lupus erythematosus M32.19
- sensory (hereditary) (idiopathic) G60.8

Polyopia H53.8

Polyorchism, polyorchidism Q55.21

Polyp, polypus
- accessory sinus J33.8
- adenoid tissue J33.0
- antrum J33.8
- anus, anal (canal) K62.0
- choanal J33.0
- colon K63.5
  - adenomatous D12.6
    - ■ sigmoid D12.5
    - ■ transverse D12.3
  - ascending K63.5
  - cecum K63.5
  - descending K63.5
  - inflammatory K51.40
    - with
      - abscess K51.414
    - complication K51.419
      - ◊ specified NEC K51.418
    - fistula K51.413
    - intestinal obstruction K51.412
    - rectal bleeding K51.411
  - sigmoid K63.5
  - transverse K63.5
- esophageal K22.81
- esophagogastric junction K22.82
- ethmoidal (sinus) J33.8
- frontal (sinus) J33.8
- maxillary (sinus) J33.8
- nares
  - anterior J33.9
  - posterior J33.0
- nasal (mucous) J33.9
  - cavity J33.0
  - septum J33.0
- nasopharyngeal J33.0
- nose (mucous) J33.9
- rectum (nonadenomatous) K62.1
- septum (nasal) J33.0
- sinus (accessory) (ethmoidal) (frontal) (maxillary) (sphenoidal) J33.8
- sphenoidal (sinus) J33.8
- turbinate, mucous membrane J33.8
- umbilical, newborn P83.6

Polyposis—*see also* Polyp
- coli (adenomatous) D12.6
- colon (adenomatous) D12.6
- familial D12.6
- intestinal (adenomatous) D12.6

Polyserositis
- due to pericarditis I31.1
- pericardial I31.1

Polysyndactyly (*see also* Syndactylism) Q70.4

Polyuria R35.89
- nocturnal R35.81
- psychogenic F45.8
- specified NEC R35.89

Pomphylox L30.1

Poor
- urinary stream R39.12
- vision NEC H54.7

ALPHABETIC INDEX

Porencephaly (congenital) (developmental) (true) Q04.6
- acquired G93.0
  - nondevelopmental G93.0
  - traumatic (post) F07.89

Porocephaliasis B88.8

Porokeratosis Q82.8

Port wine nevus, mark, or stain Q82.5

Positive
- culture (nonspecific)
  - blood R78.81
  - bronchial washings R84.5
  - cerebrospinal fluid R83.5
  - nose R84.5
    - *staphylococcus* (Methicillin susceptible) Z22.321
      - Methicillin resistant Z22.322
  - urine R82.79
- PPD (skin test) R76.11
- serology for syphilis A53.0
  - false R76.8
  - with signs or symptoms—*code as* Syphilis, by site and stage
- skin test, tuberculin (without active tuberculosis) R76.11
- test, human immunodeficiency virus (HIV) R75
- VDRL A53.0
  - with signs and symptoms—*code by* site and stage under Syphilis A53.9
- Wassermann reaction A53.0

Postcardiotomy syndrome I97.0

Postcommissurotomy syndrome I97.0

Postconcussional syndrome F07.81

Postcontusional syndrome F07.81

Post COVID-19 condition, unspecified U09.9

Posthemorrhagic anemia (chronic) D50.0
- acute D62
- newborn P61.3

Postmaturity, postmature (over 42 weeks)
- newborn P08.22

Postmeasles complication NEC (*see also* Disease, diseased) B05.89

Postnasal drip R09.82
- due to
  - allergic rhinitis—*see* Rhinitis, allergic
  - common cold J00
  - gastroesophageal reflux—*see* Reflux, gastroesophageal
  - nasopharyngitis—*see* Nasopharyngitis
  - other known condition—*code to* condition
  - sinusitis—*see* Sinusitis

Postoperative (postprocedural)—*see* Complication, postprocedural
- state NEC Z98.890

Post-term (40-42 weeks) (pregnancy) (mother)
- infant P08.21

Post-traumatic brain syndrome, nonpsychotic F07.81

Postural orthostatic tachycardia syndrome [POTS] G90.A

Postvaccinal reaction or complication—*see* Complications, vaccination

Postvalvulotomy syndrome I97.0

Potter's
- facies Q60.6
- syndrome (with renal agenesis) Q60.6

Poultryman's itch B88.0

Poverty NEC Z59.6
- extreme Z59.5

Prader-Willi syndrome Q87.11

Precocious
- adrenarche E30.1
- menarche E30.1
- menstruation E30.1
- pubarche E30.1
- puberty E30.1
  - central E22.8
- sexual development NEC E30.1

Precocity, sexual (constitutional) (female) (idiopathic) (male) E30.1
- with adrenal hyperplasia E25.9
  - congenital E25.0

Prediabetes, prediabetic R73.03

Pre-eclampsia O14.9
- with pre-existing hypertension—*see* Hypertension, complicating, pregnancy, pre-existing, with, pre-eclampsia
- mild O14.0-
- moderate O14.0-
- severe O14.1
  - with hemolysis, elevated liver enzymes and low platelet count (HELLP) O14.2-

Pre-excitation atrioventricular conduction I45.6

Pregnancy (single) (uterine)—*see also* Delivery

Note: The Tabular must be reviewed for assignment of the appropriate character indicating the trimester of the pregnancy

Note: The Tabular must be reviewed for assignment of appropriate seventh character for multiple gestation codes in Chapter 15

- abdominal (ectopic) O00.00
  - with uterine pregnancy O00.01
  - with viable fetus O36.7-
- ampullar O00.10-
- broad ligament O00.80
- cervical O00.80
- complicated by (care of) (management affected by)
  - abnormal, abnormality
    - findings on antenatal screening of mother O28.9
      - biochemical O28.1
      - chromosomal O28.5
      - cytological O28.2
      - genetic O28.5
      - hematological O28.0
      - radiological O28.4
      - specified NEC O28.8
      - ultrasonic O28.3
  - conjoined twins O30.02-
  - death of fetus (near term) O36.4
    - early pregnancy O02.1
  - decreased fetal movement O36.81-
  - diabetes (mellitus)
    - gestational (pregnancy induced—*see* Diabetes, gestational
      - type 1 O24.01-
      - type 2 O24.11-
  - edema
    - with
      - gestational hypertension, mild (*see also* Pre-eclampsia) O14.0-
  - fetal (maternal care for)
    - abnormality or damage O35.9
      - specified type NEC O35.8
    - anemia and thrombocytopenia O36.82-
    - anencephaly O35.0
    - bradycardia O36.83-
    - chromosomal abnormality (conditions in Q90 – Q99) O35.1
    - conjoined twins O30.02-
    - damage from
      - amniocentesis O35.7
      - biopsy procedures O35.7
      - drug addiction O35.5
      - hematological investigation O35.7
      - intrauterine contraceptive device O35.7
    - maternal
      - alcohol addiction O35.4
      - cytomegalovirus infection O35.3
      - disease NEC O35.8
      - drug addiction O35.5
      - listeriosis O35.8
      - rubella O35.3
      - toxoplasmosis O35.8
      - viral infection O35.3
    - medical procedure NEC O35.7
    - radiation O35.6
  - death (near term) O36.4
    - early pregnancy O02.1
  - decreased movement O36.81-
  - depressed heart rate tones O36.83-
  - excessive growth (large for dates) O36.6-
  - fetal heart rate or rhythm O36.83-

Pregnancy, *continued*
- growth retardation O36.59-
  - light for dates O36.59-
  - small for dates O36.59-
- heart rate irregularity (abnormal variability) (bradycardia) (decelerations) (tachycardia) O36.83-
- hereditary disease O35.2
- hydrocephalus O35.0
- intrauterine death O36.4
- non-reassuring heart rate or rhythm O36.83-
- poor growth O36.59-
  - light for dates O36.59-
  - small for dates O36.59-
- problem O36.9-
  - specified NEC O36.89-
- spina bifida O35.0
- thrombocytopenia O36.82-
- HELLP syndrome (hemolysis, elevated liver enzymes and low platelet count) O14.2-
- hemorrhage
  - before 20 completed weeks gestation O20.9
    - specified NEC O20.8
  - early O20.9
    - specified NEC O20.8
  - threatened abortion O20.0
- hydramnios O40.-
- hydrops
  - amnii O40.-
  - fetalis O36.2-
    - associated with isoimmunization (*see also* Pregnancy, complicated by, isoimmunization) O36.11-
- hydrorrhea O42.90
- inconclusive fetal viability O36.80
- intrauterine fetal death (near term) O36.4
  - early pregnancy O02.1
- isoimmunization O36.11-
  - anti-A sensitization O36.11-
  - anti-B sensitization O36.19-
  - Rh O36.09-
    - anti-D antibody O36.01-
    - specified NEC O36.19-
- missed
  - abortion O02.1
  - delivery O36.4
- multiple gestations
  - conjoined twins O30.02-
  - specified number of multiples NEC—*see* Pregnancy, multiple (gestation), specified NEC
  - quadruplet—*see* Pregnancy, quadruplet
  - specified complication NEC O31.8X-
  - triplet—*see* Pregnancy, triplet
  - twin—*see* Pregnancy, twin
- oligohydramnios O41.0-
  - with premature rupture of membranes (*see also* Pregnancy, complicated, premature rupture of membranes) O42.-
- placental insufficiency O36.51-
- polyhydramnios O40.-
- pre-eclampsia O14.9-
  - mild O14.0-
  - moderate O14.0-
  - severe O14.1-
    - with hemolysis, elevated liver enzymes and low platelet count (HELLP) O14.2-
- premature rupture of membranes O42.90
  - after 37 weeks gestation O42.92
  - full-term, unspec as to length of time between rupture and onset of labor O42.92
  - with onset of labor
    - within 24 hours O42.00
      - at or after 37 weeks gestation O42.02
      - pre-term (before 37 completed weeks of gestation) O42.01-
    - after 24 hours O42.10
      - at or after 37 weeks gestation O42.12
      - pre-term (before 37 completed weeks of gestation) O42.11-
  - pre-term (before 37 completed weeks of gestation) O42.91-

ALPHABETIC INDEX

Pregnancy, *continued*

- preterm labor
  - ■ second trimester
    - without delivery O60.02
  - ■ third trimester
    - without delivery O60.03
  - ■ without delivery
    - second trimester O60.02
    - third trimester O60.03
- Rh immunization, incompatibility or sensitization NEC O36.09-
  - ■ anti-D antibody O36.01-
  - threatened
    - ■ abortion O20.0
  - young mother
    - ■ multigravida O09.62-
    - ■ primigravida O09.61-
- cornual O00.8-
- ectopic (ruptured) O00.9-
  - abdominal O00.00
    - ■ with uterine pregnancy O00.01
    - ■ with viable fetus O36.7-
  - cervical O00.8-
  - cornual O00.8-
  - intraligamentous O00.8-
  - mural O00.8-
  - ovarian O00.20-
  - specified site NEC O00.8-
  - tubal (ruptured) O00.10-
    - ■ with intrauterine pregnancy O00.11
- fallopian O00.10-
  - with intrauterine pregnancy O00.11
- incidental finding Z33.1
- interstitial O00.8-
- intraligamentous O00.8-
- intramural O00.8-
- intraperitoneal O00.00
  - with intrauterine pregnancy O00.01
- isthmian O00.10-
- mesometric (mural) O00.8-
- multiple (gestation)
  - greater than quadruplets—*see* Pregnancy, multiple (gestation), specified NEC
  - specified NEC O30.80-
    - ■ number of chorions and amnions are both equal to the number of fetuses O30.83-
    - ■ two or more monoamniotic fetuses O30.82-
    - ■ two or more monochorionic fetuses O30.81-
    - ■ unable to determine number of placenta and number of amniotic sacs O30.89-
    - ■ unspecified number of placenta and unspecified number of amniotic sacs O30.80-
- mural O00.8-
- ovarian O00.2-
- quadruplet O30.20-
  - with
    - ■ two or more monoamniotic fetuses O30.22-
    - ■ two or more monochorionic fetuses O30.21-
  - quadrachorionic/quadra-amniotic O30.23-
  - two or more monoamniotic fetuses O30.22-
  - two or more monochorionic fetuses O30.21-
  - unable to determine number of placenta and number of amniotic sacs O30.29-
  - unspecified number of placenta and unspecified number of amniotic sacs O30.20-
- quintuplet—*see* Pregnancy, multiple (gestation), specified NEC
- sextuplet—*see* Pregnancy, multiple (gestation), specified NEC
- supervision of
  - young mother
    - ■ multigravida O09.62-
    - ■ primigravida O09.61-
- triplet O30.10-
  - with
    - ■ two or more monoamniotic fetuses O30.12-
    - ■ two or more monochorionic fetuses O30.11-
  - trichorionic/triamniotic O30.13-
  - two or more monoamniotic fetuses O30.12-
  - two or more monochorionic fetuses O30.11-
  - unable to determine number of placenta and number of amniotic sacs O30.19-

Pregnancy, *continued*

- unspecified number of placenta and unspecified number of amniotic sacs O30.10-
- tubal (with abortion) (with rupture) O00.10-
  - with intrauterine pregnancy O00.11
- twin O30.00-
  - conjoined O30.02-
  - dichorionic/diamniotic (two placentae, two amniotic sacs) O30.04-
  - monochorionic/diamniotic (one placenta, two amniotic sacs) O30.03-
  - monochorionic/monoamniotic (one placenta, one amniotic sac) O30.01-
  - unable to determine number of placenta and number of amniotic sacs O30.09-
  - unspecified number of placenta and unspecified number of amniotic sacs O30.00-
- unwanted Z64.0
- weeks of gestation
  - 8 weeks Z3A.08
  - 9 weeks Z3A.09
  - 10 weeks Z3A.10
  - 11 weeks Z3A.11
  - 12 weeks Z3A.12
  - 13 weeks Z3A.13
  - 14 weeks Z3A.14
  - 15 weeks Z3A.15
  - 16 weeks Z3A.16
  - 17 weeks Z3A.17
  - 18 weeks Z3A.18
  - 19 weeks Z3A.19
  - 20 weeks Z3A.20
  - 21 weeks Z3A.21
  - 22 weeks Z3A.22
  - 23 weeks Z3A.23
  - 24 weeks Z3A.24
  - 25 weeks Z3A.25
  - 26 weeks Z3A.26
  - 27 weeks Z3A.27
  - 28 weeks Z3A.28
  - 29 weeks Z3A.29
  - 30 weeks Z3A.30
  - 31 weeks Z3A.31
  - 32 weeks Z3A.32
  - 33 weeks Z3A.33
  - 34 weeks Z3A.34
  - 35 weeks Z3A.35
  - 36 weeks Z3A.36
  - 37 weeks Z3A.37
  - 38 weeks Z3A.38
  - 39 weeks Z3A.39
  - 40 weeks Z3A.40
  - 41 weeks Z3A.41
  - 42 weeks Z3A.42
  - greater than 42 weeks Z3A.49
  - less than 8 weeks Z3A.01
  - not specified Z3A.00

Premature—*see also* Disease, diseased

- beats I49.40
  - atrial I49.1
  - auricular I49.1
  - supraventricular I49.1
- birth NEC—*see* Preterm, newborn
- closure, foramen ovale Q21.8
- contraction
  - atrial I49.1
  - auricular I49.1
  - auriculoventricular I49.49
  - heart (extrasystole) I49.49
- lungs P28.0
- newborn
  - extreme (less than 28 completed weeks)—*see* Immaturity, extreme
  - less than 37 completed weeks—*see* Preterm, newborn
- puberty E30.1

Premenstrual

- dysphoric disorder (PMDD) F32.81
- tension N94.3

Prenatal

- teeth K00.6

Preponderance, left or right ventricular I51.7

Prescription of contraceptives (initial) Z30.019

- barrier Z30.018
- diaphragm Z30.018
- emergency (postcoital) Z30.012
- implantable subdermal Z30.017
- injectable Z30.013
- intrauterine contraceptive device Z30.014
- pills Z30.011
- postcoital (emergency) Z30.012
- repeat Z30.40
  - barrier Z30.49
  - diaphragm Z30.49
  - implantable subdermal Z30.46
  - injectable Z30.42
  - pills Z30.41
  - specified type NEC Z30.49
  - transdermal patch Z30.45
  - vaginal ring Z30.44
- specified type NEC Z30.018
- transdermal patch Z30.016
- vaginal ring Z30.015

Presence (of)

- arterial-venous shunt (dialysis) Z99.2
- artificial
  - heart (fully implantable) (mechanical) Z95.812
    - ■ valve Z95.2
- bladder implant (functional) Z96.0
- cardiac
  - pacemaker Z95.0
- cardioverter-defibrillator Z95.810
- cerebrospinal fluid drainage device Z98.2
- contact lens(es) Z97.3
- CSF shunt Z98.2
- endocrine implant (functional) NEC Z96.49
- external hearing-aid or device Z97.4
- functional implant Z96.9
  - specified NEC Z96.89
- heart valve implant (functional) Z95.2
  - prosthetic Z95.2
  - specified type NEC Z95.4
  - xenogenic Z95.3
- implanted device (artificial) (functional) (prosthetic) Z96.9
  - cardiac pacemaker Z95.0
  - heart valve Z95.2
    - ■ prosthetic Z95.2
    - ■ specified NEC Z95.4
    - ■ xenogenic Z95.3
  - neurostimulator Z96.82
  - skin Z96.81

Prespondylolisthesis (congenital) Q76.2

Pressure

- area, skin—*see* Ulcer, pressure, by site
- increased
  - intracranial (benign) G93.2
    - ■ injury at birth P11.0

Pre-syncope R55

Preterm

- newborn (infant) P07.30
  - gestational age
    - ■ 28 completed weeks (28 weeks, 0 days through 28 weeks, 6 days) P07.31
    - ■ 29 completed weeks (29 weeks, 0 days through 29 weeks, 6 days) P07.32
    - ■ 30 completed weeks (30 weeks, 0 days through 30 weeks, 6 days) P07.33
    - ■ 31 completed weeks (31 weeks, 0 days through 31 weeks, 6 days) P07.34
    - ■ 32 completed weeks (32 weeks, 0 days through 32 weeks, 6 days) P07.35
    - ■ 33 completed weeks (33 weeks, 0 days through 33 weeks, 6 days) P07.36
    - ■ 34 completed weeks (34 weeks, 0 days through 34 weeks, 6 days) P07.37
    - ■ 35 completed weeks (35 weeks, 0 days through 35 weeks, 6 days) P07.38
    - ■ 36 completed weeks (36 weeks, 0 days through 36 weeks, 6 days) P07.39

ALPHABETIC INDEX

Priapism N48.30
- due to
  - disease classified elsewhere N48.32
  - drug N48.33
  - specified cause NEC N48.39
  - trauma N48.31

Prickly heat L74.0

Primus varus (bilateral) Q66.21-

Pringle's disease (tuberous sclerosis) Q85.1

Problem (with) (related to)
- academic Z55.8
- acculturation Z60.3
- adopted child Z62.821
- alcoholism in family Z63.72
- atypical parenting situation Z62.9
- bankruptcy Z59.89
- behavioral (adult)
  - drug seeking Z76.5
- birth of sibling affecting child Z62.898
- care (of)
- child
  - abuse (affecting the child)—*see* Maltreatment, child
  - custody or support proceedings Z65.3
  - in
    - care of non-parental family member Z62.23
    - custody of
      - grandparent Z62.23
      - non-parental relative Z62.23
      - non-relative guardian Z62.24
    - foster care Z62.21
    - kinship care Z62.23
    - welfare
      - custody Z62.21
      - guardianship Z62.21
    - leaving living situation without permission Z62.892
  - living in
    - group home Z62.22
    - orphanage Z62.22
- conflict or discord (with)
  - classmates Z55.4
  - counselor Z64.4
  - family Z63.9
    - specified NEC Z63.8
  - probation officer Z64.4
  - social worker Z64.4
  - teachers Z55.4
- drug addict in family Z63.72
- economic Z59.9
- education Z55.9
  - specified NEC Z55.8
- enuresis, child F98.0
- failed examinations (school) Z55.2
- falling Z91.81
- family (*see also* Disruption, family) Z63.9-
  - specified NEC Z63.8
- feeding (elderly) (infant) R63.39
  - newborn P92.9
    - breast P92.5
    - overfeeding P92.4
    - slow P92.2
    - specified NEC P92.8
    - underfeeding P92.3
  - nonorganic F50.89
- finance Z59.-
- foster child Z62.822
- genital NEC
  - female N94.9
  - male N50.9
- homelessness Z59.00
- housing Z59.9
  - inadequate Z59.10
- identity (of childhood) F93.8
- intrafamilial communication Z63.8
  - isolated Z59.89
- jealousy, child F93.8
- language (developmental) F80.9
- learning (developmental) F81.9
- lifestyle Z72.9
  - gambling Z72.6
  - high-risk sexual behavior (heterosexual) Z72.51
    - bisexual Z72.53
    - homosexual Z72.5

Problem (with) (related to), *continued*
- inappropriate eating habits Z72.4
- self-damaging behavior NEC Z72.89
  - specified NEC Z72.89
    - tobacco use Z72.0
- literacy Z55.9
  - low level Z55.0
    - specified NEC Z55.8
- mental F48.9
- presence of sick or disabled person in family or household Z63.79
  - needing care Z63.6
- primary support group (family) Z63.9
  - specified NEC Z63.8
- psychosocial Z65.9
  - specified NEC Z65.8
- related to physical environment, specified NEC Z58.89
- relationship Z63.9
  - childhood F93.8
- seeking and accepting known hazardous and harmful
  - behavioral or psychological interventions Z65.8
  - chemical, nutritional or physical interventions Z65.8
- sight H54.7
- speech R47.9
  - developmental F80.9
  - specified NEC R47.89
- swallowing—*see* Dysphagia
- taste—*see* Disturbance, sensation
- tic, child F95.0
- underachievement in school Z55.3
- voice production R47.89

Procedure (surgical)
- for purpose other than remedying health state Z41.9
  - specified NEC Z41.8
- not done Z53.9
  - because of
    - administrative reasons Z53.8
    - contraindication Z53.09
      - smoking Z53.01
    - patient's decision Z53.20
      - for reasons of belief or group pressure Z53.1
      - left against medical advice (AMA) Z53.29
      - left without being seen Z53.21
        - specified reason NEC Z53.29
    - specified reason NEC Z53.8

Proctalgia K62.89

Proctitis K62.89
- amebic (acute) A06.0
- chlamydial A56.3
- gonococcal A54.6
- granulomatous—*see* Enteritis, regional, large intestine
- herpetic A60
- ulcerative (chronic) K51.20
  - with
    - complication K51.219
      - abscess K51.214
      - fistula K51.213
      - obstruction K51.212
      - rectal bleeding K51.211
      - specified NEC K51.218

Proctocele
- male K62.3

Proctocolitis
- allergic K52.29
- food-induced eosinophilic K52.29
- food protein-induced K52.29
- milk protein-induced K52.29

Proctoptosis K62.3

Proctorrhagia K62.5

Proctospasm K59.4
- psychogenic F45.8

Prolapse, prolapsed
- anus, anal (canal) (sphincter) K62.2
- bladder (mucosa) (sphincter) (acquired)
  - congenital Q79.4
- rectum (mucosa) (sphincter) K62.3

Prolonged, prolongation (of)
- bleeding (time) (idiopathic) R79.1
- coagulation (time) R79.1
- gestation (over 42 completed weeks)
  - newborn P08.22

Prolonged, prolongation, *continued*
- interval I44.0
- partial thromboplastin time (PTT) R79.1
- prothrombin time R79.1
- QT interval R94.31

Pronation
- ankle—*see* Deformity, limb, foot, specified NEC
- foot—*see also* Deformity, limb, foot, specified NEC
  - congenital Q74.2

Prophylactic
- administration of
  - antibiotics, long-term Z79.2
  - antivenin Z29.12
    - short-term use—omit code
  - drug (*see also* Long-term (current) (prophylactic) drug therapy (use of)) Z79.899-
    - fluoride varnish application Z29.3
    - other specified Z29.8
    - rabies immune therapy Z29.14
    - respiratory syncytial virus (RSV) immune globulin Z29.11
    - Rho (D) immune globulin Z29.13
    - unspecified Z29.9
  - medication Z79.899
  - vaccination Z23

Prostatitis (congestive) (suppurative) (with cystitis) N41.9
- acute N41.0

Prostration R53.83
- heat—*see also* Heat, exhaustion
  - anhydrotic T67.3
  - due to
    - salt (and water) depletion T67.4
    - water depletion T67.3

Protein
- sickness (*see also* Reaction, serum) T80.69

Proteinuria R80.9
- Bence Jones R80.3
- isolated R80.0
  - with glomerular lesion N06.9
    - membranous (diffuse) - *see also* Nephropathy, membranous N06.20
    - with diffuse membranous glomerulonephritis N06.29
  - orthostatic R80.2
    - with glomerular lesion—*see* Proteinuria, isolated, with glomerular lesion
  - postural R80.2
    - with glomerular lesion—*see* Proteinuria, isolated, with glomerular lesion
  - specified type NEC R80.8

Proteolysis, pathologic D65

Proteus (mirabilis) (morganii), **as the cause of disease classified elsewhere** B96.4

Protrusion, protrusio
- device, implant or graft (*see also* Complications, by site and type, mechanical) T85.698
  - catheter NEC T85.698
    - cystostomy T83.090
    - urinary—*see also* Complications, catheter, urinary T83.098
  - ventricular intracranial shunt T85.09

Prune belly (syndrome) Q79.4

Prurigo (ferox) (gravis) (Hebrae) (Hebra's) (mitis) (simplex) L28.2
- Besnier's L20.0
- psychogenic F45.8

Pruritus, pruritic (essential) L29.9
- ani, anus L29.0
  - psychogenic F45.8
- anogenital L29.3
  - psychogenic F45.8
- cholestatic L29.81
- hiemalis L29.89
- neurogenic (any site) F45.8
- perianal L29.0
- psychogenic (any site) F45.8
- senile, senilis L29.89
- scroti, scrotum L29.1
  - psychogenic F45.8

ALPHABETIC INDEX

Pruritus, pruritic, *continued*
- specified NEC L29.89
  - psychogenic F45.8
- Trichomonas A59.9
- vulva, vulvae L29.2
  - psychogenic F45.8

Pseudo-Hurler's polydystrophy E77.0

Pseudoangioma I81

Pseudarthrosis, pseudoarthrosis (bone)
- clavicle, congenital Q74.0

Pseudocirrhosis, liver, pericardial I31.1

Pseudocyesis F45.8

Pseudohemophilia (Bernuth's) (hereditary) (type B) D68.0

Pseudohermaphroditism Q56.3
- adrenal E25.8
- female Q56.2
  - with adrenocortical disorder E25.8
  - without adrenocortical disorder Q56.2
  - adrenal, congenital E25.0
- male Q56.1
  - with
    - androgen resistance E34.51
    - feminizing testis E34.51

Pseudohydrocephalus G93.2

Pseudohypertrophic muscular dystrophy (Erb's) G71.02

Pseudohypertrophy, muscle G71.09

Pseudoinsomnia F51.03

Pseudomeningocele (cerebral) (infective) (post-traumatic) G96.198

Pseudomonas
- aeruginosa, as cause of disease classified elsewhere B96.5
- mallei infection
  - as cause of disease classified elsewhere B96.5
- pseudomallei, as cause of disease classified elsewhere B96.5

Pseudoparalysis
- atonic, congenital P94.2

Pseudopolycythemia D75.1

Pseudopuberty, precocious
- female heterosexual E25.8
- male isosexual E25.8

Pseudorubella B08.20

Pseudosclerema, newborn P83.88

Pseudotuberculosis A28.2
- enterocolitis A04.8
- pasteurella (infection) A28.0

Pseudotumor G93.2

Pseudoxanthoma elasticum Q82.8

Psilosis (sprue) (tropical) K90.1
- nontropical K90.0

Psoriasis L40.9
- flexural L40.8
- specified NEC L40.8

Psychological and behavioral factors affecting medical condition F59

Psychoneurosis, psychoneurotic—*see also* Neurosis
- hysteria F44.9

Psychopathy, psychopathic
- autistic F84.5
- constitution, post-traumatic F07.81
- personality—*see* Disorder, personality

Psychosexual identity disorder of childhood F64.2

Psychosis, psychotic
- acute (transient)
  - hysterical F44.9
- affective—*see* Disorder, mood
- childhood F84.0
  - atypical F84.8
- exhaustive F43.0
- hysterical (acute) F44.9
- infantile F84.0
  - atypical F84.8

PTEN tumor syndrome Q85.81

Ptosis—*see also* Blepharoptosis
- brow or eyebrow H57.81-
- eyelid—*see* Blepharoptosis
  - congenital Q10.0

PTP D69.51

Ptyalism (periodic) K11.7
- hysterical F45.8

Pubarche, precocious E30.1

Pubertas praecox E30.1

Puberty (development state) Z00.3
- bleeding (excessive) N92.2
- delayed E30.0
- precocious (constitutional) (cryptogenic) (idiopathic) E30.1
  - central E22.8
  - due to
    - ovarian hyperfunction E28.1
    - estrogen E28.0
- premature E30.1
  - due to
    - adrenal cortical hyperfunction E25.8
    - pineal tumor E34.8
    - pituitary (anterior) hyperfunction E22.8

Puente's disease (simple glandular cheilitis) K13.0

Pulse
- alternating R00.8
- bigeminal R00.8
- fast R00.0
- feeble, rapid due to shock following injury T79.4
- rapid R00.0
- weak R09.89

Punch drunk F07.81

Punctum lacrimale occlusion—*see* Obstruction, lacrimal

Puncture
- abdomen, abdominal
  - wall S31.139
    - with
      - foreign body S31.149
    - epigastric region S31.132
      - with
        - ◊ foreign body S31.142
    - left
      - lower quadrant S31.134
        - ◊ with
          - » foreign body S31.144
      - upper quadrant S31.131
        - ◊ with
          - » foreign body S31.141
    - periumbillic region S31.135
      - with
        - ◊ foreign body S31.145
    - right
      - lower quadrant S31.133
        - ◊ with
          - » foreign body S31.143
      - upper quadrant S31.130
        - ◊ with
          - » foreign body S31.140
- accidental, complicating surgery—*see* Complication
- alveolar (process)—*see* Puncture, oral cavity
- ankle S91.03-
  - with
    - foreign body S91.04-
  - left S91.032
    - with
      - foreign body S91.042
  - right S91.031
    - with
      - foreign body S91.041
- anus S31.833
  - with foreign body S31.834
- arm (upper) S41.13-
  - with foreign body S41.14-
  - left S41.132
    - with foreign body S41.142
  - lower—*see* Puncture, forearm
  - right S41.131
    - with foreign body S41.141
- auditory canal (external) (meatus)—*see* Puncture, ear
- auricle, ear—*see* Puncture, ear

Puncture, *continued*
- axilla—*see* Puncture, arm
- back—*see also* Puncture, thorax, back
  - lower S31.030
    - with
      - foreign body S31.040
  - bladder (traumatic)
    - nontraumatic N32.89
- buttock S31.8-
  - with foreign body S31.8-
  - left S31.823
    - with foreign body S31.824
  - right S31.813
    - with foreign body S31.814
- by
  - device, implant or graft—*see* Complications, by site and type, mechanical
  - instrument (any) during a procedure, accidental—*see* Puncture, accidental complicating surgery
- calf—*see* Puncture, leg
- canaliculus lacrimalis—*see* Puncture, eyelid
- canthus, eye—*see* Puncture, eyelid
- cheek (external) S01.43-
  - with foreign body S01.44
  - internal—*see* Puncture, oral cavity
  - left S01.432
    - with foreign body S01.442
  - right S01.431
    - with foreign body S01.441
- chest wall—*see* Puncture, thorax
- chin—*see* Puncture, head, specified site NEC
- clitoris—*see* Puncture, vulva
- costal region—*see* Puncture, thorax
- digit(s)
  - hand—*see* Puncture, finger
  - foot—*see* Puncture, toe
- ear (canal) (external) S01.33-
  - drum S09.2-
    - with foreign body S01.34-
  - left S01.332
    - with foreign body S01.342
  - right S01.331
    - with foreign body S01.341
- elbow S51.03-
  - with
    - foreign body S51.04-
  - left S51.032
    - with
      - foreign body S51.042
  - right S51.031
    - with
      - foreign body S51.041
- epididymis—*see* Puncture
- epigastric region—*see* Puncture, abdomen, wall, epigastric region
- epiglottis S11.83
  - with foreign body S11.84
- eyebrow—*see* Puncture, eyelid
- eyelid S01.13-
  - with foreign body S01.14-
  - left S01.132
    - with foreign body S01.142
  - right S01.131
    - with foreign body S01.141
- face NEC—*see* Puncture, head, specified site NEC
- finger(s) S61.23-
  - with
    - damage to nail S61.33-
      - with
        - ◊ foreign body S61.34-
    - foreign body S61.24-
  - index S61.23-
    - with
      - damage to nail S61.33-
        - ◊ with
          - » foreign body S61.34-
        - foreign body S61.24-
  - left S61.231
    - with
      - ◊ damage to nail S61.331
        - » with
          - ◆ foreign body S61.341
        - ◊ foreign body S61.241

ALPHABETIC INDEX

Puncture, *continued*

- ■ right S61.230
  - ~ with
    - ◊ damage to nail S61.330
      - » with
        - ◆ foreign body S61.340
    - ◊ foreign body S61.240
  - – little S61.23-
    - ■ with
      - ~ damage to nail S61.33-
        - ◊ with
          - » foreign body S61.34-
          - ~ foreign body S61.24-
    - ■ left S61.237
      - ~ with
        - ◊ damage to nail S61.337
          - » with
            - ◆ foreign body S61.347
          - ◊ foreign body S61.247
    - ■ right S61.236
      - ~ with
        - ◊ damage to nail S61.336
          - » with
            - ◆ foreign body S61.346
          - ◊ foreign body S61.246
  - – middle S61.23-
    - ■ with
      - ~ damage to nail S61.33-
        - ◊ with
          - » foreign body S61.34-
          - ~ foreign body S61.24-
    - ■ left S61.233
      - ~ with
        - ◊ damage to nail S61.333
          - » with
            - ◆ foreign body S61.343
          - ◊ foreign body S61.243
    - ■ right S61.232
      - ~ with
        - ◊ damage to nail S61.332
          - » with
            - ◆ foreign body S61.342
          - ◊ foreign body S61.242
  - – ring S61.238
    - ■ with
      - ~ damage to nail S61.33-
        - ◊ with
          - » foreign body S61.34-
          - ~ foreign body S61.24-
    - ■ left S61.235
      - ~ with
        - ◊ damage to nail S61.335
          - » with
            - ◆ foreign body S61.345
          - ◊ foreign body S61.245
    - ■ right S61.234
      - ~ with
        - ◊ damage to nail S61.334
          - » with
            - ◆ foreign body S61.344
          - ◊ foreign body S61.244
- flank S31.139
  - ~ with foreign body S31.149
- foot (except toe(s) alone) S91.33-
  - ~ with foreign body S91.34-
  - ■ left S91.332
    - ■ with foreign body S91.342
  - – right S91.331
    - ■ with foreign body S91.341
  - – toe—*see* Puncture, toe
- forearm S51.83-
  - ~ with
    - ■ foreign body S51.84-
  - – elbow only—*see* Puncture, elbow
  - – left S51.832
    - ■ with
      - ~ foreign body S51.842
  - – right S51.831
    - ■ with
      - ~ foreign body S51.841
- forehead—*see* Puncture, head, specified site NEC

Puncture, *continued*

- genital organs, external
  - – female (*code to* Puncture by specific site for vagina or vulva)
  - – male (*code to* Puncture by specific site for penis, scrotum, or testis)
- groin—*see* Puncture, abdomen, wall
- gum—*see* Puncture, oral cavity
- hand (*code to* Puncture by specific site for finger or thumb) S61.43-
  - ~ with
    - ■ foreign body S61.44-
  - – left S61.432
    - ■ with
      - ~ foreign body S61.442
  - – right S61.431
    - ■ with
      - ~ foreign body S61.441
- head (*code to* Puncture by specific site for cheek/ temporomandibular area, ear, eyelid, nose, or oral cavity) S01.93
  - ~ with foreign body S01.94
  - – scalp S01.03
    - ■ with foreign body S01.04
  - – specified site NEC S01.83
    - ■ with foreign body S01.84
- heel—*see* Puncture, foot
- hip S71.03-
  - ~ with foreign body S71.04-
  - – left S71.032
    - ■ with foreign body S71.042
  - – right S71.031
    - ■ with foreign body S71.041
- hypochondrium—*see* Puncture, abdomen, wall
- hypogastric region—*see* Puncture, abdomen, wall
- inguinal region—*see* Puncture, abdomen, wall
- instep—*see* Puncture, foot
- interscapular region—*see* Puncture, thorax, back
- jaw—*see* Puncture, head, specified site NEC
- knee S81.03-
  - ~ with foreign body S81.04-
  - – left S81.032
    - ■ with foreign body S81.042
  - – right S81.031
    - ■ with foreign body S81.041
- leg (lower) (*code to* Puncture by specified site for foot, knee, or upper leg/thigh) S81.83-
  - ~ with foreign body S81.84-
  - – left S81.832
    - ■ with foreign body S81.842
  - – right S81.831
    - ■ with foreign body S81.841
- lip S01.531
  - ~ with foreign body S01.541
- loin—*see* Puncture, abdomen, wall
- lower back—*see* Puncture, back, lower
- lumbar region—*see* Puncture, back, lower
- malar region—*see* Puncture, head, specified site NEC
- mastoid region—*see* Puncture, head, specified site NEC
- mouth—*see* Puncture, oral cavity
- nail
  - – finger—*see* Puncture, finger, with, damage to nail
  - – toe—*see* Puncture, toe, with, damage to nail
- nasal (septum) (sinus)—*see* Puncture, nose
- nasopharynx—*see* Puncture, head, specified site NEC
- neck S11.93
  - ~ with foreign body S11.94
- nose (septum) (sinus) S01.23
  - ~ with foreign body S01.24
- oral cavity S01.532
  - ~ with foreign body S01.542
- palate—*see* Puncture, oral cavity
- palm—*see* Puncture, hand
- penis S31.23
  - ~ with foreign body S31.24
- perineum
  - – female S31.43
    - ■ with foreign body S31.44
  - – male S31.139
    - ■ with foreign body S31.149
- phalanges
  - – finger—*see* Puncture, finger
  - – toe—*see* Puncture, toe

Puncture, *continued*

- pinna—*see* Puncture, ear
- popliteal space—*see* Puncture, knee
- scalp S01.03
  - ~ with foreign body S01.04
- scapular region—*see* Puncture, shoulder
- scrotum S31.33
  - ~ with foreign body S31.34
- shin—*see* Puncture, leg
- shoulder S41.03-
  - ~ with foreign body S41.04-
  - – left S41.032
    - ■ with foreign body S41.042
  - – right S41.031
    - ■ with foreign body S41.041
- subungual
  - – finger(s)—*see* Puncture, finger, with, damage to nail
  - – toe—*see* Puncture, toe, with, damage to nail
- testis S31.33
- thigh S71.13-
  - ~ with foreign body S71.14-
  - – left S71.132
    - ■ with foreign body S71.142
  - – right S71.131
    - ■ with foreign body S71.141
- thorax, thoracic (wall) S21.93
  - ~ with foreign body S21.94
  - – back S21.23-
    - ■ with
      - ~ foreign body S21.24-
  - – front S21.13-
    - ■ with
      - ~ foreign body S21.14-
- throat—*see* Puncture, neck
- thumb S61.03-
  - ~ with
    - ■ damage to nail S61.13-
      - ~ with
        - ◊ foreign body S61.14-
    - ■ foreign body S61.04-
  - – left S61.032
    - ■ with
      - ~ damage to nail S61.132
        - ◊ with
          - » foreign body S61.142
      - ~ foreign body S61.042
  - – right S61.031
    - ■ with
      - ~ damage to nail S61.131
        - ◊ with
          - » foreign body S61.141
      - ~ foreign body S61.041
- toe(s) S91.13-
  - ~ with
    - ■ damage to nail S91.23-
      - ■ with
        - ◊ foreign body S91.24-
      - ■ foreign body S91.14-
  - – great S91.13-
    - ■ with
      - ~ damage to nail S91.23-with
        - » foreign body S91.24-
      - ~ foreign body S91.14-
    - ■ left S91.132
      - ~ with
        - ◊ damage to nail S91.232
          - » with
            - ◆ foreign body S91.242
          - ◊ foreign body S91.142
    - ■ right S91.131
      - ~ with
        - ◊ damage to nail S91.231
          - » with
            - ◆ foreign body S91.241
          - ◊ foreign body S91.141
  - – lesser S91.13-
    - ■ with
      - ~ damage to nail S91.23-
        - ◊ with
          - » foreign body S91.24-
      - ~ foreign body S91.14-

Puncture, *continued*
- ■ left S91.135
  - – with
    - ◊ damage to nail S91.235
      - » with
        - ◊ foreign body S91.245
    - ◊ foreign body S91.145
- ■ right S91.134
  - – with
    - ◊ damage to nail S91.234
      - » with
        - ◊ foreign body S91.244
    - ◊ foreign body S91.144
- tympanum, tympanic membrane S09.2-
- umbilical region S31.135
  - – with foreign body S31.145
- vagina S31.43
  - – with foreign body S31.44
- vulva S31.43
  - – with foreign body S31.44
- wrist S61.53-
  - ■ with
    - ■ foreign body S61.54-
  - – left S61.532
    - ■ with
      - – foreign body S61.542
  - – right S61.531
    - ■ with
      - – foreign body S61.541

PUO (pyrexia of unknown origin) R50.9

Purpura D69.2
- abdominal D69.0
- allergic D69.0
- anaphylactoid D69.0
- arthritic D69.0
- autoerythrocyte sensitization D69.2
- autoimmune D69.0
- bacterial D69.0
- Bateman's (senile) D69.2
- capillary fragility (hereditary) (idiopathic) D69.8
- Devil's pinches D69.2
- fibrinolytic—*see* Fibrinolysis
- fulminans, fulminous D65
- gangrenous D65
- hemorrhagic, hemorrhagica D69.3
  - – not due to thrombocytopenia D69.0
- Henoch (-Schönlein) (allergic) D69.0
- idiopathic (thrombocytopenic) D69.3
  - – nonthrombocytopenic D69.0
- immune thrombocytopenic D69.3
- infectious D69.0
- malignant D69.0
- neonatorum P54.5
- nervosa D69.0
- newborn P54.5
- nonthrombocytopenic D69.2
  - – hemorrhagic D69.0
  - – idiopathic D69.0
- nonthrombopenic D69.2
- peliosis rheumatica D69.0
- posttransfusion (post-transfusion) (from (fresh) whole blood or blood products) D69.51
- primary D69.49
- red cell membrane sensitivity D69.2
- rheumatica D69.0
- Schönlein (-Henoch) (allergic) D69.0
- senile D69.2
- simplex D69.2
- symptomatica D69.0
- telangiectasia annularis L81.7
- thrombocytopenic D69.49
  - – congenital D69.42
  - – hemorrhagic D69.3
  - – hereditary D69.42
  - – idiopathic D69.3
  - – immune D69.3
  - – neonatal, transitory P61.0
  - – thrombotic M31.19
- thrombohemolytic—*see* Fibrinolysis
- thrombolytic—*see* Fibrinolysis
- thrombopenic D69.49
- thrombotic, thrombocytopenic M31.19

Purpura, *continued*
- toxic D69.0
- vascular D69.0
- visceral symptoms D69.0

Purpuric spots R23.3

Purulent—*see* Disease, diseased

Pus
- in
  - – stool R19.5
  - – urine N39.0
- tube (rupture)—*see* Salpingo-oophoritis

Pustular rash L08.0

Pustule (nonmalignant) L08.9
- malignant A22.0

Pyelectasis—*see* Hydronephrosis

Pyelitis (congenital) (uremic)—*see also* Pyelonephritis
- with
  - – calculus—*see* category N20
    - ■ with hydronephrosis N13.6
- acute N10
- chronic N11.9
  - – with calculus—*see* category N20
    - ■ with hydronephrosis N13.6

Pyelonephritis—*see also* Nephritis, tubulo-interstitial
- with
  - – calculus—*see* category N20
    - ■ with hydronephrosis N13.6
- acute N10
- calculous—*see* category N20
  - – with hydronephrosis N13.6
- chronic N11.9
  - – with calculus—*see* category N20
    - ■ with hydronephrosis N13.6
- in (due to)
  - – lymphoma NEC C85.90 /N16/
  - – sarcoidosis D86.84
  - – sepsis A41.9 /N16/
  - – transplant rejection T86.- /N16/

Pyelophlebitis I80.8

Pyemia, pyemic (fever) (infection) (purulent)—*see also* Sepsis
- pneumococcal
- specified organism NEC A41.89

Pyloritis K29.90
- with bleeding K29.91

Pylorospasm (reflex) NEC K31.3
- congenital or infantile Q40.0
- newborn Q40.0
- neurotic F45.8
- psychogenic F45.8

Pylorus, pyloric—*see* Disease, diseased

Pyoarthrosis—*see* Arthritis, pyogenic or pyemic

Pyocele
- sinus (accessory)—*see* Sinusitis
- turbinate (bone) J32.9

Pyoderma, pyodermia L08.0
- gangrenosum L88
- newborn P39.4
- phagedenic L88

Pyodermatitis L08.0

Pyopericarditis, pyopericardium I30.1

Pyopneumopericardium I30.1

Pyopneumothorax (infective) J86.9
- with fistula J86.0

Pyothorax J86.9
- with fistula J86.0

Pyrexia (of unknown origin) R50.9
- atmospheric T67.01
- heat T67.01
- newborn P81.9
  - – environmentally-induced P81.0
- persistent R50.9

Pyroglobulinemia NEC E88.09

Pyrosis R12

Pyuria
- abnormal laboratory finding R82.81
- bacterial N39.0

Pityriasis (capitis) L21.0
- furfuracea L21.0

Q

Quadricuspid aortic valve Q23.88

Quadriparesis—*see* Quadriplegia
- meaning muscle weakness M62.81

Quadriplegia G82.50
- complete
  - – C1–C4 level G82.51
  - – C5–C7 level G82.53
- incomplete
  - – C1–C4 level G82.52
  - – C5–C7 level G82.54
- traumatic *code to* injury with seventh character S
  - – current episode—*see* Injury, spinal (cord), cervical

Quervain's disease M65.4
- thyroid E06.1

Quincke's disease or edema T78.3

Quinsy (gangrenous) J36

R

Rabies A82.9
- contact Z20.3
- exposure to Z20.3
- inoculation reaction—*see* Complications, vaccination

Radiation
- therapy, encounter for Z51.0

Radiotherapy session Z51.0

Rag picker's disease A22.1

Rag sorter's disease A22.1

Rales R09.89

Ramsay-Hunt disease or syndrome (*see also* Hunt's)
- meaning dyssynergia cerebellaris myoclonica G11.19

Rape
- alleged, observation or examination, ruled out
  - – child Z04.42
- child
  - – confirmed T74.22
  - – suspected T76.22

Rapid
- feeble pulse, due to shock, following injury T79.4
- heart (beat) R00.0
  - – psychogenic F45.8

Rash (toxic) R21
- canker A38.9
- diaper L22
- drug (internal use) L27.0
  - – contact (*see also* Dermatitis, due to, drugs and medicaments) L25.1
- following immunization T88.1-
- food—*see* Dermatitis, due to, food
- heat L74.0
- napkin (psoriasiform) L22
- nettle—*see* Urticaria
- pustular L08.0
- rose R21
  - – epidemic B06.9
- scarlet A38.9
- serum (*see also* Reaction, serum) T80.69
- wandering tongue K14.1

Rat-bite fever A25.9
- due to Streptobacillus moniliformis A25.1
- spirochetal (morsus muris) A25.0

RDS (newborn) (type I) P22.0
- type II P22.1

Reaction—*see also* Disorder
- adverse
  - – food (any) (ingested) NEC T78.1
    - ■ anaphylactic—*see* Shock, anaphylactic, due to food
- allergic—*see* Allergy
- anaphylactic—*see* Shock, anaphylactic
- anaphylactoid—*see* Shock, anaphylactic

ALPHABETIC INDEX

Reaction, *continued*

- antitoxin (prophylactic) (therapeutic)—*see* Complications, vaccination
- combat and operational stress F43.0
- compulsive F42.8
- conversion F44.9
- crisis, acute F43.0
- deoxyribonuclease (DNA) (DNase) hypersensitivity D69.2
- depressive (single episode) F32.9
  - psychotic F32.3
  - recurrent—*see* Disorder, depressive, recurrent
- dissociative F44.9
- drug NEC T88.7
  - allergic—*see* Allergy, drug
  - newborn P93.8
    - gray baby syndrome P93.0
  - overdose or poisoning (by accident)—*see* Table of Drugs and Chemicals, by drug, poisoning
  - photoallergic L56.1
  - phototoxic L56.0
  - withdrawal—*see* Dependence, by drug, with, withdrawal
    - infant of dependent mother P96.1
    - newborn P96.1
  - wrong substance given or taken (by accident)—*see* Table of Drugs and Chemicals, by drug, poisoning
- fear F40.9
  - child (abnormal) F93.8
- febrile nonhemolytic transfusion (FNHTR) R50.84
- hypoglycemic, due to insulin E16.0
  - therapeutic misadventure—*see* subcategory T38.3
- hysterical F44.9
- immunization—*see* Complications, vaccination
- insulin T38.3-
- leukemoid D72.823
  - basophilic D72.823
  - lymphocytic D72.823
  - monocytic D72.823
  - myelocytic D72.823
  - neutrophilic D72.823
- neurogenic—*see* Neurosis
- neurotic F48.9
- nonspecific
  - to
    - cell mediated immunity measurement of gamma interferon antigen response without active tuberculosis R76.12
    - QuantiFERON-TB test (QFT) without active tuberculosis R76.12
    - tuberculin test (*see also* Reaction) R76.11
- obsessive-compulsive F42.8
- phobic F40.9
- psychoneurotic—*see also* Neurosis
  - compulsive F42
  - obsessive F42
- psychophysiologic—*see* Disorder, somatoform
- psychosomatic—*see* Disorder, somatoform
- psychotic—*see* Psychosis
- scarlet fever toxin—*see* Complications, vaccination
- serum T80.69-
  - anaphylactic (immediate) (*see also* Shock, anaphylactic) T80.59-
  - specified reaction NEC
    - due to
      - administration of blood and blood products T80.61-
      - immunization T80.62-
      - serum specified NEC T80.69-
      - vaccination T80.62-
- spinal puncture G97.1
  - dural G97.1
- stress (severe) F43.9
  - acute (agitation) ("daze") (disorientation) (disturbance of consciousness) (flight reaction) (fugue) F43.0
  - specified NEC F43.8
- surgical procedure—*see* Complications, surgical procedure
- tetanus antitoxin—*see* Complications, vaccination
- toxic, to local anesthesia T81.89
- toxin-antitoxin—*see* Complications, vaccination
- tuberculin skin test, abnormal R76.11
- withdrawing, child or adolescent F93.8

Reactive airway disease—*see* Asthma

Reactive depression—*see* Reaction, depressive

Recklinghausen disease Q85.01

Rectalgia K62.89

Rectitis K62.89

Rectocele

- male K62.3

Rectosigmoiditis K63.89

- ulcerative (chronic) K51.30
  - with
    - complication K51.319
      - abscess K51.314
      - fistula K51.313
      - obstruction K51.312
      - rectal bleeding K51.311
      - specified NEC K51.318

Red bugs B88.0

Reduced

- mobility Z74.09
- ventilatory or vital capacity R94.2

Redundant, redundancy

- foreskin (congenital) N47.8
- prepuce (congenital) N47.8

Reflex R29.2

- vasovagal R55

Reflux K21.9

- acid K21.9
- esophageal K21.9
  - with esophagitis K21.0-
  - newborn P78.83
- gastroesophageal K21.9
  - with esophagitis K21.0-
- vesicoureteral (with scarring) N13.70
  - without nephropathy N13.71

Refusal of

- food, psychogenic F50.89
- treatment (because of) Z53.20
  - left against medical advice (AMA) Z53.29
  - left without being seen Z53.21

Regurgitation R11.10

- aortic (valve)—*see* Insufficiency, aortic
- food—*see also* Vomiting
  - with reswallowing—*see* Rumination
  - newborn P92.1
- gastric contents—*see* Vomiting
- heart—*see* Endocarditis
- mitral (valve)—*see* Insufficiency, mitral
  - congenital Q23.3
- myocardial—*see* Endocarditis
- pulmonary (valve) (heart) I37.1
  - congenital Q22.2
  - syphilitic A52.03
- tricuspid—*see* Insufficiency, tricuspid
- valve, valvular—*see* Endocarditis
  - congenital Q24.8

Reifenstein syndrome E34.52

Reinsertion

- implantable subdermal contraceptive Z30.46
- intrauterine contraceptive device Z30.433

Rejection

- food, psychogenic F50.89
- transplant
  - bone
    - marrow T86.01
  - heart T86.21
    - with lung(s) T86.31
  - kidney T86.11
  - liver T86.41
  - lung(s) T86.810
    - with heart T86.31
  - organ (immune or nonimmune cause) T86.-
  - stem cell (peripheral blood) (umbilical cord) T86.5

Relapsing fever A68.9

- louse-borne (epidemic) A68.0
- Novy's (American) A68.1
- tick borne (endemic) A68.1

Relaxation

- anus (sphincter) K62.89
  - psychogenic F45.8
- cardioesophageal K21.9
- diaphragm J98.6
- posture R29.3
- rectum (sphincter) K62.89

Remittent fever (malarial) B54

Remnant

- fingernail L60.8
  - congenital Q84.6
- thyroglossal duct Q89.2
- tonsil J35.8
  - infected (chronic) J35.01

Removal (from) (of)

- device
  - contraceptive Z30.432
    - implantable subdermal Z30.46
- dressing (nonsurgical) Z48.00
  - surgical Z48.01
- home in childhood (to foster home or institution) Z62.29
- staples Z48.02
- suture Z48.02

Rendu-Osler-Weber disease or syndrome I78.0

Renon-Delille syndrome E23.3

Replacement by artificial or mechanical device or prosthesis of

- heart Z95.812
  - valve Z95.2
    - prosthetic Z95.2
    - specified NEC Z95.4
    - xenogenic Z95.3
- organ replacement
  - by artificial or mechanical device or prosthesis of
    - heart Z95.812
      - valve Z95.2

Request for expert evidence Z04.89

Residing

- in place not meant for human habitation (abandoned building) (car) (park) (sidewalk) (street) Z59.02

Residual—*see also* Disease, diseased

- urine R39.198

Resistance, resistant (to)

- insulin E88.819
  - specified type NEC E88.818
- organism(s)
  - to
    - drug Z16.30
      - aminoglycosides Z16.29
      - amoxicillin Z16.11
      - ampicillin Z16.11
      - antibiotic(s) Z16.20
        - ◊ multiple Z16.24
        - ◊ specified NEC Z16.29
      - antimicrobial (single) Z16.30
        - ◊ multiple Z16.35
        - ◊ specified NEC Z16.39
      - beta lactam antibiotics Z16.10
        - ◊ specified NEC Z16.19
      - carbapenem Z16.13
      - cephalosporins Z16.19
      - extended beta lactamase (ESBL) Z16.12
      - macrolides Z16.29
      - methicillin—*see* MRSA
      - multiple drugs (MDRO)
        - ◊ antibiotics Z16.24
        - ◊ antimycobacterial (single) Z16.341
      - penicillins Z16.11
      - sulfonamides Z16.29
      - tetracyclines Z16.29
      - vancomycin Z16.21
        - ◊ related antibiotics Z16.22

Respiration

- Cheyne-Stokes R06.3
- decreased due to shock, following injury T79.4
- disorder of, psychogenic F45.8
- insufficient, or poor R06.89
  - newborn P28.5
- painful R07.1
- sighing, psychogenic F45.8

ALPHABETIC INDEX

Respiratory—*see also* Disease, diseased
- distress syndrome (newborn) (type I) P22.0
  - type II P22.1
- syncytial virus (RSV), as cause of disease classified elsewhere B97

Restless legs (syndrome) G25.81

Restriction of housing space Z59.19

Rests, ovarian, in fallopian tube Q50.6

Retained—*see also* Retention
- foreign body fragments (type of) Z18.9
  - acrylics Z18.2
  - animal quill(s) or spines Z18.31
  - cement Z18.83
  - concrete Z18.83
  - crystalline Z18.83
  - diethylhexylphthalates Z18.2
  - glass Z18.81
  - isocyanate Z18.2
  - magnetic metal Z18.11
  - metal Z18.10
  - nonmagnetic metal Z18.12
  - organic NEC Z18.39
  - plastic Z18.2
  - quill(s) (animal) Z18.31
  - specified NEC Z18.89
  - spine(s) (animal) Z18.31
  - stone Z18.83
  - tooth (teeth) Z18.32
  - wood Z18.33
- fragments (type of) Z18.9
  - acrylics Z18.2
  - animal quill(s) or spines Z18.31
  - cement Z18.83
  - concrete Z18.83
  - crystalline Z18.83
  - diethylhexylphthalates Z18.2
  - glass Z18.81
  - isocyanate Z18.2
  - magnetic metal Z18.11
  - metal Z18.10
  - nonmagnetic metal Z18.12
  - organic NEC Z18.39
  - plastic Z18.2
  - quill(s) (animal) Z18.31
  - specified NEC Z18.89
  - spine(s) (animal) Z18.31
  - stone Z18.83
  - tooth (teeth) Z18.32
  - wood Z18.33

Retardation
- development, developmental, specific—*see* Disorder, developmental
- growth R62.50
  - due to malnutrition E45
- mental—*see* Disability, intellectual
- motor function, specific F82
- physical (child) R62.52
  - due to malnutrition E45
- reading (specific) F81.0
- spelling (specific) (without reading disorder) F81.81

Retching—*see* Vomiting

Retention—*see also* Retained
- cyst—*see* Cyst
- dead
  - fetus (at or near term) (mother) O36.4
  - deciduous tooth K00.6
- fetus
  - dead O36.4
- fluid R60.9
- foreign body
  - current trauma—*code as* Foreign body, by site or type
- menses N94.89
- urine R33.9
  - psychogenic F45.8

Reticulocytosis R70.1

Reticulohistiocytoma (giant-cell) D76.3

Reticulosis (skin)
- hemophagocytic, familial D76.1

Retina, retinal—*see also* Disease, diseased

Retinoblastoma C69.2-
- differentiated C69.2-
- undifferentiated C69.2-

Retinopathy (background) H35.00
- in (due to)
  - diabetes—*see* Diabetes, retinopathy
  - sickle-cell disorders
    - nonproliferative D57.- *[H36.81-]*
    - proliferative D57.- *[H36.82-]*
- of prematurity H35.10-
  - stage 0 H35.11-
  - stage 1 H35.12-
  - stage 2 H35.13-
  - stage 3 H35.14-
  - stage 4 H35.15-
  - stage 5 H35.16-
- proliferative NEC H35.2-
  - Diabetic—*see* Diabetes, retinopathy, proliferative
  - Sickle-cell—*[H36.82-]*
  - thalassemia H35.2

Retractile testis Q55.22

Retraction
- nipple N64.53
  - associated with
  - congenital Q83.8

Retrograde menstruation N92.5

Retrosternal thyroid (congenital) Q89.2

Retroversion, retroverted
- testis (congenital) Q55.29

Rett's disease or syndrome F84.2

Rh (factor)
- hemolytic disease (newborn) P55.0
- incompatibility, immunization or sensitization
  - affecting management of pregnancy NEC O36.09-
    - anti-D antibody O36.01-
  - newborn P55.0
  - transfusion reaction—*see* Complication(s), transfusion, incompatibility reaction
- negative mother affecting newborn P55.0
- titer elevated—*see* Complication(s), transfusion, incompatibility reaction
- transfusion reaction—*see* Complication(s), transfusion, incompatibility reaction

Rhabdomyolysis (idiopathic) NEC M62.82

Rheumatic (acute) (subacute)
- chronic I09.89
- coronary arteritis I01.8
- fever (acute)—*see* Fever, rheumatic
- heart—*see* Disease, heart, rheumatic
- myocardial degeneration—*see* Degeneration, myocardium
- myocarditis (chronic) (inactive) (with chorea) I09.0
  - active or acute I01.2
  - with chorea (acute) (rheumatic) (Sydenham's) I02.0
- pancarditis, acute I01.8
  - with chorea (acute (rheumatic) Sydenham's) I02.0
- pericarditis (active) (acute) (with effusion) (with pneumonia) I01.0
  - with chorea (acute) (rheumatic) (Sydenham's) I02.0
  - chronic or inactive I09.2
- pneumonia I00 *[J17]*
- torticollis M43.6

Rheumatism (articular) (neuralgic) (nonarticular) M79.0
- intercostal, meaning Tietze's disease M94.0
- sciatic M54.4-

Rhinitis (atrophic) (catarrhal) (chronic) (croupous) (fibrinous) (granulomatous) (hyperplastic) (hypertrophic) (membranous) (obstructive) (purulent) (suppurative) (ulcerative) J31.0
- with
  - sore throat—*see* Nasopharyngitis
  - acute J00
  - allergic J30.9
  - with asthma J45.909
    - with
      - exacerbation (acute) J45.901
      - status asthmaticus J45.902
  - due to
    - food J30.5

Rhinitis, *continued*
  - pollen J30.1
  - nonseasonal J30.89
  - perennial J30.89
  - seasonal NEC J30.2
  - specified NEC J30.89
- infective J00
- pneumococcal J00
- vasomotor J30.0

Rhinoantritis (chronic)—*see* Sinusitis, maxillary

Rhinolith (nasal sinus) J34.89

Rhinomegaly J34.89

Rhinopharyngitis (acute) (subacute)—*see also* Nasopharyngitis

Rhinorrhea J34.89
- cerebrospinal (fluid) G96.01
  - postoperative G96.08
  - specified NEC G96.08
  - spontaneous G96.01
  - traumatic G96.08
- paroxysmal—*see* Rhinitis, allergic
- spasmodic—*see* Rhinitis, allergic

Rhinovirus infection NEC B34.8

Rhizomelic chondrodysplasia punctata E71.540

Rhythm
- disorder I49.9
- escape I49.9
- heart, abnormal I49.9
- idioventricular I44.2
- sleep, inversion G47.2-

Rhytidosis facialis L98.8

Rickets (active) (acute) (adolescent) (chest wall) (congenital) (current) (infantile) (intestinal) E55.0
- celiac K90.0
- hypophosphatemic with nephrotic-glycosuric dwarfism E72.09

Rickettsial disease A79.9
- specified type NEC A79.89

Rickettsialpox (rickettsia akari) A79.1

Rickettsiosis A79.9
- due to
  - Rickettsia akari (rickettsialpox) A79.1
- specified type NEC A79.89
- tick-borne A77.9
- vesicular A79.1

Riedel's
- lobe, liver Q44.79
- struma, thyroiditis or disease E06.5

Rieger anomaly or syndrome Q13.81

Riehl's melanosis L81.4

Rietti-Greppi-Micheli anemia D56.9

Rieux's hernia—*see* Hernia

Riga (-Fede) **disease** K14.0

Right middle lobe syndrome J98.11

Rigid, rigidity—*see also* Disease, diseased
- abdominal R19.30
  - with severe abdominal pain R10.0
- nuchal R29.1

Rigors R68.89
- with fever R50.9

Ringworm B35.9
- beard B35.0
- black dot B35.0
- body B35.4
- corporeal B35.4
- foot B35.3
- groin B35.6
- hand B35.2
- honeycomb B35.0
- nails B35.1
- perianal (area) B35.6
- scalp B35.0
- specified NEC B35.8

ALPHABETIC INDEX

Risk
- for
  - dental caries Z91.849
    - high Z91.843
    - low Z91.841
    - moderate Z91.842
  - homelessness, imminent Z59.811
- suicidal
  - meaning personal history of attempted suicide Z91.51
  - meaning suicidal ideation—*see* Ideation, suicidal

Ritter's disease L00

Robert's pelvis Q74.2

Robin (-Pierre) syndrome Q87.0

Robinow-Silverman-Smith syndrome Q87.19

Rocky Mountain (spotted) fever A77.0

Roger's disease Q21.0

Rolando's fracture (displaced) S62.22-
- nondisplaced S62.22-

Romano-Ward (prolonged QT interval) **syndrome** I45.81

Romberg's disease or syndrome G51.8

Roof, mouth—*see* Disease, diseased

Rosary, rachitic E55.0

Rose
- cold J30.1
- fever J30.1
- rash R21
  - epidemic B06.9

Rosenthal's disease or syndrome D68.1

Roseola B09
- infantum B08.20
  - due to human herpesvirus 6 B08.21
  - due to human herpesvirus 7 B08.22

Rossbach's disease K31.89
- psychogenic F45.8

Rothmund (-Thomson) syndrome Q82.8

Rotor's disease or syndrome E80.6

Round
- worms (large) (infestation) NEC B82.0
  - Ascariasis (*see also* Ascariasis) B77.9

Rubella (German measles) B06.9
- complication NEC B06.09
  - neurological B06.00
- congenital P35.0
- contact Z20.4
- exposure to Z20.4
- maternal
  - care for (suspected) damage to fetus O35.3
  - manifest rubella in infant P35.0
  - suspected damage to fetus affecting management of pregnancy O35.3
- specified complications NEC B06.89

Rubeola (meaning measles)—*see* Measles
- meaning rubella—*see* Rubella

Rudimentary (congenital)—*see also* Agenesis
- bone Q79.9

Ruled out condition—*see* Observation, suspected

Rumination R11.10
- with nausea R11.2
- disorder of infancy F98.21
- disorder of infancy or childhood (in remission) F98.21
- neurotic F42.8
- newborn P92.1
- obsessional F42.8
- psychogenic F42.8

Runaway [from current living environment] Z62.892

Runny nose R09.89

Rupture, ruptured
- abscess (spontaneous)—*code by site under* Abscess
- aorta, aortic I71.8
  - arch I71.12
  - ascending I71.11
    - thoracic I71.13
  - thorax, thoracic I71.10
  - valve or cusp (*see also* Endocarditis, aortic) I35.8

Rupture, ruptured, *continued*
- appendix (with peritonitis) K35.32
  - with localized peritonitis K35.32
- arteriovenous fistula, brain I60.8-
- cardiac (auricle) (ventricle) (wall) I23.3
  - with hemopericardium I23.0
  - infectional I40.9
- cecum (with peritonitis) K65.0
  - with peritoneal abscess K35.33
- cerebral aneurysm (congenital) (*see* Hemorrhage, intracranial, subarachnoid)
- circle of Willis I60.6
- corpus luteum (infected) (ovary) N83.1-
- cyst—*see* Cyst
- ear drum (nontraumatic)—*see also* Perforation, tympanum
  - traumatic S09.2-
- fallopian tube NEC (nonobstetric) (nontraumatic) N83.8
  - due to pregnancy O00.10
- gastric
  - vessel K92.2
- graafian follicle (hematoma) N83.0-
- hymen (nontraumatic) (nonintentional) N89.8
- kidney (traumatic) birth injury P15.8
- meningeal artery I60.8-
- ovary, ovarian N83.8
  - corpus luteum cyst N83.1-
  - follicle (graafian) N83.0-
- oviduct (nonobstetric) (nontraumatic) N83.8
  - due to pregnancy O00.10
- pulmonary
  - valve (heart) I37.8
- rotator cuff (nontraumatic) M75.10-
  - complete M75.12-
  - incomplete M75.11-
- spleen (traumatic) S36.03-
  - birth injury P15.1
- tonsil J35.8
- traumatic
  - spleen S36.03-
- tricuspid (heart) (valve) I07.8
- tube, tubal (nonobstetric) (nontraumatic) N83.8
  - abscess—*see* Salpingitis
  - due to pregnancy O00.10
- tympanum, tympanic (membrane) (nontraumatic) (*see also* Perforation, tympanic membrane) H72.9-
  - traumatic—*see* Rupture, ear drum, traumatic
- viscus R19.8

Russell-Silver syndrome Q87.19

Ruvalcaba-Myhre-Smith syndrome E71.440

Rytand-Lipsitch syndrome I44.2

S

Saccharomyces infection B37.9

Sachs' amaurotic familial idiocy or disease E75.02

Sachs-Tay disease E75.02

Sacks-Libman disease M32.11

Sacralgia M53.3

Sacrodynia M53.3

Saint
- Anthony's fire—*see* Erysipelas

Salmonella—*see* Infection, Salmonella

Salmonellosis A02.0

Salpingitis (catarrhal) (fallopian tube) (nodular) (pseudofollicular) (purulent) (septic) N70.91
- with oophoritis N70.93
- acute N70.01
  - with oophoritis N70.03
- chlamydial A56.11
- chronic N70.11
  - with oophoritis N70.13
- gonococcal (acute) (chronic) A54.24
- specific (gonococcal) (acute) (chronic) A54.24
- venereal (gonococcal) (acute) (chronic) A54.24

Salpingo-oophoritis (catarrhal) (purulent) (ruptured) (septic) (suppurative) N70.93
- acute N70.03
  - gonococcal A54.24
  - chronic N70.13

Salpingo-oophoritis, *continued*
- gonococcal (acute) (chronic) A54.24
- specific (gonococcal) (acute) (chronic) A54.24
- venereal (gonococcal) (acute) (chronic) A54.24

Sandhoff's disease E75.01

Sanfilippo (Type B) (Type C) (Type D) **syndrome** E76.22

Sanger-Brown ataxia G11.2

Sao Paulo fever or typhus A77.0

Sarcoepiplocele—*see* Hernia

Sarcoepiplomphalocele Q79.2

Sarcoid—*see also* Sarcoidosis
- arthropathy D86.86
- Boeck's D86.9
- Darier-Roussy D86.3
- iridocyclitis D86.83
- meningitis D86.81
- myocarditis D86.85
- myositis D86.87
- pyelonephritis D86.84

Sarcoidosis D86.9
- with
  - cranial nerve palsies D86.82
  - hepatic granuloma D86.89
  - polyarthritis D86.86
  - tubulo-interstitial nephropathy D86.84
- combined sites NEC D86.89
- lung D86.0
  - and lymph nodes D86.2
- lymph nodes D86.1
  - and lung D86.2
- meninges D86.81
- skin D86.3
- specified type NEC D86.89

Sarcoma (of)—*see also* Neoplasm, connective tissue, malignant in Table of Neoplasms in the complete *ICD-10-CM* manual
- cerebellar C71.6
  - circumscribed (arachnoidal) C71.6
- circumscribed (arachnoidal) cerebellar C71.6
- clear cell—*see also* Neoplasm, connective tissue, malignant in Table of Neoplasms in the complete *ICD-10-CM* manual
  - kidney C64.-
- monstrocellular
  - specified site—*see* Neoplasm, malignant, by site in Table of Neoplasms in the complete *ICD-10-CM* manual
  - unspecified site C71.9

SARS-CoV-2— *see also* COVID-19
- sequelae (post acute) U09.9

SBE (subacute bacterial endocarditis) I33.0

Scabies (any site) B86

Scaglietti-Dagnini syndrome E22.0

Scald—*see* Burn

Scaphocephaly, non-deformational Q75.01

Scapulohumeral myopathy G71.02

Scar, scarring (*see also* Cicatrix) L90.5
- adherent L90.5
- atrophic L90.5
- cheloid L91.0
- hypertrophic L91.0
- keloid L91.0
- painful L90.5
- vagina N89.8
  - postoperative N99.2
- vulva N90.89

Scarabiasis B88.2

Scarlatina (anginosa) (maligna) A38.9
- myocarditis (acute) A38.1
  - old—*see* Myocarditis
- otitis media A38.0
- ulcerosa A38.8

Scarlet fever (albuminuria) (angina) A38.9

Schaumann's
- benign lymphogranulomatosis D86.1
- disease or syndrome—*see* Sarcoidosis

Schistosomiasis B65.9
- cutaneous B65.3

Schizencephaly Q04.6

Schizophrenia, schizophrenic
- childhood type F84.5
  - syndrome of childhood F84.5

Schlatter-Osgood disease or osteochondrosis M92.52-

Schlatter's tibia M92.52-

Schmorl's disease or nodes
- sacrococcygeal region M53.3

Scholte's E34.09

Schönlein (-Henoch) disease or purpura (primary) (rheumatic) D69.0

Schultze's type acroparesthesia, simple I73.89

Schwannomatosis Q85.03

Schwartz-Bartter syndrome E22.2

Sciatica (infective)
- with lumbago M54.4-

Scleredema
- newborn P83.0

Sclerema (adiposum) (edematosum) (neonatorum) (newborn) P83.0

Sclerocystic ovary syndrome E28.2

Scleroderma, sclerodermia (acrosclerotic) (diffuse) (generalized) (progressive) (pulmonary) (*see also* Sclerosis)
- newborn P83.88

Sclérose en plaques G35

Sclerosis, sclerotic
- ascending multiple G35
- brain (generalized) (lobular) G37.9
  - disseminated G35
  - insular G35
  - miliary G35
  - multiple G35
  - stem, multiple G35
  - tuberous Q85.1
- bulbar, multiple G35
- cerebrospinal (disseminated) (multiple) G35
- disseminated G35
- dorsal G35
- extrapyramidal G25.9
- Friedreich's (spinal cord) G11.11
- hereditary
  - spinal (Friedreich's ataxia) G11.11
- hippocampal G93.81
- insular G35
- mesial temporal G93.81
- mitral I05.8
- multiple (brain stem) (cerebral) (generalized) (spinal cord) G35
- plaques G35
- pulmonary
  - artery I27.0
- spinal (cord) (progressive) G95.89
  - hereditary (Friedreich's) (mixed form) G11.11
- temporal (mesial) G93.81
- tricuspid (heart) (valve) I07.8
- tuberous (brain) Q85.1

Scoliosis (acquired) (postural) M41.9
- adolescent (idiopathic)—*see* Scoliosis, idiopathic, juvenile
- congenital Q67.5
  - due to bony malformation Q76.3
- idiopathic M41.20
  - adolescent M41.129
    - cervical region M41.122
    - cervicothoracic region M41.123
    - lumbar region M41.126
    - lumbosacral region M41.127
    - thoracic region M41.124
    - thoracolumbar region M41.125
  - cervical region M41.22
  - cervicothoracic region M41.23
  - infantile M41.00
    - cervical region M41.02
    - cervicothoracic region M41.03
    - lumbar region M41.06
    - lumbosacral region M41.07

Scoliosis, *continued*
    - sacrococcygeal region M41.08
    - thoracic region M41.04
    - thoracolumbar region M41.05
  - juvenile M41.119
    - cervical region M41.112
    - cervicothoracic region M41.113
    - lumbar region M41.116
    - lumbosacral region M41.117
    - thoracic region M41.114
    - thoracolumbar region M41.115
  - lumbar M41.26
    - lumbosacral M41.27
    - thoracic M41.24
    - thoracolumbar M41.25
- sciatic M54.4-

Scratch—*see* Abrasion

Scratchy throat R09.89

Screening (for) Z13.9
- alcoholism Z13.89
- anemia Z13.0
- autism Z13.41
- behavioral disorders Z13.30
- cardiovascular disorder Z13.6
- chlamydial diseases Z11.8
- chromosomal abnormalities (nonprocreative) NEC Z13.79
- congenital
  - dislocation of hip Z13.89
  - eye disorder Z13.5
  - malformation or deformation Z13.89
- cystic fibrosis Z13.228
- depression (adult) (adolescent) (child) Z13.31
  - maternal or perinatal Z13.32
- developmental
  - delays Z13.40
    - global (milestones) Z13.42
    - specified NEC Z13.49
  - handicap Z13.42
    - in early childhood Z13.42
- diabetes mellitus Z13.1
- disability, intellectual Z13.39
  - infant Z13.41
- disease or disorder Z13.9
  - bacterial NEC Z11.2
    - intestinal infectious Z11.0
    - respiratory tuberculosis Z11.1
  - behavioral Z13.30
    - specified NEC Z13.49
  - blood or blood-forming organ Z13.0
  - cardiovascular Z13.6
  - chlamydial Z11.8
  - coronavirus (novel) 2019 Z11.52
  - dental Z13.89
  - developmental delays Z13.40
    - global (milestones) Z13.42
    - specified NEC Z13.49
  - endocrine Z13.29
  - heart Z13.6
  - human immunodeficiency virus (HIV) infection Z11.4
  - immunity Z13.0
  - infectious Z11.9
  - mental health and behavioral Z13.30
  - metabolic Z13.228
  - neurological Z13.89
  - nutritional Z13.21
    - metabolic Z13.228
    - lipoid disorders Z13.220
  - respiratory Z13.83
  - rheumatic Z13.828
  - rickettsial Z11.8
  - sexually-transmitted NEC Z11.3
    - human immunodeficiency virus (HIV) Z11.4
  - sickle cell trait Z13.0
  - spirochetal Z11.8
  - thyroid Z13.29
  - venereal Z11.3
  - viral NEC Z11.59
    - human immunodeficiency virus (HIV) Z11.4
- elevated titer Z13.89
- galactosemia Z13.228
- gonorrhea Z11.3

Screening, *continued*
- hematopoietic malignancy Z12.89
- hemoglobinopathies Z13.0
- Hodgkin disease Z12.89
- human immunodeficiency virus (HIV) Z11.4
- human papillomavirus (HPV) Z11.51
- hypertension Z13.6
- immunity disorders Z13.0
- infant or child (over 28 days old) Z00.12-
- infection
  - mycotic Z11.8
  - parasitic Z11.8
- intellectual disability Z13.39
- leukemia Z12.89
- lymphoma Z12.89
- malaria Z11.6
- measles Z11.59
- mental health disorder Z13.30
- metabolic errors, inborn Z13.228
- musculoskeletal disorder Z13.828
- mycoses Z11.8
- neoplasm (malignant) (of) Z12.9
  - blood Z12.89
  - breast Z12.39
    - routine mammogram Z12.31
  - cervix Z12.4
  - hematopoietic system Z12.89
  - lymph (glands) Z12.89
  - nervous system Z12.82
- nephropathy Z13.89
- nervous system disorders NEC Z13.858
- neurological condition Z13.89
- parasitic infestation Z11.9
  - specified NEC Z11.8
- phenylketonuria Z13.228
- poisoning (chemical) (heavy metal) Z13.88
- postnatal, chromosomal abnormalities Z13.89
- rheumatoid arthritis Z13.828
- sexually-transmitted disease NEC Z11.3
  - human immunodeficiency virus (HIV) Z11.4
- sickle-cell disease or trait Z13.0
- special Z13.9
  - specified NEC Z13.89
- syphilis Z11.3
- traumatic brain injury Z13.850
- tuberculosis, respiratory
  - active Z11.1
  - latent Z11.7
- venereal disease Z11.3
- viral encephalitis (mosquito- or tick-borne) Z11.59
- whooping cough Z11.2

Scrofula, scrofulosis (tuberculosis of cervical lymph glands) A18.2

Scurvy, scorbutic
- anemia D53.2
- rickets E55.0 [M90.80]

Seasickness T75.3

Seatworm (infection) (infestation) B80

Seborrhea, seborrheic L21.9
- capillitii R23.8
- capitis L21.0
- dermatitis L21.9
  - infantile L21.1
- eczema L21.9
  - infantile L21.1
- sicca L21.0

Seckel's syndrome Q87.19

Second hand tobacco smoke exposure (acute) (chronic) Z77.22
- in the perinatal period P96.81

Secretion
- antidiuretic hormone, inappropriate E22.2
- hormone
  - antidiuretic, inappropriate (syndrome) E22.2
  - by
    - carcinoid tumor (*see also* Tumor, carcinoid) E34.09
  - urinary
    - excessive R35.89
    - suppression R34

Seitelberger's syndrome (infantile neuraxonal dystrophy) G31.89

ALPHABETIC INDEX

Seizure(s) (*see also* Convulsions) R56.9
- akinetic—*see* Epilepsy, generalized, specified NEC
- atonic—*see* Epilepsy, generalized, specified NEC
- convulsive—*see* Convulsions
- disorder (*see also* Epilepsy) G40.909
- epileptic—*see* Epilepsy
- febrile (simple) R56.00
  - with status epilepticus G40.901
  - complex (atypical) (complicated) R56.01
    - with status epilepticus G40.901
- newborn P90
- nonspecific epileptic
  - atonic—*see* Epilepsy, generalized, specified NEC
  - clonic—*see* Epilepsy, generalized, specified NEC
  - myoclonic—*see* Epilepsy, generalized, specified NEC
  - tonic—*see* Epilepsy, generalized, specified NEC
  - tonic-clonic—*see* Epilepsy, generalized, specified NEC
- partial, developing into secondarily generalized seizures
  - complex—*see* Epilepsy, localization-related, symptomatic, with complex partial seizures
  - simple—*see* Epilepsy, localization-related, symptomatic
- petit mal G40.A-
  - intractable G40.A1-
    - with status epilepticus G40.A11
    - without status epilepticus G40.A19
  - not intractable G40.A0-
    - with status epilepticus G40.A01
    - without status epilepticus G40.A09
- post traumatic R56.1
- recurrent G40.909
- specified NEC G40.89

Self-damaging behavior (life-style) Z72.89

Self-harm (attempted)
- history (personal)
  - in family Z81.8
  - nonsuicidal Z91.52
  - suicidal Z91.51
- nonsuicidal R45.88

Self-injury, nonsuicidal R45.88
- personal history Z91.52

Self-mutilation (attempted)
- history (personal)
  - in family Z81.8
  - nonsuicidal Z91.52
  - suicidal Z91.51
- nonsuicidal R45.88

Self-poisoning
- history (personal) Z91.51
  - in family Z81.8
- observation following (alleged) attempt Z03.6

Semicoma R40.1

Sensation
- foreign body R09.A0
  - eye H57.8A-
  - globus R09.A2
  - nose R09.A1
  - specified site NEC R09.A9
  - throat R09.A2

Sensitive, sensitivity—*see also* Allergy
- child (excessive) F93.8
- cold, autoimmune D59.12
- dentin K03.89
- gluten (non-celiac) K90.41
- methemoglobin D74.8
- tuberculin, without clinical or radiological symptoms R76.11

Sensitization, auto-erythrocytic D69.2

Separation
- anxiety, abnormal (of childhood) F93.0
- apophysis, traumatic—*code as* Fracture, by site
- epiphysis, epiphyseal
  - nontraumatic—*see also* Osteochondropathy
    - upper femoral—*see* Slipped, epiphysis, upper femoral
  - traumatic—*code as* Fracture, by site

Sepsis (generalize) (unspecified organism) A41.9
- with
  - organ dysfunction (acute) (multiple) R65.20
    - with septic shock R65.21
  - anaerobic A41.4
  - candidal B37.7
  - cryptogenic A41.9
- due to device, implant or graft T85.79
  - catheter NEC T85.79
    - dialysis (renal) T82.7
    - infusion NEC T82.7
    - urethral indwelling T83.511
      - urinary T83.518
    - vascular T82.7
  - Enterococcus A41.81
  - Escherichia coli (E. coli) A41.51
  - following
    - immunization T88.0
    - infusion, therapeutic injection or transfusion NEC T80.29
  - gangrenous A41.9
  - Gram-negative (organism) A41.5-
    - anaerobic A41.4
  - Haemophilus influenzae A41.3
  - localized—code to specific localized infection
    - in operation wound T81.49
    - postprocedural T81.44
  - meningeal—*see* Meningitis
  - meningococcal A39.4
    - acute A39.2
    - chronic A39.3
  - MSSA (Methicillin susceptible Staphylococcus aureus) A41.01
  - newborn P36.9
    - due to
      - anaerobes NEC P36.5
      - Escherichia coli P36.4
      - Staphylococcus P36.30
        - aureus P36.2
        - specified NEC P36.39
      - Streptococcus P36.10
        - group B P36.0
        - specified NEC P36.19
    - specified NEC P36.8
  - Pasteurella multocida A28.0
  - pneumococcal A40.3
  - severe R65.20
    - with septic shock R65.21
  - Shigella (*see also* Dysentery, bacillary) A03.9
  - skin, localized—*see* Abscess
  - specified organism NEC A41.89
  - Staphylococcus, staphylococcal A41.2
    - aureus (methicillin susceptible) (MSSA) A41.01
      - methicillin resistant (MRSA) A41.02
    - coagulase-negative A41.1
    - specified NEC A41.1
  - Streptococcus, streptococcal A40.9
    - group
      - D A41.81
    - neonatal P36.10
      - group B P36.0
      - specified NEC P36.19
    - pneumoniae A40.3

Septic—*see* Disease, diseased
- gallbladder (acute) K81.0
- sore—*see also* Abscess
  - throat J02.0
    - streptococcal J02.0
  - tonsils, chronic J35.01
    - with adenoiditis J35.03

Septicemia A41.9
- meaning sepsis—*see* Sepsis

Septum, septate (congenital)—*see also* Anomaly, by site
- anal Q42.3
  - with fistula Q42.2
- aqueduct of Sylvius Q03.0
  - with spina bifida—*see* Spina bifida, by site, with hydrocephalus
- uterus Q51.2-
- vaginal, longitudinal Q52.129

Septum, septate, *continued*
- microperforate
  - left side Q52.124
  - right side Q52.123
- nonobstructing Q52.120
- obstructing
  - left side Q52.122
  - right side Q52.121

Sequelae (of)—*see also* Disease, diseased
- COVID-19 (post acute) U09.9
- encephalitis or encephalomyelitis (conditions in G04)
  G09
  - in infectious disease NEC B94.8
  - viral B94.1
- hepatitis, viral B94.2
- infectious disease B94.9
  - specified NEC B94.8
- parasitic disease B94.9
- SARS-CoV-2 (post acute) U09.9
- viral
  - encephalitis B94.1
  - hepatitis B94.2

Serology for syphilis
- doubtful
  - with signs or symptoms—*code by site and stage under* Syphilis
- reactivated A53.0
- positive A53.0

Serositis, multiple K65.8
- pericardial I31.1

Serum
- allergy, allergic reaction (*see also* Reaction, serum) T80.69
  - shock (*see also* Shock, anaphylactic) T80.59
- arthritis (*see also* Reaction, serum) T80.69
- complication or reaction NEC (*see also* Reaction, serum) T80.69
- disease NEC (*see also* Reaction, serum) T80.69
- hepatitis—*see also* Hepatitis, viral, type B
  - carrier (suspected) of B18.1
- intoxication (*see also* Reaction, serum) T80.69
- neuritis (*see also* Reaction, serum) T80.69
- poisoning NEC (*see also* Reaction, serum) T80.69
- rash NEC (*see also* Reaction, serum) T80.69
- reaction NEC (*see also* Reaction, serum) T80.69
- sickness NEC (*see also* Reaction, serum) T80.69
- urticaria (*see also* Reaction, serum) T80.69

Severe sepsis R65.20
- with septic shock R65.21

Sexual
- immaturity (female) (male) E30.0
- precocity (constitutional) (cryptogenic) (female) (idiopathic) (male) E30.1

Shadow lung R91.8

Shedding
- nail L60.8
- premature, primary (deciduous) teeth K00.6

Sheehan's disease or syndrome E23.0

Shelf, rectal K62.89

Shellshock (current) F43.0
- lasting state—*see* Disorder, post-traumatic stress

Shigellosis A03.9
- Group A A03.0
- Group B A03.1
- Group C A03.2
- Group D A03.3

Shock R57.9
- adverse food reaction (anaphylactic)—*see* Shock, anaphylactic, due to food
- allergic—*see* Shock, anaphylactic
- anaphylactic T78.2
  - chemical—*see* Table of Drugs and Chemicals
  - due to drug or medicinal substance
    - correct substance properly administered T88.6-
    - overdose or wrong substance given or taken (by accident)—*see* Table of Drugs and Chemicals, by drug, poisoning
  - due to food (nonpoisonous) T78.00
    - additives T78.06
    - dairy products T78.07

ALPHABETIC INDEX

Shock, *continued*
- ■ eggs T78.08
- ■ fish T78.03
  - ~ shellfish T78.02
- ■ fruit T78.04
- ■ milk T78.07
- ■ nuts T78.05
  - ~ peanuts T78.01
- ■ peanuts T78.01
- ■ seeds T78.05
- ■ specified type NEC T78.09
- ■ vegetable T78.04
- – following sting(s)—*see* Table of Drugs and Chemicals, by animal or substance, poisoning
- – immunization T80.52-
- – serum T80.59-
  - ■ blood and blood products T80.51-
  - ■ immunization T80.52-
  - ■ specified NEC T80.59-
  - ■ vaccination T80.52-
- anaphylactoid—*see* Shock, anaphylactic
- cardiogenic R57.0
- chemical substance—*see* Table of Drugs and Chemicals
- culture—*see* Disorder, adjustment
- drug
  - – due to correct substance properly administered T88.6
  - – overdose or wrong substance given or taken (by accident)—*see* Table of Drugs and Chemicals, by drug, poisoning
- electric T75.4
  - – (taser) T75.4
- endotoxic R65.21
- postprocedural (during or resulting from a procedure, not elsewhere classified) T81.12-
- following
  - – injury (immediate) (delayed) T79.4
- food (anaphylactic)—*see* Shock, anaphylactic, due to food
- from electroshock gun (taser) T75.4
- gram-negative R65.21
  - – postprocedural (during or resulting from a procedure, NEC) T81.12
- hematologic R57.8
- hemorrhagic R57.8
  - – surgery (intraoperative) (postoperative) T81.19
  - – trauma T79.4
- hypovolemic R57.1
  - – surgical T81.19
  - – traumatic T79.4
- insulin E15
  - – therapeutic misadventure—*see* subcategory T38.3
- kidney N17.0
- lung J80
- pleural (surgical) T81.19
  - – due to trauma T79.4
- postprocedural (postoperative) T81.10
  - – cardiogenic T81.11
  - – endotoxic T81.12-
  - – gram-negative T81.12-
  - – hypovolemic T81.19
  - – septic T81.12-
  - – specified type NEC T81.19
- psychic F43.0
- septic (due to severe sepsis) R65.21
- specified NEC R57.8
- surgical T81.10
- taser gun (taser) T75.4
- therapeutic misadventure NEC T81.10
- toxic, syndrome A48.3
- transfusion—*see* Complications, transfusion
- traumatic (immediate) (delayed) T79.4

Short, shortening, shortness
- arm (acquired)—*see also* Deformity, limb length
  - – congenital Q71.81-
- breath R06.02
- bowel syndrome K91.2
- common bile duct, congenital Q44.5
- cystic duct, congenital Q44.5
- frenum, frenulum, linguae (congenital) Q38.1
- hip (acquired)—*see also* Deformity, limb
  - – congenital Q65.89
- leg (acquired)—*see also* Deformity, limb
  - – congenital Q72.81-

Short, shortening, shortness, *continued*
- lower limb (acquired)—*see also* Deformity, limb
  - – congenital Q72.81-
- rib syndrome Q77.2
- stature (child) (hereditary) (idiopathic) NEC R62.52
  - – constitutional E34.31
  - – due to endocrine disorder E34.3
  - – insulin-like growth factor-1 (IGF-1) resistance E34.322
  - – Laron-type E34.3
  - – other genetic causes of short stature E34.328
  - – other short stature due to endocrine disorder E34.39
  - – primary insulin-like growth factor-1 (IGF-1) deficiency E34.321
  - – unspecified genetic causes of short stature E34.329
- tendon—*see also* Contraction
  - – with contracture of joint—*see* Contraction, joint
  - – Achilles (acquired) M67.0-
    - ■ congenital Q66.89
  - – congenital Q79.8

Shunt
- arterial-venous (dialysis) Z99.2
- arteriovenous, pulmonary (acquired) I28.0
  - – congenital Q25.72
- cerebral ventricle (communicating) in situ Z98.2

Sialitis, silitis (any gland) (chronic) (suppurative)—*see* Sialoadenitis

Sialoadenitis (any gland) (periodic) (suppurative) K11.20
- acute K11.21
  - – recurrent K11.22
- chronic K11.23

Sialidosis E77.1

Sibling rivalry Z62.891

Sicard's syndrome G52.7

Sick R69
- or handicapped person in family Z63.79
  - – needing care at home Z63.6
- sinus (syndrome) I49.5

Sickle-cell
- anemia—*see* Disease, sickle-cell
- beta plus—*see* Disease, sickle-cell, thalassemia, beta plus
- beta zero—*see* Disease, sickle-cell, thalassemia, beta zero
- trait D57.3

Sicklemia—*see also* Disease, sickle-cell
- trait D57.3

Sickness
- air (travel) T75.3
- airplane T75.3
- car T75.3
- green D50.8
- milk—*see* Poisoning, food, noxious
- motion T75.3
- mountain T70.29
  - – acute D75.1
- protein (*see also* Reaction, serum) T80.69
- roundabout (motion) T75.3
- sea T75.3
- serum NEC (*see also* Reaction, serum) T80.69
- swing (motion) T75.3
- train (railway) (travel) T75.3
- travel (any vehicle) T75.3

Siemens' syndrome (ectodermal dysplasia) Q82.8

Sighing R06.89
- psychogenic F45.8

Sigmoiditis (*see also* Enteritis) K52.9
- infectious A09
- noninfectious K52.9

Silver's syndrome Q87.19

Simple, simplex—*see* Disease, diseased

Simulation, conscious (of illness) Z76.5

Single
- atrium Q21.2
- umbilical artery Q27.0

Sinus—*see also* Fistula
- bradycardia R00.1
- dermal (congenital) Q06.8
  - – with abscess Q06.8
- pilonidal (infected) (rectum) L05.92
  - – with abscess L05.02
- preauricular Q18.1
- tachycardia R00.0
  - – paroxysmal I47.19
- tarsi syndrome M25.57-

Sinusitis (accessory) (chronic) (hyperplastic) (nasal) (nonpurulent) (purulent) J32.9
- acute J01.90
  - – ethmoidal J01.20
    - ■ recurrent J01.21
  - – frontal J01.10
    - ■ recurrent J01.11
  - – involving more than one sinus, other than pansinusitis J01.80
    - ■ recurrent J01.81
  - – maxillary J01.00
    - ■ recurrent J01.01
  - – pansinusitis J01.40
    - ■ recurrent J01.41
  - – recurrent J01.91
  - – specified NEC J01.80
    - ■ recurrent J01.81
  - – sphenoidal J01.30
    - ■ recurrent J01.31
- allergic—*see* Rhinitis, allergic
- ethmoidal J32.2
  - – acute J01.20
    - ■ recurrent J01.21
- frontal J32.1
  - – acute J01.10
    - ■ recurrent J01.11
- influenzal—*see* Influenza, with, respiratory manifestations NEC
- involving more than one sinus but not pansinusitis J32.8
  - – acute J01.80
    - ■ recurrent J01.81
- maxillary J32.0
  - – acute J01.00
    - ■ recurrent J01.01
- sphenoidal J32.3
  - – acute J01.30
    - ■ recurrent J01.31

Sinusitis-bronchiectasis-situs inversus (syndrome) (triad) Q89.3

Siriasis T67.01

Situation, psychiatric F99

Situational
- disturbance (transient)—*see* Disorder, adjustment
  - – acute F43.0
- maladjustment—*see* Disorder, adjustment
- reaction—*see* Disorder, adjustment
  - – acute F43.0

Situs inversus or transversus (abdominalis) (thoracis) Q89.3

Sixth disease B08.20
- due to human herpesvirus 6 B08.21
- due to human herpesvirus 7 B08.22

Sjögren-Larsson syndrome Q87.19

Skin—*see also* Disease, diseased
- clammy R23.1
- dry L85.3

Sleep
- disorder or disturbance G47.9
  - – child F51.9
  - – nonorganic origin F51.9
  - – specified NEC G47.8
- disturbance G47.9
  - – nonorganic origin F51.9
- drunkenness F51.9
- rhythm inversion G47.2-
- risk of suffocation (smothering) under another while sleeping Z72.823
- terrors F51.4
- walking F51.3
  - – hysterical F44.89

Sleep-wake schedule disorder G47.20

Slim disease (in HIV infection) B20

Slipped, slipping
- epiphysis (traumatic)—*see also* Osteochondropathy
  - capital femoral (traumatic)
    - acute (on chronic) S79.01-
  - current traumatic—*code as* Fracture, by site
  - upper femoral (nontraumatic) M93.0-
    - acute M93.01-
    - on chronic M93.03-
    - chronic M93.02-
- ligature, umbilical P51.8

Slow
- feeding, newborn P92.2
- heart (beat) R00.1

Slowing, urinary stream R39.198

Small(ness)
- for gestational age—*see* Small for dates
- introitus, vagina N89.6
- kidney (unknown cause)
  - bilateral N27.1
  - unilateral N27.0
- ovary (congenital) Q50.39
- uterus N85.8
- white kidney N03.9

Small-and-light-for-dates—*see* Small for dates

Small-for-dates (infant) P05.10
- with weight of
  - 499 grams or less P05.11
  - 500–749 grams P05.12
  - 750–999 grams P05.13
  - 1000–1249 grams P05.14
  - 1250–1499 grams P05.15
  - 1500–1749 grams P05.16
  - 1750–1999 grams P05.17
  - 2000–2499 grams P05.18
  - 2500 grams and over P05.19

Smearing, fecal R15.1

SMEI (severe myoclonic epilepsy in infancy) G40.83-

Smith's fracture S52.54-

Smoker—*see* Dependence, drug, nicotine

Smoking
- passive Z77.22

Smothering spells R06.81

Sneezing (intractable) R06.7

Sniffing
- cocaine
  - abuse—*see* Abuse, drug, cocaine
  - dependence—*see* Dependence, drug, cocaine
- gasoline
  - abuse—*see* Abuse, drug, inhalant
  - dependence—*see* Dependence, drug, inhalant
- glue (airplane)
  - abuse—*see* Abuse, drug, inhalant
  - drug dependence—*see* Dependence, drug, inhalant

Sniffles
- newborn P28.89

Snoring R06.83

Snuffles (non-syphilitic) R06.5
- newborn P28.89

Social
- exclusion Z60.4
- migrant Z59.0
  - acculturation difficulty Z60.3
- rejection Z60.4
- skills inadequacy NEC Z73.4
- transplantation Z60.3

Sodoku A25.0

Softening
- brain (necrotic) (progressive) G93.89
  - congenital Q04.8
- cartilage M94.2-
  - patella M22.4-

Soldier's
- heart F45.8
- patches I31.0

Solitary
- cyst, kidney N28.1
- kidney, congenital Q60.0

Soor B37.0

Sore
- mouth K13.79
  - canker K12.0
- muscle M79.10
- skin L98.9
- throat (acute)—*see also* Pharyngitis
  - with influenza, flu, or grippe—*see* Influenza, with, respiratory manifestations NEC
  - chronic J31.2
  - coxsackie (virus) B08.5
  - herpesviral B00.2
  - influenzal—*see* Influenza, with, respiratory manifestations NEC
  - septic J02.0
  - streptococcal (ulcerative) J02.0
  - viral NEC J02.8
    - coxsackie B08.5

Soto's syndrome (cerebral gigantism) Q87.3

Spading nail L60.8
- congenital Q84.6

Spanish collar N47.1

Spasm(s), spastic, spasticity (*see also* Disease, diseased) R25.2
- artery I73.9
  - cerebral G45.9
- anus, ani (sphincter) (reflex) K59.4
  - psychogenic F45.8
- bladder (sphincter, external or internal) N32.89
  - psychogenic F45.8
- bronchus, bronchiole J98.01
- cerebral (arteries) (vascular) G45.9
- colon K58.9
  - with constipation K58.1
  - with diarrhea K58.0
  - mixed K58.2
  - other K58.8
  - psychogenic F45.8
- diaphragm (reflex) R06.6
  - psychogenic F45.8
- esophagus (diffuse) K22.4
  - psychogenic F45.8
- gastrointestinal (tract) K31.89
  - psychogenic F45.8
- glottis J38.5
  - hysterical F44.4
  - psychogenic F45.8
    - conversion reaction F44.4
  - reflex through recurrent laryngeal nerve J38.5
- habit—*see* Tic
- hysterical F44.4
- intestinal (*see also* Syndrome, irritable, bowel) K58.9
  - psychogenic F45.8
- larynx, laryngeal J38.5
  - hysterical F44.4
  - psychogenic F45.8
    - conversion reaction F44.4
- muscle NEC M62.838
  - back M62.830
- nerve, trigeminal G51.0
- nervous F45.8
- nodding F98.4
- oculogyric H51.8
  - psychogenic F45.8
- perineal, female N94.89
- pharynx (reflex) J39.2
  - hysterical F45.8
  - psychogenic F45.8
- psychogenic F45.8
- pylorus NEC K31.3
  - congenital or infantile Q40.0
  - psychogenic F45.8
- rectum (sphincter) K59.4
  - psychogenic F45.8
- sigmoid (*see also* Syndrome, irritable, bowel) K58.9
  - psychogenic F45.8
- stomach K31.89
  - neurotic F45.8

Spasm(s), spastic, spasticity, *continued*
- throat J39.2
  - hysterical F45.8
  - psychogenic F45.8
- tic F95.9
  - chronic F95.1
  - transient of childhood F95.0
- urethra (sphincter) N35.919

Spasmodic—*see* Disease, diseased

Spasmus nutans F98.4

Spastic, spasticity—*see also* Spasm
- child (cerebral) (congenital) (paralysis) G80.1

Specific, specified—*see* Disease, diseased

Speech
- defect, disorder, disturbance, impediment R47.9
  - psychogenic, in childhood and adolescence F98.8
  - slurring R47.81
  - specified NEC R47.89

Spens' syndrome (syncope with heart block) I45.9

Spermatocele N43.40
- congenital Q55.4
- multiple N43.42
- single N43.41

Sphericity, increased, lens (congenital) Q12.4

Spherocytosis (congenital) (familial) (hereditary) D58.0
- hemoglobin disease D58.0
- sickle-cell (disease) D57.8-

Spherophakia Q12.4

Spider
- bite—*see* Table of Drugs and Chemicals, by animal or substance, poisoning
- fingers—*see* Syndrome, Marfans
- nevus I78.1
- toes—*see* Syndrome, Marfans
- vascular I78.1

Spiegler-Fendt
- benign lymphocytoma L98.8

Spina bifida (aperta) Q05.9
- with hydrocephalus NEC Q05.4
- cervical Q05.5
  - with hydrocephalus Q05.0
- dorsal Q05.6
  - with hydrocephalus Q05.1
- lumbar Q05.7
  - with hydrocephalus Q05.2
- lumbosacral Q05.7
  - with hydrocephalus Q05.2
- occulta Q76.0
- sacral Q05.8
  - with hydrocephalus Q05.3
- thoracic Q05.6
  - with hydrocephalus Q05.1
- thoracolumbar Q05.6
  - with hydrocephalus Q05.1

Spirillosis A25.0

Splenitis (interstitial) (malignant) (nonspecific) D73.89
- malarial (*see also* Malaria) B54 *[D77]*
- tuberculous A18.85

Splenomegaly, splenomegalia (Bengal) (cryptogenic) (idiopathic) (tropical) R16.1
- with hepatomegaly R16.2
- malarial (*see also* Malaria) B54 *[D77]*
- neutropenic D73.81

Spondylolisthesis (acquired) (degenerative) M43.1-
- congenital Q76.2

Spondylolysis (acquired) M43.0-
- congenital Q76.2

Spongioblastoma (any type)—*see* Neoplasm, malignant, by site in Table of Neoplasms in the complete *ICD-10-CM* manual
- specified site—*see* Neoplasm, malignant, by site in Table of Neoplasms in the complete *ICD-10-CM* manual
- unspecified site C71.9

Spongioneuroblastoma—*see* Neoplasm, malignant, by site in Table of Neoplasms in the complete *ICD-10-CM* manual

Sporadic—*see* Disease, diseased

ALPHABETIC INDEX

Spots, spotting (in) (of)
- café au lait L81.3
- Cayenne pepper I78.1
- de Morgan's (senile angiomas) I78.1
- intermenstrual (regular) N92.0
  - irregular N92.1
- liver L81.4
- purpuric R23.3
- ruby I78.1

Sprain (joint) (ligament)
- ankle S93.40-
  - calcaneofibular ligament S93.41-
  - deltoid ligament S93.42-
  - internal collateral ligament S93.49-
  - specified ligament NEC S93.49-
  - talofibular ligament S93.49-
  - tibiofibular ligament S93.43-
- anterior longitudinal, cervical S13.4
- atlas, atlanto-axial, atlanto-occipital S13.4
- cervical, cervicodorsal, cervicothoracic S13.4
- elbow S53.40-
  - radial collateral ligament S53.43-
  - radiohumeral S53.41-
  - specified type NEC S53.49-
  - ulnar collateral ligament S53.44-
  - ulnohumeral S53.42-
- finger(s) S63.61-
  - index S63.61-
  - interphalangeal (joint) S63.63-
    - index S63.63-
      - ■ little S63.63-
      - ■ middle S63.63-
      - ■ ring S63.63-
  - little S63.61-
  - middle S63.61-
  - ring S63.61-
  - metacarpophalangeal (joint) S63.65-
  - specified site NEC S63.69-
    - ■ index S63.69-
    - ■ little S63.69-
    - ■ middle S63.69-
    - ■ ring S63.69-
- foot S93.60-
  - specified ligament NEC S93.69-
  - tarsal ligament S93.61-
  - tarsometatarsal ligament S93.62-
- hand S63.9-
  - specified site NEC—*see* subcategory S63.8
- innominate
  - sacral junction S33.6
- jaw (articular disc) (cartilage) (meniscus) S03.4-
  - old M26.69
- knee S83.9-
  - collateral ligament S83.40-
    - ■ lateral (fibular) S83.42-
    - ■ medial (tibial) S83.41-
  - cruciate ligament S83.50-
    - ■ anterior S83.51-
    - ■ posterior S83.52-
- lumbar (spine) S33.5
- lumbosacral S33.9
- mandible (articular disc) S03.4-
  - old M26.69
- meniscus
  - jaw S03.4-
    - old M26.69
  - mandible S03.4
    - ■ old M26.69
- neck S13.9
  - anterior longitudinal cervical ligament S13.4
  - atlanto-axial joint S13.4
  - atlanto-occipital joint S13.4
  - cervical spine S13.4
- pelvis NEC S33.8
- rotator cuff (capsule) S43.42-
- sacroiliac (region)
  - joint S33.6
- spine
  - cervical S13.4
  - lumbar S33.5

Sprain (joint) (ligament), *continued*
- symphysis
  - jaw S03.4-
    - ■ old M26.69
  - mandibular S03.4-
    - ■ old M26.69
- talofibular S93.49-
- tarsal—see Sprain, foot, specified site NEC
- tarsometatarsal—see Sprain, foot, specified site NEC
- temporomandibular S03.4-
  - old M26.69
- thumb S63.60-
  - interphalangeal (joint) S63.62-
  - metacarpophalangeal (joint) S63.64-
  - specified site NEC S63.68-
- toe(s) S93.50-
  - great S93.50-
  - interphalangeal joint S93.51-
    - ■ great S93.51-
    - ■ lesser S93.51-
  - lesser S93.50-
  - metatarsophalangeal joint S93.52-
    - ■ great S93.52-
    - ■ lesser S93.52-
- wrist S63.50-
  - carpal S63.51-
  - radiocarpal S63.52-
  - specified site NEC S63.59-

Sprengel's deformity (congenital) Q74.0

Sprue (tropical) K90.1
- celiac K90.0
- idiopathic K90.49
- meaning thrush B37.0
- nontropical K90.0

Spur, bone—*see also* Enthesopathy
- iliac crest M76.2-
- nose (septum) J34.89

Spurway's syndrome Q78.0

Sputum
- abnormal (amount) (color) (odor) (purulent) R09.3
- blood-stained R04.2
- excessive (cause unknown) R09.3

Squashed nose M95.0
- congenital Q67.4

SSADHD (succinic semialdehyde dehydrogenase deficiency) E72.81

St. Hubert's disease A82.9

Staggering gait R26.0
- hysterical F44.4

Stain, staining
- meconium (newborn) P96.83
- port wine Q82.5

Stammering (*see also* Disorder, fluency) F80.81

Staphylitis (acute) (catarrhal) (chronic) (gangrenous) (membranous) (suppurative) (ulcerative) K12.2

Staphylococcal scalded skin syndrome L00

Staphylococcemia A41.2

Staphylococcus, staphylococcal—*see also* Disease, diseased
- as cause of disease classified elsewhere B95.8
  - aureus (methicillin susceptible) (MSSA) B95.61
    - ■ methicillin resistant (MRSA) B95.62
- specified NEC, as the cause of disease classified elsewhere B95.7

Stasis
- renal N19
  - tubular N17.0

State (of)
- agitated R45.1
  - acute reaction to stress F43.0
- compulsive F42.8
  - mixed with obsessional thoughts F42.2
- crisis F43.0
- depressive F32.A
- dissociative F44.9
- neurotic F48.9
- obsessional F42.8
- panic F41.0

State (of), *continued*
- persistent vegetative R40.3
- phobic F40.9
- pregnant, incidental Z33.1
- tension (mental) F48.9
  - specified NEC F48.8
- vegetative, persistent R40.3
- withdrawal—*see* Withdrawal state

Status (post)—*see also* Presence (of)
- absence, epileptic—*see* Epilepsy, by type, with status epilepticus
- asthmaticus—*see* Asthma, by type, with status asthmaticus
- awaiting organ transplant Z76.82
- colectomy (complete) (partial) Z90.49
- colonization—*see* Carrier (suspected) of
- delinquent immunization Z28.3
- dialysis (hemodialysis) (peritoneal) Z99.2
- do not resuscitate (DNR) Z66
- epileptic, epilepticus (*see also* Epilepsy, by type, with status epilepticus) G40.901
- gastrostomy Z93.1
- human immunodeficiency virus (HIV) infection, asymptomatic Z21
- ileostomy (ileal pouch) (Koch pouch) Z93.2
- lapsed immunization schedule Z28.3
- nephrectomy (unilateral) (bilateral) Z90.5
- pacemaker
  - cardiac Z95.0
- physical restraint Z78.1
- postcommotio cerebri F07.81
- postoperative (postprocedural) NEC Z98.890
- postsurgical (postprocedural) NEC Z98.890
- pregnant, incidental Z33.1
- renal dialysis (hemodialysis) (peritoneal) Z99.2
- retained foreign body—*see* Retained, foreign body fragments (type of)
- shunt
  - arteriovenous (for dialysis) Z99.2
  - cerebrospinal fluid Z98.2
- transplant—*see* Transplant
  - organ removed Z98.85
- underimmunization Z28.3
  - other underimmunization status Z28.39
  - partially vaccinated for COVID-19 Z28.311
  - unvaccinated for COVID-19 Z28.310
- ventricular (communicating) (for drainage) Z98.2

Stealing
- child problem F91.8
  - in company with others Z72.810

Steam burn—*see* Burn

Steatoma L72.3
- eyelid (cystic)—*see* Dermatitis
  - infected—*see* Hordeolum

Steatorrhea (chronic) K90.49
- idiopathic (adult) (infantile) K90.9
- primary K90.0

Steinbrocker's syndrome G90.89

Stein-Leventhal syndrome E28.2

Stein's syndrome E28.2

Stenocephaly Q75.8

Stenosis, stenotic (cicatricial)—*see also* Stricture
- anus, anal (canal) (sphincter) K62.4
  - and rectum K62.4
  - congenital Q42.3
    - ■ with fistula Q42.2
- aorta (ascending) (supraventricular) (congenital) Q25.1
- aortic (valve) I35.0
  - with insufficiency I35.2
  - congenital Q23.0
  - rheumatic I06.0
    - ■ with
      - incompetency, insufficiency or regurgitation I06.2
      - ◊ with mitral (valve) disease I08.0
        - ▪ with tricuspid (valve) disease I08.3
    - mitral (valve) disease I08.0
      - ◊ with tricuspid (valve) disease I08.3
    - tricuspid (valve) disease I08.2
      - ◊ with mitral (valve) disease I08.3

ALPHABETIC INDEX

Stenosis, stenotic, *continued*

- specified cause NEC I35.0
- aqueduct of Sylvius (congenital) Q03.0
  - with spina bifida—*see* Spina bifida, by site, with hydrocephalus
  - acquired G91.1
- bile duct (common) (hepatic) K83.1
  - congenital Q44.3
- brain G93.89
- colon—*see also* Obstruction, intestine
  - congenital Q42.9
    - specified NEC Q42.8
- common (bile) duct K83.1
  - congenital Q44.3
- heart valve (see also endocarditis) I38
  - congenital Q24.8
    - pulmonary Q22.1
    - tricuspid Q22.4
  - hypertrophic subaortic (idiopathic) I42.1
- intestine—*see also* Obstruction, intestine
  - congenital (small) Q41.9
    - large Q42.9
      - specified NEC Q42.8
      - specified NEC Q41.8
- lacrimal (passage)
  - congenital Q10.5
  - duct H04.55-
  - sac H04.57-
- lacrimonasal duct—*see* Stenosis, lacrimal, duct
  - congenital Q10.5
- mitral (chronic) (inactive) (valve) I05.0
  - with
    - aortic valve disease I08.0
    - incompetency, insufficiency or regurgitation I05.2
  - active or acute I01.1
    - with rheumatic or Sydenham's chorea I02.0
  - congenital Q23.2
  - specified cause, except rheumatic I34.2
- myocardium, myocardial—*see also* Degeneration, myocardial
  - hypertrophic subaortic (idiopathic) I42.1
- nares (anterior) (posterior) J34.89
  - congenital Q30.0
- nasal duct—*see also* Stenosis, lacrimal, duct
  - congenital Q10.5
- nasolacrimal duct—*see also* Stenosis, lacrimal, duct
  - congenital Q10.5
- pulmonary (artery) (congenital) Q25.6
  - with ventricular septal defect, transposition of aorta, and hypertrophy of right ventricle Q21.3
  - in tetralogy of Fallot Q21.3
  - infundibular Q24.3
  - subvalvular Q24.3
  - supravalvular Q25.6
  - valve I37.0
    - with insufficiency I37.2
    - congenital Q22.1
    - rheumatic I09.89
    - with aortic, mitral or tricuspid (valve) disease I08.8
- pulmonic (congenital) Q22.1
- pylorus (hypertrophic) (acquired) K31.1
  - congenital Q40.0
  - infantile Q40.0
- spinal M48.0-
- subaortic (congenital) Q24.4
  - hypertrophic (idiopathic) I42.1
- tricuspid (valve) I07.0
  - with
    - aortic (valve) disease I08.2
    - incompetency, insufficiency or regurgitation I07.2
      - with aortic (valve) disease I08.2
      - ◊ with mitral (valve) disease I08.3
    - mitral (valve) disease I08.1
      - with aortic (valve) disease I08.3
  - congenital Q22.4
  - nonrheumatic I36.0
    - with insufficiency I36.2
- ureteropelvic junction, congenital Q62.11
- ureterovesical orifice, congenital Q62.12
- vagina N89.5
  - congenital Q52.4

Stenosis, stenotic, *continued*

- valve (cardiac) (heart) (*see also* Endocarditis) I38
  - congenital Q24.8
    - aortic Q23.0
    - pulmonary Q22.1

Stercolith (impaction) K56.41

Stercoraceous, stercoral ulcer K63.3

- anus or rectum K62.6

Stereotypies NEC F98.4

Steroid

- effects (adverse) (adrenocortical) (iatrogenic)
  - cushingoid E24.2
  - correct substance properly administered—*see* Table of Drugs and Chemicals, by drug, adverse effect
  - overdose or wrong substance given or taken—*see* Table of Drugs and Chemicals, by drug, poisoning

Stevens-Johnson disease or syndrome L51.1

- toxic epidermal necrolysis overlap L51.3

Sticker's disease B08.3

Stiffness, joint NEC M25.60-

- ankle M25.67-
- contracture—*see* Contraction, joint
- elbow M25.62-
- foot M25.67-
- hand M25.64-
- hip M25.65-
- knee M25.66-
- shoulder M25.61-
- wrist M25.63-

Stillbirth P95

Still's disease or syndrome (juvenile) M08.20

- specified site NEC M08.2A

Stitch

- abscess T81.41

Stokes-Adams disease or syndrome I45.9

Stomatitis (denture) (ulcerative) K12.1

- angular K13.0
- aphthous K12.0
- candidal B37.0
- catarrhal K12.1
- due to
  - thrush B37.0
- follicular K12.1
- herpesviral, herpetic B00.2
- herpetiformis K12.0
- malignant K12.1
- membranous acute K12.1
- monilial B37.0
- mycotic B37.0
- parasitic B37.0
- septic K12.1
- suppurative (acute) K12.2
- vesicular K12.1
  - with exanthem (enteroviral) B08.4

Stomatocytosis D58.8

Stomatomycosis B37.0

Stomatorrhagia K13.79

Stovkis (-Talma) **disease** D74.8

Strabismus (congenital) (nonparalytic) H50.9

- concomitant H50.40
  - convergent—*see* Strabismus, convergent concomitant
  - divergent—*see* Strabismus, divergent concomitant
- convergent concomitant H50.00
  - accommodative component H50.43
  - alternating H50.05
    - with
      - A pattern H50.06
      - specified nonconcomitances NEC H50.08
      - V pattern H50.07
  - monocular H50.01-
    - with
      - A pattern H50.02-
      - specified nonconcomitances NEC H50.04-
      - V pattern H50.03-
    - intermittent H50.31-
      - alternating H50.32

Strabismus, *continued*

- cyclotropia H50.41
- divergent concomitant H50.10
  - alternating H50.15
    - with
      - A pattern H50.16
      - specified noncomitances NEC H50.18
      - V pattern H50.17
  - monocular H50.11-
    - with
      - A pattern H50.12-
      - specified noncomitances NEC H50.14-
      - V pattern H50.13-
    - intermittent H50.33
      - alternating H50.34
- Duane's syndrome H50.81-
- due to adhesions, scars H50.69
- heterophoria H50.50
  - alternating H50.55
  - cyclophoria H50.54
  - esophoria H50.51
  - exophoria H50.52
  - vertical H50.53
- heterotropia H50.40
  - intermittent H50.30
  - hypertropia H50.2-
  - hypotropia—*see* Strabismus, Hypertropia
- latent H50.50
- mechanical H50.60
  - Brown's sheath syndrome H50.61-
  - specified type NEC H50.69
- monofixation syndrome H50.42
- paralytic H49.9
  - abducens nerve H49.2-
  - fourth nerve H49.1-
  - Kearns-Sayre syndrome H49.81-
  - ophthalmoplegia (external)
    - progressive H49.4-
      - with pigmentary retinopathy H49.81-
    - total H49.3-
  - sixth nerve H49.2-
  - specified type NEC H49.88-
  - third nerve H49.0-
  - trochlear nerve H49.1-
  - specified type NEC H50.89
  - vertical H50.2-

Strain

- cervical S16.1
- neck S16.1

Strangulation, strangulated—*see also* Asphyxia, traumatic

- bladder-neck N32.0
- bowel or colon K56.2
- intestine (large) (small) K56.2
  - with hernia—*see also* Hernia, by site, with, obstruction
    - with gangrene—*see* Hernia, by site, with, gangrene
- mesentery K56.2
- omentum K56.2
- organ or site, congenital NEC—*see* Atresia, by site
- vesicourethral orifice N32.0

Strangury R30.0

Strawberry

- mark Q82.5

Straw itch B88.0

Strephosymbolia F81.0

- secondary to organic lesion R48.8

Streptobacillary fever A25.1

Streptococcus, streptococcal—*see also* Disease, diseased

- as cause of disease classified elsewhere B95.5
- group
  - A, as cause of disease classified elsewhere B95.0
  - B, as cause of disease classified elsewhere B95.1
  - D, as cause of disease classified elsewhere B95.2
- pneumoniae, as cause of disease classified elsewhere B95.3
- specified NEC, as cause of disease classified elsewhere B95.4

ALPHABETIC INDEX

Stress F43.9
- family—*see* Disruption, family
- fetal P84
- polycythemia D75.1
- reaction (see also Reaction, stress) F43.9

Stricture—*see also* Stenosis
- anus (sphincter) K62.4
  - congenital Q42.3
    - with fistula Q42.2
  - infantile Q42.3
    - with fistula Q42.3
- aorta (ascending) (congenital) Q25.1
- aortic (valve)—*see* Stenosis, aortic
- aqueduct of Sylvius (congenital) Q03.0
  - with spina bifida—*see* Spina bifida, by site, with hydrocephalus
  - acquired G91.1
- artery I77.1
  - congenital (peripheral) Q27.8
    - umbilical Q27.0
- bile duct (common) (hepatic) K83.1
  - congenital Q44.3
- bladder N32.89
  - neck N32.0
- brain G93.89
- colon—*see also* Obstruction, intestine
  - congenital Q42.9
    - specified NEC Q42.8
- digestive organs NEC, congenital Q45.8
- fallopian tube N97.1
  - gonococcal A54.24
- heart—*see also* Disease, heart
  - valve (see also Endocarditis) I38
    - aortic Q23.0
    - mitral Q23.4
    - pulmonary Q22.1
- intestine—*see also* Obstruction, intestine
  - congenital (small) Q41.9
    - large Q42.9
      - specified NEC Q42.8
      - specified NEC Q41.8
  - ischemic K55.1
- myocardium, myocardial I51.5
  - hypertrophic subaortic (idiopathic) I42.1
- nares (anterior) (posterior) J34.89
  - congenital Q30.0
- nose J34.89
  - congenital Q30.0
- nostril (anterior) (posterior) J34.89
  - congenital Q30.0
- pelviureteric junction (congenital) Q62.11
- pulmonary, pulmonic
  - artery (congenital) Q25.6
  - infundibulum (congenital) Q24.3
  - valve I37.0
    - congenital Q22.1
- punctum lacrimale
  - congenital Q10.5
- pylorus (hypertrophic) K31.1
  - congenital Q40.0
  - infantile Q40.0
- rectum (sphincter) K62.4
  - congenital Q42.1
    - with fistula Q42.0
  - gonococcal A54.6
- subaortic Q24.4
  - hypertrophic (acquired) (idiopathic) I42.1
- ureter (postoperative) N13.5
  - with
    - hydronephrosis N13.1
- ureteropelvic junction N13.0
  - congenital Q62.11
- urethra (organic) (spasmodic) N35.9-
  - congenital Q64.39
    - valvular (posterior) Q64.2
  - female N35.92
  - gonococcal, gonorrheal A54.01
  - male N35.919
    - anterior urethra N35.914
    - bulbous urethra N35.912
    - meatal N35.911
    - membranous urethra N35.913
    - overlapping sites N35.116

Stricture, *continued*
- postinfective NEC
  - female N35.12
  - male N35.119
    - anterior urethra N35.114
    - bulbous urethra N35.112
    - meatal N35.111
    - membranous urethra N35.113
    - overlapping sites N35.116
- post-traumatic
  - female N35.028
  - male N35.014
    - anterior urethra N35.013
    - bulbous urethra N35.011
    - meatal N35.010
    - membranous urethra N35.012
    - overlapping sites N35.016
- specified cause NEC
  - female N35.82
  - male N35.819
    - anterior urethra N35.814
    - bulbous urethra N35.812
    - meatal N35.811
    - membranous urethra N35.813
    - overlapping sites N35.816
- valve (cardiac) (heart)—*see also* Endocarditis
  - congenital
    - aortic Q23.0
    - pulmonary Q22.1
- vesicourethral orifice N32.0
  - congenital Q64.31

Stridor R06.1
- congenital (larynx) P28.89

Stroke (apoplectic) (brain) (embolic) (ischemic) (paralytic) (thrombotic)
- cerebral, perinatal P91.82-
- epileptic—*see* Epilepsy
- heat T67.01
  - exertional T67.02
  - specified NEC T67.09
- ischemic, perinatal arterial P91.82-
- neonatal P91.82-
- sun T67.01
  - specified NEC T67.09

Struma—*see also* Goiter
- Hashimoto E06.3
- lymphomatosa E06.3
- nodosa (simplex) E04.9
  - endemic E01.2
    - multinodular E01.1
- Riedel's E06.5

Stupor (catatonic) R40.1
- reaction to exceptional stress (transient) F43.0

Sturge (-Weber) (-Dimitri) (-Kalischer) **disease or syndrome** Q85.8

Stuttering F80.81
- childhood onset F80.81
- in conditions classified elsewhere R47.82

Sty, stye (external) (internal) (meibomian) (zeisian)—*see* Hordeolum

Subacidity, gastric K31.89
- psychogenic F45.8

Subacute—*see* Disease, diseased

Subarachnoid—*see* Disease, diseased

Subcortical—*see* Disease, diseased

Subglossitis—*see* Glossitis

Subhemophilia D66

Subluxation—*see also* Dislocation
- finger S63.20-
  - index S63.20-
  - interphalangeal S63.2-
    - distal S63.24-
      - index S63.24-
      - little S63.24-
      - middle S63.24-
      - ring S63.24-
    - index S63.2-
    - little S63.2-
    - middle S63.2-

Subluxation, *continued*
- proximal S63.23-
  - index S63.23-
  - little S63.23-
  - middle S63.23-
  - ring S63.23-
- ring S63.2-
- thumb S63.12-
- knee S83.10-
  - cap—*see* Subluxation, patella
  - patella—*see* Subluxation, patella
  - proximal tibia
    - anteriorly S83.11-
    - laterally S83.14-
    - medially S83.13-
    - posteriorly S83.12-
    - specified type NEC S83.19-
- metacarpal (bone)
  - proximal end S63.06-
- metacarpophalangeal (joint)
  - finger S63.21-
    - index S63.21-
    - little S63.21-
    - middle S63.21-
    - ring S63.21-
  - thumb S63.11-
- patella S83.00-
  - lateral S83.01-
  - recurrent (nontraumatic) M22.1-
  - specified type NEC S83.09-
- radial head S53.00-
  - nursemaid's elbow S53.03-
  - specified type NEC S53.09-
- thumb S63.10-
  - interphalangeal joint—*see* Subluxation, interphalangeal (joint), thumb
  - metacarpophalangeal joint S63.11-

Submersion (fatal) (nonfatal) T75.1

Substernal thyroid E04.9
- congenital Q89.2

Substitution disorder F44.9

Subthyroidism (acquired)—*see also* Hypothyroidism
- congenital E03.1

Sucking thumb, child (excessive) F98.8

Sudamen, sudamina L74.1

Sugar
- blood
  - high (transient) R73.9
  - low (transient) E16.2
- in urine R81

PEDIATRIC ICD-10-CM 2025: A MANUAL FOR PROVIDER-BASED CODING

ALPHABETIC INDEX

Suicide, suicidal (attempted) T14.91
- by poisoning—*see* Table of Drugs and Chemicals
- history of (personal) Z91.51
  - in family Z81.8
- ideation—*see* Ideation, suicidal
- risk
  - meaning personal history of attempted suicide Z91.51
  - meaning suicidal ideation—see Ideation, suicidal
- tendencies
  - meaning personal history of attempted suicide Z91.51
  - meaning suicidal ideation—*see* Ideation, suicidal
- trauma—*see* nature of injury by site

Sulfhemoglobinemia, sulphemoglobinemia (acquired) (with methemoglobinemia) D74.8

Sunburn L55.9
- due to
  - tanning bed (acute) L56.8
- first degree L55.0
- second degree L55.1
- third degree L55.2

Sunstroke T67.01

Supernumerary (congenital)
- aortic cusps Q23.88
- cusps, heart valve NEC Q24.8
  - aortic Q23.88
- carpal bones Q74.0
- fallopian tube Q50.6
- finger Q69.0
- lacrimonasal duct Q10.6
- lobule (ear) Q17.0
- nipple(s) Q83.3
- ovary Q50.31
- oviduct Q50.6.
- ossicles, auditory Q16.3
- tarsal bones Q74.2
- testis Q55.29
- thumb Q69.1
- toe Q69.2
- uterus Q51.28

Supervision (of)
- contraceptive—*see* Prescription of contraceptives
- dietary (for) Z71.3
  - allergy (food) Z71.3
  - colitis Z71.3
  - diabetes mellitus Z71.3
  - food allergy or intolerance Z71.3
  - gastritis Z71.3
  - hypercholesterolemia Z71.3
  - hypoglycemia Z71.3
  - intolerance (food) Z71.3
  - obesity Z71.3
  - specified NEC Z71.3
- healthy infant or child Z76.2
  - foundling Z76.1
- lactation Z39.1

Suppression
- menstruation N94.89
- urine, urinary secretion R34

Suppuration, suppurative—*see also* Disease, diseased
- accessory sinus (chronic)—*see* Sinusitis
- antrum (chronic)—*see* Sinusitis, maxillary
- bladder—*see* Cystitis
- brain G06.0
  - sequelae G09
- breast N61.1
- ear (middle)—*see also* Otitis, media
  - external NEC—*see* Otitis, externa, infective
  - internal—*see* subcategory H83.0
- ethmoidal (chronic) (sinus)—*see* Sinusitis, ethmoidal
- frontal (chronic) (sinus)—*see* Sinusitis, frontal
- gallbladder (acute) K81.0
- intracranial G06.0
- joint—*see* Arthritis, pyogenic or pyemic
- labyrinthine—*see* subcategory H83.0
- mammary gland N61.1
- maxilla, maxillary M27.2
  - sinus (chronic)—*see* Sinusitis, maxillary
- muscle—*see* Myositis, infective
- nasal sinus (chronic)—*see* Sinusitis

Suppuration, suppurative, *continued*
- pelvis, pelvic
  - female—*see* Disease, pelvis, inflammatory
  - male K65.0
- sinus (accessory) (chronic) (nasal)—*see* Sinusitis
- sphenoidal sinus (chronic)—*see* Sinusitis, sphenoidal
- thyroid (gland) E06.0
- tonsil—*see* Tonsillitis
- uterus—*see* Endometritis

Supraglottitis J04.30
- with obstruction J04.31

Surgical
- shock T81.10

Surveillance (of) (for)—*see also* Observation
- alcohol abuse Z71.41
- contraceptive—*see* Prescription of contraceptives
- dietary Z71.3
- drug abuse Z71.51

Suspected condition, ruled out—*see also* Observation, suspected
- fetal anomaly Z03.73
- fetal growth Z03.74
- newborn—*see* Observation, newborn (for suspected condition, ruled out) Z05-

Suture
- burst (in operation wound) T81.31
  - external operation wound T81.31
- removal Z48.02

Swearing, compulsive F42.8
- in Gilles de la Tourette's syndrome F95.2

Sweat, sweats
- night R61

Sweating, excessive R61

Swelling (of) R60.9
- abdomen, abdominal (not referable to any particular organ)—*see* Mass, abdominal
- ankle—*see* Effusion, joint, ankle
- arm M79.89
  - forearm M79.89
- breast (*see also*, Lump, breast) N63.0
- chest, localized R22.2
- extremity (lower) (upper)—*see* Disorder
  - finger M79.89
- foot M79.89
- glands R59.9
  - generalized R59.1
  - localized R59.0
- hand M79.89
- head (localized) R22.0
- inflammatory—*see* Inflammation
- intra-abdominal—*see* Mass, abdominal
- joint—*see* Effusion, joint
- leg M79.89
  - lower M79.89
- limb—*see* Disorder
- localized (skin) R22.9
  - chest R22.2
  - head R22.0
  - limb
    - lower—*see* Mass, localized, limb, lower
    - upper—*see* Mass, localized, limb, upper
  - neck R22.1
  - trunk R22.2
- neck (localized) R22.1
- pelvic—*see* Mass, abdominal
- scrotum N50.89
- splenic—*see* Splenomegaly
- testis N50.89
- toe M79.89
- umbilical R19.09

Swimmer's
- cramp T75.1
- ear H60.33-
- itch B65.3

Swimming in the head R42

Swollen—*see* Swelling

Sycocis L73.8
- barbae (not parasitic) L73.8
- contagiosa (mycotic) B35.0

Sycocis, *continued*
- lupoides L73.8
- mycotic B35.0
- parasitic B35.0
- vulgaris L73.8

Symblepharon
- congenital Q10.3

Symond's syndrome G93.2

Sympathetic—*see* Disease, diseased

Sympathicoblastoma
- specified site—*see* Neoplasm, malignant, by site in Table of Neoplasms in the complete *ICD-10-CM* manual
- unspecified site C74.90

Sympathogonioma—*see* Sympathicoblastoma

Symphalangy (fingers) (toes) Q70.9

Symptoms NEC R68.89
- breast NEC N64.59
- cold J00
- development NEC R63.8
- genital organs, female R10.2
- involving
  - abdomen NEC R19.8
  - awareness R41.9
    - altered mental status R41.82
  - cardiovascular system NEC R09.89
  - chest NEC R09.89
  - circulatory system NEC R09.89
  - cognitive functions R41.9
    - altered mental status R41.82
  - development NEC R62.50
  - digestive system R19.8
  - food and fluid intake R63.8
  - general perceptions and sensations R44.9
    - specified NEC R44.8
  - musculoskeletal system R29.91
    - specified NEC R29.898
  - nervous system R29.90
    - specified NEC R29.818
  - pelvis R19.8
  - respiratory system NEC R09.89
- metabolism NEC R63.8
- of infancy R68.19
- pelvis NEC, female R10.2
- viral syndrome J00

Sympus Q74.2

Syncope (near) (pre-) R55
- bradycardia R00.1
- cardiac R55
- heart R55
- heat T67.1
- laryngeal R05.4
- psychogenic F48.8
- tussive R05.8
- vasoconstriction R55
- vasodepressor R55
- vasomotor R55
- vasovagal R55

Syndactylism, syndactyly Q70.9
- complex (with synostosis)
  - fingers Q70.0-
  - toes Q70.2-
- simple (without synostosis)
  - fingers Q70.1-
  - toes Q70.3-

Syndrome—*see also* Disease
- 4H G11.5
- 22q13.3 deletion Q93.52
- abdominal
  - acute R10.0
  - muscle deficiency Q79.4
- abstinence, neonatal P96.1
- acquired immunodeficiency—*see* Human, immunodeficiency virus (HIV) disease
- activated phosphoinositide 3-kinase delta syndrome [APDS] D81.82
- acute abdominal R10.0
- acute respiratory distress (adult) (child) J80
- Adair-Dighton Q78.0
- Adams-Stokes (-Morgagni) I45.9
- adrenocortical—*see* Cushing's, syndrome

ALPHABETIC INDEX

Syndrome, *continued*

- adrenogenital E25.9
  - congenital, associated with enzyme deficiency E25.0
- Alder's D72.0
- Aldrich (-Wiskott) D82.0
- Alagille (-Watson) Q44.71
- Alport Q87.81
- alveolar hypoventilation E66.2
- androgen insensitivity E34.50
  - complete E34.51
  - partial E34.52
- androgen resistance (*see also* Syndrome, androgen insensitivity) E34.50
- Angelman Q93.51
- ankyloglossia superior Q38.1
- antibody deficiency D80.9
  - agammaglobulinemic D80.1
    - hereditary D80.0
  - congenital D80.0
  - hypogammaglobulinemic D80.1
    - hereditary D80.0
- argentaffin, arginatfinoma E34.09
- Arnold-Chiari—*see* Arnold-Chiari disease
- Arrillaga-Ayerza I27.0
- arterial tortuosity Q87.82
- aspiration, of newborn—*see* Aspiration, by substance, with, pneumonia
  - meconium P24.01
- ataxia-telangiectasia G11.3
- autoerythrocyte sensitization (Gardner-Diamond) D69.2
- autoimmune lymphoproliferative [ALPS] D89.82
- Axenfeld-Rieger Q13.81
- Ayerza (-Arrillaga) I27.0
- Bardet-Biedl Q87.83
- Beals Q87.40
- bilateral polycystic ovarian E28.2
- black
  - widow spider bite—*see* Table of Drugs and Chemicals, by animal or substance, poisoning
- Blackfan-Diamond D61.01
- blind loop K90.2
  - congenital Q43.8
  - postsurgical K91.2
- blue sclera Q78.0
- Boder-Sedgewick G11.3
- Borjeson Forssman Lehmann Q89.8
- Bouillaud's I01.9
- Bourneville (-Pringle) Q85.1
- bradycardia-tachycardia I49.5
- brain (nonpsychotic) F09
  - with psychosis, psychotic reaction F09
  - acute or subacute—*see* Delirium
  - congenital—*see* Disability, intellectual
  - organic F09
    - post-traumatic (nonpsychotic) F07.81
  - postcontusional F07.81
  - post-traumatic, nonpsychotic F07.81
- Brock's J98.11
- bronchiolitis obliterans—*see also* Bronchiolitis, obliterative J44.81
- bronze baby P83.88
- Burnett's (milk-alkali) E83.52
- carbohydrate-deficient glycoprotein (CDGS) E77.8
- carcinoid E34.00
  - heart E34.01
  - specified NEC E34.09
- cardiacos negros I27.0
- cardiopulmonary-obesity E66.2
- cardiorespiratory distress (idiopathic), newborn P22.0
- Cassidy (-Scholte) E34.09
- cat cry Q93.4
- celiac K90.0
- cerebral
  - gigantism E22.0
- CHARGE Q89.8
- child maltreatment—*see* Maltreatment, child
- chondrocostal junction M94.0
- chondroectodermal dysplasia Q77.6
- chromosome 5 short arm deletion Q93.4
- Clerambault's automatism G93.89
- clumsiness, clumsy child F82

Syndrome, *continued*

- cluster headache G44.009
  - intractable G44.001
  - not intractable G44.009
- Coffin-Lowry Q89.8
- combined immunity deficiency D81.9
- concussion F07.81
- congenital
  - facial diplegia Q87.0
  - oculo-auriculovertebral Q87.0
  - oculofacial diplegia (Moebius) Q87.0
  - rubella (manifest) P35.0
- congestive dysmenorrhea N94.6
- Costen's (complex) M26.69
- costochondral junction M94.0
- costovertebral E22.0
- Cowden Q85.8
- cri-du-chat Q93.4
- crib death R99
- croup J05.0
- Cushing's E24.9
  - due to
    - drugs E24.2
    - overproduction of pituitary ACTH E24.0
  - drug-induced E24.2
  - overdose or wrong substance given or taken—*see* Table of Drugs and Chemicals, by drug, poisoning
  - pituitary-dependent E24.0
  - specified type NEC E24.8
- cryptophthalmos Q87.0
- cytokine release D89.839
  - grade 1 D89.831
  - grade 2 D89.832
  - grade 3 D89.833
  - grade 4 D89.834
  - grade 5 D89.835
- Dandy-Walker Q03.1
  - with spina bifida Q07.01
- defibrination—*see also* Fibrinolysis
  - newborn P60
- dependence—*see* F10-F19 with fourth character .2
- De Quervain E34.51
- de Vivo syndrome E74.810
- diabetes mellitus in newborn infant P70.2
- Diamond-Blackfan D61.01
- Diamond-Gardener D69.2
- DIC (diffuse or disseminated intravascular coagulopathy) D65
- di George's D82.1
- Dighton's Q78.0
- disequilibrium E87.8
- Döhle body-panmyelopathic D72.0
- Down (*see also* Down syndrome) Q90.9
- Dravet (intractable) G40.834
  - with status epilepticus G40.833
  - without status epilepticus G40.834
- DRESS (drug rash with eosinophilia and systemic symptoms) D72.12
- Dressler's (postmyocardial infarction) I24.1
  - postcardiotomy I97.0
- drug rash with eosinophilia and systemic symptoms (DRESS) D72.12
- drug withdrawal, infant of dependent mother P96.1
- dry eye H04.12-
- due to abnormality
  - chromosomal Q99.9
    - sex
      - female phenotype Q97.9
      - male phenotype Q98.9
    - specified NEC Q99.8
- Dupré's (meningism) R29.1
- dysmetabolic X E88.810
- dyspraxia, developmental F82
- Eagle-Barrett Q79.4
- eczema-thrombocytopenia D82.0
- Eddowes' Q78.0
- effort (psychogenic) F45.8
- Ehlers-Danlos Q79.60
  - classical Ehlers-Danlos syndrome Q79.61
  - hypermobile Ehlers-Danlos syndrome Q79.62
  - other Ehlers-Danlos syndromes Q79.69
  - vascular Ehlers-Danlos syndrome Q79.63
- Eisenmenger's I27.83

Syndrome *continued*

- Ekman's Q78.0
- Ellis-van Creveld Q77.6
- eosinophilia-myalgia M35.8
- epileptic—*see* Epilepsy, by type
- Erdheim's E22.0
- Evans D69.41
- eye retraction—*see* Strabismus
- eyelid-malar-mandible Q87.0
- facet M47.89-
- Fallot's Q21.3
- familial eczema-thrombocytopenia (Wiskott-Aldrich) D82.0
- fatigue
  - chronic R53.82
- faulty bowel habit K59.39
- fetal
  - alcohol (dysmorphic) Q86.0
- Fiedler's I40.1
- first arch Q87.0
- fish odor E72.89
- floppy
  - baby P94.2
- food protein-induced enterocolitis (FPIES) K52.21
- fragile X Q99.2
- Fukuhara E88.49
- functional
  - bowel K59.9
- Gaisböck's D75.1
- Gardner-Diamond D69.2
- Gee-Herter-Heubner K90.0
- Gianotti-Crosti L44.4
- Gilles de la Tourette's F95.2
- Gleich's D72.118
- Goldberg Q89.8
- Goldberg-Maxwell E34.51
- Good's D83.8
- Gouley's I31.1
- Gower's R55
- hand-foot L27.1
- Hegglin's D72.0
- hemolytic-uremic D59.3
- hemophagocytic, infection-associated D76.2
- Henoch-Schönlein D69.0
- hepatopulmonary K76.81
- hereditary alpha tryptasemia D89.44
- Herter (-Gee) (nontropical sprue) K90.0
- Heubner-Herter K90.0
- histamine-like (fish poisoning)—*see* Poisoning, food, noxious or naturally toxic, fish
- histiocytic D76.3
- histiocytosis NEC D76.3
- HIV infection, acute B20
- Hoffmann-Werdnig G12.0
- hypereosinophilic (HES) D72.119
  - idiopathic (IHES) D72.110
  - lymphocytic variant (LHES) D72.111
  - myeloid D72.118
  - specified NEC D72.118
- hyperkinetic—*see* Hyperkinesia
- hypermobility M35.7
- hypernatremia E87.0
- hyperosmolarity E87.0
- hypertransfusion, newborn P61.1
- hyperventilation F45.8
- hyperviscosity (of serum)
  - polycythemic D75.1
- hypoglycemic (familial) (neonatal) E16.2
- hyponatremic E87.1
- hypoplastic left-heart Q23.4
- hyposmolality E87.1
- hypothenar hammer I73.89
- ICF (intravascular coagulation-fibrinolysis) D65
- idiopathic
  - cardiorespiratory distress, newborn P22.0
  - nephrotic (infantile) N04.9
- immune effector cell-associated neurotoxicity (ICANS) G92.00
  - grade
    - 1 G92.01
    - 2 G92.02
    - 3 G92.03
    - 4 G92.04

ALPHABETIC INDEX

Syndrome, *continued*
- 5 G92.05
- unspecified G92.00
- immunity deficiency, combined D81.9
- immunodeficiency
  - acquired—*see* Human, immunodeficiency virus (HIV) disease
  - combined D81.9
- inappropriate secretion of antidiuretic hormone E22.2
- inspissated bile (newborn) P59.1
- insulin resistance
  - type A E88.811
  - type B E88.818
- intestinal
  - carcinoid E34.09
  - knot K56.2
- intravascular coagulation-fibrinolysis (ICF) D65
- iodine-deficiency, congenital E00.-
- IRDS (idiopathic respiratory distress, newborn) P22.0
- irritable
  - bowel K58.9
    - with constipation K58.1
    - with diarrhea K58.0
    - mixed K58.2
    - other K58.8
  - psychogenic F45.8
  - heart (psychogenic) F45.8
- IVC (intravascular coagulopathy) D65
- Jervell-Lange-Nielsen I45.81
- Job's D71
- Joseph-Diamond-Blackfan D61.01
- jugular foramen G52.7
- Kabuki Q‾ ¬1
- Kanner's (ism) F84.0
- Kartagener's Q89.3
- Kleefstra Q87.86
- Kostmann's D70.0
- Lambert-E
  - in neoplastic disease G73.1
- Launois' E22.0
- Laurence-Moon Q87.84
- lazy
  - leukocyte D70.8
- Lemierre I80.88
- Lennox-Gastaut G40.812
  - intractable G40.814
    - with status epilepticus G40.813
    - without status epilepticus G40.814
  - not intractable G40.812
    - with status epilepticus G40.811
    - without status epilepticus G40.812
- Leopold-Levi's E05.90
- Lev's I44.2
- long arm 18 or 21 deletion Q93.89
- long QT I45.81
- Louis-Barré G11.3
- low
  - back M54.50
  - output (cardiac) I50.9
- Luetscher's (dehydration) E86.0
- Lutembacher's Q21.1
- macrophage activation D76.1
  - due to infection D76.2
- Mal de Debarquement R42
- malabsorption K90.9
  - postsurgical K91.2
- malformation, congenital, due to
  - alcohol Q86.0
- malignant
  - carcinoid E34.00
- maple-syrup-urine E71.0
- Marfans Q87.40
  - with
    - cardiovascular manifestations Q87.418
      - aortic dilation Q87.410
    - ocular manifestations Q87.42
    - skeletal manifestations Q87.43
- Marie's E22.0
- mast cell activation D89.40
  - idiopathic D89.42
  - monoclonal D89.41
  - other D89.49
  - secondary D89.43

Syndrome, *continued*
- May (-Hegglin) D72.0
- McQuarrie's E16.2
- meconium plug (newborn) P76.0
- MED13L (mediator complex subunit 13L) Q87.85
- mediator complex subunit 13L (MED13L) Q87.85
- Meekeren-Ehlers-Danlos Q79.6-
- MELAS E88.41
- membranous (diffuse) N06.20
  - with
    - nephrotic syndrome N04.20
    - primary N04.21
    - secondary N04.22
  - idiopathic, with nephrotic syndrome N04.21
  - primary N06.21
    - with nephrotic syndrome N04.21
  - secondary N06.22
    - with nephrotic syndrome N04.22
- MERRF (myoclonic epilepsy associated with ragged-red fibers) E88.42
- metabolic E88.810
- metastatic carcinoid E34.00
- micrognathia-glossoptosis Q87.0
- midbrain NEC G93.89
- migraine—*see also* Migraine G43.909
- milk-alkali E83.52
- Miller-Dieker Q93.88
- Minkowski-Chauffard D58.0
- MNGIE (Mitochondrial Neurogastrointestinal Encephalopathy) E88.49
- Morgagni-Adams-Stokes I45.9
- mucocutaneous lymph node (acute febrile) (MCLS) M30.3
- myasthenic G70.9
  - in
    - diabetes mellitus—*see* Diabetes, type 1, with, amyotrophy
    - endocrine disease NEC E34.9 [G73.3]
    - neoplastic disease (*see also* Table of Neoplasms in the complete *ICD-10-CM* manual) D49.9 [G73.3]
    - thyrotoxicosis (hyperthyroidism) E05.90 [G73.3]
    - with thyroid storm E05.91 [G73.3]
- myelodysplastic D46.9
  - with
    - multilineage dysplasia D46.A
    - with ringed sideroblasts D46.B
  - myeloid hypereosinophilic D72.118
- myofascial pain M79.18
- NARP (Neuropathy, Ataxia and Retinitis pigmentosa) E88.49
- neonatal abstinence P96.1
- nephritic—*see also* Nephritis
  - with edema—*see* Nephrosis
  - acute N00.9
  - chronic N03.9
- nephrotic (congenital) (*see also* Nephrosis) N04.9
  - with
    - C3
      - glomerulonephritis N04.A
      - glomerulopathy N04.A
        - ◊ with dense deposit disease N04.6
    - dense deposit disease N04.6
    - diffuse
      - crescentic glomerulonephritis N04.7
      - endocapillary proliferative glomerulonephritis N04.4
      - membranous glomerulonephritis N04.20
      - mesangial proliferative glomerulonephritis N04.3
      - mesangiocapillary glomerulonephritis N04.5
    - focal and segmental glomerular lesions N04.1
    - minor glomerular abnormality N04.0
    - specified morphological changes NEC N04.8
    - specified type NEC with diffuse membranous glomerulonephritis N04.29
- Nothnagel's vasomotor acroparesthesia I73.89
- obliterans
  - bronchiolitis—*see also* Bronchiolitis, obliterative J44.81
- Ogilvie K59.81
- ophthalmoplegia-cerebellar ataxia—*see* Strabismus, paralytic, third nerve
- oral-facial-digital Q87.0

Syndrome, *continued*
- oro-facial-digital Q87.0
- Osler-Weber-Rendu I78.0
- oto-palatal-digital Q87.0
- outlet (thoracic) (*see also* Syndrome, thoracic outlet) G54.0
- ovary
  - polycystic E28.2
  - sclerocystic E28.2
- pain—*see also* Pain
  - complex regional I G90.5-
    - lower limb G90.52-
    - specified site NEC G90.59
    - upper limb G90.51-
  - painful
    - bruising D69.2
  - paralytic G83.9
- pediatric autoimmune neuropsychiatric disorders associated with streptococcal infections (PANDAS) D89.89
- pharyngeal pouch D82.1
- Phelan-McDermid Q93.52
- Pick's (heart) (liver) I31.1
- Pickwickian E66.2
- pituitary E22.0
- pontine NEC G93.89
- postcardiac injury
  - postcardiotomy I97.0
  - postcommissurotomy I97.0
  - postconcussional F07.81
  - postcontusional F07.81
- post-COVID (-19) U09.9
- postvalvulotomy I97.0
- prune belly Q79.4
- pseudoparalytica G70.00
  - with exacerbation (acute) G70.01
  - in crisis G70.01
- pseudo-Turner's Q87.19
- pulmonary
  - arteriosclerosis I27.0
  - dysmaturity (Wilson-Mikity) P27.0
  - hypoperfusion (idiopathic) P22.0
- QT interval prolongation I45.81
- RDS (respiratory distress syndrome, newborn) P22.0
- Reifenstein E34.52
- Rendu-Osler-Weber I78.0
- respiratory
  - distress
    - acute J80
    - child J80
  - newborn (idiopathic) (type I) P22.0
    - type II P22.1
- retinoblastoma (familial) C69.2
  - retroperitoneal fibrosis K68.2
- retroviral seroconversion (acute) Z21
- Romano-Ward (prolonged QT interval) I45.81
- rubella (congenital) P35.0
- Ruvalcaba-Myhre-Smith E71.440
- Rytand-Lipsitch I44.2
- salt
  - depletion E87.1
    - due to heat NEC T67.8
      - causing heat exhaustion or prostration T67.4
    - low E87.1
- Scaglietti-Dagnini E22.0
- scapuloperoneal G71.09
- schizophrenic, of childhood NEC F84.5
- Scholte's E34.09
- Schwachman (-Diamond) D61.02
- Schwartz-Bartter E22.2
- sclerocystic ovary E28.2
- Seitelberger's G31.89
- seroconversion, retroviral (acute) Z21
- serotonin G90.81
- serous meningitis G93.2
- severe acute respiratory (SARS) J12.81
- shaken infant T74.4
- shock (traumatic) T79.4
  - kidney N17.0
  - toxic A48.3
- shock-lung J80
- short
  - bowel K90.829

SYNDROME–SYNDROME

ALPHABETIC INDEX

Syndrome, *continued*

- ■ with
  - ~ colon in continuity K90.821
  - ~ ileocolonic anastomosis K90.821
  - ■ without colon in continuity K90.822
- ~ rib Q77.2
- Shwachman (-Diamond) D61.02
- sick
  - ~ cell E87.1
  - ~ sinus I49.5
- sinus tarsi M25.57-
- sinusitis-bronchiectasis-situs inversus Q89.3
- Smith-Magenis Q93.88
- Soto's Q87.3
- Spen's I45.9
- splenic
  - ~ neutropenia D73.81
- Spurway's Q78.0
- staphylococcal scalded skin L00
- Stein-Leventhal E28.2
- Stein's E28.2
- Stevens-Johnson syndrome L51.1
  - ~ toxic epidermal necrolysis overlap L51.3
- Stickler Q89.8
- stiff baby Q89.8
- Stokes (-Adams) I45.9
- swallowed blood P78.2
- sweat retention L74.0
- Symond's G93.2
- systemic inflammatory response (SIRS), of non-infectious origin (without organ dysfunction) R65.10
  - ~ with acute organ dysfunction R65.11
- tachycardia-bradycardia I49.5
- teething K00.7
- tegmental G93.89
- telangiectasia-pigmentation-cataract Q82.8
- temporal pyramidal apex—*see* Otitis, media, suppurative, acute
- temporomandibular joint-pain-dysfunction M26.62-
- testicular feminization (*see also* Syndrome, androgen insensitivity) E34.51
- Tietze's M94.0
- toxic shock A48.3
- triple X, female Q97.0
- trisomy Q92.9
  - ~ 13 Q91.7
    - ■ meiotic nondisjunction Q91.4
  - ~ 18 Q91.3
    - ■ meiotic nondisjunction Q91.0
  - ~ 21 Q90.9
- tumor lysis (following antineoplastic chemotherapy) (spontaneous) NEC E88.3
- uremia, chronic (*see also* Disease, kidney, chronic) N18.9
- vago-hypoglossal G52.7
- van der Hoeve's Q78.0
- vasovagal R55
- velo-cardio-facial Q93.81
- visual disorientation H53.8
- von Willebrand (-Jürgens) D68.0
- wasting (syndrome) due to underlying condition E88.A
- Werdnig-Hoffman G12.0
- wet
  - ~ lung, newborn P22.1
- whiplash S13.4
- whistling face Q87.0
- Willebrand (-Jürgens) D68.0
- Williams Q93.82
- Wiskott-Aldrich D82.0
- withdrawal—*see* Withdrawal state
  - ~ drug
    - ■ infant of dependent mother P96.1
    - ■ therapeutic use, newborn P96.2
- Yao M04.8
- Zahorsky's B08.5
- Zellweger syndrome E71.510
- Zellweger-like syndrome E71.541

Synostosis (congenital) Q78.8

- astragalo-scaphoid Q74.2
- radioulnar Q74.0

Synovitis (*see also* Tenosynovitis) M65.90

- ankle and foot M65.97-
- arm, upper M65.92-
- forearm M65.93-
- hand M65.94-
- leg, lower M65.96-
- multiple sites, unspecified type M65.99
- shoulder M65.91-
- specified site, unspecified type M65.98
- thigh M65.95-

Syphilis, syphilitic (acquired) A52.79

- age under 2 years NOS—*see also* Syphilis, congenital, early
  - ~ acquired A51.9
- anemia (late) A52.79 [D63.8]
- asymptomatic—*see* Syphilis, latent
- bubo (primary) A51.0
- chancre (multiple) A51.0
  - ~ extragenital A51.2
  - ~ Rollet's A51.0
- congenital A50.9
  - ~ early, or less than 2 years after birth NEC A50.2
    - ■ with manifestations—see Syphilis, congenital, early
  - ~ contact Z20.2
- cutaneous A51.39
- early A51.9
  - ~ symptomatic A51.9
    - ■ extragenital chancre A51.2
    - ■ primary, except extragenital chancre A51.0
- exposure to Z20.2
- genital (primary) A51.0
- inactive—*see* Syphilis, latent
- infantum—*see* Syphilis, congenital
- inherited—*see* Syphilis, congenital
- latent A53.0
  - ~ with signs or symptoms—*code by site and stage under* Syphilis
  - ~ date of infection unspecified A53.0
  - ~ early, or less than 2 years after infection A51.5
  - ~ follow-up of latent syphilis A53.0
    - ■ date of infection unspecified A53.0
    - ■ late, or 2 years or more after infection A52.8
  - ~ late, or 2 years or more after infection A52.8
  - ~ positive serology (only finding) A53.0
    - ■ date of infection unspecified A53.0
    - ■ early, or less than 2 years after infection A51.5
    - ■ late, or 2 years or more after infection A52.8
- lip A51.39
  - ~ chancre (primary) A51.2
  - ~ late A52.79
- penis (chancre) A51.0
- primary A51.0
  - ~ extragenital chancre NEC A51.2
  - ~ fingers A51.2
  - ~ genital A51.0
  - ~ lip A51.2
  - ~ specified site NEC A51.2
  - ~ tonsils A51.2
- skin (with ulceration) (early) (secondary) A51.39
- tonsil (lingual) (late) A52.76
  - ~ primary A51.2
- vagina A51.0
  - ~ late A52.76
- vulva A51.0
  - ~ late A52.76
  - ~ secondary A51.39

System, systemic—*see also* Disease, diseased

- inflammatory response syndrome (SIRS) of non-infectious origin (without organ dysfunction) R65.10
  - ~ with acute organ dysfunction R65.11
- lupus erythematosus M32.9

T

Tachyalimentation K91.2

Tachyarrhythmia, tachyrhythmia—*see* Tachycardia

Tachycardia R00.0

- atrial (paroxysmal) I47.19
- auricular I47.19
- AV nodal re-entry (re-entrant) I47.19
- junctional (paroxysmal) I47.19

Tachycardia, *continued*

- newborn P29.11
- nodal (paroxysmal) I47.19
- paroxysmal (sustained) (nonsustained) I47.9
  - ~ atrial (PAT) I47.1
  - ~ with sinus bradycardia I49.5
  - ~ atrioventricular (AV) (re-entrant) I47.19
    - ■ psychogenic F54
  - ~ junctional I47.19
    - ■ ectopic I47.19
  - ~ nodal I47.19
  - ~ supraventricular (sustained) I47.10
- psychogenic F45.8
- sick sinus I49.5
- sinoauricular NOS R00.0
  - ~ paroxysmal I47.19
- sinus [sinusal] NOS R00.0
  - ~ inappropriate, so stated (IST) I47.11
  - ~ paroxysmal I47.19
- supraventricular I47.10
- ventricular (paroxysmal) (sustained) I47.2

Tachypnea R06.82

- hysterical F45.8
- newborn (idiopathic) (transitory) P22.1
- psychogenic F45.8
- transitory, of newborn P22.1

TACO (transfusion associated circulatory overload) E87.71

Tag (hypertrophied skin) (infected) L91.8

- adenoid J35.8
- anus K64.4
- hemorrhoidal K64.4
- sentinel K64.4
- skin L91.8
  - ~ accessory (congenital) Q82.8
  - ~ anus K64.4
  - ~ congenital Q82.8
  - ~ preauricular Q17.0
- tonsil J35.8

Talipes (congenital) Q66.89

- acquired, planus—*see* Deformity, limb, flat foot
- asymmetric Q66.89
- calcaneovalgus Q66.4-
- calcaneovarus Q66.1-
- calcaneus Q66.89
- cavus Q66.7-
- equinovalgus Q66.6
- equinovarus Q66.0-
- equinus Q66.89
- percavus Q66.7-
- planovalgus Q66.6
- planus (acquired) (any degree)—*see also* Deformity, limb, flat foot
  - ~ congenital Q66.5-
- valgus Q66.6
- varus Q66.3-

Tall stature, constitutional E34.4

Tamponade, heart I31.4

Tantrum, child problem F91.8

Tapeworm (infection) (infestation)—*see* Infestation, tapeworm

Tapia's syndrome G52.7

Tattoo (mark) L81.8

Tay-Sachs amaurotic familial idiocy or disease E75.02

TBI (traumatic brain injury) S06.9

Tear, torn (traumatic)—*see also* Laceration

- anus, anal (sphincter) S31.831
  - ~ nontraumatic (healed) (old) K62.81
- rotator cuff (nontraumatic) M75.10-
  - ~ complete M75.12-
  - ~ incomplete M75.11-
  - ~ traumatic S46.01-
    - ■ capsule S43.42-
- vagina—*see* Laceration, vagina

Teeth—*see also* Disease, diseased

- grinding
  - ~ psychogenic F45.8
  - ~ sleep related G47.63

Teething (syndrome) K00.7

ALPHABETIC INDEX

Telangiectasia, telangiectasis (verrucous) I78.1
- ataxic (cerebellar) (Louis-Bar) G11.3
- familial I78.0
- hemorrhagic, hereditary (congenital) (senile) I78.0
- hereditary, hemorrhagic (congenital) (senile) I78.0
- spider I78.1

Telescoped bowel or intestine K56.1
- congenital Q43.8

Temperature
- body, high (of unknown origin) R50.9
- cold, trauma from
  - newborn P80.0

Temporomandibular joint pain-dysfunction syndrome M26.62-

Tendency
- bleeding—*see* Defect, coagulation
- suicide
  - meaning personal history of attempted suicide Z91.51
  - meaning suicidal ideation—*see* Ideation, suicidal

Tenderness, abdominal R10.819
- epigastric R10.816
- generalized R10.817
- left lower quadrant R10.814
- left upper quadrant R10.812
- periumbillic R10.815
- right lower quadrant R10.813
- right upper quadrant R10.811
- rebound R10.829
  - epigastric R10.826
  - generalized R10.827
  - left lower quadrant R10.824
  - left upper quadrant R10.822
  - periumbillic R10.825
  - right lower quadrant R10.823
  - right upper quadrant R10.821

Tendinitis, tendonitis—*see also* Enthesopathy
- Achilles M76.6-

Tenesmus (rectal) R19.8

Tennis elbow—*see* Epicondylitis, lateral

Tenosynovitis M65.90
- adhesive—*see* Tenosynovitis, specified type NEC
- shoulder region M65.81-
  - adhesive—*see* Capsulitis, adhesive
- specified type NEC M65.88
  - ankle M65.87-
  - foot M65.87-
  - forearm M65.83-
  - hand M65.84-
  - lower leg M65.86-
  - multiple sites M65.89
  - pelvic region M65.85-
  - shoulder region M65.81-
  - specified site NEC M65.88
  - thigh M65.85-
  - upper arm M65.82-

Tension
- arterial, high—*see also* Hypertension
  - without diagnosis of hypertension R03.0
- headache G44.209
  - intractable G44.201
  - not intractable G44.209
- nervous R45.0
- pneumothorax J93.0
- state (mental) F48.9

Tentorium—*see* Disease, diseased

Teratencephalus Q89.8

Teratism Q89.7

Terror(s) night (child) F51.4

Test, tests, testing (for)
- blood-alcohol Z02.83
  - positive—*see* Findings
- blood-drug Z02.83
  - positive—*see* Findings
- hearing Z01.10
  - with abnormal findings NEC Z01.118
  - infant or child (over 28 days old) Z00.129
    - with abnormal findings Z00.121

Test, tests, testing, *continued*
- HIV (human immunodeficiency virus)
  - nonconclusive (in infants) R75
  - positive Z21
  - seropositive Z21
- immunity status Z01.84
- laboratory (as part of a general medical examination) Z00.00
  - with abnormal finding Z00.01
  - for medicolegal reason NEC Z04.89
- Mantoux (for tuberculosis) Z11.1
  - abnormal result R76.11
- skin, diagnostic
  - allergy Z01.82
    - special screening examination—*see* Screening, by name of disease
  - Mantoux Z11.1
  - tuberculin Z11.1
  - specified NEC Z01.89
- tuberculin Z11.1
  - abnormal result R76.11
- vision Z01.00
  - with abnormal findings Z01.01
  - after failed exam Z01.02-
  - infant or child (over 28 days old) Z00.129
    - with abnormal findings Z00.121
- Wassermann Z11.3
  - positive—*see* Serology for syphilis

Testicle, testicular, testes—*see also* Disease, diseased
- feminization syndrome (*see also* Syndrome, androgen insensitivity) E34.51
- migrans Q55.29

Tetanus, tetanic (cephalic) (convulsions) A35

Tetany (due to) R29.0
- associated with rickets E55.0
- hyperpnea R06.4
  - hysterical F44.5
  - psychogenic F45.8
- hyperventilation (*see also* Hyperventilation) R06.4
  - hysterical F44.5
- neonatal (without calcium or magnesium deficiency) P71.3
- psychogenic (conversion reaction) F44.5

Tetralogy of Fallot Q21.3

Tetraplegia (chronic) (*see also* Quadriplegia) G82.50

Thalassemia (anemia) (disease) D56.9
- with other hemoglobinopathy D56.8
- alpha (major) (severe) (triple gene defect) D56.0
  - minor D56.3
  - silent carrier D56.3
  - trait D56.3
- beta (severe) D56.1
  - homozygous D56.1
  - major D56.1
  - minor D56.3
  - trait D56.3
- delta-beta (homozygous) D56.2
  - minor D56.3
  - trait D56.3
- dominant D56.8
- hemoglobin
  - C D56.8
  - E-beta D56.5
- intermedia D56.1
- major D56.1
- minor D56.3
- mixed D56.8
- sickle-cell—*see* Disease, sickle-cell, thalassemia
- specified type NEC D56.8
- trait D56.3
- variants D56.8

Thanatophoric dwarfism or short stature Q77.1

Thaysen-Gee disease (nontropical sprue) K90.0

Thaysen's disease K90.0

Thelitis N61.0

Therapy
- drug, long-term (current) (prophylactic)
  - antibiotics Z79.2
  - anti-inflammatory Z79.1
  - aspirin Z79.82

Therapy, *continued*
- drug, specified NEC Z79.899
  - hypoglycemic drugs, oral Z79.84
  - insulin Z79.4
  - steroids
    - inhaled Z79.51
    - systemic Z79.52

Thermoplegia T67.0

Thickening
- breast N64.59

Thirst, excessive R63.1
- due to deprivation of water T73.1

Thomsen disease G71.12

Thoracic—*see also* condition
- outlet syndrome (*see also* Syndrome, thoracic outlet) G54.0

Threadworm (infection) (infestation) B80

Threatened
- abortion O20.0
  - with subsequent abortion O03.9
  - miscarriage O20.0

Thrombocythemia (essential) (hemorrhagic) (idiopathic) (primary) D47.3
- essential D47.3
- idiopathic D47.3
- primary D47.3

Thrombocytopenia, thrombocytopenic D69.6
- with absent radius (TAR) Q87.2
- congenital D69.42
- dilutional D69.59
- due to
  - drugs D69.59
    - heparin induced (HIT) D75.82
      - heparin-induced (HIT), unspecified D75.829
      - immune-mediated heparin induced (HIT) D75.822
      - non-immune heparin induced (HIT) D75.821
  - extracorporeal circulation of blood D69.59
  - (massive) blood transfusion D69.59
  - platelet alloimmunization D69.59
- essential D69.3
- heparin induced (HIT) D75.82
- hereditary D69.42
- idiopathic D69.3
- neonatal, transitory P61.0
  - due to
    - exchange transfusion P61.0
    - idiopathic maternal thrombocytopenia P61.0
    - isoimmunization P61.0
- other platelet-activating anti-PF4 disorders D75.84
- primary NEC D69.49
  - idiopathic D69.3
- secondary D69.59
- transient neonatal P61.0

Thrombocytosis, essential D47.3
- essential D47.3
- idiopathic D47.3
- primary D47.3
- reactive D75.838
- secondary D75.838
- specified NEC D75.838

Thromboembolism—*see* Embolism

Thrombopathy (Bernard-Soulier) D69.1
- constitutional D68.0
- Willebrand-Jürgens D68.0

Thrombophlebitis I80.9
- calf muscular vein (NOS) I80.25-
- femoral vein (superficial) I80.1-
- femoropopliteal vein I80.0-
- gastrocnemial vein I80.25-
- hepatic (vein) I80.8
- iliac vein (common) (external) (internal) I80.21-
- iliofemoral I80.1-
- leg I80.3
  - superficial I80.0-
- lower extremity I80.299
- peroneal vein I80.24-
- popliteal vein—*see* Phlebitis, leg
- saphenous (greater) (lesser) I80.0-

ALPHABETIC INDEX

Thrombophlebitis, *continued*
- soleal vein I80.25-
- specified site NEC I80.8
- tibial vein (anterior) (posterior) I80.23-

Thrombosis, thrombotic (bland) (multiple) (progressive) (silent) (vessel) I82.90
- anus K64.5
- artery, arteries (postinfectional) I74.9
- genital organ
  - female NEC N94.89
- liver (venous) I82.0
  - artery I74.8
  - portal vein I81
- mesenteric (artery) (with gangrene) K55.0
  - vein (inferior) (superior) I81
- perianal venous K64.5
- portal I81
- renal (artery) N28.0
  - vein I82.3
- tricuspid I07.8
- vein (acute) I82.90
  - perianal K64.5
  - renal I82.3
- venous, perianal K64.5

Thrombus—*see* Thrombosis

Thrush—*see also* Candidiasis
- oral B37.0
- newborn P37.5
- vagina B37.3

Thumb—*see also* Disease, diseased
- sucking (child problem) F98.8

Thyroglossal—*see also* Disease, diseased
- cyst Q89.2
- duct, persistent Q89.2

Thyroid (gland) (body)—*see also* Disease, diseased
- lingual Q89.2

Thyroiditis E06.9
- acute (nonsuppurative) (pyogenic) (suppurative) E06.0
- autoimmune E06.3
- chronic (nonspecific) (sclerosing) E06.5
  - with thyrotoxicosis, transient E06.2
  - fibrous E06.5
  - lymphadenoid E06.3
  - lymphocytic E06.3
  - lymphoid E06.3
- de Quervain's E06.1
- drug-induced E06.4
- fibrous (chronic) E06.5
- giant-cell (follicular) E06.1
- granulomatous (de Quervain) (subacute) E06.1
- Hashimoto's (struma lymphomatosa) E06.3
- iatrogenic E06.4
- ligneous E06.5
- lymphocytic (chronic) E06.3
- lymphoid E06.3
- lymphomatous E06.3
- nonsuppurative E06.1
- pseudotuberculous E06.1
- pyogenic E06.0
- radiation E06.4
- Riedel's E06.5
- subacute (granulomatous) E06.1
- suppurative E06.0
- viral E06.1
- woody E06.5

Thyrolyngual duct, persistent Q89.2

Thyrotoxic
- crisis—*see* Thyrotoxicosis
- heart disease or failure (*see also* Thyrotoxicosis) E05.90 [I43]
  - with thyroid storm E05.91 [I43]
- storm—*see* Thyrotoxicosis

Thyrotoxicosis (recurrent) E05.90
- with
  - goiter (diffuse) E05.00
    - with thyroid storm E05.01
  - heart E05.90 [I43]
    - with thyroid storm E05.91 [I43]
    - failure E05.90 [I43]

Thyrotoxicosis, *continued*
- neonatal (transient) P72.1
- transient with chronic thyroiditis E06.2

Tibia vara M92.51-

Tic (disorder) F95.9
- child problem F95.0
- compulsive F95.1
- de la Tourette F95.2
- disorder
  - chronic
    - motor F95.1
    - vocal F95.1
  - combined vocal and multiple motor F95.2
  - transient F95.0
- habit F95.9
  - transient of childhood F95.0
- lid, transient of childhood F95.0
- motor-verbal F95.2
- orbicularis F95.8
  - transient of childhood F95.0
- provisional F95.0
- spasm (motor or vocal) F95.9
  - chronic F95.1
  - transient of childhood F95.0

Tick-borne—*see* Disease, diseased

Tietze's disease or syndrome M94.0

Tight, tightness
- anus K62.89
- foreskin (congenital) N47.1
- rectal sphincter K62.89
- urethral sphincter N35.919

Timidity, child F93.8

Tinea (intersecta) (tarsi) B35.9
- asbestina B35.0
- barbae B35.0
- beard B35.0
- black dot B35.0
- capitis B35.0
- corporis B35.4
- cruris B35.6
- flava B36.0
- foot B35.3
- furfuracea B36.0
- imbricata (Tokelau) B35.5
- kerion B35.0
- microsporic—*see* Dermatophytosis
- nodosa B36.-
- pedis B35.3
- scalp B35.0
- specified NEC B35.8
- sycosis B35.0
- tonsurans B35.0
- trichophytic—*see* Dermatophytosis
- unguium B35.1
- versicolor B36.0

Tinnitus NOS H93.1-
- audible H93.1-
- aurium H93.1-
- pulsatile H93.A-
- subjective H93.1-

Tiredness R53.83

Tobacco (nicotine)
- abuse—*see* Tobacco, use
- dependence—*see* Dependence, drug, nicotine
- harmful use Z72.0
- heart—*see* Tobacco, toxic effect
- maternal use, affecting newborn P04.2
- toxic effect—*see* Table of Drugs and Chemicals, by substance, poisoning
  - chewing tobacco—*see* Table of Drugs and Chemicals, by substance, poisoning
  - cigarettes—*see* Table of Drugs and Chemicals, by substance, poisoning
- use Z72.0
  - counseling and surveillance Z71.6
  - history Z87.891
- withdrawal state—*see* Dependence, drug, nicotine F17.203

Tongue—*see also* Disease, diseased
- tie Q38.1

Tonsillitis (acute) (catarrhal) (croupous) (follicular) (gangrenous) (infective) (lacunar) (lingual) (malignant) (membranous) (parenchymatous) (phlegmonous) (pseudomembranous) (purulent) (septic) (subacute) (suppurative) (toxic) (ulcerative) (vesicular) (viral) J03.90
- chronic J35.01
  - with adenoiditis J35.03
- hypertrophic J35.01
  - with adenoiditis J35.03
- recurrent J03.91
- specified organism NEC J03.80
  - recurrent J03.81
- staphylococcal J03.80
  - recurrent J03.81
- streptococcal J03.00
  - recurrent J03.01

Tooth, teeth—*see* Disease, diseased

TORCH infection—*see* Infection, congenital
- without active infection P00.2

Torsion
- appendix epididymis N44.04
- appendix testis N44.03
- bile duct (common) (hepatic) K83.8
  - congenital Q44.5
- bowel, colon or intestine K56.2
- epididymis (appendix) N44.04
- gallbladder K82.8
  - congenital Q44.1
- hydatid of Morgagni
  - male N44.03
- Meckel's diverticulum (congenital) Q43.0
- mesentery K56.2
- omentum K56.2
- organ or site, congenital NEC—*see* Anomaly, by site
- ovary (pedicle) N83.51-
  - with fallopian tube N83.53
  - congenital Q50.2
- penis (acquired) N48.82
  - congenital Q55.63
- spermatic cord N44.02
  - extravaginal N44.01
  - intravaginal N44.02
- testis, testicle N44.00
  - appendix N44.03
- tibia—*see* Deformity, limb, specified type NEC, lower leg

Torticollis (intermittent) (spastic) M43.6
- congenital (sternomastoid) Q68.0
- due to birth injury P15.8
- hysterical F44.4
- ocular R29.891
- psychogenic F45.8
  - conversion reaction F44.4
- rheumatic M43.6
- traumatic, current S13.4

Tortuous
- ureter N13.8

Tourette's syndrome F95.2

Tourniquet syndrome—*see* Constriction, external, by site

Tower skull Q75.009
- with exophthalmos Q87.0

Toxemia
- erysipelatous—*see* Erysipelas
- food—*see* Poisoning, food
- staphylococcal, due to food A05.0

Toxic (poisoning) (*see also* Disease, diseased) T65.91
- effect—*see* Table of Drugs and Chemicals, by substance, poisoning
- shock syndrome A48.3

Toxicity—*see* Table of Drugs and Chemicals, by substance, poisoning
- fava bean D55.0
- food, noxious—*see* Poisoning, food
- from drug or nonmedicinal substance—*see* Table of Drugs and Chemicals, by drug

Toxicosis—*see also* Toxemia
- capillary, hemorrhagic D69.0

ALPHABETIC INDEX

Toxoplasma, toxoplasmosis (acquired) B58.9
- with
  - meningoencephalitis B58.2
  - ocular involvement B58.00
  - other organ involvement B58.89
  - pneumonia, pneumonitis B58.3
- congenital (acute) (subacute) (chronic) P37.1
- maternal, manifest toxoplasmosis in infant (acute) (subacute) (chronic) P37.1

Tracheitis (catarrhal) (infantile) (membranous) (plastic) (septal) (suppurative) (viral) J04.10
- with
  - bronchitis (15 years of age and above) J40
    - acute or subacute—*see* Bronchitis, acute
      - under 15 years of age J20.9
  - laryngitis (acute) J04.2
    - chronic J37.1
- acute J04.10
  - with obstruction J04.11
- chronic J42
  - with
    - laryngitis (chronic) J37.1

Tracheomalacia J39.8
- congenital Q32.0

Tracheopharyngitis (acute) J06.9
- chronic J42

Trachoma, trachomatous A71.9
- Türck's J37.0

Train sickness T75.3

Trait
- Hb-S D57.3
- hemoglobin
  - abnormal NEC D58.2
    - with thalassemia D56.3
  - C—*see* Disease, hemoglobin or Hb
  - S (Hb-S) D57.3
- Lepore D56.3
- sickle-cell D57.3
  - with elliptocytosis or spherocytosis D57.3

Transaminasemia R74.01

Transfusion
- associated (red blood cell) hemochromatosis E83.111
- reaction (adverse)—*see* Complications, transfusion
- related acute lung injury (TRALI) J95.84

Transient (meaning homeless) (*see also* Disease, diseased) Z59.00

Translocation
- balanced autosomal Q95.9
  - in normal individual Q95.0
- chromosomes NEC Q99.8
  - balanced and insertion in normal individual Q95.0
- Down syndrome Q90.2
- trisomy
  - 13 Q91.6
  - 18 Q91.2
  - 21 Q90.2

Transplant (ed) (status) Z94.9
- awaiting organ Z76.82
- bone Z94.6
  - marrow Z94.81
- candidate Z76.82
- heart Z94.1
  - valve Z95.2
    - prosthetic Z95.2
    - specified NEC Z95.4
    - xenogenic Z95.3
- intestine Z94.82
- kidney Z94.0
- liver Z94.4
- lung(s) Z94.2
  - and heart Z94.3
- organ (failure) (infection) (rejection) Z94.9
  - removal status Z98.85
- pancreas Z94.83
- skin Z94.5
- social Z60.3
- specified organ or tissue NEC Z94.89
- stem cells Z94.84
- tissue Z94.9

Transposition (congenital)—*see also* Malposition, congenital
- abdominal viscera Q89.3
- aorta (dextra) Q20.3
- great vessels (complete) (partial) Q20.3
- heart Q24.0
  - with complete transposition of viscera Q89.3
- scrotum Q55.23
- stomach Q40.2
  - with general transposition of viscera Q89.3
- vessels, great (complete) (partial) Q20.3
- viscera (abdominal) (thoracic) Q89.3

Transsexualism F64.0

Transvestism, transvestitism (dual-role) F64.1

Trauma, traumatism—*see also* Injury
- acoustic—*see* subcategory H83.3
- occlusal
  - primary K08.81
  - secondary K08.82

Tremor(s) R25.1
- hysterical F44.4
- psychogenic (conversion reaction) F44.4

Triad
- Kartagener's Q89.3

Trichocephaliasis, trichocephalosis B79

Trichocephalus infestation B79

Trichomoniasis A59.9
- bladder A59.03
- cervix A59.09
- seminal vesicles A59.09
- specified site NEC A59.8
- urethra A59.03
- urogenitalis A59.00
- vagina A59.01
- vulva A59.01

Trigger finger (acquired)
- congenital Q74.0

Trigonocephaly Q75.03

Triphalangeal thumb Q74.0

Triple—*see also* Accessory
- X, female Q97.0

Trismus R25.2

Trisomy (syndrome) Q92.9
- 13 (partial) Q91.7
  - meiotic nondisjunction Q91.4
- 18 (partial) Q91.3
  - meiotic nondisjunction Q91.0
- 21 (partial) Q90.9

Trombiculosis, trombiculiasis, trombidiosis B88.0

Trophoneurosis NEC G96.89

Trouble—*see also* Disease
- nervous R45.0

Truancy, childhood
- from school Z72.810

Truncus
- arteriosus (persistent) Q20.0
- communis Q20.0

Trunk—*see* Disease, diseased

Tryptasemia, hereditary alpha D89.44

Tuberculoma—*see also* Tuberculosis
- brain A17.81
- meninges (cerebral) (spinal) A17.1
- spinal cord A17.81

Tuberculosis, tubercular, tuberculous (calcification) (calcified) (caseous) (chromogenic acid-fast bacilli) (degeneration) (fibrocaseous) (fistula) (interstitial) (isolated circumscribed lesions) (necrosis) (parenchymatous) (ulcerative) A15.9
- abscess (respiratory) A15.9
  - latent Z22.7
  - meninges (cerebral) (spinal) A17.0
  - scrofulous A18.2
- arachnoid A17.0
- axilla, axillary (gland) A18.2
- cachexia A15.9
- cerebrospinal A17.81
  - meninges A17.0
- cervical (lymph gland or node) A18.2

Tuberculosis, tubercular, tuberculous, *continued*
- contact Z20.1
- dura (mater) (cerebral) (spinal) A17.0
  - abscess (cerebral) (spinal) A17.81
- exposure (to) Z20.1
- glandular, general A18.2
- immunological findings only A15.7
- infection A15.9
  - without clinical manifestation A15.7
- infraclavicular gland A18.2
- inguinal gland A18.2
- inguinalis A18.2
- latent Z22.7
- leptomeninges, leptomeningitis (cerebral) (spinal) A17.0
- lymph gland or node (peripheral) A18.2
  - cervical A18.2
- marasmus A15.9
- neck gland A18.2
- meninges, meningitis (basilar) (cerebral) (cerebrospinal) (spinal) A17.0
- pachymeningitis A17.0
- respiratory A15.9
  - primary A15.7
  - specified site NEC A15.8
- scrofulous A18.2
- senile A15.9
- spine, spinal (column) A18.01
  - cord A17.81
  - medulla A17.81
  - membrane A17.0
  - meninges A17.0
- supraclavicular gland A18.2
- unspecified site A15.9

Tuberous sclerosis (brain) Q85.1

Tumefaction—*see also* Swelling
- liver—*see* Hypertrophy, liver

Tumor—*see also* Neoplasm, unspecified behavior, by site in Table of Neoplasms in the complete *ICD-10-CM* manual
- carcinoid D3A.00
  - benign D3A.00
    - appendix D3A.020
    - ascending colon D3A.022
    - bronchus (lung) D3A.090
    - cecum D3A.021
    - colon D3A.029
    - descending colon D3A.024
    - duodenum D3A.010
    - foregut NOS D3A.094
    - hindgut NOS D3A.096
    - ileum D3A.012
    - jejunum D3A.011
    - kidney D3A.093
    - large intestine D3A.029
    - lung (bronchus) D3A.090
    - midgut NOS D3A.095
    - rectum D3A.026
    - sigmoid colon D3A.025
    - small intestine D3A.019
    - specified NEC D3A.098
    - stomach D3A.092
    - thymus D3A.091
    - transverse colon D3A.023
- Cock's peculiar L72.3
- glomus D18.00
  - skin D18.01
  - specified site NEC D18.09
- Grawitz's C64.-
- neuroectodermal (peripheral)—*see* Neoplasm, malignant, by site in Table of Neoplasms in the complete *ICD-10-CM* manual
  - primitive
    - specified site—*see* Neoplasm, malignant, by site in Table of Neoplasms in the complete *ICD-10-CM* manual
    - unspecified site C71.9
- neuroendocrine D3A.8
- phantom F45.8
- sternomastoid (congenital) Q68.0
- turban D23.4
- Wilms' C64.-

Tumor lysis syndrome (following antineoplastic chemotherapy) (spontaneous) NEC E88.3

Tungiasis B88.1
Tunica vasculosa lentis Q12.2
Turban tumor D23.4
Türck's trachoma J37.0
Turner-like syndrome Q87.19
Turner's syndrome Q96.9
Turner-Ullrich syndrome Q96.9
Twist, twisted
- bowel, colon or intestine K56.2
- mesentery K56.2
- omentum K56.2
- organ or site, congenital NEC—*see* Anomaly, by site
Tylosis (acquired) L84
- palmaris et plantaris (congenital) (inherited) Q82.8
  - acquired L85.1
Tympanism R14.0
Tympanites (abdominal) (intestinal) R14.0
Tympanitis—*see* Myringitis
Tympany
- abdomen R14.0
- chest R09.89
Typhus (fever)
- Sao Paulo A77.0

U

Ulcer, ulcerated, ulcerating, ulceration, ulcerative
- anorectal K62.6
- anus (sphincter) (solitary) K62.6
- aphthous (oral) (recurrent) K12.0
- bleeding K27.4
- breast N61.1
- buccal (cavity) (traumatic) K12.1
- cervix (uteri) (decubitus) (trophic) N86
  - with cervicitis N72
- Dieulafoy's K25.0
- duodenum, duodenal (eroded) (peptic) K26.9
  - with
    - hemorrhage K26.4
      - and perforation K26.6
    - perforation K26.5
  - acute K26.3
    - with
      - hemorrhage K26.0
        - ◊ and perforation K26.2
      - perforation K26.1
  - chronic K26.7
    - with
      - hemorrhage K26.4
        - ◊ and perforation K26.6
      - perforation K26.5
- dysenteric A09
- esophagus (peptic) K22.10
  - due to
    - gastrointestinal reflux disease K21.0-
- frenum (tongue) K14.0
- hemorrhoid (*see also* Hemorrhoids, by degree) K64.8
- intestine, intestinal K63.3
  - rectum K62.6
- lip K13.0
- meatus (urinarius) N34.2
- Meckel's diverticulum Q43.0
- oral mucosa (traumatic) K12.1
- palate (soft) K12.1
- peptic (site unspecified) K27.9
  - with
    - hemorrhage K27.4
      - and perforation K27.6
    - perforation K27.5
  - acute K27.3
    - with
      - hemorrhage K27.0
        - ◊ and perforation K27.2
      - perforation K27.1
  - chronic K27.7
    - with
      - hemorrhage K27.4
        - ◊ and perforation K27.6
      - perforation K27.5

Ulcer, ulcerated, ulcerating, ulceration, ulcerative, *continued*
  - esophagus K22.10
    - with bleeding K22.11
  - newborn P78.82
- perforating K27.5
- peritonsillar J35.8
- pressure (pressure area) L89.9-
  - ankle L89.5-
  - back L89.1-
  - buttock L89.3-
  - coccyx L89.15-
  - contiguous site of back, buttock, hip L89.4-
  - elbow L89.0-
  - face L89.81-
  - head L89.81-
  - heel L89.6-
  - hip L89.2-
  - sacral region (tailbone) L89.15-
  - specified site NEC L89.89-
  - stage 1 (healing) (pre-ulcer skin changes limited to persistent focal edema)
    - ankle L89.5-
    - back L89.1-
    - buttock L89.3-
    - coccyx L89.15-
    - contiguous site of back, buttock, hip L89.4-
    - elbow L89.0-
    - face L89.81-
    - head L89.81-
    - heel L89.6-
    - hip L89.2-
    - sacral region (tailbone) L89.15-
    - specified site NEC L89.89-
  - stage 2 (healing) (abrasion, blister, partial thickness skin loss involving epidermis and/or dermis)
    - ankle L89.5-
    - back L89.1-
    - buttock L89.3-
    - coccyx L89.15-
    - contiguous site of back, buttock, hip L89.4-
    - elbow L89.0-
    - face L89.81-
    - head L89.81-
    - heel L89.6-
    - hip L89.2-
    - sacral region (tailbone) L89.15-
    - specified site NEC L89.89-
  - stage 3 (healing) (full thickness skin loss involving damage or necrosis of subcutaneous tissue)
    - ankle L89.5-
    - back L89.1-
    - buttock L89.3-
    - coccyx L89.15-
    - contiguous site of back, buttock, hip L89.4-
    - elbow L89.0-
    - face L89.81-
    - head L89.81-
    - heel L89.6-
    - hip L89.2-
    - sacral region (tailbone) L89.15-
    - specified site NEC L89.89-
  - stage 4 (healing) (necrosis of soft tissues through to underlying muscle, tendon, or bone)
    - ankle L89.5-
    - back L89.1-
    - buttock L89.3-
    - coccyx L89.15-
    - contiguous site of back, buttock, hip L89.4-
    - elbow L89.0-
    - face L89.81-
    - head L89.81-
    - heel L89.6-
    - hip L89.2-
    - sacral region (tailbone) L89.15-
    - specified site NEC L89.89-
- rectum (sphincter) (solitary) K62.6
  - stercoraceous, stercoral K62.6
- scrofulous (tuberculous) A18.2
- scrotum N50.89
  - varicose I86.1
- solitary, anus or rectum (sphincter) K62.6

Ulcer, ulcerated, ulcerating, ulceration, ulcerative, *continued*
- sore throat J02.9
  - streptococcal J02.0
- stercoraceous, stercoral K63.3
  - anus or rectum K62.6
- stomach (eroded) (peptic) (round) K25.9
  - with
    - hemorrhage K25.4
      - and perforation K25.6
    - perforation K25.5
  - acute K25.3
    - with
      - hemorrhage K25.0
        - ◊ and perforation K25.2
      - perforation K25.1
  - chronic K25.7
    - with
      - hemorrhage K25.4
        - ◊ and perforation K25.6
      - perforation K25.5
- stomatitis K12.1
- strumous (tuberculous) A18.2
- tongue (traumatic) K14.0
- tonsil J35.8
- turbinate J34.89
- uterus N85.8
  - cervix N86
    - with cervicitis N72
  - neck N86
    - with cervicitis N72
- valve, heart I33.0
- varicose (lower limb, any part)—*see also* Varix
  - scrotum I86.1

Ulcerosa scarlatina A38.8
Ulcus—*see also* Ulcer
- durum (syphilitic) A51.0
  - extragenital A51.2
Ulerythema
- ophryogenes, congenital Q84.2
- sycosiforme L73.8
Ullrich (-Bonnevie) (-Turner) syndrome Q87.19
Ullrich-Feichtiger syndrome Q87.0
Unable to
- obtain
  - adequate
    - childcare due to limited financial resources, specified NEC Z59.87
    - clothing due to limited financial resources, specified NEC Z59.87
    - utilities due to limited financial resources, specified NEC Z59.87
  - basic
    - needs due to limited financial resources, specified NEC Z59.87
    - services in physical environment Z58.81
  - internet service, due to unavailability in geographic area Z58.81
  - telephone service, due to unavailability in geographic area Z58.81
  - utilities, due to inadequate physical environment Z58.81
Unavailability (of)
- medical facilities (at) Z75.3
  - due to
    - lack of services at home Z75.0
  - home Z75.0
Underdevelopment—*see also* Undeveloped
- sexual E30.0
Underdosing (*see also* Table of Drugs and Chemicals, categories T36–T50, with final character 6) Z91.14
- intentional NEC Z91.128
  - due to financial hardship of patient Z91.120
- unintentional NEC Z91.138
Underimmunization status Z28.3
Underweight R63.6
- for gestational age—*see* Light for dates
Underwood's disease P83.0

ALPHABETIC INDEX

Undeveloped, undevelopment—*see also* Hypoplasia
- brain (congenital) Q02
- cerebral (congenital) Q02
- heart Q24.8
- lung Q33.6
- uterus E30.0

Undiagnosed (disease) R69

Unguis incarnatus L60.0

Unicuspid aortic valve (at birth) (congenital) Q23.81

Unsatisfactory
- surroundings Z59.19

Unstable
- hip (congenital) Q65.6

Unsteadiness on feet R26.81

Untruthfulness, child problem F91.8

Upbringing, institutional Z62.22
- away from parents NEC Z62.29
- in care of non-parental family member Z62.21
- in foster care Z62.21
- in orphanage or group home Z62.22
- in welfare custody Z62.21

Upper respiratory—*see* Disease, diseased

Upset
- gastric K30
- gastrointestinal K30
  - psychogenic F45.8
- intestinal (large) (small) K59.9
  - psychogenic F45.8
- mental F48.9
- stomach K30
  - psychogenic F45.8

Uremia, uremic N19
- chronic NOS (*see also* Disease, kidney, chronic) N18.9
  - due to hypertension—*see* Hypertensive, kidney
- congenital P96.0

Ureteralgia N23

Ureteritis N28.89
- due to calculus N20.1
  - with calculus, kidney N20.2
    - with hydronephrosis N13.2
  - nonspecific N28.89

Ureterocele N28.89
- congenital (orthotopic) Q62.31

Urethralgia R39.89

Urethritis (anterior) (posterior) N34.2
- candidal B37.41
- chlamydial A56.01
- diplococcal (gonococcal) A54.01
  - with abscess (accessory gland) (periurethral) A54.1
- gonococcal A54.01
  - with abscess (accessory gland) (periurethral) A54.1
- nongonococcal N34.1
- nonspecific N34.1
- nonvenereal N34.1
- specified NEC N34.2
- trichomonal or due to Trichomonas (vaginalis) A59.03

Urethrorrhea R36.9

Urgency
- fecal R15.2
- urinary R39.15

Uric acid in blood (increased) E79.0

Uricacidemia (asymptomatic) E79.0

Uricemia (asymptomatic) E79.0

Uricosuria R82.998

Urination
- frequent R35.0

Urine
- blood in—*see* Hematuria
- discharge, excessive R35.89
- enuresis, nonorganic origin F98.0
- frequency R35.0
- incontinence R32
  - nonorganic origin F98.0
- intermittent stream R39.198
- pus in N39.0
- retention or stasis R33.9
  - psychogenic F45.8

Urine, *continued*
- secretion
  - deficient R34
  - excessive R35.89
  - frequency R35.0
- stream
  - intermittent R39.198
  - slowing R39.198
  - weak R39.12

Urodialysis R34

Uropathy N39.9
- obstructive N13.9
  - specified NEC N13.8
- reflux N13.9
  - specified NEC N13.8

Urticaria L50.9
- with angioneurotic edema T78.3
- allergic L50.0
- cholinergic L50.5
- chronic L50.8
- due to
  - cold or heat L50.2
  - drugs L50.0
  - food L50.0
  - inhalants L50.0
  - plants L50.6
  - serum (*see also* Reaction, serum) T80.69
- factitial L50.3
- giant T78.3
- gigantea T78.3
- idiopathic L50.1
- larynx T78.3
- neonatorum P83.88
- pigmentosa D47.01
  - congenital Q82.2
  - of neonatal onset Q82.2
- nonallergic L50.1
- pigmentosa D47.01
  - congenital Q82.2
  - of neonatal onset Q82.2
- recurrent periodic L50.8
- serum (*see also* Reaction, serum) T80.69
- specified type NEC L50.8
- thermal (cold) (heat) L50.2
- vibratory L50.4

Use (of)
- alcohol (*see also* Alcohol, alcoholic, by disorder) F10.90
- caffeine—*see* Use, stimulant NEC
- cannabis F12.90
  - withdrawal F12.93
- inhalants F18.9-
- stimulant NEC F15.90
  - with
    - other, unspecified, in remission F15.91
    - withdrawal F15.93
  - harmful—*see* Abuse, drug, stimulant NEC
- tobacco Z72.0
  - with dependence—*see* Dependence, drug, nicotine
- volatile solvents (*see also* Use, inhalant) F18.90
  - harmful—*see* Abuse, drug, inhalant

Uveitis (anterior)
- due to toxoplasmosis (acquired) B58.09
  - congenital P37.1

Uveoparotitis D86.89

Uvulitis (acute) (catarrhal) (chronic) (membranous) (suppurative) (ulcerative) K12.2

V

Vaccination (prophylactic)
- complication or reaction—*see* Complications, vaccination
- delayed Z28.9
- encounter for Z23
- not done—*see* Immunization, not done, because (of)

Vaccinia (generalized) (localized) T88.1
- congenital P35.8

Vacuum, in sinus (accessory) (nasal) J34.89

Vagabond's disease B85.1

Vaginitis (acute) (circumscribed) (diffuse) (emphysematous) (nonvenereal) (ulcerative) N76.0
- with abscess (accessory gland) (periurethral) A54.1
- bacterial N76.0
- blennorrhagic (gonococcal) A54.02
- candidal B37.3
- chlamydial A56.02
- chronic N76.1
- due to Trichomonas (vaginalis) A59.01
- gonococcal A54.02
- in (due to)
  - candidiasis B37.3
  - herpesviral (herpes simplex) infection A60.04
  - pinworm infection B80 [N77.1]
- monilial B37.3
- mycotic (candidal) B37.3
- syphilitic (early) A51.0
  - late A52.76
- trichomonal A59.01

Vaginosis—*see* Vaginitis

Valve, valvular (formation)—*see also* Disease, diseased
- cerebral ventricle (communicating) in situ Z98.2

Van der Hoeve (-de Kleyn) **syndrome** Q78.0

Vanishing lung J44.89

Vapor asphyxia or suffocation
- specified agent—*see* Table of Drugs and Chemicals

Variants, thalassemic D56.8

Varicella B01.9
- with
  - complications NEC B01.89
  - encephalitis B01.11
  - encephalomyelitis B01.11
  - meningitis B01.0
  - myelitis B01.12
  - pneumonia B01.2
- congenital P35.8

Varices—*see* Varix

Varicocele (scrotum) (thrombosed) I86.1
- spermatic cord (ulcerated) I86.1

Varicose
- ulcer
  - anus (*see also* Hemorrhoids) K64.8
  - scrotum I86.1

Varix (lower limb) I83.9-
- esophagus (idiopathic) (primary) (ulcerated) I85.00
  - bleeding I85.01
  - congenital Q27.8
- scrotum (ulcerated) I86.1

Vascular—*see also* Disease, diseased
- spider I78.1

Vasculitis I77.6
- allergic D69.0
- antineutrophilic cytoplasmic antibody [ANCA] I77.82
- systemic M31.8

Vasovagal attack (paroxysmal) R55
- psychogenic F45.8

Vegetation, vegetative
- adenoid (nasal fossa) J35.8
- endocarditis (acute) (any valve) (subacute) I33.0
- heart (mycotic) (valve) I33.0

Venereal
- disease A64

Venom, venomous—*see* Table of Drugs and Chemicals, by animal or substance, poisoning

Ventricular tachycardia
- other I47.29
- torsades de pointes I47.21
- unspecified I47.20

Ventriculitis (cerebral) (*see also* Encephalitis) G04.90

Ventriculostomy status Z98.2

Vernet's syndrome G52.7

Verruca (due to HPV) (filiformis) (simplex) (viral) (vulgaris) B07.9
- acuminata A63.0
- plana B07.8
- plantaris B07.0
- venereal A63.0

ALPHABETIC INDEX

Vertigo R42
- aural H81.31-
- benign paroxysmal (positional) H81.1-
- central (origin) H81.4
- cerebral H81.4
- laryngeal R05.4
- peripheral NEC H81.39-
  - malignant H81.4

Vesiculitis (seminal) N49.0
- trichomonal A59.09

Vestibulitis (ear) (*see also* subcategory) H83.0
- nose (external) J34.89
- vulvar N94.810

Villaret's syndrome G52.7

Virilism (adrenal) E25.9
- congenital E25.0

Virilization (female) (suprarenal) E25.9
- congenital E25.0
- isosexual E28.2

Virus, viral—*see also* Disease, diseased
- as cause of disease classified elsewhere B97.89
- cytomegalovirus B25.9
- human immunodeficiency (HIV)—*see* Human, immunodeficiency virus (HIV) disease
- infection—*see* Infection, virus
- respiratory syncytial (RSV)
  - as cause of disease classified elsewhere B97.4
  - bronchiolitis J21.0
  - bronchitis J20.5
  - bronchopneumonia J12.1
  - otitis media H65.- [B97.4]
  - pneumonia J12.1
  - upper respiratory infection J06.9 [B97.4]
- specified NEC B34.8
- swine influenza (viruses that normally cause infections in pigs) (*see also* Influenza, due to, identified novel influenza A virus) J09.X2
- West Nile (fever) A92.30
  - with
    - complications NEC A92.39
    - cranial nerve disorders A92.32
    - encephalitis A92.31
    - encephalomyelitis A92.31
    - neurologic manifestation NEC A92.32
    - optic neuritis A92.32
    - polyradiculitis A92.32
- Zika virus disease A92.5

Vision, visual
- blurred, blurring H53.8
  - hysterical F44.6
- defect, defective NEC H54.7
- disorientation (syndrome) H53.8
- disturbance H53.9
  - hysterical F44.6
- double H53.2
- examination Z01.00
  - with abnormal findings Z01.01
  - after failed exam Z01.02-
- hallucinations R44.1

Vitality, lack or want of R53.83
- newborn P96.89

Vitamin deficiency—*see* Deficiency, vitamin

Vitelline duct, persistent Q43.0

Vitiligo L80

Volvulus (bowel) (colon) (intestine) K56.2
- with perforation K56.2
- congenital Q43.8
- duodenum K31.5
  - without refractory migraine G43.A0

Vomiting R11.10
- with nausea R11.2
- bilious (cause unknown) R11.14
  - in newborn P92.01
- cyclical, in migraine G43.A0
  - with refractory migraine G43.A1
- intractable G43.A1
- not intractable G43.A0
- psychogenic F50.89
  - without refractory migraine G43.A0

Vomiting, *continued*
- cyclical syndrome NOS (unrelated to migraine) R11.1
- fecal matter R11.13
- following gastrointestinal surgery K91.0
  - psychogenic F50.89
- functional K31.89
- hysterical F50.89
- nervous F50.89
- neurotic F50.89
- newborn NEC P92.09
  - bilious P92.01
- periodic R11.10
  - psychogenic F50.89
- projectile R11.12
  - psychogenic F50.89
- without nausea R11.11

Von Hippel (-Lindau) **disease or syndrome** Q85.83

Von Recklinghausen
- disease (neurofibromatosis) Q85.01

Von Willebrand disease D68.0
- acquired D68.04
- other D68.09
- type 1C D68.01
- type 2, unspecified D68.029
- type 2A D68.020
- type 2B D68.021
- type 2M D68.022
- type 2N D68.023
- type 3 D68.03
- unspecified D68.00

Vrolik's disease Q78.0

Vulvitis (acute) (allergic) (atrophic) (hypertrophic) (intertriginous) (senile) N76.2
- adhesive, congenital Q52.79
- blennorrhagic (gonococcal) A54.02
- candidal B37.3
- chlamydial A56.02
- gonococcal A54.02
  - with abscess (accessory gland) (periurethral) A54.1
- monilial B37.3
- syphilitic (early) A51.0
  - late A52.76
- trichomonal A59.01

Vulvodynia N94.819
- specified NEC N94.818

Vulvorectal—*see* Disease, diseased

Vulvovaginitis (acute)—*see* Vaginitis

W

Waiting list
- for organ transplant Z76.82

Waldenstrom
- syndrome or macroglobulinemia C88.0-

Walking
- difficulty R26.2
  - psychogenic F44.4
- sleep F51.3
  - hysterical F44.89

Wall, abdominal—*see* Disease, diseased

Wandering
- gallbladder, congenital Q44.1
- in diseases classified elsewhere Z91.83

Wart (due to HPV) (filiform) (infectious) (viral) B07.9
- anogenital region (venereal) A63.0
- common B07.8
- external genital organs (venereal) A63.0
- flat B07.8
- plantar B07.0
- venereal A63.0

Wasting
- disease (syndrome) E88.A
  - due to
    - underlying condition E88.A

Water
- lack of T73.1
  - safe drinking Z58.6

Waterbrash R12

Weak, weakening, weakness (generalized) R53.1
- bladder (sphincter) R32
- mind F70
- muscle M62.81
- newborn P96.89
- urinary stream R39.12

Weaver's syndrome Q87.3

Web, webbed (congenital)
- fingers Q70.1-
- toes Q70.3-

Weber-Cockayne syndrome (epidermolysis bullosa) Q81.8

Weber-Osler syndrome I78.0

Weight
- 1000–2499 grams at birth (low)—*see* Low, birthweight
- 999 grams or less at birth (extremely low)—*see* Low, birthweight, extreme
- and length below 10th percentile for gestational age P05.1-
- below 10th percentile but length above 10th percentile P05.0-
- gain (abnormal) (excessive) R63.5
- loss (abnormal) (cause unknown) R63.4

Weil (l)-Marchesani syndrome Q87.19

Wen—*see* Cyst, sebaceous

Wenckebach's block or phenomenon I44.1

Werdnig-Hoffmann syndrome (muscular atrophy) G12.0

Werlhof's disease D69.3

Wernicke's
- developmental aphasia F80.2

West's syndrome—*see* Epilepsy, spasms

Wet
- lung (syndrome), newborn P22.1

Wheal—*see* Urticaria

Wheezing R06.2

Whiplash injury S13.4

Whipple's disease (*see also* subcategory M14.8-) K90.81

Whistling face Q87.0

White—*see also* Disease, diseased
- kidney, small N03.9
- mouth B37.0

Whitehead L70.0

Whitlow—*see also* Cellulitis
- with lymphangitis—*see* Lymphangitis, digit
- herpesvirai B00.89

Whooping cough A37.90
- with pneumonia A37.91

Williams syndrome Q93.82

Wilms' tumor C64.-

Wiskott-Aldrich syndrome D82.0

Withdrawal state—*see also* Dependence, drug by type, with withdrawal
- newborn
  - correct therapeutic substance properly administered P96.2
  - infant of dependent mother P96.1
  - therapeutic substance, neonatal P96.2

Witts' anemia D50.8

Wolff-Parkinson-White syndrome I45.6

Wool sorter's disease A22.1

Word
- blindness (congenital) (developmental) F81.0
- deafness (congenital) (developmental) H93.25

Worries R45.82

Wound, open T14.8

See Bite, Laceration, or Puncture by site for types of wounds not referenced here.
- abdomen, abdominal
  - wall S31.109
- ankle S91.0-
- antecubital space S51.0-
- anterior chamber, eye—*see* Wound, open, ocular
- anus S31.83-
  - bite S31.835
- arm (upper) S41.1-
  - forearm S51.8-

Wound, open, *continued*

- axilla S41.10-
- back—*see also* Wound, open, thorax, back
  - lower S31.000
- buttock S31.8-
  - left S31.82-
  - right S31.81-
- calf S81.8-
- canaliculus lacrimalis S01.10-
- canthus, eye S01.10-
- cheek (external) S01.4-
- chest wall—*see* Wound, open, thorax
- chin S01.8-
- choroid—*see* Wound, open, ocular
- ciliary body (eye)—*see* Wound, open, ocular
- clitoris S31.4-
  - bite S31.45
- conjunctiva—*see* Wound, open, ocular
- cornea—*see* Wound, open, ocular
- costal region—*see* Wound, open, thorax
- Descemet's membrane—*see* Wound, open, ocular
- digit(s)
  - foot—*see* Wound, open, toe
  - hand—*see* Wound, open, finger
- ear (canal) (external)
  - with amputation—*see* Amputation, traumatic, ear
  - drum S09.2-
- elbow S51.0-
- epididymis—*see* Wound, open, testis
- epiglottis S11.80
- eye—*see* Wound, open, ocular
- eyeball—*see* Wound, open, ocular
- eyebrow S01.10-
- eyelid S01.10-
- face NEC—*see* Wound, open, head, specified site NEC
- finger(s) S61.2-
  - with
    - amputation—*see* Amputation, traumatic, finger
    - damage to nail S61.3-
  - index S61.2-
    - with
      - damage to nail S61.3-
    - left S61.2-
      - with
        - ◊ damage to nail S61.3-
    - right S61.2-
      - with
        - ◊ damage to nail S61.3-
  - little S61.2-
    - with
      - damage to nail S61.3-
    - left S61.2-
      - with damage to nail S61.3-
    - right S61.2-
      - with damage to nail S61.3-
  - middle S61.2-
    - with
      - damage to nail S61.3-
    - left S61.2-
      - with damage to nail S61.3-
    - right S61.2-
      - with damage to nail S61.3-
  - ring S61.2-
    - with
      - damage to nail S61.3-
    - left S61.2-
      - with damage to nail S61.3-
    - right S61.2-
      - with damage to nail S61.3-
- flank—*see* Wound, open
- foot (except toe(s) alone) S91.3-
  - toe—*see* Wound, open, toe
- forearm S51.8-
  - elbow only S51.0-
- forehead S01.8-
- genital organs, external
  - female
    - vagina S31.4-
    - vulva S31.4-
  - male
    - penis S31.2-
    - scrotum S31.3-
    - testes S31.3-

Wound, open, *continued*

- globe (eye)—*see* Wound, open, ocular
- groin—*see* Wound, open
- gum—*see* Wound, open, oral cavity
- hand S61.4-
  - finger(s)—*see* Wound, open, finger
  - thumb—*see* Wound, open, thumb
- head S01.90
  - cheek S01.4-
  - ear S01.3-
  - eyelid S01.10-
  - lip S01.5-
  - nose S01.2-
  - oral cavity—*see* Wound, open, oral cavity
  - scalp—*see* Wound, open, scalp
  - specified site NEC S01.8-
  - temporomandibular area S01.4-
- heel S91.3-
- hip S71.0-
- hymen S31.4-
- instep S91.3-
- interscapular region—*see* Wound, open, thorax, back
- intraocular—*see* Wound, open, ocular
- iris—*see* Wound, open, ocular
- jaw S01.8-
- knee S81.0-
- labium (majus) (minus)—*see* Wound, open, vulva
- lacrimal duct S01.10-
- leg (lower) S81.8-
  - ankle S91.0-
  - foot S91.3-
  - knee S81.0-
  - toe—*see* Wound, open, toe
  - upper S71.1-
- lip S01.5-
- lower back—*see* Wound, open, back, lower
- lumbar region—*see* Wound, open, back, lower
- malar region—*see* Wound, open, head, specified site NEC
- mastoid region—*see* Wound, open, head, specified site NEC
- mouth—*see* Wound, open, oral cavity
- nail
  - finger—*see* Wound, open, finger, with, damage to nail
  - toe—*see* Wound, open, toe, with, damage to nail
- nape (neck)—*see* Wound, open, neck
- nasal (septum) (sinus) S01.20
- nasopharynx S01.8-
- neck S11.9-
  - involving
    - specified site NEC S11.80
- nose (septum) (sinus) S01.20
- ocular S05.9-
  - periocular area S01.10-
  - specified NEC S05.8X-
- oral cavity S01.5-
  - bite S01.552
- orbit—*see* Wound, open, ocular, orbit
- palate—*see* Wound, open, oral cavity
- palm S61.4-
- pelvis, pelvic—*see also* Wound, open, back, lower
  - girdle—*see* Wound, open, hip
- penetrating—*see* Puncture, by site
- penis S31.2-
  - bite S31.25
- periocular area (with or without lacrimal passages) S01.10-
- phalanges
  - finger—*see* Wound, open, finger
  - toe—*see* Wound, open, toe
- pinna S01.3-
- popliteal space S81.0-
- prepuce—*see* Wound, open, penis
- pubic region—*see* Wound, open, back, lower
- pudendum—*see* Wound, open, genital organs, external
- rectovaginal septum—*see* Wound, open, vagina
- sacral region—*see* Wound, open, back, lower
- sacroiliac region—*see* Wound, open, back, lower
- salivary gland—*see* Wound, open, oral cavity
- scalp S01.0-
  - bite S01.05
- scalpel, newborn (birth injury) P15.8

Wound, open, *continued*

- scapular region S41.0-
- sclera—*see* Wound, open, ocular
- scrotum S31.3-
  - bite S31.35
- shin S81.80-
- shoulder S41.0-
- skin NOS T14.8
- spermatic cord—*see* Wound, open, testis
- sternal region—*see* Wound, open, thorax, front
- submaxillary region S01.8-
- submental region S01.8-
- subungual
  - finger(s)—*see* Wound, open, finger
  - toe(s)—*see* Wound, open, toe
- supraclavicular region—*see* Wound, open, neck, specified site NEC
- temple, temporal region S01.8-
- temporomandibular area—*see* Wound, open, cheek
- testis S31.3-
  - bite S31.35
- thigh S71.10-
- thorax, thoracic (wall) S21.9-
  - back S21.2-
  - front S21.1-
- throat—*see* Wound, open, neck
- thumb S61.0
  - with
    - damage to nail S61.1-
  - left S61.0-
    - with
      - damage to nail S61.1-
  - right S61.0-
    - with
      - damage to nail S61.1-
- toe(s) S91.1-
  - with
    - damage to nail S91.2-
  - bite—*see* Bite, toe
  - great S91.1-
    - with
      - damage to nail S91.2-
    - left S91.1-
      - with
        - ◊ damage to nail S91.2-
    - right S91.1-
      - with
        - ◊ damage to nail S91.2-
  - lesser S91.1-
    - with
      - damage to nail S91.2-
    - left S91.1-
      - with
        - ◊ damage to nail S91.2-
    - right S91.1-
      - with
        - ◊ damage to nail S91.2-
- tongue—*see* Wound, open, oral cavity
- tunica vaginalis—*see* Wound, open, testis
- tympanum, tympanic membrane S09.2-
- umbilical region—*see* Wound, open, abdomen
- uvula—*see* Wound, open, oral cavity
- vagina S31.4-
  - bite S31.45
- vitreous (humor)—*see* Wound, open, ocular
- vulva S31.4-
  - bite S31.45
- wrist S61.5-

Wound, superficial—*see* Injury—*see also* specified injury type

X

Xanthelasmatosis (essential) E78.2

Xanthinuria, hereditary E79.8

Xanthoastrocytoma

- specified site—*see* Neoplasm, malignant, by in Table of Neoplasms in the complete *ICD-10-CM* manual
- unspecified site C71.9

Xanthogranuloma D76.3

Xanthoma(s), xanthomatosis (primary) (familial) (hereditary)
- with
  - hyperlipoproteinemia
    - Type III E78.2
- disseminatum (skin) E78.2
- eruptive E78.2
- hypercholesterinemic E78.00
- hypercholesterolemic E78.00
- hyperlipidemic E78.5
- multiple (skin) E78.2
- tuberosum E78.2
- tuberous E78.2
- tubo-eruptive E78.2

Xerosis
- cutis (dry skin) L85.3

XO syndrome Q96.9

X-ray (of)
- abnormal findings—Abnormal, diagnostic imaging
- breast (mammogram) (routine) Z12.31
- chest
  - routine (as part of a general medical examination) Z00.00
    - with abnormal findings Z00.01
- routine (as part of a general medical examination) Z00.00
  - with abnormal findings Z00.01

Y

Yawning R06.89
- psychogenic F45.8

Yeast infection (*see also* Candidiasis) B37.9

Z

Zahorsky's syndrome (herpangina) B08.5

Zika virus NOS A92.5
- congential P35.4

Chapter 1. Certain infectious and parasitic diseases (A00–B99)

GUIDELINES

COVID-19 Infection (Infection Due to SARS-CoV-2)

See category U07.

HIV Infections

See category B20.

Coding of Sepsis and Severe Sepsis

SEPSIS

For a diagnosis of sepsis, assign the appropriate code for the underlying systemic infection. If the type of infection or causal organism is not further specified, assign code A41.9, Sepsis, unspecified organism. A code from subcategory R65.2, Severe sepsis, should not be assigned unless severe sepsis or an associated acute organ dysfunction is documented.

Negative or inconclusive blood cultures and sepsis

Negative or inconclusive blood cultures do not preclude a diagnosis of sepsis in patients with clinical evidence of the condition, however, the provider should be queried.

Urosepsis

The term urosepsis is a nonspecific term. It is not to be considered synonymous with sepsis. It has no default code in the Alphabetic Index. Should a provider use this term, he/she must be queried for clarification.

Sepsis with organ dysfunction

If a patient has sepsis and associated acute organ dysfunction or multiple organ dysfunction (MOD), follow the instructions for coding severe sepsis.

Acute organ dysfunction that is not clearly associated with the sepsis

If a patient has sepsis and an acute organ dysfunction, but the medical record documentation indicates that the acute organ dysfunction is related to a medical condition other than the sepsis, do not assign a code from subcategory R65.2, Severe sepsis. An acute organ dysfunction must be associated with the sepsis in order to assign the severe sepsis code. If the documentation is not clear as to whether an acute organ dysfunction is related to the sepsis or another medical condition, query the provider.

SEVERE SEPSIS

The coding of severe sepsis requires a minimum of 2 codes: first a code for the underlying systemic infection, followed by a code from subcategory R65.2, Severe sepsis. If the causal organism is not documented, assign code A41.9, Sepsis, unspecified organism, for the infection. Additional code(s) for the associated acute organ dysfunction are also required.

Due to the complex nature of severe sepsis, some cases may require querying the provider prior to assignment of the codes.

Septic shock

Septic shock generally refers to circulatory failure associated with severe sepsis, and therefore, it represents a type of acute organ dysfunction. For cases of septic shock, the code for the systemic infection should be sequenced first, followed by code R65.21, Severe sepsis with septic shock or code T81.12, Postprocedural septic shock. Any additional codes for the other acute organ dysfunctions should also be assigned. As noted in the sequencing instructions in the Tabular List, the code for septic shock cannot be assigned as a principal diagnosis.

Sequencing of severe sepsis

If severe sepsis is present on admission, and meets the definition of principal diagnosis, the underlying systemic infection should be assigned as principal diagnosis followed by the appropriate code from subcategory R65.2 as required by the sequencing rules in the Tabular List. A code from subcategory R65.2 can never be assigned as a principal diagnosis. When severe sepsis develops during an encounter (it was not present on admission) the underlying systemic infection and the appropriate code from subcategory R65.2 should be assigned as secondary diagnoses. Severe sepsis may be present on admission but the diagnosis may not be confirmed until sometime after admission. If the documentation is not clear whether severe sepsis was present on admission, the provider should be queried.

Sepsis *or* severe sepsis with a localized infection

If the reason for admission is sepsis or severe sepsis and a localized infection, such as pneumonia or cellulitis, a code(s) for the underlying systemic infection should be assigned first and the code for the localized infection should be assigned as a secondary diagnosis. If the patient has severe sepsis, a code from subcategory

R65.2 should also be assigned as a secondary diagnosis. If the patient is admitted with a localized infection, such as pneumonia, and sepsis/severe sepsis doesn't develop until after admission, the localized infection should be assigned first, followed by the appropriate sepsis/severe sepsis codes.

SEPSIS DUE TO A POSTPROCEDURAL INFECTION

Documentation of causal relationship

As with all postprocedural complications, code assignment is based on the provider's documentation of the relationship between the infection and the procedure.

Sepsis due to a postprocedural infection

For sepsis following a **postprocedural wound (surgical site) infection**, a code from T81.41 to T81.43, Infection following a procedure, or a code from O86.00 to O86.03, Infection of obstetric surgical wound, that identifies the site of the infection should be **sequenced** first, if known. Assign an additional code for sepsis following a procedure (T81.44) or sepsis following an obstetrical procedure (O86.04). Use an additional code to identify the infectious agent. If the patient has severe sepsis, the appropriate code from subcategory R65.2 should also be assigned with the additional code(s) for any acute organ dysfunction.

For infections following infusion, transfusion, therapeutic injection, or immunization, a code from subcategory T80.2, Infections following infusion, transfusion, and therapeutic injection, or code T88.0-, Infection following immunization, should be coded first, followed by the code for the specific infection. If the patient has severe sepsis, the appropriate code from subcategory R65.2 should also be assigned, with the additional codes(s) for any acute organ dysfunction.

Postprocedural infection and postprocedural septic shock

If a postprocedural infection has resulted in postprocedural septic shock, assign the codes indicated above for sepsis due to a postprocedural infection, followed by code T81.12-, Postprocedural septic shock. Do not assign code R65.21, Severe sepsis with septic shock. Additional code(s) should be assigned for any acute organ dysfunction.

SEPSIS AND SEVERE SEPSIS ASSOCIATED WITH A NONINFECTIOUS PROCESS (CONDITION)

In some cases, a noninfectious process (condition), such as trauma, may lead to an infection which can result in sepsis or severe sepsis. If sepsis or severe sepsis is documented as associated with a noninfectious condition, such as a burn or serious injury, and this condition meets the definition for principal diagnosis, the code for the noninfectious condition should be sequenced first, followed by the code for the resulting infection. If severe sepsis is present, a code from subcategory R65.2 should also be assigned with any associated organ dysfunction(s) codes. It is not necessary to assign a code from subcategory R65.1, Systemic inflammatory response syndrome (SIRS) of non-infectious origin, for these cases.

If the infection meets the definition of principal diagnosis, it should be sequenced before the non-infectious condition. When both the associated non-infectious condition and the infection meet the definition of principal diagnosis, either may be assigned as principal diagnosis.

Only one code from category R65, Symptoms and signs specifically associated with systemic inflammation and infection, should be assigned. Therefore, when a non-infectious condition leads to an infection resulting in severe sepsis, assign the appropriate code from subcategory R65.2, Severe sepsis. Do not additionally assign a code from subcategory R65.1, SIRS of non-infectious origin.

Methicillin Resistant *Staphylococcus aureus* (MRSA) Conditions

See code A49.0.

Zika virus infections

See code A92.5.

(A00–A09) INTESTINAL INFECTIOUS DISEASES

Includes: diseases generally recognized as communicable or transmissible
Use additional code to identify resistance to antimicrobial drugs (Z16.-)
Excludes1: certain localized infections — see body system-related chapters
Excludes2: carrier or suspected carrier of infectious disease (Z22.-)
infectious and parasitic diseases specific to the perinatal period (P35 – P39)
influenza and other acute respiratory infections (J00 – J22)

A02 OTHER SALMONELLA INFECTIONS

Includes: infection or foodborne intoxication due to any Salmonella species other than S. typhi and S. paratyphi

A02.0 Salmonella enteritis
Salmonellosis

A02.1 Salmonella sepsis

A02.2 Localized salmonella infections

A02.20 Localized salmonella infection, unspecified

A02.21 Salmonella meningitis

A02.22 Salmonella pneumonia

A02.23 Salmonella arthritis

A02.24 Salmonella osteomyelitis

A02.25 Salmonella pyelonephritis
Salmonella tubulointerstitial nephropathy

A02.29 Salmonella with other localized infection

A02.8 Other specified salmonella infections

A02.9 Salmonella infection, unspecified

A03 SHIGELLOSIS

A03.0 Shigellosis due to Shigella dysenteriae
Group A shigellosis [Shiga-Kruse dysentery]

A03.1 Shigellosis due to Shigella flexneri
Group B shigellosis

A03.2 Shigellosis due to Shigella boydii
Group C shigellosis

A03.3 Shigellosis due to Shigella sonnei
Group D shigellosis

A03.8 Other shigellosis

A03.9 Shigellosis, unspecified
Bacillary dysentery NOS

A04 OTHER BACTERIAL INTESTINAL INFECTIONS

Excludes1: bacterial foodborne intoxications, NEC (A05.-)
tuberculous enteritis (A18.32)

A04.0 Enteropathogenic E. coli infection

A04.1 Enterotoxigenic E. coli infection

A04.2 Enteroinvasive E. coli infection

A04.3 Enterohemorrhagic E. coli infection

A04.4 Other intestinal E. coli infections
E. coli enteritis NOS

A04.5 Campylobacter enteritis

A04.6 Enteritis due to Yersinia enterocolitica
Excludes1: extraintestinal yersiniosis (A28.2)

A04.7 Enterocolitis due to Clostridium difficile
Foodborne intoxication by Clostridium difficile
Pseudomembranous colitis
Clostridioides difficile colitis

A04.71 Enterocolitis due to Clostridium difficile, recurrent

A04.72 Enterocolitis due to Clostridium difficile, not specified as recurrent

A04.8 Other specified bacterial intestinal infections
H. pylori

A04.9 Bacterial intestinal infection, unspecified
Bacterial enteritis NOS

A05 OTHER BACTERIAL FOODBORNE INTOXICATIONS, NOT ELSEWHERE CLASSIFIED

Excludes1: Clostridium difficile foodborne intoxication and infection (A04.7-)
E. coli infection (A04.0-A04.4)
listeriosis (A32.-)
salmonella foodborne intoxication and infection (A02.-)
toxic effect of noxious foodstuffs (T61-T62)

A05.0 Foodborne staphylococcal intoxication

A05.1 Botulism food poisoning
Botulism NOS
Classical foodborne intoxication due to Clostridium botulinum
Excludes1: infant botulism (A48.51)
wound botulism (A48.52)

A05.2 Foodborne Clostridium perfringens [Clostridium welchii] intoxication
Enteritis necroticans
Pigbel

A05.3 Foodborne Vibrio parahaemolyticus intoxication

A05.4 Foodborne Bacillus cereus intoxication

A05.5 Foodborne Vibrio vulnificus intoxication

A05.8 Other specified bacterial foodborne intoxications

A05.9 Bacterial foodborne intoxication, unspecified

A06 AMEBIASIS

Includes: infection due to Entamoeba histolytica
Excludes1: other protozoal intestinal diseases (A07.-)
Excludes2: acanthamebiasis (B60.1-)
Naegleriasis (B60.2)

A06.0 Acute amebic dysentery
Acute amebiasis
Intestinal amebiasis NOS

A07 OTHER PROTOZOAL INTESTINAL DISEASES

A07.1 Giardiasis [lambliasis]

A07.2 Cryptosporidiosis

A08 VIRAL AND OTHER SPECIFIED INTESTINAL INFECTIONS

Excludes1: influenza with involvement of gastrointestinal tract (J09.X3, J10.2, J11.2)

A08.0 Rotaviral enteritis

A08.3 Other viral enteritis

A08.39 Other viral enteritis
Coxsackie virus enteritis
Echovirus enteritis
Enterovirus enteritis NEC
Torovirus enteritis

A08.4 Viral intestinal infection, unspecified
Viral enteritis NOS
Viral gastroenteritis NOS
Viral gastroenteropathy NOS

A08.8 Other specified intestinal infections

A09 INFECTIOUS GASTROENTERITIS AND COLITIS, UNSPECIFIED

Infectious colitis NOS
Infectious enteritis NOS
Infectious gastroenteritis NOS
Excludes1: colitis NOS (K52.9)
diarrhea NOS (R19.7)
enteritis NOS (K52.9)
gastroenteritis NOS (K52.9)
noninfective gastroenteritis and colitis, unspecified (K52.9)

(A15-A19) TUBERCULOSIS

Includes: infections due to Mycobacterium tuberculosis and Mycobacterium bovis
Excludes1: congenital tuberculosis (P37.0)
nonspecific reaction to test for tuberculosis without active tuberculosis (R76.1-)
pneumoconiosis associated with tuberculosis, any type in A15 (J65)
positive PPD (R76.11)
positive tuberculin skin test without active tuberculosis (R76.11)
sequelae of tuberculosis (B90.-)
silicotuberculosis (J65)

A15 RESPIRATORY TUBERCULOSIS

A15.0 Tuberculosis of lung
Tuberculous bronchiectasis
Tuberculous fibrosis of lung
Tuberculous pneumonia
Tuberculous pneumothorax

A15.4 Tuberculosis of intrathoracic lymph nodes
Tuberculosis of hilar lymph nodes
Tuberculosis of mediastinal lymph nodes
Tuberculosis of tracheobronchial lymph nodes
Excludes1: tuberculosis specified as primary (A15.7)

A15.5 Tuberculosis of larynx, trachea and bronchus
Tuberculosis of bronchus
Tuberculosis of glottis
Tuberculosis of larynx
Tuberculosis of trachea

A15.6 Tuberculous pleurisy
Tuberculosis of pleura Tuberculous empyema
Excludes1: primary respiratory tuberculosis (A15.7)

A15.7 Primary respiratory tuberculosis

A15.8 Other respiratory tuberculosis
Mediastinal tuberculosis
Nasopharyngeal tuberculosis
Tuberculosis of nose
Tuberculosis of sinus [any nasal]

A15.9 Respiratory tuberculosis unspecified

A17 TUBERCULOSIS OF NERVOUS SYSTEM

A17.0 Tuberculous meningitis
Tuberculosis of meninges (cerebral)(spinal)
Tuberculous leptomeningitis
Excludes1: tuberculous meningoencephalitis (A17.82)

A17.1 Meningeal tuberculoma
Tuberculoma of meninges (cerebral) (spinal)
Excludes2: tuberculoma of brain and spinal cord (A17.81)

A17.8 Other tuberculosis of nervous system

A17.81 Tuberculoma of brain and spinal cord
Tuberculous abscess of brain and spinal cord

A17.82 Tuberculous meningoencephalitis
Tuberculous myelitis

A17.83 Tuberculous neuritis
Tuberculous mononeuropathy

A17.89 Other tuberculosis of nervous system
Tuberculous polyneuropathy

A17.9 Tuberculosis of nervous system, unspecified

A18 TUBERCULOSIS OF OTHER ORGANS

A18.0 Tuberculosis of bones and joints

A18.01 Tuberculosis of spine
Pott's disease or curvature of spine
Tuberculous arthritis
Tuberculous osteomyelitis of spine
Tuberculous spondylitis

A18.02 Tuberculous arthritis of other joints
Tuberculosis of hip (joint)
Tuberculosis of knee (joint)

A18.03 Tuberculosis of other bones
Tuberculous mastoiditis
Tuberculous osteomyelitis

A18.09 Other musculoskeletal tuberculosis
Tuberculous myositis
Tuberculous synovitis
Tuberculous tenosynovitis

A18.2 Tuberculous peripheral lymphadenopathy
Tuberculous adenitis
Excludes2: tuberculosis of bronchial and mediastinal lymph nodes (A15.4)
tuberculosis of mesenteric and retroperitoneal lymph nodes (A18.39)
tuberculous tracheobronchial adenopathy (A15.4)

A18.3 Tuberculosis of intestines, peritoneum and mesenteric glands

A18.31 Tuberculous peritonitis
Tuberculous ascites

A18.32 Tuberculous enteritis
Tuberculosis of anus and rectum
Tuberculosis of intestine (large) (small)

A18.39 Retroperitoneal tuberculosis
Tuberculosis of mesenteric glands
Tuberculosis of retroperitoneal (lymph glands)

A18.4 Tuberculosis of skin and subcutaneous tissue
Erythema induratum, tuberculous
Lupus exedens
Lupus vulgaris NOS
Lupus vulgaris of eyelid
Scrofuloderma
Tuberculosis of external ear
Excludes2: lupus erythematosus (L93.-)
lupus NOS (M32.9)
systemic lupus erythematosus (M32.-)

A18.6 Tuberculosis of (inner) (middle) ear
Tuberculous otitis media
Excludes2: tuberculosis of external ear (A18.4)
tuberculous mastoiditis (A18.03)

A18.8 Tuberculosis of other specified organs

A18.84 Tuberculosis of heart
Tuberculous cardiomyopathy
Tuberculous endocarditis
Tuberculous myocarditis
Tuberculous pericarditis

A18.85 Tuberculosis of spleen

A18.89 Tuberculosis of other sites
Tuberculosis of muscle
Tuberculous cerebral arteritis

A19 MILIARY TUBERCULOSIS

Includes: disseminated tuberculosis
generalized tuberculosis
tuberculous polyserositis

A19.0 Acute miliary tuberculosis of a single specified site

A19.1 Acute miliary tuberculosis of multiple sites

A19.2 Acute miliary tuberculosis, unspecified

A19.8 Other miliary tuberculosis

A19.9 Miliary tuberculosis, unspecified

(A20–A28) CERTAIN ZOONOTIC BACTERIAL DISEASES

A22 ANTHRAX

Includes: infection due to Bacillus anthracis

A22.0 Cutaneous anthrax
Malignant carbuncle
Malignant pustule

A22.1 Pulmonary anthrax
Inhalation anthrax
Rag picker's disease
Wool sorter's disease

A22.2 Gastrointestinal anthrax

A22.9 Anthrax, unspecified

A25 RAT-BITE FEVERS

A25.0 Spirillosis

A25.1 Streptobacillosis

A25.9 Rat-bite fever, unspecified

A26 ERYSIPELOID

A26.0 Cutaneous erysipeloid

A26.7 Erysipelothrix sepsis

A26.8 Other forms of erysipeloid

A26.9 Erysipeloid, unspecified

A27 LEPTOSPIROSIS

A27.0 Leptospirosis icterohemorrhagica

A27.8 Other forms of leptospirosis

A27.81 Aseptic meningitis in leptospirosis

A27.89 Other forms of leptospirosis

A27.9 Leptospirosis, unspecified

A28 OTHER ZOONOTIC BACTERIAL DISEASES, NEC

A28.0 Pasteurellosis

A28.1 Cat-scratch disease
Cat-scratch fever

A28.2 Extraintestinal yersiniosis
Excludes1: enteritis due to Yersinia enterocolitica (A04.6)

(A30–A49) OTHER BACTERIAL DISEASES

A31 INFECTION DUE TO OTHER MYCOBACTERIA

Excludes2: tuberculosis (A15–A19)

A31.0 Pulmonary mycobacterial infection

A31.1 Cutaneous mycobacterial infection

A31.2 Disseminated mycobacterium avium-intracellulare complex (DMAC)

A31.8 Other mycobacterial infections

A31.9 Mycobacterial infection, unspecified

A32 LISTERIOSIS

Includes: listerial foodborne infection
Excludes1: neonatal (disseminated) listeriosis (P37.2)

A32.0 Cutaneous listeriosis

A32.1 Listerial meningitis and meningoencephalitis

A32.11 Listerial meningitis

A32.12 Listerial meningoencephalitis

A32.7 Listerial sepsis

A32.8 Other forms of listeriosis

5th **A32.81 Oculoglandular listeriosis**

A32.82 Listerial endocarditis

A32.89 Other forms of listeriosis

Listerial cerebral arteritis

A32.9 Listeriosis, unspecified

A35 OTHER TETANUS

✔

A36 DIPHTHERIA

4th

A36.0 Pharyngeal diphtheria

A36.1 Nasopharyngeal diphtheria

A36.2 Laryngeal diphtheria

A36.8 Other diphtheria

5th **A36.89 Other diphtheritic complications**

A36.9 Diphtheria, unspecified

A37 WHOOPING COUGH

4th

A37.0 Whooping cough due to Bordetella pertussis;

5th **A37.00 without pneumonia**

Paroxysmal cough due to Bordetella pertussis without pneumonia

A37.01 with pneumonia

Paroxysmal cough due to Bordetella pertussis with pneumonia

A37.1 Whooping cough due to Bordetella parapertussis;

5th **A37.10 without pneumonia**

A37.11 with pneumonia

A37.8 Whooping cough due to other Bordetella species;

5th **A37.80 without pneumonia**

A37.81 with pneumonia

A37.9 Whooping cough, unspecified species;

5th **A37.90 without pneumonia**

A37.91 with pneumonia

A38 SCARLET FEVER

4th

Includes: scarlatina

Excludes2: streptococcal sore throat (J02.0)

A38.0 Scarlet fever with otitis media

A38.1 Scarlet fever with myocarditis

A38.8 Scarlet fever with other complications

A38.9 Scarlet fever, uncomplicated

Scarlet fever, NOS

A39 MENINGOCOCCAL INFECTION

4th

A39.0 Meningococcal meningitis

A39.1 Waterhouse-Friderichsen syndrome

Meningococcal hemorrhagic adrenalitis

Meningococcic adrenal syndrome

A39.2 Acute meningococcemia

A39.3 Chronic meningococcemia

A39.4 Meningococcemia, unspecified

A39.5 Meningococcal heart disease

5th **A39.50 Meningococcal carditis, unspecified**

A39.51 Meningococcal endocarditis

A39.52 Meningococcal myocarditis

A39.53 Meningococcal pericarditis

A39.8 Other meningococcal infections

5th **A39.89 Other meningococcal infections**

Meningococcal conjunctivitis

A39.9 Meningococcal infection, unspecified

Meningococcal disease NOS

A40 STREPTOCOCCAL SEPSIS

4th

GUIDELINES

See Chapter 1 guidelines.

Code first, if applicable, postprocedural sepsis (T81.44-)

sepsis due to central venous catheter (T80.211-)

streptococcal sepsis during labor (O75.3)

streptococcal sepsis following abortion or ectopic or molar pregnancy (O03.37, O03.87, O04.87, O07.37, O08.82)

streptococcal sepsis following immunization (T88.0-)

streptococcal sepsis following infusion, transfusion or therapeutic injection (T80.22-, T80.29-)

Excludes1: neonatal (P36.0-P36.1)

puerperal sepsis (O85)

sepsis due to Streptococcus, group D (A41.81)

A40.0 Sepsis due to streptococcus, group A

A40.1 Sepsis due to streptococcus, group B

A40.3 Sepsis due to Streptococcus pneumoniae

Pneumococcal sepsis

A40.8 Other streptococcal sepsis

A40.9 Streptococcal sepsis, unspecified

A41 OTHER SEPSIS

4th

GUIDELINES

See Chapter 1 guidelines.

Code first, if applicable, postprocedural sepsis (T81.44-)

sepsis due to central venous catheter (T80.211-), during labor (O75.3), following abortion, ectopic or molar pregnancy (O03.37, O03.87, O04.87, O07.37, O08.82), following immunization (T88.0-), following infusion, transfusion or therapeutic injection (T80.22-, T80.29-)

Excludes1: bacteremia NOS (R78.81)

neonatal (P36.-)

puerperal sepsis (O85)

streptococcal sepsis (A40.-)

Excludes2: sepsis (due to) (in) actinomycotic (A42.7), anthrax (A22.7), candidal (B37.7), Erysipelothrix (A26.7), extraintestinal yersiniosis (A28.2), gonococcal (A54.86), herpesviral (B00.7), listerial (A32.7), melioidosis (A24.1), meningococcal (A39.2-A39.4), plague (A20.7), tularemia (A21.7), toxic shock syndrome (A48.3)

A41.0 Sepsis due to Staphylococcus aureus

5th **A41.01 Sepsis due to**

MSSA

MSSA sepsis

Staphylococcus aureus sepsis NOS

A41.02 Sepsis due to MRSA

A41.1 Sepsis due to other specified staphylococcus

Coagulase negative staphylococcus sepsis

A41.2 Sepsis due to unspecified staphylococcus

A41.3 Sepsis due to H. influenzae

A41.4 Sepsis due to anaerobes

Excludes1: gas gangrene (A48.0)

A41.5 Sepsis due to other Gram-negative organisms

5th **A41.50 Gram-negative sepsis, unspecified**

Gram-negative sepsis NOS

A41.51 Sepsis due to E. coli

A41.52 Sepsis due to Pseudomonas

Pseudomonas aeruginosa

A41.53 Sepsis due to Serratia

A41.59 Other Gram-negative sepsis

A41.8 Other specified sepsis

5th **A41.81 Sepsis due to Enterococcus**

A41.89 Other specified sepsis

If the type of infection or causal organism is not further specified for sepsis, assign code A41.9

A41.9 Sepsis, unspecified organism

Septicemia NOS

A42 ACTINOMYCOSIS

4th

Excludes1: actinomycetoma (B47.1)

A42.0 Pulmonary actinomycosis

A42.1 Abdominal actinomycosis

A42.2 Cervicofacial actinomycosis

A42.7 Actinomycotic sepsis

A42.8 Other forms of actinomycosis

5th **A42.81 Actinomycotic meningitis**

A42.82 Actinomycotic encephalitis

A42.89 Other forms of actinomycosis

A42.9 Actinomycosis, unspecified

A43 NOCARDIOSIS

4th

A43.0 Pulmonary nocardiosis

A43.1 Cutaneous nocardiosis

A43.8 Other forms of nocardiosis

A43.9 Nocardiosis, unspecified

A44 BARTONELLOSIS

4th

A44.0 Systemic bartonellosis

A44.1 Cutaneous and mucocutaneous bartonellosis
A44.8 Other forms of bartonellosis
A44.9 Bartonellosis, unspecified

A46 ERYSIPELAS

✓ *Excludes1:* postpartum or puerperal erysipelas (O86.89)

A48 OTHER BACTERIAL DISEASES, NOT ELSEWHERE CLASSIFIED

4th

Excludes1: actinomycetoma (B47.1)

A48.1 Legionnaires' disease
A48.2 Nonpneumonic Legionnaires' disease [Pontiac fever]
A48.3 Toxic shock syndrome
Use additional code to identify the organism (B95, B96)
Excludes1: endotoxic shock NOS (R57.8)
sepsis NOS (A41.9)
A48.5 Other specified botulism
5th Non-foodborne intoxication due to toxins of Clostridium botulinum [C. botulinum]
Excludes1: food poisoning due to toxins of Clostridium botulinum (A05.1)
A48.51 Infant botulism
A48.52 Wound botulism
Non-foodborne botulism NOS
Use additional code for associated wound
A48.8 Other specified bacterial diseases

A49 BACTERIAL INFECTION OF UNSPECIFIED SITE

4th *Excludes1:* bacterial agents as the cause of diseases classified elsewhere (B95–B96)
chlamydial infection NOS (A74.9)
meningococcal infection NOS (A39.9)
rickettsial infection NOS (A79.9)
spirochetal infection NOS (A69.9)

A49.0 Staphylococcal infection, unspecified site

5th **GUIDELINES**

Methicillin susceptible Staphylococcus aureus (MSSA) and MRSA colonization

The condition or state of being colonized or carrying MSSA or MRSA is called colonization or carriage, while an individual person is described as being colonized or being a carrier. Colonization means that MSSA or MSRA is present on or in the body without necessarily causing illness. A positive MRSA colonization test might be documented by the provider as "MRSA screen positive" or "MRSA nasal swab positive". Assign code Z22.322, Carrier or suspected carrier of MRSA, for patients documented as having MRSA colonization. Assign code Z22.321, Carrier or suspected carrier of MSSA, for patient documented as having MSSA colonization. Colonization is not necessarily indicative of a disease process or as the cause of a specific condition the patient may have unless documented as such by the provider.

MRSA colonization and infection

If a patient is documented as having both MRSA colonization and infection during a hospital admission, code Z22.322, and a code for the MRSA infection may both be assigned.

A49.01 MSSA infection, unspecified site
MSSA infection
Staphylococcus aureus infection NOS
A49.02 MRSA infection, unspecified site
MRSA infection
A49.1 Streptococcal infection, unspecified site
A49.2 H. influenzae infection, unspecified site
A49.3 Mycoplasma infection, unspecified site
A49.8 Other bacterial infections of unspecified site
A49.9 Bacterial infection, unspecified
Excludes1: bacteremia NOS (R78.81)

(A50–A64) INFECTIONS WITH A PREDOMINANTLY SEXUAL MODE OF TRANSMISSION

Excludes1: HIV disease (B20)
nonspecific and nongonococcal urethritis (N34.1)
Reiter's disease (M02.3-)

A50 CONGENITAL SYPHILIS

4th

A50.0 Early congenital syphilis, symptomatic
5th Any congenital syphilitic condition specified as early or manifest less than two years after birth.
A50.01 Early congenital syphilitic; oculopathy
A50.02 osteochondropathy
A50.03 pharyngitis
Early congenital syphilitic laryngitis
A50.04 pneumonia
A50.05 rhinitis
A50.06 Early cutaneous congenital syphilis
A50.07 Early mucocutaneous congenital syphilis
A50.08 Early visceral congenital syphilis
A50.09 Other early congenital syphilis, symptomatic

A50.1 Early congenital syphilis, latent
Congenital syphilis without clinical manifestations, with positive serological reaction and negative spinal fluid test, less than two years after birth.

A50.2 Early congenital syphilis, unspecified
Congenital syphilis NOS less than two years after birth.

A50.3 Late congenital syphilitic oculopathy
5th *Excludes1:* Hutchinson's triad (A50.53)
A50.30 Late congenital syphilitic oculopathy, unspecified
A50.31 Late congenital syphilitic interstitial keratitis
A50.32 Late congenital syphilitic chorioretinitis
A50.39 Other late congenital syphilitic oculopathy

A50.4 Late congenital neurosyphilis [juvenile neurosyphilis]
5th Use additional code to identify any associated mental disorder
Excludes1: Hutchinson's triad (A50.53)
A50.40 Late congenital neurosyphilis, unspecified
Juvenile neurosyphilis NOS
A50.41 Late congenital syphilitic meningitis
A50.42 Late congenital syphilitic encephalitis
A50.43 Late congenital syphilitic polyneuropathy
A50.44 Late congenital syphilitic optic nerve atrophy
A50.45 Juvenile general paresis
Dementia paralytica juvenilis
Juvenile taboparetic neurosyphilis
A50.49 Other late congenital neurosyphilis
Juvenile tabes dorsalis

A50.5 Other late congenital syphilis, symptomatic
5th Any congenital syphilitic condition specified as late or manifest two years or more after birth.
A50.51 Clutton's joints
A50.52 Hutchinson's teeth
A50.53 Hutchinson's triad
A50.54 Late congenital cardiovascular syphilis
A50.55 Late congenital syphilitic arthropathy
A50.56 Late congenital syphilitic osteochondropathy
A50.57 Syphilitic saddle nose
A50.59 Other late congenital syphilis, symptomatic

A50.6 Late congenital syphilis, latent
Congenital syphilis without clinical manifestations, with positive serological reaction and negative spinal fluid test, two years or more after birth.

A50.7 Late congenital syphilis, unspecified
Congenital syphilis NOS two years or more after birth.

A50.9 Congenital syphilis, unspecified

A51 EARLY SYPHILIS

4th

A51.0 Primary genital syphilis
Syphilitic chancre NOS
A51.1 Primary anal syphilis
A51.2 Primary syphilis of other sites
A51.3 Secondary syphilis of skin and mucous membranes
5th **A51.31** Condyloma latum
A51.32 Syphilitic alopecia
A51.39 Other secondary syphilis of skin
A51.5 Early syphilis, latent
Syphilis (acquired) without clinical manifestations, with positive serological reaction and negative spinal fluid test, less than two years after infection.
A51.9 Early syphilis, unspecified

A52 LATE SYPHILIS

- **A52.0 Cardiovascular and cerebrovascular syphilis**
  - A52.00 Cardiovascular syphilis, unspecified
  - A52.03 Syphilitic endocarditis
    - Syphilitic aortic valve incompetence or stenosis
    - Syphilitic mitral valve stenosis
    - Syphilitic pulmonary valve regurgitation
  - A52.06 Other syphilitic heart involvement
    - Syphilitic coronary artery disease
    - Syphilitic myocarditis
    - Syphilitic pericarditis
  - A52.09 Other cardiovascular syphilis
- **A52.7 Other symptomatic late syphilis**
  - A52.76 Other genitourinary symptomatic late syphilis
  - A52.79 Other symptomatic late syphilis
- **A52.8 Late syphilis, latent**
  - Syphilis (acquired) without clinical manifestations, with positive serological reaction and negative spinal fluid test, two years or more after infection
- **A52.9 Late syphilis, unspecified**

A53 OTHER AND UNSPECIFIED SYPHILIS

- **A53.0 Latent syphilis, unspecified as early or late**
  - Latent syphilis NOS
  - Positive serological reaction for syphilis
- **A53.9 Syphilis, unspecified**
  - Infection due to Treponema pallidum NOS
  - Syphilis (acquired) NOS
  - *Excludes1:* syphilis NOS under two years of age (A50.2)

A54 GONOCOCCAL INFECTION

- **A54.0 Gonococcal infection of lower genitourinary tract without periurethral or accessory gland abscess**
  - *Excludes1:* gonococcal infection with genitourinary gland abscess (A54.1)
  - gonococcal infection with periurethral abscess (A54.1)
  - A54.00 Gonococcal infection of lower genitourinary tract, unspecified
  - A54.01 Gonococcal cystitis and urethritis, unspecified
  - A54.02 Gonococcal vulvovaginitis, unspecified
  - A54.03 Gonococcal cervicitis, unspecified
  - A54.09 Other gonococcal infection of lower genitourinary tract
- **A54.1 Gonococcal infection of lower genitourinary tract with periurethral and accessory gland abscess**
  - Gonococcal Bartholin's gland abscess
- **A54.2 Gonococcal pelviperitonitis and other gonococcal genitourinary infection**
  - A54.21 Gonococcal infection of kidney and ureter
  - A54.22 Gonococcal prostatitis
  - A54.23 Gonococcal infection of other male genital organs
    - Gonococcal epididymitis
    - Gonococcal orchitis
  - A54.24 Gonococcal female pelvic inflammatory disease
    - Gonococcal pelviperitonitis
    - *Excludes1:* gonococcal peritonitis (A54.85)
  - A54.29 Other gonococcal genitourinary infections
- **A54.3 Gonococcal infection of eye**
  - A54.30 Gonococcal infection of eye, unspecified
  - A54.31 Gonococcal conjunctivitis
    - Ophthalmia neonatorum due to gonococcus
  - A54.32 Gonococcal iridocyclitis
  - A54.33 Gonococcal keratitis
  - A54.39 Other gonococcal eye infection
    - Gonococcal endophthalmia
- **A54.4 Gonococcal infection of musculoskeletal system**
  - A54.40 Gonococcal infection of musculoskeletal system, unspecified
  - A54.41 Gonococcal spondylopathy
    - *Excludes2:* gonococcal infection of spine (A54.41)
  - A54.49 Gonococcal infection of other musculoskeletal tissue
    - Gonococcal bursitis
    - Gonococcal myositis
    - Gonococcal synovitis
    - Gonococcal tenosynovitis
- **A54.5 Gonococcal pharyngitis**
- **A54.6 Gonococcal infection of anus and rectum**
- **A54.8 Other gonococcal infections**
  - A54.84 Gonococcal pneumonia
  - A54.85 Gonococcal peritonitis
    - *Excludes1:* gonococcal pelviperitonitis (A54.24)
  - A54.86 Gonococcal sepsis
  - A54.89 Other gonococcal infections
    - Gonococcal keratoderma
    - Gonococcal lymphadenitis
- **A54.9 Gonococcal infection, unspecified**

A56 OTHER SEXUALLY TRANSMITTED CHLAMYDIAL DISEASES

Includes: sexually transmitted diseases due to Chlamydia trachomatis

Excludes1: neonatal chlamydial conjunctivitis (P39.1) neonatal chlamydial pneumonia (P23.1)

Excludes2: chlamydial lymphogranuloma (A55) conditions classified to A74.-

- **A56.0 Chlamydial infection of lower genitourinary tract**
  - A56.00 Chlamydial infection of lower genitourinary tract, unspecified
  - A56.01 Chlamydial cystitis and urethritis
  - A56.02 Chlamydial vulvovaginitis
  - A56.09 Other chlamydial infection of lower genitourinary tract
    - Chlamydial cervicitis
- **A56.1 Chlamydial infection of pelviperitoneum and other genitourinary organs**
  - A56.11 Chlamydial female pelvic inflammatory disease
  - A56.19 Other chlamydial genitourinary infection
    - Chlamydial epididymitis
    - Chlamydial orchitis
- **A56.2 Chlamydial infection of genitourinary tract, unspecified**
- **A56.3 Chlamydial infection of anus and rectum**
- **A56.4 Chlamydial infection of pharynx**
- **A56.8 Sexually transmitted chlamydial infection of other sites**

A59 TRICHOMONIASIS

Excludes2: intestinal trichomoniasis (A07.8)

- **A59.0 Urogenital trichomoniasis**
  - A59.00 Urogenital trichomoniasis, unspecified
    - Fluor (vaginalis) due to Trichomonas
    - Leukorrhea (vaginalis) due to Trichomonas
  - A59.01 Trichomonal vulvovaginitis
  - A59.02 Trichomonal prostatitis
  - A59.03 Trichomonal cystitis and urethritis
  - A59.09 Other urogenital trichomoniasis
    - Trichomonas cervicitis
- **A59.8 Trichomoniasis of other sites**
- **A59.9 Trichomoniasis, unspecified**

A60 ANOGENITAL HERPESVIRAL [HERPES SIMPLEX] INFECTIONS

- **A60.0 Herpesviral infection of genitalia and urogenital tract**
  - A60.00 Herpesviral infection of urogenital system, unspecified
  - A60.01 Herpesviral infection of penis
  - A60.02 Herpesviral infection of other male genital organs
  - A60.03 Herpesviral cervicitis
  - A60.04 Herpesviral vulvovaginitis
    - Herpesviral [herpes simplex] ulceration
    - Herpesviral [herpes simplex] vaginitis
    - Herpesviral [herpes simplex] vulvitis
  - A60.09 Herpesviral infection of other urogenital tract
- **A60.1 Herpesviral infection of perianal skin and rectum**
- **A60.9 Anogenital herpesviral infection, unspecified**

A63 OTHER PREDOMINANTLY SEXUALLY TRANSMITTED DISEASES, NEC

Excludes2: molluscum contagiosum (B08.1) papilloma of cervix (D26.0)

- **A63.0 Anogenital (venereal) warts**
  - Anogenital warts due to (human) papillomavirus [HPV]
  - Condyloma acuminatum

A63.8 Other specified predominantly sexually transmitted diseases

A64 UNSPECIFIED SEXUALLY TRANSMITTED DISEASE

✓ Other spirochetal diseases (A65–A69)
Excludes2: leptospirosis (A27.-)
syphilis (A50–A53)

(A65–A69) OTHER SPIROCHETAL DISEASES

A68 RELAPSING FEVERS

4th *Includes:* recurrent fever
Excludes2: Lyme disease (A69.2-)

A68.0 Louse-borne relapsing fever
Relapsing fever due to Borrelia recurrentis

A68.1 Tick-borne relapsing fever
Relapsing fever due to any Borrelia species other than Borrelia recurrentis

A68.9 Relapsing fever, unspecified

A69 OTHER SPIROCHETAL INFECTIONS

4th **A69.2 Lyme disease**

5th Erythema chronicum migrans due to Borrelia burgdorferi

A69.20 Lyme disease, unspecified

A69.21 Meningitis due to Lyme disease

A69.22 Other neurologic disorders in Lyme disease
Cranial neuritis
Meningoencephalitis
Polyneuropathy

A69.23 Arthritis due to Lyme disease

A69.29 Other conditions associated with Lyme disease
Myopericarditis due to Lyme disease

A69.8 Other specified spirochetal infections

A69.9 Spirochetal infection, unspecified
Other diseases caused by chlamydiae (A70–A74)
Excludes1: sexually transmitted chlamydial diseases (A55–A56)

(A70–A74) OTHER DISEASES CAUSED BY CHLAMYDIAE

A71 TRACHOMA

4th **A71.0 Initial stage of trachoma**
Trachoma dubium

A71.1 Active stage of trachoma
Granular conjunctivitis (trachomatous)
Trachomatous follicular conjunctivitis
Trachomatous pannus

A71.9 Trachoma, unspecified

A74 OTHER DISEASES CAUSED BY CHLAMYDIAE

4th *Excludes1:* neonatal chlamydial conjunctivitis (P39.1)
neonatal chlamydial pneumonia (P23.1)
Reiter's disease (M02.3-)
sexually transmitted chlamydial diseases (A55–A56)
Excludes2: chlamydial pneumonia (J16.0)

A74.0 Chlamydial conjunctivitis
Paratrachoma

A74.8 Other chlamydial diseases

5th **A74.81 Chlamydial peritonitis**

A74.89 Other chlamydial diseases

A74.9 Chlamydial infection, unspecified
Chlamydiosis NOS

(A75–A79) RICKETTSIOSES

A77 SPOTTED FEVER [TICK-BORNE RICKETTSIOSES]

4th **A77.0 Spotted fever due to Rickettsia rickettsii**
Rocky Mountain spotted fever
Sao Paulo fever

A77.4 Ehrlichiosis

5th *Excludes1:* anaplasmosis [A. phagocytophilum] (A79.82)
rickettsiosis due to Ehrlichia sennetsu (A79.81)

A77.40 Ehrlichiosis, unspecified

▲A77.41 Ehrlichiosis chaffeensis [E. chaffeensis]

A77.49 Other ehrlichiosis
Ehrlichiosis due to E. ewingii
Ehrlichiosis due to E. muris euclairensis

A77.8 Other spotted fevers
Rickettsia 364D/R. philipii (Pacific Coast tick fever)
Spotted fever due to Rickettsia africae (African tick bite fever)
Spotted fever due to Rickettsia parkeri

A77.9 Spotted fever, unspecified
Tick-borne typhus NOS

A79 OTHER RICKETTSIOSES

4th **A79.1 Rickettsialpox due to Rickettsia akari**
Kew Garden fever
Vesicular rickettsiosis

A79.8 Other specified rickettsioses

5th **A79.82 Anaplasmosis [A. phagocytophilum]**
Transfusion transmitted A. phagocytophilum

A79.89 Other specified rickettsioses

A79.9 Rickettsiosis, unspecified
Rickettsial infection NOS

(A80–A89) VIRAL AND PRION INFECTIONS OF THE CENTRAL NERVOUS SYSTEM

Excludes1: postpolio syndrome (G14)
sequelae of poliomyelitis (B91)
sequelae of viral encephalitis (B94.1)

A80 ACUTE POLIOMYELITIS

4th *Excludes1:* acute flaccid myelitis (G04.82)

A80.1 Acute paralytic poliomyelitis, wild virus, imported

A80.2 Acute paralytic poliomyelitis, wild virus, indigenous

A80.3 Acute paralytic poliomyelitis, other and unspecified

5th **A80.30 Acute paralytic poliomyelitis, unspecified**

A80.39 Other acute paralytic poliomyelitis

A80.9 Acute poliomyelitis, unspecified

A82 RABIES

4th **A82.0 Sylvatic rabies**

A82.1 Urban rabies

A82.9 Rabies, unspecified

A83 MOSQUITO-BORNE VIRAL ENCEPHALITIS

4th *Includes:* mosquito-borne viral meningoencephalitis
Excludes2: Venezuelan equine encephalitis (A92.2)
West Nile fever (A92.3-)
West Nile virus (A92.3-)

A83.2 Eastern equine encephalitis

A83.3 St Louis encephalitis

A83.5 California encephalitis
California meningoencephalitis
La Crosse encephalitis

A83.8 Other mosquito-borne viral encephalitis

A83.9 Mosquito-borne viral encephalitis, unspecified

A84 TICK-BORNE VIRAL ENCEPHALITIS

4th *Includes:* tick-borne viral meningoencephalitis

A84.8 Other tick-borne viral encephalitis

5th **A84.81 Powassan virus disease**

A84.89 Other tick-borne viral encephalitis
Louping ill
Code first, if applicable, transfusion related infection (T80.22-)

A84.9 Tick-borne viral encephalitis, unspecified

A85 OTHER VIRAL ENCEPHALITIS, NEC

4th *Includes:* specified viral encephalomyelitis NEC
specified viral meningoencephalitis NEC
Excludes1: benign myalgic encephalomyelitis (G93.3)
encephalitis due to cytomegalovirus (B25.8)
encephalitis due to herpesvirus NEC (B10.0-)
encephalitis due to herpesvirus [herpes simplex] (B00.4)
encephalitis due to measles virus (B05.0)
encephalitis due to mumps virus (B26.2)
encephalitis due to poliomyelitis virus (A80.-)
encephalitis due to zoster (B02.0)
lymphocytic choriomeningitis (A87.2)

A85.0 Enteroviral encephalitis
Enteroviral encephalomyelitis

- **A85.1 Adenoviral encephalitis**
  - Adenoviral meningoencephalitis
- **A85.2 Arthropod-borne viral encephalitis, unspecified**
  - *Excludes1:* West nile virus with encephalitis (A92.31)
- **A85.8 Other specified viral encephalitis**
  - Encephalitis lethargica
  - Von Economo-Cruchet disease

A86 UNSPECIFIED VIRAL ENCEPHALITIS
✓
- Viral encephalomyelitis NOS
- Viral meningoencephalitis NOS

A87 VIRAL MENINGITIS
4th
- *Excludes1:* meningitis due to herpesvirus [herpes simplex] (B00.3)
  - meningitis due to herpesvirus [herpes simplex] (B00.3)
  - meningitis due to measles virus (B05.1)
  - meningitis due to mumps virus (B26.1)
  - meningitis due to poliomyelitis virus (A80.-)
  - meningitis due to zoster (B02.1)
- **A87.0 Enteroviral meningitis**
  - Coxsackievirus meningitis
  - Echovirus meningitis
- **A87.1 Adenoviral meningitis**
- **A87.8 Other viral meningitis**
- **A87.9 Viral meningitis, unspecified**

A88 OTHER VIRAL INFECTIONS OF CENTRAL NERVOUS SYSTEM, NEC
4th
- *Excludes1:* viral encephalitis NOS (A86)
  - viral meningitis NOS (A87.9)
- **A88.0 Enteroviral exanthematous fever [Boston exanthem]**
- **A88.1 Epidemic vertigo**
- **A88.8 Other specified viral infections of central nervous system**

A89 UNSPECIFIED VIRAL INFECTION OF CENTRAL NERVOUS SYSTEM
✓

(A90–A99) ARTHROPOD-BORNE VIRAL FEVERS AND VIRAL HEMORRHAGIC FEVERS

A92 OTHER MOSQUITO-BORNE VIRAL FEVERS
4th
- *Excludes1:* Ross River disease (B33.1)
- **A92.3 West Nile virus infection**
  - 5th West Nile fever
  - **A92.30 West Nile virus infection, unspecified**
    - West Nile fever NOS
    - West Nile fever without complications
    - West Nile virus NOS
  - **A92.31 West Nile virus infection with encephalitis**
    - West Nile encephalitis
    - West Nile encephalomyelitis
  - **A92.32 West Nile virus infection with other neurologic manifestation**
    - **Use additional code** to specify the neurologic manifestation
  - **A92.39 West Nile virus infection with other complications**
    - **Use additional code** to specify the other conditions
- **A92.5 Zika virus disease**

  GUIDELINE

  Code only confirmed cases
  Code only a confirmed diagnosis of Zika virus (A92.5, Zika virus disease) as documented by the provider. This is an exception to the hospital inpatient guideline Section II, H. In this context, "confirmation" does not require documentation of the type of test performed; the provider's diagnostic statement that the condition is confirmed is sufficient. This code should be assigned regardless of the stated mode of transmission.

  If the provider documents "suspected", "possible" or "probable" Zika, do not assign code A92.5. Assign a code(s) explaining the reason for encounter (such as fever, rash, or joint pain) or Z20.821, Contact with and (suspected) exposure to Zika virus.

  - Zika virus fever
  - Zika virus infection
  - Zika, NOS
  - *Excludes1:* congenital Zika virus disease (P35.4)
- **A92.8 Other specified mosquito-borne viral fevers**
- **A92.9 Mosquito-borne viral fever, unspecified**

A93 OTHER ARTHROPOD-BORNE VIRAL FEVERS, NOT ELSEWHERE CLASSIFIED
4th
- **A93.0 Oropouche virus disease**
  - Oropouche fever
- **A93.1 Sandfly fever**
  - Pappataci fever
  - Phlebotomus fever
- **A93.2 Colorado tick fever**
- **A93.8 Other specified arthropod-borne viral fevers**
  - Piry virus disease
  - Vesicular stomatitis virus disease [Indiana fever]

A94 UNSPECIFIED ARTHROPOD-BORNE VIRAL FEVER
✓
- Arboviral fever NOS
- Arbovirus infection NOS

A95 YELLOW FEVER
4th
- **A95.0 Sylvatic yellow fever**
  - Jungle yellow fever
- **A95.1 Urban yellow fever**
- **A95.9 Yellow fever, unspecified**

A96 ARENAVIRAL HEMORRHAGIC FEVER
4th
- **A96.0 Junin hemorrhagic fever**
  - Argentinian hemorrhagic fever
- **A96.1 Machupo hemorrhagic fever**
  - Bolivian hemorrhagic fever
- **A96.2 Lassa fever**
- **A96.8 Other arenaviral hemorrhagic fevers**
- **A96.9 Arenaviral hemorrhagic fever, unspecified**

A98 OTHER VIRAL HEMORRHAGIC FEVERS, NOT ELSEWHERE CLASSIFIED
4th
- *Excludes1:* chikungunya hemorrhagic fever (A92.0)
  - dengue hemorrhagic fever (A91)
- **A98.4 Ebola virus disease**
- **A98.5 Hemorrhagic fever with renal syndrome**
  - Epidemic hemorrhagic fever
  - Korean hemorrhagic fever
  - Russian hemorrhagic fever
  - Hantaan virus disease
  - Hantavirus disease with renal manifestations
  - Nephropathia epidemica
  - Songo fever
  - *Excludes1:* hantavirus (cardio)-pulmonary syndrome (B33.4)
- **A98.8 Other specified viral hemorrhagic fevers**

A99 UNSPECIFIED VIRAL HEMORRHAGIC FEVER
✓

(B00–B09) VIRAL INFECTIONS CHARACTERIZED BY SKIN AND MUCOUS MEMBRANE LESIONS

B00 HERPESVIRAL [HERPES SIMPLEX] INFECTIONS
4th
- *Excludes1:* congenital herpesviral infections (P35.2)
- *Excludes2:* anogenital herpesviral infection (A60.-)
  - gammaherpesviral mononucleosis (B27.0-)
  - herpangina (B08.5)
- **B00.0 Eczema herpeticum**
  - Kaposi's varicelliform eruption
- **B00.1 Herpesviral vesicular dermatitis**
  - Herpes simplex facialis
  - Herpes simplex labialis
  - Herpes simplex otitis externa
  - Vesicular dermatitis of ear
  - Vesicular dermatitis of lip
- **B00.2 Herpesviral gingivostomatitis and pharyngotonsillitis**
  - Herpesviral pharyngitis
- **B00.3 Herpesviral meningitis**

B00.4 Herpesviral encephalitis
Herpesviral meningoencephalitis
Simian B disease
Excludes1: herpesviral encephalitis due to herpesvirus 6 and 7 (B10.01, B10.09)
non-simplex herpesviral encephalitis (B10.0-)

B00.5 Herpesviral ocular disease

5th **B00.50 Herpesviral ocular disease, unspecified**

B00.51 Herpesviral iridocyclitis
Herpesviral iritis
Herpesviral uveitis, anterior

B00.52 Herpesviral keratitis
Herpesviral keratoconjunctivitis

B00.53 Herpesviral conjunctivitis

B00.59 Other herpesviral disease of eye
Herpesviral dermatitis of eyelid

B00.7 Disseminated herpesviral disease
Herpesviral sepsis

B00.8 Other forms of herpesviral infections

5th **B00.81 Herpesviral hepatitis**

B00.82 Herpes simplex myelitis

B00.89 Other herpesviral infection
Herpesviral whitlow

B00.9 Herpesviral infection, unspecified
Herpes simplex infection NOS

B01 VARICELLA [CHICKENPOX]

4th

B01.0 Varicella meningitis

B01.1 Varicella encephalitis, myelitis and encephalomyelitis
Postchickenpox encephalitis, myelitis and encephalomyelitis

5th **B01.11 Varicella encephalitis and encephalomyelitis**
Postchickenpox encephalitis and encephalomyelitis

B01.12 Varicella myelitis
Postchickenpox myelitis

B01.2 Varicella pneumonia

B01.8 Varicella with other complications

5th **B01.81 Varicella keratitis**

B01.89 Other varicella complications

B01.9 Varicella without complication
Varicella NOS

B04 MONKEYPOX

Mpox

B05 MEASLES

4th

Includes: morbilli
Excludes1: subacute sclerosing panencephalitis (A81.1)

B05.0 Measles complicated by encephalitis
Postmeasles encephalitis

B05.1 Measles complicated by meningitis
Postmeasles meningitis

B05.2 Measles complicated by pneumonia
Postmeasles pneumonia

B05.3 Measles complicated by otitis media
Postmeasles otitis media

B05.4 Measles with intestinal complications

B05.8 Measles with other complications

5th **B05.81 Measles keratitis and keratoconjunctivitis**

B05.89 Other measles complications

B05.9 Measles without complication
Measles NOS

B06 RUBELLA [GERMAN MEASLES]

4th

Excludes1: congenital rubella (P35.0)

B06.0 Rubella with neurological complications

5th **B06.00 Rubella with neurological complication, unspecified**

B06.09 Other neurological complications of rubella

B06.8 Rubella with other complications

5th **B06.81 Rubella pneumonia**

B06.89 Other rubella complications

B06.9 Rubella without complication
Rubella NOS

B07 VIRAL WARTS

4th

Includes: verruca simplex
verruca vulgaris
viral warts due to human papillomavirus
Excludes2: anogenital (venereal) warts (A63.0)
papilloma of bladder (D41.4)
papilloma of cervix (D26.0)
papilloma larynx (D14.1)

B07.0 Plantar wart
Verruca plantaris

B07.8 Other viral warts
Common wart
Flat wart
Verruca plana

B07.9 Viral wart, unspecified

B08 OTHER VIRAL INFECTIONS CHARACTERIZED BY SKIN AND MUCOUS MEMBRANE LESIONS, NEC

4th

Excludes1: vesicular stomatitis virus disease (A93.8)

B08.1 Molluscum contagiosum

B08.2 Exanthema subitum [sixth disease]
Roseola infantum

5th **B08.20 Exanthema subitum [sixth disease], unspecified**
Roseola infantum, unspecified

B08.21 Exanthema subitum [sixth disease] due to human herpesvirus 6
Roseola infantum due to human herpesvirus 6

B08.22 Exanthema subitum [sixth disease] due to human herpesvirus 7
Roseola infantum due to human herpesvirus 7

B08.3 Erythema infectiosum [fifth disease]

B08.4 Enteroviral vesicular stomatitis with exanthem
Hand, foot and mouth disease

B08.5 Enteroviral vesicular pharyngitis
Herpangina

B08.8 Other specified viral infections characterized by skin and mucous membrane lesions
Enteroviral lymphonodular pharyngitis
Foot-and-mouth disease
Poxvirus NEC

B09 UNSPECIFIED VIRAL INFECTION CHARACTERIZED BY SKIN AND MUCOUS MEMBRANE LESIONS

✓

Viral enanthema NOS
Viral exanthema NOS

(B10) OTHER HUMAN HERPESVIRUSES

B10 OTHER HUMAN HERPESVIRUSES

4th

Excludes2: cytomegalovirus (B25.9)
Epstein-Barr virus (B27.0-)
herpes NOS (B00.9)
herpes simplex (B00.-)
herpes zoster (B02.-)
human herpesvirus NOS (B00.-)
human herpesvirus 1 and 2 (B00.-)
human herpesvirus 3 (B01.-, B02.-)
human herpesvirus 4 (B27.0-)
human herpesvirus 5 (B25.-)
varicella (B01.-)
zoster (B02.-)

B10.0 Other human herpesvirus encephalitis

5th *Excludes2:* herpes encephalitis NOS (B00.4)
herpes simplex encephalitis (B00.4)
human herpesvirus encephalitis (B00.4)
simian B herpes virus encephalitis (B00.4)

B10.01 Human herpesvirus 6 encephalitis

B10.09 Other human herpesvirus encephalitis
Human herpesvirus 7 encephalitis

B10.8 Other human herpesvirus infection

5th **B10.81 Human herpesvirus 6 infection**

B10.82 Human herpesvirus 7 infection

B10.89 Other human herpesvirus infection
Human herpesvirus 8 infection
Kaposi's sarcoma-associated herpesvirus infection

●=New Code
▲=Revised Code

Excludes1—Not coded here, do not use together
Excludes2—Not included here

(B15–B19) VIRAL HEPATITIS

Excludes1: sequelae of viral hepatitis (B94.2)
Excludes2: cytomegaloviral hepatitis (B25.1)
herpesviral [herpes simplex] hepatitis (B00.81)

B15 ACUTE HEPATITIS A

4th B15.9 Hepatitis A without hepatic coma
Hepatitis A (acute)(viral) NOS

B16 ACUTE HEPATITIS B

4th B16.9 Acute hepatitis B without delta-agent and without hepatic coma
Hepatitis B (acute) (viral) NOS

B17 OTHER ACUTE VIRAL HEPATITIS

4th B17.1 Acute hepatitis C
5th B17.10 Acute hepatitis C without hepatic coma
Acute hepatitis C NOS
B17.9 **Acute viral hepatitis, unspecified**
Acute infectious hepatitis NOS

B18 CHRONIC VIRAL HEPATITIS

4th *Includes:* Carrier of viral hepatitis
B18.1 Chronic viral hepatitis B without delta-agent
Carrier of viral hepatitis B
B18.2 Chronic viral hepatitis C
Carrier of viral hepatitis C
B18.8 Other chronic viral hepatitis
Carrier of other viral hepatitis
B18.9 Chronic viral hepatitis, unspecified
Carrier of unspecified viral hepatitis

B19 UNSPECIFIED VIRAL HEPATITIS

4th B19.1 Unspecified viral hepatitis B
5th B19.10 Unspecified viral hepatitis B without hepatic coma
Unspecified viral hepatitis B NOS
B19.2 Unspecified viral hepatitis C
5th B19.20 Unspecified viral hepatitis C without hepatic coma
Viral hepatitis C NOS
B19.9 Unspecified viral hepatitis without hepatic coma
Viral hepatitis NOS

(B20) HIV DISEASE

GUIDELINES

Refer to your *ICD-10-CM* resource for complete guidelines.

Code only confirmed cases

In this context, "confirmation" does not require documentation of positive serology or culture for HIV; the provider's diagnostic statement that the patient is HIV positive or has an HIV-related illness is sufficient.

Asymptomatic HIV

Z21, Asymptomatic HIV infection status, is to be applied when the patient without any documentation of symptoms is listed as being "HIV positive," "known HIV," "HIV test positive," or similar terminology. Do not use this code if the term "AIDS" or "HIV Disease" is used or if the patient is treated for any HIV-related illness or is described as having any condition(s) resulting from his/her HIV positive status; use B20 in these cases.

Patients with inconclusive HIV serology

Patients with inconclusive HIV serology, but no definitive diagnosis or manifestations of the illness, may be assigned code R75, Inconclusive laboratory evidence of HIV.

Encounters for testing for HIV

If a patient is being seen to determine his/her HIV status, use code Z11.4, Encounter for screening for human immunodeficiency virus [HIV]. Use additional codes for any associated high-risk behavior, if applicable.

If a patient with signs or symptoms is being seen for HIV testing, code the signs and symptoms. An additional counseling code Z71.7, Human immunodeficiency virus [HIV] counseling, may be used if counseling is provided during the encounter for the test.

When a patient returns to be informed of his/her HIV test results and the test result is negative, use code Z71.7, Human immunodeficiency virus [HIV] counseling.

If the results are positive, see previous guidelines and assign codes as appropriate.

(i) HIV managed by antiretroviral medication

If a patient with documented history of HIV disease, HIV-related illness or AIDS is currently managed on antiretroviral medications, assign code B20, Human immunodeficiency virus [HIV] disease. Code Z79.899, Other long term (current) drug therapy, may be assigned as an additional code to identify the long-term (current) use of antiretroviral medications.

B20 HIV DISEASE

✔ *Includes:* acquired immune deficiency syndrome [AIDS]
AIDS-related complex [ARC]
HIV infection, symptomatic
Use additional code(s) to identify all manifestations of HIV infection
Excludes1: asymptomatic HIV infection status (Z21)
exposure to HIV virus (Z20.6)
inconclusive serologic evidence of HIV (R75)
Other viral diseases (B25–B34)

(B25–B34) OTHER VIRAL DISEASES

B25 CYTOMEGALOVIRAL DISEASE

4th *Excludes1:* congenital cytomegalovirus infection (P35.1)
cytomegaloviral mononucleosis (B27.1-)
B25.0 Cytomegaloviral pneumonitis
B25.8 Other cytomegaloviral diseases
Cytomegaloviral encephalitis
B25.9 Cytomegaloviral disease, unspecified

B26 MUMPS

4th *Includes:* epidemic parotitis
infectious parotitis
B26.0 Mumps orchitis
B26.1 Mumps meningitis
B26.2 Mumps encephalitis
B26.8 Mumps with other complications
5th B26.89 Other mumps complications
B26.9 Mumps without complication
Mumps NOS
Mumps parotitis NOS

B27 INFECTIOUS MONONUCLEOSIS

4th *Includes:* glandular fever
monocytic angina
Pfeiffer's disease
B27.0 Gammaherpesviral mononucleosis;
5th Mononucleosis due to Epstein-Barr virus
B27.00 without complication
B27.01 with polyneuropathy
B27.02 with meningitis
B27.09 with other complications
Hepatomegaly in gammaherpesviral mononucleosis
B27.1 Cytomegaloviral mononucleosis;
5th B27.10 without complications
B27.11 with polyneuropathy
B27.12 with meningitis
B27.19 with other complication
Hepatomegaly in cytomegaloviral mononucleosis
B27.8 Other infectious mononucleosis;
5th B27.80 **without complication**
B27.81 **with polyneuropathy**
B27.82 **with meningitis**
B27.89 **with other complication**
Hepatomegaly in other infectious mononucleosis
B27.9 Infectious mononucleosis, unspecified;
5th B27.90 **without complication**
B27.91 **with polyneuropathy**
B27.92 **with meningitis**
B27.99 **with other complication**
Hepatomegaly in unspecified infectious mononucleosis

B30 VIRAL CONJUNCTIVITIS

Excludes1: herpesviral [herpes simplex] ocular disease (B00.5) ocular zoster (B02.3)

B30.0 Keratoconjunctivitis due to adenovirus Epidemic keratoconjunctivitis Shipyard eye

B30.1 Conjunctivitis due to adenovirus Acute adenoviral follicular conjunctivitis Swimming-pool conjunctivitis

B30.2 Viral pharyngoconjunctivitis

B30.3 Acute epidemic hemorrhagic conjunctivitis (enteroviral) Conjunctivitis due to coxsackievirus 24 Conjunctivitis due to enterovirus 70 Hemorrhagic conjunctivitis (acute)(epidemic)

B30.8 Other viral conjunctivitis Newcastle conjunctivitis

B30.9 Viral conjunctivitis, unspecified

B33 OTHER VIRAL DISEASES, NEC

B33.2 Viral carditis

Coxsackie (virus) carditis

B33.20 Viral carditis, unspecified

B33.21 Viral endocarditis

B33.22 Viral myocarditis

B33.23 Viral pericarditis

B33.24 Viral cardiomyopathy

B33.3 Retrovirus infections, NEC Retrovirus infection NOS

B33.8 Other specified viral diseases *Excludes1:* anogenital human papillomavirus infection (A63.0) viral warts due to human papillomavirus infection (B07)

B34 VIRAL INFECTION OF UNSPECIFIED SITE

Excludes1: anogenital human papillomavirus infection (A63.0) cytomegaloviral disease NOS (B25.9) herpesvirus [herpes simplex] infection NOS (B00.9) retrovirus infection NOS (B33.3) viral agents as the cause of diseases classified elsewhere (B97.-) viral warts due to human papillomavirus infection (B07)

B34.0 Adenovirus infection, unspecified

B34.1 Enterovirus infection, unspecified Coxsackievirus infection NOS Echovirus infection NOS

B34.2 Coronavirus infection, unspecified *Excludes1:* COVID-19 (U07.1) pneumonia due to SARS-associated coronavirus (J12.81)

B34.3 Parvovirus infection, unspecified

B34.4 Papovavirus infection, unspecified

B34.8 Other viral infections of unspecified site

B34.9 Viral infection, unspecified Viremia NOS

(B35–B49) MYCOSES

Excludes2: hypersensitivity pneumonitis due to organic dust (J67.-) mycosis fungoides (C84.0-)

B35 DERMATOPHYTOSIS

Includes: favus infections due to species of Epidermophyton, Micro-sporum and Trichophyton tinea, any type except those in B36.-

B35.0 Tinea barbae and tinea capitis Beard ringworm Kerion Scalp ringworm Sycosis, mycotic

B35.1 Tinea unguium Dermatophytic onychia Dermatophytosis of nail Onychomycosis Ringworm of nails

B35.2 Tinea manuum Dermatophytosis of hand Hand ringworm

B35.3 Tinea pedis Athlete's foot Dermatophytosis of foot Foot ringworm

B35.4 Tinea corporis Ringworm of the body

B35.5 Tinea imbricata Tokelau

B35.6 Tinea cruris Dhobi itch Groin ringworm Jock itch

B35.8 Other dermatophytoses Disseminated dermatophytosis Granulomatous dermatophytosis

B35.9 Dermatophytosis, unspecified Ringworm NOS

B36 OTHER SUPERFICIAL MYCOSES

B36.0 Pityriasis versicolor Tinea flava Tinea versicolor

B36.8 Other specified superficial mycoses

B36.9 Superficial mycosis, unspecified

B37 CANDIDIASIS

Includes: candidosis moniliasis

Excludes1: neonatal candidiasis (P37.5)

B37.0 Candidal stomatitis Oral thrush

B37.1 Pulmonary candidiasis Candidal bronchitis Candidal pneumonia

B37.2 Candidiasis of skin and nail Candidal onychia Candidal paronychia *Excludes2:* diaper dermatitis (L22)

B37.3 Candidiasis of vulva and vagina Candidal vulvovaginitis Monilial vulvovaginitis Vaginal thrush

B37.31 Acute candidiasis of vulva and vagina

B37.32 Chronic candidiasis of vulva and vagina

B37.4 Candidiasis of other urogenital sites

B37.41 Candidal cystitis and urethritis

B37.42 Candidal balanitis

B37.49 Other urogenital candidiasis Candidal pyelonephritis

B37.5 Candidal meningitis

B37.6 Candidal endocarditis

B37.7 Candidal sepsis Disseminated candidiasis Systemic candidiasis

B37.8 Candidiasis of other sites

B37.81 Candidal esophagitis

B37.82 Candidal enteritis Candidal proctitis

B37.83 Candidal cheilitis

B37.84 Candidal otitis externa

B37.89 Other sites of candidiasis Candidal osteomyelitis

B37.9 Candidiasis, unspecified Thrush NOS

B39 HISTOPLASMOSIS

Code first associated AIDS (B20)

Use additional code for any associated manifestations, such as: endocarditis (I39) meningitis (G02) pericarditis (I32) retinitis (H32)

B39.0 Acute pulmonary histoplasmosis capsulati

B39.1 Chronic pulmonary histoplasmosis capsulati

B39.2 Pulmonary histoplasmosis capsulati, unspecified

B39.3 Disseminated histoplasmosis capsulati
Generalized histoplasmosis capsulati

B39.4 Histoplasmosis capsulati, unspecified
American histoplasmosis

B39.9 Histoplasmosis, unspecified

B40 BLASTOMYCOSIS

4th

Excludes1: Brazilian blastomycosis (B41.-)
keloidal blastomycosis (B48.0)

B40.0 Acute pulmonary blastomycosis

B40.1 Chronic pulmonary blastomycosis

B40.2 Pulmonary blastomycosis, unspecified

B40.3 Cutaneous blastomycosis

B40.7 Disseminated blastomycosis
Generalized blastomycosis

B40.8 Other forms of blastomycosis

5th **B40.81 Blastomycotic meningoencephalitis**
Meningomyelitis due to blastomycosis

B40.89 Other forms of blastomycosis

B40.9 Blastomycosis, unspecified

B44 ASPERGILLOSIS

4th

Includes: aspergilloma

B44.8 Other forms of aspergillosis

5th **B44.81 Allergic bronchopulmonary aspergillosis**

B44.89 Other forms of aspergillosis

B44.9 Aspergillosis, unspecified

B49 UNSPECIFIED MYCOSIS

✓ Fungemia NOS

(B50–B64) PROTOZOAL DISEASES

Excludes1: amebiasis (A06.-)
other protozoal intestinal diseases (A07.-)

B54 UNSPECIFIED MALARIA

✓

B58 TOXOPLASMOSIS

4th

Includes: infection due to Toxoplasma gondii
Excludes1: congenital toxoplasmosis (P37.1)

B58.0 Toxoplasma oculopathy

5th **B58.00 Toxoplasma oculopathy, unspecified**

B58.01 Toxoplasma chorioretinitis

B58.09 Other toxoplasma oculopathy
Toxoplasma uveitis

B58.2 Toxoplasma meningoencephalitis

B58.3 Pulmonary toxoplasmosis

B58.8 Toxoplasmosis with other organ involvement

5th **B58.83 Toxoplasma tubulo-interstitial nephropathy**
Toxoplasma pyelonephritis

B58.89 Toxoplasmosis with other organ involvement

B58.9 Toxoplasmosis, unspecified

B60 OTHER PROTOZOAL DISEASES, NOT ELSEWHERE CLASSIFIED

4th

Excludes1: cryptosporidiosis (A07.2)
intestinal microsporidiosis (A07.8)
isosporiasis (A07.3)

B60.0 Babesiosis

5th **B60.00 Babesiosis, unspecified**
Babesiosis due to unspecified Babesia species
Piroplasmosis, unspecified

B60.01 Babesiosis due to Babesia microti
Infection due to B. microti

B60.02 Babesiosis due to Babesia duncani
Infection due to B. duncani and B. duncani-type species

B60.03 Babesiosis due to Babesia divergens
Babesiosis due to Babesia MO-1
Infection due to B. divergens and B. divergens-like strains

B60.09 Other babesiosis
Babesiosis due to Babesia KO-1
Babesiosis due to Babesia venatorum
Infection due to other Babesia species
Infection due to other protozoa of the order Piroplasmida
Other piroplasmosis

B60.1 Acanthamebiasis

5th **B60.10 Acanthamebiasis, unspecified**

B60.11 Meningoencephalitis due to Acanthamoeba (culbertsoni)

B60.12 Conjunctivitis due to Acanthamoeba

B60.13 Keratoconjunctivitis due to Acanthamoeba

B60.19 Other acanthamebic disease

B64 UNSPECIFIED PROTOZOAL DISEASE

✓

(B65–B83) HELMINTHIASES

B65 SCHISTOSOMIASIS [BILHARZIASIS]

4th

Includes: snail fever

B65.3 Cercarial dermatitis
Swimmer's itch

B65.8 Other schistosomiasis
Infection due to Schistosoma intercalatum
Infection due to Schistosoma mattheei
Infection due to Schistosoma mekongi

B65.9 Schistosomiasis, unspecified

B66 OTHER FLUKE INFECTIONS

4th

B66.8 Other specified fluke infections
Echinostomiasis
Heterophyiasis
Metagonomiasis
Nanophyetiasis
Watsoniasis

B66.9 Fluke infection, unspecified

B69 CYSTICERCOSIS

4th

Includes: cysticerciasis infection due to larval form of Taenia solium

B69.0 Cysticercosis of central nervous system

B69.8 Cysticercosis of other sites

5th **B69.89 Cysticercosis of other sites**

B69.9 Cysticercosis, unspecified

B71 OTHER CESTODE INFECTIONS

4th

B71.0 Hymenolepiasis
Dwarf tapeworm infection
Rat tapeworm (infection)

B71.8 Other specified cestode infections
Coenurosis

B71.9 Cestode infection, unspecified
Tapeworm (infection) NOS

B76 HOOKWORM DISEASES

4th

Includes: uncinariasis

B76.9 Hookworm disease, unspecified
Cutaneous larva migrans NOS

B77 ASCARIASIS

4th

Includes: ascaridiasis
roundworm infection

B77.0 Ascariasis with intestinal complications

B77.8 Ascariasis with other complications

5th **B77.81 Ascariasis pneumonia**

B77.89 Ascariasis with other complications

B77.9 Ascariasis, unspecified

B79 TRICHURIASIS

✓

Includes: trichocephaliasis
whipworm (disease)(infection)

B80 ENTEROBIASIS

✓

Includes: oxyuriasis
pinworm infection
threadworm infection

B82 UNSPECIFIED INTESTINAL PARASITISM

4th

B82.0 Intestinal helminthiasis, unspecified

B82.9 Intestinal parasitism, unspecified

(B85–B89) PEDICULOSIS, ACARIASIS AND OTHER INFESTATIONS

B85 PEDICULOSIS AND PHTHIRIASIS

- **B85.0 Pediculosis due to Pediculus humanus capitis**
  - Head-louse infestation
- **B85.1 Pediculosis due to Pediculus humanus corporis**
  - Body-louse infestation
- **B85.2 Pediculosis, unspecified**
- **B85.3 Phthiriasis**
  - Infestation by crab-louse
  - Infestation by Phthirus pubis
- **B85.4 Mixed pediculosis and phthiriasis**
  - Infestation classifiable to more than one of the categories B85.0–B85.3

B86 SCABIES

Sarcoptic itch

B88 OTHER INFESTATIONS

- **B88.0 Other acariasis**
  - Acarine dermatitis
  - Dermatitis due to Demodex species
  - Dermatitis due to Dermanyssus gallinae
  - Dermatitis due to Liponyssoides sanguineus
  - Trombiculosis
  - *Excludes2:* scabies (B86)
- **B88.1 Tungiasis [sandflea infestation]**
- **B88.2 Other arthropod infestations**
  - Scarabiasis
- **B88.3 External hirudiniasis**
  - Leech infestation NOS
  - *Excludes2:* internal hirudiniasis (B83.4)
- **B88.8 Other specified infestations**
  - Ichthyoparasitism due to Vandellia cirrhosa
  - Linguatulosis
  - Porocephaliasis
- **B88.9 Infestation, unspecified**
  - Infestation (skin) NOS
  - Infestation by mites NOS
  - Skin parasites NOS

B89 UNSPECIFIED PARASITIC DISEASE

(B90–B94) SEQUELAE OF INFECTIOUS AND PARASITIC DISEASES

Note: Categories B90–B94 are to be used to indicate conditions in categories A00–B89 as the cause of sequelae, which are themselves classified elsewhere. The 'sequelae' include conditions specified as such; they also include residuals of diseases classifiable to the above categories if there is evidence that the disease itself is no longer present. Codes from these categories are not to be used for chronic infections. Code chronic current infections to active infectious disease as appropriate.

Code first condition resulting from (sequela) the infectious or parasitic disease

B90 SEQUELAE OF TUBERCULOSIS

- **B90.0 Sequelae of central nervous system tuberculosis**
- **B90.1 Sequelae of genitourinary tuberculosis**
- **B90.2 Sequelae of tuberculosis of bones and joints**
- **B90.8 Sequelae of tuberculosis of other organs**
  - *Excludes2:* sequelae of respiratory tuberculosis (B90.9)
- **B90.9 Sequelae of respiratory and unspecified tuberculosis**
  - Sequelae of tuberculosis NOS

B94 SEQUELAE OF OTHER AND UNSPECIFIED INFECTIOUS AND PARASITIC DISEASES

- **B94.1 Sequelae of viral encephalitis**
- **B94.2 Sequelae of viral hepatitis**
- **B94.8 Sequelae of other specified infectious and parasitic diseases**
- **B94.9 Sequelae of unspecified infectious and parasitic disease**
  - *Excludes2:* post COVID-19 condition (U09.9)

(B95–B97) BACTERIAL AND VIRAL INFECTIOUS AGENTS

Note: These categories are provided for use as supplementary or additional codes to identify the infectious agent(s) in diseases classified elsewhere.

B95 STREPTOCOCCUS, STAPHYLOCOCCUS, AND ENTEROCOCCUS AS THE CAUSE OF DISEASES CLASSIFIED ELSEWHERE

- **B95.0 Streptococcus, group A, as the cause of diseases classified elsewhere**
- **B95.1 Streptococcus, group B, as the cause of diseases classified elsewhere**
- **B95.2 Enterococcus as the cause of diseases classified elsewhere**
- **B95.3 Streptococcus pneumoniae as the cause of diseases classified elsewhere**
- **B95.4 Other streptococcus as the cause of diseases classified elsewhere**
- **B95.5 Unspecified streptococcus as the cause of diseases classified elsewhere**
- **B95.6 Staphylococcus aureus as the cause of diseases classified elsewhere**
  - **B95.61 MSSA infection as the cause of diseases classified elsewhere**
    - MSSA infection as the cause of diseases classified elsewhere
    - Staphylococcus aureus infection NOS as the cause of diseases classified elsewhere
  - **B95.62 MRSA infection as the cause of diseases classified elsewhere**
    - MRSA infection as the cause of diseases classified elsewhere
- **B95.7 Other staphylococcus as the cause of diseases classified elsewhere**
- **B95.8 Unspecified staphylococcus as the cause of diseases classified elsewhere**

B96 OTHER BACTERIAL AGENTS AS THE CAUSE OF DISEASES CLASSIFIED ELSEWHERE

- **B96.0 M. pneumoniae as the cause of diseases classified elsewhere**
  - Pleuro-pneumonia-like-organism [PPLO]
- **B96.1 K. pneumoniae as the cause of diseases classified elsewhere**
- **B96.2 E. coli as the cause of diseases classified elsewhere**
  - **B96.20 Unspecified E. coli as the cause of diseases classified elsewhere**
    - E. coli NOS
  - **B96.21 STEC 0157 as the cause of diseases classified elsewhere**
    - E. coli O157:H- (nonmotile) with confirmation of Shiga toxin
    - E. coli O157 with confirmation of Shiga toxin when H antigen is unknown, or is not H7
    - O157:H7 E. coli with or without confirmation of Shiga toxin-production
    - STEC O157:H7 with or without confirmation of Shiga toxin-production
    - STEC O157:H7 with or without confirmation of Shiga toxin-production
  - **B96.22 Other specified STEC as the cause of diseases classified elsewhere**
    - Non-O157 STEC
    - Non-O157 STEC with known O group
  - **B96.23 STEC as the cause of diseases classified elsewhere**
    - STEC with unspecified O group
    - STEC NOS
  - **B96.29 Other E. coli as the cause of diseases classified elsewhere**
    - Non-STEC
- **B96.3 H. influenzae as the cause of diseases classified elsewhere**
- **B96.4 Proteus (mirabilis) (morganii) as the cause of diseases classified elsewhere**
- **B96.5 Pseudomonas (aeruginosa) (mallei) (pseudomallei) as the cause of diseases classified elsewhere**
- **B96.8 Other specified bacterial agents as the cause of diseases classified elsewhere**

B96.81 H. pylori as the cause of diseases classified elsewhere

B96.82 Vibrio vulnificus as the cause of diseases classified elsewhere

B96.83 Acinetobacter baumannii as the cause of diseases classified elsewhere

B96.89 Other specified bacterial agents as the cause of diseases classified elsewhere

B97 VIRAL AGENTS AS THE CAUSE OF DISEASES CLASSIFIED ELSEWHERE

B97.0 Adenovirus as the cause of diseases classified elsewhere

B97.1 Enterovirus as the cause of diseases classified elsewhere

B97.10 Unspecified enterovirus as the cause of diseases classified elsewhere

B97.11 Coxsackievirus as the cause of diseases classified elsewhere

B97.12 Echovirus as the cause of diseases classified elsewhere

B97.19 Other enterovirus as the cause of diseases classified elsewhere

B97.2 Coronavirus as the cause of diseases classified elsewhere

B97.21 SARS-associated coronavirus as the cause of diseases classified elsewhere

Excludes1: pneumonia due to SARS-associated coronavirus (J12.81)

B97.29 Other coronavirus as the cause of diseases classified elsewhere

B97.4 Respiratory syncytial virus as the cause of diseases classified elsewhere

RSV as the cause of diseases classified elsewhere

Code first related disorders, such as:

otitis media (H65.-)

upper respiratory infection (J06.9)

Excludes1: acute bronchiolitis due to respiratory syncytial virus (RSV) (J21.0)

acute bronchitis due to respiratory syncytial virus (RSV) (J20.5)

respiratory syncytial virus (RSV) pneumonia (J12.1)

B97.6 Parvovirus as the cause of diseases classified elsewhere

B97.8 Other viral agents as the cause of diseases classified elsewhere

B97.89 Other viral agents as the cause of diseases classified elsewhere

(B99) OTHER INFECTIOUS DISEASES

B99 OTHER AND UNSPECIFIED INFECTIOUS DISEASES

B99.8 Other infectious disease

B99.9 Unspecified infectious disease

Chapter 2. Neoplasms (C00–D49)

GUIDELINES

Chapter 2 of the *ICD-10-CM* contains the codes for most benign and all malignant neoplasms. Certain benign neoplasms, such as prostatic adenomas, may be found in the specific body system chapters. To properly code a neoplasm, it is necessary to determine from the record if the neoplasm is benign, in-situ, malignant, or of uncertain histologic behavior. If malignant, any secondary (metastatic) sites should also be determined.

Primary malignant neoplasms overlapping site boundaries

A primary malignant neoplasm that overlaps two or more contiguous (next to each other) sites should be classified to the subcategory/code .8 ('overlapping lesion'), unless the combination is specifically indexed elsewhere. For multiple neoplasms of the same site that are not contiguous such as tumors in different quadrants of the same breast, codes for each site should be assigned.

Malignant neoplasm of ectopic tissue

Malignant neoplasms of ectopic tissue are to be coded to the site of origin mentioned, e.g., ectopic pancreatic malignant neoplasms involving the stomach are coded to malignant neoplasm of pancreas, unspecified (C25.9).

The neoplasm table in the Alphabetic Index should be referenced first. However, if the histological term is documented, that term should be referenced first, rather than going immediately to the Neoplasm Table, in order to determine which column in the Neoplasm Table is appropriate. For example, if the documentation indicates "adenoma," refer to the term in the Alphabetic Index to review the entries under this term and the instructional note to "see also neoplasm, by site, benign." The table provides the proper code based on the type of neoplasm and the site. It is important to select the proper column in the table that corresponds to the type of neoplasm. The Tabular List should then be referenced to verify that the correct code has been selected from the table and that a more specific site code does not exist.

Refer to the *ICD-10-CM* manual for information regarding Z15.0, codes for genetic susceptibility to cancer.

ADMISSION/ENCOUNTER FOR TREATMENT OF PRIMARY SITE

If the malignancy is chiefly responsible for occasioning the patient admission/ encounter and treatment is directed at the primary site, designate the primary malignancy as the principal/first-listed diagnosis.

The only exception to this guideline is if the administration of chemotherapy, immunotherapy or external beam radiation therapy is chiefly responsible for occasioning the admission/encounter. In that case, assign the appropriate Z51.-- code as the first-listed or principal diagnosis, and the underlying diagnosis or problem for which the service is being performed as a secondary diagnosis.

ADMISSION/ENCOUNTER FOR TREATMENT OF SECONDARY SITE

When a patient is admitted because of a primary neoplasm with metastasis and treatment is directed toward the secondary site only, the secondary neoplasm is designated as the principal diagnosis even though the primary malignancy is still present.

CODING AND SEQUENCING OF COMPLICATIONS

Coding and sequencing of complications associated with the malignancies or with the therapy thereof are subject to the following guidelines:

Anemia associated with malignancy

When admission/encounter is for management of an anemia associated with the malignancy, and the treatment is only for anemia, the appropriate code for the malignancy is sequenced as the principal or first-listed diagnosis followed by the appropriate code for the anemia (such as code D63.0, Anemia in neoplastic disease).

Anemia associated with chemotherapy, immunotherapy, and radiation therapy

When the admission/encounter is for management of an anemia associated with an adverse effect of the administration of chemotherapy or immunotherapy and the only treatment is for the anemia, the anemia code is sequenced first followed by the appropriate codes for the neoplasm and the adverse effect (T45.1X5, Adverse effect of antineoplastic and immunosuppressive drugs).

When the admission/encounter is for management of an anemia associated with an adverse effect of radiotherapy, the anemia code should be sequenced first, followed by the appropriate neoplasm code and code Y84.2, Radiological procedure

and radiotherapy as the cause of abnormal reaction of the patient, or of later complication, without mention of misadventure at the time of the procedure.

Management of dehydration due to the malignancy

When the admission/encounter is for management of dehydration due to the malignancy and only the dehydration is being treated (intravenous rehydration), the dehydration is sequenced first, followed by the code(s) for the malignancy.

Treatment of a complication resulting from a surgical procedure

When the admission/encounter is for treatment of a complication resulting from a surgical procedure, designate the complication as the principal or first-listed diagnosis if treatment is directed at resolving the complication.

PRIMARY MALIGNANCY PREVIOUSLY EXCISED

When a primary malignancy has been previously excised or eradicated from its site and there is no further treatment directed to that site and there is no evidence of any existing primary malignancy at that site, a code from category Z85, Personal history of malignant neoplasm, should be used to indicate the former site of the malignancy. Any mention of extension, invasion, or metastasis to another site is coded as a secondary malignant neoplasm to that site. The secondary site may be the principal or first-listed a diagnosis with the Z85 code used as a secondary code. *See "Secondary malignant neoplasm of lymphoid tissue."*

ADMISSIONS/ENCOUNTERS INVOLVING CHEMOTHERAPY, IMMUNO-THERAPY AND RADIATION THERAPY

Episode of care involves surgical removal of neoplasm

When an episode of care involves the surgical removal of a neoplasm, primary or secondary site, followed by adjunct chemotherapy or radiation treatment during the same episode of care, the code for the neoplasm should be assigned as principal or first-listed diagnosis.

Patient admission/encounter solely for administration of chemotherapy, immunotherapy and radiation therapy

If a patient admission/encounter is **chiefly** for the administration of chemotherapy, immunotherapy or external beam radiation therapy assign code Z51.0, Encounter for antineoplastic radiation therapy, or Z51.11, Encounter for antineoplastic chemotherapy, or Z51.12, Encounter for antineoplastic immunotherapy as the first-listed or principal diagnosis. If a patient receives more than one of these therapies during the same admission more than one of these codes may be assigned, in any sequence. The malignancy for which the therapy is being administered should be assigned as a secondary diagnosis.

If a patient admission/encounter is for the insertion or implantation of radioactive elements (e.g., brachytherapy) the appropriate code for the malignancy is sequenced as the principal or first-listed diagnosis. Code Z51.0 should not be assigned.

Patient admitted for radiation therapy, chemotherapy or immunotherapy and develops complications

When a patient is admitted for the purpose of external beam radiotherapy, immunotherapy or chemotherapy and develops complications such as uncontrolled nausea and vomiting or dehydration, the principal or first-listed diagnosis is Z51.0, Encounter for antineoplastic radiation therapy, or Z51.11, Encounter for antineoplastic chemotherapy, or Z51.12, Encounter for antineoplastic immunotherapy followed by any codes for the complications. When a patient is admitted for the purpose of insertion or implantation of radioactive elements (e.g., brachytherapy) and develops complications such as uncontrolled nausea and vomiting or dehydration, the principal or first-listed diagnosis is the appropriate code for the malignancy followed by any codes for the complications.

ADMISSION/ENCOUNTER TO DETERMINE EXTENT OF MALIGNANCY

When the reason for admission/encounter is to determine the extent of the malignancy, or for a procedure such as paracentesis or thoracentesis, the primary malignancy or appropriate metastatic site is designated as the principal or first-listed diagnosis, even though chemotherapy or radiotherapy is administered.

SYMPTOMS, SIGNS, AND ABNORMAL FINDINGS LISTED IN CHAPTER 18 ASSOCIATED WITH NEOPLASMS

Symptoms, signs, and ill-defined conditions listed in Chapter 18 characteristic of, or associated with, an existing primary or secondary site malignancy cannot be used to replace the malignancy as principal or first-listed diagnosis, regardless of the number of admissions or encounters for treatment and care of the neoplasm.

ADMISSION/ENCOUNTER FOR PAIN CONTROL/MANAGEMENT

See category G89 for information on coding admission/encounter for pain control/ management.

MALIGNANCY IN TWO OR MORE NONCONTIGUOUS SITES

A patient may have more than one malignant tumor in the same organ. These tumors may represent different primaries or metastatic disease, depending on the site. Should the documentation be unclear, the provider should be queried as to the status of each tumor so that the correct codes can be assigned.

DISSEMINATED MALIGNANT NEOPLASM, UNSPECIFIED

See code C80.0.

MALIGNANT NEOPLASM WITHOUT SPECIFICATION OF SITE

See code C80.1.

SEQUENCING OF NEOPLASM CODES

Encounter for treatment of primary malignancy

If the reason for the encounter is for treatment of a primary malignancy, assign the malignancy as the principal/first-listed diagnosis. The primary site is to be sequenced first, followed by any metastatic sites.

Encounter for treatment of secondary malignancy

When an encounter is for a primary malignancy with metastasis and treatment is directed toward the metastatic (secondary) site(s) only, the metastatic site(s) is designated as the principal/first-listed diagnosis. The primary malignancy is coded as an additional code.

Encounter for complication associated with a neoplasm

When an encounter is for management of a complication associated with a neoplasm, such as dehydration, and the treatment is only for the complication, the complication is coded first, followed by the appropriate code(s) for the neoplasm.

The exception to this guideline is anemia. When the admission/encounter is for management of an anemia associated with the malignancy, and the treatment is only for anemia, the appropriate code for the malignancy is sequenced as the principal or first-listed diagnosis followed by code D63.0, Anemia in neoplastic disease.

Complication from surgical procedure for treatment of a neoplasm

When an encounter is for treatment of a complication resulting from a surgical procedure performed for the treatment of the neoplasm, designate the complication as the principal/first-listed diagnosis. See the guideline regarding the coding of a current malignancy versus personal history to determine if the code for the neoplasm should also be assigned.

Pathologic fracture due to a neoplasm

When an encounter is for a pathological fracture due to a neoplasm, and the focus of treatment is the fracture, a code from subcategory M84.5, Pathological fracture in neoplastic disease, should be sequenced first, followed by the code for the neoplasm.

If the focus of treatment is the neoplasm with an associated pathological fracture, the neoplasm code should be sequenced first, followed by a code from M84.5 for the pathological fracture.

CURRENT MALIGNANCY VERSUS PERSONAL HISTORY OF MALIGNANCY

When a primary malignancy has been excised but further treatment, such as additional surgery for the malignancy, radiation therapy or chemotherapy is directed to that site, the primary malignancy code should be used until treatment is completed.

When a primary malignancy has been previously excised or eradicated from its site, there is no further treatment (of the malignancy) directed to that site, and there is no evidence of any existing primary malignancy at that site, a code from category Z85, Personal history of malignant neoplasm, should be used to indicate the former site of the malignancy.

Codes from subcategories Z85.0–Z85.85 should only be assigned for the former site of a primary malignancy, not the site of a secondary malignancy. Code Z85.89 may be assigned for the former site(s) of either a primary or secondary malignancy.

See Chapter 21, Factors influencing health status and contact with health services, History (of).

LEUKEMIA, MULTIPLE MYELOMA, AND MALIGNANT PLASMA CELL NEOPLASMS IN REMISSION VERSUS PERSONAL HISTORY

The categories for leukemia, and category C90, Multiple myeloma and malignant plasma cell neoplasms, have codes indicating whether or not the leukemia has achieved remission. There are also codes Z85.6, Personal history of leukemia, and Z85.79, Personal history of other malignant neoplasms of lymphoid, hematopoietic and related tissues. If the documentation is unclear, as to whether the leukemia has achieved remission, the provider should be queried.

See Chapter 21, Factors influencing health status and contact with health services, History (of)

AFTERCARE FOLLOWING SURGERY FOR NEOPLASM

See Chapter 21, Factors influencing health status and contact with health services, Aftercare

FOLLOW-UP CARE FOR COMPLETED TREATMENT OF A MALIGNANCY

See Chapter 21, Factors influencing health status and contact with health services, Follow-up

PROPHYLACTIC ORGAN REMOVAL FOR PREVENTION OF MALIGNANCY

See Chapter 21, Factors influencing health

MALIGNANT NEOPLASM ASSOCIATED WITH TRANSPLANTED ORGAN

A malignant neoplasm of a transplanted organ should be coded as a transplant complication. Assign first the appropriate code from category T86.-, Complications of transplanted organs and tissue, followed by code C80.2, Malignant neoplasm associated with transplanted organ. Use an additional code for the specific malignancy.

SECONDARY MALIGNANT NEOPLASM OF LYMPHOID TISSUE

When a malignant neoplasm of lymphoid tissue metastasizes beyond the lymph nodes, a code from categories C81-C85 with a final character "9" should be assigned identifying "extranodal and solid organ sites" rather than a code for the secondary neoplasm of the affected solid organ. For example, for metastasis of B-cell lymphoma to the lung, brain and left adrenal gland, assign code C83.39, Diffuse large B-cell lymphoma, extranodal and solid organ sites.

NEOPLASMS (C00–D49)

Note: Functional activity
All neoplasms are classified in this chapter, whether they are functionally active or not. An additional code from Chapter 4 may be used, to identify functional activity associated with any neoplasm.

Morphology [Histology]
Chapter 2 classifies neoplasms primarily by site (topography), with broad groupings for behavior, malignant, in situ, benign, etc. The Table of Neoplasms should be used to identify the correct topography code. In a few cases, such as for malignant melanoma and certain neuroendocrine tumors, the morphology (histologic type) is included in the category and codes.

Primary malignant neoplasms overlapping site boundaries
A primary malignant neoplasm that overlaps two or more contiguous (next to each other) sites should be classified to the subcategory/code .8 ('overlapping lesion'), unless the combination is specifically indexed elsewhere. For multiple neoplasms of the same site that are not contiguous, such as tumors in different quadrants of the same breast, codes for each site should be assigned.

Malignant neoplasm of ectopic tissue
Malignant neoplasms of ectopic tissue are to be coded to the site mentioned, e.g., ectopic pancreatic malignant neoplasms are coded to pancreas, unspecified (C25.9).

(C00–C96) MALIGNANT NEOPLASMS

Includes: Malignant neoplasms, stated or presumed to be primary (of specified sites), and certain specified histologies, except neuroendocrine, and of lymphoid, hematopoietic and related tissue (C00–C75)

(C00–C14) MALIGNANT NEOPLASMS OF LIP, ORAL CAVITY AND PHARYNX

(C15–C26) MALIGNANT NEOPLASMS OF DIGESTIVE ORGANS

Excludes1: Kaposi's sarcoma of gastrointestinal sites (C46.4)

(C30–C39) MALIGNANT NEOPLASMS OF RESPIRATORY AND INTRATHORACIC ORGANS

Includes: malignant neoplasm of middle ear
Excludes1: mesothelioma (C45.-)

(C40–C41) MALIGNANT NEOPLASMS OF BONE AND ARTICULAR CARTILAGE

Includes: malignant neoplasm of cartilage (articular) (joint)
malignant neoplasm of periosteum
Excludes1: malignant neoplasm of bone marrow NOS (C96.9)
malignant neoplasm of synovia (C49.-)

C40 MALIGNANT NEOPLASM OF BONE AND ARTICULAR CARTILAGE OF LIMBS

Use additional code to identify major osseous defect, if applicable (M89.7-)

- **C40.0** Malignant neoplasm of scapula and long bones of upper limb
  - C40.01 right upper limb
  - C40.02 left upper limb
- **C40.1** Malignant neoplasm of short bones of; upper limb
  - C40.11 right upper limb
  - C40.12 left upper limb
- **C40.2** Malignant neoplasm of long bones of; lower limb
  - C40.21 right lower limb
  - C40.22 left lower limb
- **C40.3** Malignant neoplasm of short bones of; lower limb
  - C40.31 right lower limb
  - C40.32 left lower limb
- **C40.8** Malignant neoplasm of overlapping sites of bone and articular cartilage of; limb
  - C40.81 right limb
  - C40.82 left limb
- **C40.9** Malignant neoplasm of unspecified bones and articular cartilage of; limb
  - C40.91 right limb
  - C40.92 left limb

C41 MALIGNANT NEOPLASM OF BONE AND ARTICULAR CARTILAGE OF OTHER AND UNSPECIFIED SITES

Excludes1: malignant neoplasm of bones of limbs (C40.-)
malignant neoplasm of cartilage of ear (C49.0)
malignant neoplasm of cartilage of eyelid (C49.0)
malignant neoplasm of cartilage of larynx (C32.3)
malignant neoplasm of cartilage of limbs (C40.-)
malignant neoplasm of cartilage of nose (C30.0)

- **C41.0** Malignant neoplasm of bones of skull and face
  - Malignant neoplasm of maxilla (superior)
  - Malignant neoplasm of orbital bone
  - *Excludes2:* carcinoma, any type except intraosseous or odontogenic of:
    - maxillary sinus (C31.0)
    - upper jaw (C03.0)
    - malignant neoplasm of jaw bone (lower) (C41.1)
- **C41.1** Malignant neoplasm of mandible
  - Malignant neoplasm of inferior maxilla
  - Malignant neoplasm of lower jaw bone
  - *Excludes2:* carcinoma, any type except intraosseous or odontogenic of:
    - jaw NOS (C03.9)
    - lower (C03.1)
    - malignant neoplasm of upper jaw bone (C41.0)
- **C41.2** Malignant neoplasm of vertebral column
  - *Excludes1:* malignant neoplasm of sacrum and coccyx (C41.4)
- **C41.3** Malignant neoplasm of ribs, sternum and clavicle
- **C41.4** Malignant neoplasm of pelvic bones, sacrum and coccyx
- **C41.9** Malignant neoplasm of bone and articular cartilage, unspecified

(C43–C44) MELANOMA AND OTHER MALIGNANT NEOPLASMS OF SKIN

C43 MALIGNANT MELANOMA OF SKIN

Excludes1: melanoma in situ (D03.-)
Excludes2: malignant melanoma of skin of genital organs (C51-C52, C60.-, C63.-)
Merkel cell carcinoma (C4A.-)
sites other than skin-code to malignant neoplasm of the site

- **C43.0** Malignant melanoma of lip
  - *Excludes1:* malignant neoplasm of vermilion border of lip (C00.0-C00.2)
- **C43.1** Malignant melanoma of eyelid, including canthus;
  - C43.10 unspecified eyelid
  - C43.11 right eyelid
    - C43.111 right upper eyelid
    - C43.112 right lower eyelid
  - C43.12 Malignant melanoma of left eyelid, including canthus;
    - C43.121 left upper eyelid
    - C43.122 left lower eyelid
- **C43.2** Malignant melanoma of ear and external auricular canal;
  - C43.21 right ear
  - C43.22 left ear
- **C43.3** Malignant melanoma of other and unspecified parts of face
  - C43.30 Malignant melanoma of unspecified part of face
  - C43.31 Malignant melanoma of nose
  - C43.39 Malignant melanoma of other parts of face
- **C43.4** Malignant melanoma of scalp and neck
- **C43.5** Malignant melanoma of trunk
  - *Excludes2:* malignant neoplasm of anus NOS (C21.0) malignant neoplasm of scrotum (C63.2)
  - C43.51 Malignant melanoma of anal skin
    - Malignant melanoma of anal margin
    - Malignant melanoma of perianal skin
  - C43.52 Malignant melanoma of skin of breast
  - C43.59 Malignant melanoma of other part of trunk
- **C43.6** Malignant melanoma of upper limb, including shoulder
  - C43.61 Malignant melanoma of right upper limb, including shoulder
  - C43.62 Malignant melanoma of left upper limb, including shoulder
- **C43.7** Malignant melanoma of lower limb, including hip
  - C43.71 Malignant melanoma of right lower limb, including hip
  - C43.72 Malignant melanoma of left lower limb, including hip
- **C43.8** Malignant melanoma of overlapping sites of skin
- **C43.9** Malignant melanoma of skin, unspecified
  - Malignant melanoma of unspecified site of skin
  - Melanoma (malignant) NOS

C4A MERKEL CELL CARCINOMA

- **C4A.0** Merkel cell carcinoma of lip
  - *Excludes1:* malignant neoplasm of vermilion border of lip (C00.0-C00.2)
- **C4A.1** Merkel cell carcinoma of eyelid
  - C4A.10 unspecified eyelid
  - C4A.11 right eyelid
    - C4A.111 right upper eyelid
    - C4A.112 right lower eyelid
  - C4A.12 left eyelid, including canthus
    - C4A.121 left upper eyelid
    - C4A.122 left lower eyelid
- **C4A.2** Merkel cell carcinoma of ear and external auricular canal;
  - C4A.20 unspecified ear and external auricular canal
  - C4A.21 right ear and external auricular canal
  - C4A.22 left ear and external auricular canal
- **C4A.3** Merkel cell carcinoma of other and unspecified parts of face
  - C4A.30 Merkel cell carcinoma of unspecified part of face
  - C4A.31 Merkel cell carcinoma of nose
  - C4A.39 Merkel cell carcinoma of other parts of face
- **C4A.4** Merkel cell carcinoma of scalp and neck
- **C4A.5** Merkel cell carcinoma of trunk
  - *Excludes2:* malignant neoplasm of anus NOS (C21.0) malignant neoplasm of scrotum (C63.2)
  - C4A.51 Merkel cell carcinoma of anal skin
    - Merkel cell carcinoma of anal margin
    - Merkel cell carcinoma of perianal skin
  - C4A.52 Merkel cell carcinoma of skin of breast
  - C4A.59 Merkel cell carcinoma of other part of trunk
- **C4A.6** Merkel cell carcinoma of upper limb, including shoulder;
  - C4A.61 right upper limb
  - C4A.62 left upper limb

C4A.7 Merkel cell carcinoma of lower limb, including hip;
C4A.71 right lower limb, including hip
C4A.72 left lower limb, including hip
C4A.8 Merkel cell carcinoma of overlapping sites
C4A.9 Merkel cell carcinoma, unspecified
Merkel cell carcinoma of unspecified site
Merkel cell carcinoma NOS

C44 OTHER AND UNSPECIFIED MALIGNANT NEOPLASM OF SKIN

Includes: malignant neoplasm of sebaceous glands
malignant neoplasm of sweat glands
Excludes1: Kaposi's sarcoma of skin (C46.0)
malignant melanoma of skin (C43.-)
malignant neoplasm of skin of genital organs (C51-C52, C60.-, C63.2)
Merkel cell carcinoma (C4A.-)

C44.0 Other and unspecified malignant neoplasm of skin of lip
Excludes1: malignant neoplasm of lip (C00.-)
- C44.00 Unspecified malignant neoplasm of skin of lip
- C44.01 Basal cell carcinoma of skin of lip
- C44.02 Squamous cell carcinoma of skin of lip
- C44.09 Other specified malignant neoplasm of skin of lip

C44.1 Other and unspecified malignant neoplasm of skin of eyelid, including canthus
Excludes1: connective tissue of eyelid (C49.0)
- C44.10 Unspecified malignant neoplasm of skin of eyelid, including canthus;
  - C44.101 unspecified eyelid
  - C44.102 right eyelid
    - C44.1021 right upper eyelid
    - C44.1022 right lower eyelid
  - C44.109 left eyelid
    - C44.1091 left upper eyelid
    - C44.1092 left lower eyelid
- C44.11 Basal cell carcinoma of skin of eyelid, including canthus;
  - C44.111 unspecified eyelid
  - C44.112 right eyelid
    - C44.1121 right upper eyelid
    - C44.1122 right lower eyelid
  - C44.119 left eyelid
    - C44.1191 left upper eyelid
    - C44.1192 left lower eyelid
- C44.12 Squamous cell carcinoma of skin of eyelid, including canthus;
  - C44.121 unspecified eyelid
  - C44.122 right eyelid
    - C44.1221 right upper eyelid
    - C44.1222 right lower eyelid
  - C44.129 left eyelid
    - C44.1291 left upper eyelid
    - C44.1292 left lower eyelid
- C44.13 Sebaceous cell carcinoma of skin of eyelid, including canthus;
  - C44.131 unspecified eyelid
  - C44.132 right eyelid
    - C44.1321 right upper eyelid
    - C44.1322 right lower eyelid
  - C44.139 left eyelid
    - C44.1391 left upper eyelid
    - C44.1392 left lower eyelid
- C44.19 Other specified malignant neoplasm of skin of eyelid, including canthus;
  - C44.191 unspecified eyelid
  - C44.192 right eyelid, including canthus
    - C44.1921 right upper eyelid
    - C44.1922 right lower eyelid
  - C44.199 left eyelid
    - C44.1991 left upper eyelid
    - C44.1992 left lower eyelid

C44.2 Other and unspecified malignant neoplasm of skin of ear and external auricular canal
Excludes1: connective tissue of ear (C49.0)
- C44.20 Unspecified malignant neoplasm of skin of ear and external auricular canal;
  - C44.201 unspecified ear
  - C44.202 right ear
  - C44.209 left ear
- C44.21 Basal cell carcinoma of skin of ear and external auricular canal;
  - C44.212 right ear
  - C44.219 left ear
- C44.22 Squamous cell carcinoma of skin of ear and external auricular canal;
  - C44.222 right ear
  - C44.229 left ear
- C44.29 Other specified malignant neoplasm of skin of ear and external auricular canal;
  - C44.292 right ear
  - C44.299 left ear

C44.3 Other and unspecified malignant neoplasm of skin of other and unspecified parts of face
- C44.30 Unspecified malignant neoplasm of skin of other and unspecified parts of face;
  - C44.300 unspecified part of face
  - C44.301 nose
  - C44.309 other parts of face
- C44.31 Basal cell carcinoma of skin of other and unspecified parts of face;
  - C44.310 unspecified parts of face
  - C44.311 nose
  - C44.319 other parts of face
- C44.32 Squamous cell carcinoma of skin of other and unspecified parts of face;
  - C44.320 unspecified parts of face
  - C44.321 nose
  - C44.329 other parts of face
- C44.39 Other specified malignant neoplasm of skin of other and unspecified parts of face;
  - C44.390 unspecified parts of face
  - C44.391 skin of nose
  - C44.399 skin of other parts of face

C44.4 Other and unspecified malignant neoplasm of skin of scalp and neck
- C44.40 Unspecified malignant neoplasm of skin of scalp and neck
- C44.41 Basal cell carcinoma of skin of scalp and neck
- C44.42 Squamous cell carcinoma of skin of scalp and neck
- C44.49 Other specified malignant neoplasm of skin of scalp and neck

C44.5 Other and unspecified malignant neoplasm of skin of trunk
Excludes1: anus NOS (C21.0)
scrotum (C63.2)
- C44.50 Unspecified malignant neoplasm of skin of trunk;
  - C44.500 anal skin
    - Unspecified malignant neoplasm of anal margin
    - Unspecified malignant neoplasm of perianal skin
  - C44.501 breast
  - C44.509 other part of trunk
- C44.51 Basal cell carcinoma of skin of trunk;
  - C44.510 anal skin
    - Basal cell carcinoma of anal margin
    - Basal cell carcinoma of perianal skin
  - C44.511 breast
  - C44.519 other part of trunk
- C44.52 Squamous cell carcinoma of skin of trunk;
  - C44.520 anal skin
    - Squamous cell carcinoma of anal margin
    - Squamous cell carcinoma of perianal skin
  - C44.521 breast
  - C44.529 other part of trunk
- C44.59 Other specified malignant neoplasm of skin of trunk;

C44.590 anal skin
Other specified malignant neoplasm of anal margin
Other specified malignant neoplasm of perianal skin
C44.591 breast
C44.599 other part of trunk

C44.6 Other and unspecified malignant neoplasm of skin of upper limb, including shoulder

C44.60 Unspecified malignant neoplasm of skin of upper limb, including shoulder;
C44.602 right upper limb
C44.609 left upper limb

C44.61 Basal cell carcinoma of skin of upper limb
C44.612 right upper limb
C44.619 left upper limb

C44.62 Squamous cell carcinoma of skin of upper limb, including shoulder;
C44.622 right upper limb
C44.629 left upper limb

C44.69 Other specified malignant neoplasm of skin of upper limb, including shoulder;
C44.692 right upper limb
C44.699 left upper limb

C44.7 Other and unspecified malignant neoplasm of skin of lower limb, including hip

C44.70 Unspecified malignant neoplasm of skin of lower limb, including hip;
C44.702 right lower limb
C44.709 left lower limb

C44.71 Basal cell carcinoma of skin of lower limb, including hip;
C44.712 right lower limb
C44.719 left lower limb

C44.72 Squamous cell carcinoma of skin of lower limb, including hip;
C44.722 right lower limb
C44.729 left lower limb

C44.79 Other specified malignant neoplasm of skin of lower limb, including hip;
C44.792 right upper limb
C44.799 left lower limb

C44.8 Other and unspecified malignant neoplasm of overlapping sites of skin

C44.80 Unspecified malignant neoplasm of overlapping sites of skin
C44.81 Basal cell carcinoma of overlapping sites of skin
C44.82 Squamous cell carcinoma of overlapping sites of skin
C44.89 Other specified malignant neoplasm of overlapping sites of skin

C44.9 Other and unspecified malignant neoplasm of skin, unspecified

C44.90 Unspecified malignant neoplasm of skin, unspecified
Malignant neoplasm of unspecified site of skin
C44.91 Basal cell carcinoma of skin, unspecified
C44.92 Squamous cell carcinoma of skin, unspecified
C44.99 Other specified malignant neoplasm of skin, unspecified

(C45–C49) MALIGNANT NEOPLASMS OF MESOTHELIAL AND SOFT TISSUE

(C50) MALIGNANT NEOPLASMS OF BREAST

(C51–C58) MALIGNANT NEOPLASMS OF FEMALE GENITAL ORGANS

Includes: malignant neoplasm of skin of female genital organs

(C60–C63) MALIGNANT NEOPLASMS OF MALE GENITAL ORGANS

Includes: malignant neoplasm of skin of male genital organs

(C64–C68) MALIGNANT NEOPLASMS OF URINARY TRACT

C64 MALIGNANT NEOPLASM OF KIDNEY, EXCEPT RENAL PELVIS

Excludes1: malignant carcinoid tumor of the kidney (C7A.093)
malignant neoplasm of renal calyces (C65.-)
malignant neoplasm of renal pelvis (C65.-)

C64.1 Malignant neoplasm of right kidney, except renal pelvis
C64.2 Malignant neoplasm of left kidney, except renal pelvis

(C69–C72) MALIGNANT NEOPLASMS OF EYE, BRAIN AND OTHER PARTS OF CENTRAL NERVOUS SYSTEM

C69 MALIGNANT NEOPLASM OF EYE AND ADNEXA

Excludes1: malignant neoplasm of connective tissue of eyelid (C49.0)
malignant neoplasm of eyelid (skin) (C43.1-, C44.1-)
malignant neoplasm of optic nerve (C72.3-)

C69.2 Malignant neoplasm of retina
Excludes1: dark area on retina (D49.81)
neoplasm of unspecified behavior of retina and choroid (D49.81)
retinal freckle (D49.81)
C69.21 Malignant neoplasm of right retina
C69.22 Malignant neoplasm of left retina

C71 MALIGNANT NEOPLASM OF BRAIN

Excludes1: malignant neoplasm of cranial nerves (C72.2-C72.5)
retrobulbar malignant neoplasm (C69.6-)

C71.0 Malignant neoplasm of; cerebrum, except lobes and ventricles
Malignant neoplasm of supratentorial NOS
C71.1 frontal lobe
C71.2 temporal lobe
C71.3 parietal lobe
C71.4 occipital lobe
C71.5 cerebral ventricle
Excludes1: malignant neoplasm of fourth cerebral ventricle (C71.7)
C71.6 cerebellum
C71.7 brain stem
Malignant neoplasm of fourth cerebral ventricle
Infratentorial malignant neoplasm NOS
C71.8 overlapping sites of brain
C71.9 brain, unspecified

(C73–C75) MALIGNANT NEOPLASMS OF THYROID AND OTHER ENDOCRINE GLANDS

C74 MALIGNANT NEOPLASM OF ADRENAL GLAND

C74.0 Malignant neoplasm of cortex of; adrenal gland
C74.01 right adrenal gland
C74.02 left adrenal gland
C74.1 Malignant neoplasm of medulla of; adrenal gland
C74.11 right adrenal gland
C74.12 left adrenal gland
C74.9 Malignant neoplasm of unspecified part of; adrenal gland
C74.91 right adrenal gland
C74.92 left adrenal gland

(C7A) MALIGNANT NEUROENDOCRINE TUMORS

(C7B) SECONDARY NEUROENDOCRINE TUMORS

(C76–C80) MALIGNANT NEOPLASMS OF ILL-DEFINED, OTHER SECONDARY AND UNSPECIFIED SITES

C80 MALIGNANT NEOPLASM WITHOUT SPECIFICATION OF SITE

Excludes1: malignant carcinoid tumor of unspecified site (C7A.00)
malignant neoplasm of specified multiple sites- code to each site

C80.0 Disseminated malignant neoplasm, unspecified

GUIDELINES

Use only in those cases where the patient has advanced metastatic disease and no known primary or secondary sites are specified. It should be used in place of assigning codes for the primary site and all known secondary sites.

Carcinomatosis NOS
Generalized cancer, unspecified site (primary) (secondary)
Generalized malignancy, unspecified site (primary) (secondary)

C80.1 Malignant (primary) neoplasm, unspecified

GUIDELINES

Equates to Cancer, unspecified. Use only when no determination can be made as to the primary site of a malignancy. This code should rarely be used in the inpatient setting.

Cancer NOS
Cancer unspecified site (primary)
Carcinoma unspecified site (primary)
Malignancy unspecified (primary)
Excludes1: secondary malignant neoplasm of unspecified site (C79.9)

C80.2 Malignant neoplasm associated with transplanted organ
Code first complication of transplanted organ (T86.-)
Use additional **code** to identify the specific malignancy

(C81–C96) MALIGNANT NEOPLASMS OF LYMPHOID, HEMATOPOIETIC AND RELATED TISSUE

Excludes2: Kaposi's sarcoma of lymph nodes (C46.3)
secondary and unspecified neoplasm of lymph nodes (C77.-)
secondary neoplasm of bone marrow (C79.52)
secondary neoplasm of spleen (C78.89)

C81 HODGKIN LYMPHOMA

Excludes1: personal history of Hodgkin lymphoma (Z85.71)

C81.0 Nodular lymphocyte predominant Hodgkin lymphoma;

Code	Description
C81.00	unspecified site
C81.01	lymph nodes of head, face, and neck
C81.02	intrathoracic lymph nodes
C81.03	intra-abdominal lymph nodes
C81.04	lymph nodes of axilla and upper limb
C81.05	lymph nodes of inguinal region and lower limb
C81.06	intrapelvic lymph nodes
C81.07	spleen
C81.08	lymph nodes of multiple sites
C81.09	extranodal and solid organ sites
•C81.0A	Nodular lymphocyte predominant Hodgkin lymphoma, in remission

C81.1 Nodular sclerosis Hodgkin lymphoma
Nodular sclerosis classical Hodgkin lymphoma

C81.10	Nodular sclerosis Hodgkin lymphoma, unspecified site
C81.11	lymph nodes of head, face, and neck
C81.12	intrathoracic lymph nodes
C81.13	intra-abdominal lymph nodes
C81.14	lymph nodes of axilla and upper limb
C81.15	lymph nodes of inguinal region and lower limb
C81.16	intrapelvic lymph nodes
C81.17	spleen
C81.18	lymph nodes of multiple sites
C81.19	extranodal and solid organ sites
•C81.1A	Nodular sclerosis Hodgkin lymphoma, in remission

C81.2 Mixed cellularity Hodgkin lymphoma
Mixed cellularity classical Hodgkin lymphoma

C81.20	Mixed cellularity Hodgkin lymphoma, unspecified site
C81.21	lymph nodes of head, face, and neck
C81.22	intrathoracic lymph nodes
C81.23	intra-abdominal lymph nodes
C81.24	lymph nodes of axilla and upper limb
C81.25	lymph nodes of inguinal region and lower limb
C81.26	intrapelvic lymph nodes
C81.27	spleen
C81.28	lymph nodes of multiple sites
C81.29	extranodal and solid organ sites
•C81.2A	Mixed cellularity Hodgkin lymphoma, in remission

C81.3 Lymphocyte depleted Hodgkin lymphoma

Code	Description
•C81.3A	Lymphocyte depleted Hodgkin lymphoma, in remission

C81.9 Hodgkin lymphoma, unspecified

Code	Description
C81.91	Hodgkin lymphoma, unspecified; lymph nodes of head, face, and neck
C81.92	intrathoracic lymph nodes
C81.93	intra-abdominal lymph nodes
C81.94	lymph nodes of axilla and upper limb
C81.95	lymph nodes of inguinal region and lower limb
C81.96	intrapelvic lymph nodes
C81.97	spleen
C81.98	lymph nodes of multiple sites
C81.99	extranodal and solid organ sites
•C81.9A	Hodgkin lymphoma, unspecified, in remission

C82 FOLLICULAR LYMPHOMA

Includes: follicular lymphoma with or without diffuse areas
Excludes1: mature T/NK-cell lymphomas (C84.-)
personal history of non-Hodgkin lymphoma (Z85.72)

C82.0 Follicular lymphoma grade I

Code	Description
C82.00	Follicular lymphoma grade I, unspecified site
C82.01	lymph nodes of head, face, and neck
C82.02	intrathoracic lymph nodes
C82.03	intra-abdominal lymph nodes
C82.04	lymph nodes of axilla and upper limb
C82.05	lymph nodes of inguinal region and lower limb
C82.06	intrapelvic lymph nodes
C82.07	spleen
C82.08	lymph nodes of multiple sites
C82.09	extranodal and solid organ sites
•C82.0A	Follicular lymphoma grade I, in remission

C82.1 Follicular lymphoma grade II

Code	Description
C82.10	Follicular lymphoma grade II, unspecified site
C82.11	lymph nodes of head, face, and neck
C82.12	intrathoracic lymph nodes
C82.13	intra-abdominal lymph nodes
C82.14	lymph nodes of axilla and upper limb
C82.15	lymph nodes of inguinal region and lower limb
C82.16	intrapelvic lymph nodes
C82.17	spleen
C82.18	lymph nodes of multiple sites
C82.19	extranodal and solid organ sites
•C82.1A	Follicular lymphoma grade II, in remission

C82.2 Follicular lymphoma grade III, unspecified

Code	Description
C82.20	Follicular lymphoma grade III, unspecified, unspecified site
C82.21	lymph nodes of head, face, and neck
C82.22	unspecified, intrathoracic lymph nodes
C82.23	intra-abdominal lymph nodes
C82.24	lymph nodes of axilla and upper limb
C82.25	lymph nodes of inguinal region and lower limb
C82.26	intrapelvic lymph nodes
C82.27	spleen
C82.28	lymph nodes of multiple sites
C82.29	extranodal and solid organ sites
•C82.2A	Follicular lymphoma grade III, unspecified, in remission

C82.3 Follicular lymphoma grade IIIa

Code	Description
C82.30	Follicular lymphoma grade IIIa, unspecified site
C82.31	lymph nodes of head, face, and neck
C82.32	intrathoracic lymph nodes
C82.33	intra-abdominal lymph nodes
C82.34	lymph nodes of axilla and upper limb
C82.35	lymph nodes of inguinal region and lower limb
C82.36	intrapelvic lymph nodes
C82.37	spleen
C82.38	lymph nodes of multiple sites
C82.39	extranodal and solid organ sites

- **C82.3A** Follicular lymphoma grade IIIa, in remission
- **C82.4** Follicular lymphoma grade IIIb
  - **C82.40** Follicular lymphoma grade IIIb, unspecified site
  - **C82.41** lymph nodes of head, face, and neck
  - **C82.42** intrathoracic lymph nodes
  - **C82.43** intra-abdominal lymph nodes
  - **C82.44** lymph nodes of axilla and upper limb
  - **C82.45** lymph nodes of inguinal region and lower limb
  - **C82.46** intrapelvic lymph nodes
  - **C82.47** spleen
  - **C82.48** lymph nodes of multiple sites
  - **C82.49** extranodal and solid organ sites
  - **C82.4A** Follicular lymphoma grade IIIb, in remission
- **C82.5** Diffuse follicle center lymphoma
  - **C82.50** Diffuse follicle center lymphoma, unspecified site
  - **C82.51** lymph nodes of head, face, and neck
  - **C82.52** intrathoracic lymph nodes
  - **C82.53** intra-abdominal lymph nodes
  - **C82.54** lymph nodes of axilla and upper limb
  - **C82.55** lymph nodes of inguinal region and lower limb
  - **C82.56** intrapelvic lymph nodes
  - **C82.57** spleen
  - **C82.58** lymph nodes of multiple sites
  - **C82.59** extranodal and solid organ sites
  - **C82.5A** Diffuse follicle center lymphoma, in remission
- **C82.6** Cutaneous follicle center lymphoma
  - **C82.60** Cutaneous follicle center lymphoma, unspecified site
  - **C82.61** lymph nodes of head, face, and neck
  - **C82.62** intrathoracic lymph nodes
  - **C82.63** intra-abdominal lymph nodes
  - **C82.64** lymph nodes of axilla and upper limb
  - **C82.65** lymph nodes of inguinal region and lower limb
  - **C82.66** intrapelvic lymph nodes
  - **C82.67** spleen
  - **C82.68** lymph nodes of multiple sites
  - **C82.69** extranodal and solid organ sites
  - **C82.6A** Cutaneous follicle center lymphoma, in remission
- **C82.8** Other types of follicular lymphoma
  - **C82.80** Other types of follicular lymphoma, unspecified site
  - **C82.81** lymph nodes of head, face, and neck
  - **C82.82** intrathoracic lymph nodes
  - **C82.83** intra-abdominal lymph nodes
  - **C82.84** lymph nodes of axilla and upper limb
  - **C82.85** lymph nodes of inguinal region and lower limb
  - **C82.86** intrapelvic lymph nodes
  - **C82.87** spleen
  - **C82.88** lymph nodes of multiple sites
  - **C82.89** extranodal and solid organ sites
  - **C82.8A** Other types of follicular lymphoma, in remission
- **C82.9** Follicular lymphoma, unspecified
  - **C82.90** Follicular lymphoma, unspecified, unspecified site
  - **C82.91** lymph nodes of head, face, and neck
  - **C82.92** intrathoracic lymph nodes
  - **C82.93** intra-abdominal lymph nodes
  - **C82.94** lymph nodes of axilla and upper limb
  - **C82.95** lymph nodes of inguinal region and lower limb
  - **C82.96** intrapelvic lymph nodes
  - **C82.97** spleen
  - **C82.98** lymph nodes of multiple sites
  - **C82.99** extranodal and solid organ sites
  - **C82.9A** Follicular lymphoma, unspecified, in remission

C83 NON-FOLLICULAR LYMPHOMA

Excludes1: personal history of non-Hodgkin lymphoma (Z85.72)

- **C83.0** Small cell B-cell lymphoma
  - *Excludes1:* Waldenstrom macroglobulinemia (C88.00)
  - **C83.0A** Small cell B-cell lymphoma, in remission
- **C83.3** Diffuse large B-cell lymphoma
  - Anaplastic diffuse large B-cell lymphoma
  - CD30-positive diffuse large B-cell lymphoma
  - Centroblastic diffuse large B-cell lymphoma
  - Immunoblastic diffuse large B-cell lymphoma
  - Plasmablastic diffuse large B-cell lymphoma

Diffuse large B-cell lymphoma, subtype not specified

T-cell rich diffuse large B-cell lymphoma

Excludes1: mediastinal (thymic) large B-cell lymphoma (C85.2-) mature T/NK-cell lymphomas (C84.-)

- **C83.30** Diffuse large B-cell lymphoma; unspecified site
- **C83.31** lymph nodes of head, face, and neck
- **C83.32** intrathoracic lymph nodes
- **C83.33** intra-abdominal lymph nodes
- **C83.34** lymph nodes of axilla and upper limb
- **C83.35** lymph nodes of inguinal region and lower limb
- **C83.36** intrapelvic lymph nodes
- **C83.37** spleen
- **C83.38** lymph nodes of multiple sites
- **C83.39** extranodal and solid organ sites
- **C83.390** Primary central nervous system lymphoma
  - PCNSL of brain
  - PCNSL of meninges
  - PCNSL of spinal cord
  - PCNSL NOS
  - *Excludes1:* primary central nervous system lymphoma, Burkitt (C83.79)
  - primary central nervous system lymphoma, lymphoblastic (C83.59)
  - primary central nervous system lymphoma, other (C83.89)
  - primary central nervous system lymphoma, peripheral T-cell (C84.49)
- **C83.398** Diffuse large B-cell lymphoma of other extranodal and solid organ sites
- **C83.3A** Diffuse large B-cell lymphoma, in remission
- **C83.5** Lymphoblastic (diffuse) lymphoma
  - **C83.5A** Lymphoblastic (diffuse) lymphoma, in remission
- **C83.7** Burkitt lymphoma
  - Atypical Burkitt lymphoma
  - Burkitt-like lymphoma
  - *Excludes1:* mature B-cell leukemia Burkitt type (C91.A-)
  - **C83.70** Burkitt lymphoma, unspecified site
  - **C83.71** Burkitt lymphoma, lymph nodes of head, face, and neck
  - **C83.72** Burkitt lymphoma, intrathoracic lymph nodes
  - **C83.73** Burkitt lymphoma, intra-abdominal lymph nodes
  - **C83.74** Burkitt lymphoma, lymph nodes of axilla and upper limb
  - **C83.75** Burkitt lymphoma, lymph nodes of inguinal region and lower limb
  - **C83.76** Burkitt lymphoma, intrapelvic lymph nodes
  - **C83.77** Burkitt lymphoma, spleen
  - **C83.78** Burkitt lymphoma, lymph nodes of multiple sites
  - **C83.79** Burkitt lymphoma, extranodal and solid organ sites
  - **C83.7A** Burkitt lymphoma, in remission
- **C83.8** Other non-follicular lymphoma
  - **C83.8A** Other non-follicular lymphoma, in remission
- **C83.9** Non-follicular (diffuse) lymphoma, unspecified
  - **C83.9A** Non-follicular (diffuse) lymphoma, unspecified, in remission

C84 MATURE T/NK-CELL LYMPHOMAS

Excludes1: personal history of non-Hodgkin lymphoma (Z85.72)

- **C84.0** Mycosis fungoides
  - **C84.0A** Mycosis fungoides, in remission
- **C84.4** Peripheral T-cell lymphoma, not elsewhere classified
  - Lennert's lymphoma
  - Lymphoepithelioid lymphoma
  - Mature T-cell lymphoma, not elsewhere classified
  - **C84.41** Peripheral T-cell lymphoma, not elsewhere classified; lymph nodes of head, face, and neck
  - **C84.42** intrathoracic lymph nodes
  - **C84.43** intra-abdominal lymph nodes
  - **C84.44** lymph nodes of axilla and upper limb
  - **C84.45** lymph nodes of inguinal region and lower limb
  - **C84.46** intrapelvic lymph nodes
  - **C84.47** spleen
  - **C84.48** lymph nodes of multiple sites

C84.49 extranodal and solid organ sites

•C84.4A Peripheral T-cell lymphoma, not elsewhere classified, in remission

C84.6 Anaplastic large cell lymphoma, ALK-positive

•C84.6A Anaplastic large cell lymphoma, ALK-positive, in remission

C84.Z Other mature T/NK-cell lymphomas

Excludes1: angioimmunoblastic T-cell lymphoma (C86.50)
blastic NK-cell lymphoma (C86.40)
enteropathy-type T-cell lymphoma (C86.20)
extranodal NK-cell lymphoma, nasal type (C86.00)
hepatosplenic T-cell lymphoma (C86.10)
primary cutaneous CD30-positive T-cell proliferations (C86.60)
subcutaneous panniculitis-like T-cell lymphoma (C86.30)

•C84.ZA Other mature T/NK-cell lymphomas, in remission

C85 OTHER SPECIFIED AND UNSPECIFIED TYPES OF NON-HODGKIN LYMPHOMA

Excludes1: other specified types of T/NK-cell lymphoma (C86.-)
personal history of non-Hodgkin lymphoma (Z85.72)

C85.9 Non-Hodgkin lymphoma, unspecified

5th Lymphoma NOS
Malignant lymphoma NOS
Non-Hodgkin lymphoma NOS

C85.90 Non-Hodgkin lymphoma, unspecified, unspecified site

C85.91 Non-Hodgkin lymphoma, unspecified; lymph nodes of head, face, and neck

- **C85.92 intrathoracic lymph nodes**
- **C85.93 intra-abdominal lymph nodes**
- **C85.94 lymph nodes of axilla and upper limb**
- **C85.95 lymph nodes of inguinal region and lower limb**
- **C85.96 intrapelvic lymph nodes**
- **C85.97 spleen**
- **C85.98 lymph nodes of multiple sites**
- **C85.99 extranodal and solid organ sites**

•C85.9A Non-Hodgkin lymphoma, unspecified, in remission

C86 OTHER SPECIFIED TYPES OF T/NK-CELL LYMPHOMA

Excludes1: anaplastic large cell lymphoma, ALK negative (C84.7-)
anaplastic large cell lymphoma, ALK positive (C84.6-)
mature T/NK-cell lymphomas (C84.-)
other specified types of non-Hodgkin lymphoma (C85.8-)

C86.1 Hepatosplenic T-cell lymphoma

Alpha-beta and gamma delta types

•C86.10 Hepatosplenic T-cell lymphoma not having achieved remission

Hepatosplenic T-cell lymphoma NOS
Hepatosplenic T-cell lymphoma with failed remission

•C86.11 Hepatosplenic T-cell lymphoma, in remission

C88 MALIGNANT IMMUNOPROLIFERATIVE DISEASES AND CERTAIN OTHER B-CELL LYMPHOMAS

Excludes1: B-cell lymphoma, unspecified (C85.1-)
personal history of other malignant neoplasms of lymphoid,
hematopoietic and related tissues (Z85.79)

C88.2 Heavy chain disease

Franklin disease
Gamma heavy chain disease
Mu heavy chain disease

•C88.20 Heavy chain disease not having achieved remission

Franklin disease NOS
Franklin disease not having achieved remission
Franklin disease with failed remission
Gamma heavy chain disease NOS
Gamma heavy chain disease not having achieved remission
Gamma heavy chain disease with failed remission
Heavy chain disease NOS
Heavy chain disease with failed remission
Mu heavy chain disease not having achieved remission
Mu heavy chain disease NOS
Mu heavy chain disease not having achieved remission
Mu heavy chain disease with failed remission

•C88.21 Heavy chain disease, in remission

C91 LYMPHOID LEUKEMIA

Excludes1: personal history of leukemia (Z85.6)

C91.0 Acute lymphoblastic leukemia [ALL]

5th **Note:** Codes in subcategory C91.0- should only be used for T-cell and B-cell precursor leukemia

C91.00 ALL, not having achieved remission

ALL with failed remission
ALL NOS

- **C91.01 ALL, in remission**
- **C91.02 ALL, in relapse**

C91.9 Lymphoid leukemia, unspecified

5th **C91.90 Lymphoid leukemia, unspecified; not having achieved remission**

Lymphoid leukemia with failed remission
Lymphoid leukemia NOS

- **C91.91 in remission**
- **C91.92 in relapse**

C92 MYELOID LEUKEMIA

Includes: granulocytic leukemia
myelogenous leukemia

Code also, if applicable, pancytopenia (acquired) (D61.818)

Excludes1: personal history of leukemia (Z85.6)

C92.0 Acute myeloblastic leukemia

5th Acute myeloblastic leukemia, minimal differentiation
Acute myeloblastic leukemia (with maturation)
Acute myeloblastic leukemia 1/ETO
Acute myeloblastic leukemia M0 or M1 or M2
Acute myeloblastic leukemia with t(8;21)
Acute myeloblastic leukemia (without a FAB classification) NOS
Refractory anemia with excess blasts in transformation [RAEB T]

Excludes1: acute exacerbation of chronic myeloid leukemia (C92.10)
refractory anemia with excess of blasts not in transformation (D46.2-)

C92.00 Acute myeloblastic leukemia; not having achieved remission

Acute myeloblastic leukemia with failed remission
Acute myeloblastic leukemia NOS

- **C92.01 in remission**
- **C92.02 in relapse**

C92.1 Chronic myeloid leukemia, BCR/ABL-positive

5th Chronic myelogenous leukemia, Philadelphia chromosome (Ph1) positive
Chronic myelogenous leukemia, t(9;22) (q34:q11)
Chronic myelogenous leukemia with crisis of blast cells

Excludes1: atypical chronic myeloid leukemia BCR/ABL-negative (C92.2-)
CMML (C93.1-)
chronic myeloproliferative disease (D47.1)

C92.10 Chronic myeloid leukemia, BCR/ABL-positive; not having achieved remission

Chronic myeloid leukemia, BCR/ABL-positive with failed remission
Chronic myeloid leukemia, BCR/ABL-positive NOS

- **C92.11 in remission**
- **C92.12 in relapse**

C92.2 Atypical chronic myeloid leukemia, BCR/ABL-negative

5th **C92.20 Atypical chronic myeloid leukemia, BCR/ABL-negative; not having achieved remission**

Atypical chronic myeloid leukemia, BCR/ABL-negative with failed remission
Atypical chronic myeloid leukemia, BCR/ABL-negative NOS

- **C92.21 in remission**
- **C92.22 in relapse**

C92.9 Myeloid leukemia, unspecified

5th **C92.90 Myeloid leukemia, unspecified; not having achieved remission**

Myeloid leukemia, unspecified with failed remission
Myeloid leukemia, unspecified NOS

- **C92.91 in remission**
- **C92.92 unspecified in relapse**

C93 MONOCYTIC LEUKEMIA

Includes: monocytoid leukemia
Excludes1: personal history of leukemia (Z85.6)

C93.0 Acute monoblastic/monocytic leukemia

AML M5 or AML M5a or AML M5b

C93.00 Acute monoblastic/monocytic leukemia; not having achieved remission

Acute monoblastic/monocytic leukemia with failed remission

Acute monoblastic/monocytic leukemia NOS

- **C93.01** in remission
- **C93.02** in relapse

C93.1 Chronic myelomonocytic leukemia [CMML]

Chronic monocytic leukemia

CMML-1 or CMML-2

CMML with eosinophilia

Code also, if applicable, eosinophilia (D72.18)

C93.10 CMML not having achieved remission

CMML with failed remission

CMML NOS

- **C93.11** CMML, in remission
- **C93.12** CMML, in relapse

C93.3 Juvenile myelomonocytic leukemia

C93.30 Juvenile myelomonocytic leukemia; not having achieved remission

Juvenile myelomonocytic leukemia with failed remission

Juvenile myelomonocytic leukemia NOS

- **C93.31** in remission
- **C93.32** in relapse

C93.Z Other monocytic leukemia

C93.Z0 Other monocytic leukemia; not having achieved remission

Other monocytic leukemia NOS

- **C93.Z1** in remission
- **C93.Z2** in relapse

C93.9 Monocytic leukemia, unspecified

C93.90 Monocytic leukemia, unspecified; not having achieved remission

Monocytic leukemia, unspecified with failed remission

leukemia, unspecified NOS

- **C93.91** in remission
- **C93.92** in relapse

C94 OTHER LEUKEMIAS OF SPECIFIED CELL TYPE

Excludes1: leukemic reticuloendotheliosis (C91.4-)

myelodysplastic syndromes (D46.-)

personal history of leukemia (Z85.6)

plasma cell leukemia (C90.1-)

C94.0 Acute erythroid leukemia

Acute myeloid leukemia M6(a)(b)

Erythroleukemia

C94.00 Acute erythroid leukemia, not having achieved remission

Acute erythroid leukemia with failed remission

Acute erythroid leukemia NOS

- **C94.01** Acute erythroid leukemia, in remission
- **C94.02** Acute erythroid leukemia, in relapse

C94.3 Mast cell leukemia

C94.30 Mast cell leukemia not having achieved remission

Mast cell leukemia with failed remission

Mast cell leukemia NOS

- **C94.31** Mast cell leukemia, in remission
- **C94.32** Mast cell leukemia, in relapse

C95 LEUKEMIA OF UNSPECIFIED CELL TYPE

Excludes1: personal history of leukemia (Z85.6)

C95.9 Leukemia, unspecified

C95.90 Leukemia, unspecified not having achieved remission

Leukemia, unspecified with failed remission

Leukemia NOS

- **C95.91** Leukemia, unspecified, in remission
- **C95.92** Leukemia, unspecified, in relapse

C96 OTHER AND UNSPECIFIED MALIGNANT NEOPLASMS OF LYMPHOID, HEMATOPOIETIC AND RELATED TISSUE

Excludes1: personal history of other malignant neoplasms of lymphoid, hematopoietic and related tissues (Z85.79)

C96.2 Malignant mast cell neoplasm

Excludes1: indolent mastocytosis (D47.02)

mast cell leukemia (C94.30)

mastocytosis (congenital) (cutaneous) (Q82.2)

- **C96.20** Malignant mast cell neoplasm, unspecified
- **C96.21** Aggressive systemic mastocytosis
- **C96.22** Mast cell sarcoma
- **C96.29** Other malignant mast cell neoplasm

C96.A Histiocytic sarcoma

Malignant histiocytosis

(D00–D09) IN SITU NEOPLASMS

Includes: Bowen's disease

erythroplasia

grade III intraepithelial neoplasia

Queyrat's erythroplasia

(D10–D36) BENIGN NEOPLASMS, EXCEPT BENIGN NEUROENDOCRINE TUMORS

D12 BENIGN NEOPLASM OF COLON, RECTUM, ANUS AND ANAL CANAL

Excludes2: benign carcinoid tumors of the large intestine and rectum (D3A.02-)

polyp of colon NOS (K63.5)

- **D12.0** Benign neoplasm of; cecum
  Benign neoplasm of ileocecal valve
- **D12.1** **appendix**
  Excludes1: benign carcinoid tumor of the appendix (D3A.020)
- **D12.2** **ascending colon**
- **D12.3** **transverse colon**
  Benign neoplasm of hepatic flexure or splenic flexure
- **D12.4** **descending colon**
- **D12.5** **sigmoid colon**
- **D12.6** **colon, unspecified**
  Adenomatosis of colon
  Benign neoplasm of large intestine NOS
  Polyposis (hereditary) of colon
  Excludes1: inflammatory polyp of colon (K51.4-)
- **D12.7** **rectosigmoid junction**
- **D12.8** **rectum**
  Excludes1: benign carcinoid tumor of the rectum (D3A.026)
- **D12.9** Benign neoplasm of anus and anal canal
  Benign neoplasm of anus NOS
  Excludes1: benign neoplasm of anal margin (D22.5, D23.5)
  benign neoplasm of anal skin (D22.5, D23.5)
  benign neoplasm of perianal skin (D22.5, D23.5)

D15 BENIGN NEOPLASM OF OTHER AND UNSPECIFIED INTRATHORACIC ORGANS

Excludes1: benign neoplasm of mesothelial tissue (D19.-)

D15.1 Benign neoplasm of heart

Excludes1: benign neoplasm of great vessels (D21.3)

D17 BENIGN LIPOMATOUS NEOPLASM

- **D17.0** Benign lipomatous neoplasm of skin and subcutaneous tissue of; head, face and neck
- **D17.1** trunk
- **D17.2** Benign lipomatous neoplasm of skin and subcutaneous tissue of; limb
  - **D17.21** right arm
  - **D17.22** left arm
  - **D17.23** right leg
  - **D17.24** left leg
- **D17.3** Benign lipomatous neoplasm of skin and subcutaneous tissue of; other and unspecified sites
  - **D17.30** unspecified sites
  - **D17.39** other sites
- **D17.4** Benign lipomatous neoplasm of intrathoracic organs

D17.5 Benign lipomatous neoplasm of intra-abdominal organs
Excludes1: benign lipomatous neoplasm of peritoneum and retroperitoneum (D17.79)

D17.6 Benign lipomatous neoplasm of spermatic cord

D17.7 Benign lipomatous neoplasm of other sites
- D17.71 Benign lipomatous neoplasm of; kidney
- D17.72 other genitourinary organ
- D17.79 other sites
  - Benign lipomatous neoplasm of peritoneum or retroperitoneum

D17.9 Benign lipomatous neoplasm, unspecified
Lipoma NOS

D18 HEMANGIOMA AND LYMPHANGIOMA, ANY SITE

Excludes1: benign neoplasm of glomus jugulare (D35.6)
blue or pigmented nevus (D22.-)
nevus NOS (D22.-)
vascular nevus (Q82.5)

D18.0 Hemangioma
- Angioma NOS
- Cavernous nevus
- D18.00 Hemangioma unspecified site
- D18.01 Hemangioma of skin and subcutaneous tissue
- D18.02 Hemangioma of intracranial structures
- D18.03 Hemangioma of intra-abdominal structures
- D18.09 Hemangioma of other sites

D18.1 Lymphangioma, any site

D22 MELANOCYTIC NEVI

Includes: atypical nevus
blue hairy pigmented nevus
nevus NOS

D22.0 Melanocytic nevi of lip

D22.1 Melanocytic nevi of eyelid, including canthus
- D22.10 Melanocytic nevi of unspecified eyelid, including canthus
- D22.11 Melanocytic nevi of right eyelid, including canthus
  - D22.111 Melanocytic nevi of right upper eyelid, including canthus
  - D22.112 Melanocytic nevi of right lower eyelid, including canthus
- D22.12 Melanocytic nevi of left eyelid, including canthus
  - D22.121 Melanocytic nevi of left upper eyelid, including canthus
  - D22.122 Melanocytic nevi of left lower eyelid, including canthus

D22.2 Melanocytic nevi of ear and external auricular canal
- D22.21 Melanocytic nevi of right ear and external auricular canal
- D22.22 Melanocytic nevi of left ear and external auricular canal

D22.3 Melanocytic nevi of other and unspecified parts of face
- D22.30 Melanocytic nevi of unspecified part of face
- D22.39 Melanocytic nevi of other parts of face

D22.4 Melanocytic nevi of scalp and neck

D22.5 Melanocytic nevi of trunk
Melanocytic nevi of anal margin
Melanocytic nevi of anal skin
Melanocytic nevi of perianal skin
Melanocytic nevi of skin of breast

D22.6 Melanocytic nevi of upper limb, including shoulder
- D22.61 Melanocytic nevi of right upper limb, including shoulder
- D22.62 Melanocytic nevi of left upper limb, including shoulder

D22.7 Melanocytic nevi of lower limb, including hip
- D22.71 Melanocytic nevi of right lower limb, including hip
- D22.72 Melanocytic nevi of left lower limb, including hip

D22.9 Melanocytic nevi, unspecified

D23 OTHER BENIGN NEOPLASMS OF SKIN

Includes: benign neoplasm of hair follicles or sebaceous glands or sweat glands

Excludes1: benign lipomatous neoplasms of skin (D17.0-D17.3)
Excludes 2: melanocytic nevi (D22.-)

D23.0 Other benign neoplasm of skin of lip
Excludes1: benign neoplasm of vermilion border of lip (D10.0)

D23.1 Other benign neoplasm of skin of; eyelid, including canthus
- D23.11 right eyelid, including canthus
  - D23.111 Other benign neoplasm of skin of right upper eyelid, including canthus
  - D23.112 Other benign neoplasm of skin of right lower eyelid, including canthus
- D23.12 left eyelid, including canthus
  - D23.121 Other benign neoplasm of skin of left upper eyelid, including canthus
  - D23.122 Other benign neoplasm of skin of left lower eyelid, including canthus

D23.2 Other benign neoplasm of skin of; ear and external auricular canal
- D23.21 right ear and external auricular canal
- D23.22 left ear and external auricular canal

D23.3 Other benign neoplasm of skin of; other and unspecified parts of face
- D23.30 unspecified part of face
- D23.39 other parts of face

D23.4 Other benign neoplasm of skin of scalp and neck

D23.5 Other benign neoplasm of skin of trunk
Other benign neoplasm of anal margin or anal skin or perianal skin
Other benign neoplasm of skin of breast
Excludes1: benign neoplasm of anus NOS (D12.9)

D23.6 Other benign neoplasm of skin of; upper limb, including shoulder
- D23.61 right upper limb, including shoulder
- D23.62 left upper limb, including shoulder

D23.7 Other benign neoplasm of skin of; lower limb, including hip
- D23.71 right lower limb, including hip
- D23.72 left lower limb, including hip

D23.9 Other benign neoplasm of skin, unspecified

D24 BENIGN NEOPLASM OF BREAST

Includes: benign neoplasm of connective tissue of breast
benign neoplasm of soft parts of breast
fibroadenoma of breast

Excludes2: adenofibrosis of breast (N60.2)
benign cyst of breast (N60.-)
benign mammary dysplasia (N60.-)
benign neoplasm of skin of breast (D22.5, D23.5)
fibrocystic disease of breast (N60.-)

D24.1 Benign neoplasm of right breast

D24.2 Benign neoplasm of left breast

(D3A) BENIGN NEUROENDOCRINE TUMORS

D3A BENIGN NEUROENDOCRINE TUMORS

Code also any associated multiple endocrine neoplasia [MEN] syndromes (E31.2-)

Use additional code to identify any associated endocrine syndrome, such as:
carcinoid syndrome (E34.00)

Excludes2: benign pancreatic islet cell tumors (D13.7)

D3A.0 Benign carcinoid tumors
- D3A.00 Benign carcinoid tumor of unspecified site
  Carcinoid tumor NOS
- D3A.01 Benign carcinoid tumors of the small intestine
  - D3A.010 Benign carcinoid tumor of the duodenum
  - D3A.011 Benign carcinoid tumor of the jejunum
  - D3A.012 Benign carcinoid tumor of the ileum
  - D3A.019 Benign carcinoid tumor of the small intestine, unspecified portion
- D3A.02 Benign carcinoid tumors of the appendix, large intestine, and rectum
  - D3A.020 Benign carcinoid tumor of the appendix
  - D3A.021 Benign carcinoid tumor of the cecum
  - D3A.022 Benign carcinoid tumor of the ascending colon
  - D3A.023 Benign carcinoid tumor of the transverse colon

D3A.024 Benign carcinoid tumor of the descending colon

D3A.025 Benign carcinoid tumor of the sigmoid colon

D3A.026 Benign carcinoid tumor of the rectum

D3A.029 Benign carcinoid tumor of the large intestine, unspecified portion

Benign carcinoid tumor of the colon NOS

D3A.09 Benign carcinoid tumors of other sites

6th D3A.090 Benign carcinoid tumor of the bronchus and lung

D3A.091 Benign carcinoid tumor of the thymus

D3A.092 Benign carcinoid tumor of the stomach

D3A.093 Benign carcinoid tumor of the kidney

D3A.094 Benign carcinoid tumor of the foregut, unspecified

D3A.095 Benign carcinoid tumor of the midgut, unspecified

D3A.096 Benign carcinoid tumor of the hindgut, unspecified

D3A.098 Benign carcinoid tumors of other sites

D3A.8 Other benign neuroendocrine tumors

Neuroendocrine tumor NOS

(D37–D48) NEOPLASMS OF UNCERTAIN BEHAVIOR, POLYCYTHEMIA VERA AND MYELODYSPLASTIC SYNDROMES

Note: Categories D37–D44, and D48 classify by site neoplasms of uncertain behavior, i.e., histologic confirmation whether the neoplasm is malignant or benign cannot be made.

Excludes1: neoplasms of unspecified behavior (D49.-)

D47 OTHER NEOPLASMS OF UNCERTAIN BEHAVIOR OF LYMPHOID, HEMATOPOIETIC AND RELATED TISSUE

D47.0 Mast cell neoplasms of uncertain behavior

5th *Excludes1:*

congenital cutaneous mastocytosis (Q82.2)

histiocytic neoplasms of uncertain behavior (D47.Z9)

malignant mast cell neoplasm (C96.2-)

D47.01 Cutaneous mastocytosis

Diffuse cutaneous mastocytosis

Maculopapular cutaneous mastocytosis

Solitary mastocytoma

Telangiectasia macularis eruptiva perstans

Urticaria pigmentosa

Excludes1: congenital (diffuse) (maculopapular) cutaneous mastocytosis (Q82.2)

congenital urticaria pigmentosa (Q82.2)

extracutaneous mastocytoma (D47.09)

D47.02 Systemic mastocytosis

Indolent systemic mastocytosis

Isolated bone marrow mastocytosis

Smoldering systemic mastocytosis

Systemic mastocytosis, with an associated hematological non-mast cell lineage disease (SM-AHNMD)

Code also, if applicable, any associated hematological non-mast cell lineage disease

Excludes1: aggressive systemic mastocytosis (C96.21) mast cell leukemia (C94.3-)

D47.09 Other mast cell neoplasms of uncertain behavior

Extracutaneous mastocytoma

Mast cell tumor NOS

Mastocytoma NOS

Mastocytosis NOS

Mastocytosis NOS

D47.3 Essential (hemorrhagic) thrombocythemia

Essential thrombocytosis

Idiopathic hemorrhagic thrombocythemia

Primary thrombocytosis

Excludes2: reactive thrombocytosis (D75.838)

secondary thrombocytosis (D75.838)

thrombocythemia NOS (D75.839)

thrombocytosis NOS (D75.839)

D47.Z Other specified neoplasms of uncertain behavior of lymphoid, hematopoietic and related tissue

5th

D47.Z1 Post-transplant lymphoproliferative disorder (PTLD)

Code first complications of transplanted organs and tissue (T86.-)

D47.Z9 Other specified neoplasms of uncertain behavior of lymphoid, hematopoietic and related tissue

Histiocytic tumors of uncertain behavior

Use for kaposiform lymphangiomatosis

D47.9 Neoplasm of uncertain behavior of lymphoid, hematopoietic and related tissue, unspecified

Lymphoproliferative disease NOS

(D49) NEOPLASMS OF UNSPECIFIED BEHAVIOR

D49 NEOPLASMS OF UNSPECIFIED BEHAVIOR

4th **Note:** Category D49 classifies by site neoplasms of unspecified morphology and behavior. *The term 'mass', unless otherwise stated, is not to be regarded as a neoplastic growth.*

Includes: 'growth' NOS or neoplasm NOS or new growth NOS or tumor NOS

Excludes1: neoplasms of uncertain behavior (D37–D44, D48)

D49.0 Neoplasm of unspecified behavior of; digestive system

Excludes1: neoplasm of unspecified behavior of margin of anus or perianal skin or skin of anus (D49.2)

D49.1 respiratory system

D49.2 bone, soft tissue, and skin

Excludes1: neoplasm of unspecified behavior of anal canal or anus NOS (D49.0)

bone marrow (D49.89)

cartilage of larynx or nose (D49.1)

connective tissue of breast (D49.3)

skin of genital organs (D49.59)

vermilion border of lip (D49.0)

D49.3 breast

Excludes1: neoplasm of unspecified behavior of skin of breast (D49.2)

D49.4 bladder

D49.5 other genitourinary organs

5th **D49.51 Neoplasm of unspecified behavior of kidney**

6th D49.511 right kidney

D49.512 left kidney

D49.59 Neoplasm unspecified behavior of other genitourinary organ

D49.6 brain

Excludes1: neoplasm of unspecified behavior of cerebral meninges (D49.7)

neoplasm of unspecified behavior of cranial nerves (D49.7)

D49.7 endocrine glands and other parts of nervous system

Excludes1: neoplasm of unspecified behavior of peripheral, sympathetic, and parasympathetic nerves and ganglia (D49.2)

D49.8 other specified sites

Excludes1: neoplasm of unspecified behavior of eyelid (skin) (D49.2)

D49.9 unspecified site

Chapter 3. Diseases of the blood and blood-forming organs and certain disorders involving the immune mechanism (D50–D89)

GUIDELINES

None currently. Reserved for future guideline expansion.
Excludes2: autoimmune disease (systemic) NOS (M35.9)
certain conditions originating in the perinatal period (P00–P96)
complications of pregnancy, childbirth and the puerperium (O00–O9A)
congenital malformations, deformations and chromosomal abnormalities (Q00–Q99)
endocrine, nutritional and metabolic diseases (E00–E88)
HIV disease (B20)
injury, poisoning and certain other consequences of external causes (S00–T88)
neoplasms (C00–D49)
symptoms, signs and abnormal clinical and laboratory findings, NEC (R00–R94)

(D50–D53) NUTRITIONAL ANEMIAS

D50 IRON DEFICIENCY ANEMIA

Includes: asiderotic anemia
hypochromic anemia

D50.0 Iron deficiency anemia secondary to blood loss (chronic)
Posthemorrhagic anemia (chronic)
Excludes1: acute posthemorrhagic anemia (D62)
congenital anemia from fetal blood loss (P61.3)

D50.1 Sideropenic dysphagia
Kelly-Paterson syndrome
Plummer-Vinson syndrome

D50.8 Other iron deficiency anemias
Iron deficiency anemia due to inadequate dietary iron intake

D50.9 Iron deficiency anemia, unspecified

D51 VITAMIN B12 DEFICIENCY ANEMIA

Excludes1: vitamin B12 deficiency (E53.8)

D51.0 Vitamin B12 deficiency anemia due to intrinsic factor deficiency
Addison anemia
Biermer anemia
Pernicious (congenital) anemia
Congenital intrinsic factor deficiency

D51.1 Vitamin B12 deficiency anemia due to selective vitamin B12 malabsorption with proteinuria
Imerslund (Gräsbeck) syndrome
Megaloblastic hereditary anemia

D51.2 Transcobalamin II deficiency

D51.3 Other dietary vitamin B12 deficiency anemia
Vegan anemia

D51.8 Other vitamin B12 deficiency anemias

D51.9 Vitamin B12 deficiency anemia, unspecified

D52 FOLATE DEFICIENCY ANEMIA

Excludes1: folate deficiency without anemia (E53.8)

D52.0 Dietary folate deficiency anemia
Nutritional megaloblastic anemia

D52.1 Drug-induced folate deficiency anemia
Use additional code for adverse effect, if applicable, to identify drug (T36–T50 with fifth or sixth character 5)

D52.8 Other folate deficiency anemias

D52.9 Folate deficiency anemia, unspecified
Folic acid deficiency anemia NOS

D53 OTHER NUTRITIONAL ANEMIAS

Includes: megaloblastic anemia unresponsive to vitamin B12 or folate therapy

D53.0 Protein deficiency anemia
Amino-acid deficiency anemia
Orotaciduric anemia
Excludes1: Lesch-Nyhan syndrome (E79.1)

D53.1 Other megaloblastic anemias, NEC
Megaloblastic anemia NOS
Excludes1: Di Guglielmo's disease (C94.0)

D53.2 Scorbutic anemia
Excludes1: scurvy (E54)

D53.8 Other specified nutritional anemias
Anemia associated with deficiency of copper
Anemia associated with deficiency of molybdenum
Anemia associated with deficiency of zinc
Excludes1: nutritional deficiencies without anemia, such as:
copper deficiency NOS (E61.0)
molybdenum deficiency NOS (E61.5)
zinc deficiency NOS (E60)

D53.9 Nutritional anemia, unspecified
Simple chronic anemia
Excludes1: anemia NOS (D64.9)

(D55–D59) HEMOLYTIC ANEMIAS

D55 ANEMIA DUE TO ENZYME DISORDERS

Excludes1: drug-induced enzyme deficiency anemia (D59.2)

D55.0 Anemia due to glucose-6-phosphate dehydrogenase [G6PD] deficiency
Excludes1: G6PD deficiency without anemia (D75.A)
Favism
G6PD deficiency anemia

D55.1 Anemia due to other disorders of glutathione metabolism
Anemia (due to) enzyme deficiencies, except G6PD, related to the hexose monophosphate [HMP] shunt pathway
Anemia (due to) hemolytic nonspherocytic (hereditary), type I

D55.2 Anemia due to disorders of glycolytic enzymes
Excludes1: disorders of glycolysis not associated with anemia (E74.81-)

D55.21 Anemia due to pyruvate kinase deficiency
PK deficiency anemia
Pyruvate kinase deficiency anemia

D55.29 Anemia due to other disorders of glycolytic enzymes
Hexokinase deficiency anemia
Triose-phosphate isomerase deficiency anemia

D55.3 Anemia due to disorders of nucleotide metabolism

D55.8 Other anemias due to enzyme disorders

D55.9 Anemia due to enzyme disorder, unspecified

D56 THALASSEMIA

Excludes1: sickle-cell thalassemia (D57.4-)

D56.0 Alpha thalassemia
Alpha thalassemia major
Hemoglobin H Constant Spring
Hemoglobin H disease
Hydrops fetalis due to alpha thalassemia
Severe alpha thalassemia
Triple gene defect alpha thalassemia
Use additional code, if applicable, for hydrops fetalis due to alpha thalassemia (P56.99)
Excludes1: alpha thalassemia trait or minor (D56.3)
asymptomatic alpha thalassemia (D56.3)
hydrops fetalis due to isoimmunization (P56.0)
hydrops fetalis not due to immune hemolysis (P83.2)

D56.1 Beta thalassemia
Beta thalassemia major
Cooley's anemia
Homozygous beta thalassemia
Severe beta thalassemia
Thalassemia intermedia
Thalassemia major
Excludes1: beta thalassemia minor (D56.3)
beta thalassemia trait (D56.3)
delta-beta thalassemia (D56.2)
hemoglobin E-beta thalassemia (D56.5)
sickle-cell beta thalassemia (D57.4-)

D56.2 Delta-beta thalassemia
Homozygous delta-beta thalassemia
Excludes1: delta-beta thalassemia minor (D56.3)
delta-beta thalassemia trait (D56.3)

D56.3 Thalassemia minor
Alpha thalassemia minor
Alpha thalassemia silent carrier
Alpha thalassemia trait
Beta thalassemia minor
Beta thalassemia trait
Delta-beta thalassemia minor
Delta-beta thalassemia trait
Thalassemia trait NOS
Excludes1: alpha thalassemia (D56.0)
beta thalassemia (D56.1)
delta-beta thalassemia (D56.2)
hemoglobin E-beta thalassemia (D56.5)
sickle-cell trait (D57.3)

D56.4 Hereditary persistence of fetal hemoglobin [HPFH]

D56.5 Hemoglobin E-beta thalassemia
Excludes1: beta thalassemia (D56.1)
beta thalassemia minor (D56.3)
beta thalassemia trait (D56.3)
delta-beta thalassemia (D56.2)
delta-beta thalassemia trait (D56.3)
hemoglobin E disease (D58.2)
other hemoglobinopathies (D58.2)
sickle-cell beta thalassemia (D57.4-)

D56.8 Other thalassemias
Dominant thalassemia
Hemoglobin C thalassemia
Mixed thalassemia
Thalassemia with other hemoglobinopathy
Excludes1: hemoglobin C disease (D58.2)
hemoglobin E disease (D58.2)
other hemoglobinopathies (D58.2)
sickle-cell anemia (D57.-)
sickle-cell thalassemia (D57.4)

D56.9 Thalassemia, unspecified
Mediterranean anemia (with other hemoglobinopathy)

D57 SICKLE-CELL DISORDERS

4th

Use additional code for any associated fever (R50.81)
Excludes1: other hemoglobinopathies (D58.-)

D57.0 Hb-SS disease with crisis

5th Sickle-cell disease with crisis
Hb-SS disease with vaso-occlusive pain

D57.00 Hb-SS disease with crisis, unspecified
Hb-SS with (painful) crisis NOS
Hb-SS disease with vaso-occlusive pain NOS

D57.01 Hb-SS disease with acute chest syndrome

D57.02 Hb-SS disease with splenic sequestration

D57.03 Hb-SS disease with cerebral vascular involvement
Code also, if applicable, cerebral infarction (I63.-)

D57.04 Hb-SS disease with dactylitis

D57.09 Hb-SS disease with crisis with other specified complication
Use additional code to identify complications, such as:
cholelithiasis (K80.-)
priapism (N48.32)

D57.1 Sickle-cell disease without crisis
Hb-SS disease without crisis
Sickle-cell anemia NOS
Sickle-cell disease NOS
Sickle-cell disorder NOS

D57.2 Sickle-cell/Hb-C disease

5th Hb-SC disease
Hb-S/Hb-C disease

D57.20 Sickle-cell/Hb-C disease without crisis

D57.21 Sickle-cell/Hb-C disease with crisis

6th **D57.211 Sickle-cell/Hb-C disease with acute chest syndrome**

D57.212 Sickle-cell/Hb-C disease with splenic sequestration

D57.213 Sickle-cell/Hb-C disease with cerebral vascular involvement
Code also, if applicable, cerebral infarction (I63.-)

D57.214 Sickle-cell/Hb-C disease with dactylitis

D57.218 Sickle-cell/Hb-C disease with crisis with other specified complication
Use additional code to identify complications, such as:
cholelithiasis (K80.-)
priapism (N48.32)

D57.219 Sickle-cell/Hb-C disease with crisis, unspecified
Sickle-cell/Hb-C disease with vaso-occlusive pain NOS

D57.3 Sickle-cell trait
Hb-S trait
Heterozygous hemoglobin S

D57.4 Sickle-cell thalassemia

5th Sickle-cell beta thalassemia
Thalassemia Hb-S disease

D57.40 Sickle-cell thalassemia without crisis
Microdrepanocytosis
Sickle-cell thalassemia NOS

D57.41 Sickle-cell thalassemia, unspecified, with crisis

6th Sickle-cell thalassemia with (painful) crisis NOS
Sickle-cell thalassemia with vaso-occlusive pain NOS

D57.411 Sickle-cell thalassemia, unspecified, with acute chest syndrome

D57.412 Sickle-cell thalassemia, unspecified, with splenic sequestration

D57.413 Sickle-cell thalassemia, unspecified, with cerebral vascular involvement
Code also, if applicable, cerebral infarction (I63.-)

D57.414 Sickle-cell thalassemia, unspecified, with dactylitis

D57.418 Sickle-cell thalassemia, unspecified, with crisis with other specified complication
Use additional code to identify complications, such as:
cholelithiasis (K80.-)
priapism (N48.32)

D57.419 Sickle-cell thalassemia, unspecified, with crisis
Sickle-cell thalassemia with (painful) crisis NOS
Sickle-cell thalassemia with vaso-occlusive pain NOS

D57.42 Sickle-cell thalassemia beta zero without crisis
HbS-beta zero without crisis
Sickle-cell beta zero without crisis

D57.43 Sickle-cell thalassemia beta zero

6th HbS-beta zero with crisis
Sickle-cell beta zero with crisis

D57.431 Sickle-cell thalassemia beta zero with acute chest syndrome
HbS-beta zero with acute chest syndrome
Sickle-cell beta zero with acute chest syndrome

D57.432 Sickle-cell thalassemia beta zero with splenic sequestration
HbS-beta zero with splenic sequestration
Sickle-cell beta zero with splenic sequestration

D57.433 Sickle-cell thalassemia beta zero with cerebral vascular involvement
HbS-beta zero with cerebral vascular involvement
Sickle-cell beta zero with cerebral vascular involvement
Code also, if applicable, cerebral infarction (I63.-)

D57.434 Sickle-cell thalassemia beta zero with dactylitis

D57.438 Sickle-cell thalassemia beta zero with crisis with other specified complication
HbS-beta zero with other specified complication
Sickle-cell beta zero with other specified complication
Use additional code to identify complications, such as:
cholelithiasis (K80.-)
priapism (N48.32)

D57.439 Sickle-cell thalassemia beta zero with crisis, unspecified
HbS-beta zero with other specified complication
Sickle-cell beta zero with crisis unspecified
Sickle-cell thalassemia beta zero with (painful) crisis NOS
Sickle-cell thalassemia beta zero with vaso-occlusive pain NOS

D57.44 Sickle-cell thalassemia beta plus without crisis
HbS-beta plus without crisis
Sickle-cell beta plus without crisis

D57.45 Sickle-cell thalassemia beta plus
HbS-beta plus with crisis
Sickle-cell beta plus with crisis

D57.451 Sickle-cell thalassemia beta plus with acute chest syndrome
HbS-beta plus with acute chest syndrome
Sickle-cell beta plus with acute chest syndrome

D57.452 Sickle-cell thalassemia beta plus with splenic sequestration
HbS-beta plus with splenic sequestration
Sickle-cell beta plus with splenic sequestration

D57.453 Sickle-cell thalassemia beta plus with cerebral vascular involvement
HbS-beta plus with cerebral vascular involvement
Sickle-cell beta plus with cerebral vascular involvement
Code also, if applicable, cerebral infarction (I63.-)

D57.454 Sickle-cell thalassemia beta plus with dactylitis

D57.458 Sickle-cell thalassemia beta plus with crisis with other specified complication
HbS-beta plus with crisis with other specified complication
Sickle-cell beta plus with crisis with other specified complication
Use additional code to identify complications, such as:
cholelithiasis (K80.-)
priapism (N48.32)

D57.459 Sickle-cell thalassemia beta plus with crisis, unspecified
HbS-beta plus with crisis with unspecified complication
Sickle-cell beta plus with crisis with unspecified complication
Sickle-cell thalassemia beta plus with (painful) crisis NOS
Sickle-cell thalassemia beta plus with vaso-occlusive pain NOS

D57.8 Other sickle-cell disorders
Hb-SD disease
Hb-SE disease

D57.80 Other sickle-cell disorders without crisis

D57.81 Other sickle-cell disorders with crisis

D57.811 Other sickle-cell disorders with acute chest syndrome

D57.812 Other sickle-cell disorders with splenic sequestration

D57.813 Other sickle-cell disorders with cerebral vascular involvement
Code also, if applicable: cerebral infarction (I63.-)

D57.814 Other sickle-cell disorders with dactylitis

D57.818 Other sickle-cell disorders with crisis with other specified complication
Use additional code to identify complications, such as:
cholelithiasis (K80.-)
priapism (N48.32)

D57.819 Other sickle-cell disorders with crisis, unspecified
Other sickle-cell disorders with (vasoocclusive pain) crisis NOS

D58 OTHER HEREDITARY HEMOLYTIC ANEMIAS

Excludes1: hemolytic anemia of the newborn (P55.-)

D58.0 Hereditary spherocytosis
Acholuric (familial) jaundice
Congenital (spherocytic) hemolytic icterus
Minkowski-Chauffard syndrome

D58.1 Hereditary elliptocytosis
Elliptocytosis (congenital)
Ovalocytosis (congenital) (hereditary)

D58.2 Other hemoglobinopathies
Abnormal hemoglobin NOS
Congenital Heinz body anemia
Hb-C disease
Hb-D disease
Hb-E disease
Hemoglobinopathy NOS
Unstable hemoglobin hemolytic disease
Excludes1: familial polycythemia (D75.0)
Hb-M disease (D74.0)
hemoglobin E-beta thalassemia (D56.5)
hereditary persistence of fetal hemoglobin [HPFH] (D56.4)
high-altitude polycythemia (D75.1)
methemoglobinemia (D74.-)
other hemoglobinopathies with thalassemia (D56.8)

D58.8 Other specified hereditary hemolytic anemias
Stomatocytosis

D58.9 Hereditary hemolytic anemia, unspecified

D59 ACQUIRED HEMOLYTIC ANEMIA

D59.0 Drug-induced autoimmune hemolytic anemia
Use additional code for adverse effect, if applicable, to identify drug (T36-T50 with fifth or sixth character 5)

D59.1 Other autoimmune hemolytic anemias
Excludes2: Evans syndrome (D69.41)
hemolytic disease of newborn (P55.-)
paroxysmal cold hemoglobinuria (D59.6)

D59.10 Autoimmune hemolytic anemia, unspecified

D59.11 Warm autoimmune hemolytic anemia
Warm type (primary) (secondary) (symptomatic) autoimmune hemolytic anemia
Warm type autoimmune hemolytic disease

D59.12 Cold autoimmune hemolytic anemia
Chronic cold hemagglutinin disease
Cold agglutinin disease
Cold agglutinin hemoglobinuria
Cold type (primary) (secondary) (symptomatic) autoimmune hemolytic anemia
Cold type autoimmune hemolytic disease

D59.13 Mixed type autoimmune hemolytic anemia
Mixed type autoimmune hemolytic disease
Mixed type, cold and warm, (primary) (secondary) (symptomatic) autoimmune hemolyticanemia

D59.19 Other autoimmune hemolytic anemia

D59.2 Drug-induced nonautoimmune hemolytic anemia
Drug-induced enzyme deficiency anemia
Use additional code for adverse effect, if applicable, to identify drug (T36-T50 with fifth or sixth character 5)

D59.3 Hemolytic-uremic syndrome
5th **Use additional code** to identify associated:
E. coli infection (B96.2-)
Pneumococcal pneumonia (J13)
Shigella dysenteriae (A03.9)
D59.30 Hemolytic-uremic syndrome, unspecified
D59.31 Infection-associated hemolytic-uremic syndrome
D59.32 Hereditary hemolytic-uremic syndrome
D59.39 Other hemolytic-uremic syndrome

D59.4 Other nonautoimmune hemolytic anemias
Mechanical hemolytic anemia
Microangiopathic hemolytic anemia
Toxic hemolytic anemia

D59.5 Paroxysmal nocturnal hemoglobinuria [Marchiafava-Micheli]
Excludes1: hemoglobinuria NOS (R82.3)

D59.6 Hemoglobinuria due to hemolysis from other external causes
Hemoglobinuria from exertion
March hemoglobinuria
Paroxysmal cold hemoglobinuria
Use additional code (Chapter 20) to identify external cause
Excludes1: hemoglobinuria NOS (R82.3)

D59.8 Other acquired hemolytic anemias

D59.9 Acquired hemolytic anemia, unspecified
Idiopathic hemolytic anemia, chronic

(D60–D64) APLASTIC AND OTHER ANEMIAS AND OTHER BONE MARROW FAILURE SYNDROMES

D60 ACQUIRED PURE RED CELL APLASIA [ERYTHROBLASTOPENIA]
4th
Includes: red cell aplasia (acquired) (adult) (with thymoma)
Excludes1: congenital red cell aplasia (D61.01)
D60.0 Chronic acquired pure red cell aplasia
D60.1 Transient acquired pure red cell aplasia
D60.8 Other acquired pure red cell aplasias
D60.9 Acquired pure red cell aplasia, unspecified

D61 OTHER APLASTIC ANEMIAS AND OTHER BONE MARROW FAILURE SYNDROMES
4th
Excludes2: neutropenia (D70.-)

D61.0 Constitutional aplastic anemia
5th **D61.01 Constitutional (pure) red blood cell aplasia**
Blackfan-Diamond syndrome
Congenital (pure) red cell aplasia
Familial hypoplastic anemia
Primary (pure) red cell aplasia
Red cell (pure) aplasia of infants
Excludes1: acquired red cell aplasia (D60.9)
D61.02 Shwachman-Diamond syndrome
Code also, if applicable, associated conditions such as:
acute myeloblastic leukemia (C92.0-)
exocrine pancreatic insufficiency (K86.81)
myelodysplastic syndrome (D46.-)
Use additional code, if applicable, for genetic susceptibility to other malignant neoplasm (Z15.09)
●D61.03 Fanconi anemia
Fanconi pancytopenia
Fanconi's anemia
Excludes1: Fanconi syndrome (E72.0-)
D61.09 Other constitutional aplastic anemia
Pancytopenia with malformations

D61.1 Drug-induced aplastic anemia
Use additional code for adverse effect, if applicable, to identify drug (T36-T50 with fifth or sixth character 5)

D61.2 Aplastic anemia due to other external agents
Code first, if applicable, toxic effects of substances chiefly nonmedicinal as to source (T51-T65)

D61.3 Idiopathic aplastic anemia

D61.8 Other specified aplastic anemias and other bone marrow failure syndromes
5th
D61.81 Pancytopenia
6th *Excludes1:* pancytopenia (due to) (with) aplastic anemia (D61.9)
pancytopenia (due to) (with) bone marrow infiltration (D61.82)
pancytopenia (due to) (with) congenital (pure) red cell aplasia (D61.01)
pancytopenia (due to) (with) hairy cell leukemia (C91.4-)
pancytopenia (due to) (with) HIV disease (B20.-)
pancytopenia (due to) (with) leukoerythroblastic anemia (D61.82)
pancytopenia (due to) (with) myeloproliferative disease (D47.1)
Excludes2: pancytopenia (due to) (with) myelodysplastic syndromes (D46.-)
D61.810 Antineoplastic chemotherapy induced pancytopenia
Excludes2: aplastic anemia due to antineoplastic chemotherapy (D61.1)
D61.811 Other drug-induced pancytopenia
Excludes2: aplastic anemia due to drugs (D61.1)
D61.818 Other pancytopenia

D61.82 Myelophthisis
Leukoerythroblastic anemia
Myelophthisic anemia
Panmyelophthisis
Code also the underlying disorder, such as: malignant neoplasm of breast (C50.-)
tuberculosis (A15.-)
Excludes1: idiopathic myelofibrosis (D47.1)
myelofibrosis NOS (D75.81)
myelofibrosis with myeloid metaplasia (D47.4)
primary myelofibrosis (D47.1)
secondary myelofibrosis (D75.81)

D61.89 Other specified aplastic anemias and other bone marrow failure syndromes

D61.9 Aplastic anemia, unspecified
Hypoplastic anemia NOS
Medullary hypoplasia

D62 ACUTE POSTHEMORRHAGIC ANEMIA
✓
Excludes1: anemia due to chronic blood loss (D50.0)
blood loss anemia NOS (D50.0)
congenital anemia from fetal blood loss (P61.3)

D63 ANEMIA IN CHRONIC DISEASES CLASSIFIED ELSEWHERE
4th

D63.0 Anemia in neoplastic disease
Code first neoplasm (C00-D49)
Excludes1: aplastic anemia due to antineoplastic chemotherapy (D61.1)
Excludes2: anemia due to antineoplastic chemotherapy (D64.81)

D63.1 Anemia in chronic kidney disease
Erythropoietin-resistant anemia (EPO-resistant anemia)
Code first underlying chronic kidney disease (CKD) (N18.-)

D63.8 Anemia in other chronic diseases classified elsewhere
Code first underlying disease

D64 OTHER ANEMIAS
4th
Excludes1: refractory anemia (D46.-)
refractory anemia with excess blasts in transformation [RAEB T] (C92.0-)

D64.0 Hereditary sideroblastic anemia
Sex-linked hypochromic sideroblastic anemia

D64.1 Secondary sideroblastic anemia due to disease
Code first underlying disease

D64.2 Secondary sideroblastic anemia due to drugs and toxins
Code first poisoning due to drug or toxin, if applicable (T36 -T65 with fifth or sixth character 1-4)
Use additional code for adverse effect, if applicable, to identify drug (T36-T50 with fifth or sixth character 5)

4th **5th** **6th** **7th** Additional Character Required **✓** 3-character code

●=New Code *Excludes1*—Not coded here, do not use together
▲=Revised Code *Excludes2*—Not included here

D64.3 Other sideroblastic anemias
Sideroblastic anemia NOS
Pyridoxine-responsive sideroblastic anemia NEC

D64.4 Congenital dyserythropoietic anemia
Dyshematopoietic anemia (congenital)
Excludes1: Blackfan-Diamond syndrome (D61.01)
Di Guglielmo's disease (C94.0)

D64.8 Other specified anemias

D64.81 Anemia due to antineoplastic chemotherapy
Antineoplastic chemotherapy induced anemia
Excludes2: aplastic anemia due to antineoplastic chemotherapy (D61.1)
anemia in neoplastic disease (D63.0)

D64.89 Other specified anemias
Infantile pseudoleukemia

D64.9 Anemia, unspecified

(D65–D69) COAGULATION DEFECTS, PURPURA AND OTHER HEMORRHAGIC CONDITIONS

D65 DISSEMINATED INTRAVASCULAR COAGULATION [DEFIBRINATION SYNDROME] ✓
Afibrinogenemia, acquired
Consumption coagulopathy
Diffuse or disseminated intravascular coagulation [DIC]
Fibrinolytic hemorrhage, acquired
Fibrinolytic purpura
Purpura fulminans
Code also, if applicable, associated condition
Excludes1: disseminated intravascular coagulation (complicating):
abortion or ectopic or molar pregnancy (O00–O07, O08.1)
in newborn (P60)
pregnancy, childbirth and the puerperium (O45.0, O46.0, O67.0, O72.3)

D66 HEREDITARY FACTOR VIII DEFICIENCY ✓
Classical hemophilia
Deficiency factor VIII (with functional defect)
Hemophilia NOS
Hemophilia A
Excludes1: factor VIII deficiency with vascular defect (D68.0)

D67 HEREDITARY FACTOR IX DEFICIENCY ✓
Christmas disease
Factor IX deficiency (with functional defect)
Hemophilia B
Plasma thromboplastin component [PTC] deficiency

D68 OTHER COAGULATION DEFECTS
Excludes1: abnormal coagulation profile (R79.1)
Excludes2: coagulation defects complicating abortion or ectopic or molar pregnancy (O00–O07, O08.1)
coagulation defects complicating pregnancy, childbirth and the puerperium (O45.0, O46.0, O67.0, O72.3)

D68.0 Von Willebrand's disease
Excludes1: capillary fragility (hereditary) (D69.8)
factor VIII deficiency NOS (D66)
factor VIII deficiency with functional defect (D66)

D68.00 Von Willebrand disease, unspecified

D68.01 Von Willebrand disease, type 1C
Partial quantitative deficiency of von Willebrand factor
Type 1C von Willebrand disease

D68.02 Von Willebrand disease, type 2
Qualitative defects of von Willebrand factor

D68.020 Von Willebrand disease, type 2A
Qualitative defects of von Willebrand factor with decreased platelet adhesion and selective deficiency of high-molecular-weight multimers

D68.021 Von Willebrand disease, type 2B
Qualitative defects of von Willebrand factor with high-molecular-weight von Willebrand factor loss

Qualitative defects of von Willebrand factor with hyper-adhesive forms

Qualitative defects of von Willebrand factor with increased affinity for platelet glycoprotein Ib

D68.022 Von Willebrand disease, type 2M
Qualitative defects of von Willebrand factor with defective platelet adhesion with a normal size distribution of von Willebrand factor multimers

D68.023 Von Willebrand disease, type 2N
Qualitative defects of von Willebrand factor with defective von Willebrand factor to factor VIII binding
Qualitative defects of von Willebrand factor with markedly decreased affinity for factor VIII

D68.029 Von Willebrand disease, type 2, unspecified
Qualitative defect in von Willebrand factor function, with no further subtyping

D68.03 Von Willebrand disease, type 3
(Near) complete absence of von Willebrand factor
Total quantitative deficiency of von Willebrand factor

D68.04 Acquired von Willebrand disease
Acquired von Willebrand syndrome

D68.09 Other von Willebrand disease
Platelet-type von Willebrand disease
Pseudo-von Willebrand disease
Code also, if applicable, qualitative platelet defects (D69.1)

D68.1 Hereditary factor XI deficiency
Hemophilia C
Plasma thromboplastin antecedent [PTA] deficiency
Rosenthal's disease

D68.2 Hereditary deficiency of other clotting factors
AC globulin deficiency
Congenital afibrinogenemia
Deficiency of factor I [fibrinogen]
Deficiency of factor II [prothrombin]
Deficiency of factor V [labile]
Deficiency of factor VII [stable]
Deficiency of factor X [Stuart-Prower]
Deficiency of factor XII [Hageman]
Deficiency of factor XIII [fibrin stabilizing]
Dysfibrinogenemia (congenital)
Hypoproconvertinemia
Owren's disease
Proaccelerin deficiency

D68.3 Hemorrhagic disorder due to circulating anticoagulants

D68.31 Hemorrhagic disorder due to intrinsic circulating anticoagulants, antibodies, or inhibitors

D68.311 Acquired hemophilia
Autoimmune hemophilia
Autoimmune inhibitors to clotting factors
Secondary hemophilia

D68.312 Antiphospholipid antibody with hemorrhagic disorder
LAC with hemorrhagic disorder
SLE inhibitor with hemorrhagic disorder
Excludes1: antiphospholipid antibody, finding without diagnosis (R76.0)
antiphospholipid antibody syndrome (D68.61)
antiphospholipid antibody with hypercoagulable state (D68.61)
LAC finding without diagnosis (R76.0)
LAC with hypercoagulable state (D68.62)
SLE inhibitor finding without diagnosis (R76.0)
SLE inhibitor with hypercoagulable state (D68.62)

D68.318 Other hemorrhagic disorder due to intrinsic circulating anticoagulants, antibodies, or inhibitors

Antithromboplastinemia

Antithromboplastinogenemia

Hemorrhagic disorder due to intrinsic increase in antithrombin

Hemorrhagic disorder due to intrinsic increase in anti-VIIIa

Hemorrhagic disorder due to intrinsic increase in anti-IXa

Hemorrhagic disorder due to intrinsic increase in anti-XIa

D68.32 Hemorrhagic disorder due to extrinsic circulating anticoagulants

Drug-induced hemorrhagic disorder

Hemorrhagic disorder due to increase in anti-IIa

Hemorrhagic disorder due to increase in anti-Xa

Hyperheparinemia

Use additional code for adverse effect, if applicable, to identify drug (T45.515, T45.525)

D68.4 Acquired coagulation factor deficiency

Deficiency of coagulation factor due to liver disease

Deficiency of coagulation factor due to vitamin K deficiency

Excludes1: vitamin K deficiency of newborn (P53)

D68.5 Primary thrombophilia

5th

Primary hypercoagulable states

Excludes1: antiphospholipid syndrome (D68.61)

LAC (D68.62)

secondary activated protein C resistance (D68.69)

secondary antiphospholipid antibody syndrome (D68.69)

secondary LAC with hypercoagulable state (D68.69)

SLE inhibitor with hypercoagulable state (D68.69)

SLE inhibitor finding without diagnosis (R76.0)

SLE inhibitor with hemorrhagic disorder (D68.312)

thrombotic thrombocytopenic purpura (M31.19)

D68.51 Activated protein C resistance

Factor V Leiden mutation

D68.52 Prothrombin gene mutation

D68.59 Other primary thrombophilia

Antithrombin III deficiency

Hypercoagulable state NOS

Primary hypercoagulable state NEC

Primary thrombophilia NEC

Protein C deficiency

Protein S deficiency

Thrombophilia NOS

D68.6 Other thrombophilia

5th

Other hypercoagulable states

Excludes1: diffuse or disseminated intravascular coagulation [DIC] (D65)

heparin induced thrombocytopenia (HIT) (D75.82)

hyperhomocysteinemia (E72.11)

D68.61 Antiphospholipid syndrome

Anticardiolipin syndrome

Antiphospholipid antibody syndrome

Excludes1: anti-phospholipid antibody, finding without diagnosis (R76.0)

anti-phospholipid antibody with hemorrhagic disorder (D68.312)

LAC syndrome (D68.62)

D68.62 LAC syndrome

LAC

Presence of SLE inhibitor

Excludes1: anticardiolipin syndrome (D68.61)

antiphospholipid syndrome (D68.61)

LAC finding without diagnosis (R76.0)

LAC with hemorrhagic disorder (D68.312)

D68.69 Other thrombophilia

Hypercoagulable states NEC

Secondary hypercoagulable state NOS

D68.8 Other specified coagulation defects

Excludes1: hemorrhagic disease of newborn (P53)

D68.9 Coagulation defect, unspecified

D69 PURPURA AND OTHER HEMORRHAGIC CONDITIONS

4th

Excludes1: benign hypergammaglobulinemic purpura (D89.0)

cryoglobulinemic purpura (D89.1)

essential (hemorrhagic) thrombocythemia (D47.3)

hemorrhagic thrombocythemia (D47.3)

purpura fulminans (D65)

thrombotic thrombocytopenic purpura (M31.19)

Waldenström hypergammaglobulinemic purpura (D89.0)

D69.0 Allergic purpura

Allergic vasculitis

Nonthrombocytopenic hemorrhagic purpura

Nonthrombocytopenic idiopathic purpura

Purpura anaphylactoid

Purpura Henoch(-Schönlein)

Purpura rheumatica

Vascular purpura

Excludes1: thrombocytopenic hemorrhagic purpura (D69.3)

D69.1 Qualitative platelet defects

Bernard-Soulier [giant platelet] syndrome

Glanzmann's disease

Grey platelet syndrome

Thromboasthenia (hemorrhagic) (hereditary)

Thrombocytopathy

Excludes1: von Willebrand's disease (D68.0)

D69.2 Other nonthrombocytopenic purpura

Purpura NOS

Purpura simplex

Senile purpura

D69.3 Immune thrombocytopenic purpura

Hemorrhagic (thrombocytopenic) purpura

Idiopathic thrombocytopenic purpura

Tidal platelet dysgenesis

D69.4 Other primary thrombocytopenia

5th

Excludes1: transient neonatal thrombocytopenia (P61.0)

Wiskott-Aldrich syndrome (D82.0)

D69.41 Evans syndrome

D69.42 Congenital and hereditary thrombocytopenia purpura

Congenital thrombocytopenia

Hereditary thrombocytopenia

Code first congenital or hereditary disorder, such as:

TAR syndrome (Q87.2)

D69.49 Other primary thrombocytopenia

Megakaryocytic hypoplasia

Primary thrombocytopenia NOS

D69.5 Secondary thrombocytopenia

5th

Excludes1: heparin induced thrombocytopenia (HIT) (D75.82)

transient thrombocytopenia of newborn (P61.0)

D69.51 Posttransfusion purpura

Posttransfusion purpura from whole blood (fresh) or blood products

PTP

D69.59 Other secondary thrombocytopenia

D69.6 Thrombocytopenia, unspecified

D69.8 Other specified hemorrhagic conditions

Capillary fragility (hereditary)

Vascular pseudohemophilia

D69.9 Hemorrhagic condition, unspecified

(D70–D77) OTHER DISORDERS OF BLOOD AND BLOOD-FORMING ORGANS

D70 NEUTROPENIA

4th

Includes: agranulocytosis

decreased absolute neutrophil count (ANC)

Use additional code for any associated: fever (R50.81)

Code also, if applicable, mucositis (J34.81, K12.3-, K92.81, N76.81)

Excludes1: neutropenic splenomegaly (D73.81)

transient neonatal neutropenia (P61.5)

D70.0 Congenital agranulocytosis

Congenital neutropenia

Infantile genetic agranulocytosis

Kostmann's disease

- **D70.1 Agranulocytosis secondary to cancer chemotherapy**
  Use additional code for adverse effect, if applicable, to identify drug (T45.1X5)
  Code also underlying neoplasm
- **D70.2 Other drug-induced agranulocytosis**
  Use additional code for adverse effect, if applicable, to identify drug (T36–T50 with fifth or sixth character 5)
- **D70.3 Neutropenia due to infection**
- **D70.4 Cyclic neutropenia**
  Cyclic hematopoiesis
  Periodic neutropenia
- **D70.8 Other neutropenia**
- **D70.9 Neutropenia, unspecified**

D71 FUNCTIONAL DISORDERS OF POLYMORPHONUCLEAR NEUTROPHILS

Cell membrane receptor complex [CR3] defect
Chronic (childhood) granulomatous disease
Congenital dysphagocytosis
Progressive septic granulomatosis

D72 OTHER DISORDERS OF WHITE BLOOD CELLS

Excludes1: basophilia (D72.824)
immunity disorders (D80–D89)
neutropenia (D70)
preleukemia (syndrome) (D46.9)

D72.0 Genetic anomalies of leukocytes

Alder syndrome
Hereditary leukocytic hyper/hypo segmentation
Hereditary leukomelanopathy
May-Hegglin syndrome
Pelger-Huët syndrome

D72.1 Eosinophilia

Excludes2: Löffler's syndrome (J82.89)
pulmonary eosinophilia (J82.-)

- **D72.10 Eosinophilia, unspecified**
  - **D72.110 Idiopathic hypereosinophilic syndrome [IHES]**
  - **D72.111 Lymphocytic Variant Hypereosinophilic Syndrome [LHES]**
    Lymphocyte variant hypereosinophilia
    Code also, if applicable, any associated lymphocytic neoplastic disorder
  - **D72.118 Other hypereosinophilic syndrome**
    Episodic angioedema with eosinophilia
    Gleich's syndrome
  - **D72.119 Hypereosinophilic syndrome [HES], unspecified**
- **D72.12 Drug rash with eosinophilia and systemic symptoms syndrome**
  DRESS syndrome
  Use additional code for adverse effect, if applicable, to identify drug (T36–T50 with fifth or sixth character 5)
- **D72.18 Eosinophilia in diseases classified elsewhere**
  Code first underlying disease, such as:
  chronic myelomonocytic leukemia (C93.1-)
- **D72.19 Other eosinophilia**
  Familial eosinophilia
  Hereditary eosinophilia

D72.8 Other specified disorders of white blood cells

Excludes1: leukemia (C91–C95)

- **D72.81 Decreased white blood cell count**
  Excludes1: neutropenia (D70.-)
  - **D72.810 Lymphocytopenia**
    Decreased lymphocytes
  - **D72.818 Other decreased white blood cell count**
    Basophilic leukopenia
    Eosinophilic leukopenia
    Monocytopenia
    Other decreased leukocytes
    Plasmacytopenia
  - **D72.819 Decreased white blood cell count, unspecified**
    Decreased leukocytes, unspecified
    Leukocytopenia, unspecified
    Leukopenia
    Excludes1: malignant leukopenia (D70.9)

- **D72.82 Elevated white blood cell count**
  Excludes1: eosinophilia (D72.1)
  - **D72.820 Lymphocytosis (symptomatic)**
    Elevated lymphocytes
  - **D72.821 Monocytosis (symptomatic)**
    Excludes1: infectious mononucleosis (B27.-)
  - **D72.822 Plasmacytosis**
  - **D72.823 Leukemoid reaction**
    Basophilic leukemoid reaction
    Leukemoid reaction NOS
    Lymphocytic leukemoid reaction
    Monocytic leukemoid reaction
    Myelocytic leukemoid reaction
    Neutrophilic leukemoid reaction
  - **D72.824 Basophilia**
  - **D72.825 Bandemia**
    Bandemia without diagnosis of specific infection
    Excludes1: confirmed infection—code to infection
    leukemia (C91.-, C92.-, C93.-, C94.-, C95.-)
  - **D72.828 Other elevated white blood cell count**
  - **D72.829 Elevated white blood cell count, unspecified**
    Elevated leukocytes, unspecified
    Leukocytosis, unspecified

D72.89 Other specified disorders of white blood cells

Abnormality of white blood cells NEC

D72.9 Disorder of white blood cells, unspecified

Abnormal leukocyte differential NOS

D73 DISEASES OF SPLEEN

D73.0 Hyposplenism

Atrophy of spleen
Excludes1: asplenia (congenital) (Q89.01)
postsurgical absence of spleen (Z90.81)

D73.1 Hypersplenism

Excludes1: neutropenic splenomegaly (D73.81)
primary splenic neutropenia (D73.81)
splenitis, splenomegaly in late syphilis (A52.79)
splenitis, splenomegaly in tuberculosis (A18.85)
splenomegaly NOS (R16.1)
splenomegaly congenital (Q89.0)

D73.2 Chronic congestive splenomegaly

D73.3 Abscess of spleen

D73.4 Cyst of spleen

D73.5 Infarction of spleen

Splenic rupture, nontraumatic
Torsion of spleen
Excludes1: rupture of spleen due to Plasmodium vivax malaria (B51.0)
traumatic rupture of spleen (S36.03-)

D73.8 Other diseases of spleen

- **D73.81 Neutropenic splenomegaly**
  Werner-Schultz disease
- **D73.89 Other diseases of spleen**
  Fibrosis of spleen NOS
  Perisplenitis
  Splenitis NOS

D74 METHEMOGLOBINEMIA

D74.0 Congenital methemoglobinemia

Congenital NADH-methemoglobin reductase deficiency
Hemoglobin-M [Hb-M] disease
Methemoglobinemia, hereditary

D74.8 Other methemoglobinemias

Acquired methemoglobinemia (with sulfhemoglobinemia)
Toxic methemoglobinemia

D74.9 Methemoglobinemia, unspecified

D75 OTHER AND UNSPECIFIED DISEASES OF BLOOD AND BLOOD-FORMING ORGANS

Excludes2: acute lymphadenitis (L04.-)
chronic lymphadenitis (I88.1)
enlarged lymph nodes (R59.-)
hypergammaglobulinemia NOS (D89.2)
lymphadenitis NOS (I88.9)
mesenteric lymphadenitis (acute) (chronic) (I88.0)

D75.0 Familial erythrocytosis
Benign polycythemia
Familial polycythemia
Excludes1: hereditary ovalocytosis (D58.1)

D75.1 Secondary polycythemia
Acquired polycythemia
Emotional polycythemia
Erythrocytosis NOS
Hypoxemic polycythemia
Nephrogenous polycythemia
Polycythemia due to erythropoietin
Polycythemia due to fall in plasma volume
Polycythemia due to high altitude
Polycythemia due to stress
Polycythemia NOS
Relative polycythemia
Excludes1: polycythemia neonatorum (P61.1)
polycythemia vera (D45)

D75.8 Other specified diseases of blood and blood-forming organs

D75.81 Myelofibrosis
Myelofibrosis NOS
Secondary myelofibrosis NOS
Code first the underlying disorder
Use additional code, if applicable, for associated therapy-related myelodysplastic syndrome (D46.-)
Use additional code for adverse effect, if applicable, to identify drug (T45.1X5)
Excludes1: acute myelofibrosis (C94.4-)
idiopathic myelofibrosis (D47.1)
leukoerythroblastic anemia (D61.82)
myelofibrosis with myeloid metaplasia (D47.4)
myelophthisic anemia (D61.82)
myelophthisis (D61.82)
primary myelofibrosis (D47.1)

D75.82 Heparin-induced thrombocytopenia (HIT)

D75.821 Non-immune heparin-induced thrombocytopenia

D75.822 Immune-mediated heparin-induced thrombocytopenia

D75.828 Other heparin-induced thrombocytopenia syndrome

D75.829 Heparin-induced thrombocytopenia, unspecified

D75.83 Thrombocytosis
Excludes2: essential thrombocythemia (D47.3)

D75.838 Other thrombocytosis
Reactive thrombocytosis
Secondary thrombocytosis
Code also underlying condition, if known and applicable

D75.839 Thrombocytosis, unspecified
Thrombocythemia NOS
Thrombocytosis NOS

D75.84 Other platelet-activating anti-PF4 disorders

D75.89 Other specified diseases of blood and blood-forming organs

D75.9 Disease of blood and blood-forming organs, unspecified

D75.A Glucose-6-phosphate dehydrogenase (G6PD) deficiency without anemia
Excludes1: G6PD deficiency with anemia (D55.0)

D76 OTHER SPECIFIED DISEASES WITH PARTICIPATION OF LYMPHORETICULAR AND RETICULOHISTIOCYTIC TISSUE

Excludes1: (Abt-) Letterer-Siwe disease (C96.0)
eosinophilic granuloma (C96.6)
Hand-Schüller-Christian disease (C96.5)
histiocytic medullary reticulosis (C96.9)
histiocytic sarcoma (C96.A)
histiocytosis X, multifocal (C96.5)
histiocytosis X, unifocal (C96.6)
Langerhans-cell histiocytosis, multifocal (C96.5)
Langerhans-cell histiocytosis NOS (C96.6)
Langerhans-cell histiocytosis, unifocal (C96.6)
leukemic reticuloendotheliosis (C91.4-)
lipomelanotic reticulosis (I89.8)
malignant histiocytosis (C96.A)
malignant reticulosis (C86.0)
nonlipid reticuloendotheliosis (C96.0)

D76.1 Hemophagocytic lymphohistiocytosis
Familial hemophagocytic reticulosis
Histiocytoses of mononuclear phagocytes

D76.2 Hemophagocytic syndrome, infection-associated
Use additional code to identify infectious agent or disease.

D76.3 Other histiocytosis syndromes
Reticulohistiocytoma (giant-cell)
Sinus histiocytosis with massive lymphadenopathy
Xanthogranuloma

D77 OTHER DISORDERS OF BLOOD AND BLOOD-FORMING ORGANS IN DISEASES CLASSIFIED ELSEWHERE

Code first underlying disease, such as:
amyloidosis (E85.-)
congenital early syphilis (A50.0-)
echinococcosis (B67.0-B67.9)
malaria (B50.0-B54)
schistosomiasis [bilharziasis] (B65.0-B65.9)
vitamin C deficiency (E54)
Excludes1: rupture of spleen due to Plasmodium vivax malaria (B51.0)
splenitis, splenomegaly in late syphilis (A52.79)
splenitis, splenomegaly in tuberculosis (A18.85)

(D78) INTRAOPERATIVE AND POSTPROCEDURAL COMPLICATIONS OF THE SPLEEN

(D80-D89) CERTAIN DISORDERS INVOLVING THE IMMUNE MECHANISM

Includes: defects in the complement system
immunodeficiency disorders, except HIV disease
sarcoidosis
Excludes1: autoimmune disease (systemic) NOS (M35.9)
functional disorders of polymorphonuclear neutrophils (D71)
HIV disease (B20)

D80 IMMUNODEFICIENCY WITH PREDOMINANTLY ANTIBODY DEFECTS

D80.0 Hereditary hypogammaglobulinemia
Autosomal recessive agammaglobulinemia (Swiss type)
X-linked agammaglobulinemia [Bruton] (with growth hormone deficiency)

D80.1 Nonfamilial hypogammaglobulinemia
Agammaglobulinemia with immunoglobulin-bearing B-lymphocytes
Common variable agammaglobulinemia [CVAgamma]
Hypogammaglobulinemia NOS

D80.2 Selective deficiency of immunoglobulin A [IgA]

D80.3 Selective deficiency of immunoglobulin G [IgG] subclasses

D80.4 Selective deficiency of immunoglobulin M [IgM]

D80.5 Immunodeficiency with increased immunoglobulin M [IgM]

D80.6 Antibody deficiency with near-normal immunoglobulins or with hypogammaglobulinemia

D80.7 Transient hypogammaglobulinemia of infancy

D80.8 Other immunodeficiencies with predominantly antibody defects
Kappa light chain deficiency

D80.9 Immunodeficiency with predominantly antibody defects, unspecified

D81 COMBINED IMMUNODEFICIENCIES

Excludes1: autosomal recessive agammaglobulinemia (Swiss type) (D80.0)

- **D81.0** SCID with reticular dysgenesis
- **D81.1** SCID with low T- and B-cell numbers
- **D81.2** SCID with low or normal B-cell numbers
- **D81.3** Adenosine deaminase [ADA] deficiency
  - **D81.30** Adenosine deaminase deficiency, unspecified
    - ADA deficiency NOS
  - **D81.31** SCID due to adenosine deaminase deficiency
    - ADA deficiency with SCID
    - Adenosine deaminase [ADA] deficiency with SCID
  - **D81.32** Adenosine deaminase 2 deficiency
    - ADA2 deficiency
    - Adenosine deaminase deficiency type 2
    - **Code also**, if applicable, any associated manifestations, such as:
      - polyarteritis nodosa (M30.0)
      - stroke (I63.-)
- **D81.39** Other adenosine deaminase deficiency
  - Adenosine deaminase [ADA] deficiency type 1, NOS
  - Adenosine deaminase [ADA] deficiency type 1, without SCID
  - Partial adenosine deaminase deficiency (type 1)
- **D81.4** Nezelof's syndrome
- **D81.5** Purine nucleoside phosphorylase [PNP] deficiency
- **D81.6** Major histocompatibility complex class I deficiency
  - Bare lymphocyte syndrome
- **D81.7** Major histocompatibility complex class II deficiency
- **D81.8** Other combined immunodeficiencies
  - **D81.81** Biotin-dependent carboxylase deficiency
    - Multiple carboxylase deficiency
    - *Excludes1:* biotin-dependent carboxylase deficiency due to dietary deficiency of biotin (E53.8)
    - **D81.810** Biotinidase deficiency
    - **D81.818** Other biotin-dependent carboxylase deficiency
      - Holocarboxylase synthetase deficiency
      - Other multiple carboxylase deficiency
    - **D81.819** Biotin-dependent carboxylase deficiency, unspecified
      - Multiple carboxylase deficiency, unspecified
  - **D81.82** Activated Phosphoinositide 3-kinase Delta Syndrome [APDS] p110d-activating mutation causing senescent T cells, lymphadenopathy, and immunodeficiency [PASLI] disease
    - **Code also**, if applicable, any associated manifestations, such as:
      - bronchiectasis (J47.-)
      - herpes virus infections (B00.-)
      - other acute respiratory tract infections (J00–J06; J20–J22)
      - other infections (A00–B99)
      - pneumonia (J12–J18)
  - **D81.89** Other combined immunodeficiencies
- **D81.9** Combined immunodeficiency, unspecified
  - SCID NOS

D82 IMMUNODEFICIENCY ASSOCIATED WITH OTHER MAJOR DEFECTS

Excludes1: ataxia telangiectasia [Louis-Bar] (G11.3)

- **D82.0** Wiskott-Aldrich syndrome
  - Immunodeficiency with thrombocytopenia and eczema
- **D82.1** Di George's syndrome
  - Pharyngeal pouch syndrome
  - Thymic alymphoplasia
  - Thymic aplasia or hypoplasia with immunodeficiency
- **D82.2** Immunodeficiency with short-limbed stature
- **D82.3** Immunodeficiency following hereditary defective response to Epstein-Barr virus
  - X-linked lymphoproliferative disease
- **D82.4** Hyperimmunoglobulin E [IgE] syndrome

- **D82.9** Immunodeficiency associated with major defect, unspecified

D83 COMMON VARIABLE IMMUNODEFICIENCY

- **D83.0** Common variable immunodeficiency with predominant abnormalities of B-cell numbers and function
- **D83.1** Common variable immunodeficiency with predominant immunoregulatory T-cell disorders
  - Code first underlying condition, such as:
    - chromosomal abnormalities (Q90–Q99)
    - diabetes mellitus (E08–E13)
    - malignant neoplasms (C00–C96)
  - *Excludes1:* certain disorders involving the immune mechanism (D80-D83, D84.0, D84.1,D84.9)
    - human immunodeficiency virus [HIV] disease (B20)
- **D83.2** Common variable immunodeficiency with autoantibodies to B- or T-cells
- **D83.8** Other common variable immunodeficiencies
- **D83.9** Common variable immunodeficiency, unspecified

D84 OTHER IMMUNODEFICIENCIES

- **D84.0** Lymphocyte function antigen-1 [LFA-1] defect
- **D84.1** Defects in the complement system
  - C1 esterase inhibitor [C1-INH] deficiency
- **D84.8** Other specified immunodeficiencies
  - **D84.81** Immunodeficiency due to conditions classified elsewhere
    - **Code first** underlying condition, such as:
      - chromosomal abnormalities (Q90–Q99)
      - diabetes mellitus (E08–E13)
      - malignant neoplasms (C00–C96)
    - *Excludes1:* certain disorders involving the immune mechanism (D80–D83, D84.0, D84.1,D84.9)
      - human immunodeficiency virus [HIV] disease (B20)
  - **D84.82** Immunodeficiency due to other causes
    - **D84.821** Immunodeficiency due to drugs
      - Immunodeficiency due to (current or past) medication
      - **Use additional code** for adverse effect, if applicable, to identify adverse effect of drug (T36–T50 with fifth or six character 5)
      - **Use additional code**, if applicable, for associated long term (current) drug therapy drug or medication such as:
        - long term (current) drug therapy systemic steroids (Z79.52)
        - other long term (current) drug therapy (Z79.899)
    - **D84.822** Immunodeficiency due to external causes
      - **Code also**, if applicable, radiological procedure and radiotherapy (Y84.2)
      - **Use additional code** for external cause such as:
        - exposure to ionizing radiation (W88)
  - **D84.89** Other immunodeficiencies
- **D84.9** Immunodeficiency, unspecified
  - Immunocompromised NOS
  - Immunodeficient NOS
  - Immunosuppressed NOS

D86 SARCOIDOSIS

- **D86.0** Sarcoidosis of lung
- **D86.1** Sarcoidosis of lymph nodes
- **D86.2** Sarcoidosis of lung with sarcoidosis of lymph nodes
- **D86.3** Sarcoidosis of skin
- **D86.8** Sarcoidosis of other sites
  - **D86.81** Sarcoid meningitis
  - **D86.82** Multiple cranial nerve palsies in sarcoidosis
  - **D86.83** Sarcoid iridocyclitis
  - **D86.84** Sarcoid pyelonephritis
    - Tubulo-interstitial nephropathy in sarcoidosis
  - **D86.85** Sarcoid myocarditis
  - **D86.86** Sarcoid arthropathy
    - Polyarthritis in sarcoidosis
  - **D86.87** Sarcoid myositis

D86.89 Sarcoidosis of other sites
Hepatic granuloma
Uveoparotid fever [Heerfordt]

D86.9 Sarcoidosis, unspecified

D89 OTHER DISORDERS INVOLVING THE IMMUNE MECHANISM, NEC

4th

Excludes1: hyperglobulinemia NOS (R77.1)
monoclonal gammopathy (of undetermined significance) (D47.2)

Excludes2: transplant failure and rejection (T86.-)

D89.0 Polyclonal hypergammaglobulinemia
Benign hypergammaglobulinemic purpura
Polyclonal gammopathy NOS

D89.1 Cryoglobulinemia
Cryoglobulinemic purpura
Cryoglobulinemic vasculitis
Essential cryoglobulinemia
Idiopathic cryoglobulinemia
Mixed cryoglobulinemia
Primary cryoglobulinemia
Secondary cryoglobulinemia

D89.2 Hypergammaglobulinemia, unspecified

D89.3 Immune reconstitution syndrome
Immune reconstitution inflammatory syndrome [IRIS]
Use additional code for adverse effect, if applicable, to identify drug (T36-T50 with fifth or sixth character 5)

D89.4 Mast cell activation syndrome and related disorders

5th *Excludes1:* aggressive systemic mastocytosis (C96.21)
congenital cutaneous mastocytosis (Q82.2)
indolent systemic mastocytosis (D47.02)
malignant mast cell neoplasm (C96.2-)
mast cell leukemia (C94.3-)
malignant mastocytoma (C96.29)
systemic mastocytosis associated with a clonal hematologic
non-mast cell lineage disease (SM-AHNMD) (D47.02)
mast cell sarcoma (C96.22)
mastocytoma NOS (D47.09)
other mast cell neoplasms of uncertain behavior (D47.09)

D89.40 Mast cell activation disorder, unspecified or NOS

D89.41 Monoclonal mast cell activation syndrome

D89.42 Idiopathic mast cell activation syndrome

D89.43 Secondary mast cell activation syndrome
Secondary mast cell activation syndrome
Code also underlying etiology, if known

D89.44 Hereditary alpha tryptasemia
Use additional code, if applicable, for:
allergy status, other than to drugs and biological
substances (Z91.0-)
personal history of anaphylaxis (Z87.892)

D89.49 Other mast cell activation disorder

D89.8 Other specified disorders involving the immune mechanism, NEC

5th **D89.81 Graft-versus-host disease**

6th **Code first** underlying cause, such as:
complications of transplanted organs and tissue (T86.-)
complications of blood transfusion (T80.89)
Use additional code to identify associated
manifestations, such as:
desquamative dermatitis (L30.8)
diarrhea (R19.7)
elevated bilirubin (R17)
hair loss (L65.9)

D89.810 Acute graft-versus-host disease

D89.811 Chronic graft-versus-host disease

D89.812 Acute on chronic graft-versus-host disease

D89.813 Graft-versus-host disease, unspecified

D89.82 Autoimmune lymphoproliferative syndrome [ALPS]

D89.83 Cytokine release syndrome

6th **Code first** underlying cause, such as:
complications following infusion, transfusion and
therapeutic injection (T80.89-)
complications of transplanted organs and tissue (T86.-)
Use additional code to identify associated
manifestations
Use additional code for adverse effect, if applicable,
to identify immune checkpoint
inhibitors and immunostimulant drugs (T45.AX5)

D89.831 Cytokine release syndrome, grade 1

D89.832 Cytokine release syndrome, grade 2

D89.833 Cytokine release syndrome, grade 3

D89.834 Cytokine release syndrome, grade 4

D89.835 Cytokine release syndrome, grade 5

D89.839 Cytokine release syndrome, grade unspecified

D89.84 IgG4-related disease
Immunoglobulin G4-related disease

D89.89 Other specified disorders involving the immune mechanism, NEC
Excludes1: HIV disease (B20)

D89.9 Disorder involving the immune mechanism, unspecified
Immune disease NOS

Chapter 4. Endocrine, nutritional and metabolic diseases (E00–E89)

GUIDELINES

Diabetes Mellitus (DM)

See categories E08–E13.

Note: All neoplasms, whether functionally active or not, are classified in Chapter 2. Appropriate codes in this chapter (ie, E05.8, E07.0, E16–E31, E34.-) may be used as additional codes to indicate either functional activity by neoplasms and ectopic endocrine tissue or hyperfunction and hypofunction of endocrine glands associated with neoplasms and other conditions classified elsewhere.

TYPE OF DIABETES
See categories E08–E13

TYPE OF DIABETES MELLITUS NOT DOCUMENTED
See categories E08–E13

DIABETES MELLITUS AND THE USE OF INSULIN, ORAL HYPOGLYCEMICS, AND INJECTABLE NON-INSULIN DRUGS
See categories E08–E13

COMPLICATIONS DUE TO INSULIN PUMP MALFUNCTION
See categories E08–E13

SECONDARY DM
See categories E08–E13
Excludes1: transitory endocrine and metabolic disorders specific to newborn (P70–P74)

(E00–E07) DISORDERS OF THYROID GLAND

E00 CONGENITAL IODINE-DEFICIENCY SYNDROME

Use additional code (F70–F79) to identify associated intellectual disabilities.

Excludes1: subclinical iodine-deficiency hypothyroidism (E02)

- **E00.0 Congenital iodine-deficiency syndrome, neurological type** Endemic cretinism, neurological type
- **E00.1 Congenital iodine-deficiency syndrome, myxedematous type** Endemic hypothyroid cretinism Endemic cretinism, myxedematous type
- **E00.2 Congenital iodine-deficiency syndrome, mixed type** Endemic cretinism, mixed type
- **E00.9 Congenital iodine-deficiency syndrome, unspecified** Congenital iodine-deficiency hypothyroidism NOS Endemic cretinism NOS

E01 IODINE-DEFICIENCY RELATED THYROID DISORDERS AND ALLIED CONDITIONS

Excludes1: congenital iodine-deficiency syndrome (E00.-) subclinical iodine-deficiency hypothyroidism (E02)

- **E01.0 Iodine-deficiency related diffuse (endemic) goiter**
- **E01.1 Iodine-deficiency related multinodular (endemic) goiter** Iodine-deficiency related nodular goiter
- **E01.2 Iodine-deficiency related (endemic) goiter, unspecified** Endemic goiter NOS
- **E01.8 Other iodine-deficiency related thyroid disorders and allied conditions** Acquired iodine-deficiency hypothyroidism NOS

E02 SUBCLINICAL IODINE-DEFICIENCY HYPOTHYROIDISM

E03 OTHER HYPOTHYROIDISM

Excludes1: iodine-deficiency related hypothyroidism (E00–E02) postprocedural hypothyroidism (E89.0)

- **E03.0 Congenital hypothyroidism with diffuse goiter** Congenital parenchymatous goiter (nontoxic) Congenital goiter (nontoxic) NOS *Excludes1:* transitory congenital goiter with normal function (P72.0)
- **E03.1 Congenital hypothyroidism without goiter** Aplasia of thyroid (with myxedema) Congenital atrophy of thyroid Congenital hypothyroidism NOS

- **E03.2 Hypothyroidism due to medicines/drugs and other exogenous substances** **Code first** poisoning due to drug or toxin, if applicable (T36–T65 with fifth or sixth character 1–4) **Use additional code** for adverse effect, if applicable, to identify drug (T36–T50 with fifth or sixth character 5)
- **E03.3 Postinfectious hypothyroidism**
- **E03.4 Atrophy of thyroid (acquired)** *Excludes1:* congenital atrophy of thyroid (E03.1)
- **E03.8 Other specified hypothyroidism**
- **E03.9 Hypothyroidism, unspecified** Myxedema NOS

E04 OTHER NONTOXIC GOITER

Excludes1: congenital goiter (NOS) (diffuse) (parenchymatous) (E03.0) iodine-deficiency related goiter (E00–E02)

- **E04.0 Nontoxic diffuse goiter** Diffuse (colloid) nontoxic goiter Simple nontoxic goiter
- **E04.1 Nontoxic single thyroid nodule** Colloid nodule (cystic) (thyroid) Nontoxic uninodular goiter Thyroid (cystic) nodule NOS
- **E04.2 Nontoxic multinodular goiter** Cystic goiter NOS Multinodular (cystic) goiter NOS
- **E04.8 Other specified nontoxic goiter**
- **E04.9 Nontoxic goiter, unspecified** Goiter NOS Nodular goiter (nontoxic) NOS

E05 THYROTOXICOSIS [HYPERTHYROIDISM]

Excludes1: chronic thyroiditis with transient thyrotoxicosis (E06.2) neonatal thyrotoxicosis (P72.1)

- **E05.0 Thyrotoxicosis with diffuse goiter** Exophthalmic or toxic goiter NOS Graves' disease Toxic diffuse goiter
  - **E05.00 Thyrotoxicosis with diffuse goiter without thyrotoxic crisis or storm**
  - **E05.01 Thyrotoxicosis with diffuse goiter with thyrotoxic crisis or storm**
- **E05.9 Thyrotoxicosis, unspecified** Hyperthyroidism NOS
  - **E05.90 Thyrotoxicosis, unspecified without thyrotoxic crisis or storm**
  - **E05.91 Thyrotoxicosis, unspecified with thyrotoxic crisis or storm**

E06 THYROIDITIS

Excludes1: postpartum thyroiditis (O90.5)

- **E06.0 Acute thyroiditis** Abscess of thyroid Pyogenic thyroiditis Suppurative thyroiditis **Use additional code** (B95–B97) to identify infectious agent.
- **E06.1 Subacute thyroiditis** de Quervain thyroiditis Giant-cell thyroiditis Granulomatous thyroiditis Nonsuppurative thyroiditis Viral thyroiditis *Excludes1:* autoimmune thyroiditis (E06.3)
- **E06.2 Chronic thyroiditis with transient thyrotoxicosis** *Excludes1:* autoimmune thyroiditis (E06.3)
- **E06.3 Autoimmune thyroiditis** Hashimoto's thyroiditis Hashitoxicosis (transient) Lymphadenoid goiter Lymphocytic thyroiditis Struma lymphomatosa

---

4th 5th 6th 7th Additional Character Required ✓ 3-character code

●=New Code *Excludes1*—Not coded here, do not use together
▲=Revised Code *Excludes2*—Not included here

E06.4 Drug-induced thyroiditis
Use additional code for adverse effect, if applicable, to identify drug (T36-T50 with fifth or sixth character 5)

E06.5 Other chronic thyroiditis
Chronic fibrous thyroiditis
Chronic thyroiditis NOS
Ligneous thyroiditis
Riedel thyroiditis

E06.9 Thyroiditis, unspecified

E07 OTHER DISORDERS OF THYROID

4th **E07.8 Other specified disorders of thyroid**

5th **E07.89 Other specified disorders of thyroid**
Abnormality of thyroid-binding globulin
Hemorrhage of thyroid
Infarction of thyroid

E07.9 Disorder of thyroid, unspecified

(E08–E13) DIABETES MELLITUS

GUIDELINES

The DM codes are combination codes that include the type of DM, the body system affected, and the complications affecting that body system. As many codes within a particular category as are necessary to describe all of the complications of the disease may be used. They should be sequenced based on the reason for a particular encounter. Assign as many codes from categories E08–E13 as needed to identify all of the associated conditions that the patient has.

Type of diabetes

The age of a patient is not the sole determining factor, though most type 1 diabetics develop the condition before reaching puberty. For this reason type 1 DM is also referred to as juvenile diabetes.

Type of DM not documented

If the type of DM is not documented in the medical record the default is E11.-, Type 2 DM.

DM and the use of insulin, oral hypoglycemics, and injectable non-insulin drugs

If the documentation in a medical record does not indicate the type of diabetes but does indicate that the patient uses insulin, code E11-, Type 2 DM, should be assigned. Additional codes should be assigned from category Z79 to identify the long-term (current) use of insulin, oral hypoglycemic drugs, or injectable non-insulin antidiabetic, as follows: If the patient is treated with both oral hypoglycemic drugs and insulin, both code Z79.4, Long term (current) use of insulin, and code Z79.84, Long term (current) use of oral hypoglycemic drugs, should be assigned. If the patient is treated with both insulin and an injectable non-insulin antidiabetic drug, assign codes Z79.4, Long term (current) use of insulin, and Z79.85, Long-term (current) use of injectable non-insulin antidiabetic drugs. If the patient is treated with both oral hypoglycemic drugs and an injectable non-insulin antidiabetic drug, assign codes Z79.84, Long-term (current) use of oral hypoglycemic drugs, and Z79.85, Long-term (current) use of injectable non-insulin antidiabetic drugs. Code Z79.4 should not be assigned if insulin is given temporarily to bring a type 2 patient's blood sugar under control during an encounter.

Complications due to insulin pump malfunction

UNDERDOSE OF INSULIN DUE TO INSULIN PUMP FAILURE

An underdose of insulin due to an insulin pump failure should be assigned to a code from subcategory T85.6, Mechanical complication of other specified internal and external prosthetic devices, implants and grafts, that specifies the type of pump malfunction, as the principal or first-listed code, followed by code T38.3x6-, Underdosing of insulin and oral hypoglycemic [antidiabetic] drugs. Additional codes for the type of DM and any associated complications due to the underdosing should also be assigned.

OVERDOSE OF INSULIN DUE TO INSULIN PUMP FAILURE

The principal or first-listed code for an encounter due to an insulin pump malfunction resulting in an overdose of insulin, should also be T85.6-, Mechanical complication of other specified internal and external prosthetic devices, implants and grafts, followed by code T38.3x1-, Poisoning by insulin and oral hypoglycemic [antidiabetic] drugs, accidental (unintentional).

Secondary DM

Codes under categories E08, DM due to underlying condition, E09, Drug or chemical induced DM, and E13, Other specified DM, identify complications/ manifestations associated with secondary DM. Secondary diabetes is always caused by another condition or event (e.g., cystic fibrosis, malignant neoplasm of pancreas, pancreatectomy, adverse effect of drug, or poisoning).

SECONDARY DM AND THE USE OF INSULIN, ORAL HYPOGLYCEMIC DRUGS, OR INJECTABLE NON-INSULIN DRUGS

For patients with secondary diabetes mellitus who routinely use insulin, oral hypoglycemic drugs, or injectable non-insulin drugs, additional code(s) from category Z79 should be assigned to identify the long-term (current) use of insulin, oral hypoglycemic drugs, or non-injectable non-insulin drugs as follows:

If the patient is treated with both oral hypoglycemic drugs and insulin, both code Z79.4, Long term (current) use of insulin, and code Z79.84, Long term (current) use of oral hypoglycemic drugs, should be assigned.

If the patient is treated with both insulin and an injectable non-insulin antidiabetic drug, assign codes Z79.4, Long-term (current) use of insulin, and **Z79.85, Long-term (current) use of injectable non-insulin antidiabetic drugs.**

If the patient is treated with both oral hypoglycemic drugs and an injectable non-insulin antidiabetic drug, assign codes Z79.84, Long-term (current) use of oral hypoglycemic drugs, and **Z79.85, Long-term (current) use of injectable non-insulin antidiabetic drugs.** Code Z79.4 should not be assigned if insulin is given temporarily to bring a secondary diabetic patient's blood sugar under control during an encounter.

ASSIGNING AND SEQUENCING SECONDARY DIABETES CODES AND ITS CAUSES

The sequencing of the secondary diabetes codes in relationship to codes for the cause of the diabetes is based on the Tabular List instructions for categories E08, E09 and E13.

Secondary DM due to pancreatectomy

For postpancreatectomy DM (lack of insulin due to the surgical removal of all or part of the pancreas), assign code E89.1, Postprocedural hypoinsulinemia. Assign a code from category E13 and a code from subcategory Z90.41-, Acquired absence of pancreas, as additional codes.

Secondary diabetes due to drugs

Secondary diabetes may be caused by an adverse effect of correctly administered medications, poisoning or sequela of poisoning.

See categories T36–T50 for coding of adverse effects and poisoning.

Note for hyperglycemia not caused by DM or for transient hyperglycemia, refer to code R73.9, hyperglycemia, NOS

E08 DM DUE TO UNDERLYING CONDITION

4th **Code first** the underlying condition, such as:
congenital rubella (P35.0)
Cushing's syndrome (E24.-)
cystic fibrosis (E84.-)
malignant neoplasm (C00–C96)
malnutrition (E40–E46)
pancreatitis and other diseases of the pancreas (K85-K86.-)

Use additional code to identify control using:
insulin (Z79.4)
oral antidiabetic drugs (Z79.84)
oral hypoglycemic drugs (Z79.84)

Use additional injectable non-insulin antidiabetic drugs (Z79.85)

Excludes1: drug or chemical induced DM (E09.-)
gestational diabetes (O24.4-)
neonatal DM (transient) (P70.2)
postpancreatectomy DM (E13.-)
postprocedural DM (E13.-)
secondary DM NEC (E13.-)
type 1 DM (E10.-)
type 2 DM (E11.-)

E08.0 DM due to underlying condition with hyperosmolarity;

5th **E08.00 without NKHHC**
E08.01 with coma

E08.1 DM due to underlying condition with ketoacidosis;

5th **E08.10 without coma**
E08.11 with coma

E08.2 DM due to underlying condition with; kidney complications

5th

E08.21 diabetic nephropathy or intercapillary glomerulosclerosis or intracapillary glomerulonephrosis or Kimmelstiel-Wilson disease

E08.22 diabetic CKD
Use additional code to identify stage of CKD (N18.1–N18.6)

E08.29 other diabetic kidney complication
Renal tubular degeneration in DM due to underlying condition

E08.3 DM due to underlying condition with ophthalmic complications

E08.31 DM due to underlying condition with unspecified diabetic retinopathy;

E08.311- with macular edema

E08.319- without macular edema

E08.32 DM due to underlying condition with mild nonproliferative diabetic retinopathy (NOS);

E08.321- with macular edema

E08.329- without macular edema

E08.33 DM due to underlying condition with moderate nonproliferative diabetic retinopathy;

E08.331- with macular edema

E08.339- without macular edema

E08.34 DM due to underlying condition with severe nonproliferative diabetic retinopathy;

E08.341- with macular edema

E08.349- without macular edema

E08.35 DM due to underlying condition with proliferative diabetic retinopathy;

E08.351- with macular edema

E08.359- without macular edema

E08.36 DM due to underlying condition with diabetic cataract

E08.39 DM due to underlying condition with other diabetic ophthalmic complication
Use additional code to identify manifestation, such as: diabetic glaucoma (H40–H42)

E08.4 DM due to underlying condition with; neurological complications

E08.40 diabetic neuropathy, unspecified

E08.41 diabetic mononeuropathy

E08.42 diabetic polyneuropathy
diabetic neuralgia

E08.43 diabetic autonomic (poly)neuropathy
diabetic gastroparesis

E08.44 diabetic amyotrophy

E08.49 other diabetic neurological complication

E08.5 DM due to underlying condition with; circulatory complications

E08.51 diabetic peripheral angiopathy without gangrene

E08.52 diabetic peripheral angiopathy with gangrene
diabetic gangrene

E08.59 other circulatory complications

E08.6 DM due to underlying condition with other specified complications

E08.61 DM due to underlying condition with; diabetic arthropathy

E08.610 diabetic neuropathic arthropathy
Charcôt's joints

E08.618 other diabetic arthropathy

E08.62 DM due to underlying condition with; skin complications

E08.620 diabetic dermatitis
diabetic necrobiosis lipoidica

E08.621 foot ulcer
Use additional code to identify site of ulcer (L97.4-, L97.5-)

E08.622 other skin ulcer
Use additional code to identify site of ulcer (L97.1–L97.9, L98.41–L98.49)

E08.628 other skin complications

E08.63 DM due to underlying condition with; oral complications

E08.630 periodontal disease

E08.638 other oral complications

E08.64 DM due to underlying condition with hypoglycemia;
Use additional code for hypoglycemia level, if applicable (E16.A-)

E08.641 with coma

E08.649 without coma

E08.65 DM due to underlying condition with hyperglycemia

E08.69 DM due to underlying condition with other specified complication
Use additional code to identify complication

E08.8 DM due to underlying condition with unspecified complications

E08.9 DM due to underlying condition without complications

E09 DRUG OR CHEMICAL INDUCED DM

See category E08 for guidelines
Code first poisoning due to drug or toxin, if applicable (T36–T65 with fifth or sixth character 1–4)
Use additional code for adverse effect, if applicable, to identify drug (T36–T50 with fifth or sixth character 5)
Use additional code to identify control using:
insulin (Z79.4)
oral antidiabetic drugs (Z79.84)
oral hypoglycemic drugs (Z79.84)
Excludes1: DM due to underlying condition (E08.-)
gestational diabetes (O24.4-)
neonatal DM (P70.2)
postpancreatectomy DM (E13.-)
postprocedural DM (E13.-)
secondary DM NEC (E13.-)
type 1 DM (E10.-)
type 2 DM (E11.-)

E09.0 Drug or chemical induced DM with hyperosmolarity

E09.00 Drug or chemical induced DM with hyperosmolarity without NKHHC

E09.01 Drug or chemical induced DM with hyperosmolarity with coma

E09.1 Drug or chemical induced DM with ketoacidosis;

E09.10 without coma

E09.11 with coma

E09.2 Drug or chemical induced DM with; kidney complications

E09.21 diabetic nephropathy
Drug or chemical induced DM with intercapillary glomerulosclerosis or intracapillary glomerulonephrosis or Kimmelstiel-Wilson disease

E09.22 diabetic CKD
Use additional code to identify stage of CKD (N18.1–N18.6)

E09.29 other diabetic kidney complication
Drug or chemical induced DM with renal tubular degeneration

E09.3 Drug or chemical induced DM with ophthalmic complications

E09.31 Drug or chemical induced DM with unspecified diabetic retinopathy;

E09.311 with macular edema

E09.319 without macular edema

E09.32 **Drug or chemical induced DM with mild nonproliferative diabetic retinopathy;**

Drug or chemical induced DM with nonproliferative diabetic retinopathy NOS

E09.321- with macular edema

E09.329- without macular edema

E09.33 **Drug or chemical induced DM with moderate nonproliferative diabetic retinopathy;**

E09.331- with macular edema

E09.339- without macular edema

E09.34 **Drug or chemical induced DM with severe nonproliferative diabetic retinopathy;**

E09.341- with macular edema

E09.349- without macular edema

E09.35 **Drug or chemical induced DM with proliferative diabetic retinopathy;**

E09.351- with macular edema

E09.353- with traction retinal detachment not involving the macula

E09.354- with combined traction retinal detachment and rhegmatogenous retinal detachment

E09.355- stable

E09.359- without macular edema

E09.36 **Drug or chemical induced DM with diabetic cataract**

E09.39 **Drug or chemical induced DM with other diabetic ophthalmic complication**

Use additional code to identify manifestation, such as: diabetic glaucoma (H40–H42)

E09.4 Drug or chemical induced DM with neurological complications;

E09.40 with diabetic neuropathy, unspecified

E09.41 with diabetic mononeuropathy

E09.42 with diabetic polyneuropathy with diabetic neuralgia

E09.43 with diabetic autonomic (poly)neuropathy with diabetic gastroparesis

E09.44 diabetic amyotrophy

E09.49 with other diabetic neurological complication

E09.5 Drug or chemical induced DM with; circulatory complications

E09.51 diabetic peripheral angiopathy without gangrene

E09.52 diabetic peripheral angiopathy with gangrene diabetic gangrene

E09.59 other circulatory complications

E09.6 Drug or chemical induced DM with other specified complications

E09.61 **Drug or chemical induced DM with; diabetic arthropathy**

E09.610 diabetic neuropathic arthropathy Charcôt's joints

E09.618 other diabetic arthropathy

E09.62 **Drug or chemical induced DM with; skin complications**

E09.620 diabetic dermatitis diabetic necrobiosis lipoidica

E09.621 foot ulcer **Use additional code** to identify site of ulcer (L97.4-, L97.5-)

E09.622 other skin ulcer **Use additional code** to identify site of ulcer (L97.1–L97.9, L98.41–L98.49)

E09.628 other skin complications

E09.63 **Drug or chemical induced DM with; oral complications**

E09.630 periodontal disease

E09.638 other oral complications

E09.64 **Drug or chemical induced DM with hypoglycemia;**

Use additional code for hypoglycemia level, if applicable (E16.A-)

E09.641 with coma

E09.649 without coma

E09.65 **Drug or chemical induced DM with hyperglycemia**

E09.69 **Drug or chemical induced DM with other specified complication**

Use additional code to identify complication

E09.8 Drug or chemical induced DM with unspecified complications

E09.9 Drug or chemical induced DM without complications

E10 TYPE 1 DM

See category E08 for guidelines

Includes: brittle diabetes (mellitus)
diabetes (mellitus) due to autoimmune process
diabetes (mellitus) due to immune mediated pancreatic islet beta-cell destruction
idiopathic diabetes (mellitus)
juvenile onset diabetes (mellitus)
ketosis-prone diabetes (mellitus)

Excludes1: DM due to underlying condition (E08.-)
drug or chemical induced DM (E09.-)
gestational diabetes (O24.4-)
hyperglycemia NOS (R73.9)
neonatal DM (P70.2)
postpancreatectomy DM (E13.-)
postprocedural DM (E13.-)
secondary DM NEC (E13.-)
type 2 DM (E11.-)

E10.1 Type 1 DM with ketoacidosis;

E10.10 Type 1 DM with ketoacidosis without coma

E10.11 Type 1 DM with ketoacidosis with coma

E10.2 Type 1 DM with kidney complications

E10.21 Type 1 DM with diabetic nephropathy Type 1 DM with intercapillary glomerulosclerosis or intracapillary glomerulonephrosis or Kimmelstiel-Wilson disease

E10.22 Type 1 DM with diabetic CKD **Use additional code** to identify stage of CKD (N18.1–N18.6)

E10.29 Type 1 DM with other diabetic kidney complication Type 1 DM with renal tubular degeneration

E10.3 Type 1 DM with ophthalmic complications

E10.31 Type 1 DM with unspecified diabetic retinopathy;

E10.311 with macular edema

E10.319 without macular edema

E10.32 Type 1 DM with mild nonproliferative diabetic retinopathy; diabetic retinopathy NOS

E10.321- with macular edema

E10.329- without macular edema

E10.33 Type 1 DM with moderate nonproliferative diabetic retinopathy;

E10.331- with macular edema

E10.339- without macular edema

E10.34 Type 1 DM with severe nonproliferative diabetic retinopathy;

E10.341- with macular edema

E10.349- without macular edema

E10.35 Type 1 DM with proliferative diabetic retinopathy;
- **6th** **E10.351-** with macular edema
  - **7th**
- **E10.359-** without macular edema
  - **7th**

E10.36 Type 1 DM with diabetic cataract

E10.39 Type 1 DM with other diabetic ophthalmic complication
- **Use additional code** to identify manifestation, such as: diabetic glaucoma (H40–H42)

E10.4 Type 1 DM with neurological complications
- **5th** **E10.40** Type 1 DM with diabetic neuropathy, unspecified
- **E10.41** Type 1 DM with diabetic mononeuropathy
- **E10.42** Type 1 DM with diabetic polyneuropathy
  - Type 1 DM with diabetic neuralgia
- **E10.43** Type 1 DM with diabetic autonomic (poly)neuropathy
- **E10.44** Type 1 DM with diabetic amyotrophy
- **E10.49** Type 1 DM with other diabetic neurological complication

E10.5 Type 1 DM with circulatory complications
- **5th** **E10.51** Type 1 DM with diabetic peripheral angiopathy without gangrene
- **E10.52** Type 1 DM with diabetic peripheral angiopathy with gangrene
  - Type 1 DM with diabetic gangrene
- **E10.59** Type 1 DM with other circulatory complications

E10.6 Type 1 DM with other specified complications
- **5th** **E10.61** Type 1 DM with diabetic arthropathy
  - **6th** **E10.610** Type 1 DM with diabetic neuropathic arthropathy
    - Type 1 DM with Charcôt's joints
  - **E10.618** Type 1 DM with other diabetic arthropathy
- **E10.62** Type 1 DM with skin complications
  - **6th** **E10.620** Type 1 DM with diabetic dermatitis
    - Type 1 DM with diabetic necrobiosis lipoidica
  - **E10.621** Type 1 DM with foot ulcer
    - **Use additional code** to identify site of ulcer (L97.4-, L97.5-)
  - **E10.622** Type 1 DM with other skin ulcer
    - **Use additional code** to identify site of ulcer (L97.1–L97.9, L98.41–L98.49)
  - **E10.628** Type 1 DM with other skin complications
- **E10.63** Type 1 DM with oral complications
  - **6th** **E10.630** Type 1 DM with periodontal disease
  - **E10.638** Type 1 DM with other oral complications
- **E10.64** Type 1 DM with hypoglycemia
  - **6th** **Use additional code** for hypoglycemia level, if applicable (E16.A-)
  - **E10.641** Type 1 DM with hypoglycemia with coma
  - **E10.649** Type 1 DM with hypoglycemia without coma
- **E10.65** Type 1 DM with hyperglycemia
- **E10.69** Type 1 DM with other specified complication
  - **Use additional code** to identify complication

E10.8 Type 1 DM with unspecified complications

E10.9 Type 1 DM without complications

•E10.A Type 1 diabetes mellitus, presymptomatic
- **5th** Early-stage type 1 diabetes mellitus
- **•E10.A0** Type 1 diabetes mellitus, presymptomatic, unspecified
- **•E10.A1** Type 1 diabetes mellitus, presymptomatic, Stage 1
  - Multiple confirmed islet autoantibodies with normoglycemia
- **•E10.A2** Type 1 diabetes mellitus, presymptomatic, Stage 2
  - Confirmed islet autoimmunity with dysglycemia

E11 TYPE 2 DM

4th

See category E08 for guidelines.

If the type of DM is not documented in the medical record the default is E11.-, Type 2 DM.

Includes: diabetes (mellitus) due to insulin secretory defect
diabetes NOS
insulin resistant diabetes (mellitus)

Use additional code to identify control using:
injectable non-insulin antidiabetic drugs (Z79.85)
insulin (Z79.4)
oral antidiabetic drugs (Z79.84)
oral hypoglycemic drugs (Z79.84)

Excludes1: DM due to underlying condition (E08.-)
drug or chemical induced DM (E09.-)
gestational diabetes (O24.4-)
neonatal DM (P70.2)
postpancreatectomy DM (E13.-)
postprocedural DM (E13.-)
secondary DM NEC (E13.-)
type 1 DM (E10.-)

E11.0 Type 2 DM with hyperosmolarity;
- **5th** **E11.00** without NKHHC
- **E11.01** with coma

E11.1 Type 2 diabetes mellitus with ketoacidosis
- **5th** **E11.10** Type 2 diabetes mellitus with ketoacidosis without coma
- **E11.11** Type 2 diabetes mellitus with ketoacidosis with coma

E11.2 Type 2 DM with kidney complications
- **5th** **E11.21** Type 2 DM with diabetic nephropathy or intercapillary glomerulosclerosis or intracapillary glomerulonephrosis or Kimmelstiel-Wilson disease
- **E11.22** Type 2 DM with diabetic CKD
  - **Use additional code** to identify stage of CKD (N18.1–N18.6)
- **E11.29** Type 2 DM with other diabetic kidney complication
  - Type 2 DM with renal tubular degeneration

E11.3 Type 2 DM with ophthalmic complications
- **5th** **E11.31** Type 2 DM with unspecified diabetic retinopathy;
  - **6th** **E11.311** with macular edema
  - **E11.319** without macular edema
- **E11.32** Type 2 DM with mild nonproliferative diabetic retinopathy;
  - **6th** Type 2 DM with nonproliferative diabetic retinopathy NOS

  - **E11.321-** with macular edema
    - **7th**
  - **E11.329-** without macular edema
    - **7th**

- **E11.33** Type 2 DM with moderate nonproliferative diabetic retinopathy;
  - **6th** **E11.331-** with macular edema
    - **7th**
  - **E11.339-** without macular edema
    - **7th**

- **E11.34** Type 2 DM with severe nonproliferative diabetic retinopathy;
  - **6th** **E11.341-** with macular edema
    - **7th**
  - **E11.349-** without macular edema
    - **7th**

- **E11.35** Type 2 DM with proliferative diabetic retinopathy;
  - **6th** **E11.351-** with macular edema
    - **7th**
  - **E11.359-** without macular edema
    - **7th**

- **E11.36** Type 2 DM with diabetic cataract
- **E11.39** Type 2 DM with other diabetic ophthalmic complication
  - **Use additional code** to identify manifestation, such as: diabetic glaucoma (H40–H42)

E11.4 Type 2 DM with neurological complications
- **5th** **E11.40** Type 2 DM with diabetic neuropathy, unspecified
- **E11.41** Type 2 DM with diabetic mononeuropathy
- **E11.42** Type 2 DM with diabetic polyneuropathy
  - Type 2 DM with diabetic neuralgia
- **E11.43** Type 2 DM with diabetic autonomic (poly)neuropathy
  - Type 2 DM with diabetic gastroparesis
- **E11.44** Type 2 DM with diabetic amyotrophy

•=New Code *Excludes1*—Not coded here, do not use together
▲=Revised Code *Excludes2*—Not included here

E11.49 Type 2 DM with other diabetic neurological complication

E11.5 Type 2 DM with circulatory complications

E11.51 Type 2 DM with diabetic peripheral angiopathy without gangrene

E11.52 Type 2 DM with diabetic peripheral angiopathy with gangrene
Type 2 DM with diabetic gangrene

E11.59 Type 2 DM with other circulatory complications

E11.6 Type 2 DM with other specified complications

E11.61 Type 2 DM with diabetic arthropathy

E11.610 Type 2 DM with diabetic neuropathic arthropathy
Type 2 DM with Charcôt's joints

E11.618 Type 2 DM with other diabetic arthropathy

E11.62 Type 2 DM with skin complications

E11.620 Type 2 DM with diabetic dermatitis
Type 2 DM with diabetic necrobiosis lipoidica

E11.621 Type 2 DM with foot ulcer
Use additional code to identify site of ulcer (L97.4-, L97.5-)

E11.622 Type 2 DM with other skin ulcer
Use additional code to identify site of ulcer (L97.1-L97.9, L98.41-L98.49)

E11.628 Type 2 DM with other skin complications

E11.63 Type 2 DM with oral complications

E11.630 Type 2 DM with periodontal disease

E11.638 Type 2 DM with other oral complications

E11.64 Type 2 DM with hypoglycemia

Use additional code for hypoglycemia level, if applicable (E16.A-)

E11.641 Type 2 DM with hypoglycemia with coma

E11.649 Type 2 DM with hypoglycemia without coma

E11.65 Type 2 DM with hyperglycemia

E11.69 Type 2 DM with other specified complication
Use additional code to identify complication

E11.8 Type 2 DM with unspecified complications

E11.9 Type 2 DM without complications

(E15-E16) OTHER DISORDERS OF GLUCOSE REGULATION AND PANCREATIC INTERNAL SECRETION

E15 NONDIABETIC HYPOGLYCEMIC COMA

Includes: drug-induced insulin coma in nondiabetic
hyperinsulinism with hypoglycemic coma
hypoglycemic coma NOS

E16 OTHER DISORDERS OF PANCREATIC INTERNAL SECRETION

E16.0 Drug-induced hypoglycemia without coma
Excludes1: diabetes with hypoglycemia without coma (E09.649)
Use additional code for adverse effect, if applicable, to identify drug (T36-T50 with fifth or sixth character 5)
Use additional code for hypoglycemia level, if applicable (E16.A-)

E16.1 Other hypoglycemia
Functional hyperinsulinism
Functional nonhyperinsulinemic hypoglycemia
Hyperinsulinism NOS
Hyperplasia of pancreatic islet beta cells NOS
Excludes1: diabetes with hypoglycemia (E08.649, E10.649, E11.649)
hypoglycemia in infant of diabetic mother (P70.1)
neonatal hypoglycemia (P70.4)

E16.2 Hypoglycemia, unspecified
Excludes 1: diabetes with hypoglycemia (E08.649, E10.649, E11.649)
Use additional code for hypoglycemia level, if applicable (E16.A-)

E16.8 Other specified disorders of pancreatic internal secretion
Increased secretion from endocrine pancreas of growth hormone-releasing hormone or pancreatic polypeptide or somatostatin or vasoactive-intestinal polypeptide

E16.9 Disorder of pancreatic internal secretion, unspecified
Islet-cell hyperplasia NOS
Pancreatic endocrine cell hyperplasia NOS

•E16.A Hypoglycemia level

•E16.A1 Hypoglycemia level 1
Decreased blood glucose level 1

•E16.A2 Hypoglycemia level 2
Decreased blood glucose level 2

•E16.A3 Hypoglycemia level 3
Decreased blood glucose level 3

(E20-E35) DISORDERS OF OTHER ENDOCRINE GLANDS

Excludes1: galactorrhea (N64.3)
gynecomastia (N62)

E20 HYPOPARATHYROIDISM

Excludes1: Di George's syndrome (D82.1)
postprocedural hypoparathyroidism (E89.2)
tetany NOS (R29.0)
transitory neonatal hypoparathyroidism (P71.4)

E20.0 Idiopathic hypoparathyroidism

E20.1 Pseudohypoparathyroidism

E20.8 Other hypoparathyroidism

E20.810 Autosomal dominant hypocalcemia
Autosomal dominant hypocalcemia type 1 (ADH1)
Autosomal dominant hypocalcemia type 2 (ADH2)
Code also, if applicable, any associated conditions, such as:
calculus of kidney (N20.0)
chronic kidney disease (N18.-)
respiratory distress (J80, R06.-)
seizure disorder (G40.-, R56.9)

E20.811 Secondary hypoparathyroidism in diseases classified elsewhere
Code first underlying condition, if known

E20.812 Autoimmune hypoparathyroidism
Code first, if applicable, underlying condition such as:
autoimmune polyglandular failure (E31.0)
Schmidt's syndrome (E31.0)

E20.818 Other specified hypoparathyroidism due to impaired parathyroid hormone secretion
Familial isolated hypoparathyroidism

E20.819 Hypoparathyroidism due to impaired parathyroid hormone secretion, unspecified

E20.89 Other specified hypoparathyroidism
Familial hypoparathyroidism

E20.9 Hypoparathyroidism, unspecified
Parathyroid tetany

E22 HYPERFUNCTION OF PITUITARY GLAND

Excludes1: Cushing's syndrome (E24.-)
Nelson's syndrome (E24.1)
overproduction of ACTH not associated with Cushing's disease (E27.0)
overproduction of pituitary ACTH (E24.0)
overproduction of thyroid-stimulating hormone (E05.8-)

E22.0 Acromegaly and pituitary gigantism
Overproduction of growth hormone
Excludes1: constitutional gigantism (E34.4)
constitutional tall stature (E34.4)
increased secretion from endocrine pancreas of growth hormone-releasing hormone (E16.8)

E22.2 Syndrome of inappropriate secretion of antidiuretic hormone

E22.8 Other hyperfunction of pituitary gland
Central precocious puberty

E22.9 Hyperfunction of pituitary gland, unspecified

E23 HYPOFUNCTION AND OTHER DISORDERS OF THE PITUITARY GLAND

4th

Includes: the listed conditions whether the disorder is in the pituitary or the hypothalamus

Excludes1: postprocedural hypopituitarism (E89.3)

- **E23.0 Hypopituitarism**
- **E23.1 Drug-induced hypopituitarism**
  - **Use additional code** for adverse effect, if applicable, to identify drug (T36–T50 with fifth or sixth character 5)
- **E23.2 Diabetes insipidus**
  - *Excludes1:* nephrogenic diabetes insipidus (N25.1)
- **E23.3 Hypothalamic dysfunction, not elsewhere classified**
  - *Excludes1:* Prader-Willi syndrome (Q87.11)
  - Russell-Silver syndrome (Q87.1)
- **E23.6 Other disorders of pituitary gland**
  - Abscess of pituitary
  - Adiposogenital dystrophy
- **E24.8 Other Cushing's syndrome**
- **E23.7 Disorder of pituitary gland, unspecified**

E24 CUSHING'S SYNDROME

4th

Excludes1: congenital adrenal hyperplasia (E25.0)

- **E24.0 Pituitary-dependent Cushing's disease**
  - Overproduction of pituitary ACTH
  - Pituitary-dependent hypercorticalism
- **E24.2 Drug-induced Cushing's syndrome**
  - **Use additional code** for adverse effect, if applicable, to identify drug (T36–T50 with fifth or sixth character 5)
- **E24.8 Other Cushing's syndrome**
- **E24.9 Cushing's syndrome, unspecified**

E25 ADRENOGENITAL DISORDERS

4th

Includes: adrenogenital syndromes, virilizing or feminizing, whether acquired or due to adrenal hyperplasia consequent on inborn enzyme defects in hormone synthesis

Female adrenal pseudohermaphroditism

Female heterosexual precocious pseudopuberty

Male isosexual precocious pseudopuberty

Male macrogenitosomia praecox

Male sexual precocity with adrenal hyperplasia

Male virilization (female)

Excludes1: indeterminate sex and pseudohermaphroditism (Q56) chromosomal abnormalities (Q90–Q99)

- **E25.0 Congenital adrenogenital disorders associated with enzyme deficiency**
  - Congenital adrenal hyperplasia
  - 21-Hydroxylase deficiency
  - Salt-losing congenital adrenal hyperplasia
- **E25.8 Other adrenogenital disorders**
  - Idiopathic adrenogenital disorder
  - **Use additional code** for adverse effect, if applicable, to identify drug (T36–T50 with fifth or sixth character 5)
- **E25.9 Adrenogenital disorder, unspecified**
  - Adrenogenital syndrome NOS

E27 OTHER DISORDERS OF ADRENAL GLAND

4th

- **E27.0 Other adrenocortical overactivity**
  - Overproduction of ACTH, not associated with Cushing's disease
  - Premature adrenarche
  - *Excludes1:* Cushing's syndrome (E24.-)
- **E27.1 Primary adrenocortical insufficiency**
  - Addison's disease
  - Autoimmune adrenalitis
  - *Excludes1:* Addison only phenotype adrenoleukodystrophy (E71.528)
  - amyloidosis (E85.-)
  - tuberculous Addison's disease (A18.7)
  - Waterhouse-Friderichsen syndrome (A39.1)
- **E27.2 Addisonian crisis**
  - Adrenal crisis
  - Adrenocortical crisis
- **E27.3 Drug-induced adrenocortical insufficiency**
  - **Use additional code** for adverse effect, if applicable, to identify drug (T36–T50 with fifth or sixth character 5)

E27.4 Other and unspecified adrenocortical insufficiency

- **E27.40 Unspecified adrenocortical insufficiency**
  - Adrenocortical insufficiency NOS
- **E27.49 Other adrenocortical insufficiency**
  - Adrenal hemorrhage
  - Adrenal infarction
- **E27.8 Other specified disorders of adrenal gland**
  - Abnormality of cortisol-binding globulin
- **E27.9 Disorder of adrenal gland, unspecified**
  - *Excludes1:* adrenoleukodystrophy [Addison-Schilder] (E71.528)
  - Waterhouse-Friderichsen syndrome (A39.1)

E28 OVARIAN DYSFUNCTION

4th

Excludes1: isolated gonadotropin deficiency (E23.0)

postprocedural ovarian failure (E89.4-)

- **E28.0 Estrogen excess**
  - **Use additional code** for adverse effect, if applicable, to identify drug (T36–T50 with fifth or sixth character 5)
- **E28.1 Androgen excess**
  - Hypersecretion of ovarian androgens
  - **Use additional code** for adverse effect, if applicable, to identify drug (T36–T50 with fifth or sixth character 5)
- **E28.2 Polycystic ovarian syndrome**
  - Sclerocystic ovary syndrome
  - Stein-Leventhal syndrome
- **E28.3 Primary ovarian failure**

5th

  - *Excludes1:* pure gonadal dysgenesis (Q99.1)
  - Turner's syndrome (Q96.-)
  - **E28.39 Other primary ovarian failure**
    - Decreased estrogen
    - Resistant ovary syndrome

E30 DISORDERS OF PUBERTY, NEC

4th

- **E30.0 Delayed puberty**
  - Constitutional delay of puberty
  - Delayed sexual development
- **E30.1 Precocious puberty**
  - Precocious menstruation
  - *Excludes1:* Albright (-McCune) (-Sternberg) syndrome (Q78.1)
  - central precocious puberty (E22.8)
  - congenital adrenal hyperplasia (E25.0)
  - female heterosexual precocious pseudopuberty (E25.-)
  - male isosexual precocious pseudopuberty (E25.-)
- **E30.8 Other disorders of puberty**
  - Premature thelarche
- **E30.9 Disorder of puberty, unspecified**

E31 POLYGLANDULAR DYSFUNCTION

4th

Excludes1: ataxia telangiectasia [Louis-Bar] (G11.3)

dystrophia myotonica [Steinert] (G71.11)

pseudohypoparathyroidism (E20.1)

- **E31.2 Multiple endocrine neoplasia [MEN] syndromes**

5th

  - Multiple endocrine adenomatosis
  - *Code also* any associated malignancies and other conditions associated with the syndromes
  - **E31.20 Multiple endocrine neoplasia [MEN] syndrome, unspecified**
    - Multiple endocrine adenomatosis NOS
    - Multiple endocrine neoplasia [MEN] syndrome NOS
  - **E31.21 Multiple endocrine neoplasia [MEN] type I**
    - Wermer's syndrome
  - **E31.22 Multiple endocrine neoplasia [MEN] type IIA**
    - Sipple's syndrome
  - **E31.23 Multiple endocrine neoplasia [MEN] type IIB**

E34 OTHER ENDOCRINE DISORDERS

4th

Excludes1: pseudohypoparathyroidism (E20.1)

- **E34.0 Carcinoid syndrome**
  - **Code also** the underlying disorder, such as:
  - primary neuroendocrine tumors (C7A.-)
  - secondary neuroendocrine tumors (C7B.-)
  - •**E34.00 Carcinoid syndrome, unspecified**
    - Carcinoid disease, unspecified
  - •**E34.01 Carcinoid heart syndrome**
    - Carcinoid heart disease
    - Hedinger syndrome

4th **5th** **6th** **7th** Additional Character Required ✓ 3-character code

•=New Code **Excludes1**—Not coded here, do not use together

▲=Revised Code **Excludes2**—Not included here

*E34.09 Other carcinoid syndrome
Carcinoid disease NEC
Carcinoid syndrome NEC
Other carcinoid disease

E34.3 Short stature due to endocrine disorder
5th Constitutional short stature
Laron-type short stature
Excludes1: achondroplastic short stature (Q77.4)
hypochondroplastic short stature (Q77.4)
nutritional short stature (E45)
pituitary short stature (E23.0)
progeria (E34.8)
renal short stature (N25.0)
Russell-Silver syndrome (Q87.19)
short-limbed stature with immunodeficiency (D82.2)
short stature in specific dysmorphic syndromes — **code to syndrome — see** Alphabetical Index
short stature NOS (R62.52)

E34.31 Constitutional short stature

6th **E34.321 Primary insulin-like growth factor-1 (IGF-1) deficiency**

E34.322 Insulin-like growth factor-1 (IGF-1) resistance

E34.328 Other genetic causes of short stature

E34.329 Unspecified genetic causes of short stature

E34.39 Other short stature due to endocrine disorder

E34.4 Constitutional tall stature

E34.5 Androgen insensitivity syndrome

5th **E34.50 Androgen insensitivity syndrome, unspecified**
Androgen insensitivity NOS

E34.51 Complete androgen insensitivity syndrome
Complete androgen insensitivity
de Quervain syndrome
Goldberg-Maxwell syndrome

E34.52 Partial androgen insensitivity syndrome
Partial androgen insensitivity
Reifenstein syndrome

E34.8 Other specified endocrine disorders
Pineal gland dysfunction
Progeria
Excludes2: pseudohypoparathyroidism (E20.1)

E34.9 Endocrine disorder, unspecified
Endocrine disturbance NOS
Hormone disturbance NOS

(E36) INTRAOPERATIVE COMPLICATIONS OF ENDOCRINE SYSTEM

(E40–E46) MALNUTRITION

E40 KWASHIORKOR
✓ Severe malnutrition with nutritional edema with dyspigmentation of skin and hair
Excludes1: marasmic kwashiorkor (E42)

E44 PROTEIN-CALORIE MALNUTRITION OF MODERATE AND MILD DEGREE
4th

E44.0 Moderate protein-calorie malnutrition

E44.1 Mild protein-calorie malnutrition
Nutritional short stature
Nutritional stunting
Physical retardation due to malnutrition

E45 RETARDED DEVELOPMENT FOLLOWING PROTEIN-CALORIE MALNUTRITION
✓

E46 UNSPECIFIED PROTEIN-CALORIE MALNUTRITION
✓ Malnutrition NOS
Protein-calorie imbalance NOS
Excludes1: nutritional deficiency NOS (E63.9)

(E50–E64) OTHER NUTRITIONAL DEFICIENCIES

E55 VITAMIN D DEFICIENCY
4th *Excludes1:* adult osteomalacia (M83.-)
osteoporosis (M80.-)
sequelae of rickets (E64.3)

E55.0 Rickets, active
Infantile osteomalacia
Juvenile osteomalacia
Excludes1: celiac rickets (K90.0)
Crohn's rickets (K50.-)
hereditary vitamin D-dependent rickets (E83.32)
inactive rickets (E64.3)
renal rickets (N25.0)
sequelae of rickets (E64.3)
vitamin D-resistant rickets (E83.31)

E55.9 Vitamin D deficiency, unspecified
Avitaminosis D

E56 OTHER VITAMIN DEFICIENCIES
4th *Excludes1:* sequelae of other vitamin deficiencies (E64.8)

E56.0 Deficiency of vitamin E

E56.1 Deficiency of vitamin K
Excludes1: deficiency of coagulation factor due to vitamin K deficiency (D68.4)
vitamin K deficiency of newborn (P53)

E56.8 Deficiency of other vitamins

E56.9 Vitamin deficiency, unspecified

E58 DIETARY CALCIUM DEFICIENCY
✓ *Excludes1:* disorders of calcium metabolism (E83.5-)
sequelae of calcium deficiency (E64.8)

E63 OTHER NUTRITIONAL DEFICIENCIES
4th *Excludes2:* dehydration (E86.0)
failure to thrive, adult (R62.7)
failure to thrive, child (R62.51)
feeding problems in newborn (P92.-)
sequelae of malnutrition and other nutritional deficiencies (E64.-)

E63.0 Essential fatty acid [EFA] deficiency

E63.1 Imbalance of constituents of food intake

E63.8 Other specified nutritional deficiencies

E63.9 Nutritional deficiency, unspecified

(E65–E68) OVERWEIGHT, OBESITY AND OTHER HYPERALIMENTATION

E66 OVERWEIGHT AND OBESITY
4th **Use additional code** to identify body mass index (BMI), if known, for adults (Z68.1–Z68.45) or pediatrics (Z68.5-)
Excludes2: adipogenital dystrophy (E23.6)
lipomatosis dolorosa [Dercum] (E88.2)
lipomatosis NOS (E88.2)
Prader-Willi syndrome (Q87.11)

E66.0 Obesity due to excess calories
5th **E66.01 Morbid (severe) obesity due to excess calories**
Excludes1: morbid (severe) obesity with alveolar hypoventilation (E66.2)

E66.09 Other obesity due to excess calories

E66.1 Drug-induced obesity
Use additional code for adverse effect, if applicable, to identify drug (T36-T50 with fifth or sixth character 5)

E66.2 Morbid (severe) obesity with alveolar hypoventilation
obesity hypoventilation syndrome (OHS)
Pickwickian syndrome

E66.3 Overweight

E66.8 Other obesity
*E66.81 Obesity class
6th *E66.811 Obesity, class 1
*E66.812 Obesity, class 2
*E66.813 Obesity, class 3
*E66.89 Other obesity not elsewhere classified

E66.9 Obesity, unspecified
Obesity NOS

(E70–E88) METABOLIC DISORDERS

Excludes1: androgen insensitivity syndrome (E34.5-)
congenital adrenal hyperplasia (E25.0)
hemolytic anemias attributable to enzyme disorders (D55.-)
Marfan's syndrome (Q87.4)
5-alpha-reductase deficiency (E29.1)
Excludes2: Ehlers-Danlos syndromes (Q79.6-)

E70 DISORDERS OF AROMATIC AMINO-ACID METABOLISM

- **E70.0** Classical phenylketonuria
- **E70.1** Other hyperphenylalaninemias
- **E70.8** Disorders of aromatic amino-acid metabolism
  - **E70.81** Aromatic L-amino acid decarboxylase deficiency
    - AADC deficiency
  - **E70.89** Other disorders of aromatic amino-acid metabolism

E71 DISORDERS OF BRANCHED-CHAIN AMINO-ACID METABOLISM AND FATTY-ACID METABOLISM

- **E71.0** Maple-syrup-urine disease
- **E71.1** Other disorders of branched-chain amino-acid metabolism
  - **E71.11** Branched-chain organic acidurias
    - **E71.110** Isovaleric acidemia
    - **E71.111** 3-methylglutaconic aciduria
    - **E71.118** Other branched-chain organic acidurias
  - **E71.12** Disorders of propionate metabolism
    - **E71.120** Methylmalonic acidemia
    - **E71.121** Propionic acidemia
    - **E71.128** Other disorders of propionate metabolism
  - **E71.19** Other disorders of branched-chain amino-acid metabolism
    - Hyperleucine-isoleucinemia
    - Hypervalinemia
- **E71.2** Disorder of branched-chain amino-acid metabolism, unspecified
- **E71.3** Disorders of fatty-acid metabolism
  - *Excludes1:* peroxisomal disorders (E71.5)
    - Refsum's disease (G60.1)
    - Schilder's disease (G37.0)
  - *Excludes2:* carnitine deficiency due to inborn error of metabolism (E71.42)
  - **E71.30** Disorder of fatty-acid metabolism, unspecified
  - **E71.31** Disorders of fatty-acid oxidation
    - **E71.310** Long chain/very long chain acyl CoA dehydrogenase deficiency
      - LCAD deficiency
      - VLCAD deficiency
    - **E71.311** Medium chain acyl CoA dehydrogenase deficiency
      - MCAD deficiency
    - **E71.312** Short chain acyl CoA dehydrogenase deficiency
      - SCAD deficiency
    - **E71.313** Glutaric aciduria type II
      - Glutaric aciduria type II A
      - Glutaric aciduria type II B
      - Glutaric aciduria type II C
      - *Excludes1:* glutaric aciduria (type 1) NOS (E72.3)
    - **E71.314** Muscle carnitine palmitoyltransferase deficiency
    - **E71.318** Other disorders of fatty-acid oxidation
  - **E71.32** Disorders of ketone metabolism
  - **E71.39** Other disorders of fatty-acid metabolism
- **E71.4** Disorders of carnitine metabolism
  - *Excludes1:* Muscle carnitine palmitoyltransferase deficiency (E71.314)
  - **E71.40** Disorder of carnitine metabolism, unspecified
  - **E71.41** Primary carnitine deficiency
  - **E71.42** Carnitine deficiency due to inborn errors of metabolism
    - **Code also** associated inborn error or metabolism
  - **E71.43** Iatrogenic carnitine deficiency
    - Carnitine deficiency due to hemodialysis
    - Carnitine deficiency due to Valproic acid therapy
  - **E71.44** Other secondary carnitine deficiency
    - **E71.440** Ruvalcaba-Myhre-Smith syndrome
    - **E71.448** Other secondary carnitine deficiency
- **E71.5** Peroxisomal disorders
  - *Excludes1:* Schilder's disease (G37.0)
  - **E71.50** Peroxisomal disorder, unspecified
  - **E71.51** Disorders of peroxisome biogenesis
    - Group 1 peroxisomal disorders
    - *Excludes1:* Refsum's disease (G60.1)
    - **E71.510** Zellweger syndrome
    - **E71.511** Neonatal adrenoleukodystrophy
      - *Excludes1:* X-linked adrenoleukodystrophy (E71.42-)
    - **E71.518** Other disorders of peroxisome biogenesis
  - **E71.52** X-linked adrenoleukodystrophy
    - **E71.520** Childhood cerebral X-linked adrenoleukodystrophy
    - **E71.521** Adolescent X-linked adrenoleukodystrophy
    - **E71.522** Adrenomyeloneuropathy
    - **E71.528** Other X-linked adrenoleukodystrophy
      - Addison only phenotype adrenoleukodystrophy
      - Addison-Schilder adrenoleukodystrophy
    - **E71.529** X-linked adrenoleukodystrophy, unspecified type
  - **E71.53** Other group 2 peroxisomal disorders
  - **E71.54** Other peroxisomal disorders
    - **E71.540** Rhizomelic chondrodysplasia punctata
      - *Excludes1:* chondrodysplasia punctata NOS (Q77.3)
    - **E71.541** Zellweger-like syndrome
    - **E71.542** Other group 3 peroxisomal disorders
    - **E71.548** Other peroxisomal disorders

E72 OTHER DISORDERS OF AMINO-ACID METABOLISM

Excludes1: disorders of aromatic amino-acid metabolism (E70.-)
branched-chain amino-acid metabolism (E71.0–E71.2)
fatty-acid metabolism (E71.3)
purine and pyrimidine metabolism (E79.-)
gout (M1A.-, M10.-)

- **E72.0** Disorders of amino-acid transport
  - *Excludes1:* disorders of tryptophan metabolism (E70.5)
  - **E72.00** Disorders of amino-acid transport, unspecified
  - **E72.01** Cystinuria
  - **E72.02** Hartnup's disease
  - **E72.03** Lowe's syndrome
    - **Use additional code** for associated glaucoma (H42)
  - **E72.04** Cystinosis
  - **E72.09** Other disorders of amino-acid transport
    - Fanconi (-de Toni) (-Debré) syndrome, unspecified
- **E72.5** Disorders of glycine metabolism
  - **E72.50** Disorder of glycine metabolism, unspecified
  - **E72.51** Non-ketotic hyperglycinemia
  - **E72.52** Trimethylaminuria
  - **E72.53** Primary hyperoxaluria
    - Oxalosis
    - Oxaluria
  - **E72.59** Other disorders of glycine metabolism
    - D-glycericacidemia
    - Hyperhydroxyprolinemia
    - Hyperprolinemia (types I, II)
    - Sarcosinemia
- **E72.8** Other specified disorders of amino-acid metabolism
  - **E72.81** Disorders of gamma aminobutyric acid metabolism
    - 4-hydroxybutyric aciduria
    - Disorders of GABA metabolism
    - GABA metabolic defect
    - GABA transaminase deficiency
    - GABA-T deficiency
    - Gamma-hydroxybutyric aciduria
    - SSADHD
    - Succinic semialdehyde dehydrogenase deficiency

E72.89 Other specified disorders of amino-acid metabolism
Disorders of beta-amino-acid metabolism
Disorders of gamma-glutamyl cycle

E72.9 Disorder of amino-acid metabolism, unspecified

E73 LACTOSE INTOLERANCE

4th

E73.0 Congenital lactase deficiency

E73.1 Secondary lactase deficiency

E73.8 Other lactose intolerance

E73.9 Lactose intolerance, unspecified

E74 OTHER DISORDERS OF CARBOHYDRATE METABOLISM

4th

Excludes1: DM (E08–E13)
hypoglycemia NOS (E16.2)
increased secretion of glucagon (E16.3)
mucopolysaccharidosis (E76.0–E76.3) E74.1

E74.0 Glycogen storage disease

5th **E74.05 Lysosome-associated membrane protein 2 [LAMP2] deficiency**
Danon disease
Code also, if applicable, associated manifestations such as:
dilated cardiomyopathy (I42.0)
obstructive hypertrophic cardiomyopathy (I42.1)

E74.1 Disorders of fructose metabolism

5th *Excludes1:* muscle phosphofructokinase deficiency (E74.09)

E74.10 Disorder of fructose metabolism, unspecified

E74.11 Essential fructosuria
Fructokinase deficiency

E74.12 Hereditary fructose intolerance
Fructosemia

E74.19 Other disorders of fructose metabolism
Fructose-1, 6-diphosphatase deficiency

E74.2 Disorders of galactose metabolism

5th **E74.20 Disorders of galactose metabolism, unspecified**

E74.21 Galactosemia

E74.29 Other disorders of galactose metabolism
Galactokinase deficiency

E74.3 Other disorders of intestinal carbohydrate absorption

5th *Excludes2:* lactose intolerance (E73.-)

E74.31 Sucrase-isomaltase deficiency

E74.39 Other disorders of intestinal carbohydrate absorption
Disorder of intestinal carbohydrate absorption NOS
Glucose-galactose malabsorption
Sucrase deficiency

E74.4 Disorders of pyruvate metabolism and gluconeogenesis
Deficiency of phosphoenolpyruvate carboxylkinase
Deficiency of pyruvate carboxylase
Deficiency of pyruvate dehydrogenase
Excludes1: disorders of pyruvate metabolism and gluconeogenesis with anemia (D55.-)
Leigh's syndrome (G31.82)

E74.8 Disorders of carbohydrate metabolism

5th **E74.81 Disorders of glucose transport**

6th **E74.810 Glucose transporter protein type 1 deficiency**
De Vivo syndrome
Glucose transport defect, blood-brain barrier
Glut1 deficiency
GLUT1 deficiency syndrome 1, infantile onset
GLUT1 deficiency syndrome 2, childhood onset

E74.818 Other disorders of glucose transport
(Familial) renal glycosuria

E74.819 Disorders of glucose transport, unspecified

●**E74.82 Disorders of citrate metabolism**

6th ●**E74.820 SLC13A5 Citrate Transporter Disorder**

●**E74.829 Other disorders of citrate metabolism**

E74.89 Other specified disorders of carbohydrate metabolism
Essential pentosuria

E75 DISORDERS OF SPHINGOLIPID METABOLISM AND OTHER LIPID STORAGE DISORDERS

4th

Excludes1: mucolipidosis, types I-III (E77.0-E77.1)
Refsum's disease (G60.1)

E75.0 GM2 gangliosidosis

5th **E75.00 GM2 gangliosidosis, unspecified**

E75.01 Sandhoff disease

E75.02 Tay-Sachs disease

E75.2 Other sphingolipidosis

5th *Excludes1:* adrenoleukodystrophy [Addison-Schilder] (E71.528)

E75.21 Fabry (-Anderson) disease

E75.22 Gaucher disease

E75.23 Krabbe disease

E75.24 Niemann-Pick disease

6th **E75.240 Niemann-Pick disease type A**
Acid sphingomyelinase deficiency type A (ASMD type A)
Infantile neurovisceral acid sphingomyelinase deficiency

E75.241 Niemann-Pick disease type B
Acid sphingomyelinase deficiency type B (ASMD type B)
Chronic visceral acid sphingomyelinase deficiency

E75.242 Niemann-Pick disease type C

E75.243 Niemann-Pick disease type D

E75.244 Niemann-Pick disease type A/B
Acid sphingomyelinase deficiency type A/B (ASMD type A/B)
Chronic neurovisceral acid sphingomyelinase deficiency

E75.248 Other Niemann-Pick disease

E75.249 Niemann-Pick disease, unspecified
Acid sphingomyelinase deficiency (ASMD) NOS

E75.25 Metachromatic leukodystrophy

E75.26 Sulfatase deficiency
Multiple sulfatase deficiency (MSD)

E75.27 Pelizaeus-Merzbacher disease

E75.28 Canavan disease

E75.29 Other sphingolipidosis
Farber's syndrome
Sulfatide lipidosis

E76 DISORDERS OF GLYCOSAMINOGLYCAN METABOLISM

4th

E76.0 Mucopolysaccharidosis, type I

5th **E76.01 Hurler's syndrome**

E76.02 Hurler-Scheie syndrome

E76.03 Scheie's syndrome

E76.1 Mucopolysaccharidosis, type II
Hunter's syndrome

E76.2 Other mucopolysaccharidoses

5th **E76.21 Morquio mucopolysaccharidosis**

6th **E76.210 Morquio A mucopolysaccharidoses**
Classic Morquio syndrome
Morquio syndrome A
Mucopolysaccharidosis, type IVA

E76.211 Morquio B mucopolysaccharidoses
Morquio-like mucopolysaccharidoses
Morquio-like syndrome
Morquio syndrome B
Mucopolysaccharidosis, type IVB

E76.219 Morquio mucopolysaccharidoses, unspecified
Morquio syndrome
Mucopolysaccharidosis, type IV

E76.22 Sanfilippo mucopolysaccharidoses
Mucopolysaccharidosis, type III (A) (B) (C) (D)
Sanfilippo A syndrome
Sanfilippo B syndrome
Sanfilippo C syndrome
Sanfilippo D syndrome

E76.29 Other mucopolysaccharidoses
beta-Glucuronidase deficiency
Maroteaux-Lamy (mild) (severe) syndrome
Mucopolysaccharidosis, types VI, VII

E76.3 Mucopolysaccharidosis, unspecified

E76.8 Other disorders of glucosaminoglycan metabolism

E76.9 Glucosaminoglycan metabolism disorder, unspecified

E77 DISORDERS OF GLYCOPROTEIN METABOLISM

E77.0 Defects in post-translational modification of lysosomal enzymes
Mucolipidosis II [I-cell disease]
Mucolipidosis III [pseudo-Hurler polydystrophy]

E77.1 Defects in glycoprotein degradation
Aspartylglucosaminuria
Fucosidosis
Mannosidosis
Sialidosis [mucolipidosis I]

E77.8 Other disorders of glycoprotein metabolism

E77.9 Disorder of glycoprotein metabolism, unspecified

E78 DISORDERS OF LIPOPROTEIN METABOLISM AND OTHER LIPIDEMIAS

Excludes1: sphingolipidosis (E75.0–E75.3)

E78.0 Pure hypercholesterolemia

E78.00 Pure hypercholesterolemia, unspecified
Fredrickson's hyperlipoproteinemia, type IIa
Hyperbetalipoproteinemia
(Pure) hypercholesterolemia NOS

E78.01 Familial hypercholesterolemia

E78.1 Pure hyperglyceridemia
Elevated fasting triglycerides
Endogenous hyperglyceridemia
Fredrickson's hyperlipoproteinemia, type IV
Hyperlipidemia, group B
Hyperprebetalipoproteinemia
Very-low-density-lipoprotein-type [VLDL] hyperlipoproteinemia

E78.2 Mixed hyperlipidemia
Broad- or floating-betalipoproteinemia
Combined hyperlipidemia NOS
Elevated cholesterol with elevated triglycerides NEC
Fredrickson's hyperlipoproteinemia, type IIb or III
Hyperbetalipoproteinemia with prebetalipoproteinemia
Hypercholesteremia with endogenous hyperglyceridemia
Hyperlipidemia, group C
Tubo-eruptive xanthoma
Xanthoma tuberosum
Excludes1: cerebrotendinous cholesterosis [van Bogaert-Scherer-Epstein] (E75.5)
familial combined hyperlipidemia (E78.49)

E78.3 Hyperchylomicronemia
Chylomicron retention disease
Fredrickson's hyperlipoproteinemia, type I or V
Hyperlipidemia, group D
Mixed hyperglyceridemia

E78.4 Other hyperlipidemia

E78.41 Elevated Lipoprotein(a)
Elevated Lp(a)

E78.49 Other hyperlipidemia
Familial combined hyperlipidemia

E78.5 Hyperlipidemia, unspecified

E78.6 Lipoprotein deficiency
Abetalipoproteinemia
Depressed HDL cholesterol
High-density lipoprotein deficiency
Hypoalphalipoproteinemia
Hypobetalipoproteinemia (familial)
Lecithin cholesterol acyltransferase deficiency
Tangier disease

E78.7 Disorders of bile acid and cholesterol metabolism
Excludes1: Niemann-Pick disease type C (E75.242)

E78.70 Disorder of bile acid and cholesterol metabolism, unspecified

E78.71 Barth syndrome

E78.72 Smith-Lemli-Opitz syndrome

E78.79 Other disorders of bile acid and cholesterol metabolism

E78.8 Other disorders of lipoprotein metabolism

E78.81 Lipoid dermatoarthritis

E78.89 Other lipoprotein metabolism disorders

E78.9 Disorder of lipoprotein metabolism, unspecified

E79 DISORDERS OF PURINE AND PYRIMIDINE METABOLISM

Excludes1: Ataxia-telangiectasia (Q87.19)
Bloom's syndrome (Q82.8)
Cockayne's syndrome (Q87.19)
calculus of kidney (N20.0)
combined immunodeficiency disorders (D81.-)
Fanconi's anemia (D61.09)
gout (M1A.-, M10.-)
orotaciduric anemia (D53.0)
progeria (E34.8)
Werner's syndrome (E34.8)
xeroderma pigmentosum (Q82.1)

E79.0 Hyperuricemia without signs of inflammatory arthritis and tophaceous disease
Asymptomatic hyperuricemia

E79.1 Lesch-Nyhan syndrome
HGPRT deficiency

E79.2 Myoadenylate deaminase deficiency

E79.8 Other disorders of purine and pyrimidine metabolism

E79.81 Aicardi-Goutières syndrome

E79.82 Hereditary xanthinuria

E79.89 Other specified disorders of purine and pyrimidine metabolism

E79.9 Disorder of purine and pyrimidine metabolism, unspecified

E80 DISORDERS OF PORPHYRIN AND BILIRUBIN METABOLISM

Includes: defects of catalase and peroxidase

E80.0 Hereditary erythropoietic porphyria
Congenital erythropoietic porphyria
Erythropoietic protoporphyria

E80.2 Other and unspecified porphyria

E80.20 Unspecified porphyria
Porphyria NOS

E80.21 Acute intermittent (hepatic) porphyria

E80.29 Other porphyria
Hereditary coproporphyria

E80.4 Gilbert syndrome

E80.5 Crigler-Najjar syndrome

E80.6 Other disorders of bilirubin metabolism
Dubin-Johnson syndrome
Rotor's syndrome

E80.7 Disorder of bilirubin metabolism, unspecified

E83 DISORDERS OF MINERAL METABOLISM

Excludes1: dietary mineral deficiency (E58–E61)
parathyroid disorders (E20–E21)
vitamin D deficiency (E55.-)

E83.0 Disorders of copper metabolism

E83.00 Disorder of copper metabolism, unspecified

E83.01 Wilson's disease
Code also associated Kayser Fleischer ring (H18.04-)

E83.09 Other disorders of copper metabolism
Menkes' (kinky hair) (steely hair) disease

E83.1 Disorders of iron metabolism
Excludes1: iron deficiency anemia (D50.-)
sideroblastic anemia (D64.0–D64.3)

E83.10 Disorder of iron metabolism, unspecified

E83.11 Hemochromatosis
Excludes1: Gestational alloimmune liver disease/GALD (P78.84)
Neonatal hemochromatosis (P78.84)

E83.110 Hereditary hemochromatosis
Bronzed diabetes
Pigmentary cirrhosis (of liver)
Primary (hereditary) hemochromatosis

E83.111 Hemochromatosis due to repeated red blood cell transfusions
Iron overload due to repeated red blood cell transfusions
Transfusion (red blood cell) associated hemochromatosis

E83.118 Other hemochromatosis

E83.119 Hemochromatosis, unspecified

E83.19 Other disorders of iron metabolism
Use additional code, if applicable, for idiopathic pulmonary hemosiderosis (J84.03)

E83.2 Disorders of zinc metabolism
Acrodermatitis enteropathica

E83.3 Disorders of phosphorus metabolism and phosphatases

5th *Excludes1:* adult osteomalacia (M83.-)
osteoporosis (M80.-)

E83.30 Disorder of phosphorus metabolism, unspecified

E83.31 Familial hypophosphatemia
Vitamin D-resistant osteomalacia
Vitamin D-resistant rickets
Excludes1: vitamin D-deficiency rickets (E55.0)

E83.32 Hereditary vitamin D-dependent rickets (type 1) (type 2)
25-hydroxyvitamin D 1-alpha-hydroxylase deficiency
Pseudovitamin D deficiency
Vitamin D receptor defect

E83.39 Other disorders of phosphorus metabolism
Acid phosphatase deficiency
Hyperphosphatemia
Hypophosphatasia

E83.4 Disorders of magnesium metabolism

5th *See Category P71 for transitory neonatal disorders of magnesium metabolism*

E83.40 Disorders of magnesium metabolism, unspecified

E83.41 Hypermagnesemia

E83.42 Hypomagnesemia

E83.49 Other disorders of magnesium metabolism

E83.5 Disorders of calcium metabolism

5th *Excludes1:* autoimmune hypoparathyroidism (E20.812)
autosomal dominant hypocalcemia (E20.810)
chondrocalcinosis (M11.1–M11.2)
hungry bone syndrome (E83.81)
hyperparathyroidism (E21.0–E21.3)
secondary hypoparathyroidism in diseases classified elsewhere (E20.811)

E83.50 Unspecified disorder of calcium metabolism

E83.51 Hypocalcemia

E83.52 Hypercalcemia
Familial hypocalciuric hypercalcemia

E83.59 Other disorders of calcium metabolism

E83.8 Other disorders of mineral metabolism

5th **E83.81 Hungry bone syndrome**

E83.89 Other disorders of mineral metabolism

E83.9 Disorder of mineral metabolism, unspecified

E84 CYSTIC FIBROSIS

4th *Includes:* mucoviscidosis
Code also exocrine pancreatic insufficiency (K86.81)

E84.0 Cystic fibrosis with pulmonary manifestations
Use additional code to identify any infectious organism present, such as: Pseudomonas (B96.5)

E84.1 Cystic fibrosis with intestinal manifestations

5th **E84.11 Meconium ileus in cystic fibrosis**
Excludes1: meconium ileus not due to cystic fibrosis (P76.0)

E84.19 Cystic fibrosis with other intestinal manifestations
Distal intestinal obstruction syndrome

E84.8 Cystic fibrosis with other manifestations

E84.9 Cystic fibrosis, unspecified

E86 VOLUME DEPLETION

4th **Use additional code(s)** for any associated disorders of electrolyte and acid-base balance (E87.-)

Excludes1: dehydration of newborn (P74.1)
postprocedural hypovolemic shock (T81.19)
traumatic hypovolemic shock (T79.4)

Excludes 2: hypovolemic shock NOS (R57.1)

E86.0 Dehydration

E86.1 Hypovolemia
Depletion of volume of plasma

E86.9 Volume depletion, unspecified

E87 OTHER DISORDERS OF FLUID, ELECTROLYTE AND ACID-BASE BALANCE

4th *Excludes1:* diabetes insipidus (E23.2)
electrolyte imbalance associated with hyperemesis gravidarum (O21.1)
electrolyte imbalance following ectopic or molar pregnancy (O08.5)
familial periodic paralysis (G72.3)
metabolic acidemia in newborn, unspecified (P19.9)

E87.0 Hyperosmolality and hypernatremia
Sodium [Na] excess
Sodium [Na] overload
Excludes2: diabetes with hyperosmolarity (E08, E09, E11, E13 with final characters .00 or .01)

E87.1 Hypo-osmolality and hyponatremia
Sodium [Na] deficiency
Excludes1: syndrome of inappropriate secretion of antidiuretic hormone (E22.2)

E87.2 Acidosis

5th *Excludes1:* diabetic acidosis — see categories E08–E10, E11, E13 with ketoacidosis

E87.20 Acidosis, unspecified
Lactic acidosis NOS
Metabolic acidosis NOS
Code also, if applicable, respiratory failure with hypercapnia (J96. with 5th character 2)

E87.21 Acute metabolic acidosis
Acute lactic acidosis

E87.22 Chronic metabolic acidosis
Chronic lactic acidosis
Code first underlying etiology, if applicable

E87.29 Other acidosis
Respiratory acidosis NOS
Excludes2: acute respiratory acidosis (J96.02)
chronic respiratory acidosis (J96.12)

E87.3 Alkalosis
Alkalosis NOS
Metabolic alkalosis
Respiratory alkalosis

E87.4 Mixed disorder of acid-base balance

E87.5 Hyperkalemia
Potassium [K] excess
Potassium [K] overload

E87.6 Hypokalemia
Potassium [K] deficiency

E87.7 Fluid overload

5th *Excludes1:* edema NOS (R60.9)
fluid retention (R60.9)

E87.70 Fluid overload, unspecified

E87.71 Transfusion associated circulatory overload
Fluid overload due to transfusion (blood) (blood components)
TACO

E87.79 Other fluid overload

E87.8 Other disorders of electrolyte and fluid balance, NEC
Electrolyte imbalance NOS
Hyperchloremia
Hypochloremia

E88 OTHER AND UNSPECIFIED METABOLIC DISORDERS

4th **Use additional codes** for associated conditions
Excludes1: histiocytosis X (chronic) (C96.6)

E88.0 Disorders of plasma-protein metabolism, NEC

5th *Excludes1:* monoclonal gammopathy (of undetermined significance) (D47.2)
polyclonal hypergammaglobulinemia (D89.0)
Waldenström macroglobulinemia (C88.00)
Excludes2: disorder of lipoprotein metabolism (E78.-)

E88.01 Alpha-1-antitrypsin deficiency
AAT deficiency

E88.02 Plasminogen deficiency
Dysplasminogenemia
Hypoplasminogenemia
Type 1 plasminogen deficiency
Type 2 plasminogen deficiency
Code also, if applicable, ligneous conjunctivitis (H10.51)
Use additional code for associated findings, such as:
hydrocephalus (G91.4)
ligneous conjunctivitis (H10.51)
otitis media (H67.-)
respiratory disorder related to plasminogen deficiency (J99)

E88.09 Other disorders of plasma-protein metabolism, NEC
Bisalbuminemia

E88.1 Lipodystrophy, NEC
Lipodystrophy NOS

E88.2 Lipomatosis, NEC
Lipomatosis NOS
Lipomatosis (Check) dolorosa [Dercum]

E88.3 Tumor lysis syndrome
Tumor lysis syndrome (spontaneous)
Tumor lysis syndrome following antineoplastic drug chemotherapy
Use additional code for adverse effect, if applicable, to identify drug (T45.1X5)

E88.4 Mitochondrial metabolism disorders
5th *Excludes1:* disorders of pyruvate metabolism (E74.4)
Kearns-Sayre syndrome (H49.81)
Leber's disease (H47.22)
Leigh's encephalopathy (G31.82)
Mitochondrial myopathy, NEC (G71.3)
Reye's syndrome (G93.7)

E88.40 Mitochondrial metabolism disorder, unspecified

E88.41 MELAS syndrome
Mitochondrial myopathy, encephalopathy, lactic acidosis and stroke-like episodes

E88.42 MERRF syndrome
Myoclonic epilepsy associated with ragged-red fibers
Code also progressive myoclonic epilepsy (G40.3-)

E88.49 Other mitochondrial metabolism disorders

E88.8 Other specified metabolic disorders

5th **E88.81 Metabolic syndrome and other insulin resistance**
6th Dysmetabolic syndrome X
Use additional codes for associated manifestations, such as: obesity (E66.-)

E88.810 Metabolic syndrome
Dysmetabolic syndrome

E88.811 Insulin resistance syndrome, Type A

E88.818 Other insulin resistance
Insulin resistance syndrome, Type B

E88.819 Insulin resistance, unspecified

E88.89 Other specified metabolic disorders
Launois-Bensaude adenolipomatosis
Excludes1: adult pulmonary Langerhans cell histiocytosis (J84.82)

E88.9 Metabolic disorder, unspecified

E88.A Wasting disease (syndrome) due to underlying condition
Cachexia due to underlying condition
Code first underlying condition
Excludes1: cachexia NOS (R64)
nutritional marasmus (E41)
Excludes2: failure to thrive (R62.51, R62.7)

(E89) POSTPROCEDURAL ENDOCRINE AND METABOLIC COMPLICATIONS AND DISORDERS, NOT ELSEWHERE CLASSIFIED

E89 POSTPROCEDURAL ENDOCRINE AND METABOLIC COMPLICATIONS AND DISORDERS, NOT ELSEWHERE CLASSIFIED

4th

Excludes2: intraoperative complications of endocrine system organ or structure (E36.0-, E36.1-, E36.8)

E89.0 Postprocedural hypothyroidism
Postirradiation hypothyroidism
Postsurgical hypothyroidism

E89.1 Postprocedural hypoinsulinemia
Postpancreatectomy hyperglycemia
Postsurgical hypoinsulinemia
Code first, if applicable, diabetes mellitus (postpancreatectomy) (postprocedural) (E13.-)
Use additional code, if applicable, to identify:
acquired absence of pancreas (Z90.41-)
insulin use (Z79.4)
Excludes1: transient postprocedural hyperglycemia (R73.9)
transient postprocedural hypoglycemia (E16.2)

E89.2 Postprocedural hypoparathyroidism
Parathyroprival tetany

E89.3 Postprocedural hypopituitarism
Postirradiation hypopituitarism

E89.8 Other postprocedural endocrine and metabolic complications and disorders

5th

E89.89 Other postprocedural endocrine and metabolic complications and disorders
Use additional code, if applicable, to further specify disorder

Chapter 5. Mental, behavioral, and neurodevelopmental disorders (F01–F99)

GUIDELINES

Pain disorders related to psychological factors

See category F45.

Mental and behavioral disorders due to psychoactive substance use

See categories F10–F19
Includes: disorders of psychological development
Excludes2: symptoms, signs and abnormal clinical laboratory findings, not elsewhere classified (R00–R99)

(F01–F09) MENTAL DISORDERS DUE TO KNOWN PHYSIOLOGICAL CONDITIONS

Note: This block comprises a range of mental disorders grouped together on the basis of their having in common a demonstrable etiology in cerebral disease, brain injury, or other insult leading to cerebral dysfunction. The dysfunction may be primary, as in diseases, injuries, and insults that affect the brain directly and selectively; or secondary, as in systemic diseases and disorders that attack the brain only as one of the multiple organs or systems of the body that are involved.

F06 OTHER MENTAL DISORDERS DUE TO KNOWN PHYSIOLOGICAL CONDITION

Includes: mental disorders due to endocrine disorder
mental disorders due to exogenous hormone
mental disorders due to exogenous toxic substance
mental disorders due to primary cerebral disease
mental disorders due to somatic illness
mental disorders due to systemic disease affecting the brain

Code first the underlying physiological condition

Excludes1: unspecified dementia (F03)

Excludes2: delirium due to known physiological condition dementia as classified in F01–F02
other mental disorders associated with alcohol and other psychoactive substances (F10–F19)

F06.7 Mild neurocognitive disorder due to known physiological condition

Mild neurocognitive impairment due to a known physiological condition

Code first the underlying physiological condition, such as:
Alzheimer's disease (G30.-)
human immunodeficiency virus [HIV] disease (B20)
Huntington's disease (G10)
Neurocognitive disorder with Lewy bodies (G31.83)
Parkinson's disease (G20.-)
other frontotemporal neurocognitive disorder (G31.09)
systemic lupus erythematosus (M32.-)
traumatic brain injury (S06.-)
vitamin B deficiency (E53.-)

Excludes1: age related cognitive decline (R41.81)
altered mental status (R41.82)
cerebral degeneration (G31.9)
change in mental status (R41.82)
cognitive deficits following (sequelae of) cerebral hemorrhage or infarction (I69.01–I69.11-, I69.21–I69.31-, I69.81–I69.91-)
dementia (F01.-, F02.-, F03.-)
mild cognitive impairment due to unknown or unspecified etiology (G31.84)
neurologic neglect syndrome (R41.4)
personality change, nonpsychotic (F68.8)

F06.70 Mild neurocognitive disorder due to known physiological condition without behavioral disturbance

Mild neurocognitive disorder due to known physiological condition, NOS

F06.71 Mild neurocognitive disorder due to known physiological condition with behavioral disturbance

F07 PERSONALITY AND BEHAVIORAL DISORDERS DUE TO KNOWN PHYSIOLOGICAL CONDITION

Code first the underlying physiological condition

F07.8 Other personality and behavioral disorders due to known physiological condition

F07.81 Postconcussional syndrome
Postcontusional syndrome (encephalopathy)
Post-traumatic brain syndrome, nonpsychotic
Use additional code to identify associated post-traumatic headache, if applicable (G44.3-)
Excludes1: current concussion (brain) (S06.0-)
postencephalitic syndrome (F07.89)

F07.89 Other personality and behavioral disorders due to known physiological condition
Postencephalitic syndrome
Right hemispheric organic affective disorder

F07.9 Unspecified personality and behavioral disorder due to known physiological condition
Organic p syndrome

F09 UNSPECIFIED MENTAL DISORDER DUE TO KNOWN PHYSIOLOGICAL CONDITION

Mental disorder NOS due to known physiological condition
Organic brain syndrome NOS
Organic mental disorder NOS
Organic psychosis NOS
Symptomatic psychosis NOS

Code first the underlying physiological condition

Excludes1: psychosis NOS (F29)

(F10–F19) MENTAL AND BEHAVIORAL DISORDERS DUE TO PSYCHOACTIVE SUBSTANCE USE

GUIDELINES

Mental and behavioral disorders due to psychoactive substance use

IN REMISSION

Selection of codes describing "in remission" for categories F10–F19, Mental and behavioral disorders due to psychoactive substance use (categories F10–F19 with -.11, -.21, -.91) requires the provider's clinical judgment and are assigned only on the basis of provider documentation (as defined in the Official Guidelines for Coding and Reporting), unless otherwise instructed by the classification. Mild substance use disorders in early or sustained remission are classified to the appropriate codes for substance abuse in remission, and moderate or severe substance use disorders in early or sustained remission are classified to the appropriate codes for substance dependence in remission.

PSYCHOACTIVE SUBSTANCE USE, ABUSE, AND DEPENDENCE

When the provider documentation refers to use, abuse and dependence of the same substance (e.g. alcohol, opioid, cannabis, etc.), only one code should be assigned to identify the pattern of use based on the following hierarchy:

- If both use and abuse are documented, assign only the code for abuse
- If both abuse and dependence are documented, assign only the code for dependence
- If use, abuse and dependence are all documented, assign only the code for dependence
- If both use and dependence are documented, assign only the code for dependence.

PSYCHOACTIVE SUBSTANCE USE, UNSPECIFIED

As with all other unspecified diagnoses, the codes for unspecified psychoactive substance use (F10.9-, F11.9-, F12.9-, F13.9-, F14.9-, F15.9-, F16.9-, F18.9-, F19.9-) should only be assigned based on provider documentation and when they meet the definition of a reportable diagnosis (see Section III, Reporting Additional Diagnoses). The codes are to be used only when the psychoactive substance use is associated with a substance related disorder (chapter 5 disorders such as sexual dysfunction, sleep disorder, or a mental or behavioral disorder) or medical condition, and when such a relationship is documented by the provider.

MEDICAL CONDITIONS DUE TO PSYCHOACTIVE SUBSTANCE USE, ABUSE AND DEPENDENCE

Medical conditions due to substance use, abuse, and dependence are not classified as substance-induced disorders. Assign the diagnosis code for the medical condition as directed by the Alphabetical Index along with the appropriate psychoactive substance use, abuse or dependence code. For example, for alcoholic pancreatitis due to alcohol dependence, assign the appropriate code from subcategory K85.2, Alcohol induced acute pancreatitis, and the appropriate code from subcategory F10.2, such as code F10.20, Alcohol dependence, uncomplicated. It would not be appropriate to assign code F10.288, Alcohol dependence with other alcohol-induced disorder.

BLOOD ALCOHOL LEVEL

A code from category Y90, Evidence of alcohol involvement determined by blood alcohol level, may be assigned when this information is documented and the patient's provider has documented a condition classifiable to category F10, Alcohol related disorders. The blood alcohol level does not need to be documented by the patient's provider in order for it to be coded.

F10 ALCOHOL RELATED DISORDERS

4th Use additional code for blood alcohol level, if applicable (Y90.-)

- **F10.1 Alcohol abuse**
  - **5th** *Excludes1:* alcohol dependence (F10.2-)
    - alcohol use, unspecified (F10.9-)
  - **F10.10 Alcohol abuse, uncomplicated**
    - Alcohol use disorder, mild
  - **F10.11 Alcohol abuse, in remission**
    - Alcohol use disorder, mild, in early remission
    - Alcohol use disorder, mild, in sustained remission
  - **F10.12 Alcohol abuse with intoxication**
    - **6th**
    - **F10.120 Alcohol abuse with intoxication, uncomplicated**
    - **F10.121 Alcohol abuse with intoxication delirium**
    - **F10.129 Alcohol abuse with intoxication, unspecified**
  - **F10.13 Alcohol abuse with withdrawal**
    - **6th**
    - **F10.130 Alcohol abuse with withdrawal, uncomplicated**
    - **F10.131 Alcohol abuse with withdrawal delirium**
    - **F10.132 Alcohol abuse with withdrawal with perceptual disturbance**
    - **F10.139 Alcohol abuse with withdrawal, unspecified**
- **F10.2 Alcohol dependence**
  - **5th** *Excludes1:* alcohol abuse (F10.1-)
    - alcohol use, unspecified (F10.9-)
  - *Excludes2:* toxic effect of alcohol (T51.0-)
  - **F10.20 Alcohol dependence, uncomplicated**
    - Alcohol use disorder, moderate
    - Alcohol use disorder, severe
  - **F10.21 Alcohol dependence, in remission**
    - Alcohol use disorder, moderate or severe, in early remission
    - Alcohol use disorder, moderate or severe, in sustained remission
  - **F10.22 Alcohol dependence with intoxication**
    - **6th** Acute drunkenness (in alcoholism)
    - *Excludes2:* alcohol dependence with withdrawal (F10.23-)
    - **F10.220 Alcohol dependence with intoxication, uncomplicated**
    - **F10.221 Alcohol dependence with intoxication delirium**
    - **F10.229 Alcohol dependence with intoxication, unspecified**
  - **F10.23 Alcohol dependence with withdrawal**
    - **6th** *Excludes2:* Alcohol dependence with intoxication (F10.22-)
    - **F10.230 Alcohol dependence with withdrawal, uncomplicated**
    - **F10.231 Alcohol dependence with withdrawal delirium**

- **F10.232 Alcohol dependence with withdrawal with perceptual disturbance**
- **F10.239 Alcohol dependence with withdrawal, unspecified**
- **F10.24 Alcohol dependence with alcohol-induced mood disorder**
  - Alcohol use disorder, moderate or severe, with alcohol-induced bipolar or related disorder
  - Alcohol use disorder, moderate or severe, with alcohol-induced depressive disorder
- **F10.28 Alcohol dependence with other alcohol-induced disorders**
  - **6th**
  - **F10.280 Alcohol dependence with alcohol-induced anxiety disorder**
  - **F10.282 Alcohol dependence with alcohol-induced sleep disorder**
  - **F10.288 Alcohol dependence with other alcohol-induced disorder**
    - Alcohol use disorder, moderate or severe, with alcohol-induced mild neurocognitive disorder
- **F10.9 Alcohol use, unspecified**
  - **5th** *Excludes1:* alcohol abuse (F10.1-)
    - alcohol dependence (F10.2-)
  - **F10.90 Alcohol use, unspecified, uncomplicated**
  - **F10.91 Alcohol use, unspecified, in remission**
  - **F10.92 Alcohol use, unspecified with intoxication;**
    - **6th**
    - **F10.920 uncomplicated**
    - **F10.921 delirium**
    - **F10.929 unspecified**
  - **F10.93 Alcohol use, unspecified with withdrawal**
    - **6th**
    - **F10.930 Alcohol use, unspecified with withdrawal, uncomplicated**
    - **F10.931 Alcohol use, unspecified with withdrawal delirium**
    - **F10.932 Alcohol use, unspecified with withdrawal with perceptual disturbance**
    - **F10.939 Alcohol use, unspecified with withdrawal, unspecified**

F11 OPIOID RELATED DISORDERS

4th

- **F11.1 Opioid abuse**
  - **5th** *Excludes1:* opioid dependence (F11.2-)
    - opioid use, unspecified (F11.9-)
  - **F11.10 Opioid abuse, uncomplicated**
    - Opioid use disorder, mild
  - **F11.11 Opioid abuse, in remission**
    - Opioid use disorder, mild, in early or sustained remission
  - **F11.13 Opioid abuse with withdrawal**
- **F11.9 Opioid use, unspecified**
  - **5th** *Excludes1:* opioid abuse (F11.1-)
    - opioid dependence (F11.2-)
  - **F11.90 Opioid use, unspecified, uncomplicated**
  - **F11.91 Opioid use, unspecified, in remission**
  - **F11.92 Opioid use, unspecified with intoxication**
    - **6th** *Excludes1:* opioid use, unspecified with withdrawal (F11.93)
    - **F11.920 Opioid use, unspecified with intoxication, uncomplicated**
    - **F11.921 Opioid use, unspecified with intoxication delirium**
      - Opioid-induced delirium
    - **F11.922 Opioid use, unspecified with intoxication with perceptual disturbance**
    - **F11.929 Opioid use, unspecified with intoxication, unspecified**
  - **F11.93 Opioid use, unspecified with withdrawal**
    - *Excludes1:* opioid use, unspecified with intoxication (F11.92-)
  - **F11.94 Opioid use, unspecified with opioid-induced mood disorder**
    - Opioid induced depressive disorder, without use disorder
  - **F11.95 Opioid use, unspecified with opioid-induced**
    - **6th** psychotic disorder

F11.950 Opioid use, unspecified with opioid-induced psychotic disorder with delusions

F11.951 Opioid use, unspecified with opioid-induced psychotic disorder with hallucinations

F11.959 Opioid use, unspecified with opioid-induced psychotic disorder, unspecified

F11.98 Opioid use, unspecified with other specified opioid-induced disorder

F11.981 Opioid use, unspecified with opioid-induced sexual dysfunction Opioid induced sexual dysfunction, without use disorder

F11.982 Opioid use, unspecified with opioid-induced sleep disorder Opioid induced sleep disorder, without use disorder

F11.988 Opioid use, unspecified with other opioid-induced disorder Opioid-associated amnestic syndrome without use disorder Opioid induced anxiety disorder, without use disorder

F11.99 Opioid use, unspecified with unspecified opioid-induced disorder

F12 CANNABIS RELATED DISORDERS

Includes: marijuana

F12.1 Cannabis abuse

Excludes1: cannabis dependence (F12.2-) cannabis use, unspecified (F12.9-)

F12.10 Cannabis abuse, uncomplicated cannabis use disorder, mild

F12.11 Cannabis abuse, in remission Cannabis use disorder, mild, in early or sustained remission

F12.13 Cannabis abuse with withdrawal

F12.2 Cannabis dependence

Excludes1: cannabis abuse (F12.1-) cannabis use, unspecified (F12.9-)

Excludes2: cannabis poisoning (T40.7-)

F12.20 Cannabis dependence, uncomplicated

F12.21 Cannabis dependence, in remission Cannabis use disorder, moderate or severe, in early remission Cannabis use disorder, moderate or severe, in sustained remission

F12.22 Cannabis dependence with intoxication;

F12.220 uncomplicated Cannabis use disorder, moderate Cannabis use disorder, severe

F12.221 delirium

F12.222 with perceptual disturbance

F12.229 unspecified

F12.23 Cannabis dependence with withdrawal

F12.9 Cannabis use, unspecified

Excludes1: cannabis abuse (F12.1-) cannabis dependence (F12.2-)

F12.90 Cannabis use, unspecified, uncomplicated Amphetamine type substance use disorder, moderate or severe, in early or sustained remission Other or unspecified stimulant use disorder, moderate or severe, in early or sustained remission

F12.91 Cannabis use, unspecified, in remission

F12.93 Cannabis use, unspecified with withdrawal

F13 SEDATIVE, HYPNOTIC, OR ANIOLYTIC RELATED DISORDERS

F13.1 Sedative, hypnotic or anxiolytic-related abuse

Excludes1: sedative, hypnotic or anxiolytic-related dependence (F13.2-) sedative, hypnotic, or anxiolytic use, unspecified (F13.9-)

F13.10 Sedative, hypnotic or anxiolytic abuse, uncomplicated Sedative, hypnotic, or anxiolytic use disorder, mild

F13.11 Sedative, hypnotic or anxiolytic abuse, in remission Sedative, hypnotic or anxiolytic use disorder, mild, in early or sustained remission

F13.13 Sedative, hypnotic or anxiolytic abuse with withdrawal

F13.130 Sedative, hypnotic or anxiolytic abuse with withdrawal, uncomplicated

F13.131 Sedative, hypnotic or anxiolytic abuse with withdrawal delirium

F13.132 Sedative, hypnotic or anxiolytic abuse with withdrawal with perceptual disturbance

F13.139 Sedative, hypnotic or anxiolytic abuse with withdrawal, unspecified

F13.9 Sedative, hypnotic or anxiolytic-related use, unspecified

Excludes1: sedative, hypnotic or anxiolytic-related abuse (F13.1-) sedative, hypnotic or anxiolytic-related dependence (F13.2-)

F13.91 Sedative, hypnotic or anxiolytic use, unspecified, in remission

F14 COCAINE RELATED DISORDERS

Excludes2: other stimulant-related disorders (F15.-)

F14.1 Cocaine abuse

Excludes1: cocaine dependence (F14.2-) cocaine use, unspecified (F14.9-)

F14.10 Cocaine abuse, uncomplicated Cocaine use disorder, mild

F14.11 Cocaine abuse, in remission Cocaine use disorder, mild, in early or sustained remission

F14.12 Cocaine abuse with intoxication;

F14.120 uncomplicated

F14.121 delirium

F14.122 with perceptual disturbance

F14.129 unspecified

F14.13 Cocaine abuse, unspecified with withdrawal

F14.2 Cocaine dependence

Excludes1: cocaine abuse (F14.1-) cocaine use, unspecified (F14.9-)

Excludes2: cocaine poisoning (T40.5-)

F14.20 Cocaine dependence, uncomplicated Cocaine use disorder, moderate Cocaine use disorder, severe

F14.21 Cocaine dependence, in remission Cocaine use disorder, moderate, in early or sustained remission Cocaine use disorder, severe, in early or sustained remission

F14.22 Cocaine dependence with intoxication;

Excludes1: cocaine dependence with withdrawal (F14.23)

F14.220 uncomplicated

F14.221 delirium

F14.222 with perceptual disturbance

F14.229 unspecified

F14.23 Cocaine dependence with withdrawal *Excludes1:* cocaine dependence with intoxication (F14.22-)

F14.9 Cocaine use, unspecified

Excludes1: cocaine abuse (F14.1-) cocaine dependence (F14.2-)

F14.90 Cocaine use, unspecified, uncomplicated

F14.91 Cocaine use, unspecified, in remission

F14.92 Cocaine use, unspecified with intoxication;

F14.920 uncomplicated

F14.921 delirium

F14.922 with perceptual disturbance

F14.929 unspecified

F14.93 Cocaine use, unspecified with withdrawal

F15 OTHER STIMULANT RELATED DISORDERS

4th

Includes: amphetamine-related disorders
caffeine

Excludes2: cocaine-related disorders (F14.-)

F15.1 Other stimulant abuse

5th *Excludes1:* other stimulant dependence (F15.2-)
other stimulant use, unspecified (F15.9-)

F15.10 Other stimulant abuse, uncomplicated
Amphetamine type substance use disorder, mild
Other or unspecified stimulant use disorder, mild
Cocaine use disorder, moderate, in early or sustained remission
Cocaine use disorder, severe, in early or sustained remission

F15.11 Other stimulant abuse, in remission
Amphetamine type substance use disorder, mild, in early or sustained remission
Other or unspecified stimulant use disorder, mild, in early or sustained remission

F15.12 Other stimulant abuse with intoxication;

6th **F15.120 uncomplicated**

F15.121 delirium

F15.122 perceptual disturbance
Amphetamine or other stimulant use disorder, mild, with amphetamine or other stimulant intoxication, with perceptual disturbances

F15.129 unspecified
Amphetamine or other stimulant use disorder, mild, with amphetamine or other stimulant intoxication, without perceptual disturbances

F15.13 Other stimulant abuse with withdrawal

F15.2 Other stimulant dependence

5th *Excludes1:* other stimulant abuse (F15.1-)
other stimulant use, unspecified (F15.9-)

F15.20 Other stimulant dependence, uncomplicated
Amphetamine type substance use disorder, moderate or severe
Other or unspecified stimulant use disorder, moderate or severe

F15.21 Other stimulant dependence, in remission
Amphetamine type substance use disorder, moderate or severe, in early or sustained remission
Other or unspecified stimulant use disorder, moderate or severe, in early or sustained remission

F15.22 Other stimulant dependence with intoxication;

6th *Excludes1:* other stimulant dependence with withdrawal (F15.23)

F15.220 uncomplicated

F15.221 delirium

F15.222 with perceptual disturbance
Amphetamine or other stimulant use disorder, moderate, with amphetamine or other stimulant intoxication, with perceptual disturbances

F15.229 unspecified
Amphetamine or other stimulant use disorder, severe, with amphetamine or other stimulant intoxication, with perceptual disturbances

F15.23 Other stimulant dependence with withdrawal
Amphetamine or other stimulant withdrawal
Excludes1: other stimulant dependence with intoxication (F15.22-)

F15.9 Other stimulant use, unspecified

5th *Excludes1:* other stimulant abuse (F15.1-)
other stimulant dependence (F15.2-)

F15.90 Other stimulant use, unspecified, uncomplicated

F15.91 Other stimulant use, unspecified, in remission

F15.93 Other stimulant use, unspecified with withdrawal
Caffeine withdrawal

F16 HALLUCINOGEN RELATED DISORDERS

4th

Includes: ecstasy
PCP
phencyclidine

F16.1 Hallucinogen abuse

5th *Excludes1:* hallucinogen dependence (F16.2-)
hallucinogen use, unspecified (F16.9-)

F16.10 Hallucinogen abuse, uncomplicated
Other hallucinogen use disorder, mild
Phencyclidine use disorder, mild

F16.11 Hallucinogen abuse, in remission
Other hallucinogen use disorder, mild, in early or sustained remission
Phencyclidine use disorder, mild, in early or sustained remission

F16.2 Hallucinogen dependence

5th *Excludes1:* hallucinogen abuse (F16.1-)
hallucinogen use, unspecified (F16.9-)

F16.20 Hallucinogen dependence, uncomplicated
Other hallucinogen use disorder, moderate
Other hallucinogen use disorder, severe
Phencyclidine use disorder, moderate
Phencyclidine use disorder, severe

F16.9 Hallucinogen use, unspecified

5th *Excludes1:* hallucinogen abuse (F16.1-)
hallucinogen dependence (F16.2-)

F16.91 Hallucinogen use, unspecified, in remission

F17 NICOTINE DEPENDENCE

4th

Excludes1: history of tobacco dependence (Z87.891)
tobacco use NOS (Z72.0)

Excludes2: tobacco use (smoking) during pregnancy, childbirth and the puerperium (O99.33-)
toxic effect of nicotine (T65.2-)

F17.2 Nicotine dependence

5th **F17.20 Nicotine dependence, unspecified**

6th **F17.200 Nicotine dependence, unspecified; uncomplicated**
Tobacco use disorder, mild
Tobacco use disorder, moderate
Tobacco use disorder, severe

F17.201 in remission
Tobacco use disorder, mild, in early or sustained remission
Tobacco use disorder, moderate, in early or sustained remission
Tobacco use disorder, severe, in early or sustained remission

F17.203 with withdrawal
Tobacco withdrawal

F17.208 with other nicotine-induced disorders

F17.209 with unspecified nicotine-induced disorders

F17.21 Nicotine dependence, cigarettes

6th **F17.210 Nicotine dependence, cigarettes; uncomplicated**

F17.211 in remission
Tobacco use disorder, cigarettes, mild or moderate or severe in early or sustained remission

F17.213 with withdrawal

F17.218 with other nicotine-induced disorders

F17.219 with unspecified nicotine-induced disorders

F17.22 Nicotine dependence, chewing tobacco

6th **F17.220 Nicotine dependence, chewing tobacco; uncomplicated**

F17.221 in remission
Tobacco use disorder, chewing tobacco, mild or moderate or severe in early or sustained remission

F17.223 with withdrawal

F17.228 with other nicotine-induced disorders
F17.229 with unspecified nicotine-induced disorders
F17.29 Nicotine dependence, other tobacco product
- 6th
  - F17.290 Nicotine dependence, other tobacco product; uncomplicated
  - F17.291 in remission
    - Tobacco use disorder, other product, mild or moderate or severe in early or sustained remission
  - F17.293 with withdrawal
  - F17.298 with other nicotine-induced disorders
  - F17.299 with unspecified nicotine-induced disorders

F18 INHALANT RELATED DISORDERS

Includes: volatile solvents

F18.1 Inhalant abuse
- *Excludes1:* inhalant dependence (F18.2-)
  - inhalant use, unspecified (F18.9-)

F18.10 Inhalant abuse, uncomplicated
- Inhalant use disorder, mild

F18.11 Inhalant abuse, in remission
- Inhalant use disorder, mild, in early or sustained remission

F18.12 Inhalant abuse with intoxication
- F18.120 Inhalant abuse with intoxication; uncomplicated
- F18.121 delirium
- F18.129 unspecified

F18.2 Inhalant dependence
- *Excludes1:* inhalant abuse (F18.1-)
  - inhalant use, unspecified (F18.9-)

F18.20 Inhalant dependence, uncomplicated
- Inhalant use disorder, moderate
- Inhalant use disorder, severe

F18.21 Inhalant dependence, in remission

F18.22 Inhalant dependence with intoxication
- F18.220 Inhalant dependence with intoxication; uncomplicated
- F18.221 delirium
- F18.229 unspecified

F18.9 Inhalant use, unspecified
- *Excludes1:* inhalant abuse (F18.1-)
  - inhalant dependence (F18.2-)

F18.90 Inhalant use, unspecified, uncomplicated

F18.91 Inhalant use, unspecified, in remission

F18.92 Inhalant use, unspecified with intoxication
- F18.920 Inhalant use, unspecified with intoxication, uncomplicated
- F18.921 Inhalant use, unspecified with intoxication with delirium
- F18.929 Inhalant use, unspecified with intoxication, unspecified

F19 OTHER PSYCHOACTIVE SUBSTANCE RELATED DISORDERS

Includes: polysubstance drug use (indiscriminate drug use)

F19.1 Other psychoactive substance abuse
- *Excludes1:* other psychoactive substance dependence (F19.2-)
  - other psychoactive substance use, unspecified (F19.9-)

F19.10 Other psychoactive substance abuse, uncomplicated
- Other (or unknown) substance use disorder, mild

F19.12 Other psychoactive substance abuse with intoxication
- F19.120 Other psychoactive substance abuse with intoxication; uncomplicated
- F19.121 delirium
- F19.122 with perceptual disturbances
- F19.129 unspecified

F19.13 Other psychoactive substance abuse
- F19.130 Other psychoactive substance abuse with withdrawal, uncomplicated

F19.131 Other psychoactive substance abuse with withdrawal delirium

F19.132 Other psychoactive substance abuse with withdrawal with perceptual disturbance

F19.139 Other psychoactive substance abuse with withdrawal, unspecified

F19.2 Other psychoactive substance dependence
- *Excludes1:* other psychoactive substance abuse (F19.1-)
  - other psychoactive substance use, unspecified (F19.9-)

F19.20 Other psychoactive substance dependence, uncomplicated
- Other (or unknown) substance use disorder, moderate
- Other (or unknown) substance use disorder, severe

F19.21 Other psychoactive substance dependence, in remission
- Other (or unknown) substance use disorder, moderate, in early remission or in sustained remission
- Other (or unknown) substance use disorder, severe, in early remission or in sustained remission

F19.22 Other psychoactive substance dependence with intoxication
- *Excludes1:* psychoactive other substance dependence with withdrawal (F19.23-)

F19.220 Other psychoactive substance dependence with intoxication; uncomplicated

F19.221 delirium

F19.222 with perceptual disturbance

F19.229 unspecified

F19.23 Other psychoactive substance dependence with withdrawal
- *Excludes1:* other psychoactive substance dependence with intoxication (F19.22-)

F19.230 Other psychoactive substance dependence with withdrawal; uncomplicated

F19.231 delirium

F19.232 with perceptual disturbance

F19.239 unspecified

F19.9 Other psychoactive substance use, unspecified
- *Excludes1:* other psychoactive substance abuse (F19.1-)
  - other psychoactive substance dependence (F19.2-)

F19.90 Other psychoactive substance use, unspecified, uncomplicated

F19.91 Other psychoactive substance use, unspecified, in remission

F19.92 Other psychoactive substance use, unspecified with intoxication
- *Excludes1:* other psychoactive substance use, unspecified with withdrawal (F19.93)

F19.920 Other psychoactive substance use, unspecified with intoxication; uncomplicated

F19.921 with delirium
- Other (or unknown) substance-induced delirium

F19.922 with perceptual disturbance

F19.929 unspecified

(F20–F29) SCHIZOPHRENIA, SCHIZOTYPAL, DELUSIONAL, AND OTHER NON-MOOD PSYCHOTIC DISORDERS

(F30–F39) MOOD [AFFECTIVE] DISORDERS

F31 BIPOLAR DISORDER

Includes: bipolar I disorder
bipolar type I disorder manic-depressive illness manic-depressive psychosis manic-depressive reaction

Excludes1: bipolar disorder, single manic episode (F30.-)
major depressive disorder, single episode (F32.-)
major depressive disorder, recurrent (F33.-)

F31.0 Bipolar disorder, current episode hypomanic

F31.1 Bipolar disorder, current episode manic without psychotic features

F31.10 Bipolar disorder, current episode manic without psychotic features, unspecified

F31.11 Bipolar disorder, current episode manic without psychotic features, mild

F31.12 Bipolar disorder, current episode manic without psychotic features, moderate

F31.13 Bipolar disorder, current episode manic without psychotic features, severe

F31.3 Bipolar disorder, current episode depressed, mild or moderate severity

F31.30 Bipolar disorder, current episode depressed, mild or moderate severity, unspecified

F31.31 Bipolar disorder, current episode depressed, mild

F31.32 Bipolar disorder, current episode depressed, moderate

F31.4 Bipolar disorder, current episode depressed, severe, without psychotic features

F31.6 Bipolar disorder, current episode mixed

F31.60 Bipolar disorder, current episode mixed, unspecified

F31.61 Bipolar disorder, current episode mixed, mild

F31.62 Bipolar disorder, current episode mixed, moderate

F31.63 Bipolar disorder, current episode mixed, severe, without psychotic features

F31.8 Other bipolar disorders

F31.81 Bipolar II disorder

Bipolar disorder, type 2

F31.89 Other bipolar disorder

Recurrent manic episodes NOS

F31.9 Bipolar disorder, unspecified

Manic depression

F32 DEPRESSIVE EPISODE

Includes: single episode of agitated depression

single episode of depressive reaction

single episode of major depression

single episode of psychogenic depression

single episode of reactive depression

single episode of vital depression

Excludes1: bipolar disorder (F31.-)

manic episode (F30.-)

recurrent depressive disorder (F33.-)

Excludes2: adjustment disorder (F43.2)

F32.0 Major depressive disorder, single episode, mild

F32.1 Major depressive disorder, single episode, moderate

F32.2 Major depressive disorder, single episode, severe without psychotic features

F32.3 Major depressive disorder, single episode, severe with psychotic features

Single episode of major depression with mood-congruent psychotic symptoms

Single episode of major depression with mood-incongruent psychotic symptoms

Single episode of major depression with psychotic symptoms

Single episode of psychogenic depressive psychosis

Single episode of psychotic depression

Single episode of reactive depressive psychosis

F32.4 Major depressive disorder, single episode, in partial remission

F32.5 Major depressive disorder, single episode, in full remission

F32.8 Other depressive episodes

F32.81 Premenstrual dysphoric disorder

Excludes1: premenstrual tension syndrome (N94.3)

F32.89 Other specified depressive episodes

Atypical depression

Post-schizophrenic depression

Single episode of 'masked' depression NOS

F32.9 Major depressive disorder, single episode, unspecified

Major depression NOS

F32.A Depression, unspecified

Depression NOS

Depressive disorder NOS

F33 MAJOR DEPRESSIVE DISORDER, RECURRENT

Includes: recurrent episodes of depressive reaction

recurrent episodes of endogenous depression

recurrent episodes of major depression

recurrent episodes of psychogenic depression

recurrent episodes of reactive depression

recurrent episodes of seasonal depressive disorder

recurrent episodes of vital depression

Excludes1: bipolar disorder (F31.-)

manic episode (F30.-)

F33.0 Major depressive disorder, recurrent, mild

F33.1 Major depressive disorder, recurrent, moderate

F33.2 Major depressive disorder, recurrent severe without psychotic features

F33.3 Major depressive disorder, recurrent, severe with psychotic symptoms

Major depressive disorder, recurrent, with psychotic features

Endogenous depression with psychotic symptoms

Recurrent severe episodes of major depression with mood-congruent psychotic symptoms

Major depression with mood-incongruent psychotic symptoms

Major depression with psychotic symptoms

Psychogenic depressive psychosis

Psychotic depression

Reactive depressive psychosis

F33.4 Major depressive disorder, recurrent, in remission

F33.40 Major depressive disorder, recurrent, in remission, unspecified

F33.41 in partial remission

F33.42 in full remission

F33.8 Other recurrent depressive disorders

Recurrent brief depressive episodes

F33.9 Major depressive disorder, recurrent, unspecified

Monopolar depression NOS

F34 PERSISTENT MOOD [AFFECTIVE] DISORDERS

F34.0 Cyclothymic disorder

Affective personality disorder

Cycloid personality

Cyclothymia

Cyclothymic personality

F34.1 Dysthymic disorder

Depressive neurosis

Depressive personality disorder

Dysthymia

Neurotic depression

Persistent anxiety depression

Persistent depressive disorder

Excludes2: anxiety depression (mild or not persistent) (F41.8)

F34.8 Other persistent mood [affective] disorders

F34.81 **Disruptive mood dysregulation disorder**

F34.89 **Other specified persistent mood disorders**

F34.9 Persistent mood [affective] disorder, unspecified

F39 UNSPECIFIED MOOD [AFFECTIVE] DISORDER

Affective psychosis NOS

(F40–F48) ANXIETY, DISSOCIATIVE, STRESS-RELATED, SOMATOFORM AND OTHER NONPSYCHOTIC MENTAL DISORDERS

F40 PHOBIC ANXIETY DISORDERS

F40.0 Agoraphobia

F40.00 **Agoraphobia, unspecified**

F40.01 **Agoraphobia with panic disorder**

Panic disorder with agoraphobia

Excludes1: panic disorder without agoraphobia (F41.0)

F40.02 **Agoraphobia without panic disorder**

F40.1 Social phobias

Anthropophobia

Social anxiety disorder

Social anxiety disorder of childhood

Social neurosis

F40.10 Social phobia, unspecified
F40.11 Social phobia, generalized
F40.8 Other phobic anxiety disorders
Phobic anxiety disorder of childhood
F40.9 Phobic anxiety disorder, unspecified
Phobia NOS
Phobic state NOS

F41 OTHER ANXIETY DISORDERS

Excludes2: anxiety in: acute stress reaction (F43.0)
transient adjustment reaction (F43.2)
neurasthenia (F48.8)
psychophysiologic disorders (F45.-)
separation anxiety (F93.0)

F41.0 **Panic disorder [episodic paroxysmal anxiety]**
Panic attack
Panic state
Excludes1: panic disorder with agoraphobia (F40.01)

F41.1 **Generalized anxiety disorder**
Anxiety neurosis
Anxiety reaction
Anxiety state
Overanxious disorder
Excludes2: neurasthenia (F48.8)

F41.3 Other mixed anxiety disorders

F41.8 **Other specified anxiety disorders**
Anxiety depression (mild or not persistent)
Anxiety hysteria
Mixed anxiety and depressive disorder

F41.9 **Anxiety disorder, unspecified**
Anxiety NOS

F42 OBSESSIVE-COMPULSIVE DISORDER

Excludes2: obsessive-compulsive personality (disorder) (F60.5)
obsessive-compulsive symptoms occurring in depression (F32–F33)
obsessive-compulsive symptoms occurring in schizophrenia (F20.-)

F42.2 **Mixed obsessional thoughts and acts**

F42.3 **Hoarding disorder**

F42.4 **Excoriation (skin-picking) disorder**
Excludes1: factitial dermatitis (L98.1)
other specified behavioral and emotional disorders with onset usually occurring in early childhood and adolescence (F98.8)

F42.8 **Other obsessive compulsive disorder**
Anancastic neurosis
Obsessive-compulsive neurosis

F42.9 **Obsessive-compulsive disorder, unspecified**

F43 REACTION TO SEVERE STRESS, AND ADJUSTMENT DISORDERS

F43.0 **Acute stress reaction**
Acute crisis reaction
Acute reaction to stress
Combat and operational stress reaction
Combat fatigue
Crisis state
Psychic shock

F43.1 **Post-traumatic stress disorder (PTSD)**
Traumatic neurosis
F43.10 **Post-traumatic stress disorder, unspecified**
F43.11 **Post-traumatic stress disorder, acute**
F43.12 **Post-traumatic stress disorder, chronic**

F43.2 **Adjustment disorders**
Culture shock
Grief reaction
Hospitalism in children
Excludes2: separation anxiety disorder of childhood (F93.0)
F43.20 **Adjustment disorder, unspecified**
F43.21 **Adjustment disorder with depressed mood**
F43.22 **Adjustment disorder with anxiety**
F43.23 **Adjustment disorder with mixed anxiety and depressed mood**
F43.24 **Adjustment disorder with disturbance of conduct**
F43.25 **Adjustment disorder with mixed disturbance of emotions and conduct**

F43.29 **Adjustment disorder with other symptoms**

F43.8 **Other reactions to severe stress**
Other specified trauma and stressor-related disorder
F43.81 **Prolonged grief disorder**
F43.89 **Other reactions to severe stress**

F43.9 **Reaction to severe stress, unspecified**
Trauma and stressor-related disorder, NOS

F44 DISSOCIATIVE AND CONVERSION DISORDERS

Includes: conversion hysteria
conversion reaction
hysteria
hysterical psychosis

Excludes2: malingering [conscious simulation] (Z76.5)

F44.4 **Conversion disorder with motor symptom or deficit**
Conversion disorder with abnormal movement
Conversion disorder with speech symptoms
Conversion disorder with swallowing symptoms
Conversion disorder with weakness/paralysis
Psychogenic aphonia
Psychogenic dysphonia

F44.5 **Conversion disorder with seizures or convulsions**
Conversion disorder with attacks or seizures
Dissociative convulsions

F44.6 **Conversion disorder with sensory symptom or deficit**
Conversion disorder with anesthesia or sensory loss or with special sensory symptoms
Dissociative anesthesia and sensory loss
Psychogenic deafness

F44.7 **Conversion disorder with mixed symptom presentation**

F44.8 **Other dissociative and conversion disorders**
F44.81 **Dissociative identity disorder**
Multiple personality disorder
F44.89 **Other dissociative and conversion disorders**
Ganser's syndrome
Psychogenic confusion
Psychogenic twilight state
Trance and possession disorders

F44.9 **Dissociative and conversion disorder, unspecified**
Dissociative disorder NOS

F45 SOMATOFORM DISORDERS

GUIDELINES

Pain disorders related to psychological factors
Assign code F45.41, for pain that is exclusively related to psychological disorders. As indicated by the *Excludes1* note under category G89, a code from category G89 should not be assigned with code F45.41

Code F45.42, Pain disorders with related psychological factors, should be used with a code from category G89, Pain, not elsewhere classified, if there is documentation of a psychological component for a patient with acute or chronic pain.

See Chapter 6

Excludes2: dissociative and conversion disorders (F44.-)
factitious disorders (F68.1-, F68.A)
hair-plucking (F63.3)
lalling (F80.0)
lisping (F80.0)
malingering [conscious simulation] (Z76.5)
nail-biting (F98.8)
psychological or behavioral factors associated with disorders or diseases classified elsewhere (F54)
sexual dysfunction, not due to a substance or known physiological condition (F52.-)
thumb-sucking (F98.8)
tic disorders (in childhood and adolescence) (F95.-)
Tourette's syndrome (F95.2)
trichotillomania (F63.3)

F45.0 **Somatization disorder**
Briquet's disorder
Multiple psychosomatic disorders

F45.1 **Undifferentiated somatoform disorder**
Somatic symptom disorder
Undifferentiated psychosomatic disorder

F45.2 Hypochondriacal disorders

5th *Excludes2:* delusional dysmorphophobia (F22) fixed delusions about bodily functions or shape (F22)

F45.20 Hypochondriacal disorder, unspecified

F45.21 Hypochondriasis
Hypochondriacal neurosis
Illness anxiety disorder

F45.22 Body dysmorphic disorder
Bigorexia
Dysmorphophobia (nondelusional)
Muscle dysmorphia
Nosophobia

F45.29 Other hypochondriacal disorders

F45.4 Pain disorders related to psychological factors

5th *Excludes1:* pain NOS (R52)

F45.41 Pain disorder exclusively related to psychological factors
Somatoform pain disorder (persistent)

F45.42 Pain disorder with related psychological factors
Code also associated acute or chronic pain (G89.-)

F45.8 Other somatoform disorders
Psychogenic dysmenorrhea
Psychogenic dysphagia, including 'globus hystericus'
Psychogenic pruritus
Psychogenic torticollis
Somatoform autonomic dysfunction
Teeth grinding
Excludes1: sleep related teeth grinding (G47.63)

F45.9 Somatoform disorder, unspecified
Psychosomatic disorder NOS

F48 OTHER NONPSYCHOTIC MENTAL DISORDERS

4th

F48.8 Other specified nonpsychotic mental disorders
Dhat syndrome
Neurasthenia
Occupational neurosis, including writer's cramp
Psychasthenia
Psychasthenic neurosis
Psychogenic syncope

F48.9 Nonpsychotic mental disorder, unspecified
Neurosis NOS

(F50–F59) BEHAVIORAL SYNDROMES ASSOCIATED WITH PHYSIOLOGICAL DISTURBANCES AND PHYSICAL FACTORS

F50 EATING DISORDERS

4th *Excludes1:* anorexia NOS (R63.0) polyphagia (R63.2)
Excludes2: feeding difficulties (R63.3-)
Excludes2: feeding disorder in infancy or childhood (F98.2-)

F50.0 Anorexia nervosa

5th *Excludes1:* loss of appetite (R63.0) psychogenic loss of appetite (F50.89)

F50.00 Anorexia nervosa, unspecified

F50.01 Anorexia nervosa, restricting type

6th •**F50.010 Anorexia nervosa, restricting type, mild**
Anorexia nervosa, restricting type, with a body mass index greater than or equal to 17 kg/m2

•**F50.011 Anorexia nervosa, restricting type, moderate**
Anorexia nervosa, restricting type, with a body mass index of 16.0–16.99 kg/m2

•**F50.012 Anorexia nervosa, restricting type, severe**
Anorexia nervosa, restricting type, with a body mass index of 15.0–15.99 kg/m2

•**F50.013 Anorexia nervosa, restricting type, extreme**
Anorexia nervosa, restricting type, with a body mass index of less than 15.0 kg/m2

•**F50.014 Anorexia nervosa, restricting type, in remission**
Anorexia nervosa, restricting type, in full remission
Anorexia nervosa, restricting type, in partial remission

•**F50.019 Anorexia nervosa, restricting type, unspecified**

F50.02 Anorexia nervosa, binge eating/purging type
Excludes1: bulimia nervosa (F50.2-)

•**F50.020 Anorexia nervosa, binge eating/purging type, mild**
Anorexia nervosa, binge eating/purging type, with a body mass index greater than or equal to 17kg/m2

•**F50.021 Anorexia nervosa, binge eating/purging type, moderate**
Anorexia nervosa, binge eating/purging type, with a body mass index of 16.0–16.99 kg/m2

•**F50.022 Anorexia nervosa, binge eating/purging type, severe**
Anorexia nervosa, binge eating/purging type, with a body mass index of 15.0–15.99 kg/m2

•**F50.023 Anorexia nervosa, binge eating/purging type, extreme**
Anorexia nervosa, binge eating/purging type, with a body mass index of less than 15.0 kg/m2

•**F50.024 Anorexia nervosa, binge eating/purging type, in remission**
Anorexia nervosa, binge eating/purging type, in full remission
Anorexia nervosa, binge eating/purging type, in partial remission

•**F50.029 Anorexia nervosa, binge eating/purging type, unspecified**

F50.2 Bulimia nervosa

5th Bulimia NOS
Hyperorexia nervosa
Excludes1: anorexia nervosa, binge eating/purging type (F50.02-)

•**F50.20 Bulimia nervosa, unspecified**

•**F50.21 Bulimia nervosa, mild**
Bulimia nervosa with 1–3 episodes of inappropriate compensatory behavior per week

•**F50.22 Bulimia nervosa, moderate**
Bulimia nervosa with 4–7 episodes of inappropriate compensatory behavior per week

•**F50.23 Bulimia nervosa, severe**
Bulimia nervosa with 8–13 episodes of inappropriate compensatory behavior per week

•**F50.24 Bulimia nervosa, extreme**
Bulimia nervosa with 14 or more episodes of inappropriate compensatory behavior per week

•**F50.25 Bulimia nervosa, in remission**
Bulimia nervosa, in full remission
Bulimia nervosa, in partial remission

F50.8 Other eating disorders

5th **F50.81 Binge eating disorder**

6th •**F50.810 Binge eating disorder, mild**
Binge eating disorder with 1–3 binge eating episodes per week

•**F50.811 Binge eating disorder, moderate**
Binge eating disorder with 4–7 binge eating episodes per week

•**F50.812 Binge eating disorder, severe**
Binge eating disorder with 8–13 binge eating episodes per week

•**F50.813 Binge eating disorder, extreme**
Binge eating disorder with 14 or more eating episodes per week

•F50.814 Binge eating disorder, in remission
Binge eating disorder, in full remission
Binge eating disorder, in partial remission

•F50.819 **Binge eating disorder, unspecified**

F50.82 **Avoidant/restrictive food intake disorder**
Avoidant/restrictive food intake disorder, in remission

•F50.83 **Pica in adults**
Pica in adults, in remission
Excludes1: pica in infancy and childhood (F98.3)

•F50.84 **Rumination disorder in adults**
Rumination disorder in adults, in remission
Excludes1: rumination disorder in infancy and childhood (F98.21)

F50.89 **Other specified eating disorder**
Psychogenic loss of appetite

F50.9 **Eating disorder, unspecified**
Atypical anorexia nervosa
Atypical bulimia nervosa

Feeding or eating disorder, unspecified
Other specified feeding disorder

F51 SLEEP DISORDERS NOT DUE TO A SUBSTANCE OR KNOWN PHYSIOLOGICAL CONDITION

Excludes2: organic sleep disorders (G47.-)

F51.0 **Insomnia not due to a substance or known physiological condition**

Excludes2: alcohol related insomnia
drug-related insomnia
insomnia NOS (G47.0-)
insomnia due to known physiological condition (G47.0-)
organic insomnia (G47.0-)
sleep deprivation (Z72.820)

F51.01 **Primary insomnia**
Idiopathic insomnia

F51.02 **Adjustment insomnia**

F51.03 **Paradoxical insomnia**

F51.04 **Psychophysiological insomnia**

F51.05 **Insomnia due to other mental disorder**
Code also associated mental disorder

F51.09 **Other insomnia not due to a substance or known physiological condition**

F51.3 **Sleepwalking [somnambulism]**
Non-rapid eye movement sleep arousal disorders, sleepwalking type

F51.4 **Sleep terrors [night terrors]**
Non-rapid eye movement sleep arousal disorders, sleep terror type

F51.5 **Nightmare disorder**
Dream anxiety disorder

F51.8 **Other sleep disorders not due to a substance or known physiological condition**

F51.9 **Sleep disorder not due to a substance or known physiological condition, unspecified**
Emotional sleep disorder NOS

F54 PSYCHOLOGICAL AND BEHAVIORAL FACTORS ASSOCIATED WITH DISORDERS OR DISEASES CLASSIFIED ELSEWHERE

Psychological factors affecting physical conditions
Code first the associated physical disorder, such as:
asthma (J45.-)
dermatitis (L23-L25)
gastric ulcer (K25.-)
mucous colitis (K58.-)
ulcerative colitis (K51.-)
urticaria (L50.-)
Excludes2: tension-type headache (G44.2)

F55 ABUSE OF NON-PSYCHOACTIVE SUBSTANCES

Excludes2: abuse of psychoactive substances (F10-F19)

F55.0 **Abuse of antacids**

F55.1 **Abuse of herbal or folk remedies**

F55.2 **Abuse of laxatives**

F55.3 **Abuse of steroids or hormones**

F55.4 **Abuse of vitamins**

F55.8 **Abuse of other non-psychoactive substances**

F59 UNSPECIFIED BEHAVIORAL SYNDROMES ASSOCIATED WITH PHYSIOLOGICAL DISTURBANCES AND PHYSICAL FACTORS

Psychogenic physiological dysfunction NOS

(F60–F69) DISORDERS OF ADULT PERSONALITY AND BEHAVIOR

F60 SPECIFIC PERSONALITY DISORDERS

F60.0 **Paranoid personality disorder**
Expansive paranoid personality (disorder)
Fanatic personality (disorder)
Paranoid personality (disorder)
Sensitive paranoid personality (disorder)
Excludes2: paranoia (F22)
paranoid schizophrenia (F20.0)

F60.1 **Schizoid personality disorder**
Excludes2: Asperger's syndrome (F84.5)
delusional disorder (F22)
schizoid disorder of childhood (F84.5)
schizophrenia (F20.-)
schizotypal disorder (F21)

F60.2 **Antisocial personality disorder**
Dissocial personality disorder
Excludes1: conduct disorders (F91.-)
Excludes2: borderline personality disorder (F60.3)

F60.3 **Borderline personality disorder**
Aggressive personality (disorder)
Explosive personality (disorder)
Excludes2: antisocial personality disorder (F60.2)

F60.4 **Histrionic personality disorder**

F60.5 **Obsessive-compulsive personality disorder**
Excludes2: obsessive-compulsive disorder (F42.-)

F60.6 **Avoidant personality disorder**
Anxious personality disorder

F60.9 **Personality disorder, unspecified**
Character disorder NOS
Character neurosis NOS
Pathological personality NOS

F63 IMPULSE DISORDERS

Excludes2: habitual excessive use of alcohol or psychoactive substances (F10–F19)
impulse disorders involving sexual behavior (F65.-)

F63.0 **Pathological gambling**
Compulsive gambling
Excludes1: gambling and betting NOS (Z72.6)
Excludes2: excessive gambling by manic patients (F30, F31)
gambling in antisocial personality disorder (F60.2)

F63.1 **Pyromania**
Pathological fire-setting
Excludes2: fire-setting (by) (in):
adult with antisocial personality disorder (F60.2)
alcohol or psychoactive substance intoxication (F10–F19)
conduct disorders (F91.-)
mental disorders due to known physiological condition (F01–F09)
schizophrenia (F20.-)

F63.2 **Kleptomania**
Pathological stealing
Excludes1: shoplifting as the reason for observation for suspected mental disorder (Z03.8)
Excludes2: depressive disorder with stealing (F31–F33)
stealing due to underlying mental condition-code to mental condition
stealing in mental disorders due to known physiological condition (F01–F09)

F63.3 **Trichotillomania**
Hair plucking
Excludes2: other stereotyped movement disorder (F98.4)

F63.8 Other impulse disorders

F63.81 Intermittent explosive disorder

F63.89 Other impulse disorders

F63.9 Impulse disorder, unspecified

Impulse control disorder NOS

F64 GENDER IDENTITY DISORDERS

F64.0 Transsexualism

Gender dysphoria in adolescents and adults
Gender identity disorder in adolescence and adulthood
Gender incongruence in adolescents and adults
Transgender
Excludes1: gender identity disorder of childhood (F64.2)

F64.1 Dual role transvestism

Use additional code to identify sex reassignment status (Z87.890)
Excludes1: gender identity disorder in childhood (F64.2)
Excludes2: fetishistic transvestism (F65.1)

F64.2 Gender identity disorder of childhood

Gender dysphoria in children
Gender incongruence of childhood
Excludes1: gender identity disorder in adolescence and adulthood (F64.0)
Excludes2: sexual maturation disorder (F66)

F64.8 Other gender identity disorders

Other specified gender dysphoria

F64.9 Gender identity disorder, unspecified

Gender dysphoria, unspecified
Gender incongruence, unspecified
Gender-role disorder NOS

F66 OTHER SEXUAL DISORDERS

☑ Sexual maturation disorder
Sexual relationship disorder

(F70–F79) INTELLECTUAL DISABILITIES

Code first any associated physical or developmental disorders
Excludes1: borderline intellectual functioning, IQ above 70 to 84 (R41.83)

F70 MILD INTELLECTUAL DISABILITIES

☑ IQ level 50–55 to approximately 70
Mild mental subnormality

F71 MODERATE INTELLECTUAL DISABILITIES

☑ IQ level 35–40 to 50–55
Moderate mental subnormality

F72 SEVERE INTELLECTUAL DISABILITIES

☑ IQ level 20–25 to 35–40
Severe mental subnormality

F73 PROFOUND INTELLECTUAL DISABILITIES

☑ IQ level below 20–25
Profound mental subnormality

F78 OTHER INTELLECTUAL DISABILITIES

F78.A Genetic related intellectual disability

F78.A1 SYNGAP1-related intellectual disability

Code also, if applicable, any associated:
autism spectrum disorder (F84.0)
autistic disorder (F84.0)
encephalopathy (G93.4-)
epilepsy and recurrent seizures (G40.-)
other pervasive developmental disorders (F84.8)
pervasive developmental disorder, NOS (F84.9)

F78.A9 Other genetic related intellectual disability

Code also, if applicable, any associated disorders

F79 UNSPECIFIED INTELLECTUAL DISABILITIES

☑ Mental deficiency NOS
Mental subnormality NOS

(F80–F89) PERVASIVE AND SPECIFIC DEVELOPMENTAL DISORDERS

F80 SPECIFIC DEVELOPMENTAL DISORDERS OF SPEECH AND LANGUAGE

F80.0 Phonological disorder

Dyslalia
Functional speech articulation disorder
Lalling
Lisping
Phonological developmental disorder
Speech articulation developmental disorder
Speech-sound disorder
Excludes1: speech articulation impairment due to aphasia NOS (R47.01)
speech articulation impairment due to apraxia (R48.2)
Excludes2: speech articulation impairment due to hearing loss (F80.4)
speech articulation impairment due to intellectual disabilities (F70–F79)
speech articulation impairment with expressive language developmental disorder (F80.1)
speech articulation impairment with mixed receptive expressive language developmental disorder (F80.2)

F80.1 Expressive language disorder

Developmental dysphasia or aphasia, expressive type
Excludes1: mixed receptive-expressive language disorder (F80.2)
dysphasia and aphasia NOS (R47.-)
Excludes2: acquired aphasia with epilepsy [Landau-Kleffner] (G40.80-)
selective mutism (F94.0)
intellectual disabilities (F70–F79)
pervasive developmental disorders (F84.-)

F80.2 Mixed receptive-expressive language disorder

Developmental dysphasia or aphasia, receptive type
Developmental Wernicke's aphasia
Excludes1: central auditory processing disorder (H93.25)
dysphasia or aphasia NOS (R47.-)
expressive language disorder (F80.1)
expressive type dysphasia or aphasia (F80.1)
word deafness (H93.25)
Excludes2: acquired aphasia with epilepsy [Landau-Kleffner] (G40.80-)
pervasive developmental disorders (F84.-)
selective mutism (F94.0)
intellectual disabilities (F70–F79)

F80.4 Speech and language development delay due to hearing loss

Code also type of hearing loss (H90.-, H91.-)

F80.8 Other developmental disorders of speech and language

F80.81 Childhood onset fluency disorder

Cluttering NOS
Stuttering NOS
Excludes1: adult onset fluency disorder (F98.5)
fluency disorder in conditions classified elsewhere (R47.82)
fluency disorder (stuttering) following cerebrovascular disease (I69. with final characters -23)

F80.82 Social pragmatic communication disorder

Excludes1: Asperger's syndrome (F84.5)
autistic disorder (F84.0)

F80.89 Other developmental disorders of speech and language

F80.9 Developmental disorder of speech and language, unspecified

Communication disorder NOS
Language disorder NOS

F81 SPECIFIC DEVELOPMENTAL DISORDERS OF SCHOLASTIC SKILLS

F81.0 Specific reading disorder

'Backward reading'
Developmental dyslexia
Specific learning disorder, with impairment in reading
Excludes1: alexia NOS (R48.0)
dyslexia NOS (R48.0)

F81.2 Mathematics disorder

Developmental acalculia

Developmental arithmetical disorder

Developmental Gerstmann's syndrome

Specific learning disorder, with impairment in mathematics

Excludes1: acalculia NOS (R48.8)

Excludes2: arithmetical difficulties associated with a reading disorder (F81.0)

arithmetical difficulties associated with a spelling disorder (F81.81)

arithmetical difficulties due to inadequate teaching (Z55.8)

F81.8 Other developmental disorders of scholastic skills

F81.81 Disorder of written expression

Specific spelling disorder

Specific learning disorder, with impairment in written expression

F81.89 Other developmental disorders of scholastic skills

F81.9 Developmental disorder of scholastic skills, unspecified

Knowledge acquisition disability NOS

Learning disability NOS

Learning disorder NOS

F82 SPECIFIC DEVELOPMENTAL DISORDER OF MOTOR FUNCTION

Clumsy child syndrome

Developmental coordination disorder

Developmental dyspraxia

Excludes1: abnormalities of gait and mobility (R26.-)

lack of coordination (R27.-)

Excludes2: lack of coordination secondary to intellectual disabilities (F70–F79)

F84 PERVASIVE DEVELOPMENTAL DISORDERS

Code also to identify any associated medical condition and intellectual disabilities.

F84.0 Autistic disorder

Autism spectrum disorder

Infantile autism

Infantile psychosis

Kanner's syndrome

Excludes1: Asperger's syndrome (F84.5)

F84.2 Rett's syndrome

Excludes1: Asperger's syndrome (F84.5)

Autistic disorder (F84.0)

Other childhood disintegrative disorder (F84.3)

F84.3 Other childhood disintegrative disorder

Dementia infantilis

Disintegrative psychosis

Heller's syndrome

Symbiotic psychosis

Use additional code to identify any associated neurological condition.

Excludes1: Asperger's syndrome (F84.5)

Autistic disorder (F84.0)

Rett's syndrome (F84.2)

F84.5 Asperger's syndrome

Asperger's disorder

Autistic psychopathy

Schizoid disorder of childhood

F84.8 Other pervasive developmental disorders

Overactive disorder associated with intellectual disabilities and stereotyped movements

F84.9 Pervasive developmental disorder, unspecified

Atypical autism

F88 OTHER DISORDERS OF PSYCHOLOGICAL DEVELOPMENT

Developmental agnosia

Global developmental delay

Other specified neurodevelopmental disorder

F89 UNSPECIFIED DISORDER OF PSYCHOLOGICAL DEVELOPMENT

Developmental disorder NOS

Neurodevelopmental disorder NOS

(F90–F98) BEHAVIORAL AND EMOTIONAL DISORDERS WITH ONSET USUALLY OCCURRING IN CHILDHOOD AND ADOLESCENCE

Note: Codes within categories F90–F98 may be used regardless of the age of a patient. These disorders generally have onset within the childhood or adolescent years, but may continue throughout life or not be diagnosed until adulthood

F90 ATTENTION-DEFICIT HYPERACTIVITY DISORDERS

Includes: attention deficit disorder with hyperactivity

attention deficit syndrome with hyperactivity

Excludes2: anxiety disorders (F40.-, F41.-)

mood [affective] disorders (F30–F39)

pervasive developmental disorders (F84.-)

schizophrenia (F20.-)

F90.0 Attention-deficit hyperactivity disorder, predominantly inattentive type

ADD without hyperactivity

F90.1 Attention-deficit hyperactivity disorder, predominantly hyperactive type

F90.2 Attention-deficit hyperactivity disorder, combined type

F90.8 Attention-deficit hyperactivity disorder, other type

F90.9 Attention-deficit hyperactivity disorder, unspecified type

Attention-deficit hyperactivity disorder of childhood or adolescence NOS

Attention-deficit hyperactivity disorder NOS

F91 CONDUCT DISORDERS

Excludes1: antisocial behavior (Z72.81-)

antisocial personality disorder (F60.2)

Excludes2: conduct problems associated with attention-deficit hyperactivity disorder (F90.-)

mood [affective] disorders (F30–F39)

pervasive developmental disorders (F84.-)

schizophrenia (F20.-)

F91.0 Conduct disorder confined to family context

F91.1 Conduct disorder, childhood-onset type

Unsocialized conduct disorder

Conduct disorder, solitary aggressive type

Unsocialized aggressive disorder

F91.2 Conduct disorder, adolescent-onset type

Socialized conduct disorder

Conduct disorder, group type

F91.3 Oppositional defiant disorder

F91.8 Other conduct disorders

Other specified conduct disorder

Other specified disruptive disorder

F91.9 Conduct disorder, unspecified

Behavioral disorder NOS

Conduct disorder NOS

Disruptive behavior disorder NOS

F93 EMOTIONAL DISORDERS WITH ONSET SPECIFIC TO CHILDHOOD

F93.0 Separation anxiety disorder of childhood

Excludes2: mood [affective] disorders (F30–F39)

nonpsychotic mental disorders (F40–F48)

phobic anxiety disorder of childhood (F40.8)

social phobia (F40.1)

F93.8 Other childhood emotional disorders

Identity disorder

Excludes2: gender identity disorder of childhood (F64.2)

F93.9 Childhood emotional disorder, unspecified

F94 DISORDERS OF SOCIAL FUNCTIONING WITH ONSET SPECIFIC TO CHILDHOOD AND ADOLESCENCE

F94.0 Selective mutism

Elective mutism

Excludes2: pervasive developmental disorders (F84.-)

schizophrenia (F20.-)

specific developmental disorders of speech and language (F80.-)

transient mutism as part of separation anxiety in young children (F93.0)

- **F94.1 Reactive attachment disorder of childhood**
  Use additional code to identify any associated failure to thrive or growth retardation
  Excludes1: disinhibited attachment disorder of childhood (F94.2) normal variation in pattern of selective attachment
  Excludes2: Asperger's syndrome (F84.5) maltreatment syndromes (T74.-) sexual or physical abuse in childhood, resulting in psychosocial problems (Z62.81-)
- **F94.2 Disinhibited attachment disorder of childhood**
  Affectionless psychopathy
  Institutional syndrome
  Excludes1: reactive attachment disorder of childhood (F94.1)
  Excludes2: Asperger's syndrome (F84.5) attention-deficit hyperactivity disorders (F90.-) hospitalism in children (F43.2-)
- **F94.8 Other childhood disorders of social functioning**
- **F94.9 Childhood disorder of social functioning, unspecified**

F95 TIC DISORDER

- **F95.0 Transient tic disorder**
  Provisional tic disorder
- **F95.1 Chronic motor or vocal tic disorder**
- **F95.2 Tourette's disorder**
  Combined vocal and multiple motor tic disorder [de la Tourette] Tourette's syndrome
- **F95.8 Other tic disorders**
- **F95.9 Tic disorder, unspecified**
  Tic NOS

F98 OTHER BEHAVIORAL AND EMOTIONAL DISORDERS WITH ONSET USUALLY OCCURRING IN CHILDHOOD AND ADOLESCENCE

Excludes2: breath-holding spells (R06.89) gender identity disorder of childhood (F64.2) Kleine-Levin syndrome (G47.13) obsessive-compulsive disorder (F42.-) sleep disorders not due to a substance or known physiological condition (F51.-)

- **F98.0 Enuresis not due to a substance or known physiological condition**
  Enuresis (primary) (secondary) of nonorganic origin
  Functional enuresis
  Psychogenic enuresis
  Urinary incontinence of nonorganic origin
  Excludes1: enuresis NOS (R32)

- **F98.1 Encopresis not due to a substance or known physiological condition**
  Functional encopresis
  Incontinence of feces of nonorganic origin
  Psychogenic encopresis
  Use additional code to identify the cause of any coexisting constipation.
  Excludes1: encopresis NOS (R15.-)

- **F98.2 Other feeding disorders of infancy and childhood**
  Excludes2: feeding difficulties (R63.3-) anorexia nervosa and other eating disorders (F50.-) feeding problems of newborn (P92.-) pica of infancy or childhood (F98.3)
  - **F98.21 Rumination disorder of infancy**
    Rumination disorder in infancy or childhood, in remission
    Excludes1: rumination disorder in adults (F50.84)
  - **F98.29 Other feeding disorders of infancy and early childhood**

- **F98.3 Pica of infancy and childhood**
  Pica in infancy or childhood, in remission
  Excludes1: pica in adults (F50.83)

- **F98.4 Stereotyped movement disorders**
  Stereotype/habit disorder
  Excludes1: abnormal involuntary movements (R25.-)
  Excludes2: compulsions in obsessive-compulsive disorder (F42.-) hair plucking (F63.3) movement disorders of organic origin (G20–G25) nail-biting (F98.8) nose-picking (F98.8) stereotypies that are part of a broader psychiatric condition (F01–F95) thumb-sucking (F98.8) tic disorders (F95.-) trichotillomania (F63.3)

- **F98.8 Other specified behavioral and emotional disorders with onset usually occurring in childhood and adolescence**
  Excessive masturbation Nail-biting
  Nose-picking
  Thumb-sucking

- **F98.9 Unspecified behavioral and emotional disorders with onset usually occurring in childhood and adolescence**

(F99) UNSPECIFIED MENTAL DISORDER

F99 MENTAL DISORDER, NOT OTHERWISE SPECIFIED

Mental illness NOS
Excludes1: unspecified mental disorder due to known physiological condition (F09)

Chapter 6. Diseases of the nervous system (G00–G99)

GUIDELINES

Dominant/nondominant side

See category G81 and subcategories G83.1 and G83.2.

Pain

See category G89.

Excludes2: certain conditions originating in the perinatal period (P04–P96)
certain infectious and parasitic diseases (A00–B99)
complications of pregnancy, childbirth and the puerperium (O00–O9A)
congenital malformations, deformations, and chromosomal abnormalities (Q00–Q99)
endocrine, nutritional and metabolic diseases (E00–E88)
injury, poisoning and certain other consequences of external causes (S00–T88)
neoplasms (C00–D49)
symptoms, signs and abnormal clinical and laboratory findings, not elsewhere classified (R00–R94)

(G00–G09) INFLAMMATORY DISEASES OF THE CENTRAL NERVOUS SYSTEM

G00 BACTERIAL MENINGITIS, NOT ELSEWHERE CLASSIFIED

Includes: bacterial arachnoiditis
bacterial leptomeningitis
bacterial meningitis
bacterial pachymeningitis

Excludes1: bacterial meningoencephalitis (G04.2)
bacterial meningomyelitis (G04.2)

- **G00.0 Hemophilus meningitis**
Meningitis due to H. influenzae
- **G00.1 Pneumococcal meningitis**
Meningitis due to streptococcus pneumoniae
- **G00.2 Streptococcal meningitis**
Use additional code to further identify organism (B95.0–B95.5)
- **G00.3 Staphylococcal meningitis**
Use additional code to further identify organism (B95.61–B95.8)
- **G00.8 Other bacterial meningitis**
Meningitis due to E. coli
Meningitis due to Friedländer's bacillus
Meningitis due to Klebsiella
Use additional code to further identify organism (B96.-)
- **G00.9 Bacterial meningitis, unspecified**
Meningitis due to gram-negative bacteria, unspecified
Purulent meningitis NOS
Pyogenic meningitis NOS
Suppurative meningitis NOS

G01 MENINGITIS IN BACTERIAL DISEASES CLASSIFIED ELSEWHERE

Code first underlying disease

Excludes1: meningitis (in): gonococcal (A54.81)
leptospirosis (A27.81)
listeriosis (A32.11)
Lyme disease (A69.21)
meningococcal (A39.0)
neurosyphilis (A52.13)
tuberculosis (A17.0)
meningoencephalitis and meningomyelitis in bacterial diseases classified elsewhere (G05)

G02 MENINGITIS IN OTHER INFECTIOUS AND PARASITIC DISEASES CLASSIFIED ELSEWHERE

Code first underlying disease, such as: African trypanosomiasis (B56.-)
poliovirus infection (A80.-)

Excludes1: candidal meningitis (B37.5)
coccidioidomycosis meningitis (B38.4)
cryptococcal meningitis (B45.1)
herpesviral [herpes simplex] meningitis (B00.3)
infectious mononucleosis complicated by meningitis (B27.- with 5th character 2)

measles complicated by meningitis (B05.1)
meningoencephalitis and meningomyelitis in other infectious and parasitic diseases classified elsewhere (G05)
mumps meningitis (B26.1)
rubella meningitis (B06.02)
varicella [chickenpox] meningitis (B01.0)
zoster meningitis (B02.1)

G03 MENINGITIS DUE TO OTHER AND UNSPECIFIED CAUSES

Includes: arachnoiditis NOS
leptomeningitis NOS
meningitis NOS
pachymeningitis NOS

Excludes1: meningoencephalitis (G04.-)
meningomyelitis (G04.-)

- **G03.0 Nonpyogenic meningitis**
Aseptic meningitis
Nonbacterial meningitis
- **G03.1 Chronic meningitis**
- **G03.2 Benign recurrent meningitis [Mollaret]**
- **G03.8 Meningitis due to other specified causes**
- **G03.9 Meningitis, unspecified**
Arachnoiditis (spinal) NOS

G04 ENCEPHALITIS, MYELITIS AND ENCEPHALOMYELITIS

Includes: acute ascending myelitis
meningoencephalitis
meningomyelitis

Excludes1: encephalopathy NOS (G93.40)

Excludes2: acute transverse myelitis (G37.3)
alcoholic encephalopathy (G31.2)
benign myalgic encephalomyelitis (G93.3)
multiple sclerosis (G35)
subacute necrotizing myelitis (G37.4)
toxic encephalitis (G92.8)
toxic encephalopathy (G92.8)

- **G04.0 Acute disseminated encephalitis and encephalomyelitis (ADEM)**

Excludes1: acute necrotizing hemorrhagic encephalopathy (G04.3-)
other noninfectious acute disseminated encephalomyelitis (noninfectious ADEM) (G04.81)

  - **G04.00 Acute disseminated encephalitis and encephalomyelitis, unspecified**
  - **G04.01 Postinfectious acute disseminated encephalitis and encephalomyelitis (postinfectious ADEM)**
Excludes1: post chickenpox encephalitis (B01.1)
post measles encephalitis (B05.0)
post measles myelitis (B05.1)
  - **G04.02 Postimmunization acute disseminated encephalitis, myelitis and encephalomyelitis**
Encephalitis, post immunization
Encephalomyelitis, post immunization
Use additional code to identify the vaccine (T50.A-, T50.B-, T50.Z-)

- **G04.2 Bacterial meningoencephalitis and meningomyelitis, not elsewhere classified**

- **G04.3 Acute necrotizing hemorrhagic encephalopathy**

Excludes1: acute disseminated encephalitis and encephalomyelitis (G04.0-)

  - **G04.30 Acute necrotizing hemorrhagic encephalopathy, unspecified**
  - **G04.31 Postinfectious acute necrotizing hemorrhagic encephalopathy**
  - **G04.32 Postimmunization acute necrotizing hemorrhagic encephalopathy**
Use additional code to identify the vaccine (T50.A-, T50.B-, T50.Z-)
  - **G04.39 Other acute necrotizing hemorrhagic encephalopathy**
Code also underlying etiology, if applicable

- **G04.8 Other encephalitis, myelitis and encephalomyelitis**
Code also any associated seizure (G40.-, R56.9)

G04.81 Other encephalitis and encephalomyelitis
Noninfectious acute disseminated encephalomyelitis (noninfectious ADEM)

G04.82 Acute flaccid myelitis
Excludes1: transverse myelitis (G37.3)

G04.89 Other myelitis

G04.9 Encephalitis, myelitis and encephalomyelitis, unspecified

5th **G04.90 Encephalitis and encephalomyelitis, unspecified**
Ventriculitis (cerebral) NOS

G04.91 Myelitis, unspecified

G05 ENCEPHALITIS, MYELITIS AND ENCEPHALOMYELITIS IN DISEASES CLASSIFIED ELSEWHERE

4th

Code first underlying disease, such as:
congenital toxoplasmosis encephalitis, myelitis and encephalomyelitis (P37.1)
cytomegaloviral encephalitis, myelitis and encephalomyelitis (B25.8)
encephalitis, myelitis and encephalomyelitis (in) SLE (M32.19)
eosinophilic meningoencephalitis (B83.2)
HIV disease (B20)
poliovirus (A80.-)
suppurative otitis media (H66.01–H66.4)
systemic lupus erythematosus (M32.19)
trichinellosis (B75)

Excludes1: adenoviral encephalitis, myelitis and encephalomyelitis (A85.1)
encephalitis, myelitis and encephalomyelitis (in) measles (B05.0)
enteroviral encephalitis, myelitis and encephalomyelitis (A85.0)
herpesviral [herpes simplex] encephalitis, myelitis and encephalomyelitis (B00.4)
listerial encephalitis, myelitis and encephalomyelitis (A32.12)
meningococcal encephalitis, myelitis and encephalomyelitis (A39.81)
mumps encephalitis, myelitis and encephalomyelitis (B26.2)
postchickenpox encephalitis, myelitis and encephalomyelitis (B01.1-)
rubella encephalitis, myelitis and encephalomyelitis (B06.01)
toxoplasmosis encephalitis, myelitis and encephalomyelitis (B58.2)
zoster encephalitis, myelitis and encephalomyelitis (B02.0)

G05.3 Encephalitis and encephalomyelitis in diseases classified elsewhere
Meningoencephalitis in diseases classified elsewhere
Code first underlying disease

G05.4 Myelitis in diseases classified elsewhere
Meningomyelitis in diseases classified elsewhere

G06 INTRACRANIAL AND INTRASPINAL ABSCESS AND GRANULOMA

4th

Use additional code (B95–B97) to identify infectious agent.

G06.0 Intracranial abscess and granuloma
Brain [any part] abscess (embolic)
Cerebellar abscess (embolic)
Cerebral abscess (embolic)
Intracranial epidural abscess or granuloma
Intracranial extradural abscess or granuloma
Intracranial subdural abscess or granuloma
Otogenic abscess (embolic)
Excludes1: tuberculous intracranial abscess and granuloma (A17.81)

G06.1 Intraspinal abscess and granuloma
Abscess (embolic) of spinal cord [any part]
Intraspinal epidural abscess or granuloma
Intraspinal extradural abscess or granuloma
Intraspinal subdural abscess or granuloma
Excludes1: tuberculous intraspinal abscess and granuloma (A17.81)

G06.2 Extradural and subdural abscess, unspecified

G08 INTRACRANIAL AND INTRASPINAL PHLEBITIS AND THROMBOPHLEBITIS

✓

Septic embolism of intracranial or intraspinal venous sinuses and veins
Septic endophlebitis of intracranial or intraspinal venous sinuses and veins
Septic phlebitis of intracranial or intraspinal venous sinuses and veins
Septic thrombophlebitis of intracranial or intraspinal venous sinuses and veins
Septic thrombosis of intracranial or intraspinal venous sinuses and veins

Excludes1: intracranial phlebitis and thrombophlebitis complicating: abortion, ectopic or molar pregnancy (O00-O07, O08.7) pregnancy, childbirth and the puerperium (O22.5, O87.3) nonpyogenic intracranial phlebitis and thrombophlebitis (I67.6)

Excludes2: intracranial phlebitis and thrombophlebitis complicating nonpyogenic intraspinal phlebitis and thrombophlebitis (G95.1)

G09 SEQUELAE OF INFLAMMATORY DISEASES OF CENTRAL NERVOUS SYSTEM

✓

Note: Category G09 is to be used to indicate conditions whose primary classification is to G00-G08 as the cause of sequelae, themselves classifiable elsewhere. The 'sequelae' include conditions specified as residuals.

Code first condition resulting from (sequela) of inflammatory diseases of central nervous system

(G10–G14) SYSTEMIC ATROPHIES PRIMARILY AFFECTING THE CENTRAL NERVOUS SYSTEM

G11 HEREDITARY ATAXIA

4th

Excludes2: cerebral palsy (G80.-)
hereditary and idiopathic neuropathy (G60.-)
metabolic disorders (E70–E88)

G11.0 Congenital nonprogressive ataxia

G11.1 Early-onset cerebellar ataxia

5th **G11.10 Early-onset cerebellar ataxia, unspecified**

G11.11 Friedreich ataxia
Autosomal recessive Friedreich ataxia
Friedreich ataxia with retained reflexes

G11.19 Other early-onset cerebellar ataxia
Early-onset cerebellar ataxia with essential tremor
Early-onset cerebellar ataxia with myoclonus [Hunt's ataxia]
Early-onset cerebellar ataxia with retained tendon reflexes
X-linked recessive spinocerebellar ataxia

G11.2 Late-onset cerebellar ataxia

G11.3 Cerebellar ataxia with defective DNA repair
Ataxia telangiectasia [Louis-Bar]
Excludes2: Cockayne's syndrome (Q87.19)
other disorders of purine and pyrimidine metabolism (E79.-)
xeroderma pigmentosum (Q82.1)

G11.5 Hypomyelination—hypogonadotropic hypogonadism—hypodontia
4H syndrome
Pol III-related leukodystrophy

G11.6 Leukodystrophy with vanishing white matter disease

G11.9 Hereditary ataxia, unspecified
Hereditary cerebellar ataxia NOS
Hereditary cerebellar degeneration
Hereditary cerebellar disease
Hereditary cerebellar syndrome

G12 SPINAL MUSCULAR ATROPHY AND RELATED SYNDROMES

4th

G12.0 Infantile spinal muscular atrophy, type I [Werdnig-Hoffman]

G12.2 Motor neuron disease

5th **G12.20 Motor neuron disease, unspecified**

G12.21 Amyotrophic lateral sclerosis

G12.22 Progressive bulbar palsy

G12.25 Progressive spinal muscle atrophy

G12.29 Other motor neuron disease

G12.9 Spinal muscular atrophy, unspecified

G13 SYSTEMIC ATROPHIES PRIMARILY AFFECTING CENTRAL NERVOUS SYSTEM IN DISEASES CLASSIFIED ELSEWHERE

4th

G13.0 Paraneoplastic neuromyopathy and neuropathy
Carcinomatous neuromyopathy
Sensorial paraneoplastic neuropathy [Denny Brown]
Code first underlying neoplasm (C00-D49)

G13.1 Other systemic atrophy primarily affecting central nervous system in neoplastic disease
Paraneoplastic limbic encephalopathy
Code first underlying neoplasm (C00-D49)

G13.2 Systemic atrophy primarily affecting the central nervous system in myxedema
Code first underlying disease, such as:
hypothyroidism (E03.-)
myxedematous congenital iodine deficiency (E00.1)

G13.8 Systemic atrophy primarily affecting central nervous system in other diseases classified elsewhere
Code first underlying disease

(G20–G26) EXTRAPYRAMIDAL AND MOVEMENT DISORDERS

G23 OTHER DEGENERATIVE DISEASES OF BASAL GANGLIA

Excludes2: multi-system degeneration of the autonomic nervous system (G90.3)

G23.3 Hypomyelination with atrophy of the basal ganglia and cerebellum
H-ABC

G24 DYSTONIA

Includes: dyskinesia
Excludes2: athetoid cerebral palsy (G80.3)

G24.0 Drug induced dystonia
Use additional code for adverse effect, if applicable, to identify drug (T36-T50 with fifth or sixth character 5)

G24.01 Drug induced subacute dyskinesia
Drug induced blepharospasm
Drug induced orofacial dyskinesia
Neuroleptic induced tardive dyskinesia
Tardive dyskinesia

G24.02 Drug induced acute dystonia
Acute dystonic reaction to drugs
Neuroleptic induced acute dystonia

G24.09 Other drug induced dystonia

G24.1 Genetic torsion dystonia
Dystonia deformans progressiva
Dystonia musculorum deformans
Familial torsion dystonia
Idiopathic familial dystonia
Idiopathic (torsion) dystonia NOS
(Schwalbe-) Ziehen-Oppenheim disease

G24.2 Idiopathic nonfamilial dystonia

G24.8 Other dystonia
Acquired torsion dystonia NOS

G24.9 Dystonia, unspecified
Dyskinesia NOS

G25 OTHER EXTRAPYRAMIDAL AND MOVEMENT DISORDERS

Excludes2: sleep related movement disorders (G47.6-)

G25.0 Essential tremor
Familial tremor
Excludes1: tremor NOS (R25.1)

G25.1 Drug-induced tremor
Use additional code for adverse effect, if applicable, to identify drug (T36-T50 with fifth or sixth character 5)

G25.2 Other specified forms of tremor
Intention tremor

G25.3 Myoclonus
Drug-induced myoclonus
Palatal myoclonus
Use additional code for adverse effect, if applicable, to identify drug (T36–T50 with fifth or sixth character 5)
Excludes1: facial myokymia (G51.4)
myoclonic epilepsy (G40.-)

G25.4 Drug-induced chorea
Use additional code for adverse effect, if applicable, to identify drug (T36-T50 with fifth or sixth character 5)

G25.5 Other chorea
Chorea NOS
Excludes1: chorea NOS with heart involvement (I02.-)
Huntington's chorea (G10)

G25.6 Drug induced tics and other tics of organic origin

G25.61 Drug induced tics
Use additional code for adverse effect, if applicable, to identify drug (T36-T50 with fifth or sixth character 5)

G25.69 Other tics of organic origin
Excludes1: habit spasm (F95.9)
tic NOS (F95.9)
Tourette's syndrome (F95.2)

G25.7 Other and unspecified drug induced movement disorders
Use additional code for adverse effect, if applicable, to identify drug (T36-T50 with fifth or sixth character 5)

G25.70 Drug induced movement disorder, unspecified

G25.71 Drug induced akathisia
Drug induced acathisia
Neuroleptic induced acute akathisia
Tardive akathisia

G25.79 Other drug induced movement disorders

G25.8 Other specified extrapyramidal and movement disorders

G25.81 Restless legs syndrome

G25.83 Benign shuddering attacks

G25.89 Other specified extrapyramidal and movement disorders

G25.9 Extrapyramidal and movement disorder, unspecified

(G30–G32) OTHER DEGENERATIVE DISEASES OF THE NERVOUS SYSTEM

G31 OTHER DEGENERATIVE DISEASES OF NERVOUS SYSTEM, NOT ELSEWHERE CLASSIFIED

For codes G31.0-G31.83, G31.85-G31.9, **use additional code** to identify:
dementia with anxiety (F02.84, F02.A4, F02.B4, F02.C4)
dementia with behavioral disturbance (F02.81-, F02.A1-, F02.B1-, F02.C1-)
dementia with mood disturbance (F02.83, F02.A3, F02.B3, F02.C3)
dementia with psychotic disturbance (F02.82, F02.A2, F02.B2, F02.C2)
dementia without behavioral disturbance (F02.80, F02.A0, F02.B0, F02.C0)
mild neurocognitive disorder due to known physiological condition (F06.7-)

Excludes2: Reye's syndrome (G93.7)

G31.8 Other specified degenerative diseases of nervous system

G31.80 Leukodystrophy, unspecified

G31.86 Alexander disease

G31.89 Other specified degenerative diseases of nervous system

G31.9 Degenerative disease of nervous system, unspecified

G32 OTHER DEGENERATIVE DISORDERS OF NERVOUS SYSTEM IN DISEASES CLASSIFIED ELSEWHERE

G32.0 Subacute combined degeneration of spinal cord in diseases classified elsewhere
Dana-Putnam syndrome
Sclerosis of spinal cord (combined) (dorsolateral) (posterolateral)
Code first underlying disease, such as:
other dietary vitamin B12 deficiency anemia (D51.3)
vitamin B12 deficiency anemia due to intrinsic factor deficiency (D51.0)
vitamin B12 deficiency anemia, unspecified (D51.8)
vitamin B12 deficiency (E53.8)
Excludes1: syphilitic combined degeneration of spinal cord (A52.11)

G32.8 Other specified degenerative disorders of nervous system in diseases classified elsewhere
Code first underlying disease, such as:
amyloidosis cerebral degeneration (E85.-)
cerebral degeneration (due to) hypothyroidism (E00.0-E03.9)
cerebral degeneration (due to) neoplasm (C00-D49)
cerebral degeneration (due to) vitamin B deficiency, except thiamine (E52-E53.-)
Excludes1: superior hemorrhagic polioencephalitis [Wernicke's encephalopathy] (E51.2)

G32.81 Cerebellar ataxia in diseases classified elsewhere
Code first underlying disease, such as:
celiac disease (with gluten ataxia) (K90.0)
cerebellar ataxia (in) neoplastic disease (paraneoplastic cerebellar degeneration) (C00-D49)
non-celiac gluten ataxia (M35.9)

Excludes1: systemic atrophy primarily affecting the central nervous system in alcoholic cerebellarataxia (G31.2)

systemic atrophy primarily affecting the central nervous system in myxedema (G13.2)

G32.89 Other specified degenerative disorders of nervous system in diseases classified elsewhere

Degenerative encephalopathy in diseases classified elsewhere

(G35–G37) DEMYELINATING DISEASES OF THE CENTRAL NERVOUS SYSTEM

G35 **MULTIPLE SCLEROSIS**

✓

Disseminated multiple sclerosis
Generalized multiple sclerosis
Multiple sclerosis NOS
Multiple sclerosis of brain stem
Multiple sclerosis of cord

G36 **OTHER ACUTE DISSEMINATED DEMYELINATION**

4th

Excludes1: postinfectious encephalitis and encephalomyelitis NOS (G04.01)

- G36.0 Neuromyelitis optica [Devic]
  Demyelination in optic neuritis
  Excludes1: optic neuritis NOS (H46)
- G36.1 Acute and subacute hemorrhagic leukoencephalitis [Hurst]
- G36.8 Other specified acute disseminated demyelination
- G36.9 Acute disseminated demyelination, unspecified

G37 **OTHER DEMYELINATING DISEASES OF CENTRAL NERVOUS SYSTEM**

4th

- G37.1 Central demyelination of corpus callosum
- G37.8 Other specified demyelinating diseases of central nervous system

  5th

  - G37.81 Myelin oligodendrocyte glycoprotein antibody disease
    MOG antibody disease
    Code also associated manifestations, if known, such as: noninfectious acute disseminated encephalomyelitis (G04.81)
    neuromyelitis optica (G36.0)
  - G37.89 Other specified demyelinating diseases of central nervous system
- G37.9 Demyelinating disease of central nervous system, unspecified

(G40–G47) EPISODIC AND PAROXYSMAL DISORDERS

G40 **EPILEPSY AND RECURRENT SEIZURES**

4th

Note: the following terms are to be considered equivalent to intractable: pharmacoresistant (pharmacologically resistant), treatment resistant, refractory (medically) and poorly controlled

Excludes1: conversion disorder with seizures (F44.5)
convulsions NOS (R56.9)
post traumatic seizures (R56.1)
seizure (convulsive) NOS (R56.9)
seizure of newborn (P90)

Excludes2: hippocampal sclerosis (G93.81)
mesial temporal sclerosis (G93.81)
temporal sclerosis (G93.81)
Todd's paralysis (G83.8)

G40.0 Localization-related (focal) (partial) idiopathic epilepsy and epileptic syndromes with seizures of localized onset

5th

Benign childhood epilepsy with centrotemporal EEG spikes
Childhood epilepsy with occipital EEG paroxysms
Excludes1: adult onset localization-related epilepsy (G40.1-, G40.2-)

- **G40.00- Localization-related (focal) (partial) idiopathic epilepsy and epileptic syndromes with seizures of localized onset, not intractable (without intractability)**

  6th

- **G40.01- Localization-related (focal) (partial) idiopathic epilepsy and epileptic syndromes with seizures of localized onset, intractable**

  6th

G40.1 Localization-related (focal) (partial) symptomatic epilepsy and epileptic syndromes with simple partial seizures

5th

Attacks without alteration of consciousness
Epilepsia partialis continua [Kozhevnikof]
Simple partial seizures developing into secondarily generalized seizures

- **G40.10- Localization-related (focal) (partial) symptomatic epilepsy and epileptic syndromes with simple partial seizures, not intractable (without intractability)**

  6th

- **G40.11- Localization-related (focal) (partial) symptomatic epilepsy and epileptic syndromes with simple partial seizures, intractable**

  6th

G40.2 Localization-related (focal) (partial) symptomatic epilepsy and epileptic syndromes with complex partial seizures

5th

Attacks with alteration of consciousness, often with automatisms
Complex partial seizures developing into secondarily generalized seizures

- **G40.20- Localization-related (focal) (partial) symptomatic epilepsy and epileptic syndromes with complex partial seizures, not intractable (without intractability)**

  6th

- **G40.21- Localization-related (focal) (partial) symptomatic epilepsy and epileptic syndromes with complex partial seizures, intractable**

  6th

G40.3 Generalized idiopathic epilepsy and epileptic syndromes

5th

Code also MERRF syndrome, if applicable (E88.42)

- **G40.30- Generalized idiopathic epilepsy and epileptic syndromes, not intractable (without intractability)**

  6th

- **G40.31- Generalized idiopathic epilepsy and epileptic syndromes, intractable**

  6th

G40.A Absence epileptic syndrome

5th

Childhood absence epilepsy [pyknolepsy]
Juvenile absence epilepsy
Absence epileptic syndrome, NOS

- **G40.A0- Absence epileptic syndrome, not intractable**

  6th

- **G40.A1- Absence epileptic syndrome, intractable**

  6th

G40.B Juvenile myoclonic epilepsy [impulsive petit mal]

5th

- **G40.B0- Juvenile myoclonic epilepsy, not intractable**

  6th

- **G40.B1- Juvenile myoclonic epilepsy, intractable**

  6th

G40.C Lafora progressive myoclonus epilepsy

5th

Lafora body disease **Code also**, if applicable, associated conditions such as dementia (F02.8-)

- **G40.C0 Lafora progressive myoclonus epilepsy, not intractable**

  6th

  - G40.C01 Lafora progressive myoclonus epilepsy, not intractable, with status epilepticus
  - G40.C09 Lafora progressive myoclonus epilepsy, not intractable, without status epilepticus
    Lafora progressive myoclonus epilepsy NOS

- **G40.C11 Lafora progressive myoclonus epilepsy, intractable, with status epilepticus**

- **G40.C19 Lafora progressive myoclonus epilepsy, intractable, without status epilepticus**

G40.4 Other generalized epilepsy and epileptic syndromes

5th

Epilepsy with grand mal seizures on awakening
Epilepsy with myoclonic absences
Epilepsy with myoclonic-astatic seizures
Grand mal seizure NOS
Nonspecific atonic epileptic seizures
Nonspecific clonic epileptic seizures
Nonspecific myoclonic epileptic seizures
Nonspecific tonic epileptic seizures
Nonspecific tonic-clonic epileptic seizures
Symptomatic early myoclonic encephalopathy

G40.40- Other generalized epilepsy and epileptic syndromes, not intractable

Other generalized epilepsy and epileptic syndromes without intractability

Other generalized epilepsy and epileptic syndromes NOS

G40.41- Other generalized epilepsy and epileptic syndromes, intractable

G40.42 Cyclin-Dependent Kinase-Like 5 Deficiency Disorder

CDKL5

Use additional code, if known, to identify associated manifestations, such as:

cortical blindness (H47.61-)

global developmental delay (F88)

G40.5 Epileptic seizures related to external causes

Epileptic seizures related to alcohol

Epileptic seizures related to drugs

Epileptic seizures related to hormonal changes

Epileptic seizures related to sleep deprivation

Epileptic seizures related to stress

Code also, if applicable, associated epilepsy and recurrent seizures (G40.-)

Use additional code for adverse effect, if applicable, to identify drug (T36–T50 with fifth or sixth character 5)

G40.50 Epileptic seizures related to external causes, not intractable

G40.501 Epileptic seizures related to external causes, not intractable, with status epilepticus

G40.509 Epileptic seizures related to external causes, not intractable, without status epilepticus

Epileptic seizures related to external causes, NOS

G40.8 Other epilepsy and recurrent seizures

Epilepsies and epileptic syndromes undetermined as to whether they are focal or generalized

Landau-Kleffner syndrome

G40.80 Other epilepsy

G40.801 Other epilepsy, not intractable, with status epilepticus

Other epilepsy without intractability with status epilepticus

G40.802 Other epilepsy, not intractable, without status epilepticus

Other epilepsy NOS

Other epilepsy without intractability without status epilepticus

G40.803 Other epilepsy, intractable, with status epilepticus

G40.804 Other epilepsy, intractable, without status epilepticus

G40.81 Lennox-Gastaut syndrome

G40.811 Lennox-Gastaut syndrome, not intractable, with status epilepticus

G40.812 Lennox-Gastaut syndrome, not intractable, without status epilepticus

G40.813 Lennox-Gastaut syndrome, intractable, with status epilepticus

G40.814 Lennox-Gastaut syndrome, intractable, without status epilepticus

G40.82 Epileptic spasms

Infantile spasms

Salaam attacks

West's syndrome

G40.821 Epileptic spasms, not intractable, with status epilepticus

G40.822 Epileptic spasms, not intractable, without status epilepticus

G40.823 Epileptic spasms, intractable, with status epilepticus

G40.824 Epileptic spasms, intractable, without status epilepticus

G40.83 Dravet syndrome

Polymorphic epilepsy in infancy (PMEI)

Severe myoclonic epilepsy in infancy (SMEI)

G40.833 Dravet syndrome, intractable, with status epilepticus

G40.834 Dravet syndrome, intractable, without status epilepticus

Dravet syndrome NOS

●G40.84 KCNQ2-related epilepsy

●G40.841 KCNQ2-related epilepsy, not intractable, with status epilepticus

●G40.842 KCNQ2-related epilepsy, not intractable, without status epilepticus

KCNQ2-related epilepsy NOS

●G40.843 KCNQ2-related epilepsy, intractable, with status epilepticus

●G40.844 KCNQ2-related epilepsy, intractable, without status epilepticus

G40.89 Other seizures

Excludes1: post traumatic seizures (R56.1)

recurrent seizures NOS (G40.909)

seizure NOS (R56.9)

G40.9 Epilepsy, unspecified

G40.90 Epilepsy, unspecified, not intractable

Epilepsy, unspecified, without intractability

G40.901 Epilepsy, unspecified, not intractable, with status epilepticus

G40.909 Epilepsy, unspecified, not intractable, without status epilepticus

Epilepsy NOS

Epileptic convulsions NOS

Epileptic fits NOS

Epileptic seizures NOS

Recurrent seizures NOS

Seizure disorder NOS

G40.91- Epilepsy, unspecified, intractable

Intractable seizure disorder NOS

G43 MIGRAINE

Note: the following terms are to be considered equivalent to intractable: pharmacoresistant (pharmacologically resistant), treatment resistant, refractory (medically) and poorly controlled

Use additional code for adverse effect, if applicable, to identify drug (T36–T50 with fifth or sixth character 5)

Excludes1: headache NOS (R51.9)

lower half migraine (G44.00)

Excludes2: headache syndromes (G44.-)

G43.0 Migraine without aura

Common migraine

Excludes1: chronic migraine without aura (G43.7-)

G43.00 Migraine without aura, not intractable

Migraine without aura without mention of refractory migraine

G43.001 Migraine without aura, not intractable, with status migrainosus

G43.009 Migraine without aura, not intractable, without status migrainosus

Migraine without aura NOS

G43.01 Migraine without aura, intractable

Migraine without aura with refractory migraine

G43.011 Migraine without aura, intractable, with status migrainosus

G43.019 Migraine without aura, intractable, without status migrainosus

G43.1 Migraine with aura

Basilar migraine

Classical migraine

Migraine equivalents

Migraine preceded or accompanied by transient focal neurological phenomena

Migraine triggered seizures

Migraine with acute-onset aura

●=New Code
▲=Revised Code

Excludes1—Not coded here, do not use together
Excludes2—Not included here

Migraine with aura without headache (migraine equivalents)
Migraine with prolonged aura
Migraine with typical aura
Retinal migraine
Code also any associated seizure (G40.-, R56.9)
Excludes1: chronic migraine with aura (G43.E-)
persistent migraine aura (G43.5-, G43.6-)

G43.10 Migraine with aura, not intractable

6th Migraine with aura without mention of refractory migraine

G43.101 Migraine with aura, not intractable, with status migrainosus

G43.109 Migraine with aura, not intractable, without status migrainosus

Migraine with aura NOS

G43.11 Migraine with aura, intractable

6th Migraine with aura with refractory migraine

G43.111 Migraine with aura, intractable, with status migrainosus

G43.119 Migraine with aura, intractable, without status migrainosus

G43.A Cyclical vomiting

5th *Excludes 1:* cyclical vomiting syndrome unrelated to migraine (R11.15)

G43.A0 Cyclical vomiting, in migraine not intractable

Cyclical vomiting, without refractory migraine

G43.A1 Cyclical vomiting, in migraine intractable

Cyclical vomiting, with refractory migraine

G43.C Periodic headache syndromes in child or adult

5th **G43.C0 Periodic headache syndromes in child or adult, not intractable**

Periodic headache syndromes in child or adult, without refractory migraine

G43.C1 Periodic headache syndromes in child or adult, intractable

Periodic headache syndromes in child or adult, with refractory migraine

G43.8 Other migraine

5th **G43.80 Other migraine, not intractable**

6th Other migraine, without refractory migraine

G43.801 Other migraine, not intractable, with status migrainosus

G43.809 Other migraine, not intractable, without status migrainosus

G43.81 Other migraine, intractable

6th Other migraine, with refractory migraine

G43.811 Other migraine, intractable, with status migrainosus

G43.819 Other migraine, intractable, without status migrainosus

G43.82 Menstrual migraine, not intractable

6th Menstrual migraine, without refractory migraine
Menstrually related migraine, not intractable
Pre-menstrual migraine/headache, not intractable
Pure menstrual migraine, not intractable
Code also associated premenstrual tension syndrome (N94.3)

G43.821 Menstrual migraine, not intractable, with status migrainosus

G43.829 Menstrual migraine, not intractable, without status migrainosus

Menstrual migraine NOS

G43.83 Menstrual migraine, intractable

6th Menstrual headache, intractable
Menstrual migraine, with refractory migraine
Menstrually related migraine, intractable
Pre-menstrual migraine/headache, intractable
Pure menstrual migraine, intractable
Code also associated premenstrual tension syndrome (N94.3)

G43.831 Menstrual migraine, intractable, with status migrainosus

G43.839 Menstrual migraine, intractable, without status migrainosus

G43.9 Migraine, unspecified

5th **G43.90 Migraine, unspecified, not intractable**

6th Migraine, unspecified, without refractory migraine

G43.901 Migraine, unspecified, not intractable, with status migrainosus

Status migrainosus NOS

G43.909 Migraine, unspecified, not intractable, without status migrainosus

Migraine NOS

G43.91 Migraine, unspecified, intractable

6th Migraine, unspecified, with refractory migraine

G43.911 Migraine, unspecified, intractable, with status migrainosus

G43.919 Migraine, unspecified, intractable, without status migrainosus

G43.E Chronic migraine with aura

5th *Excludes1:* migraine with aura (G43.1-)

G43.E0 Chronic migraine with aura, not intractable

6th Chronic migraine with aura, without refractory migraine

G43.E01 Chronic migraine with aura, not intractable, with status migrainosus

G43.E09 Chronic migraine with aura, not intractable, without status migrainosus

G43.E1 Chronic migraine with aura, intractable

6th Chronic migraine with aura, with refractory migraine

G43.E11 Chronic migraine with aura, intractable, with status migrainosus

G43.E19 Chronic migraine with aura, intractable, without status migrainosus

G44 OTHER HEADACHE SYNDROMES

4th *Excludes1:* headache NOS (R51.9)
Excludes2: atypical facial pain (G50.1)
headache due to lumbar puncture (G97.1)
migraines (G43.-)
trigeminal neuralgia (G50.0)

G44.0 Cluster headaches and other trigeminal autonomic cephalgias (TAC)

5th **G44.00 Cluster headache syndrome, unspecified**

6th Ciliary neuralgia
Cluster headache NOS
Histamine cephalgia
Lower half migraine
Migrainous neuralgia

G44.001 Cluster headache syndrome, unspecified, intractable

G44.009 Cluster headache syndrome, unspecified, not intractable

Cluster headache syndrome NOS

G44.2 Tension-type headache

5th **G44.20 Tension-type headache, unspecified**

6th **G44.201 Tension-type headache, unspecified, intractable**

G44.209 Tension-type headache, unspecified, not intractable

Tension headache NOS

G44.21 Episodic tension-type headache

6th **G44.211 Episodic tension-type headache, intractable**

G44.219 Episodic tension-type headache, not intractable

Episodic tension-type headache NOS

G44.22 Chronic tension-type headache

6th **G44.221 Chronic tension-type headache, intractable**

G44.229 Chronic tension-type headache, not intractable

Chronic tension-type headache NOS

G44.3 Post-traumatic headache

5th **G44.30 Post-traumatic headache, unspecified**

6th **G44.301 Post-traumatic headache, unspecified, intractable**

●=New Code *Excludes1*—Not coded here, do not use together
▲=Revised Code *Excludes2*—Not included here

G44.309 Post-traumatic headache, unspecified, not intractable
Post-traumatic headache NOS

G44.31 Acute post-traumatic headache

G44.311 Acute post-traumatic headache, intractable

G44.319 Acute post-traumatic headache, not intractable
Acute post-traumatic headache NOS

G44.32 Chronic post-traumatic headache

G44.321 Chronic post-traumatic headache, intractable

G44.329 Chronic post-traumatic headache, not intractable
Chronic post-traumatic headache NOS

G44.8 Other specified headache syndromes

Excludes2: headache with orthostatic or positional component, not elsewhere classified (R51.0)

G44.81 Hypnic headache

G44.83 Primary cough headache

G44.84 Primary exertional headache

G44.85 Primary stabbing headache

G44.86 Cervicogenic headache
Code also associated cervical spinal condition, if known

G44.89 Other headache syndrome

G45 TRANSIENT CEREBRAL ISCHEMIC ATTACKS AND RELATED SYNDROMES

Excludes1: neonatal cerebral ischemia (P91.0)
transient retinal artery occlusion (H34.0-)

G45.8 Other transient cerebral ischemic attacks and related syndromes

G45.9 Transient cerebral ischemic attack, unspecified
Spasm of cerebral artery
TIA
Transient cerebral ischemia NOS

G47 SLEEP DISORDERS

Excludes2: nightmares (F51.5)
nonorganic sleep disorders (F51.-)
sleep terrors (F51.4)
sleepwalking (F51.3)

G47.0 Insomnia

Excludes2: alcohol or drug-related insomnia
idiopathic insomnia (F51.01)
insomnia due to a mental disorder (F51.05)
insomnia not due to a substance or known physiological condition (F51.0-)
nonorganic insomnia (F51.0-)
primary insomnia (F51.01)
sleep apnea (G47.3-)

G47.00 Insomnia, unspecified
Insomnia NOS

G47.01 Insomnia due to medical condition
Code **also** associated medical condition

G47.09 Other insomnia

G47.2 Circadian rhythm sleep disorders

Disorders of the sleep wake schedule
Inversion of nyctohemeral rhythm
Inversion of sleep rhythm

G47.20 Circadian rhythm sleep disorder, unspecified type
Sleep wake schedule disorder NOS

G47.21 Circadian rhythm sleep disorder, delayed sleep phase type
Delayed sleep phase syndrome

G47.22 Circadian rhythm sleep disorder, advanced sleep phase type

G47.23 Circadian rhythm sleep disorder, irregular sleep wake type
Irregular sleep-wake pattern

G47.24 Circadian rhythm sleep disorder, free running type
Circadian rhythm sleep disorder, non-24-hour sleep-wake type

G47.25 Circadian rhythm sleep disorder, jet lag type

G47.27 Circadian rhythm sleep disorder in conditions classified elsewhere
Code **first** underlying condition

G47.29 Other circadian rhythm sleep disorder

G47.3 Sleep apnea

Code **also** any associated underlying condition
Excludes1: apnea NOS (R06.81)
Cheyne-Stokes breathing (R06.3)
pickwickian syndrome (E66.2)
sleep apnea of newborn (P28.3)

G47.30 Sleep apnea, unspecified
Sleep apnea NOS

G47.31 Primary central sleep apnea
Idiopathic central sleep apnea

G47.32 High altitude periodic breathing

G47.33 Obstructive sleep apnea (adult) (pediatric)
Obstructive sleep apnea hypopnea
Excludes1: obstructive sleep apnea of newborn (P28.3)

G47.37 Central sleep apnea in conditions classified elsewhere
Code **first** underlying condition

G47.39 Other sleep apnea

G47.5 Parasomnia

Excludes1: alcohol induced parasomnia
drug induced parasomnia
parasomnia not due to a substance or known physiological condition

G47.50 Parasomnia, unspecified
Parasomnia NOS

G47.51 Confusional arousals

G47.52 REM sleep behavior disorder

G47.53 Recurrent isolated sleep paralysis

G47.54 Parasomnia in conditions classified elsewhere
Code **first** underlying condition

G47.59 Other parasomnia

G47.6 Sleep related movement disorders

Excludes2: restless legs syndrome (G25.81)

G47.61 Periodic limb movement disorder

G47.62 Sleep related leg cramps

G47.63 Sleep related bruxism
Excludes1: psychogenic bruxism (F45.8)

G47.69 Other sleep related movement disorders

G47.8 Other sleep disorders
Other specified sleep-wake disorder

G47.9 Sleep disorder, unspecified
Sleep disorder NOS

(G50–G59) NERVE, NERVE ROOT AND PLEXUS DISORDERS

Excludes1: current traumatic nerve, nerve root and plexus disorders — see Injury, nerve by body region
neuralgia NOS (M79.2)
neuritis NOS (M79.2)
peripheral neuritis in pregnancy (O26.82-)
radiculitis NOS (M54.1-)

G51 FACIAL NERVE DISORDERS

Includes: disorders of 7th cranial nerve

G51.0 Bell's palsy
Facial palsy

G51.8 Other disorders of facial nerve

G51.9 Disorder of facial nerve, unspecified

G52 DISORDERS OF OTHER CRANIAL NERVES

Excludes2: disorders of acoustic [8th] nerve (H93.3)
disorders of optic [2nd] nerve (H46, H47.0)
paralytic strabismus due to nerve palsy (H49.0–H49.2)

G52.2 Disorders of vagus nerve
Disorders of pneumogastric [10th] nerve

G52.7 Disorders of multiple cranial nerves
Polyneuritis cranialis

G52.9 Cranial nerve disorder, unspecified

G53 CRANIAL NERVE DISORDERS IN DISEASES CLASSIFIED ELSEWHERE

Code first underlying disease, such as:
neoplasm (C00-D49)

Excludes1: multiple cranial nerve palsy in sarcoidosis (D86.82)
multiple cranial nerve palsy in syphilis (A52.15)
postherpetic geniculate ganglionitis (B02.21)
postherpetic trigeminal neuralgia (B02.22)

G54 NERVE ROOT AND PLEXUS DISORDERS

Excludes1: current traumatic nerve root and plexus disorders—see nerve injury by body region
intervertebral disc disorders (M50-M51)
neuralgia or neuritis NOS (M79.2)
neuritis or radiculitis brachial NOS (M54.13)
neuritis or radiculitis lumbar NOS (M54.16)
neuritis or radiculitis lumbosacral NOS (M54.17)
neuritis or radiculitis thoracic NOS (M54.14)
radiculitis NOS (M54.10)
radiculopathy NOS (M54.10)
spondylosis (M47.-)

- **G54.0 Brachial plexus disorders**
  Thoracic outlet syndrome
- **G54.1 Lumbosacral plexus disorders**
- **G54.9 Nerve root and plexus disorder, unspecified**

G55 NERVE ROOT AND PLEXUS COMPRESSIONS IN DISEASES CLASSIFIED ELSEWHERE

Code first underlying disease, such as:
neoplasm (C00-D49)

Excludes1: nerve root compression (due to) (in) ankylosing spondylitis (M45.-)
nerve root compression (due to) (in) dorsopathies (M53.-, M54.-)
nerve root compression (due to) (in) intervertebral disc disorders (M50.1.-, M51.1.-)
nerve root compression (due to) (in) spondylopathies (M46.-, M48.-)
nerve root compression (due to) (in) spondylosis (M47.0-M47.2.-)

G58 OTHER MONONEUROPATHIES

- **G58.9 Mononeuropathy, unspecified**

(G60–G65) POLYNEUROPATHIES AND OTHER DISORDERS OF THE PERIPHERAL NERVOUS SYSTEM

Excludes1: neuralgia NOS (M79.2)
neuritis NOS (M79.2)
peripheral neuritis in pregnancy (O26.82-)
radiculitis NOS (M54.10)

G60 HEREDITARY AND IDIOPATHIC NEUROPATHY

- **G60.0 Hereditary motor and sensory neuropathy**
  Charcot-Marie-Tooth disease
  Déjérine-Sottas disease
  Hereditary motor and sensory neuropathy, types I-IV
  Hypertrophic neuropathy of infancy
  Peroneal muscular atrophy (axonal type) (hypertrophic type)
  Roussy-Levy syndrome
- **G60.3 Idiopathic progressive neuropathy**
- **G60.8 Other hereditary and idiopathic neuropathies**
  Dominantly inherited sensory neuropathy
  Morvan's disease
  Nelaton's syndrome
  Recessively inherited sensory neuropathy
- **G60.9 Hereditary and idiopathic neuropathy, unspecified**

G61 INFLAMMATORY POLYNEUROPATHY

- **G61.0 Guillain-Barre syndrome**
  Acute (post-) infective polyneuritis
  Miller Fisher Syndrome
- **G61.9 Inflammatory polyneuropathy, unspecified**

G62 OTHER AND UNSPECIFIED POLYNEUROPATHIES

- **G62.9 Polyneuropathy, unspecified**
  Neuropathy NOS

G63 POLYNEUROPATHY IN DISEASES CLASSIFIED ELSEWHERE

Code first underlying disease, such as:
amyloidosis (E85.-)
endocrine disease, except diabetes (E00-E07, E15-E16, E20-E34)
metabolic diseases (E70-E88)
neoplasm (C00-D49)
nutritional deficiency (E40-E64)

Excludes1: polyneuropathy (in):
diabetes mellitus (E08-E13 with .42)
diphtheria (A36.83)
infectious mononucleosis (B27.0-B27.9 with 5th character 1)
Lyme disease (A69.22)
mumps (B26.84)
postherpetic (B02.23)
rheumatoid arthritis (M05.5-)
scleroderma (M34.83)
systemic lupus erythematosus (M32.19)

(G70–G73) DISEASES OF MYONEURAL JUNCTION AND MUSCLE

G70 MYASTHENIA GRAVIS AND OTHER MYONEURAL DISORDERS

Excludes1: botulism (A05.1, A48.51–A48.52)
transient neonatal myasthenia gravis (P94.0)

- **G70.0 Myasthenia gravis**
  - **G70.00 Myasthenia gravis without (acute) exacerbation**
    Myasthenia gravis NOS
  - **G70.01 Myasthenia gravis with (acute) exacerbation**
    Myasthenia gravis in crisis
- **G70.1 Toxic myoneural disorders**
  Code first (T51–T65) to identify toxic agent
- **G70.2 Congenital and developmental myasthenia**
- **G70.8 Other specified myoneural disorders**
  - **G70.80 Lambert-Eaton syndrome, unspecified**
    Lambert-Eaton syndrome NOS
  - **G70.81 Lambert-Eaton syndrome in disease classified elsewhere**
    Code first underlying disease
    Excludes1: Lambert-Eaton syndrome in neoplastic disease (G73.1)
  - **G70.89 Other specified myoneural disorders**
- **G70.9 Myoneural disorder, unspecified**

G71 PRIMARY DISORDERS OF MUSCLES

Excludes2: arthrogryposis multiplex congenita (Q74.3)
metabolic disorders (E70–E88)
myositis (M60.-)

- **G71.0 Muscular dystrophy**
  - **G71.00 Muscular dystrophy, unspecified**
  - **G71.01 Duchenne or Becker muscular dystrophy**
    Autosomal recessive, childhood type, muscular dystrophy resembling Duchenne or Becker muscular dystrophy
    Benign [Becker] muscular dystrophy
    Severe [Duchenne] muscular dystrophy
  - **G71.02 Facioscapulohumeral muscular dystrophy**
    Scapulohumeral muscular dystrophy
  - **G71.03 Limb girdle muscular dystrophies**
    - **G71.031 Autosomal dominant limb girdle muscular dystrophy**
    - **G71.032 Autosomal recessive limb girdle muscular dystrophy due to calpain-3 dysfunction**
    - **G71.033 Limb girdle muscular dystrophy due to dysferlin dysfunction**
    - **G71.034 Limb girdle muscular dystrophy due to sarcoglycan dysfunction**
      - **G71.0340 Limb girdle muscular dystrophy due to sarcoglycan dysfunction, unspecified**
      - **G71.0341 Limb girdle muscular dystrophy due to alpha sarcoglycan dysfunction**

G71.0342 Limb girdle muscular dystrophy due to beta sarcoglycan dysfunction

G71.0349 Limb girdle muscular dystrophy due to other sarcoglycan dysfunction

G71.035 Limb girdle muscular dystrophy due to anoctamin-5 dysfunction

G71.038 Other limb girdle muscular dystrophy

G71.039 Limb girdle muscular dystrophy, unspecified

G71.09 **Other specified muscular dystrophies**
Benign scapuloperoneal muscular dystrophy with early contractures [Emery-Dreifuss]
Congenital muscular dystrophy NOS
Congenital muscular dystrophy with specific morphological abnormalities of the muscle fiber
Distal muscular dystrophy
Limb-girdle muscular dystrophy
Ocular muscular dystrophy
Oculopharyngeal muscular dystrophy
Scapuloperoneal muscular dystrophy

G71.1 Myotonic disorders

G71.11 Myotonic muscular dystrophy
Dystrophia myotonica [Steinert]
Myotonia atrophica

G71.12 Myotonia congenita
Acetazolamide responsive myotonia congenita
Dominant myotonia congenita [Thomsen disease]
Myotonia levior
Recessive myotonia congenita [Becker disease]

G71.13 Myotonic chondrodystrophy
Chondrodystrophic myotonia
Congenital myotonic chondrodystrophy
Schwartz-Jampel disease

G71.2 **Congenital myopathies**
Excludes2: arthrogryposis multiplex congenita (Q74.3)

G71.20 **Congenital myopathy, unspecified**

G71.21 **Nemaline myopathy**

G71.22 **Centronuclear myopathy**

G71.220 **X-linked myotubular myopathy**
Myotubular (centronuclear) myopathy

G71.228 **Other centronuclear myopathy**
Autosomal centronuclear myopathy
Autosomal dominant centronuclear myopathy
Autosomal recessive centronuclear myopathy
Centronuclear myopathy, NOS

G71.29 **Other congenital myopathy**
Central core disease
Minicore disease
Multicore disease
Multiminicore disease

G71.9 **Primary disorder of muscle, unspecified**
Hereditary myopathy NOS

G72 OTHER AND UNSPECIFIED MYOPATHIES

Excludes1: arthrogryposis multiplex congenita (Q74.3)
dermatomyositis (M33.-)
ischemic infarction of muscle (M62.2-)
myositis (M60.-)
polymyositis (M33.2-)

G72.8 **Other specified myopathies**

G72.81 **Critical illness myopathy**
Acute necrotizing myopathy
Acute quadriplegic myopathy
Intensive care (ICU) myopathy
Myopathy of critical illness

G72.89 **Other specified myopathies**

G72.9 **Myopathy, unspecified**

G73 DISORDERS OF MYONEURAL JUNCTION AND MUSCLE IN DISEASES CLASSIFIED ELSEWHERE

G73.1 Lambert-Eaton syndrome in neoplastic disease
Code first underlying neoplasm (C00–D49)
Excludes1: Lambert-Eaton syndrome not associated with neoplasm (G70.80–G70.81)

G73.3 Myasthenic syndromes in other diseases classified elsewhere
Code first underlying disease, such as:
neoplasm (C00-D49)
thyrotoxicosis (E05.-)

G73.7 **Myopathy in diseases classified elsewhere**
Code first underlying disease, such as:
glycogen storage disease (E74.0-)
hyperparathyroidism (E21.0, E21.3)
hypoparathyroidism (E20.-)
lipid storage disorders (E75.-)
Excludes1: myopathy in:
rheumatoid arthritis (M05.32)
sarcoidosis (D86.87)
scleroderma (M34.82)
Sjögren syndrome (M35.03)
systemic lupus erythematosus (M32.19)

(G80–G83) CEREBRAL PALSY AND OTHER PARALYTIC SYNDROMES

G80 CEREBRAL PALSY

Excludes1: hereditary spastic paraplegia (G11.4)

G80.0 Spastic quadriplegic cerebral palsy
Congenital spastic paralysis (cerebral)

G80.1 Spastic diplegic cerebral palsy
Spastic cerebral palsy NOS

G80.2 Spastic hemiplegic cerebral palsy

G80.3 Athetoid cerebral palsy
Double athetosis (syndrome)
Dyskinetic cerebral palsy
Dystonic cerebral palsy
Vogt disease

G80.4 Ataxic cerebral palsy

G80.8 Other cerebral palsy
Mixed cerebral palsy syndromes

G80.9 Cerebral palsy, unspecified
Cerebral palsy NOS

G81 HEMIPLEGIA AND HEMIPARESIS

GUIDELINES

Codes from category G81, Hemiplegia and hemiparesis, and subcategories G83.1, Monoplegia of lower limb, G83.2, Monoplegia of upper limb, and G83.3, Monoplegia, unspecified, identify whether the dominant or nondominant side is affected. Should the affected side be documented, but not specified as dominant or nondominant, and the classification system does not indicate a default, code selection is as follows:
For ambidextrous patients, the default should be dominant.
If the left side is affected, the default is non-dominant.
If the right side is affected, the default is dominant.

Note: This category is to be used only when hemiplegia (complete) (incomplete) is reported without further specification, or is stated to be old or longstanding but of unspecified cause. The category is also for use in multiple coding to identify these types of hemiplegia resulting from any cause.

Excludes1: congenital cerebral palsy (G80.-)
hemiplegia and hemiparesis due to sequela of cerebrovascular disease (I69.05-, I69.15-, I69.25-, I69.35-, I69.85-, I69.95-)

G81.0 Flaccid hemiplegia

G81.01 Flaccid hemiplegia affecting right dominant side

G81.02 Flaccid hemiplegia affecting left dominant side

G81.03 Flaccid hemiplegia affecting right nondominant side

G81.04 Flaccid hemiplegia affecting left nondominant side

G81.1 Spastic hemiplegia

G81.11 Spastic hemiplegia affecting right dominant side

G81.12 Spastic hemiplegia affecting left dominant side

G81.13 Spastic hemiplegia affecting right nondominant side

G81.14 Spastic hemiplegia affecting left nondominant side

●=New Code *Excludes1*—Not coded here, do not use together
▲=Revised Code *Excludes2*—Not included here

G81.9 Hemiplegia, unspecified

G81.91 Hemiplegia, unspecified affecting right dominant side

G81.92 Hemiplegia, unspecified affecting left dominant side

G81.93 Hemiplegia, unspecified affecting right nondominant side

G81.94 Hemiplegia, unspecified affecting left nondominant side

G82 PARAPLEGIA (PARAPARESIS) AND QUADRIPLEGIA (QUADRIPARESIS)

Note: This category is to be used only when the listed conditions are reported without further specification, or are stated to be old or longstanding but of unspecified cause. The category is also for use in multiple coding to identify these conditions resulting from any cause.

Excludes1: congenital cerebral palsy (G80.-)
functional quadriplegia (R53.2)
hysterical paralysis (F44.4)

G82.2 Paraplegia

Paralysis of both lower limbs NOS
Paraparesis (lower) NOS
Paraplegia (lower) NOS

G82.20 Paraplegia, unspecified

G82.21 Paraplegia, complete

G82.22 Paraplegia, incomplete

G82.5 Quadriplegia

G82.50 Quadriplegia, unspecified

G82.51 Quadriplegia, C1-C4 complete

G82.52 Quadriplegia, C1-C4 incomplete

G82.53 Quadriplegia, C5-C7 complete

G82.54 Quadriplegia, C5-C7 incomplete

G83 OTHER PARALYTIC SYNDROMES

GUIDELINES

Note: This category is to be used only when the listed conditions are reported without further specification, or are stated to be old or longstanding but of unspecified cause. The category is also for use in multiple coding to identify these conditions resulting from any cause.

Includes: paralysis (complete) (incomplete), except as in G80-G82

G83.0 Diplegia of upper limbs
Diplegia (upper)
Paralysis of both upper limbs

G83.1 Monoplegia of lower limb

Paralysis of lower limb

Excludes1: monoplegia of lower limbs due to sequela of cerebrovascular disease (I69.04-, I69.14-, I69.24-, I69.34-, I69.84-, I69.94-)

G83.10 Monoplegia of lower limb affecting; unspecified side

G83.11 right dominant side

G83.12 left dominant side

G83.13 right nondominant side

G83.14 left nondominant side

G83.2 Monoplegia of upper limb

Paralysis of upper limb

Excludes1: monoplegia of upper limbs due to sequela of cerebrovascular disease (I69.03-, I69.13-, I69.23-, I69.33-, I69.83-, I69.93-)

G83.21 Monoplegia of upper limb affecting; right dominant side

G83.22 left dominant side

G83.23 right nondominant side

G83.24 left nondominant side

G83.3 Monoplegia, unspecified

G83.31 Monoplegia, unspecified affecting; right dominant side

G83.32 left dominant side

G83.33 right nondominant side

G83.34 left nondominant side

G83.4 Cauda equina syndrome

Neurogenic bladder due to cauda equina syndrome

Excludes1: cord bladder NOS (G95.89)
neurogenic bladder NOS (N31.9)

G83.9 Paralytic syndrome, unspecified

(G89-G99) OTHER DISORDERS OF THE NERVOUS SYSTEM

G89 PAIN, NOT ELSEWHERE CLASSIFIED

GUIDELINES

General coding information

Codes in category G89, Pain, not elsewhere classified, may be used in conjunction with codes from other categories and chapters to provide more detail about acute or chronic pain and neoplasm-related pain, unless otherwise indicated below.

If the pain is not specified as acute or chronic, post-thoracotomy, post-procedural, or neoplasm-related, do not assign codes from category G89.

A code from category G89 should not be assigned if the underlying (definitive) diagnosis is known, unless the reason for the encounter is pain control/management and not management of the underlying condition.

When an admission or encounter is for a procedure aimed at treating the underlying condition (e.g., spinal fusion, kyphoplasty), a code for the underlying condition (e.g., vertebral fracture, spinal stenosis) should be assigned as the principal diagnosis. No code from category G89 should be assigned.

CATEGORY G89 CODES AS PRINCIPAL OR FIRST-LISTED DIAGNOSIS

Category G89 codes are acceptable as principal diagnosis or the first-listed code:

- When pain control or pain management is the reason for the admission/encounter. The underlying cause of the pain should be reported as an additional diagnosis, if known.
- When a patient is admitted for the insertion of a neurostimulator for pain control, assign the appropriate pain code as the principal or first-listed diagnosis.
- When an admission or encounter is for a procedure aimed at treating the underlying condition and a neurostimulator is inserted for pain control during the same admission/encounter, a code for the underlying condition should be assigned as the principal diagnosis and the appropriate pain code should be assigned as a secondary diagnosis.

USE OF CATEGORY G89 CODES IN CONJUNCTION WITH SITE-SPECIFIC PAIN CODES

Assigning Category G89 and Site-Specific Pain Codes

Codes from category G89 may be used in conjunction with codes that identify the site of pain (including codes from Chapter 18) if the category G89 code provides additional information. For example, if the code describes the site of the pain, but does not fully describe whether the pain is acute or chronic, then both codes should be assigned.

Sequencing of Category G89 Codes with Site-Specific Pain Codes

The sequencing of category G89 codes with site-specific pain codes (including Chapter 18 codes), is dependent on the circumstances of the encounter/admission as follows:

- If the encounter is for pain control or pain management, assign the code from category G89 followed by the code identifying the specific site of pain (e.g., encounter for pain management for acute neck pain from trauma is assigned code G89.11, Acute pain due to trauma, followed by code M54.2, Cervicalgia, to identify the site of pain).
- If the encounter is for any other reason except pain control or pain management, and a related definitive diagnosis has not been established (confirmed) by the provider, assign the code for the specific site of pain first, followed by the appropriate code from category G89.

Pain due to devices, implants, and grafts

See Chapter 19 for pain due to medical devices.

Postoperative Pain

The provider's documentation should be used to guide the coding of postoperative pain, as well as Section III. Reporting Additional Diagnoses and Section IV. Diagnostic Coding and Reporting in the Outpatient Setting.

The default for post-thoracotomy and other postoperative pain not specified as acute or chronic is the code for the acute form.

Routine or expected postoperative pain immediately after surgery should not be coded.

- Postoperative pain not associated with a specific postoperative complication is assigned to the appropriate postoperative pain code in category G89.
- Postoperative pain associated with a specific postoperative complication (such as painful wire sutures) is assigned to the appropriate code(s) found in Chapter 19, Injury, poisoning, and certain other consequences of external causes. If appropriate, use additional code(s) from category G89 to identify acute or chronic pain (G89.18 or G89.28).

Chronic Pain

Chronic pain is classified to subcategory G89.2. There is no time frame defining when pain becomes chronic pain. The provider's documentation should be used to guide use of these codes.

Neoplasm Related Pain

Code G89.3 is assigned to pain documented as being related, associated or due to cancer, primary or secondary malignancy, or tumor. This code is assigned regardless of whether the pain is acute or chronic. This code may be assigned as the principal or first-listed code when the stated reason for the admission/encounter is documented as pain control/pain management. The underlying neoplasm should be reported as an additional diagnosis.

When the reason for the admission/encounter is management of the neoplasm and the pain associated with the neoplasm is also documented, code G89.3 may be assigned as an additional diagnosis. It is not necessary to assign an additional code for the site of the pain.

Refer to Chapter 2 for instructions on the sequencing of neoplasms for all other stated reasons for the admission/encounter (except for pain control/pain management).

Chronic Pain Syndrome

Central pain syndrome (G89.0) and chronic pain syndrome (G89.4) are different than the term "chronic pain," and therefore codes should only be used when the provider has specifically documented this condition.

See Chapter 5 for pain disorders related to psychological factors

Code also related psychological factors associated with pain (F45.42)

Excludes1: generalized pain NOS (R52)

pain disorders exclusively related to psychological factors (F45.41)

pain NOS (R52)

Excludes2: atypical face pain (G50.1)

headache syndromes (G44.-)

localized pain, unspecified type — code to pain by site, such as:

abdomen pain (R10.-)

back pain (M54.9)

breast pain (N64.4)

chest pain (R07.1–R07.9)

ear pain (H92.0-)

eye pain (H57.1)

headache (R51.9)

joint pain (M25.5-)

limb pain (M79.6-)

lumbar region pain (M54.5-)

painful urination (R30.9)

pelvic and perineal pain (R10.2)

shoulder pain (M25.51-)

spine pain (M54.-)

throat pain (R07.0)

tongue pain (K14.6)

tooth pain (K08.8)

renal colic (N23)

migraines (G43.-)

myalgia (M79.1-)

pain from prosthetic devices, implants, and grafts (T82.84, T83.84, T84.84, T85.84-)

phantom limb syndrome with pain (G54.6)

vulvar vestibulitis (N94.810)

vulvodynia (N94.81-)

G89.1 Acute pain, not elsewhere classified

5th **G89.11 Acute pain due to trauma**

G89.12 Acute post-thoracotomy pain

Post-thoracotomy pain NOS

G89.18 Other acute postprocedural pain

Postoperative pain NOS

Postprocedural pain NOS

G89.2 Chronic pain, NEC

5th ***Excludes1:*** causalgia, lower limb (G57.7-)

causalgia, upper limb (G56.4-)

central pain syndrome (G89.0)

chronic pain syndrome (G89.4)

complex regional pain syndrome II, lower limb (G57.7-)

complex regional pain syndrome II, upper limb (G56.4-)

neoplasm related chronic pain (G89.3)

reflex sympathetic dystrophy (G90.5-)

G89.21 Chronic pain due to trauma

G89.22 Chronic post-thoracotomy pain

G89.28 Other chronic postprocedural pain

Other chronic postoperative pain

G89.3 Neoplasm related pain (acute) (chronic)

Cancer associated pain

Pain due to malignancy (primary) (secondary)

Tumor associated pain

G90 DISORDERS OF AUTONOMIC NERVOUS SYSTEM

4th ***Excludes1:*** dysfunction of the autonomic nervous system due to alcohol (G31.2)

G90.A Postural orthostatic tachycardia syndrome [POTS]

G90.B LMNB1-related autosomal dominant leukodystrophy

G90.5 Complex regional pain syndrome I (CRPS I)

5th Reflex sympathetic dystrophy

Excludes1: causalgia of lower limb (G57.7-)

causalgia of upper limb (G56.4-)

complex regional pain syndrome II of lower limb (G57.7-)

complex regional pain syndrome II of upper limb (G56.4-)

G90.51 Complex regional pain syndrome I of upper limb

6th **G90.511 Complex regional pain syndrome I of; right upper limb**

G90.512 left upper limb

G90.513 bilateral

G90.519 unspecified upper limb

G90.52 Complex regional pain syndrome I of lower limb

6th **G90.521 Complex regional pain syndrome I of; right lower limb**

G90.522 left lower limb

G90.523 bilateral

G90.529 unspecified lower limb

G90.59 Complex regional pain syndrome I of other specified site

G90.8 Other disorders of autonomic nervous system

5th **●G90.81 Serotonin syndrome**

Serotonin toxicity

Code first poisoning due to drug or toxin, such as:

linezolid (T36.8X- with sixth character 1–4)

monoamine oxidase inhibitors (T43.1X with sixth character 1–4)

selective serotonin and norepinephrine reuptake inhibitors [SSNRI] (T43.21 with sixth character 1–4)

selective serotonin reuptake inhibitors [SSRI] (T43.22 with sixth character 1–4)

Use additional code for adverse effect, if applicable, to identify drug, such as:

linezolid (T36.8X5)

monoamine oxidase inhibitors (T43.1X5)

selective serotonin and norepinephrine reuptake inhibitors [SSNRI] (T43.215)

selective serotonin reuptake inhibitors [SSRI] (T43.225)

Use additional code, if applicable, to identify:

disseminated intravascular coagulation (D65)

hypertensive crisis (I16.-)

metabolic acidosis (E87.2-)

shock, not elsewhere classified (R57.-)

toxic encephalopathy (G92.-)

ventricular tachycardia (I47.2-)

●G90.89 Other disorders of autonomic nervous system

G90.9 Disorder of the autonomic nervous system, unspecified

G91 HYDROCEPHALUS

4th ***Includes:*** acquired hydrocephalus

Excludes1: Arnold-Chiari syndrome with hydrocephalus (Q07.-)

congenital hydrocephalus (Q03.-)

spina bifida with hydrocephalus (Q05.-)

- **G91.0 Communicating hydrocephalus**
  Secondary normal pressure hydrocephalus
- **G91.1 Obstructive hydrocephalus**
- **G91.2 (Idiopathic) normal pressure hydrocephalus**
  Normal pressure hydrocephalus NOS
- **G91.3 Post-traumatic hydrocephalus, unspecified**
- **G91.4 Hydrocephalus in diseases classified elsewhere**
  Code first underlying condition, such as:
  plasminogen deficiency E88.02
  Excludes1: hydrocephalus due to congenital toxoplasmosis (P37.1)
- **G91.8 Other hydrocephalus**
- **G91.9 Hydrocephalus, unspecified**

G92 TOXIC ENCEPHALOPATHY

- **G92.0 Immune effector cell-associated neurotoxicity syndrome (ICANS)**
  Code first if applicable, drug induced (T36–T50) or use (T51–T65) to identify toxic agent
  Code also, if applicable, associated signs and symptoms, such as:
  cerebral edema (G93.6)
  unspecified convulsions (R56.9)
  - **G92.00** ICANS, grade unspecified
  - **G92.01** ICANS, grade 1
  - **G92.02** ICANS, grade 2
  - **G92.03** ICANS, grade 3
  - **G92.04** ICANS, grade 4
  - **G92.05** ICANS, grade 5
- **G92.8 Other toxic encephalopathy**
  Toxic encephalitis
  Toxic metabolic encephalopathy
  Code first poisoning due to drug or toxin, if applicable, (T36–T65 with 5th or 6th character 1–4)
  Use Additional code for adverse effect, if applicable, to identify drug (T36–T50 with 5th or 6th character 5)
- **G92.9 Unspecified toxic encephalopathy**
  Code first poisoning due to drug or toxin, if applicable, (T36–T65 with 5th or 6th character 1–4)
  Use Additional code for adverse effect, if applicable, to identify drug (T36–T50 with 5th or 6th character 5)

G93 OTHER DISORDERS OF BRAIN

- **G93.0 Cerebral cysts**
  Arachnoid cyst
  Porencephalic cyst, acquired
  Excludes1: acquired periventricular cysts of newborn (P91.1)
  congenital cerebral cysts (Q04.6)
- **G93.1 Anoxic brain damage, not elsewhere classified**
  Excludes1: cerebral anoxia due to anesthesia during labor and delivery (O74.3)
  cerebral anoxia due to anesthesia during the puerperium (O89.2)
  neonatal anoxia (P84)
- **G93.2 Benign intracranial hypertension**
  Pseudotumor
  Excludes1: hypertensive encephalopathy (I67.4)
  obstructive hydrocephalus (G91.1)
- **G93.3 Postviral fatigue syndrome**
  Benign myalgic encephalomyelitis
  Excludes1: chronic fatigue NOS (R53.82)
  - **G93.31** Postviral fatigue syndrome
  - **G93.32** Myalgic encephalomyelitis/chronic fatigue syndrome
  - **G93.39** Other post infection and related fatigue syndromes
- **G93.4 Other and unspecified encephalopathy**
  Excludes2: alcoholic encephalopathy (G31.2)
  encephalopathy in diseases classified elsewhere (G94)
  hypertensive encephalopathy (I67.4)
  toxic (metabolic) encephalopathy (G92.8)
  - **G93.40** Encephalopathy, unspecified
  - **G93.41** Metabolic encephalopathy
    Septic encephalopathy
  - **▲G93.42** **Megalencephalic leukoencephalopathy with subcortical cysts**
  - **G93.43** Leukoencephalopathy with calcifications and cysts

- **●G93.45** **Developmental and epileptic encephalopathy**
  Early infantile epileptic encephalopathy
  Code also, if applicable, associated disorders such as:
  developmental disorders of scholastic skills (F81.-)
  developmental disorder of speech and language (F80.-)
  epilepsy, by specific type (G40.-)
  intellectual disabilities (F70-F79)
  other neurodevelopmental disorder (F88)
  pervasive developmental disorders (F84.-)
- **G93.49** Other encephalopathy
  Encephalopathy NEC
- **G93.5 Compression of brain**
  Arnold-Chiari type 1 compression of brain
  Compression of brain (stem)
  Herniation of brain (stem)
  Excludes1: traumatic compression of brain (S06.A-)
- **G93.6 Cerebral edema**
  Excludes1: cerebral edema due to birth injury (P11.0)
  traumatic cerebral edema (S06.1-)
- **G93.7 Reye's syndrome**
  Code first poisoning due to salicylates, if applicable (T39.0-, with 6th character 1–4)
  Use additional code for adverse effect due to salicylates, if applicable (T39.0-, with 6th character 5)
- **G93.8 Other specified disorders of brain**
  - **G93.81** **Temporal sclerosis**
    Hippocampal sclerosis
    Mesial temporal sclerosis
  - **G93.82** **Brain death**
  - **G93.89** Other specified disorders of brain
    Post-radiation encephalopathy
- **G93.9 Disorder of brain, unspecified**

G94 OTHER DISORDERS OF BRAIN IN DISEASES CLASSIFIED ELSEWHERE

Code first underlying disease

G95 OTHER AND UNSPECIFIED DISEASES OF SPINAL CORD

Excludes2: myelitis (G04.-)

- **G95.1 Vascular myelopathies**
  Excludes2: intraspinal phlebitis and thrombophlebitis, except non-pyogenic (G08)
  - **G95.11** **Acute infarction of spinal cord (embolic) (nonembolic)**
    Anoxia of spinal cord
    Arterial thrombosis of spinal cord
  - **G95.19** **Other vascular myelopathies**
    Edema of spinal cord
    Hematomyelia
    Nonpyogenic intraspinal phlebitis and thrombophlebitis
    Subacute necrotic myelopathy
- **G95.8 Other specified diseases of spinal cord**
  Excludes1: neurogenic bladder NOS (N31.9)
  neurogenic bladder due to cauda equina syndrome (G83.4)
  neuromuscular dysfunction of bladder without spinal cord lesion (N31.-)
  - **G95.89** Other specified diseases of spinal cord
    Cord bladder NOS
    Drug-induced myelopathy
    Radiation-induced myelopathy
    Excludes1: myelopathy NOS (G95.9)
- **G95.9 Disease of spinal cord, unspecified**
  Myelopathy NOS

G96 OTHER DISORDERS OF THE CENTRAL NERVOUS SYSTEM

- **G96.0 Cerebrospinal fluid leak**
  Excludes1: cerebrospinal fluid leak from spinal puncture (G97.0)
  Code also, if applicable:
  intracranial hypotension (G96.81-)
  - **G96.00** **Cerebrospinal fluid leak, unspecified**
    Code also, if applicable:
    head injury (S00.- to S09.-)

G96.01 **Cranial cerebrospinal fluid leak, spontaneous**
Otorrhea due to spontaneous cerebrospinal fluid CSF leak
Rhinorrhea due to spontaneous cerebrospinal fluid CSF leak
Spontaneous cerebrospinal fluid leak from skull base

G96.02 **Spinal cerebrospinal fluid leak, spontaneous**
Spontaneous cerebrospinal fluid leak from spine

G96.08 **Other cranial cerebrospinal fluid leak**
Postoperative cranial cerebrospinal fluid leak
Traumatic cranial cerebrospinal fluid leak
Code also, if applicable:
head injury (S00- to S09-)

G96.09 **Other spinal cerebrospinal fluid leak**
Other spinal CSF leak
Postoperative spinal cerebrospinal fluid leak
Traumatic spinal cerebrospinal fluid leak
Code also, if applicable:
head injury (S00- to S09-)

G96.1 Disorders of meninges, not elsewhere classified

G96.11 **Dural tear**
Excludes1: accidental puncture or laceration of dura during a procedure (G97.41)
Code also intracranial hypotension, if applicable (G96.81-)

G96.12 **Meningeal adhesions (cerebral) (spinal)**

G96.19 **Other disorders of meninges, NEC**

G96.191 **Perineural cyst**
Cervical nerve root cyst
Lumbar nerve root cyst
Sacral nerve root cyst
Tarlov cyst
Thoracic nerve root cyst

G96.198 **Other disorders of meninges, not elsewhere classified**

G96.8 Other specified disorders of central nervous system

G96.81 **Intracranial hypotension**
Code also any associated diagnoses, such as:
Brachial amyotrophy (G54.5)
Cerebrospinal fluid leak from spine (G96.02)
Cranial nerve disorders in diseases classified elsewhere (G53)
Nerve root and compressions in diseases classified elsewhere (G55)
Nonpyogenic thrombosis of intracranial venous system (I67.6)
Nontraumatic intracerebral hemorrhage (I61.-)
Nontraumatic subdural hemorrhage (I62.0-)
Other and unspecified cord compression (G95.2-)
Other secondary parkinsonism (G21.8)
Reversible cerebrovascular vasoconstriction syndrome (I67.841)
Spinal cord herniation (G95.89)
Stroke (I63.-)
Syringomyelia (G95.0)

G96.810 **Intracranial hypotension, unspecified**

G96.811 **Intracranial hypotension, spontaneous**

G96.819 **Other intracranial hypotension**

G96.89 **Other specified disorders of central nervous system**

G96.9 Disorder of central nervous system, unspecified

G98 OTHER DISORDERS OF NERVOUS SYSTEM NOT ELSEWHERE CLASSIFIED

Includes: nervous system disorder NOS

G98.0 Neurogenic arthritis, not elsewhere classified
Nonsyphilitic neurogenic arthropathy NEC
Nonsyphilitic neurogenic spondylopathy NEC
Excludes1: spondylopathy (in):
syringomyelia and syringobulbia (G95.0)
tabes dorsalis (A52.11)

G98.8 Other disorders of nervous system
Nervous system disorder NOS

G99 OTHER DISORDERS OF NERVOUS SYSTEM IN DISEASES CLASSIFIED ELSEWHERE

G99.0 Autonomic neuropathy in diseases classified elsewhere
Code first underlying disease, such as:
amyloidosis (E85.-)
gout (M1A.-, M10.-)
hyperthyroidism (E05.-)
Excludes1: diabetic autonomic neuropathy (E08-E13 with .43)

G99.2 Myelopathy in diseases classified elsewhere
Code first underlying disease, such as:
neoplasm (C00–D49)
Excludes1: myelopathy in:
intervertebral disease (M50.0-, M51.0-)
spondylosis (M47.0-, M47.1-)

Chapter 7. Diseases of the eye and adnexa (H00–H59)

GUIDELINES

Blindness

See category H54.

Note: Use an external cause code following the code for the eye condition, if applicable, to identify the cause of the eye condition

Excludes2: certain conditions originating in the perinatal period (P04–P96)
certain infectious and parasitic diseases (A00–B99)
complications of pregnancy, childbirth and the puerperium (O00–O9A)
congenital malformations, deformations, and chromosomal abnormalities (Q00–Q99)
DM related eye conditions (E09.3-, E10.3-, E11.3-, E13.3-)
endocrine, nutritional and metabolic diseases (E00–E88)
injury (trauma) of eye and orbit (S05.-)
injury, poisoning and certain other consequences of external causes (S00–T88)
neoplasms (C00–D49)
symptoms, signs and abnormal clinical and laboratory findings, not elsewhere classified (R00–R94)
syphilis related eye disorders (A50.01, A50.3-, A51.43, A52.71)

(H00–H05) DISORDERS OF EYELID, LACRIMAL SYSTEM AND ORBIT

H00 HORDEOLUM AND CHALAZION

- H00.0 Hordeolum (externum) (internum) of eyelid
  - **H00.01 Hordeolum externum**
    - Hordeolum NOS
    - Stye
    - H00.011 Hordeolum externum right upper eyelid
    - H00.012 Hordeolum externum right lower eyelid
    - H00.013 Hordeolum externum right eye, unspecified eyelid
    - H00.014 Hordeolum externum left upper eyelid
    - H00.015 Hordeolum externum left lower eyelid
    - H00.016 Hordeolum externum left eye, unspecified eyelid
  - **H00.02 Hordeolum internum**
    - Infection of meibomian gland
    - H00.021 Hordeolum internum right upper eyelid
    - H00.022 Hordeolum internum right lower eyelid
    - H00.023 Hordeolum internum right eye, unspecified eyelid
    - H00.024 Hordeolum internum left upper eyelid
    - H00.025 Hordeolum internum left lower eyelid
    - H00.026 Hordeolum internum left eye, unspecified eyelid
  - **H00.03 Abscess of eyelid**
    - Furuncle of eyelid
    - H00.031 Abscess of right upper eyelid
    - H00.032 Abscess of right lower eyelid
    - H00.033 Abscess of eyelid right eye, unspecified eyelid
    - H00.034 Abscess of left upper eyelid
    - H00.035 Abscess of left lower eyelid
    - H00.036 Abscess of eyelid left eye, unspecified eyelid
- H00.1 Chalazion
  - Meibomian (gland) cyst
  - *Excludes2:* infected meibomian gland (H00.02-)
  - H00.11 Chalazion right upper eyelid
  - H00.12 Chalazion right lower eyelid
  - H00.13 Chalazion right eye, unspecified eyelid
  - H00.14 Chalazion left upper eyelid
  - H00.15 Chalazion left lower eyelid
  - H00.16 Chalazion left eye, unspecified eyelid

H01 OTHER INFLAMMATION OF EYELID

- H01.0 Blepharitis
  - *Excludes1:* blepharoconjunctivitis (H10.5-)
  - **H01.00 Unspecified blepharitis**
    - H01.001 Unspecified blepharitis right upper eyelid
    - H01.002 Unspecified blepharitis right lower eyelid
    - H01.003 Unspecified blepharitis right eye, unspecified eyelid
    - H01.004 Unspecified blepharitis left upper eyelid
    - H01.005 Unspecified blepharitis left lower eyelid
    - H01.006 Unspecified blepharitis left eye, unspecified eyelid
    - H01.00A Unspecified blepharitis right eye, upper and lower eyelids
    - H01.00B Unspecified blepharitis left eye, upper and lower eyelids
- H01.1 Noninfectious dermatoses of eyelid
  - **H01.11 Allergic dermatitis of eyelid**
    - Contact dermatitis of eyelid
    - H01.111 Allergic dermatitis of right upper eyelid
    - H01.112 Allergic dermatitis of right lower eyelid
    - H01.113 Allergic dermatitis of right eye, unspecified eyelid
    - H01.114 Allergic dermatitis of left upper eyelid
    - H01.115 Allergic dermatitis of left lower eyelid
    - H01.116 Allergic dermatitis of left eye, unspecified eyelid
- H01.8 Other specified inflammations of eyelid
- H01.9 Unspecified inflammation of eyelid
  - Inflammation of eyelid NOS

H02 OTHER DISORDERS OF EYELID

- *Excludes1:* congenital malformations of eyelid (Q10.0–Q10.3)
- H02.4 Ptosis of eyelid
  - **H02.40 Unspecified ptosis of eyelid**
    - H02.401 Unspecified ptosis of right eyelid
    - H02.402 Unspecified ptosis of left eyelid
    - H02.403 Unspecified ptosis of bilateral eyelids
    - H02.409 Unspecified ptosis of unspecified eyelid
- H02.8 Other specified disorders of eyelid
  - **H02.82 Cysts of eyelid**
    - Sebaceous cyst of eyelid
    - H02.821 Cysts of right upper eyelid
    - H02.822 Cysts of right lower eyelid
    - H02.823 Cysts of right eye, unspecified eyelid
    - H02.824 Cysts of left upper eyelid
    - H02.825 Cysts of left lower eyelid
    - H02.826 Cysts of left eye, unspecified eyelid
  - **H02.84 Edema of eyelid**
    - Hyperemia of eyelid
    - H02.841 Edema of right upper eyelid
    - H02.842 Edema of right lower eyelid
    - H02.843 Edema of right eye, unspecified eyelid
    - H02.844 Edema of left upper eyelid
    - H02.845 Edema of left lower eyelid
    - H02.846 Edema of left eye, unspecified eyelid
  - **H02.88 Meibomian gland dysfunction**
    - H02.881 Meibomian gland dysfunction right upper eyelid
    - H02.882 Meibomian gland dysfunction right lower eyelid
    - H02.883 Meibomian gland dysfunction of right eye, unspecified eyelid
    - H02.884 Meibomian gland dysfunction left upper eyelid
    - H02.885 Meibomian gland dysfunction left lower eyelid
    - H02.886 Meibomian gland dysfunction of left eye, unspecified eyelid
    - H02.889 Meibomian gland dysfunction of unspecified eye, unspecified eyelid
    - H02.88A Meibomian gland dysfunction right eye, upper and lower eyelids
    - H02.88B Meibomian gland dysfunction left eye, upper and lower eyelids
- H02.89 Other specified disorders of eyelid
  - Hemorrhage of eyelid

H02.9 Unspecified disorder of eyelid
Disorder of eyelid NOS

H04 DISORDERS OF LACRIMAL SYSTEM

4th *Excludes1:* congenital malformations of lacrimal system (Q10.4-Q10.6)

H04.1 Other disorders of lacrimal gland

5th H04.12 Dry eye syndrome

6th Tear film insufficiency, NOS

H04.121 Dry eye syndrome of right lacrimal gland

H04.122 Dry eye syndrome of left lacrimal gland

H04.123 Dry eye syndrome of bilateral lacrimal glands

H04.5 Stenosis and insufficiency of lacrimal passages

5th H04.53 Neonatal obstruction of nasolacrimal duct

6th *Excludes1:* congenital stenosis and stricture of lacrimal duct (Q10.5)

H04.531 Neonatal obstruction of right nasolacrimal duct

H04.532 Neonatal obstruction of left nasolacrimal duct

H04.533 Neonatal obstruction of bilateral nasolacrimal duct

H04.55 Acquired stenosis of nasolacrimal duct

6th H04.551 Acquired stenosis of right nasolacrimal duct

H04.552 Acquired stenosis of left nasolacrimal duct

H04.553 Acquired stenosis of bilateral nasolacrimal duct

H04.57 Stenosis of lacrimal sac

6th H04.571 Stenosis of right lacrimal sac

H04.572 Stenosis of left lacrimal sac

H04.573 Stenosis of bilateral lacrimal sac

H04.9 Disorder of lacrimal system, unspecified

H05 DISORDERS OF ORBIT

4th *Excludes1:* congenital malformation of orbit (Q10.7)

H05.0 Acute inflammation of orbit

5th H05.00 Unspecified acute inflammation of orbit

H05.01 Cellulitis of orbit

6th Abscess of orbit

H05.011 Cellulitis of right orbit

H05.012 Cellulitis of left orbit

H05.013 Cellulitis of bilateral orbits

H05.11 Granuloma of orbit

6th Pseudotumor (inflammatory) of orbit

H05.111 Granuloma of right orbit

H05.112 Granuloma of left orbit

H05.113 Granuloma of bilateral orbits

(H10–H11) DISORDERS OF CONJUNCTIVA

H10 CONJUNCTIVITIS

4th *Excludes1:* keratoconjunctivitis (H16.2-)

H10.0 Mucopurulent conjunctivitis

5th H10.01 Acute follicular conjunctivitis

6th H10.011 Acute follicular conjunctivitis, right eye

H10.012 Acute follicular conjunctivitis, left eye

H10.013 Acute follicular conjunctivitis, bilateral

H10.02 Other mucopurulent conjunctivitis

6th H10.021 Other mucopurulent conjunctivitis, right eye

H10.022 Other mucopurulent conjunctivitis, left eye

H10.023 Other mucopurulent conjunctivitis, bilateral

H10.1 Acute atopic conjunctivitis

5th Acute papillary conjunctivitis

H10.11 Acute atopic conjunctivitis, right eye

H10.12 Acute atopic conjunctivitis, left eye

H10.13 Acute atopic conjunctivitis, bilateral

H10.2 Other acute conjunctivitis

5th H10.21 Acute toxic conjunctivitis

6th Acute chemical conjunctivitis

Code first (T51–T65) to identify chemical and intent

Excludes1: burn and corrosion of eye and adnexa (T26.-)

H10.211 Acute toxic conjunctivitis, right eye

H10.212 Acute toxic conjunctivitis, left eye

H10.213 Acute toxic conjunctivitis, bilateral

H10.22 Pseudomembranous conjunctivitis

6th H10.221 Pseudomembranous conjunctivitis, right eye

H10.222 Pseudomembranous conjunctivitis, left eye

H10.223 Pseudomembranous conjunctivitis, bilateral

H10.23 Serous conjunctivitis, except viral

6th *Excludes1:* viral conjunctivitis (B30.-)

H10.231 Serous conjunctivitis, except viral, right eye

H10.232 Serous conjunctivitis, except viral, left eye

H10.233 Serous conjunctivitis, except viral, bilateral

H10.239 Serous conjunctivitis, except viral, unspecified eye

H10.3 Unspecified acute conjunctivitis

5th *Excludes1:* ophthalmia neonatorum NOS (P39.1)

H10.31 Unspecified acute conjunctivitis, right eye

H10.32 Unspecified acute conjunctivitis, left eye

H10.33 Unspecified acute conjunctivitis, bilateral

H10.5 Blepharoconjunctivitis

5th H10.50 Unspecified blepharoconjunctivitis

6th H10.501 Unspecified blepharoconjunctivitis, right eye

H10.502 Unspecified blepharoconjunctivitis, left eye

H10.503 Unspecified blepharoconjunctivitis, bilateral

H10.8 Other conjunctivitis

5th H10.82 Rosacea conjunctivitis

6th **Code first** underlying rosacea dermatitis (L71.-)

H10.821 Rosacea conjunctivitis, right eye

H10.822 Rosacea conjunctivitis, left eye

H10.823 Rosacea conjunctivitis, bilateral

H10.9 Unspecified conjunctivitis

H11 OTHER DISORDERS OF CONJUNCTIVA

4th *Excludes1:* keratoconjunctivitis (H16.2-)

H11.3 Conjunctival hemorrhage

5th Subconjunctival hemorrhage

H11.31 Conjunctival hemorrhage, right eye

H11.32 Conjunctival hemorrhage, left eye

H11.33 Conjunctival hemorrhage, bilateral

H11.4 Other conjunctival vascular disorders and cysts

5th H11.42 Conjunctival edema

6th H11.421 Conjunctival edema, right eye

H11.422 Conjunctival edema, left eye

H11.423 Conjunctival edema, bilateral

H11.9 Unspecified disorder of conjunctiva

(H15–H22) DISORDERS OF SCLERA, CORNEA, IRIS AND CILIARY BODY

H16 KERATITIS

4th H16.2 Keratoconjunctivitis

5th H16.20 Unspecified keratoconjunctivitis

6th Superficial keratitis with conjunctivitis NOS

H16.201 Unspecified keratoconjunctivitis, right eye

H16.202 Unspecified keratoconjunctivitis, left eye

H16.203 Unspecified keratoconjunctivitis, bilateral

H16.9 Unspecified keratitis

H18 OTHER DISORDERS OF CORNEA

4th H18.5 Hereditary corneal dystrophies

5th H18.50 Unspecified hereditary corneal dystrophies

6th H18.501 Unspecified hereditary corneal dystrophies, right eye

H18.502 Unspecified hereditary corneal dystrophies, left eye

4th **5th** **6th** **7th** Additional Character Required ✓ 3-character code

Unspecified laterality codes were excluded here. *=New Code *Excludes1*—Not coded here, do not use together △=Revised Code *Excludes2*—Not included here

H18.503 Unspecified hereditary corneal dystrophies, bilateral

H18.51 Endothelial corneal dystrophy

Fuchs' dystrophy

H18.511 Endothelial corneal dystrophy, right eye

H18.512 Endothelial corneal dystrophy, left eye

H18.513 Endothelial corneal dystrophy, bilateral

H18.52 Epithelial (juvenile) corneal dystrophy

H18.521 Epithelial (juvenile) corneal dystrophy, right eye

H18.522 Epithelial (juvenile) corneal dystrophy, left eye

H18.523 Epithelial (juvenile) corneal dystrophy, bilateral

H18.59 Other hereditary corneal dystrophies

H18.591 Other hereditary corneal dystrophies, right eye

H18.592 Other hereditary corneal dystrophies, left eye

H18.593 Other hereditary corneal dystrophies, bilateral

H18.79 Other corneal deformities

H18.791 Other corneal deformities, right eye

H18.792 Other corneal deformities, left eye

H18.793 Other corneal deformities, bilateral

H18.8 Other specified disorders of cornea

H18.82 Corneal disorder due to contact lens

Excludes2: corneal edema due to contact lens (H18.21-)

H18.821 Corneal disorder due to contact lens, right eye

H18.822 Corneal disorder due to contact lens, left eye

H18.823 Corneal disorder due to contact lens, bilateral

H18.9 Unspecified disorder of cornea

(H25–H28) DISORDERS OF LENS

H26 OTHER CATARACT

Excludes1: congenital cataract (Q12.0)

H26.0 Infantile and juvenile cataract

H26.00 Unspecified infantile and juvenile cataract

H26.001 Unspecified infantile and juvenile cataract, right eye

H26.002 Unspecified infantile and juvenile cataract, left eye

H26.003 Unspecified infantile and juvenile cataract, bilateral

H26.01 Infantile and juvenile cortical, lamellar, or zonular cataract

H26.011 Infantile and juvenile cortical, lamellar, or zonular cataract, right eye

H26.012 Infantile and juvenile cortical, lamellar, or zonular cataract, left eye

H26.013 Infantile and juvenile cortical, lamellar, or zonular cataract, bilateral

H26.03 Infantile and juvenile nuclear cataract

H26.031 Infantile and juvenile nuclear cataract, right eye

H26.032 Infantile and juvenile nuclear cataract, left eye

H26.033 Infantile and juvenile nuclear cataract, bilateral

H26.04 Anterior subcapsular polar infantile and juvenile cataract

H26.041 Anterior subcapsular polar infantile and juvenile cataract, right eye

H26.042 Anterior subcapsular polar infantile and juvenile cataract, left eye

H26.043 Anterior subcapsular polar infantile and juvenile cataract, bilateral

H26.05 Posterior subcapsular polar infantile and juvenile cataract

H26.051 Posterior subcapsular polar infantile and juvenile cataract, right eye

H26.052 Posterior subcapsular polar infantile and juvenile cataract, left eye

H26.053 Posterior subcapsular polar infantile and juvenile cataract, bilateral

H26.06 Combined forms of infantile and juvenile cataract

H26.061 Combined forms of infantile and juvenile cataract, right eye

H26.062 Combined forms of infantile and juvenile cataract, left eye

H26.063 Combined forms of infantile and juvenile cataract, bilateral

H26.09 Other infantile and juvenile cataract

H26.9 Unspecified cataract

H27 OTHER DISORDERS OF LENS

Excludes1: congenital lens malformations (Q12.-)

mechanical complications of intraocular lens implant (T85.2)

pseudophakia (Z96.1)

H27.0 Aphakia

Acquired absence of lens

Acquired aphakia

Aphakia due to trauma

Excludes1: cataract extraction status (Z98.4-)

congenital absence of lens (Q12.3)

congenital aphakia (Q12.3)

H27.01 Aphakia, right eye

H27.02 Aphakia, left eye

H27.03 Aphakia, bilateral

H27.1 Dislocation of lens

H27.10 Unspecified dislocation of lens

H27.11 Subluxation of lens

H27.111 Subluxation of lens, right eye

H27.112 Subluxation of lens, left eye

H27.113 Subluxation of lens, bilateral

H27.12 Anterior dislocation of lens

H27.121 Anterior dislocation of lens, right eye

H27.122 Anterior dislocation of lens, left eye

H27.123 Anterior dislocation of lens, bilateral

H27.13 Posterior dislocation of lens

H27.131 Posterior dislocation of lens, right eye

H27.132 Posterior dislocation of lens, left eye

H27.133 Posterior dislocation of lens, bilateral

H27.8 Other specified disorders of lens

H27.9 Unspecified disorder of lens

H28 CATARACT IN DISEASES CLASSIFIED ELSEWHERE

✓ **Code first** underlying disease, such as:

hypoparathyroidism (E20.-)

myotonia (G71.1-)

myxedema (E03.-)

protein-calorie malnutrition (E40-E46)

Excludes1: cataract in diabetes mellitus

(H30–H36) DISORDERS OF CHOROID AND RETINA

H32 CHORIORETINAL DISORDERS IN DISEASES CLASSIFIED ELSEWHERE

✓ **Code first** underlying disease, such as:

congenital toxoplasmosis (P37.1)

histoplasmosis (B39.-)

leprosy (A30.-)

Excludes1: chorioretinitis (in):

toxoplasmosis (acquired) (B58.01)

tuberculosis (A18.53)

H35 OTHER RETINAL DISORDERS

Excludes2: diabetic retinal disorders (E08.311–E08.359, E09.311–E09.359, E10.311–E10.359, E11.311–E11.359, E13.311–E13.359)

H35.1 Retinopathy of prematurity [ROP]

H35.10 Retinopathy of prematurity, unspecified

Retinopathy of prematurity NOS

H35.101 ROP, unspecified, right eye

H35.102 ROP, unspecified, left eye
H35.103 ROP, unspecified, bilateral

H35.11 Retinopathy of prematurity, stage 0

6th H35.111 ROP, stage 0, right eye
H35.112 ROP, stage 0, left eye
H35.113 ROP, stage 0, bilateral

H35.12 Retinopathy of prematurity, stage 1

6th H35.121 ROP, stage 1, right eye
H35.122 ROP, stage 1, left eye
H35.123 ROP, stage 1, bilateral

H35.13 Retinopathy of prematurity, stage 2

6th H35.131 ROP, stage 2, right eye
H35.132 ROP, stage 2, left eye
H35.133 ROP, stage 2, bilateral

H35.14 Retinopathy of prematurity, stage 3

6th H35.141 ROP, stage 3, right eye
H35.142 ROP, stage 3, left eye
H35.143 ROP, stage 3, bilateral

H35.15 Retinopathy of prematurity, stage 4

6th H35.151 ROP, stage 4, right eye
H35.152 ROP, stage 4, left eye
H35.153 ROP, stage 4, bilateral

H35.16 Retinopathy of prematurity, stage 5

6th H35.161 ROP, stage 5, right eye
H35.162 ROP, stage 5, left eye
H35.163 ROP, stage 5, bilateral

H35.17 Retrolental fibroplasia

6th H35.171 Retrolental fibroplasia, right eye
H35.172 Retrolental fibroplasia, left eye
H35.173 Retrolental fibroplasia, bilateral
H35.179 Retrolental fibroplasia, unspecified eye

H35.5 Hereditary retinal dystrophy

5th *Excludes1:* dystrophies primarily involving Bruch's membrane (H31.1-)

H35.50 Unspecified hereditary retinal dystrophy
H35.51 Vitreoretinal dystrophy
H35.52 Pigmentary retinal dystrophy
Albipunctate retinal dystrophy
Retinitis pigmentosa
Tapetoretinal dystrophy

H35.53 Other dystrophies primarily involving the sensory retina
Stargardt's disease

H35.54 Dystrophies primarily involving the retinal pigment epithelium
Vitelliform retinal dystrophy

H36 RETINAL DISORDERS IN DISEASES CLASSIFIED ELSEWHERE

4th **Code first** underlying disease, such as:
lipid storage disorders (E75.-)
sickle-cell disorders (D57.-)
Excludes1: arteriosclerotic retinopathy (H35.0-)
diabetic retinopathy (E08.3-, E09.3-, E10.3-, E11.3-, E13.3-)

H36.8 Other retinal disorders in diseases classified elsewhere

5th H36.81 Nonproliferative sickle-cell retinopathy

6th H36.811 Nonproliferative sickle-cell retinopathy, right eye
H36.812 Nonproliferative sickle-cell retinopathy, left eye
H36.813 Nonproliferative sickle-cell retinopathy, bilateral
H36.819 Nonproliferative sickle-cell retinopathy, unspecified eye

H36.82 Proliferative sickle-cell retinopathy

6th H36.821 Proliferative sickle-cell retinopathy, right eye
H36.822 Proliferative sickle-cell retinopathy, left eye
H36.823 Proliferative sickle-cell retinopathy, bilateral
H36.829 Proliferative sickle-cell retinopathy, unspecified eye

(H40–H42) GLAUCOMA

H40 GLAUCOMA

4th *Excludes1:* absolute glaucoma (H44.51-)
congenital glaucoma (Q15.0)
traumatic glaucoma due to birth injury (P15.3)

H40.3 Glaucoma secondary to eye

5th trauma
Code also underlying condition

H40.31X- Glaucoma secondary

7th to eye trauma, right eye

H40.32X- Glaucoma secondary

7th to eye trauma, left eye

H40.33X- Glaucoma secondary to eye trauma, bilateral

7th

H40.3 requires a 7th character:
0—stage unspecified
1—mild stage
2—moderate stage
3—severe stage
4—indeterminate stage

H42 GLAUCOMA IN DISEASES CLASSIFIED ELSEWHERE

✓ **Code first** underlying condition, such as: amyloidosis (E85.-)
aniridia (Q13.1)
Lowe's syndrome (E72.03)
glaucoma in DM (E08.39, E09.39, E10.39, E11.39, E13.39)
Rieger anomaly (Q13.81)
specified metabolic disorder (E70–E88)
Excludes1: glaucoma (in):
onchocerciasis (B73.02)
syphilis (A52.71)
tuberculous (A18.59)

(H43–H44) DISORDERS OF VITREOUS BODY AND GLOBE

(H46–H47) DISORDERS OF OPTIC NERVE AND VISUAL PATHWAYS

H47 OTHER DISORDERS OF OPTIC [2ND] NERVE AND VISUAL PATHWAYS

4th

H47.0 Disorders of optic nerve, not elsewhere classified

5th H47.03 Optic nerve hypoplasia

6th H47.031 Optic nerve hypoplasia, right eye
H47.032 Optic nerve hypoplasia, left eye
H47.033 Optic nerve hypoplasia, bilateral
H47.039 Optic nerve hypoplasia, unspecified eye

H47.1 Papilledema

5th H47.10 Unspecified papilledema
H47.11 Papilledema associated with increased intracranial pressure
H47.12 Papilledema associated with decreased ocular pressure
H47.13 Papilledema associated with retinal disorder

(H49–H52) DISORDERS OF OCULAR MUSCLES, BINOCULAR MOVEMENT, ACCOMMODATION AND REFRACTION

H49 PARALYTIC STRABISMUS

4th *Excludes2:* internal ophthalmoplegia (H52.51-)
internuclear ophthalmoplegia (H51.2-)
progressive supranuclear ophthalmoplegia (G23.1)

H49.0 Third [oculomotor] nerve palsy

5th H49.00 Third [oculomotor] nerve palsy, unspecified eye
H49.01 Third [oculomotor] nerve palsy, right eye
H49.02 Third [oculomotor] nerve palsy, left eye
H49.03 Third [oculomotor] nerve palsy, bilateral

H49.1 Fourth [trochlear] nerve palsy

5th H49.11 Fourth [trochlear] nerve palsy, right eye
H49.12 Fourth [trochlear] nerve palsy, left eye
H49.13 Fourth [trochlear] nerve palsy, bilateral

H49.2 Sixth [abducent] nerve palsy

5th H49.21 Sixth [abducent] nerve palsy, right eye
H49.22 Sixth [abducent] nerve palsy, left eye
H49.23 Sixth [abducent] nerve palsy, bilateral

H49.3 Total (external) ophthalmoplegia

5th H49.31 Total (external) ophthalmoplegia, right eye

H49.32 Total (external) ophthalmoplegia, left eye
H49.33 Total (external) ophthalmoplegia, bilateral
H49.4 Progressive external ophthalmoplegia
- **5th** *Excludes1:* Kearns-Sayre syndrome (H49.81-)
- H49.41 Progressive external ophthalmoplegia, right eye
- H49.42 Progressive external ophthalmoplegia, left eye
- H49.43 Progressive external ophthalmoplegia, bilateral

H49.8 Other paralytic strabismus
- **5th** H49.81 Kearns-Sayre syndrome
  - **6th** Progressive external ophthalmoplegia with pigmentary retinopathy
  - **Code also**, if applicable, other manifestations, such as: heart block (I45.9)
  - H49.811 Kearns-Sayre syndrome, right eye
  - H49.812 Kearns-Sayre syndrome, left eye
  - H49.813 Kearns-Sayre syndrome, bilateral
- H49.88 Other paralytic strabismus
  - **6th** External ophthalmoplegia NOS
  - H49.881 Other paralytic strabismus, right eye
  - H49.882 Other paralytic strabismus, left eye
  - H49.883 Other paralytic strabismus, bilateral

H49.9 Unspecified paralytic strabismus

H50 OTHER STRABISMUS

- **4th**

H50.0 Esotropia
- **5th** Convergent concomitant strabismus
- *Excludes1:* intermittent esotropia (H50.31-, H50.32)
- H50.00 Unspecified esotropia
- H50.01 Monocular esotropia
  - **6th** H50.011 Monocular esotropia, right eye
  - H50.012 Monocular esotropia, left eye
- H50.02 Monocular esotropia with A pattern
  - **6th** H50.021 Monocular esotropia with A pattern, right eye
  - H50.022 Monocular esotropia with A pattern, left eye
- H50.03 Monocular esotropia with V pattern
  - **6th** H50.031 Monocular esotropia with V pattern, right eye
  - H50.032 Monocular esotropia with V pattern, left eye
- H50.04 Monocular esotropia with other noncomitancies
  - **6th** H50.041 Monocular esotropia with other noncomitancies, right eye
  - H50.042 Monocular esotropia with other noncomitancies, left eye
- H50.05 Alternating esotropia
- H50.06 Alternating esotropia with A pattern
- H50.07 Alternating esotropia with V pattern
- H50.08 Alternating esotropia with other noncomitancies

H50.1 Exotropia
- **5th** Divergent concomitant strabismus
- *Excludes1:* intermittent exotropia (H50.33-, H50.34)
- H50.10 Unspecified exotropia
- H50.11 Monocular exotropia
  - **6th** H50.111 Monocular exotropia, right eye
  - H50.112 Monocular exotropia, left eye
- H50.12 Monocular exotropia with A pattern
  - **6th** H50.121 Monocular exotropia with A pattern, right eye
  - H50.122 Monocular exotropia with A pattern, left eye
- H50.13 Monocular exotropia with V pattern
  - **6th** H50.131 Monocular exotropia with V pattern, right eye
  - H50.132 Monocular exotropia with V pattern, left eye
- H50.14 Monocular exotropia with other noncomitancies
  - **6th** H50.141 Monocular exotropia with other noncomitancies, right eye
  - H50.142 Monocular exotropia with other noncomitancies, left eye
- H50.15 Alternating exotropia

H50.16 Alternating exotropia with A pattern
H50.17 Alternating exotropia with V pattern
H50.18 Alternating exotropia with other noncomitancies

H50.2 Vertical strabismus
- **5th** Hypertropia
- H50.21 Vertical strabismus, right eye
- H50.22 Vertical strabismus, left eye

H50.3 Intermittent heterotropia
- **5th** H50.30 Unspecified intermittent heterotropia
- H50.31 Intermittent monocular esotropia
  - **6th** H50.311 Intermittent monocular esotropia, right eye
  - H50.312 Intermittent monocular esotropia, left eye
- H50.32 Intermittent alternating esotropia
- H50.33 Intermittent monocular exotropia
  - **6th** H50.331 Intermittent monocular exotropia, right eye
  - H50.332 Intermittent monocular exotropia, left eye
- H50.34 Intermittent alternating exotropia

H50.4 Other and unspecified heterotropia
- **5th** H50.40 Unspecified heterotropia
- H50.41 Cyclotropia
  - **6th** H50.411 Cyclotropia, right eye
  - H50.412 Cyclotropia, left eye
- H50.42 Monofixation syndrome
- H50.43 Accommodative component in esotropia

H50.5 Heterophoria
- **5th** H50.50 Unspecified heterophoria
- H50.51 Esophoria
- H50.52 Exophoria
- H50.53 Vertical heterophoria
- H50.54 Cyclophoria
- H50.55 Alternating heterophoria

H50.6 Mechanical strabismus
- **5th** H50.60 Mechanical strabismus, unspecified
- H50.61 Brown's sheath syndrome
  - **6th** H50.611 Brown's sheath syndrome, right eye
  - H50.612 Brown's sheath syndrome, left eye
- H50.69 Other mechanical strabismus
  - Strabismus due to adhesions
  - Traumatic limitation of duction of eye muscle

H50.8 Other specified strabismus
- **5th** H50.81 Duane's syndrome
  - **6th** H50.811 Duane's syndrome, right eye
  - H50.812 Duane's syndrome, left eye
- H50.89 Other specified strabismus

H50.9 Unspecified strabismus

H51 OTHER DISORDERS OF BINOCULAR MOVEMENT

- **4th**

H51.0 Palsy (spasm) of conjugate gaze
H51.8 Other specified disorders of binocular movement
H51.9 Unspecified disorder of binocular movement

H52 DISORDERS OF REFRACTION AND ACCOMMODATION

- **4th**

H52.0 Hypermetropia
- **5th** H52.01 Hypermetropia, right eye
- H52.02 Hypermetropia, left eye
- H52.03 Hypermetropia, bilateral

H52.1 Myopia
- **5th** *Excludes1:* degenerative myopia (H44.2-)
- H52.11 Myopia, right eye
- H52.12 Myopia, left eye
- H52.13 Myopia, bilateral

H52.2 Astigmatism
- **5th** H52.20 Unspecified astigmatism
  - **6th** H52.201 Unspecified astigmatism, right eye
  - H52.202 Unspecified astigmatism, left eye
  - H52.203 Unspecified astigmatism, bilateral
- H52.21 Irregular astigmatism
  - **6th** H52.211 Irregular astigmatism, right eye
  - H52.212 Irregular astigmatism, left eye
  - H52.213 Irregular astigmatism, bilateral

H52.22 Regular astigmatism
- H52.221 Regular astigmatism, right eye
- H52.222 Regular astigmatism, left eye
- H52.223 Regular astigmatism, bilateral

H52.3 Anisometropia and aniseikonia
- 5th H52.31 Anisometropia
- H52.32 Aniseikonia

H52.4 Presbyopia

H52.5 Disorders of accommodation
- 5th H52.51 Internal ophthalmoplegia (complete) (total)
  - 6th H52.511 right eye
  - H52.512 left eye
  - H52.513 bilateral
- H52.52 Paresis of accommodation
  - 6th H52.521 Paresis of accommodation, right eye
  - H52.522 Paresis of accommodation, left eye
  - H52.523 Paresis of accommodation, bilateral
- H52.53 Spasm of accommodation
  - 6th H52.531 Spasm of accommodation, right eye
  - H52.532 Spasm of accommodation, left eye
  - H52.533 Spasm of accommodation, bilateral

H52.6 Other disorders of refraction

H52.7 Unspecified disorder of refraction

(H53–H54) VISUAL DISTURBANCES AND BLINDNESS

H53 VISUAL DISTURBANCES

4th

H53.0 Amblyopia ex anopsia
- 5th *Excludes1:* amblyopia due to vitamin A deficiency (E50.5)
- H53.00 Unspecified amblyopia
  - 6th H53.001 Unspecified amblyopia, right eye
  - H53.002 Unspecified amblyopia, left eye
  - H53.003 Unspecified amblyopia, bilateral
- H53.01 Deprivation amblyopia
  - 6th H53.011 Deprivation amblyopia, right eye
  - H53.012 Deprivation amblyopia, left eye
  - H53.013 Deprivation amblyopia, bilateral
- H53.02 Refractive amblyopia
  - 6th H53.021 Refractive amblyopia, right eye
  - H53.022 Refractive amblyopia, left eye
  - H53.023 Refractive amblyopia, bilateral
- H53.04 Amblyopia suspect
  - 6th H53.041 Amblyopia suspect, right eye
  - H53.042 Amblyopia suspect, left eye
  - H53.043 Amblyopia suspect, bilateral eye

H53.2 Diplopia
- Double vision

H53.3 Other and unspecified disorders of binocular vision
- 5th H53.30 Unspecified disorder of binocular vision
- H53.31 Abnormal retinal correspondence

H53.8 Other visual disturbances

H53.9 Unspecified visual disturbance

H54 BLINDNESS AND LOW VISION

4th

GUIDELINES

If "blindness" or "low vision" of both eyes is documented but the visual impairment category is not documented, assign code H54.3, Unqualified visual loss, both eyes. If "blindness" or "low vision" in one eye is documented but the visual impairment category is not documented, assign a code from H54.6-, Unqualified visual loss, one eye. If "blindness" or "visual loss" is documented without any information about whether one or both eyes are affected, assign code H54.7, Unspecified visual loss.

Note: For definition of visual impairment categories see table below

Code first any associated underlying cause of the blindness

Excludes1: amaurosis fugax (G45.3)

H54.0 Blindness, both eyes
- 5th Visual impairment categories 3, 4, 5 in both eyes.
- **H54.0X Blindness, both eyes, different category levels**
  - 6th **H54.0X3 Blindness right eye, category 3**
    - 7th

H54.0X33 Blindness right eye category 3, blindness left eye category 3

H54.0X34 Blindness right eye category 3, blindness left eye category 4

H54.0X35 Blindness right eye category 3, blindness left eye category 5

- **H54.0X4 Blindness right eye, category 4**
  - 7th H54.0X43 Blindness right eye category 4, blindness left eye category 3

H54.0X44 Blindness right eye category 4, blindness left eye category 4

H54.0X45 Blindness right eye category 4, blindness left eye category 5

- **H54.0X5 Blindness right eye, category 5**
  - 7th H54.0X53 Blindness right eye category 5, blindness left eye category 3

H54.0X54 Blindness right eye category 5, blindness left eye category 4

H54.0X55 Blindness right eye category 5, blindness left eye category 5

H54.1 Blindness, one eye, low vision other eye
- 5th Visual impairment categories 3, 4, 5 in one eye, with categories 1 or 2 in the other eye.

- **H54.11 Blindness, right eye, low vision left eye**
  - 6th
  - H54.113 Blindness right eye category 3, low vision left eye
    - 7th
    - H54.1131 Blindness right eye category 3, low vision left eye category 1
    - H54.1132 Blindness right eye category 3, low vision left eye category 2
  - H54.114 Blindness right eye category 4, low vision left eye
    - 7th
    - H54.1141 Blindness right eye category 4, low vision left eye category 1
    - H54.1142 Blindness right eye category 4, low vision left eye category 2
  - H54.115 Blindness right eye category 5, low vision left eye
    - 7th
    - H54.1151 Blindness right eye category 5, low vision left eye category 1
    - H54.1152 Blindness right eye category 5, low vision left eye category 2

- **H54.12 Blindness, left eye, low vision right eye**
  - 6th
  - H54.121 Low vision right eye category 1, blindness left eye
    - 7th
    - H54.1213 Low vision right eye category 1, blindness left eye category 3
    - H54.1214 Low vision right eye category 1, blindness left eye category 4
    - H54.1215 Low vision right eye category 1, blindness left eye category 5
  - H54.122 Low vision right eye category 2, blindness left eye
    - 7th
    - H54.1223 Low vision right eye category 2, blindness left eye category 3
    - H54.1224 Low vision right eye category 2, blindness left eye category 4
    - H54.1225 Low vision right eye category 2, blindness left eye category 5

H54.2 Low vision, both eyes
- 5th Visual impairment categories 1 or 2 in both eyes.
- **H54.2X Low vision, both eyes, different category levels**
  - 6th **H54.2X1 Low vision, right eye, category 1**
    - 7th H54.2X11 Low vision right eye category 1, low vision left eye category 1
    - H54.2X12 Low vision right eye category 1, low vision left eye category 2
  - **H54.2X2 Low vision, right eye, category 2**
    - 7th

H54.2X21 Low vision right eye category 2, low vision left eye category 1

H54.2X22 Low vision right eye category 2, low vision left eye category 2

H54.3 Unqualified visual loss, both eyes

Visual impairment category 9 in both eyes.

H54.4 Blindness, one eye

5th Visual impairment categories 3, 4, 5 in one eye [normal vision in other eye].

H54.41 Blindness, right eye, normal vision left eye

6th **H54.413** Blindness, right eye, category 3

7th **H54.413A** Blindness right eye category 3, normal vision left eye

H54.414 Blindness, right eye, category 4

7th **H54.414A** Blindness right eye category 4, normal vision left eye

H54.415 Blindness, right eye, category 5

7th **H54.415A** Blindness right eye category 5, normal vision left eye

H54.42 Blindness, left eye, normal vision right eye

6th **H54.42A** Blindness, left eye, category 3-5

7th **H54.42A3** Blindness left eye category 3, normal vision right eye

H54.42A4 Blindness left eye category 4, normal vision right eye

H54.42A5 Blindness left eye category 5, normal vision right eye

H54.5 Low vision, one eye

5th Visual impairment categories 1 or 2 in one eye [normal vision in other eye].

H54.51 Low vision, right eye, normal vision left eye

6th **H54.511** Low vision, right eye, category 1

7th **H54.511A** Low vision right eye category 1, normal vision left eye

H54.512 Low vision, right eye, category 2

7th **H54.512A** Low vision right eye category 2, normal vision left eye

H54.52 Low vision, left eye, normal vision right eye

6th **H54.52A** Low vision, left eye, category 1-2

7th **H54.52A1** Low vision left eye category 1, normal vision right eye

H54.52A2 Low vision left eye category 2, normal vision right eye

H54.6 Unqualified visual loss, one eye

5th Visual impairment category 9 in one eye [normal vision in other eye].

H54.61 Unqualified visual loss, right eye, normal vision left eye

H54.62 Unqualified visual loss, left eye, normal vision right eye

H54.7 Unspecified visual loss

Visual impairment category 9 NOS

H54.8 Legal blindness, as defined in USA

Blindness NOS according to USA definition

Excludes1: legal blindness with specification of impairment level (H54.0-H54.7)

Note: The term 'low vision' in category H54 comprises categories 1 and 2 of the table, the term 'blindness' categories 3, 4, and 5, and the term 'unqualified visual loss' category 9.

If the extent of the visual field is taken into account, patients with a field no greater than 10 but greater than 5 around central fixation should be placed in category 3 and patients with a field no greater than 5 around central fixation should be placed in category 4, even if the central acuity is not impaired.

Category of visual impairment	Visual acuity with best possible correction	
	Maximum less than:	Minimum equal to or better than:
	6/18	6/60
3/10 (0.3)	1/10 (0.1)	
20/70	20/200	
	6/60	3/60
1/10 (0.1)	1/20 (0.05)	
20/200	20/400	
	3/60	1/60 (finger counting at one meter)
1/20 (0.05)	1/50 (0.02)	
20/400	5/300 (20/1200)	
	1/60 (finer counting at one meter)	Light perception
1/50 (0.02)		
5/300		
	No light perception	
	Undetermined or unspecified	

(H55-H57) OTHER DISORDERS OF EYE AND ADNEXA

H55 **NYSTAGMUS AND OTHER IRREGULAR EYE MOVEMENTS**

4th **H55.0** Nystagmus

5th **H55.00** Unspecified nystagmus

H55.01 Congenital nystagmus

H55.02 Latent nystagmus

H55.03 Visual deprivation nystagmus

H55.04 Dissociated nystagmus

H55.09 Other forms of nystagmus

H57 **OTHER DISORDERS OF EYE AND ADNEXA**

4th **H57.0** Anomalies of pupillary function

5th **H57.00** Unspecified anomaly of pupillary function

Excludes1: syphilitic Argyll Robertson pupil (A52.19)

H57.02 Anisocoria

H57.09 Other anomalies of pupillary function

H57.1 Ocular pain

5th **H57.11** Ocular pain, right eye

H57.12 Ocular pain, left eye

H57.13 Ocular pain, bilateral

H57.8 Other specified disorders of eye and adnexa

5th **H57.81** Brow ptosis acquired

6th **H57.811** Brow ptosis, right

H57.812 Brow ptosis, left

H57.813 Brow ptosis, bilateral

H57.819 Brow ptosis, unspecified

H57.89 Other specified disorders of eye and adnexa

H57.8A Foreign body sensation eye (ocular)

6th **H57.8A1** Foreign body sensation, right eye

H57.8A2 Foreign body sensation, left eye

H57.8A3 Foreign body sensation, bilateral eyes

H57.8A9 Foreign body sensation, unspecified eye

H57.9 Unspecified disorder of eye and adnexa

(H59) INTRAOPERATIVE AND POSTPROCEDURAL COMPLICATIONS AND DISORDERS OF EYE AND ADNEXA, NOT ELSEWHERE CLASSIFIED

Chapter 8. Diseases of the ear and mastoid process (H60–H95)

Note: Use an external cause code following the code for the ear condition, if applicable, to identify the cause of the ear condition

Excludes2: certain conditions originating in the perinatal period (P04–P96)
certain infectious and parasitic diseases (A00–B99)
complications of pregnancy, childbirth and the puerperium (O00–O9A)
congenital malformations, deformations and chromosomal abnormalities (Q00–Q99)
endocrine, nutritional and metabolic diseases (E00–E88)
injury, poisoning and certain other consequences of external causes (S00–T88)
neoplasms (C00–D49)
symptoms, signs and abnormal clinical and laboratory findings, not elsewhere classified (R00–R94)

(H60–H62) DISEASES OF EXTERNAL EAR

H60 OTITIS EXTERNA

- **H60.0 Abscess of external ear**
  - Boil of external ear
  - Carbuncle of auricle or external auditory canal
  - Furuncle of external ear
  - **H60.01 Abscess of right external ear**
  - **H60.02 Abscess of left external ear**
  - **H60.03 Abscess of external ear, bilateral**
- **H60.1 Cellulitis of external ear**
  - Cellulitis of auricle
  - Cellulitis of external auditory canal
  - **H60.11 Cellulitis of right external ear**
  - **H60.12 Cellulitis of left external ear**
  - **H60.13 Cellulitis of external ear, bilateral**
- **H60.3 Other infective otitis externa**
  - **H60.31 Diffuse otitis externa**
    - **H60.311 Diffuse otitis externa, right ear**
    - **H60.312 Diffuse otitis externa, left ear**
    - **H60.313 Diffuse otitis externa, bilateral**
  - **H60.32 Hemorrhagic otitis externa**
    - **H60.321 Hemorrhagic otitis externa, right ear**
    - **H60.322 Hemorrhagic otitis externa, left ear**
    - **H60.323 Hemorrhagic otitis externa, bilateral**
  - **H60.33 Swimmer's ear**
    - **H60.331 Swimmer's ear, right ear**
    - **H60.332 Swimmer's ear, left ear**
    - **H60.333 Swimmer's ear, bilateral**
  - **H60.39 Other infective otitis externa**
    - **H60.391 Other infective otitis externa, right ear**
    - **H60.392 Other infective otitis externa, left ear**
    - **H60.393 Other infective otitis externa, bilateral**
- **H60.5 Acute noninfective otitis externa**
  - **H60.50 Unspecified acute noninfective otitis externa**
    - Acute otitis externa NOS
    - **H60.501 Unspecified acute noninfective otitis externa, right ear**
    - **H60.502 Unspecified acute noninfective otitis externa, left ear**
    - **H60.503 Unspecified acute noninfective otitis externa, bilateral**
- **H60.8 Other otitis externa**
  - **H60.8X Other otitis externa**
    - **H60.8X1 Other otitis externa, right ear**
    - **H60.8X2 Other otitis externa, left ear**
    - **H60.8X3 Other otitis externa, bilateral**
    - **H60.8X9 Other otitis externa, unspecified ear**
- **H60.9 Unspecified otitis externa**
  - **H60.91 Unspecified otitis externa, right ear**
  - **H60.92 Unspecified otitis externa, left ear**
  - **H60.93 Unspecified otitis externa, bilateral**

H61 OTHER DISORDERS OF EXTERNAL EAR

- **H61.0 Chondritis and perichondritis of external ear**
  - Chondrodermatitis nodularis chronica helicis
  - Perichondritis of auricle
  - Perichondritis of pinna
  - **H61.00 Unspecified perichondritis of external ear**
    - **H61.001 Unspecified perichondritis of right external ear**
    - **H61.002 Unspecified perichondritis of left external ear**
    - **H61.003 Unspecified perichondritis of external ear, bilateral**
  - **H61.01 Acute perichondritis of external ear**
    - **H61.011 Acute perichondritis of right external ear**
    - **H61.012 Acute perichondritis of left external ear**
    - **H61.013 Acute perichondritis of external ear, bilateral**
  - **H61.02 Chronic perichondritis of external ear**
    - **H61.021 Chronic perichondritis of right external ear**
    - **H61.022 Chronic perichondritis of left external ear**
    - **H61.023 Chronic perichondritis of external ear, bilateral**
- **H61.1 Noninfective disorders of pinna**
  - *Excludes2:* cauliflower ear (M95.1-)
  - gouty tophi of ear (M1A.-)
  - **H61.10 Unspecified noninfective disorders of pinna**
    - Disorder of pinna NOS
    - **H61.101 Unspecified noninfective disorders of pinna, right ear**
    - **H61.102 Unspecified noninfective disorders of pinna, left ear**
    - **H61.103 Unspecified noninfective disorders of pinna, bilateral**
  - **H61.11 Acquired deformity of pinna**
    - Acquired deformity of auricle
    - *Excludes2:* cauliflower ear (M95.1-)
    - **H61.111 Acquired deformity of pinna, right ear**
    - **H61.112 Acquired deformity of pinna, left ear**
    - **H61.113 Acquired deformity of pinna, bilateral**
  - **H61.12 Hematoma of pinna**
    - Hematoma of auricle
    - **H61.121 Hematoma of pinna, right ear**
    - **H61.122 Hematoma of pinna, left ear**
    - **H61.123 Hematoma of pinna, bilateral**
  - **H61.19 Other noninfective disorders of pinna**
    - **H61.191 Noninfective disorders of pinna, right ear**
    - **H61.192 Noninfective disorders of pinna, left ear**
    - **H61.193 Noninfective disorders of pinna, bilateral**
- **H61.2 Impacted cerumen**
  - Wax in ear
  - **H61.21 Impacted cerumen, right ear**
  - **H61.22 Impacted cerumen, left ear**
  - **H61.23 Impacted cerumen, bilateral**

H62 DISORDERS OF EXTERNAL EAR IN DISEASES CLASSIFIED ELSEWHERE

- **H62.4 Otitis externa in other diseases classified elsewhere**
  - Code first underlying disease, such as: erysipelas (A46)
  - impetigo (L01.0-)
  - *Excludes1:* otitis externa (in):
    - candidiasis (B37.84)
    - herpes viral [herpes simplex] (B00.1)
    - herpes zoster (B02.8)
  - **H62.41 Otitis externa in other diseases classified elsewhere, right ear**
  - **H62.42 Otitis externa in other diseases classified elsewhere, left ear**
  - **H62.43 Otitis externa in other diseases classified elsewhere, bilateral**

(H65–H75) DISEASES OF MIDDLE EAR AND MASTOID

H65 NONSUPPURATIVE OTITIS MEDIA

4th *Includes:* nonsuppurative otitis media with myringitis

Use additional code for any associated perforated tympanic membrane (H72.-)

Use additional code, if applicable, to identify:
exposure to environmental tobacco smoke (Z77.22)
exposure to tobacco smoke in the perinatal period (P96.81)
history of tobacco dependence (Z87.891)
infectious agent (B95-B97)
occupational exposure to environmental tobacco smoke (Z57.31)
tobacco dependence (F17.-)
tobacco use (Z72.0)

- **H65.0** Acute serous otitis media
  - 5th Acute and subacute secretory otitis
  - **H65.01** Acute serous otitis media, right ear
  - **H65.02** Acute serous otitis media, left ear
  - **H65.03** Acute serous otitis media, bilateral
  - **H65.04** Acute serous otitis media, recurrent, right ear
  - **H65.05** Acute serous otitis media, recurrent, left ear
  - **H65.06** Acute serous otitis media, recurrent, bilateral
- **H65.1** Other acute nonsuppurative otitis media
  - 5th *Excludes1:* otitic barotrauma (T70.0)
  - otitis media (acute) NOS (H66.9)
  - **H65.11** Acute and subacute allergic otitis media (mucoid) (sanguinous) (serous)
    - 6th
    - **H65.111** Acute and subacute allergic otitis media (mucoid) (sanguinous) (serous), right ear
    - **H65.112** Acute and subacute allergic otitis media (mucoid) (sanguinous) (serous), left ear
    - **H65.113** Acute and subacute allergic otitis media (mucoid) (sanguinous) (serous), bilateral
    - **H65.114** Acute and subacute allergic otitis media (mucoid) (sanguinous) (serous), recurrent, right ear
    - **H65.115** Acute and subacute allergic otitis media (mucoid) (sanguinous) (serous), recurrent, left ear
    - **H65.116** Acute and subacute allergic otitis media (mucoid) (sanguinous) (serous), recurrent, bilateral
- **H65.2** Chronic serous otitis media
  - 5th Chronic tubotympanal catarrh
  - **H65.21** Chronic serous otitis media, right ear
  - **H65.22** Chronic serous otitis media, left ear
  - **H65.23** Chronic serous otitis media, bilateral
- **H65.3** Chronic mucoid otitis media
  - 5th Chronic mucinous otitis media
  - Chronic secretory otitis media
  - Chronic transudative otitis media
  - Glue ear
  - *Excludes1:* adhesive middle ear disease (H74.1)
  - **H65.31** Chronic mucoid otitis media, right ear
  - **H65.32** Chronic mucoid otitis media, left ear
  - **H65.33** Chronic mucoid otitis media, bilateral
- **H65.4** Other chronic nonsuppurative otitis media
  - 5th **H65.41** Chronic allergic otitis media
    - 6th **H65.411** Chronic allergic otitis media, right ear
    - **H65.412** Chronic allergic otitis media, left ear
    - **H65.413** Chronic allergic otitis media, bilateral
  - **H65.49** Other chronic nonsuppurative otitis media
    - 6th Chronic exudative otitis media
    - Chronic nonsuppurative otitis media NOS
    - Chronic otitis media with effusion (nonpurulent)
    - Chronic seromucinous otitis media
    - **H65.491** Other chronic nonsuppurative otitis media, right ear
    - **H65.492** Other chronic nonsuppurative otitis media, left ear
    - **H65.493** Other chronic nonsuppurative otitis media, bilateral

- **H65.9** Unspecified nonsuppurative otitis media
  - 5th Allergic otitis media NOS
  - Catarrhal otitis media NOS
  - Exudative otitis media NOS
  - Mucoid otitis media NOS
  - Otitis media with effusion (nonpurulent) NOS
  - Secretory otitis media NOS
  - Seromucinous otitis media NOS
  - Serous otitis media NOS
  - Transudative otitis media NOS
  - **H65.91** Unspecified nonsuppurative otitis media, right ear
  - **H65.92** Unspecified nonsuppurative otitis media, left ear
  - **H65.93** Unspecified nonsuppurative otitis media, bilateral

H66 SUPPURATIVE AND UNSPECIFIED OTITIS MEDIA

4th *Includes:* suppurative and unspecified otitis media with myringitis

Use additional code to identify: exposure to environmental tobacco smoke (Z77.22)
exposure to tobacco smoke in the perinatal period (P96.81)
history of tobacco dependence (Z87.891)
occupational exposure to environmental tobacco smoke (Z57.31)
tobacco dependence (F17.-)
tobacco use (Z72.0)

- **H66.0** Acute suppurative otitis media
  - 5th **H66.00** Acute suppurative otitis media without spontaneous rupture of; ear drum
    - 6th
    - **H66.001** right ear drum
    - **H66.002** left ear drum
    - **H66.003** bilateral ear drums
    - **H66.004** recurrent, right ear drum
    - **H66.005** recurrent, left ear drum
    - **H66.006** recurrent, bilateral ear drums
  - **H66.01** Acute suppurative otitis media with spontaneous rupture of; ear drum
    - 6th
    - **H66.011** right ear drum
    - **H66.012** left ear drum
    - **H66.013** bilateral ear drums
    - **H66.014** recurrent, right ear drum
    - **H66.015** recurrent, left ear drum
    - **H66.016** recurrent, bilateral ear drums
- **H66.1** Chronic tubotympanic suppurative otitis media
  - 5th Benign chronic suppurative otitis media
  - Chronic tubotympanic disease
  - **Use additional code** for any associated perforated tympanic membrane (H72.-)
  - **H66.11** Chronic tubotympanic suppurative otitis media, right ear
  - **H66.12** Chronic tubotympanic suppurative otitis media, left ear
  - **H66.13** Chronic tubotympanic suppurative otitis media, bilateral
- **H66.2** Chronic atticoantral suppurative otitis media
  - 5th Chronic atticoantral disease
  - **Use additional code** for any associated perforated tympanic membrane(H72.-)
  - **H66.21** Chronic atticoantral suppurative otitis media, right ear
  - **H66.22** Chronic atticoantral suppurative otitis media, left ear
  - **H66.23** Chronic atticoantral suppurative otitis media, bilateral
- **H66.3** Other chronic suppurative otitis media
  - 5th Chronic suppurative otitis media NOS
  - **Use additional code** for any associated perforated tympanic membrane (H72.-)
  - *Excludes1:* tuberculous otitis media (A18.6)
  - **H66.3X** Other chronic suppurative otitis media
    - 6th **H66.3X1** Other chronic suppurative otitis media, right ear
    - **H66.3X2** Other chronic suppurative otitis media, left ear
    - **H66.3X3** Other chronic suppurative otitis media, bilateral

H66.4 Suppurative otitis media, unspecified

5th Purulent otitis media NOS

Use additional code for any associated perforated tympanic membrane (H72.-)

H66.41 Suppurative otitis media, unspecified, right ear

H66.42 Suppurative otitis media, unspecified, left ear

H66.43 Suppurative otitis media, unspecified, bilateral

H66.9 Otitis media, unspecified

5th Otitis media NOS

Acute otitis media NOS

Chronic otitis media NOS

Use additional code for any associated perforated tympanic membrane (H72.-)

H66.91 Otitis media, unspecified, right ear

H66.92 Otitis media, unspecified, left ear

H66.93 Otitis media, unspecified, bilateral

H67 OTITIS MEDIA IN DISEASES CLASSIFIED ELSEWHERE

4th **Code first** underlying disease, such as:

plasminogen deficiency (E88.02)

viral disease NEC (B00–B34)

Use additional code for any associated perforated tympanic membrane (H72.-)

Excludes1: otitis media in: influenza (J09.X9, J10.83, J11.83)

measles (B05.3)

scarlet fever (A38.0)

tuberculosis (A18.6)

H67.1 Otitis media in diseases classified elsewhere, right ear

H67.2 Otitis media in diseases classified elsewhere, left ear

H67.3 Otitis media in diseases classified elsewhere, bilateral

H69 OTHER AND UNSPECIFIED DISORDERS OF EUSTACHIAN TUBE

4th

H69.8 Other specified disorders of Eustachian tube

5th Use for Eustachian tube dysfunction

H69.81 Other specified disorders of Eustachian tube, right ear

H69.82 Other specified disorders of Eustachian tube, left ear

H69.83 Other specified disorders of Eustachian tube, bilateral

H69.9 Unspecified Eustachian tube disorder

5th **H69.91 Unspecified Eustachian tube disorder, right ear**

H69.92 Unspecified Eustachian tube disorder, left ear

H69.93 Unspecified Eustachian tube disorder, bilateral

H72 PERFORATION OF TYMPANIC MEMBRANE

4th *Includes:* persistent post-traumatic perforation of ear drum

postinflammatory perforation of ear drum

Code first any associated otitis media

Excludes1: acute suppurative otitis media with rupture of the tympanic membrane

traumatic rupture of ear drum

H72.0 Central perforation of tympanic membrane

5th **H72.01 Central perforation of tympanic membrane, right ear**

H72.02 Central perforation of tympanic membrane, left ear

H72.03 Central perforation of tympanic membrane, bilateral

H72.1 Attic perforation of tympanic membrane

5th Perforation of pars flaccida

H72.11 Attic perforation of tympanic membrane, right ear

H72.12 Attic perforation of tympanic membrane, left ear

H72.13 Attic perforation of tympanic membrane, bilateral

H72.2 Other marginal perforations of tympanic membrane

5th **H72.2X Other marginal perforations of tympanic membrane**

6th **H72.2X1 Other marginal perforations of tympanic membrane, right ear**

H72.2X2 Other marginal perforations of tympanic membrane, left ear

H72.2X3 Other marginal perforations of tympanic membrane, bilateral

H72.8 Other perforations of tympanic membrane

5th **H72.81 Multiple perforations of tympanic membrane**

6th **H72.811 Multiple perforations of tympanic membrane, right ear**

H72.812 Multiple perforations of tympanic membrane, left ear

H72.813 Multiple perforations of tympanic membrane, bilateral

H72.82 Total perforations of tympanic membrane

6th **H72.821 Total perforations of tympanic membrane, right ear**

H72.822 Total perforations of tympanic membrane, left ear

H72.823 Total perforations of tympanic membrane, bilateral

H72.9 Unspecified perforation of tympanic membrane

5th **H72.91 Unspecified perforation of tympanic membrane, right ear**

H72.92 Unspecified perforation of tympanic membrane, left ear

H72.93 Unspecified perforation of tympanic membrane, bilateral

H73 OTHER DISORDERS OF TYMPANIC MEMBRANE

4th

H73.0 Acute myringitis

5th *Excludes1:* acute myringitis with otitis media (H65, H66)

H73.00 Unspecified acute myringitis

6th Acute tympanitis NOS

H73.001 Acute myringitis, right ear

H73.002 Acute myringitis, left ear

H73.003 Acute myringitis, bilateral

H73.01 Bullous myringitis

6th **H73.011 Bullous myringitis, right ear**

H73.012 Bullous myringitis, left ear

H73.013 Bullous myringitis, bilateral

H73.1 Chronic myringitis

5th Chronic tympanitis

Excludes1: chronic myringitis with otitis media (H65, H66)

H73.11 Chronic myringitis, right ear

H73.12 Chronic myringitis, left ear

H73.13 Chronic myringitis, bilateral

H73.2 Unspecified myringitis

5th **H73.21 Unspecified myringitis, right ear**

H73.22 Unspecified myringitis, left ear

H73.23 Unspecified myringitis, bilateral

H73.8 Other specified disorders of tympanic membrane

(H80–H83) DISEASES OF INNER EAR

H81 DISORDERS OF VESTIBULAR FUNCTION

4th *Excludes1:* epidemic vertigo (A88.1)

vertigo NOS (R42)

H81.0 Ménière's disease

5th Labyrinthine hydrops

Ménière's syndrome or vertigo

H81.01 Ménière's disease, right ear

H81.02 Ménière's disease, left ear

H81.03 Ménière's disease, bilateral

H81.1 Benign paroxysmal vertigo

5th **H81.11 Benign paroxysmal vertigo, right ear**

H81.12 Benign paroxysmal vertigo, left ear

H81.13 Benign paroxysmal vertigo, bilateral

H81.3 Other peripheral vertigo

5th **H81.31 Aural vertigo**

6th **H81.311 Aural vertigo, right ear**

H81.312 Aural vertigo, left ear

H81.313 Aural vertigo, bilateral

H81.39 Other peripheral vertigo

6th Lermoyez' syndrome

Otogenic vertigo

Peripheral vertigo NOS

H81.391 Other peripheral vertigo, right ear

H81.392 Other peripheral vertigo, left ear

H81.393 Other peripheral vertigo, bilateral

H81.4 Vertigo of central origin

Central positional nystagmus

H81.8 Other disorders of vestibular function

5th **H81.8X Other disorders of vestibular function**

6th **H81.8X1 Other disorders of vestibular function, right ear**

H81.8X2 Other disorders of vestibular function, left ear

H81.8X3 Other disorders of vestibular function, bilateral

H81.9 Unspecified disorder of vestibular function

Vertiginous syndrome NOS

H81.91 Unspecified disorder of vestibular function, right ear

H81.92 Unspecified disorder of vestibular function, left ear

H81.93 Unspecified disorder of vestibular function, bilateral

H83 OTHER DISEASES OF INNER EAR

H83.0 Labyrinthitis

H83.01 Labyrinthitis, right ear

H83.02 Labyrinthitis, left ear

H83.03 Labyrinthitis, bilateral

H83.09 Labyrinthitis, unspecified ear

H83.3 Noise effects on inner ear

Acoustic trauma of inner ear

Noise-induced hearing loss of inner ear

H83.3X Noise effects on inner ear

H83.3X1 Noise effects on right inner ear

H83.3X2 Noise effects on left inner ear

H83.3X3 Noise effects on inner ear, bilateral

(H90–H94) OTHER DISORDERS OF EAR

H90 CONDUCTIVE AND SENSORINEURAL HEARING LOSS

Excludes1: deaf nonspeaking NEC (H91.3)

deafness NOS (H91.9-)

hearing loss NOS (H91.9-)

noise-induced hearing loss (H83.3-)

ototoxic hearing loss (H91.0-)

sudden (idiopathic) hearing loss (H91.2-)

H90.0 Conductive hearing loss, bilateral

H90.1 Conductive hearing loss, unilateral with unrestricted hearing on the contralateral side

H90.11 Conductive hearing loss, unilateral, right ear, with unrestricted hearing on the contralateral side

H90.12 Conductive hearing loss, unilateral, left ear, with unrestricted hearing on the contralateral side

H90.2 Conductive hearing loss, unspecified

Conductive deafness NOS

H90.3 Sensorineural hearing loss, bilateral

H90.4 Sensorineural hearing loss, unilateral with unrestricted hearing on the contralateral side

H90.41 Sensorineural hearing loss, unilateral, right ear, with unrestricted hearing on the contralateral side

H90.42 Sensorineural hearing loss, unilateral, left ear, with unrestricted hearing on the contralateral side

H90.5 Unspecified sensorineural hearing loss

Central hearing loss NOS

Congenital deafness NOS

Neural hearing loss NOS

Perceptive hearing loss NOS

Sensorineural deafness NOS

Sensory hearing loss NOS

Excludes1: abnormal auditory perception (H93.2-)

psychogenic deafness (F44.6)

H90.6 Mixed conductive and sensorineural hearing loss, bilateral

H90.7 Mixed conductive and sensorineural hearing loss, unilateral with unrestricted hearing on the contralateral side

H90.71 Mixed conductive and sensorineural hearing loss, unilateral, right ear, with unrestricted hearing on the contralateral side

H90.72 Mixed conductive and sensorineural hearing loss, unilateral, left ear, with unrestricted hearing on the contralateral side

H90.8 Mixed conductive and sensorineural hearing loss, unspecified

H90.A Hearing loss, unilateral, with restricted hearing on the contralateral side

H90.A1 Conductive hearing loss, unilateral, with restricted hearing on the contralateral side

H90.A11 Conductive hearing loss, unilateral, right ear with restricted hearing on the contralateral side

H90.A12 Conductive hearing loss, unilateral, left ear with restricted hearing on the contralateral side

H90.A2 Sensorineural hearing loss, unilateral, with restricted hearing on the contralateral side

H90.A21 Sensorineural hearing loss, unilateral, right ear, with restricted hearing on the contralateral side

H90.A22 Sensorineural hearing loss, unilateral, left ear, with restricted hearing on the contralateral side

H90.A3 Mixed conductive and sensorineural hearing loss, unilateral, with restricted hearing on the contralateral side

H90.A31 Mixed conductive and sensorineural hearing loss, unilateral, right ear with restricted hearing on the contralateral side

H90.A32 Mixed conductive and sensorineural hearing, unilateral, left ear with restricted hearing on the contralateral side

H91 OTHER AND UNSPECIFIED HEARING LOSS

Excludes1: abnormal auditory perception (H93.2-)

hearing loss as classified in H90.-

impacted cerumen (H61.2-)

noise-induced hearing loss (H83.3-)

psychogenic deafness (F44.6)

transient ischemic deafness (H93.01-)

H91.2 Sudden idiopathic hearing loss

Sudden hearing loss NOS

H91.21 Sudden idiopathic hearing loss, right ear

H91.22 Sudden idiopathic hearing loss, left ear

H91.23 Sudden idiopathic hearing loss, bilateral

H91.3 Deaf nonspeaking, not elsewhere classified

H91.8 Other specified hearing loss

H91.8X Other specified hearing loss

H91.8X1 Other specified hearing loss, right ear

H91.8X2 Other specified hearing loss, left ear

H91.8X3 Other specified hearing loss, bilateral

H91.9 Unspecified hearing loss

Deafness NOS

High frequency deafness

Low frequency deafness

H91.91 Unspecified hearing loss, right ear

H91.92 Unspecified hearing loss, left ear

H91.93 Unspecified hearing loss, bilateral

H92 OTALGIA AND EFFUSION OF EAR

H92.0 Otalgia

H92.01 Otalgia, right ear

H92.02 Otalgia, left ear

H92.03 Otalgia, bilateral

H92.1 Otorrhea

Excludes1: leakage of cerebrospinal fluid through ear (G96.0)

H92.11 Otorrhea, right ear

H92.12 Otorrhea, left ear

H92.13 Otorrhea, bilateral

H93 OTHER DISORDERS OF EAR, NOT ELSEWHERE CLASSIFIED

H93.1 Tinnitus

H93.11 Tinnitus, right ear

H93.12 Tinnitus, left ear

H93.13 Tinnitus, bilateral

H93.A Pulsatile tinnitus

H93.A1 Pulsatile tinnitus, right ear

H93.A2 Pulsatile tinnitus, left ear

H93.A3 Pulsatile tinnitus, bilateral

H93.2 Other abnormal auditory perceptions

auditory hallucinations (R44.0)

H93.25 Central auditory processing disorder
Congenital auditory imperception
Word deafness

H93.29 Other abnormal auditory perceptions

6th H93.291 Other abnormal auditory perceptions, right ear

H93.292 Other abnormal auditory perceptions, left ear

H93.293 Other abnormal auditory perceptions, bilateral

H93.8 Other specified disorders of ear

5th **H93.8X Other specified disorders of ear**

6th H93.8X1 Other specified disorders of right ear

H93.8X2 Other specified disorders of left ear

H93.8X3 Other specified disorders of ear, bilateral

(H95) INTRAOPERATIVE AND POSTPROCEDURAL COMPLICATIONS AND DISORDERS OF EAR AND MASTOID PROCESS, NOT ELSEWHERE CLASSIFIED

Chapter 9. Diseases of the circulatory system (I00–I99)

GUIDELINES

Hypertension

The classification presumes a causal relationship between hypertension and heart involvement and between hypertension and kidney involvement, as the two conditions are linked by the term "with" in the Alphabetic Index. These conditions should be coded as related even in the absence of provider documentation explicitly linking them, unless the documentation clearly states the conditions are unrelated.

For hypertension and conditions not specifically linked by relational terms such as "with," "associated with" or "due to" in the classification, provider documentation must link the conditions in order to code them as related.

HYPERTENSION WITH HEART DISEASE

Hypertension with heart conditions classified to I50.- or I51.4–I51.7, I51.89, I51.9, are assigned to a code from category I11, Hypertensive heart disease. Use additional code(s) from category I50, Heart failure, to identify the type(s) of heart failure in those patients with heart failure.

The same heart conditions (I50.-, I51.4–I51.7, I51.89, I51.9) with hypertension are coded separately if the provider has documented they are unrelated to the hypertension. Sequence according to the circumstances of the admission/encounter.

HYPERTENSIVE CHRONIC KIDNEY DISEASE

See category I12.

HYPERTENSIVE CRISIS

See category I16.

PULMONARY HYPERTENSION

See category I27.

Refer to ICD-10-CM Official Guidelines for Coding and Reporting for instructions for reporting atherosclerotic coronary artery disease, cerebrovascular accident, and/or myocardial infarction

Excludes2:

certain conditions originating in the perinatal period (P04–P96)

certain infectious and parasitic diseases (A00–B99)

complications of pregnancy, childbirth and the puerperium (O00–O9A)

congenital malformations, deformations, and chromosomal abnormalities (Q00–Q99)

endocrine, nutritional and metabolic diseases (E00–E88)

injury, poisoning and certain other consequences of external causes (S00–T88)

neoplasms (C00–D49)

symptoms, signs and abnormal clinical and laboratory findings, not elsewhere classified (R00–R94)

systemic connective tissue disorders (M30–M36)

transient cerebral ischemic attacks and related syndromes (G45.-)

(I00–I02) ACUTE RHEUMATIC FEVER

I00 RHEUMATIC FEVER WITHOUT HEART INVOLVEMENT

✓ *Includes:* arthritis, rheumatic, acute or subacute

Excludes1: rheumatic fever with heart involvement (I01.0–I01.9)

I01 RHEUMATIC FEVER WITH HEART INVOLVEMENT

4th *Excludes1:* chronic diseases of rheumatic origin (I05–I09) unless rheumatic fever is also present or there is evidence of reactivation or activity of the rheumatic process.

- **I01.0 Acute rheumatic pericarditis**
  - Any condition in I00 with pericarditis
  - Rheumatic pericarditis (acute)
  - *Excludes1:* acute pericarditis not specified as rheumatic (I30.-)
- **I01.1 Acute rheumatic endocarditis**
  - Any condition in I00 with endocarditis or valvulitis
  - Acute rheumatic valvulitis
- **I01.2 Acute rheumatic myocarditis**
  - Any condition in I00 with myocarditis
- **I01.8 Other acute rheumatic heart disease**
  - Any condition in I00 with other or multiple types of heart involvement
  - Acute rheumatic pancarditis
- **I01.9 Acute rheumatic heart disease, unspecified**
  - Any condition in I00 with unspecified type of heart involvement
  - Rheumatic carditis, acute
  - Rheumatic heart disease, active or acute

I02 RHEUMATIC CHOREA

4th *Includes:* Sydenham's chorea

Excludes1: chorea NOS (G25.5)

Huntington's chorea (G10)

- **I02.0 Rheumatic chorea with heart involvement**
  - Chorea NOS with heart involvement
  - Rheumatic chorea with heart involvement of any type classifiable under I01.-
- **I02.9 Rheumatic chorea without heart involvement**
  - Rheumatic chorea NOS
  - Rheumatic heart disease, active or acute

(I05–I09) CHRONIC RHEUMATIC HEART DISEASES

I05 RHEUMATIC MITRAL VALVE DISEASES

4th *Includes:* conditions classifiable to both I05.0 and I05.2–I05.9, whether specified as rheumatic or not

Excludes1: mitral valve disease specified as nonrheumatic (I34.-)

mitral valve disease with aortic and/or tricuspid valve involvement (I08.-)

- **I05.0 Rheumatic mitral stenosis**
  - Mitral (valve) obstruction (rheumatic)
- **I05.1 Rheumatic mitral insufficiency**
  - Rheumatic mitral incompetence
  - Rheumatic mitral regurgitation
  - *Excludes1:* mitral insufficiency not specified as rheumatic (I34.0)
- **I05.2 Rheumatic mitral stenosis with insufficiency**
  - Rheumatic mitral stenosis with incompetence or regurgitation
- **I05.8 Other rheumatic mitral valve diseases**
  - Rheumatic mitral (valve) failure
- **I05.9 Rheumatic mitral valve disease, unspecified**
  - Rheumatic mitral (valve) disorder (chronic) NOS

I06 RHEUMATIC AORTIC VALVE DISEASES

4th *Excludes1:* aortic valve disease not specified as rheumatic (I35.-)

aortic valve disease with mitral and/or tricuspid valve involvement (I08.-)

- **I06.0 Rheumatic aortic stenosis**
  - Rheumatic aortic (valve) obstruction
- **I06.1 Rheumatic aortic insufficiency**
  - Rheumatic aortic incompetence
  - Rheumatic aortic regurgitation
- **I06.2 Rheumatic aortic stenosis with insufficiency**
  - Rheumatic aortic stenosis with incompetence or regurgitation
- **I06.8 Other rheumatic aortic valve diseases**
- **I06.9 Rheumatic aortic valve disease, unspecified**
  - Rheumatic aortic (valve) disease NOS

I07 RHEUMATIC TRICUSPID VALVE DISEASES

4th *Includes:* rheumatic tricuspid valve diseases specified as rheumatic or unspecified

Excludes1: tricuspid valve disease specified as nonrheumatic (I36.-)

tricuspid valve disease with aortic and/or mitral valve involvement (I08.-)

- **I07.0 Rheumatic tricuspid stenosis**
  - Tricuspid (valve) stenosis (rheumatic)
- **I07.1 Rheumatic tricuspid insufficiency**
  - Tricuspid (valve) insufficiency (rheumatic)
- **I07.2 Rheumatic tricuspid stenosis and insufficiency**
- **I07.8 Other rheumatic tricuspid valve diseases**
- **I07.9 Rheumatic tricuspid valve disease, unspecified**
  - Rheumatic tricuspid valve disorder NOS

I08 MULTIPLE VALVE DISEASES

4th *Includes:* multiple valve diseases specified as rheumatic or unspecified

Excludes2: multiple valve disease specified as nonrheumatic (I34.-, I35.-, I36.-, I37.-, I38.-, Q22.-, Q23.-, Q24.8-)

rheumatic valve disease NOS (I09.1)

- **I08.0 Rheumatic disorders of both mitral and aortic valves**
  - Involvement of both mitral and aortic valves specified as rheumatic or unspecified
- **I08.1 Rheumatic disorders of both mitral and tricuspid valves**

●=New Code *Excludes1*—Not coded here, do not use together

▲=Revised Code *Excludes2*—Not included here

I08.2 Rheumatic disorders of both aortic and tricuspid valves
I08.3 Combined rheumatic disorders of mitral, aortic and tricuspid valves
I08.8 Other rheumatic multiple valve diseases
I08.9 Rheumatic multiple valve disease, unspecified

I09 OTHER RHEUMATIC HEART DISEASES

I09.0 Rheumatic myocarditis
Excludes1: myocarditis not specified as rheumatic (I51.4)

I09.1 Rheumatic diseases of endocardium, valve unspecified
Rheumatic endocarditis (chronic)
Rheumatic valvulitis (chronic)
Excludes1: endocarditis, valve unspecified (I38)

I09.2 Chronic rheumatic pericarditis
Adherent pericardium, rheumatic
Chronic rheumatic mediastinopericarditis
Chronic rheumatic myopericarditis
Excludes1: chronic pericarditis not specified as rheumatic (I31.-)

I09.8 Other specified rheumatic heart diseases

I09.81 Rheumatic heart failure
Use additional code to identify type of heart failure (I50.-)

I09.89 Other specified rheumatic heart diseases
Rheumatic disease of pulmonary valve

I09.9 Rheumatic heart disease, unspecified
Rheumatic carditis
Excludes1: rheumatoid carditis (M05.31)

(I10–I16) HYPERTENSIVE DISEASES

Use additional code to identify: exposure to environmental tobacco smoke (Z77.22)
history of tobacco dependence (Z87.891)
occupational exposure to environmental tobacco smoke (Z57.31)
tobacco dependence (F17.-)
tobacco use (Z72.0)
Excludes1: neonatal hypertension (P29.2)
primary pulmonary hypertension (I27.0)
Excludes2: hypertensive disease complicating pregnancy, childbirth and the puerperium (O10–O11, O13–O16)

I10 ESSENTIAL (PRIMARY) HYPERTENSION

✓ *Includes:* high blood pressure
hypertension (arterial) (benign) (essential) (malignant) (primary) (systemic)
Excludes1: hypertensive disease complicating pregnancy, childbirth and the puerperium (O10–O11, O13–O16)
Excludes2: essential (primary) hypertension involving vessels of brain (I60–I69)
essential (primary) hypertension involving vessels of eye (H35.0-)

I11 HYPERTENSIVE HEART DISEASE

Includes: any condition in I50.-, or I51.4-, I51.7, I51.89, I51.9 due to hypertension

I11.0 Hypertensive heart disease with heart failure
Hypertensive heart failure
Use additional code to identify type of heart failure (I50.-)

I11.9 Hypertensive heart disease without heart failure
Hypertensive heart disease NOS

I12 HYPERTENSIVE CHRONIC KIDNEY DISEASE

GUIDELINES

Assign codes from category I12, Hypertensive chronic kidney disease, when both hypertension and a condition classifiable to category N18, Chronic kidney disease (CKD), are present. CKD should not be coded as hypertensive if the provider indicates the CKD is not related to the hypertension.

The appropriate code from category N18 should be used as a secondary code with a code from category I12 to identify the stage of chronic kidney disease.

If a patient has hypertensive chronic kidney disease and acute renal failure, the acute renal failure should also be coded. Sequence according to the circumstances of the admission/encounter.
Includes: any condition in N18 and N26 - due to hypertension
arteriosclerosis of kidney
arteriosclerotic nephritis (chronic) (interstitial)
hypertensive nephropathy
nephrosclerosis

Excludes1: hypertension due to kidney disease (I15.0, I15.1)
renovascular hypertension (I15.0)
secondary hypertension (I15.-)
Excludes2: acute kidney failure (N17.-)

I12.0 Hypertensive chronic kidney disease with stage 5 chronic kidney disease or end stage renal disease
Use additional code to identify the stage of chronic kidney disease (N18.5, N18.6)

I12.9 Hypertensive chronic kidney disease with stage 1 through stage 4 chronic kidney disease, or unspecified chronic kidney disease
Hypertensive chronic kidney disease NOS
Hypertensive renal disease NOS
Use additional code to identify the stage of chronic kidney disease (N18.1-N18.4, N18.9)

I16 HYPERTENSIVE CRISIS

GUIDELINES

Assign a code from category I16, Hypertensive crisis, for documented hypertensive urgency, hypertensive emergency or unspecified hypertensive crisis. Code also any identified hypertensive disease (I10-I15). The sequencing is based on the reason for the encounter.
Code also any identified hypertensive disease (I10–I15, I1A)

I16.0 Hypertensive urgency

I16.1 Hypertensive emergency
Use additional code, if applicable, to identify specific organ dysfunction, such as:
acute kidney injury (N17.-)
acute myocardial infarction (I21.-)
acute pulmonary edema (left and/or right ventricular failure) (J81.0, I50.-)
aortic dissection (I71.0-)
cerebral hemorrhage (I60.-. I61.-, I62.-)
cerebral infarction (I63.-)
eclampsia (O15.-)
hypertensive encephalopathy (I67.4)
seizure (R56.9)

I16.9 Hypertensive crisis, unspecified

I1A Other hypertension

I1A.0 Resistant hypertension
Apparent treatment resistant hypertension
Treatment resistant hypertension
True resistant hypertension
Code first specific type of existing hypertension, if known, such as:
essential hypertension (I10)
secondary hypertension (I15.-)

(I20–I25) ISCHEMIC HEART DISEASES

Code also the presence of hypertension (I10–I1A)
Please see full ICD-10-CM manual for cardiovascular disease with symptoms or infarction.

I20 ANGINA PECTORIS

Use additional code to identify:
exposure to environmental tobacco smoke (Z77.22)
history of tobacco dependence (Z87.891)
occupational exposure to environmental tobacco smoke (Z57.31)
tobacco dependence (F17.-)
tobacco use (Z72.0)
Excludes1: angina pectoris with atherosclerotic heart disease of native coronary arteries (I25.1-)
atherosclerosis of coronary artery bypass graft(s) and coronary artery of transplanted heart with anginapectoris (I25.7-)
postinfarction angina (I23.7)

I20.2 Refractory angina pectoris

I20.9 Angina pectoris, unspecified
Angina NOS
Anginal syndrome
Cardiac angina
Ischemic chest pain

I23 CERTAIN CURRENT COMPLICATIONS FOLLOWING ST ELEVATION (STEMI) AND NON-ST ELEVATION (NSTEMI) MYOCARDIALINFARCTION (WITHIN THE 28 DAY PERIOD)

I23.0 Hemopericardium as current complication following acute myocardial infarction

Excludes1: hemopericardium not specified as current complication following acute myocardial infarction (I31.2)

I23.3 Rupture of cardiac wall without hemopericardium as current complication following acute myocardial infarction

I24 OTHER ACUTE ISCHEMIC HEART DISEASES

Excludes1: angina pectoris (I20.-)
transient myocardial ischemia in newborn (P29.4)

Excludes2: non-ischemic myocardial injury (I5A)

I24.1 Dressler's syndrome
Postmyocardial infarction syndrome
Excludes1: postinfarction angina (I23.7)

I24.9 Acute ischemic heart disease, unspecified
Excludes1: ischemic heart disease (chronic) NOS (I25.9)

I25 CHRONIC ISCHEMIC HEART DISEASE

Use additional code to identify:
chronic total occlusion of coronary artery (I25.82)
exposure to environmental tobacco smoke (Z77.22)
history of tobacco dependence (Z87.891)
occupational exposure to environmental tobacco smoke (Z57.31)
tobacco dependence (F17.-)
tobacco use (Z72.0)

Excludes2: non-ischemic myocardial injury (I5A)

I25.1 Atherosclerotic cardiovascular disease
Coronary (artery) atheroma
Coronary (artery) atherosclerosis
Coronary (artery) disease
Coronary (artery) sclerosis

I25.10 Atherosclerotic heart disease of native coronary artery without angina pectoris
Atherosclerotic heart disease NOS

I25.11 Atherosclerotic heart disease of native coronary artery with angina pectoris

I25.112 Atherosclerotic heart disease of native coronary artery with refractory angina pectoris

I25.7 Atherosclerosis of coronary artery bypass graft(s) and coronary artery of transplanted heart with anginapectoris

Use additional code, if applicable, to identify:
coronary atherosclerosis due to calcified coronary lesion (I25.84)
coronary atherosclerosis due to lipid rich plaque (I25.83)

Excludes1: atherosclerosis of bypass graft(s) of transplanted heart without angina pectoris (I25.812)
atherosclerosis of coronary artery bypass graft(s) without angina pectoris (I25.810)
atherosclerosis of native coronary artery of transplanted heart without angina pectoris (I25.811)

I25.702 Atherosclerosis of coronary artery bypass graft(s), unspecified, with refractory angina pectoris

I25.712 Atherosclerosis of autologous vein coronary artery bypass graft(s) with refractory angina pectoris

I25.722 Atherosclerosis of autologous artery coronary artery bypass graft(s) with refractory angina pectoris

I25.732 Atherosclerosis of nonautologous biological coronary artery bypass graft(s) with refractory angina pectoris

I25.752 Atherosclerosis of native coronary artery of transplanted heart with refractory angina pectoris

I25.762 Atherosclerosis of bypass graft of coronary artery of transplanted heart with refractory angina pectoris

I25.792 Atherosclerosis of other coronary artery bypass graft(s) with refractory angina pectoris

(I26–I28) PULMONARY HEART DISEASE AND DISEASES OF PULMONARY CIRCULATION

I27 OTHER PULMONARY HEART DISEASES

GUIDELINES

Pulmonary Hypertension

Pulmonary hypertension is classified to category I27, Other pulmonary heart diseases. For secondary pulmonary hypertension (I27.1, I27.2-), code also any associated conditions or adverse effects of drugs or toxins. The sequencing is based on the reason for the encounter, except for adverse effects of drugs.

I27.0 Primary pulmonary hypertension
Heritable pulmonary arterial hypertension
Idiopathic pulmonary arterial hypertension
Primary group 1 pulmonary hypertension
Primary pulmonary arterial hypertension

Excludes1: persistent pulmonary hypertension of newborn (P29.30)
pulmonary hypertension NOS (I27.20)
secondary pulmonary arterial hypertension (I27.21)
secondary pulmonary hypertension (I27.29)

I27.1 Kyphoscoliotic heart disease

I27.2 Other secondary pulmonary hypertension

Code also associated underlying condition

Excludes1: Eisenmenger's syndrome (I27.83)

I27.20 Pulmonary hypertension, unspecified
Pulmonary hypertension NOS

I27.21 Secondary pulmonary arterial hypertension
(Associated) (drug-induced) (toxin-induced) pulmonary arterial hypertension NOS
(Associated) (drug-induced) (toxin-induced) (secondary) group 1 pulmonary hypertension

Code also associated conditions if applicable, or adverse effects of drugs or toxins, such as:
adverse effect of appetite depressants (T50.5X5)
congenital heart disease (Q20-Q28)
human immunodeficiency virus [HIV] disease (B20)
polymyositis (M33.2-)
portal hypertension (K76.6)
rheumatoid arthritis (M05.-)
schistosomiasis (B65.-)
Sjögren syndrome (M35.0-)
systemic sclerosis (M34.-)

I27.22 Pulmonary hypertension due to left heart disease
Group 2 pulmonary hypertension

Code also associated left heart disease, if known, such as:
multiple valve disease (I08.-)
rheumatic mitral valve diseases (I05.-)
rheumatic aortic valve diseases (I06.-)

I27.23 Pulmonary hypertension due to lung diseases and hypoxia
Group 3 pulmonary hypertension

Code also associated lung disease, if known, such as:
bronchiectasis (J47.-)
cystic fibrosis with pulmonary manifestations (E84.0)
interstitial lung disease (J84.-)
pleural effusion (J90)
sleep apnea (G47.3-)

I27.24 Chronic thromboembolic pulmonary hypertension
Group 4 pulmonary hypertension

Code also associated pulmonary embolism, if applicable (I26.-, I27.82)

I27.29 Other secondary pulmonary hypertension
Group 5 pulmonary hypertension
Pulmonary hypertension with unclear multifactorial mechanisms
Pulmonary hypertension due to hematologic disorders
Pulmonary hypertension due to metabolic disorders
Pulmonary hypertension due to other systemic disorders

Code also other associated disorders, if known, such as:
chronic myeloid leukemia (C92.10–C92.22)
essential thrombocythemia (D47.3)
Gaucher disease (E75.22)
hypertensive chronic kidney disease with end stage
renal disease (I12.0, I13.11, I13.2)
hyperthyroidism (E05.-)
hypothyroidism (E00-E03)
polycythemia vera (D45)
sarcoidosis (D86.-)

- **I27.8 Other specified pulmonary heart diseases**
  - **I27.81 Cor pulmonale (chronic)**
    - Cor pulmonale NOS
    - **Code also**, if applicable, right heart failure (I50.81-)
    - *Excludes1:* acute cor pulmonale (I26.0-)
  - **I27.82 Chronic pulmonary embolism**
    - **Use additional code**, if applicable, for associated long-term (current) use of anticoagulants (Z79.01)
    - *Excludes1:* personal history of pulmonary embolism (Z86.711)
  - **I27.83 Eisenmenger's syndrome**
    - Eisenmenger's complex
    - (Irreversible) Eisenmenger's disease
    - Pulmonary hypertension with right to left shunt related to congenital heart disease
    - **Code also** underlying heart defect, if known, such as:
      - atrial septal defect (Q21.1)
      - Eisenmenger's defect (Q21.8)
      - patent ductus arteriosus (Q25.0)
      - ventricular septal defect (Q21.0)
  - **I27.89 Other specified pulmonary heart diseases**
    - *Excludes1:* Eisenmenger's defect (Q21.8)
- **I27.9 Pulmonary heart disease, unspecified**
  - Chronic cardiopulmonary disease

I28 OTHER DISEASES OF PULMONARY VESSELS

- **I28.0 Arteriovenous fistula of pulmonary vessels**
  - *Excludes1:* congenital arteriovenous fistula (Q25.72)
- **I28.1 Aneurysm of pulmonary artery**
  - *Excludes1:* congenital aneurysm (Q25.79)
  - congenital arteriovenous aneurysm (Q25.72)
- **I28.8 Other diseases of pulmonary vessels**
  - Pulmonary arteritis
  - Pulmonary endarteritis
  - Rupture of pulmonary vessels
  - Stenosis of pulmonary vessels
  - Stricture of pulmonary vessels
- **I28.9 Disease of pulmonary vessels, unspecified**

(I30–I52) OTHER FORMS OF HEART DISEASE

I30 ACUTE PERICARDITIS

Includes: acute mediastinopericarditis
acute myopericarditis
acute pericardial effusion
acute pleuropericarditis
acute pneumopericarditis

Excludes1: Dressler's syndrome (I24.1)
rheumatic pericarditis (acute) (I01.0)
viral pericarditis due to Coxsackie virus (B33.23)

- **I30.0 Acute nonspecific idiopathic pericarditis**
- **I30.1 Infective pericarditis**
  - Pneumococcal pericarditis
  - Pneumopyopericardium
  - Purulent pericarditis
  - Pyopericarditis
  - Pyopericardium
  - Pyopneumopericardium
  - Staphylococcal pericarditis
  - Streptococcal pericarditis
  - Suppurative pericarditis
  - Viral pericarditis
  - **Use additional code** (B95–B97) to identify infectious agent
- **I30.8 Other forms of acute pericarditis**
- **I30.9 Acute pericarditis, unspecified**

I31 OTHER DISEASES OF PERICARDIUM

Excludes1: diseases of pericardium specified as rheumatic (I09.2)
postcardiotomy syndrome (I97.0)
traumatic injury to pericardium (S26.-)

- **I31.0 Chronic adhesive pericarditis**
  - Accretio cordis
  - Adherent pericardium
  - Adhesive mediastinopericarditis
- **I31.1 Chronic constrictive pericarditis**
  - Concretio cordis
  - Pericardial calcification
- **I31.2 Hemopericardium, not elsewhere classified**
  - *Excludes1:* hemopericardium as current complication following acute myocardial infarction (I23.0)
- **I31.3 Pericardial effusion (noninflammatory)**
  - Chylopericardium
  - *Excludes1:* acute pericardial effusion (I30.9)
  - **I31.31 Malignant pericardial effusion in diseases classified elsewhere**
  - **I31.39 Other pericardial effusion (noninflammatory)**
- **I31.4 Cardiac tamponade**
  - Code first underlying cause
- **I31.8 Other specified diseases of pericardium**
  - Epicardial plaques
  - Focal pericardial adhesions
- **I31.9 Disease of pericardium, unspecified**
  - Pericarditis (chronic) NOS

I33 ACUTE AND SUBACUTE ENDOCARDITIS

Excludes1: acute rheumatic endocarditis (I01.1)
endocarditis NOS (I38)

- **I33.0 Acute and subacute infective endocarditis**
  - Bacterial endocarditis (acute) (subacute)
  - Infective endocarditis (acute) (subacute) NOS
  - Endocarditis lenta (acute) (subacute)
  - Malignant endocarditis (acute) (subacute)
  - Purulent endocarditis (acute) (subacute)
  - Septic endocarditis (acute) (subacute)
  - Ulcerative endocarditis (acute) (subacute)
  - Vegetative endocarditis (acute) (subacute)
  - **Use additional code** (B95–B97) to identify infectious agent
- **I33.9 Acute and subacute endocarditis, unspecified**
  - Acute endocarditis NOS
  - Acute myoendocarditis NOS
  - Acute periendocarditis NOS
  - Subacute endocarditis NOS
  - Subacute myoendocarditis NOS
  - Subacute periendocarditis NOS

I34 NONRHEUMATIC MITRAL VALVE DISORDERS

Excludes1: mitral valve disease (I05.9)
mitral valve failure (I05.8)
mitral valve stenosis (I05.0)
mitral valve disorder of unspecified cause with diseases of aortic and/or tricuspid valve(s) (I08.-)
mitral valve disorder of unspecified cause with mitral stenosis or obstruction (I05.0)
mitral valve disorder specified as congenital (Q23.2, Q23.9)
mitral valve disorder specified as rheumatic (I05.-)

- **I34.0 Nonrheumatic mitral (valve) insufficiency**
  - Nonrheumatic mitral (valve) incompetence NOS
  - Nonrheumatic mitral (valve) regurgitation NOS
- **I34.8 Other nonrheumatic mitral valve disorders**
  - **I34.81 Nonrheumatic mitral (valve) annulus calcification**
  - **I34.89 Other nonrheumatic mitral valve disorders**

I35 NONRHEUMATIC AORTIC VALVE DISORDERS

Excludes2: aortic valve disorder of unspecified cause but with diseases of mitral and/or tricuspid valve(s) (I08.-)
aortic valve disorder specified as congenital (Q23.0, Q23.1)
aortic valve disorder specified as rheumatic (I06.-)
hypertrophic subaortic stenosis (I42.1)

- **I35.0 Nonrheumatic aortic (valve) stenosis**

I35.1 Nonrheumatic aortic (valve) insufficiency
Nonrheumatic aortic (valve) incompetence NOS
Nonrheumatic aortic (valve) regurgitation NOS

I35.2 Nonrheumatic aortic (valve) stenosis with insufficiency

I35.8 Other nonrheumatic aortic valve disorders

I35.9 Nonrheumatic aortic valve disorder, unspecified

I36 NONRHEUMATIC TRICUSPID VALVE DISORDERS

Excludes1: tricuspid valve disorders of unspecified cause (I07.-)
tricuspid valve disorders specified as congenital (Q22.4, Q22.8, Q22.9)
tricuspid valve disorders specified as rheumatic (I07.-)
tricuspid valve disorders with aortic and/or mitral valve involvement (I08.-)

I36.0 Nonrheumatic tricuspid (valve) stenosis

I36.1 Nonrheumatic tricuspid (valve) insufficiency
Nonrheumatic tricuspid (valve) incompetence
Nonrheumatic tricuspid (valve) regurgitation

I36.2 Nonrheumatic tricuspid (valve) stenosis with insufficiency

I36.8 Other nonrheumatic tricuspid valve disorders

I36.9 Nonrheumatic tricuspid valve disorder, unspecified

I37 NONRHEUMATIC PULMONARY VALVE DISORDERS

Excludes1: pulmonary valve disorder specified as congenital (Q22.1, Q22.2, Q22.3)
pulmonary valve disorder specified as rheumatic (I09.89)

I37.0 Nonrheumatic pulmonary valve stenosis

I37.1 Nonrheumatic pulmonary valve insufficiency
Nonrheumatic pulmonary valve incompetence
Nonrheumatic pulmonary valve regurgitation

I37.2 Nonrheumatic pulmonary valve stenosis with insufficiency

I37.8 Other nonrheumatic pulmonary valve disorders

I37.9 Nonrheumatic pulmonary valve disorder, unspecified

I38 ENDOCARDITIS, VALVE UNSPECIFIED

Includes: endocarditis (chronic) NOS
valvular incompetence NOS
valvular insufficiency NOS
valvular regurgitation NOS
valvular stenosis NOS
valvulitis (chronic) NOS

Excludes1: congenital insufficiency of cardiac valve NOS (Q24.8)
congenital stenosis of cardiac valve NOS (Q24.8)
endocardial fibroelastosis (I42.4)
endocarditis specified as rheumatic (I09.1)

I40 ACUTE MYOCARDITIS

Includes: subacute myocarditis

Excludes1: acute rheumatic myocarditis (I01.2)

I40.0 Infective myocarditis
Septic myocarditis
Use additional code (B95–B97) to identify infectious agent

I40.8 Other acute myocarditis

I40.9 Acute myocarditis, unspecified

I42 CARDIOMYOPATHY

Includes: myocardiopathy

Code first pre-existing cardiomyopathy complicating pregnancy and puerperium (O99.4)

Excludes2: ischemic cardiomyopathy (I25.5)
peripartum cardiomyopathy (O90.3)
ventricular hypertrophy (I51.7)

I42.1 Obstructive hypertrophic cardiomyopathy
Hypertrophic subaortic stenosis (idiopathic)

I42.2 Other hypertrophic cardiomyopathy
Nonobstructive hypertrophic cardiomyopathy

I42.5 Other restrictive cardiomyopathy
Constrictive cardiomyopathy NOS

I42.9 Cardiomyopathy, unspecified
Cardiomyopathy (primary) (secondary) NOS

I43 CARDIOMYOPATHY IN DISEASES CLASSIFIED ELSEWHERE

Code first underlying disease, such as:
amyloidosis (E85.-)
glycogen storage disease (E74.0-)
gout (M10.0-)
thyrotoxicosis (E05.0-E05.9-)

Excludes1: cardiomyopathy (in):
infectious diseases
sarcoidosis (D86.85)

I44 ATRIOVENTRICULAR AND LEFT BUNDLE-BRANCH BLOCK

I44.0 Atrioventricular block, first degree

I44.1 Atrioventricular block, second degree
Atrioventricular block, type I and II
Möbitz block, type I and II
Second degree block, type I and II
Wenckebach's block

I44.2 Atrioventricular block, complete
Complete heart block NOS
Third degree block

I45 OTHER CONDUCTION DISORDERS

I45.6 Pre-excitation syndrome
Accelerated atrioventricular conduction
Accessory atrioventricular conduction
Anomalous atrioventricular excitation
Lown-Ganong-Levine syndrome
Pre-excitation atrioventricular conduction
Wolff-Parkinson-White syndrome

I45.8 Other specified conduction disorders

I45.81 Long QT syndrome

I45.89 Other specified conduction disorders
Atrioventricular [AV] dissociation
Interference dissociation
Isorhythmic dissociation
Nonparoxysmal AV nodal tachycardia

I45.9 Conduction disorder, unspecified
Heart block NOS
Stokes-Adams syndrome

I46 CARDIAC ARREST

Excludes2: cardiogenic shock (R57.0)

I46.2 Cardiac arrest due to underlying cardiac condition
Code first underlying cardiac condition

I46.8 Cardiac arrest due to other underlying condition
Code first underlying condition

I46.9 Cardiac arrest, cause unspecified

I47 PAROXYSMAL TACHYCARDIA

Code first tachycardia complicating: abortion or ectopic or molar pregnancy (O00–O07, O08.8)
obstetric surgery and procedures (O75.4)

Excludes1: tachycardia NOS (R00.0)
sinoauricular tachycardia NOS (R00.0)
sinus [sinusal] tachycardia NOS (R00.0)

I47.1 Supraventricular tachycardia

I47.10 Supraventricular tachycardia, unspecified

I47.11 Inappropriate sinus tachycardia, so stated
IST

I47.19 Other supraventricular tachycardia
Atrial (paroxysmal) tachycardia
Atrioventricular [AV] (paroxysmal) tachycardia
Atrioventricular re-entrant (nodal) tachycardia [AVNRT]
[AVRT]
Junctional (paroxysmal) tachycardia
Nodal (paroxysmal) tachycardia

I47.2 Ventricular tachycardia

I47.20 Ventricular tachycardia, unspecified

I47.21 Torsades de pointes

I47.29 Other ventricular tachycardia

I48 ATRIAL FIBRILLATION AND FLUTTER

I48.0 Paroxysmal atrial fibrillation

I48.1 Persistent atrial fibrillation

Excludes1: Permanent atrial fibrillation (I48.21)

I48.11 Longstanding persistent atrial fibrillation

I48.19 Other persistent atrial fibrillation
Chronic persistent atrial fibrillation
Persistent atrial fibrillation, NOS

I48.2 Chronic atrial fibrillation

I48.20 Chronic atrial fibrillation, unspecified
Excludes1: Chronic persistent atrial fibrillation (I48.19)

I48.21 Permanent atrial fibrillation

I48.3 Typical atrial flutter
Type I atrial flutter

I48.4 Atypical atrial flutter
Type II atrial flutter

I48.9 Unspecified atrial fibrillation and atrial flutter
- I48.91 Unspecified atrial fibrillation
- I48.92 Unspecified atrial flutter

I49 OTHER CARDIAC ARRHYTHMIAS

Code first cardiac arrhythmia complicating: abortion or ectopic or molar pregnancy (O00–O07, O08.8)
obstetric surgery and procedures (O75.4)

Excludes2: bradycardia NOS (R00.1)
neonatal dysrhythmia (P29.1-)
sinoatrial bradycardia (R00.1)
sinus bradycardia (R00.1)
vagal bradycardia (R00.1)

I49.0 **Ventricular fibrillation and flutter**
- I49.01 Ventricular fibrillation
- I49.02 Ventricular flutter

I49.1 **Atrial premature depolarization**
Atrial premature beats

I49.5 **Sick sinus syndrome**
Tachycardia-bradycardia syndrome

I49.9 **Cardiac arrhythmia, unspecified**
Arrhythmia (cardiac) NOS

I50 HEART FAILURE

Code first: heart failure complicating abortion or ectopic or molar pregnancy (O00–O07, O08.8)
heart failure due to hypertension (I11.0)
heart failure due to hypertension with CKD (I13.-)
heart failure following surgery (I97.13-)
obstetric surgery and procedures (O75.4)
rheumatic heart failure (I09.81)

Excludes1: neonatal cardiac failure (P29.0)

Excludes2: cardiac arrest (I46.-)

I50.1 **Left ventricular failure, unspecified**
Cardiac asthma
Edema of lung with heart disease NOS
Edema of lung with heart failure
Left heart failure
Pulmonary edema with heart disease NOS
Pulmonary edema with heart failure
Excludes1: edema of lung without heart disease or heart failure (J81.-)
pulmonary edema without heart disease or failure (J81.-)

I50.2 **Systolic (congestive) heart failure**
Heart failure with reduced ejection fraction [HFrEF]
Systolic left ventricular heart failure
Code also end stage heart failure, if applicable (I50.84)
Excludes1: combined systolic (congestive) and diastolic (congestive) heart failure (I50.4-)
- I50.20 Unspecified systolic (congestive) heart failure
- I50.21 Acute systolic (congestive) heart failure
- I50.22 Chronic systolic (congestive) heart failure
- I50.23 Acute on chronic systolic (congestive) heart failure

I50.3 **Diastolic (congestive) heart failure**
Diastolic left ventricular heart failure
Heart failure with normal ejection fraction
Heart failure with preserved ejection fraction [HFpEF]
Code also end stage heart failure, if applicable (I50.84)
Excludes1: combined systolic (congestive) and diastolic (congestive) heart failure (I50.4-)
- I50.30 Unspecified diastolic (congestive) heart failure
- I50.31 Acute diastolic (congestive) heart failure
- I50.32 Chronic diastolic (congestive) heart failure
- I50.33 Acute on chronic diastolic (congestive) heart failure

I50.4 **Combined systolic (congestive) and diastolic (congestive) heart failure**
- I50.40 Unspecified combined systolic (congestive) and diastolic (congestive) heart failure

I50.41 Acute combined systolic (congestive) and diastolic (congestive) heart failure

I50.42 Chronic combined systolic (congestive) and diastolic (congestive) heart failure

I50.43 Acute on chronic combined systolic (congestive) and diastolic (congestive) heart failure

I50.8 **Other heart failure**

I50.82 **Biventricular heart failure**
Code also the type of left ventricular failure as systolic, diastolic, or combined, if known (I50.2-I50.43)

I50.83 **High output heart failure**

I50.84 **End stage heart failure**
Stage D heart failure
Code also the type of heart failure as systolic, diastolic, or combined, if known (I50.2-I50.43)

I50.89 **Other heart failure**

I50.9 **Heart failure, unspecified**
Biventricular (heart) failure NOS
Cardiac, heart or myocardial failure NOS
Congestive heart disease
Congestive heart failure NOS
Right ventricular failure (secondary to left heart failure)
Excludes2: fluid overload unrelated to congestive heart failure (E87.70)

I51 COMPLICATIONS AND ILL-DEFINED DESCRIPTIONS OF HEART DISEASE

Excludes1: any condition in I51.4–I51.9 due to hypertension (I11.-)
any condition in I51.4–I51.9 due to hypertension and CKD (I13.-)
heart disease specified as rheumatic (I00–I09)

I51.4 **Myocarditis, unspecified**
Chronic (interstitial) myocarditis
Myocardial fibrosis
Myocarditis NOS
Excludes1: acute or subacute myocarditis (I40.-)

I51.5 **Myocardial degeneration**
Fatty degeneration of heart or myocardium
Myocardial disease
Senile degeneration of heart or myocardium

I51.7 **Cardiomegaly**
Cardiac dilatation
Cardiac hypertrophy
Ventricular dilatation

I51.8 **Other ill-defined heart diseases**

I51.81 **Takotsubo syndrome**
Reversible left ventricular dysfunction following sudden emotional stress
Stress induced cardiomyopathy
Takotsubo cardiomyopathy
Transient left ventricular apical ballooning syndrome

I51.89 **Other ill-defined heart diseases**
Carditis (acute)(chronic)
Pancarditis (acute)(chronic)

I51.9 **Heart disease, unspecified**

I5A NON-ISCHEMIC MYOCARDIAL INJURY (NON-TRAUMATIC)

I52 OTHER HEART DISORDERS IN DISEASES CLASSIFIED ELSEWHERE

Code first underlying disease, such as:
congenital syphilis (A50.5)
mucopolysaccharidosis (E76.3)
schistosomiasis (B65.0-B65.9)

Excludes1: heart disease (in):
gonococcal infection (A54.83)
meningococcal infection (A39.50)
rheumatoid arthritis (M05.31)
syphilis (A52.06)

(I60–I69) CEREBROVASCULAR DISEASES

Use additional code to identify presence of:
alcohol abuse and dependence (F10.-)
exposure to environmental tobacco smoke (Z77.22)
history of tobacco dependence (Z87.891)

hypertension (I10–I1A)
occupational exposure to environmental tobacco smoke (Z57.31)
tobacco dependence (F17.-)
tobacco use (Z72.0)
Excludes1: traumatic intracranial hemorrhage (S06.-)

I60 NONTRAUMATIC SUBARACHNOID HEMORRHAGE

Use **additional** code, if known, to indicate National Institutes of Health Stroke Scale (NIHSS) score (R29.7-)

Excludes1: syphilitic ruptured cerebral aneurysm (A52.05)

Excludes2: sequelae of subarachnoid hemorrhage (I69.0-)

- **I60.0** Nontraumatic subarachnoid hemorrhage from; carotid siphon and bifurcation
  - **I60.00** unspecified carotid siphon and bifurcation
  - **I60.01** right carotid siphon and bifurcation
  - **I60.02** left carotid siphon and bifurcation
- **I60.1** Nontraumatic subarachnoid hemorrhage from; middle cerebral artery
- **I60.2** Nontraumatic subarachnoid hemorrhage from; anterior communicating artery
- **I60.3** Nontraumatic subarachnoid hemorrhage from; posterior communicating artery
  - **I60.30** unspecified posterior communicating artery
  - **I60.31** right posterior communicating artery
  - **I60.32** left posterior communicating artery
- **I60.4** Nontraumatic subarachnoid hemorrhage from basilar artery
- **I60.5** Nontraumatic subarachnoid hemorrhage from; vertebral artery
  - **I60.50** unspecified vertebral artery
  - **I60.51** from right vertebral artery
  - **I60.52** from left vertebral artery
- **I60.6** Nontraumatic subarachnoid hemorrhage from other intracranial arteries
- **I60.7** Nontraumatic subarachnoid hemorrhage from unspecified intracranial artery
  - Ruptured (congenital) berry aneurysm
  - Ruptured (congenital) cerebral aneurysm
  - Subarachnoid hemorrhage (nontraumatic) from cerebral artery NOS
  - Subarachnoid hemorrhage (nontraumatic) from communicating artery NOS
  - *Excludes1:* berry aneurysm, nonruptured (I67.1)
- **I60.8** Other nontraumatic subarachnoid hemorrhage
  - Meningeal hemorrhage
  - Rupture of cerebral arteriovenous malformation
- **I60.9** Nontraumatic subarachnoid hemorrhage, unspecified

I61 NONTRAUMATIC INTRACEREBRAL HEMORRHAGE

Use **additional** code, if known, to indicate National Institutes of Health Stroke Scale (NIHSS) score (R29.7-)

Excludes2: sequelae of intracerebral hemorrhage (I69.1-)

- **I61.0** Nontraumatic intracerebral hemorrhage in hemisphere, subcortical
  - Deep intracerebral hemorrhage (nontraumatic)
- **I61.1** Nontraumatic intracerebral hemorrhage; in hemisphere, cortical
  - Cerebral lobe hemorrhage (nontraumatic)
  - Superficial intracerebral hemorrhage (nontraumatic)
- **I61.2** in hemisphere, unspecified
- **I61.3** in brain stem
- **I61.4** in cerebellum
- **I61.5** intraventricular
- **I61.6** multiple localized
- **I61.8** Other nontraumatic intracerebral hemorrhage
- **I61.9** Nontraumatic intracerebral hemorrhage, unspecified

I62 OTHER AND UNSPECIFIED NONTRAUMATIC INTRACRANIAL HEMORRHAGE

Use **additional** code, if known, to indicate National Institutes of Health Stroke Scale (NIHSS) score (R29.7-)

Excludes2: sequelae of intracranial hemorrhage (I69.2)

- **I62.0** Nontraumatic subdural hemorrhage
  - **I62.00** Nontraumatic subdural hemorrhage, unspecified
  - **I62.01** Nontraumatic acute subdural hemorrhage
  - **I62.02** Nontraumatic subacute subdural hemorrhage
  - **I62.03** Nontraumatic chronic subdural hemorrhage
- **I62.1** Nontraumatic extradural hemorrhage
  - Nontraumatic epidural hemorrhage
- **I62.9** Nontraumatic intracranial hemorrhage, unspecified

I67 OTHER CEREBROVASCULAR DISEASES

Excludes1: Occlusion and stenosis of cerebral artery causing cerebral infarction (I63.3-I63.5-)
Occlusion and stenosis of precerebral artery causing cerebral infarction (I63.2-)

Excludes2: sequelae of the listed conditions (I69.8)

- **I67.1** Cerebral aneurysm, nonruptured
  - Cerebral aneurysm NOS
  - Cerebral arteriovenous fistula, acquired
  - Internal carotid artery aneurysm, intracranial portion
  - Internal carotid artery aneurysm, NOS
  - *Excludes1:* congenital cerebral aneurysm, nonruptured (Q28.-)
  - ruptured cerebral aneurysm (I60.7)
- **I67.4** Hypertensive encephalopathy
  - **Code also**, if applicable, associated hypertensive conditions such as:
    - essential (primary) hypertension (I10)
    - hypertensive chronic kidney disease (I12.-)
    - hypertensive heart and chronic kidney disease (I13.-)
    - hypertensive heart disease (I11.-)
  - *Excludes2:* insufficiency, NOS, of precerebral arteries (G45.2)
- **I67.7** Cerebral arteritis, not elsewhere classified
  - Granulomatous angiitis of the nervous system
  - *Excludes1:* allergic granulomatous angiitis (M30.1)
- **I67.8** Other specified cerebrovascular diseases
  - **I67.81** Acute cerebrovascular insufficiency
    - Acute cerebrovascular insufficiency unspecified as to location or reversibility
  - **I67.82** Cerebral ischemia
    - Chronic cerebral ischemia
  - **I67.83** Posterior reversible encephalopathy syndrome
    - PRES
  - **I67.84** Cerebral vasospasm and vasoconstriction
    - **I67.841** Reversible cerebrovascular vasoconstriction syndrome
      - Call-Fleming syndrome
      - **Code first** underlying condition, if applicable, such as eclampsia (O15.00-O15.9)
    - **I67.848** Other cerebrovascular vasospasm and vasoconstriction
  - **I67.85** Hereditary cerebrovascular diseases
    - **I67.850** Cerebral autosomal dominant arteriopathy with subcortical infarcts and leukoencephalopathy CADASIL
      - **Code also** any associated diagnoses, such as:
        - epilepsy (G40.-)
        - stroke (I63.-)
        - vascular dementia (F01.-)
    - **I67.858** Other hereditary cerebrovascular disease
  - **I67.89** Other cerebrovascular disease
- **I67.9** Cerebrovascular disease, unspecified

(I70–I79) DISEASES OF ARTERIES, ARTERIOLES AND CAPILLARIES

I70 ATHEROSCLEROSIS

Includes: arteriolosclerosis
arterial degeneration
arteriosclerosis
arteriosclerotic vascular disease
arteriovascular degeneration
atheroma
endarteritis deformans or obliterans
senile arteritis
senile endarteritis
vascular degeneration

Use **additional** code to identify:
exposure to environmental tobacco smoke (Z77.22)
history of tobacco dependence (Z87.891)

occupational exposure to environmental tobacco smoke (Z57.31)
tobacco dependence (F17.-)
tobacco use (Z72.0)

Excludes2: arteriosclerotic cardiovascular disease (I25.1-)
arteriosclerotic heart disease (I25.1-)
atheroembolism (I75.-)
cerebral atherosclerosis (I67.2)
coronary atherosclerosis (I25.1-)
mesenteric atherosclerosis (K55.1)
precerebral atherosclerosis (I67.2)
primary pulmonary atherosclerosis (I27.0)

- I70.0 Atherosclerosis of aorta
- I70.8 Atherosclerosis of other arteries
- I70.9 Other and unspecified atherosclerosis
  - I70.90 Unspecified atherosclerosis
  - I70.91 Generalized atherosclerosis
  - I70.92 Chronic total occlusion of artery of the extremities
    Complete occlusion of artery of the extremities
    Total occlusion of artery of the extremities
    Code first atherosclerosis of arteries of the extremities (I70.2-, I70.3-, I70.4-, I70.5-, I70.6-, I70.7-)

I71 AORTIC ANEURYSM AND DISSECTION

Excludes1: aortic ectasia (I77.81-)
syphilitic aortic aneurysm (A52.01)
traumatic aortic aneurysm (S25.09, S35.09)

- I71.0 Dissection of aorta
  - I71.010 Dissection of ascending aorta
  - I71.011 Dissection of aortic arch
  - I71.012 Dissection of descending thoracic aorta
  - I71.019 Dissection of thoracic aorta, unspecified
- I71.1 Thoracic aortic aneurysm, ruptured
  - I71.10 Thoracic aortic aneurysm, ruptured, unspecifie
  - I71.11 Aneurysm of the ascending aorta, ruptured
  - I71.12 Aneurysm of the aortic arch, ruptured
  - I71.13 Aneurysm of the descending thoracic aorta, ruptured
- I71.2 Thoracic aortic aneurysm, without rupture
  - I71.20 Thoracic aortic aneurysm, without rupture, unspecified
  - I71.21 Aneurysm of the ascending aorta, without rupture
  - I71.22 Aneurysm of the aortic arch, without rupture
  - I71.23 Aneurysm of the descending thoracic aorta, without rupture
- I71.3 Abdominal aortic aneurysm, ruptured
  - I71.30 Abdominal aortic aneurysm, ruptured, unspecified
  - I71.31 Pararenal abdominal aortic aneurysm, ruptured
  - I71.32 Juxtarenal abdominal aortic aneurysm, ruptured
  - I71.33 Infrarenal abdominal aortic aneurysm, ruptured
- I71.4 Abdominal aortic aneurysm, without rupture
  - I71.40 Abdominal aortic aneurysm, without rupture, unspecified
  - I71.41 Pararenal abdominal aortic aneurysm, without rupture
  - I71.42 Juxtarenal abdominal aortic aneurysm, without rupture
  - I71.43 Infrarenal abdominal aortic aneurysm, without rupture
- I71.5 Thoracoabdominal aortic aneurysm, ruptured
  - I71.50 Thoracoabdominal aortic aneurysm, ruptured, unspecified
  - I71.51 Supraceliac aneurysm of the thoracoabdominal aorta, ruptured
  - I71.52 Paravisceral aneurysm of the thoracoabdominal aorta, ruptured
- I71.6 Thoracoabdominal aortic aneurysm, without rupture
  - I71.60 Thoracoabdominal aortic aneurysm, without rupture, unspecified
  - I71.61 Supraceliac aneurysm of the thoracoabdominal aorta, without rupture
  - I71.62 Paravisceral aneurysm of the thoracoabdominal aorta, without rupture
- I71.8 Aortic aneurysm of unspecified site, ruptured
  Rupture of aorta NOS

- I71.82 Antineutrophilic cytoplasmic antibody [ANCA] vasculitis
- I71.9 Aortic aneurysm of unspecified site, without rupture
  Aneurysm of aorta
  Dilatation of aorta
  Hyaline necrosis of aorta

I73 OTHER PERIPHERAL VASCULAR DISEASES

Excludes2: chilblains (T69.1)
frostbite (T33-T34)
immersion hand or foot (T69.0-)
spasm of cerebral artery (G45.9)

- I73.8 Other specified peripheral vascular diseases
  - **Excludes1:** diabetic (peripheral) angiopathy (E08-E13 with .51-.52)
  - I73.89 Other specified peripheral vascular diseases
    Acrocyanosis
    Erythrocyanosis
    Simple acroparesthesia [Schultze's type]
    Vasomotor acroparesthesia [Nothnagel's type]
- I73.9 Peripheral vascular disease, unspecified
  Intermittent claudication
  Peripheral angiopathy NOS
  Spasm of artery
  Excludes1: atherosclerosis of the extremities (I70.2-I70.7-)

I74 ARTERIAL EMBOLISM AND THROMBOSIS

Includes: embolic infarction
embolic occlusion
thrombotic infarction
thrombotic occlusion

Code first embolism and thrombosis complicating abortion or ectopic or molar pregnancy (O00-O07, O08.2)
embolism and thrombosis complicating pregnancy, childbirth and the puerperium (O88.-)

Excludes2: atheroembolism (I75.-)
basilar embolism and thrombosis (I63.0-I63.2, I65.1)
carotid embolism and thrombosis (I63.0-I63.2, I65.2)
cerebral embolism and thrombosis (I63.3-I63.5, I66.-)
coronary embolism and thrombosis (I21-I25)
mesenteric embolism and thrombosis (K55.0-)
ophthalmic embolism and thrombosis (H34.-)
precerebral embolism and thrombosis NOS (I63.0-I63.2, I65.9)
pulmonary embolism and thrombosis (I26.-)
renal embolism and thrombosis (N28.0)
retinal embolism and thrombosis (H34.-)
septic embolism and thrombosis (I76)
vertebral embolism and thrombosis (I63.0-I63.2, I65.0)

- I74.8 Embolism and thrombosis of other arteries
- I74.9 Embolism and thrombosis of unspecified artery

I76 SEPTIC ARTERIAL EMBOLISM

Code first underlying infection, such as:
infective endocarditis (I33.0)
lung abscess (J85.-)

Use additional code to identify the site of the embolism (I74.-)

Excludes2: septic pulmonary embolism (I26.01, I26.90)

I77 OTHER DISORDERS OF ARTERIES AND ARTERIOLES

Excludes2: collagen (vascular) diseases (M30-M36)
hypersensitivity angiitis (M31.0)
pulmonary artery (I28.-)

- I77.1 Stricture of artery
  Narrowing of artery
- I77.6 Arteritis, unspecified
  Aortitis NOS
  Endarteritis NOS
  Excludes1: arteritis or endarteritis:
  aortic arch (M31.4)
  cerebral NEC (I67.7)
  coronary (I25.89)
  deformans (I70.-)
  giant cell (M31.5, M31.6)
  obliterans (I70.-)
  senile (I70.-)

I78 DISEASES OF CAPILLARIES

- **I78.0** Hereditary hemorrhagic telangiectasia
  - Rendu-Osler-Weber disease
- **I78.1** Nevus, non-neoplastic
  - Araneus nevus
  - Senile nevus
  - Spider nevus
  - Stellar nevus
  - *Excludes1:* nevus NOS (D22.-)
    - vascular NOS (Q82.5)
  - *Excludes2:* blue nevus (D22.-)
    - flammeus nevus (Q82.5)
    - hairy nevus (D22.-)
    - melanocytic nevus (D22.-)
    - pigmented nevus (D22.-)
    - portwine nevus (Q82.5)
    - sanguineous nevus (Q82.5)
    - strawberry nevus (Q82.5)
    - verrucous nevus (Q82.5)
- **I78.8** Other diseases of capillaries
- **I78.9** Disease of capillaries, unspecified

(I80–I89) DISEASES OF VEINS, LYMPHATIC VESSELS AND LYMPH NODES, NOT ELSEWHERE CLASSIFIED

I80 PHLEBITIS AND THROMBOPHLEBITIS

Includes: endophlebitis
inflammation, vein
periphlebitis
suppurative phlebitis

Code first phlebitis and thrombophlebitis complicating abortion, ectopic or molar pregnancy (O00–O07, O08.7) phlebitis and thrombophlebitis complicating pregnancy, childbirth and the puerperium (O22.-, O87.-)

Excludes1: venous embolism and thrombosis of lower extremities (I82.4-, I82.5-, I82.81-)

- **I80.0** Phlebitis and thrombophlebitis of superficial vessels of; lower extremities
  - Phlebitis and thrombophlebitis of femoropopliteal vein
  - **I80.00** unspecified lower extremity
  - **I80.01** right lower extremity
  - **I80.02** left lower extremity
  - **I80.03** lower extremities, bilateral
- **I80.1** Phlebitis and thrombophlebitis of; femoral vein
  - Phlebitis and thrombophlebitis of common femoral vein
  - Phlebitis and thrombophlebitis of deep femoral vein
  - **I80.10** unspecified femoral vein
  - **I80.11** right femoral vein
  - **I80.12** left femoral vein
  - **I80.13** femoral vein, bilateral
- **I80.2** Phlebitis and thrombophlebitis of other and unspecified deep vessels of lower extremities
  - **I80.20** Phlebitis and thrombophlebitis of unspecified deep vessels of; lower extremities
    - **I80.201** right lower extremity
    - **I80.202** left lower extremity
    - **I80.203** lower extremities, bilateral
    - **I80.209** unspecified lower extremity
  - **I80.21** Phlebitis and thrombophlebitis of; iliac vein
    - Phlebitis and thrombophlebitis of common iliac vein
    - Phlebitis and thrombophlebitis of external iliac vein
    - Phlebitis and thrombophlebitis of internal iliac vein
    - **I80.211** right iliac vein
    - **I80.212** left iliac vein
    - **I80.213** iliac vein, bilateral
    - **I80.219** unspecified iliac vein
  - **I80.22** Phlebitis and thrombophlebitis of; popliteal vein
    - **I80.221** right popliteal vein
    - **I80.222** left popliteal vein
    - **I80.223** popliteal vein, bilateral
    - **I80.229** unspecified popliteal vein
  - **I80.23** Phlebitis and thrombophlebitis of; tibial vein
    - Phlebitis and thrombophlebitis of anterior tibial vein
    - Phlebitis and thrombophlebitis of posterior tibial vein
    - **I80.231** right tibial vein
    - **I80.232** left tibial vein
    - **I80.233** tibial vein, bilateral
    - **I80.239** unspecified tibial vein
  - **I80.24** Phlebitis and thrombophlebitis of peroneal vein
    - **I80.241** Phlebitis and thrombophlebitis of right peroneal vein
    - **I80.242** Phlebitis and thrombophlebitis of left peroneal vein
    - **I80.243** Phlebitis and thrombophlebitis of peroneal vein, bilateral
    - **I80.249** Phlebitis and thrombophlebitis of unspecified peroneal vein
  - **I80.25** Phlebitis and thrombophlebitis of calf muscular vein
    - Phlebitis and thrombophlebitis of calf muscular vein, NOS
    - Phlebitis and thrombophlebitis of gastrocnemial vein
    - Phlebitis and thrombophlebitis of soleal vein
    - **I80.251** Phlebitis and thrombophlebitis of right calf muscular vein
    - **I80.252** Phlebitis and thrombophlebitis of left calf muscular vein
    - **I80.253** Phlebitis and thrombophlebitis of calf muscular vein, bilateral
    - **I80.259** Phlebitis and thrombophlebitis of unspecified calf muscular vein
  - **I80.29** Phlebitis and thrombophlebitis of other deep vessels of; lower extremities
    - **I80.291** right lower extremity
    - **I80.292** left lower extremity
    - **I80.293** lower extremity, bilateral
    - **I80.299** unspecified lower extremity
- **I80.3** Phlebitis and thrombophlebitis of lower extremities, unspecified
- **I80.8** Phlebitis and thrombophlebitis of other sites
- **I80.9** Phlebitis and thrombophlebitis of unspecified site

I81 PORTAL VEIN THROMBOSIS

Portal (vein) obstruction

Excludes2: hepatic vein thrombosis (I82.0)
phlebitis of portal vein (K75.1)

I82 OTHER VENOUS EMBOLISM AND THROMBOSIS

Code first venous embolism and thrombosis complicating:
abortion, ectopic or molar pregnancy (O00–O07, O08.7)
pregnancy, childbirth and the puerperium (O22.-, O87.-)

Excludes2: venous embolism and thrombosis (of):
cerebral (I63.6, I67.6)
coronary (I21–I25)
intracranial and intraspinal, septic or NOS (G08)
intracranial, nonpyogenic (I67.6)
intraspinal, nonpyogenic (G95.1)
mesenteric (K55.0-)
portal (I81)
pulmonary (I26.-)

- **I82.0** **Budd-Chiari syndrome**
  - Hepatic vein thrombosis
- **I82.3** **Embolism and thrombosis of renal vein**
- **I82.9** **Embolism and thrombosis of unspecified vein**
  - **I82.90** **Acute embolism and thrombosis of unspecified vein**
    - Embolism of vein NOS
    - Thrombosis (vein) NOS

I83 VARICOSE VEINS OF LOWER EXTREMITIES

Excludes2: varicose veins complicating pregnancy (O22.0-)
varicose veins complicating the puerperium (O87.4)

- **I83.9** **Asymptomatic varicose veins of lower extremities**
  - Phlebectasia of lower extremities
  - Varicose veins of lower extremities
  - Varix of lower extremities
  - **I83.91** Asymptomatic varicose veins of right lower extremity
  - **I83.92** Asymptomatic varicose veins of left lower extremity
  - **I83.93** Asymptomatic varicose veins of bilateral lower extremities

I85 ESOPHAGEAL VARICES

Use additional code to identify:
alcohol abuse and dependence (F10.-)

I85.0 Esophageal varices

Idiopathic esophageal varices
Primary esophageal varices

I85.00 Esophageal varices without bleeding
Esophageal varices NOS

I85.01 Esophageal varices with bleeding

I86 VARICOSE VEINS OF OTHER SITES

Excludes1: varicose veins of unspecified site (I83.9-)
Excludes2: retinal varices (H35.0-)

I86.1 Scrotal varices
Varicocele

I88 NONSPECIFIC LYMPHADENITIS

Excludes1: acute lymphadenitis, except mesenteric (L04.-)
enlarged lymph nodes NOS (R59.-)
HIV disease resulting in generalized lymphadenopathy (B20)

I88.0 Nonspecific mesenteric lymphadenitis
Mesenteric lymphadenitis (acute)(chronic)

I88.1 Chronic lymphadenitis, except mesenteric
Adenitis
Lymphadenitis

I88.8 Other nonspecific lymphadenitis

I88.9 Nonspecific lymphadenitis, unspecified
Lymphadenitis NOS

I89 OTHER NONINFECTIVE DISORDERS OF LYMPHATIC VESSELS AND LYMPH NODES

Excludes1: chylocele, tunica vaginalis (nonfilarial) NOS (N50.89)
enlarged lymph nodes NOS (R59.-)
filarial chylocele (B74.-)
hereditary lymphedema (Q82.0)

I89.1 Lymphangitis
Chronic lymphangitis
Lymphangitis NOS
Subacute lymphangitis
Excludes1: acute lymphangitis (L03.-)

I89.8 Other specified noninfective disorders of lymphatic vessels and lymph nodes
Chylocele (nonfilarial)
Chylous ascites
Chylous cyst
Lipomelanotic reticulosis
Lymph node or vessel fistula
Lymph node or vessel infarction
Lymph node or vessel rupture

I89.9 Noninfective disorder of lymphatic vessels and lymph nodes, unspecified
Disease of lymphatic vessels NOS

(I95–I99) OTHER AND UNSPECIFIED DISORDERS OF THE CIRCULATORY SYSTEM

I95 HYPOTENSION

Excludes1: cardiovascular collapse (R57.9)
maternal hypotension syndrome (O26.5-)
nonspecific low blood pressure reading NOS (R03.1)

I95.1 Orthostatic hypotension
Hypotension, postural
Excludes1: neurogenic orthostatic hypotension [Shy-Drager] (G90.3)
orthostatic hypotension due to drugs (I95.2)

I95.9 Hypotension, unspecified

I97 INTRAOPERATIVE AND POSTPROCEDURAL COMPLICATIONS AND DISORDERS OF CIRCULATORY SYSTEM, NOT ELSEWHERE CLASSIFIED

Excludes2: postprocedural shock (T81.1-)

I97.0 Postcardiotomy syndrome

I97.1 Other postprocedural cardiac functional disturbances
Excludes2: acute pulmonary insufficiency following thoracic surgery (J95.1)
intraoperative cardiac functional disturbances (I97.7-)

I97.11 Postprocedural cardiac insufficiency

I97.110 Postprocedural cardiac insufficiency following cardiac surgery

I97.111 Postprocedural cardiac insufficiency following other surgery

I97.12 Postprocedural cardiac arrest

I97.120 Postprocedural cardiac arrest following cardiac surgery

I97.121 Postprocedural cardiac arrest following other surgery

I97.13 Postprocedural heart failure
Use additional code to identify the heart failure (I50.-)

I97.130 Postprocedural heart failure following cardiac surgery

I97.131 Postprocedural heart failure following other surgery

I97.19 Other postprocedural cardiac functional disturbances
Use additional code, if applicable, to further specify disorder

I97.190 Other postprocedural cardiac functional disturbances following cardiac surgery

I97.191 Other postprocedural cardiac functional disturbances following other surgery

I97.8 Other intraoperative and postprocedural complications and disorders of the circulatory system, not elsewhere classified
Use additional code, if applicable, to further specify disorder

I97.88 Other intraoperative complications of the circulatory system, NEC

I97.89 Other postprocedural complications and disorders of the circulatory system, NEC

I99 OTHER AND UNSPECIFIED DISORDERS OF CIRCULATORY SYSTEM

I99.8 Other disorder of circulatory system

I99.9 Unspecified disorder of circulatory system

Chapter 10. Diseases of the respiratory system (J00–J99)

GUIDELINES

Acute Respiratory Failure

See category J96.

ACUTE RESPIRATORY FAILURE AS PRINCIPAL DIAGNOSIS

Influenza due to certain identified influenza viruses

See categories J09–J18.

Ventilator associated Pneumonia

DOCUMENTATION OF VENTILATOR ASSOCIATED PNEUMONIA
See category J95.

VENTILATOR ASSOCIATED PNEUMONIA DEVELOPS AFTER ADMISSION
See category J95.

VAPING-RELATED DISORDERS

See code U07.0.

Note: When a respiratory condition is described as occurring in more than one site and is not specifically indexed, it should be classified to the lower anatomic site (e.g. tracheobronchitis to bronchitis in J40).

Use additional code, where applicable, to identify:
exposure to environmental tobacco smoke (Z77.22)
exposure to tobacco smoke in the perinatal period (P96.81)
history of tobacco dependence (Z87.891)
occupational exposure to environmental tobacco smoke (Z57.31)
tobacco dependence (F17.-)
tobacco use (Z72.0)

Excludes2: certain conditions originating in the perinatal period (P04–P96)
certain infectious and parasitic diseases (A00–B99)
complications of pregnancy, childbirth and the puerperium (O00–O9A)
congenital malformations, deformations and chromosomal abnormalities (Q00–Q99)
endocrine, nutritional and metabolic diseases (E00–E88)
injury, poisoning and certain other consequences of external causes (S00–T88)
neoplasms (C00–D49)
smoke inhalation (T59.81-)
symptoms, signs and abnormal clinical and laboratory findings, NEC (R00–R94)

(J00–J06) ACUTE UPPER RESPIRATORY INFECTIONS

Excludes1: COPD with acute lower respiratory infection (J44.0)

J00 ACUTE NASOPHARYNGITIS [COMMON COLD]

✓ Acute rhinitis
Coryza (acute)
Infective nasopharyngitis NOS
Infective rhinitis
Nasal catarrh, acute
Nasopharyngitis NOS

Excludes1: acute pharyngitis (J02.-)
acute sore throat NOS (J02.9)
influenza virus with other respiratory manifestations (J09.X2, J10.1, J11.1)
pharyngitis NOS (J02.9)
rhinitis NOS (J31.0)
sore throat NOS (J02.9)

Excludes2: allergic rhinitis (J30.1–J30.9)
chronic pharyngitis (J31.2)
chronic rhinitis (J31.0)
chronic sore throat (J31.2)
nasopharyngitis, chronic (J31.1)
vasomotor rhinitis (J30.0)

J01 ACUTE SINUSITIS

Includes: acute abscess of sinus
acute empyema of sinus
acute infection of sinus
acute inflammation of sinus
acute suppuration of sinus

Use additional code (B95–B97) to identify infectious agent.

Excludes1: sinusitis NOS (J32.9)

Excludes2: chronic sinusitis (J32.0–J32.8)

- **J01.0 Acute maxillary sinusitis**
  - Acute antritis
  - **J01.00** Acute maxillary sinusitis, unspecified
  - **J01.01** Acute recurrent maxillary sinusitis
- **J01.1 Acute frontal sinusitis**
  - **J01.10** Acute frontal sinusitis, unspecified
  - **J01.11** Acute recurrent frontal sinusitis
- **J01.2 Acute ethmoidal sinusitis**
  - **J01.20** Acute ethmoidal sinusitis, unspecified
  - **J01.21** Acute recurrent ethmoidal sinusitis
- **J01.3 Acute sphenoidal sinusitis**
  - **J01.30** Acute sphenoidal sinusitis, unspecified
  - **J01.31** Acute recurrent sphenoidal sinusitis
- **J01.4 Acute pansinusitis**
  - **J01.40** Acute pansinusitis, unspecified
  - **J01.41** Acute recurrent pansinusitis
- **J01.8 Other acute sinusitis**
  - **J01.80** Other acute sinusitis
    - Acute sinusitis involving more than one sinus but not pansinusitis
  - **J01.81** Other acute recurrent sinusitis
    - Acute recurrent sinusitis involving more than one sinus but not pansinusitis
- **J01.9 Acute sinusitis, unspecified**
  - **J01.90** Acute sinusitis, unspecified
  - **J01.91** Acute recurrent sinusitis, unspecified

J02 ACUTE PHARYNGITIS

Includes: acute sore throat

Excludes1: acute laryngopharyngitis (J06.0)
peritonsillar abscess (J36)
pharyngeal abscess (J39.1)
retropharyngeal abscess (J39.0)

Excludes2: chronic pharyngitis (J31.2)

- **J02.0 Streptococcal pharyngitis**
  - Septic pharyngitis
  - Streptococcal sore throat
  - ***Excludes2:*** scarlet fever (A38.-)
- **J02.8 Acute pharyngitis due to other specified organisms**
  - **Use additional code** (B95–B97) to identify infectious agent
  - ***Excludes1:*** acute pharyngitis due to coxsackie virus (B08.5)
    - acute pharyngitis due to gonococcus (A54.5)
    - acute pharyngitis due to herpes [simplex] virus (B00.2)
    - acute pharyngitis due to infectious mononucleosis (B27.-)
    - enteroviral vesicular pharyngitis (B08.5)
- **J02.9 Acute pharyngitis, unspecified**
  - Gangrenous pharyngitis (acute)
  - Infective pharyngitis (acute) NOS
  - Pharyngitis (acute) NOS
  - Sore throat (acute) NOS
  - Suppurative pharyngitis (acute)
  - Ulcerative pharyngitis (acute)
  - ***Excludes1:*** influenza virus with other respiratory manifestations (J09.X2, J10.1, J11.1)

J03 ACUTE TONSILLITIS

Excludes1: acute sore throat (J02.-)
hypertrophy of tonsils (J35.1)
peritonsillar abscess (J36)
sore throat NOS (J02.9)
streptococcal sore throat (J02.0)

Excludes2: chronic tonsillitis (J35.0)

- **J03.0 Streptococcal tonsillitis**
  - **J03.00 Acute streptococcal tonsillitis, unspecified**
  - **J03.01 Acute recurrent streptococcal tonsillitis**
- **J03.8 Acute tonsillitis due to other specified organisms**
  - Use additional code (B95–B97) to identify infectious agent.
  - *Excludes1:* diphtheritic tonsillitis (A36.0)
    - herpesviral pharyngotonsillitis (B00.2)
    - streptococcal tonsillitis (J03.0)
    - tuberculous tonsillitis (A15.8)
    - Vincent's tonsillitis (A69.1)
  - **J03.80 Acute tonsillitis due to other specified organisms**
  - **J03.81 Acute recurrent tonsillitis due to other specified organisms**
- **J03.9 Acute tonsillitis, unspecified**
  - Follicular tonsillitis (acute)
  - Gangrenous tonsillitis (acute)
  - Infective tonsillitis (acute)
  - Tonsillitis (acute) NOS
  - Ulcerative tonsillitis (acute)
  - *Excludes1:* influenza virus with other respiratory manifestations (J09.X2, J10.1, J11.1)
  - **J03.90 Acute tonsillitis, unspecified**
  - **J03.91 Acute recurrent tonsillitis, unspecified**

J04 ACUTE LARYNGITIS AND TRACHEITIS

Use additional code (B95–B97) to identify infectious agent.
Code also influenza, if present, such as:
- influenza due to identified novel influenza A virus with other respiratory manifestations (J09.X2)
- influenza due to other identified influenza virus with other respiratory manifestations (J10.1)
- influenza due to unidentified influenza virus with other respiratory manifestations (J11.1)

Excludes1: acute obstructive laryngitis [croup] and epiglottitis (J05.-)
Excludes2: laryngismus (stridulus) (J38.5)

- **J04.0 Acute laryngitis**
  - Edematous laryngitis (acute)
  - Laryngitis (acute) NOS
  - Subglottic laryngitis (acute)
  - Suppurative laryngitis (acute)
  - Ulcerative laryngitis (acute)
  - *Excludes1:* acute obstructive laryngitis (J05.0)
  - *Excludes2:* chronic laryngitis (J37.0)
- **J04.1 Acute tracheitis**
  - Acute viral tracheitis
  - Catarrhal tracheitis (acute)
  - Tracheitis (acute) NOS
  - *Excludes2:* chronic tracheitis (J42)
  - **J04.10 Acute tracheitis without obstruction**
  - **J04.11 Acute tracheitis with obstruction**
- **J04.2 Acute laryngotracheitis**
  - Laryngotracheitis NOS
  - Tracheitis (acute) with laryngitis (acute)
  - *Excludes1:* acute obstructive laryngotracheitis (J05.0)
  - *Excludes2:* chronic laryngotracheitis (J37.1)
- **J04.3 Supraglottitis, unspecified**
  - **J04.30 Supraglottitis, unspecified, without obstruction**
  - **J04.31 Supraglottitis, unspecified, with obstruction**

J05 ACUTE OBSTRUCTIVE LARYNGITIS [CROUP] AND EPIGLOTTITIS

Use additional code (B95–B97) to identify infectious agent.
Code also influenza, if present, such as:
- influenza due to identified novel influenza A virus with other respiratory manifestations (J09.X2)
- influenza due to other identified influenza virus with other respiratory manifestations (J10.1)
- influenza due to unidentified influenza virus with other respiratory manifestations (J11.1)

- **J05.0 Acute obstructive laryngitis [croup]**
  - Obstructive laryngitis (acute) NOS
  - Obstructive laryngotracheitis NOS

- **J05.1 Acute epiglottitis**
  - *Excludes2:* epiglottitis, chronic (J37.0)
  - **J05.10 Acute epiglottitis without obstruction**
    - Epiglottitis NOS
  - **J05.11 Acute epiglottitis with obstruction**

J06 ACUTE UPPER RESPIRATORY INFECTIONS OF MULTIPLE AND UNSPECIFIED SITES

Excludes1: acute respiratory infection NOS (J22)
- influenza virus with other respiratory manifestations (J09.X2, J10.1, J11.1)
- streptococcal pharyngitis (J02.0)

- **J06.0 Acute laryngopharyngitis**
- **J06.9 Acute upper respiratory infection, unspecified**
  - Use additional code (B95-B97) to identify infectious agent, if known, such as:
    - respiratory syncytial virus (RSV) (B97.4)
  - Upper respiratory disease, acute
  - Upper respiratory infection NOS

(J09–J18) INFLUENZA AND PNEUMONIA

GUIDELINES

Code only confirmed cases of influenza due to certain identified influenza viruses (category J09), and due to other identified influenza virus (category J10). This is an exception to the hospital inpatient guideline Section II, H. (Uncertain Diagnosis).

In this context, "confirmation" does not require documentation of positive laboratory testing specific for avian or other novel influenza A or other identified influenza virus. However, coding should be based on the provider's diagnostic statement that the patient has avian influenza, or other novel influenza A, for category J09, or has another particular identified strain of influenza, such as H1N1 or H3N2, but not identified as novel or variant, for category J10.

If the provider records "suspected" or "possible" or "probable" avian influenza, or novel influenza, or other identified influenza, then the appropriate influenza code from category J11, Influenza due to unidentified influenza virus, should be assigned. A code from category J09, Influenza due to certain identified influenza viruses, should not be assigned nor should a code from category J10, Influenza due to other identified influenza virus.

Use additional code, if applicable, to identify resistance to antimicrobial drugs (Z16.-)

Excludes2: allergic or eosinophilic pneumonia (J82)
- aspiration pneumonia NOS (J69.0)
- meconium pneumonia (P24.01)
- neonatal aspiration pneumonia (P24.-)
- pneumonia due to solids and liquids (J69.-)
- congenital pneumonia (P23.9)
- lipid pneumonia (J69.1)
- rheumatic pneumonia (I00)
- ventilator associated pneumonia (J95.851)

J09 INFLUENZA DUE TO CERTAIN IDENTIFIED INFLUENZA VIRUSES

Excludes1: influenza A/H1N1 (J10.-)
- influenza due to other identified influenza virus (J10.-)
- influenza due to unidentified influenza virus (J11.-)
- seasonal influenza due to other identified influenza virus (J10.-)
- seasonal influenza due to unidentified influenza virus (J11.-)

- **J09.X Influenza due to identified novel influenza A virus**
  - Avian influenza
  - Bird influenza
  - Influenza A/H5N1
  - Influenza of other animal origin, not bird or swine
  - Swine influenza virus (viruses that normally cause infections in pigs)
  - **J09.X1 Influenza due to identified novel influenza A virus with pneumonia**
    - **Code also**, if applicable, associated: lung abscess (J85.1)
    - other specified type of pneumonia

J09.X2 Influenza due to identified novel influenza A virus with other respiratory manifestations

Influenza due to identified novel influenza A virus NOS

Influenza due to identified novel influenza A virus with laryngitis

Influenza due to identified novel influenza A virus with pharyngitis

Influenza due to identified novel influenza A virus with upper respiratory symptoms

Use additional code, if applicable, for associated: pleural effusion (J91.8) sinusitis (J01.-)

J09.X3 Influenza due to identified novel influenza A virus with gastrointestinal manifestations

Influenza due to identified novel influenza A virus gastroenteritis

Excludes1: 'intestinal flu' [viral gastroenteritis] (A08.-)

J09.X9 Influenza due to identified novel influenza A virus with other manifestations

Influenza due to identified novel influenza A virus with encephalopathy

Influenza due to identified novel influenza A virus with myocarditis

Influenza due to identified novel influenza A virus with otitis media

Use additional code to identify manifestation

J10 INFLUENZA DUE TO OTHER IDENTIFIED INFLUENZA VIRUS

Includes: influenza A (non-novel)

influenza B

influenza C

Excludes1: influenza due to avian influenza virus (J09.X-)

influenza due to swine flu (J09.X-)

influenza due to unidentified influenza virus (J11.-)

J10.0 Influenza due to other identified influenza virus with pneumonia

Code also associated lung abscess, if applicable (J85.1)

J10.00 Influenza due to other identified influenza virus with unspecified type of pneumonia

J10.01 Influenza due to other identified influenza virus with the same other identified influenza virus pneumonia

J10.08 Influenza due to other identified influenza virus with other specified pneumonia

Code also other specified type of pneumonia

J10.1 Influenza due to other identified influenza virus with other respiratory manifestations

Influenza due to other identified influenza virus NOS

Influenza due to other identified influenza virus with laryngitis

Influenza due to other identified influenza virus with pharyngitis

Influenza due to other identified influenza virus with upper respiratory symptoms

Use additional code for associated pleural effusion, if applicable (J91.8)

Use additional code for associated sinusitis, if applicable (J01.-)

J10.2 Influenza due to other identified influenza virus with gastrointestinal manifestations

Influenza due to other identified influenza virus gastroenteritis

Excludes1: 'intestinal flu' [viral gastroenteritis] (A08.-)

J10.8 Influenza due to other identified influenza virus with other manifestations

J10.81 Influenza due to other identified influenza virus with encephalopathy

J10.82 Influenza due to other identified influenza virus with myocarditis

J10.83 Influenza due to other identified influenza virus with otitis media

Use additional code for any associated perforated tympanic membrane (H72.-)

J10.89 Influenza due to other identified influenza virus with other manifestations

Use additional codes to identify the manifestations

J11 INFLUENZA DUE TO UNIDENTIFIED INFLUENZA VIRUS

J11.0 Influenza due to unidentified influenza virus with pneumonia

Code also associated lung abscess, if applicable (J85.1)

J11.00 Influenza due to unidentified influenza virus with unspecified type of pneumonia

Influenza with pneumonia NOS

J11.08 Influenza due to unidentified influenza virus with specified pneumonia

Code also other specified type of pneumonia

J11.1 Influenza due to unidentified influenza virus with other respiratory manifestations

Influenza NOS

Influenzal laryngitis NOS

Influenzal pharyngitis NOS

Influenza with upper respiratory symptoms NOS

Use additional code for associated pleural effusion, if applicable (J91.8)

Use additional code for associated sinusitis, if applicable (J01.-)

J11.2 Influenza due to unidentified influenza virus with gastrointestinal manifestations

Influenza gastroenteritis NOS

Excludes1: 'intestinal flu' [viral gastroenteritis] (A08.-)

J11.8 Influenza due to unidentified influenza virus with other manifestations

J11.81 Influenza due to unidentified influenza virus with encephalopathy

Influenzal encephalopathy NOS

J11.82 Influenza due to unidentified influenza virus with myocarditis

Influenzal myocarditis NOS

J11.83 Influenza due to unidentified influenza virus with otitis media

Influenzal otitis media NOS

Use additional code for any associated perforated tympanic membrane (H72.-)

J11.89 Influenza due to unidentified influenza virus with other manifestations

Use additional codes to identify the manifestations

J12 VIRAL PNEUMONIA, NEC

Includes: bronchopneumonia due to viruses other than influenza viruses

Code first associated influenza, if applicable (J09.X1, J10.0-, J11.0-)

Code also associated abscess, if applicable (J85.1)

Excludes2: aspiration pneumonia due to anesthesia during labor and delivery (O74.0)

aspiration pneumonia due to anesthesia during pregnancy (O29)

aspiration pneumonia due to anesthesia during puerperium (O89.0)

aspiration pneumonia due to solids and liquids (J69.-)

aspiration pneumonia NOS (J69.0)

congenital pneumonia (P23.0)

congenital rubella pneumonitis (P35.0)

interstitial pneumonia NOS (J84.9)

lipid pneumonia (J69.1)

neonatal aspiration pneumonia (P24.-)

J12.0 Adenoviral pneumonia

J12.1 RSV pneumonia

J12.2 Parainfluenza virus pneumonia

J12.3 Human metapneumovirus pneumonia

J12.8 Other viral pneumonia

J12.81 Pneumonia due to SARS-associated coronavirus

SARS NOS GUIDELINE

See code U07.1 for further details.

J12.82 Pneumonia due to coronavirus disease 2019

J12.89 Other viral pneumonia

J12.9 Viral pneumonia, unspecified

J13 PNEUMONIA DUE TO STREPTOCOCCUS PNEUMONIAE

Bronchopneumonia due to S. pneumoniae

Code first, if applicable, associated influenza (J09.X1, J10.0-, J11.0-)

Code also, if applicable, any associated condition such as:

abscess (J85.1)

aspiration pneumonia (J69.-)

Excludes1: congenital pneumonia due to S. pneumoniae (P23.6)

lobar pneumonia, unspecified organism (J18.1)

pneumonia due to other streptococci (J15.3-J15.4)

J14 PNEUMONIA DUE TO H. INFLUENZAE

✓ Bronchopneumonia due to H. influenzae
Code first, if applicable, associated influenza (J09.X1, J10.0-, J11.0-)
Code also, if applicable, any associated condition such as:
abscess (J85.1)
aspiration pneumonia (J69.-)
Excludes1: congenital pneumonia due to H. influenzae (P23.6)

J15 BACTERIAL PNEUMONIA, NEC

4th ***Includes***: bronchopneumonia due to bacteria other than S. pneumoniae and H. influenzae
Code first, if applicable, associated influenza (J09.X1, J10.0-, J11.0-)
Code also, if applicable, any associated condition such as:
abscess (J85.1)
aspiration pneumonia (J69.-)
Excludes1: chlamydial pneumonia (J16.0)
congenital pneumonia (P23.-)
Legionnaires' disease (A48.1)
spirochetal pneumonia (A69.8)
J15.0 Pneumonia due to K. pneumoniae
J15.1 Pneumonia due to Pseudomonas
J15.2 Pneumonia due to staphylococcus
5th **J15.20 Pneumonia due to staphylococcus, unspecified**
J15.21 Pneumonia due to staphylococcus aureus
6th **J15.211 Pneumonia due to MSSA**
MSSA pneumonia
Pneumonia due to Staphylococcus aureus NOS
J15.212 Pneumonia due to MRSA
J15.29 Pneumonia due to other staphylococcus
J15.3 Pneumonia due to streptococcus, group B
J15.4 Pneumonia due to other streptococci
Excludes1: pneumonia due to streptococcus, group B (J15.3)
pneumonia due to Streptococcus pneumoniae (J13)
J15.5 Pneumonia due to E. coli
J15.6 Pneumonia due to other (aerobic) Gram-negative bacteria
5th **J15.61 Pneumonia due to Acinetobacter baumannii**
J15.69 Pneumonia due to other Gram-negative bacteria
Pneumonia due to other aerobic Gram-negative bacteria
Pneumonia due to Serratia marcescens
J15.7 Pneumonia due to M. pneumoniae
J15.8 Pneumonia due to other specified bacteria
J15.9 Unspecified bacterial pneumonia
Pneumonia due to gram-positive bacteria

J16 PNEUMONIA DUE TO OTHER INFECTIOUS ORGANISMS, NEC

4th **Code first**, if applicable, associated influenza (J09.X1, J10.0-, J11.0-)
Code also, if applicable, any associated condition such as:
abscess (J85.1)
aspiration pneumonia (J69.-)
Excludes1: congenital pneumonia (P23.-)
ornithosis (A70)
pneumocystosis (B59)
pneumonia NOS (J18.9)
J16.0 Chlamydial pneumonia
J16.8 Pneumonia due to other specified infectious organisms

J17 PNEUMONIA IN DISEASES CLASSIFIED ELSEWHERE

✓ **Code first** underlying disease, such as:
Q fever (A78)
rheumatic fever (I00)
schistosomiasis (B65.0–B65.9)
Code also, if applicable, any associated condition such as:
abscess (J85.1)
aspiration pneumonia (J69.-)
Excludes1: candidial pneumonia (B37.1)
chlamydial pneumonia (J16.0)
gonorrheal pneumonia (A54.84)
histoplasmosis pneumonia (B39.0–B39.2)
measles pneumonia (B05.2)
nocardiosis pneumonia (A43.0)
pneumocystosis (B59)
pneumonia due to Pneumocystis carinii (B59)

pneumonia due to Pneumocystis jiroveci (B59)
pneumonia in actinomycosis (A42.0)
pneumonia in anthrax (A22.1)
pneumonia in ascariasis (B77.81)
pneumonia in aspergillosis (B44.0–B44.1)
pneumonia in coccidioidomycosis (B38.0–B38.2)
pneumonia in cytomegalovirus disease (B25.0)
pneumonia in toxoplasmosis (B58.3)
rubella pneumonia (B06.81)
salmonella pneumonia (A02.22)
spirochetal infection NEC with pneumonia (A69.8)
tularemia pneumonia (A21.2)
typhoid fever with pneumonia (A01.03)
varicella pneumonia (B01.2)
whooping cough with pneumonia (A37 with fifth-character 1)

J18 PNEUMONIA, UNSPECIFIED ORGANISM

4th **Code first**, if applicable, associated influenza (J09.X1, J10.0-, J11.0-)
Code also, if applicable, any associated condition such as:
aspiration pneumonia (J69.-)
Excludes2: abscess of lung with pneumonia (J85.1)
aspiration pneumonia due to anesthesia during labor and delivery (O74.0)
aspiration pneumonia due to anesthesia during pregnancy (O29)
aspiration pneumonia due to anesthesia during puerperium (O89.0)
aspiration pneumonia due to solids and liquids (J69.-)
aspiration pneumonia NOS (J69.0)
lipid pneumonia (J69.1)
pneumonitis due to external agents (J67-J70)
J18.0 Bronchopneumonia, unspecified organism
Excludes1: hypostatic bronchopneumonia (J18.2)
lipid pneumonia (J69.1)
Excludes2: acute bronchiolitis (J21.-)
chronic bronchiolitis (J44.89)
other specified chronic obstructive pulmonary disease (J44.89)
J18.1 Lobar pneumonia, unspecified organism
J18.8 Other pneumonia, unspecified organism
J18.9 Pneumonia, unspecified organism

(J20–J22) OTHER ACUTE LOWER RESPIRATORY INFECTIONS

Excludes2: COPD with acute lower respiratory infection (J44.0)

J20 ACUTE BRONCHITIS

4th ***Includes***: acute and subacute bronchitis (with) bronchospasm
acute and subacute bronchitis (with) tracheitis
acute and subacute bronchitis (with) tracheobronchitis, acute
acute and subacute fibrinous bronchitis
acute and subacute membranous bronchitis
acute and subacute purulent bronchitis
acute and subacute septic bronchitis
Excludes1: bronchitis NOS (J40)
tracheobronchitis NOS
Excludes2: acute bronchitis with bronchiectasis (J47.0)
acute bronchitis with chronic obstructive asthma (J44.0)
acute bronchitis with COPD (J44.0)
allergic bronchitis NOS (J45.909-)
bronchitis due to chemicals, fumes and vapors (J68.0)
chronic bronchitis NOS (J42)
chronic mucopurulent bronchitis (J41.1)
chronic obstructive bronchitis (J44.-)
chronic obstructive tracheobronchitis (J44.-)
chronic simple bronchitis (J41.0)
chronic tracheobronchitis (J42)
J20.0 Acute bronchitis due to M. pneumoniae
J20.1 Acute bronchitis due to H. influenzae
J20.2 Acute bronchitis due to streptococcus
J20.3 Acute bronchitis due to coxsackievirus
J20.4 Acute bronchitis due to parainfluenza virus
J20.5 Acute bronchitis due to RSV
J20.6 Acute bronchitis due to rhinovirus
J20.7 Acute bronchitis due to echovirus
J20.8 Acute bronchitis due to other specified organisms
J20.9 Acute bronchitis, unspecified

J21 ACUTE BRONCHIOLITIS

Includes: acute bronchiolitis with bronchospasm
Excludes2: respiratory bronchiolitis interstitial lung disease (J84.115)

- J21.0 **Acute bronchiolitis due to RSV**
- J21.1 **Acute bronchiolitis due to human metapneumovirus**
- J21.8 **Acute bronchiolitis due to other specified organisms**
- J21.9 **Acute bronchiolitis, unspecified**
  - Bronchiolitis (acute)
  - *Excludes1:* chronic bronchiolitis (J44.89)

J22 UNSPECIFIED ACUTE LOWER RESPIRATORY INFECTION

Acute (lower) respiratory (tract) infection NOS
Excludes1: upper respiratory infection (acute) (J06.9)

(J30–J39) OTHER DISEASES OF UPPER RESPIRATORY TRACT

J30 VASOMOTOR AND ALLERGIC RHINITIS

Includes: spasmodic rhinorrhea
Excludes1: allergic rhinitis with asthma (bronchial) (J45.909)
rhinitis NOS (J31.0)

- J30.1 **Allergic rhinitis due to pollen**
  - Allergy NOS due to pollen
  - Hay fever
  - Pollinosis
- J30.2 **Other seasonal allergic rhinitis**
- J30.5 **Allergic rhinitis due to food**
- J30.8 **Other allergic rhinitis**
  - J30.81 **Allergic rhinitis due to animal (cat) (dog) hair and dander**
  - J30.89 **Other allergic rhinitis**
    - Perennial allergic rhinitis
- J30.9 **Allergic rhinitis, unspecified**

J31 CHRONIC RHINITIS, NASOPHARYNGITIS AND PHARYNGITIS

- J31.0 **Chronic rhinitis**
  - Atrophic rhinitis (chronic)
  - Granulomatous rhinitis (chronic)
  - Hypertrophic rhinitis (chronic)
  - Obstructive rhinitis (chronic)
  - Ozena
  - Purulent rhinitis (chronic)
  - Rhinitis (chronic) NOS
  - Ulcerative rhinitis (chronic)
  - *Excludes1:* allergic rhinitis (J30.1–J30.9)
    - vasomotor rhinitis (J30.0)
- J31.1 **Chronic nasopharyngitis**
  - *Excludes2:* acute nasopharyngitis (J00)
- J31.2 **Chronic pharyngitis**
  - Chronic sore throat
  - Atrophic pharyngitis (chronic)
  - Granular pharyngitis (chronic)
  - Hypertrophic pharyngitis (chronic)
  - *Excludes2* acute pharyngitis (J02.9)

J32 CHRONIC SINUSITIS

Includes: sinus abscess
sinus empyema
sinus infection
sinus suppuration

Use additional code to identify:
infectious agent (B95–B97)
Excludes2: acute sinusitis (J01.-)

- J32.0 **Chronic maxillary sinusitis**
  - Antritis (chronic)
  - Maxillary sinusitis NOS
- J32.1 **Chronic frontal sinusitis**
  - Frontal sinusitis NOS
- J32.2 **Chronic ethmoidal sinusitis**
  - Ethmoidal sinusitis NOS
  - *Excludes1:* Woakes' ethmoiditis (J33.1)
- J32.3 **Chronic sphenoidal sinusitis**
  - Sphenoidal sinusitis NOS
- J32.4 **Chronic pansinusitis**
  - Pansinusitis NOS
- J32.8 **Other chronic sinusitis**
  - Sinusitis (chronic) involving more than one sinus but not pansinusitis
- J32.9 **Chronic sinusitis, unspecified**
  - Sinusitis (chronic) NOS

J33 NASAL POLYP

Excludes1: adenomatous polyps (D14.0)

- J33.0 **Polyp of nasal cavity**
  - Choanal polyp
  - Nasopharyngeal polyp
- J33.8 **Other polyp of sinus**
  - Accessory polyp of sinus
  - Ethmoidal polyp of sinus
  - Maxillary polyp of sinus
  - Sphenoidal polyp of sinus
- J33.9 **Nasal polyp, unspecified**

J34 OTHER AND UNSPECIFIED DISORDERS OF NOSE AND NASAL SINUSES

Excludes2: varicose ulcer of nasal septum (I86.8)

- J34.0 **Abscess, furuncle and carbuncle of nose**
  - Cellulitis of nose
  - Necrosis of nose
  - Ulceration of nose
- J34.1 **Cyst and mucocele of nose and nasal sinus**
- J34.2 **Deviated nasal septum**
  - Deflection or deviation of septum (nasal) (acquired)
  - *Excludes1:* congenital deviated nasal septum (Q67.4)
- J34.3 **Hypertrophy of nasal turbinates**
- J34.8 **Other specified disorders of nose and nasal sinuses**
  - J34.81 **Nasal mucositis (ulcerative)**
    - Code also type of associated therapy, such as:
    - antineoplastic and immunosuppressive drugs (T45.1X-)
    - radiological procedure and radiotherapy (Y84.2)
    - *Excludes2:* gastrointestinal mucositis (ulcerative) (K92.81)
    - mucositis (ulcerative) of vagina and vulva (N76.81)
    - oral mucositis (ulcerative) (K12.3-)
  - •J34.82 **Nasal valve collapse**
    - Nasal valve compromise
    - Nasal valve stenosis
    - **Code first** underlying cause, such as:
    - deviated nasal septum (J34.2)
    - •J34.820 **Internal nasal valve collapse**
      - •J34.8200 **Internal nasal valve collapse, unspecified**
      - •J34.8201 **Internal nasal valve collapse, static**
        - Narrowing of the septum, head of the inferior turbinate and the upper lateral cartilage
      - •J34.8202 **Internal nasal valve collapse, dynamic**
        - Collapse or falling of the upper, middle sidewall of the nose on inspiration
    - •J34.821 **External nasal valve collapse**
      - •J34.8210 **External nasal valve collapse, unspecified**
      - •J34.8211 **External nasal valve collapse, static**
        - Add fixed narrowing of the caudal septum, lower lateral cartilage, alar rim and nasal sill
      - •J34.8212 **External nasal valve collapse, dynamic**
        - Collapse or falling of the lower sidewall or nostril of the nose on inspiration
    - •J34.829 **Nasal valve collapse, unspecified**
      - Nasal valve collapse, NOS

J34.89 Other specified disorders of nose and nasal sinuses
Perforation of nasal septum NOS
Rhinolith

J34.9 Unspecified disorder of nose and nasal sinuses

J35 CHRONIC DISEASES OF TONSILS AND ADENOIDS

J35.0 Chronic tonsillitis and adenoiditis

Excludes2: acute tonsillitis (J03.-)

J35.01 Chronic tonsillitis

J35.02 Chronic adenoiditis

J35.03 Chronic tonsillitis and adenoiditis

J35.1 Hypertrophy of tonsils
Enlargement of tonsils
Excludes1: hypertrophy of tonsils with tonsillitis (J35.0-)

J35.2 Hypertrophy of adenoids
Enlargement of adenoids
Excludes1: hypertrophy of adenoids with adenoiditis (J35.0-)

J35.3 Hypertrophy of tonsils with hypertrophy of adenoids
Excludes1: hypertrophy of tonsils and adenoids with tonsillitis and adenoiditis (J35.03)

J35.8 Other chronic diseases of tonsils and adenoids
Adenoid vegetations
Amygdalolith
Calculus, tonsil
Cicatrix of tonsil (and adenoid)
Tonsillar tag
Ulcer of tonsil

J35.9 Chronic disease of tonsils and adenoids, unspecified
Disease (chronic) of tonsils and adenoids NOS

J36 PERITONSILLAR ABSCESS

✓

Includes: abscess of tonsil
peritonsillar cellulitis
quinsy

Use additional code (B95-B97) to identify infectious agent.

Excludes1: acute tonsillitis (J03.-)
chronic tonsillitis (J35.0)
retropharyngeal abscess (J39.0)
tonsillitis NOS (J03.9-)

J37 CHRONIC LARYNGITIS AND LARYNGOTRACHEITIS

Use additional code to identify: *(See Chapter 10 guidelines for codes)*

J37.0 Chronic laryngitis
Catarrhal laryngitis
Hypertrophic laryngitis
Sicca laryngitis
Excludes2: acute laryngitis (J04.0)
obstructive (acute) laryngitis (J05.0)

J37.1 Chronic laryngotracheitis
Laryngitis, chronic, with tracheitis (chronic)
Tracheitis, chronic, with laryngitis
Excludes1: chronic tracheitis (J42)
Excludes2: acute laryngotracheitis (J04.2)
acute tracheitis (J04.1)

J38 DISEASES OF VOCAL CORDS AND LARYNX, NEC

Excludes1: congenital laryngeal stridor (P28.89)
obstructive laryngitis (acute) (J05.0)
postprocedural subglottic stenosis (J95.5)
stridor (R06.1)
ulcerative laryngitis (J04.0)

J38.0 Paralysis of vocal cords and larynx
Laryngoplegia
Paralysis of glottis

J38.00 Paralysis of vocal cords and larynx, unspecified

J38.01 Paralysis of vocal cords and larynx, unilateral

J38.02 Paralysis of vocal cords and larynx, bilateral

J38.4 Edema of larynx
Edema (of) glottis
Subglottic edema
Supraglottic edema
Excludes1: acute obstructive laryngitis [croup] (J05.0)
edematous laryngitis (J04.0)

J38.5 Laryngeal spasm
Laryngismus (stridulus)

J39 OTHER DISEASES OF UPPER RESPIRATORY TRACT

Excludes1: acute respiratory infection NOS (J22)
acute upper respiratory infection (J06.9)
upper respiratory inflammation due to chemicals, gases, fumes or vapors (J68.2)

J39.0 Retropharyngeal and parapharyngeal abscess
Peripharyngeal abscess
Excludes1: peritonsillar abscess (J36)

J39.2 Other diseases of pharynx
Cyst of pharynx
Edema of pharynx
Excludes2: chronic pharyngitis (J31.2)
ulcerative pharyngitis (J02.9)

J39.8 Other specified diseases of upper respiratory tract

J39.9 Disease of upper respiratory tract, unspecified

(J40-J4A) CHRONIC LOWER RESPIRATORY DISEASES

Excludes1: bronchitis due to chemicals, gases, fumes and vapors (J68.0)

Excludes2: cystic fibrosis (E84.-)

J40 BRONCHITIS, NOT SPECIFIED AS ACUTE OR CHRONIC

✓

Bronchitis NOS
Bronchitis with tracheitis NOS
Catarrhal bronchitis
Tracheobronchitis NOS

Use additional code to identify: *(See Chapter 10 guidelines for codes)*

Excludes1: acute bronchitis (J20.-)
allergic bronchitis NOS (J45.909-)
asthmatic bronchitis NOS (J45.9-)
bronchitis due to chemicals, gases, fumes and vapors (J68.0)

J42 UNSPECIFIED CHRONIC BRONCHITIS

✓

Chronic bronchitis NOS
Chronic tracheitis
Chronic tracheobronchitis

Use additional code to identify:
exposure to environmental tobacco smoke (Z77.22)
exposure to tobacco smoke in the perinatal period (P96.81)
history of tobacco dependence (Z87.891)
occupational exposure to environmental tobacco smoke (Z57.31)
tobacco dependence (F17.-)
tobacco use (Z72.0)

Excludes1: bronchiolitis obliterans and bronchiolitis obliterans syndrome (J44.81)
chronic asthmatic bronchitis (J44.-)
chronic bronchitis with airway obstruction (J44.-)
chronic emphysematous bronchitis (J44.-)
chronic obstructive pulmonary disease NOS (J44.9)
simple and mucopurulent chronic bronchitis (J41.-)

J44 OTHER CHRONIC OBSTRUCTIVE PULMONARY DISEASE

Includes: asthma with chronic obstructive pulmonary disease
chronic asthmatic (obstructive) bronchitis
chronic bronchitis with airway obstruction
chronic bronchitis with emphysema
chronic emphysematous bronchitis
chronic obstructive asthma
chronic obstructive bronchitis
chronic obstructive tracheobronchitis

Code also type of asthma, if applicable (J45.-)

Excludes1: chronic bronchitis NOS (J42)
chronic simple and mucopurulent bronchitis (J41.-)
chronic tracheitis (J42)
chronic tracheobronchitis (J42)

Excludes2: bronchiectasis (J47.-)
emphysema without chronic bronchitis (J43.-)

J44.8 Other specified chronic obstructive pulmonary disease

J44.81 Bronchiolitis obliterans and bronchiolitis obliterans syndrome
Obliterative bronchiolitis
Code first, if applicable:
complication of bone marrow transplant (T86.09)
complication of stem cell transplant (T86.5)
heart-lung transplant rejection (T86.31)

lung transplant rejection (T86.810)
other complications of heart-lung transplant (T86.39)
other complications of lung transplant (T86.818)

Code also, if applicable, associated conditions, such as:
chronic graft-versus-host disease (D89.811)
chronic lung allograft dysfunction (J4A.-)
chronic respiratory conditions due to chemicals, gases, fumes and vapors (J68.4)

J44.89 Other specified chronic obstructive pulmonary disease
Chronic asthmatic (obstructive) bronchitis
Chronic emphysematous bronchitis

J45 ASTHMA

Includes: allergic (predominantly) asthma
allergic bronchitis NOS
allergic rhinitis with asthma
atopic asthma
extrinsic allergic asthma
hay fever with asthma
idiosyncratic asthma
intrinsic nonallergic asthma
nonallergic asthma

Use additional code to identify: *(See Chapter 10 guidelines for codes)*
eosinophilic asthma (J82.83)

Excludes1: detergent asthma (J69.8)
miner's asthma (J60)
wheezing NOS (R06.2)
wood asthma (J67.8)

Excludes2: asthma with COPD (J44.9)
asthma with chronic obstructive pulmonary disease (J44.89)
chronic asthmatic (obstructive) bronchitis (J44.89)
chronic obstructive asthma (J44.89)
other specified chronic obstructive pulmonary disease (J44.89)

J45.2 Mild intermittent asthma

J45.20 Mild intermittent asthma, uncomplicated
Mild intermittent asthma NOS

J45.21 Mild intermittent asthma with (acute) exacerbation

J45.22 Mild intermittent asthma with status asthmaticus

J45.3 Mild persistent asthma

J45.30 Mild persistent asthma, uncomplicated
Mild persistent asthma NOS

J45.31 Mild persistent asthma with (acute) exacerbation

J45.32 Mild persistent asthma with status asthmaticus

J45.4 Moderate persistent asthma

J45.40 Moderate persistent asthma, uncomplicated
Moderate persistent asthma NOS

J45.41 Moderate persistent asthma with (acute) exacerbation

J45.42 Moderate persistent asthma with status asthmaticus

J45.5 Severe persistent asthma

J45.50 Severe persistent asthma, uncomplicated
Severe persistent asthma NOS

J45.51 Severe persistent asthma with (acute) exacerbation

J45.52 Severe persistent asthma with status asthmaticus

J45.9 Other and unspecified asthma

J45.90 Unspecified asthma
Asthmatic bronchitis NOS
Childhood asthma NOS
Late onset asthma

J45.901 Unspecified asthma with (acute) exacerbation

J45.902 Unspecified asthma with status asthmaticus

J45.909 Unspecified asthma, uncomplicated
Asthma NOS
Excludes2: lung diseases due to external agents (J60-J70)

J45.99 Other asthma

J45.990 Exercise induced bronchospasm

J45.991 Cough variant asthma

J45.998 Other asthma

(J60-J70) LUNG DISEASES DUE TO EXTERNAL AGENTS

Excludes2: asthma (J45.-)
malignant neoplasm of bronchus and lung (C34.-)

J69 PNEUMONITIS DUE TO SOLIDS AND LIQUIDS

Codes also, if applicable, other types of pneumonias
Excludes1: neonatal aspiration syndromes (P24.-)
postprocedural pneumonitis (J95.4)

J69.0 Pneumonitis due to inhalation of food and vomit
Aspiration pneumonia NOS
Aspiration pneumonia (due to) food (regurgitated)
Aspiration pneumonia (due to) gastric secretions
Aspiration pneumonia (due to) milk
Aspiration pneumonia (due to) vomit
Code also any associated FB in respiratory tract (T17.-)
Excludes1: chemical pneumonitis due to anesthesia (J95.4)

J69.1 Pneumonitis due to inhalation of oils and essences
Exogenous lipoid pneumonia
Lipid pneumonia NOS
Code first (T51-T65) to identify substance
Excludes1: endogenous lipoid pneumonia (J84.89)

J69.8 Pneumonitis due to inhalation of other solids and liquids
Pneumonitis due to aspiration of blood
Pneumonitis due to aspiration of detergent
Code first (T51-T65) to identify substance

J70 RESPIRATORY CONDITIONS DUE TO OTHER EXTERNAL AGENTS

J70.5 Respiratory conditions due to smoke inhalation
Code first smoke inhalation (T59.81-)
Excludes2: smoke inhalation due to chemicals, gases, fumes and vapors (J68.9)

J70.9 Respiratory conditions due to unspecified external agent
Code first (T51-T65) to identify the external agent

(J80-J84) OTHER RESPIRATORY DISEASES PRINCIPALLY AFFECTING THE INTERSTITIUM

J80 ACUTE RESPIRATORY DISTRESS SYNDROME

Acute respiratory distress syndrome in adult or child
Adult hyaline membrane disease
Excludes1: respiratory distress syndrome in newborn (perinatal) (P22.0)

J81 PULMONARY EDEMA

Use additional code to identify: *(See Chapter 10 guidelines for codes)*
Excludes1: chemical (acute) pulmonary edema (J68.1)
hypostatic pneumonia (J18.2)
passive pneumonia (J18.2)
pulmonary edema due to external agents (J60-J70)
pulmonary edema with heart disease NOS (I50.1)
pulmonary edema with heart failure (I50.1)

J81.0 Acute pulmonary edema
Acute edema of lung

J82 PULMONARY EOSINOPHILIA, NOT ELSEWHERE CLASSIFIED

J82.8 Pulmonary eosinophilia, NEC

J82.81 Chronic eosinophilic pneumonia
Eosinophilic pneumonia, NOS

J82.82 Acute eosinophilic pneumonia

J82.83 Eosinophilic asthma
Code first asthma, by type, such as:
mild intermittent asthma (J45.2-)
mild persistent asthma (J45.3-)
moderate persistent asthma (J45.4-)
severe persistent asthma (J45.5-)

J82.89 Other pulmonary eosinophilia, not elsewhere classified
Allergic pneumonia
Löffler's pneumonia
Tropical (pulmonary) eosinophilia NOS

J84 OTHER INTERSTITIAL PULMONARY DISEASES

4th **Code also**, if applicable, associated condition
Excludes1: drug-induced interstitial lung disorders (J70.2-J70.4)
interstitial emphysema (J98.2)
Excludes2: lung diseases due to external agents (J60-J70)

J84.0 Alveolar and parieto-alveolar conditions

5th J84.01 Alveolar proteinosis
J84.02 Pulmonary alveolar microlithiasis
J84.03 Idiopathic pulmonary hemosiderosis
Essential brown induration of lung
Code first underlying disease, such as:
disorders of iron metabolism (E83.1-)
Excludes1: acute idiopathic pulmonary hemorrhage in infants [AIPHI] (R04.81)

J84.09 Other alveolar and parieto-alveolar conditions

J84.8 Other specified interstitial pulmonary diseases

5th *Excludes1:* exogenous or unspecified lipoid pneumonia (J69.1)

J84.83 Surfactant mutations of the lung
J84.84 Other interstitial lung diseases of childhood

6th J84.841 Neuroendocrine cell hyperplasia of infancy
J84.842 Pulmonary interstitial glycogenosis
J84.843 Alveolar capillary dysplasia with vein misalignment
J84.848 Other interstitial lung diseases of childhood

J84.89 Other specified interstitial pulmonary disease

J84.9 Interstitial pulmonary disease, unspecified
Interstitial pneumonia NOS

(J85-J86) SUPPURATIVE AND NECROTIC CONDITIONS OF THE LOWER RESPIRATORY TRACT

J86 PYOTHORAX

4th Use additional code (B95-B97) to identify infectious agent.
Excludes1: abscess of lung (J85.-)
pyothorax due to tuberculosis (A15.6)

J86.0 Pyothorax with fistula
Bronchocutaneous fistula
Bronchopleural fistula
Hepatopleural fistula
Mediastinal fistula
Pleural fistula
Thoracic fistula
Any condition classifiable to J86.9 with fistula
Code also, if applicable, disruption of internal operation (surgical) wound (T81.32-)

J86.9 Pyothorax without fistula
Abscess of pleura
Abscess of thorax
Empyema (chest) (lung) (pleura)
Fibrinopurulent pleurisy
Purulent pleurisy
Pyopneumothorax
Septic pleurisy
Seropurulent pleurisy
Suppurative pleurisy

(J90-J94) OTHER DISEASES OF THE PLEURA

J90 PLEURAL EFFUSION, NEC

✓ Encysted pleurisy
Pleural effusion NOS
Pleurisy with effusion (exudative) (serous)
Excludes1: chylous (pleural) effusion (J94.0)
malignant pleural effusion (J91.0))
pleurisy NOS (R09.1)
tuberculous pleural effusion (A15.6)

J91 PLEURAL EFFUSION IN CONDITIONS CLASSIFIED ELSEWHERE

4th *Excludes2:* pleural effusion in heart failure (I50.-)
pleural effusion in SLE (M32.13)

J91.0 Malignant pleural effusion
Code first underlying neoplasm

J91.8 Pleural effusion in other conditions classified elsewhere
Code first underlying disease, such as:
filariasis (B74.0-B74.9)
influenza (J09.X2, J10.1, J11.1)

J93 PNEUMOTHORAX AND AIR LEAK

4th *Excludes1:* congenital or perinatal pneumothorax (P25.1)
postprocedural air leak (J95.812)
postprocedural pneumothorax (J95.811)
traumatic pneumothorax (S27.0)
tuberculous (current disease) pneumothorax (A15.-)
pyopneumothorax (J86.-)

J93.0 Spontaneous tension pneumothorax

J93.1 Other spontaneous pneumothorax

5th J93.11 Primary spontaneous pneumothorax
J93.12 Secondary spontaneous pneumothorax
Code first underlying condition, such as:
catamenial pneumothorax due to endometriosis (N80.8)
cystic fibrosis (E84.-)
eosinophilic pneumonia (J82.81-J82.82)
lymphangioleiomyomatosis (J84.81)
malignant neoplasm of bronchus and lung (C34.-)
Marfan's syndrome (Q87.4-)
pneumonia due to Pneumocystis carinii (B59)
secondary malignant neoplasm of lung (C78.0-)
spontaneous rupture of the esophagus (K22.3)

J93.8 Other pneumothorax and air leak

5th J93.81 Chronic pneumothorax
J93.82 Other air leak
Persistent air leak
J93.83 Other pneumothorax
Acute pneumothorax
Spontaneous pneumothorax NOS

J93.9 Pneumothorax, unspecified
Pneumothorax NOS

(J95) INTRAOPERATIVE AND POSTPROCEDURAL COMPLICATIONS AND DISORDERS OF RESPIRATORY SYSTEM, NEC

GUIDELINES

Documentation of Ventilator associated Pneumonia
As with all procedural or postprocedural complications, code assignment is based on the provider's documentation of the relationship between the condition and the procedure.

Code J95.851, Ventilator associated pneumonia (VAP), should be assigned only when the provider has documented VAP. An additional code to identify the organism (e.g., Pseudomonas aeruginosa, code B96.5) should also be assigned. Do not assign an additional code from categories J12-J18 to identify the type of pneumonia.

Code J95.851 should not be assigned for cases where the patient has pneumonia and is on a mechanical ventilator and the provider has not specifically stated that the pneumonia is ventilator-associated pneumonia. If the documentation is unclear as to whether the patient has a pneumonia that is a complication attributable to the mechanical ventilator, query the provider.

Ventilator associated Pneumonia Develops after Admission
A patient may be admitted with one type of pneumonia (e.g., code J13, Pneumonia due to Streptococcus pneumonia) and subsequently develop VAP. In this instance, the principal diagnosis would be the appropriate code from categories J12-J18 for the pneumonia diagnosed at the time of admission. Code J95.851, Ventilator associated pneumonia, would be assigned as an additional diagnosis when the provider has also documented the presence of ventilator associated pneumonia.

J95 INTRAOPERATIVE AND POSTPROCEDURAL COMPLICATIONS AND DISORDERS OF RESPIRATORY SYSTEM, NEC

4th *Excludes2:* aspiration pneumonia (J69.-)
emphysema (subcutaneous) resulting from a procedure (T81.82)
hypostatic pneumonia (J18.2)
pulmonary manifestations due to radiation (J70.0-J70.1)

J95.8 Other intraoperative and postprocedural complications and

5th **disorders of respiratory system, NEC**

4th 5th **6th** **7th** Additional Character Required ✓ 3-character code

*=New Code *Excludes1*—Not coded here, do not use together
▲=Revised Code *Excludes2*—Not included here

J95.81 Postprocedural pneumothorax and air leak

6th J95.811 Postprocedural pneumothorax

J95.812 Postprocedural air leak

J95.82 Postprocedural respiratory failure

6th *Excludes1:* Respiratory failure in other conditions (J96.-)

J95.821 Acute postprocedural respiratory failure
Postprocedural respiratory failure NOS

J95.822 Acute and chronic post-procedural respiratory failure

J95.83 Postprocedural hemorrhage of a respiratory system organ or structure; following a procedure

6th J95.830 following a respiratory system procedure

J95.831 following other procedure

J95.84 Transfusion-related acute lung injury (TRALI)

J95.85 Complication of respirator [ventilator]

6th **J95.850 Mechanical complication of respirator**

Excludes1: encounter for respirator [ventilator] dependence during power failure (Z99.12)

J95.851 Ventilator associated pneumonia
Ventilator associated pneumonitis
Use additional code to identify organism, if known (B95.-, B96.-, B97.-)
Excludes1: ventilator lung in newborn (P27.8)

J95.859 Other complication of respirator [ventilator]

J95.86 Postprocedural hematoma and seroma of a respiratory system organ or structure following a procedure

6th J95.860 Postprocedural hematoma of a respiratory system organ or structure following a respiratory system procedure

J95.861 Postprocedural hematoma of a respiratory system organ or structure following other procedure

J95.862 Postprocedural seroma of a respiratory system organ or structure following a respiratory system procedure

J95.863 Postprocedural seroma of a respiratory system organ or structure following other procedure

J95.87 Transfusion-associated dyspnea (TAD)

J95.88 Other intraoperative complications of respiratory system, NEC

J95.89 Other postprocedural complications and disorders of respiratory system, NEC

Use additional code to identify disorder, such as:
aspiration pneumonia (J69.-)
bacterial or viral pneumonia (J12-J18)
Excludes2: acute pulmonary insufficiency following thoracic surgery (J95.1)
postprocedural subglottic stenosis (J95.5)

(J96–J99) OTHER DISEASES OF THE RESPIRATORY SYSTEM

J96 RESPIRATORY FAILURE, NEC

4th **GUIDELINES**

Acute Respiratory Failure

AS PRINCIPAL DIAGNOSIS

A code from subcategory J96.0, Acute respiratory failure, or subcategory J96.2, Acute and chronic respiratory failure, may be assigned as a principal diagnosis when it is the condition established after study to be chiefly responsible for occasioning the admission to the hospital, and the selection is supported by the Alphabetic Index and Tabular List. However, chapter-specific coding guidelines (such as obstetrics, poisoning, HIV, newborn) that provide sequencing direction take precedence.

AS SECONDARY DIAGNOSIS

Respiratory failure may be listed as a secondary diagnosis if it occurs after admission, or if it is present on admission, but does not meet the definition of principal diagnosis.

SEQUENCING OF ACUTE RESPIRATORY FAILURE AND ANOTHER ACUTE CONDITION

When a patient is admitted with respiratory failure and another acute condition, (eg, myocardial infarction, cerebrovascular accident, aspiration pneumonia), the principal diagnosis will not be the same in every situation. This applies whether the other acute condition is a respiratory or nonrespiratory condition. Selection of the principal diagnosis will be dependent on the circumstances of admission. If both the respiratory failure and the other acute condition are equally responsible for occasioning the admission to the hospital, and there are no chapter-specific sequencing rules, the guideline regarding two or more diagnoses that equally meet the definition for principal diagnosis may be applied in these situations. If the documentation is not clear as to whether acute respiratory failure and another condition are equally responsible for occasioning the admission, query the provider for clarification.

Excludes1: acute respiratory distress syndrome (J80)
cardiorespiratory failure (R09.2)
newborn respiratory distress syndrome (P22.0)
postprocedural respiratory failure (J95.82-)
respiratory arrest (R09.2)
respiratory arrest of newborn (P28.81)
respiratory failure of newborn (P28.5)

J96.0 Acute respiratory failure

5th **J96.00 Acute respiratory failure, unspecified whether with hypoxia or hypercapnia**

J96.01 Acute respiratory failure with hypoxia

J96.02 Acute respiratory failure with hypercapnia

J96.1 Chronic respiratory failure

5th **J96.10 Chronic respiratory failure, unspecified whether with hypoxia or hypercapnia**

J96.11 Chronic respiratory failure with hypoxia

J96.12 Chronic respiratory failure with hypercapnia

J96.2 Acute and chronic respiratory failure

5th Acute on chronic respiratory failure

J96.20 Acute and chronic respiratory failure, unspecified whether with hypoxia or hypercapnia

J96.21 Acute and chronic respiratory failure with hypoxia

J96.22 Acute and chronic respiratory failure with hypercapnia

J96.9 Respiratory failure, unspecified

5th **J96.90 Respiratory failure, unspecified, unspecified whether with hypoxia or hypercapnia**

J96.91 Respiratory failure, unspecified with hypoxia

J96.92 Respiratory failure, unspecified with hypercapnia

J98 OTHER RESPIRATORY DISORDERS

4th **Use additional code** to identify (*See Chapter 10 guidelines for codes*)

Excludes1: newborn apnea (P28.4)
newborn sleep apnea (P28.3)
Excludes2: apnea NOS (R06.81)
sleep apnea (G47.3-)

J98.0 Diseases of bronchus, NEC

5th **J98.01 Acute bronchospasm**

Excludes1: acute bronchiolitis with bronchospasm (J21.-)
acute bronchitis with bronchospasm (J20.-)
asthma (J45.-)
exercise induced bronchospasm (J45.990)

J98.09 Other diseases of bronchus, not elsewhere classified
Broncholithiasis
Calcification of bronchus
Stenosis of bronchus
Tracheobronchial collapse
Tracheobronchial dyskinesia
Ulcer of bronchus

J98.1 Pulmonary collapse

5th *Excludes1:* therapeutic collapse of lung status (Z98.3)

J98.11 Atelectasis

Excludes1: newborn atelectasis
tuberculous atelectasis (current disease) (A15)

J98.2 Interstitial emphysema
Mediastinal emphysema
Excludes1: emphysema NOS (J43.9)
emphysema in newborn (P25.0)
surgical emphysema (subcutaneous) (T81.82)
traumatic subcutaneous emphysema (T79.7)

J98.4 Other disorders of lung
Calcification of lung
Cystic lung disease (acquired)
Lung disease NOS
Pulmolithiasis

J98.6 Disorders of diaphragm
Diaphragmatitis
Paralysis of diaphragm
Relaxation of diaphragm
Excludes1: congenital malformation of diaphragm NEC (Q79.1)
congenital diaphragmatic hernia (Q79.0)
Excludes2: diaphragmatic hernia (K44.-)

J98.8 Other specified respiratory disorders

J98.9 Respiratory disorder, unspecified
Respiratory disease (chronic) NOS

J99 RESPIRATORY DISORDERS IN DISEASES CLASSIFIED ELSEWHERE

Code first underlying disease, such as:
amyloidosis (E85.-)
ankylosing spondylitis (M45.-)
congenital syphilis (A50.-)
cryoglobulinemia (D89.1)
early congenital syphilis (A50.0-)
plasminogen deficiency (E88.02)
schistosomiasis (B65.0-B65.9)

Excludes1: respiratory disorders in:
amebiasis (A06.5)
blastomycosis (B40.0-B40.2)
candidiasis (B37.1)
coccidioidomycosis (B38.0-B38.2)
cystic fibrosis with pulmonary manifestations (E84.0)
dermatomyositis (M33.01, M33.11)
histoplasmosis (B39.0-B39.2)
late syphilis (A52.72, A52.73)
polymyositis (M33.21)
Sjögren syndrome (M35.02)
SLE (M32.13)
systemic sclerosis (M34.81)
Wegener's granulomatosis (M31.30-M31.31)

Chapter 11. Diseases of the digestive system (K00–K95)

Excludes2: certain conditions originating in the perinatal period (P04–P96)
certain infectious and parasitic diseases (A00–B99)
complications of pregnancy, childbirth and the puerperium (O00–O9A)
congenital malformations, deformations and chromosomal abnormalities (Q00–Q99)
endocrine, nutritional and metabolic diseases (E00–E88)
injury, poisoning and certain other consequences of external causes (S00–T88)
neoplasms (C00–D49)
symptoms, signs and abnormal clinical and laboratory findings, NEC (R00–R94)

(K00–K14) DISEASES OF ORAL CAVITY AND SALIVARY GLANDS

K00 DISORDERS OF TOOTH DEVELOPMENT AND ERUPTION

Excludes2: embedded and impacted teeth (K01.-)

K00.0 Anodontia
Hypodontia
Oligodontia
Excludes1: acquired absence of teeth (K08.1-)

K00.1 Supernumerary teeth
Distomolar
Fourth molar
Mesiodens
Paramolar
Supplementary teeth
Excludes2: supernumerary roots (K00.2)

K00.3 Mottled teeth
Dental fluorosis
Mottling of enamel
Nonfluoride enamel opacities
Excludes2: deposits [accretions] on teeth (K03.6)

K00.6 Disturbances in tooth eruption
Dentia praecox
Natal tooth
Neonatal tooth
Premature eruption of tooth
Premature shedding of primary [deciduous] tooth
Prenatal teeth
Retained [persistent] primary tooth
Excludes2: embedded and impacted teeth (K01.-)

K00.7 Teething syndrome

K00.8 Other disorders of tooth development
Color changes during tooth formation
Intrinsic staining of teeth NOS
Excludes2: posteruptive color changes (K03.7)

K00.9 Disorder of tooth development, unspecified
Disorder of odontogenesis NOS

K02 DENTAL CARIES

Includes: caries of dentine
early childhood caries
pre-eruptive caries
recurrent caries (dentino enamel junction) (enamel) (to the pulp)
dental cavities
tooth decay

K02.9 Dental caries, unspecified

K03 OTHER DISEASES OF HARD TISSUES OF TEETH

Excludes2: bruxism (F45.8)
dental caries (K02.-)
teeth-grinding NOS (F45.8)

K03.1 Abrasion of teeth
Dentifrice abrasion of teeth
Habitual abrasion of teeth
Occupational abrasion of teeth
Ritual abrasion of teeth
Traditional abrasion of teeth
Wedge defect NOS

K03.8 Other specified diseases of hard tissues of teeth

K03.81 Cracked tooth
Excludes1: broken or fractured tooth due to trauma (S02.5)

K03.89 Other specified diseases of hard tissues of teeth

K03.9 Disease of hard tissues of teeth, unspecified

K04 DISEASES OF PULP AND PERIAPICAL TISSUES

K04.7 Periapical abscess without sinus
Dental abscess without sinus
Dentoalveolar abscess without sinus
Periapical abscess without sinus

K04.8 Radicular cyst
Apical (periodontal) cyst
Periapical cyst
Residual radicular cyst
Excludes2: lateral periodontal cyst (K09.0)

K05 GINGIVITIS AND PERIODONTAL DISEASES

Use additional code to identify:
alcohol abuse and dependence (F10.-)
exposure to environmental tobacco smoke (Z77.22)
exposure to tobacco smoke in the perinatal period (P96.81)
history of tobacco dependence (Z87.891)
occupational exposure to environmental tobacco smoke (Z57.31)
tobacco dependence (F17.-)
tobacco use (Z72.0)

K05.0 Acute gingivitis
Excludes1: acute necrotizing ulcerative gingivitis (A69.1)
herpesviral [herpes simplex] gingivostomatitis (B00.2)

K05.00 Acute gingivitis, plaque induced
Acute gingivitis NOS
Plaque-induced gingival disease

K06 OTHER DISORDERS OF GINGIVA AND EDENTULOUS ALVEOLAR RIDGE

Excludes2: acute gingivitis (K05.0)
atrophy of edentulous alveolar ridge (K08.2)
chronic gingivitis (K05.1)
gingivitis NOS (K05.1)

K06.1 Gingival enlargement
Gingival fibromatosis

K08 OTHER DISORDERS OF TEETH AND SUPPORTING STRUCTURES

Excludes2: dentofacial anomalies [including malocclusion] (M26.-)
disorders of jaw (M27.-)

K08.1 Complete loss of teeth
Acquired loss of teeth, complete
Excludes1: congenital absence of teeth (K00.0)
exfoliation of teeth due to systemic causes (K08.0)
partial loss of teeth (K08.4-)

K08.10 Complete loss of teeth, unspecified cause

K08.101 Complete loss of teeth, unspecified cause; class I

K08.102 class II
K08.103 class III
K08.104 class IV
K08.109 unspecified class
Edentulism NOS

K08.11 Complete loss of teeth due to trauma

K08.111 Complete loss of teeth due to trauma; class I

K08.112 class II
K08.113 class III
K08.114 class IV
K08.119 unspecified class

K08.12 Complete loss of teeth due to periodontal diseases

K08.121 Complete loss of teeth due to periodontal diseases, class I

K08.122 class II
K08.123 class III
K08.124 class IV
K08.129 unspecified class

K08.13 Complete loss of teeth due to caries

K08.131 Complete loss of teeth due to caries; class I

K08.132 class II

K08.133 class III

K08.134 class IV

K08.139 unspecified class

K08.19 Complete loss of teeth due to other specified cause

K08.191 Complete loss of teeth due to other specified cause, class I

K08.192 class II

K08.193 class III

K08.194 class IV

K08.199 unspecified class

K08.4 Partial loss of teeth

Acquired loss of teeth, partial

Excludes1: complete loss of teeth (K08.1-)

congenital absence of teeth (K00.0)

Excludes2: exfoliation of teeth due to systemic causes (K08.0)

K08.40 Partial loss of teeth, unspecified cause

K08.401 Partial loss of teeth, unspecified cause; class I

K08.402 class II

K08.403 class III

K08.404 class IV

K08.409 unspecified class

Tooth extraction status NOS

K08.41 Partial loss of teeth due to trauma

K08.411 Partial loss of teeth due to trauma; class I

K08.412 class II

K08.413 class III

K08.414 class IV

K08.419 unspecified class

K08.42 Partial loss of teeth due to periodontal diseases

K08.421 Partial loss of teeth due to periodontal diseases, class I

K08.422 class II

K08.423 class III

K08.424 class IV

K08.429 unspecified class

K08.43 Partial loss of teeth due to caries

K08.431 Partial loss of teeth due to caries; class I

K08.432 class II

K08.433 class III

K08.434 class IV

K08.439 unspecified class

K08.49 Partial loss of teeth due to other specified cause

K08.491 Partial loss of teeth due to other specified cause, class I

K08.492 class II

K08.493 class III

K08.494 class IV

K08.499 unspecified class

K08.8 Other specified disorders of teeth and supporting structures

K08.81 Primary occlusal trauma

K08.82 Secondary occlusal trauma

K08.89 Other specified disorders of teeth and supporting structures

Enlargement of alveolar ridge NOS

Insufficient anatomic crown height

Insufficient clinical crown length

Irregular alveolar process

Toothache NOS

K08.9 Disorder of teeth and supporting structures, unspecified

K09 CYSTS OF ORAL REGION, NEC

Includes: lesions showing histological features both of aneurysmal cyst and of another fibro-osseous lesion

Excludes2: cysts of jaw (M27.0-, M27.4-)

radicular cyst (K04.8)

K09.0 Developmental odontogenic cysts

Dentigerous cyst

Eruption cyst

Follicular cyst

Gingival cyst

Lateral periodontal cyst

Primordial cyst

Excludes2: keratocysts (D16.4, D16.5)

odontogenic keratocystic tumors (D16.4, D16.5)

K09.1 Developmental (nonodontogenic) cysts of oral region

Cyst (of) incisive canal or palatine of papilla

Globulomaxillary cyst

Median palatal cyst

Nasoalveolar cyst

Nasolabial cyst

Nasopalatine duct cyst

K09.8 Other cysts of oral region, NEC

Dermoid cyst

Epidermoid cyst

Lymphoepithelial cyst

Epstein's pearl

K09.9 Cyst of oral region, unspecified

K11 DISEASES OF SALIVARY GLANDS

Use **additional code** to identify:

alcohol abuse and dependence (F10.-)

exposure to environmental tobacco smoke (Z77.22)

exposure to tobacco smoke in the perinatal period (P96.81)

history of tobacco dependence (Z87.891)

occupational exposure to environmental tobacco smoke (Z57.31)

tobacco dependence (F17.-)

tobacco use (Z72.0)

K11.2 Sialadenitis

Parotitis

Excludes1: epidemic parotitis (B26.-)

mumps (B26.-)

uveoparotid fever [Heerfordt] (D86.89)

K11.20 Sialadenitis, unspecified

K11.21 Acute sialadenitis

Excludes1: acute recurrent sialadenitis (K11.22)

K11.22 Acute recurrent sialadenitis

K11.23 Chronic sialadenitis

K11.3 Abscess of salivary gland

K11.4 Fistula of salivary gland

Excludes1: congenital fistula of salivary gland (Q38.4)

K11.7 Disturbances of salivary secretion

Hypoptyalism

Ptyalism

Xerostomia

Excludes2: dry mouth NOS (R68.2)

K11.8 Other diseases of salivary glands

Benign lymphoepithelial lesion of salivary gland

Mikulicz' disease

Necrotizing sialometaplasia

Sialectasia

Stenosis of salivary duct

Stricture of salivary duct

Excludes1: Sjögren syndrome (M35.0-)

K11.9 Disease of salivary gland, unspecified

Sialoadenopathy NOS

K12 STOMATITIS AND RELATED LESIONS

Use **additional code** to identify: alcohol abuse and dependence (F10.-)

exposure to environmental tobacco smoke (Z77.22)

exposure to tobacco smoke in the perinatal period (P96.81)

history of tobacco dependence (Z87.891)

occupational exposure to environmental tobacco smoke (Z57.31)

tobacco dependence (F17.-)

tobacco use (Z72.0)

Excludes1: cancrum oris (A69.0)

cheilitis (K13.0)

gangrenous stomatitis (A69.0)

herpesviral [herpes simplex] gingivostomatitis (B00.2)

noma (A69.0)

K12.0 Recurrent oral aphthae
Aphthous stomatitis (major) (minor)
Bednar's aphthae
Periadenitis mucosa necrotica recurrens
Recurrent aphthous ulcer
Stomatitis herpetiformis

K12.1 Other forms of stomatitis
Stomatitis NOS
Denture stomatitis
Ulcerative stomatitis
Vesicular stomatitis
Excludes1: acute necrotizing ulcerative stomatitis (A69.1)

K12.2 Cellulitis and abscess of mouth
Cellulitis of mouth (floor)
Submandibular abscess
Excludes2: abscess of salivary gland (K11.3)
abscess of tongue (K14.0)
periapical abscess (K04.6–K04.7)
periodontal abscess (K05.21)
peritonsillar abscess (J36)

K12.3 Oral mucositis (ulcerative)
Mucositis (oral) (oropharyngeal)
Excludes2: gastrointestinal mucositis (ulcerative) (K92.81)
mucositis (ulcerative) of vagina and vulva (N76.81)
nasal mucositis (ulcerative) (J34.81)

K12.30 Oral mucositis (ulcerative), unspecified

K13 OTHER DISEASES OF LIP AND ORAL MUCOSA

Includes: epithelial disturbances of tongue
Use additional code to identify:
alcohol abuse and dependence (F10.-)
exposure to environmental tobacco smoke (Z77.22)
exposure to tobacco smoke in the perinatal period (P96.81)
history of tobacco dependence (Z87.891)
occupational exposure to environmental tobacco smoke (Z57.31)
tobacco dependence (F17.-)
tobacco use (Z72.0)
Excludes2: certain disorders of gingiva and edentulous alveolar ridge (K05–K06)
cysts of oral region (K09.-)
diseases of tongue (K14.-)
stomatitis and related lesions (K12.-)

K13.0 Diseases of lips
Abscess of lips
Angular cheilitis
Cellulitis of lips
Cheilitis NOS
Cheilodynia
Cheilosis
Exfoliative cheilitis
Fistula of lips
Glandular cheilitis
Hypertrophy of lips
Perlèche NEC
Excludes1: ariboflavinosis (E53.0)
cheilitis due to radiation-related disorders (L55–L59)
congenital fistula of lips (Q38.0)
congenital hypertrophy of lips (Q18.6)
Perlèche due to candidiasis (B37.83)
Perlèche due to riboflavin deficiency (E53.0)

K13.1 Cheek and lip biting

K13.7 Other and unspecified lesions of oral mucosa

K13.70 Unspecified lesions of oral mucosa

K13.79 Other lesions of oral mucosa
Focal oral mucinosis

K14 DISEASES OF TONGUE

Use additional code to identify: alcohol abuse and dependence (F10.-)
exposure to environmental tobacco smoke (Z77.22)
history of tobacco dependence (Z87.891)
occupational exposure to environmental tobacco smoke (Z57.31)
tobacco dependence (F17.-)
tobacco use (Z72.0)

Excludes2: erythroplakia (K13.29)
focal epithelial hyperplasia (K13.29)
leukoedema of tongue (K13.29)
leukoplakia of tongue (K13.21)
hairy leukoplakia (K13.3)
macroglossia (congenital) (Q38.2)
submucous fibrosis of tongue (K13.5)

K14.0 Glossitis
Abscess of tongue
Ulceration (traumatic) of tongue
Excludes1: atrophic glossitis (K14.4)

K14.1 Geographic tongue
Benign migratory glossitis
Glossitis areata exfoliativa

K14.3 Hypertrophy of tongue papillae
Black hairy tongue
Coated tongue
Hypertrophy of foliate papillae
Lingua villosa nigra

K14.8 Other diseases of tongue
Atrophy of tongue
Crenated tongue
Enlargement of tongue
Glossocele
Glossoptosis
Hypertrophy of tongue

(K20–K31) DISEASES OF ESOPHAGUS, STOMACH AND DUODENUM

Excludes2: hiatus hernia (K44.-)

K20 ESOPHAGITIS

Use additional code to identify: alcohol abuse and dependence (F10.-)
Excludes1: erosion of esophagus (K22.1-)
esophagitis with gastro-esophageal reflux disease (K21.0-)
reflux esophagitis (K21.0-)
ulcerative esophagitis (K22.1-)
Excludes2: eosinophilic gastritis or gastroenteritis (K52.81)

K20.0 Eosinophilic esophagitis

K20.8 Other esophagitis

K20.80 Other esophagitis without bleeding
Abscess of esophagus
Other esophagitis NOS

K20.81 Other esophagitis with bleeding

K20.9 Esophagitis, unspecified

K20.90 Esophagitis, unspecified without bleeding
Esophagitis, NOS

K20.91 Esophagitis, unspecified with bleeding

K21 GASTRO-ESOPHAGEAL REFLUX DISEASE

Excludes1: newborn esophageal reflux (P78.83)

K21.0 Gastro-esophageal reflux disease (GERD) with esophagitis

K21.00 GERD with esophagitis, without bleeding
Reflux esophagitis

K21.01 GERD with esophagitis, with bleeding

K21.9 GERD without esophagitis
Esophageal reflux NOS

K22 OTHER DISEASES OF ESOPHAGUS

Excludes2: esophageal varices (I85.-)

K22.0 Achalasia of cardia
Achalasia NOS
Cardiospasm
Excludes1: congenital cardiospasm (Q39.5)

K22.1 Ulcer of esophagus
Barrett's ulcer
Erosion of esophagus
Fungal ulcer of esophagus
Peptic ulcer of esophagus
Ulcer of esophagus due to ingestion of chemicals
Ulcer of esophagus due to ingestion of drugs and medicaments
Ulcerative esophagitis
Code first poisoning due to drug or toxin, if applicable (T36-T65 with fifth or sixth character 1-4)

Use **additional** code for adverse effect, if applicable, to identify drug (T36-T50 with fifth or sixth character 5)

Excludes1: Barrett's esophagus (K22.7-)

- K22.10 Ulcer of esophagus without bleeding
  - Ulcer of esophagus NOS
- K22.11 Ulcer of esophagus with bleeding
  - *Excludes2:* bleeding esophageal varices (I85.01, I85.11)
- K22.4 Dyskinesia of esophagus
  - Corkscrew esophagus
  - Diffuse esophageal spasm
  - Spasm of esophagus
  - *Excludes1:* cardiospasm (K22.0)
- K22.8 Other specified diseases of esophagus
  - *Excludes2:* esophageal varices (I85.-)
  - Paterson-Kelly syndrome (D50.1)
  - K22.81 Esophageal polyp
    - *Excludes1:* benign neoplasm of esophagus (D13.0)
  - K22.82 Esophagogastric junction polyp
    - *Excludes1:* benign neoplasm of stomach (D13.1)
  - K22.89 Other specified disease of esophagus
    - Hemorrhage of esophagus NOS
- K22.9 Disease of esophagus, unspecified

K25 GASTRIC ULCER

Includes: erosion (acute) of stomach
pylorus ulcer (peptic)
stomach ulcer (peptic)

Use **additional** code to identify: alcohol abuse and dependence (F10.-)

Excludes1: acute gastritis (K29.0-)
peptic ulcer NOS (K27.-)

- K25.0 Acute gastric ulcer; with hemorrhage
- K25.1 with perforation
- K25.2 with both hemorrhage and perforation
- K25.3 without hemorrhage or perforation
- K25.4 Chronic or unspecified gastric ulcer; with hemorrhage
- K25.5 with perforation
- K25.6 with both hemorrhage and perforation
- K25.7 without hemorrhage or perforation
- K25.9 Gastric ulcer, unspecified as acute or chronic, without hemorrhage or perforation

K26 DUODENAL ULCER

Includes: erosion (acute) of duodenum
duodenum ulcer (peptic)
postpyloric ulcer (peptic)

Use **additional** code to identify: alcohol abuse and dependence (F10.-)

Excludes1: peptic ulcer NOS (K27.-)

- K26.0 Acute duodenal ulcer; with hemorrhage
- K26.1 with perforation
- K26.2 with both hemorrhage and perforation
- K26.3 without hemorrhage or perforation
- K26.4 Chronic or unspecified duodenal ulcer; with hemorrhage
- K26.5 with perforation
- K26.6 with both hemorrhage and perforation
- K26.7 without hemorrhage or perforation
- K26.9 Duodenal ulcer, unspecified as acute or chronic, without hemorrhage or perforation

K27 PEPTIC ULCER, SITE UNSPECIFIED

Includes: gastroduodenal ulcer NOS
peptic ulcer NOS

Use **additional** code to identify: alcohol abuse and dependence (F10.-)

Excludes1: peptic ulcer of newborn (P78.82)

- K27.0 Acute peptic ulcer, site unspecified; with hemorrhage
- K27.1 with perforation
- K27.2 with both hemorrhage and perforation
- K27.3 without hemorrhage or perforation
- K27.4 Chronic or unspecified peptic ulcer, site unspecified; with hemorrhage
- K27.5 with perforation
- K27.6 with both hemorrhage and perforation
- K27.7 without hemorrhage or perforation
- K27.9 Peptic ulcer, site unspecified, unspecified as acute or chronic, without hemorrhage or perforation

K29 GASTRITIS AND DUODENITIS

Excludes1: eosinophilic gastritis or gastroenteritis (K52.81)
Zollinger-Ellison syndrome (E16.4)

- K29.0 Acute gastritis
  - Use **additional** code to identify: alcohol abuse and dependence (F10.-)
  - *Excludes1:* erosion (acute) of stomach (K25.-)
  - K29.00 Acute gastritis without bleeding
  - K29.01 Acute gastritis with bleeding
- K29.7 Gastritis, unspecified
  - K29.70 Gastritis, unspecified, without bleeding
  - K29.71 Gastritis, unspecified, with bleeding
- K29.8 Duodenitis
  - K29.80 Duodenitis without bleeding
  - K29.81 Duodenitis with bleeding
- K29.9 Gastroduodenitis, unspecified
  - K29.90 Gastroduodenitis, unspecified, without bleeding
  - K29.91 Gastroduodenitis, unspecified, with bleeding

K30 FUNCTIONAL DYSPEPSIA

Indigestion

Excludes1: dyspepsia NOS (R10.13)
heartburn (R12)
nervous dyspepsia (F45.8)
neurotic dyspepsia (F45.8)
psychogenic dyspepsia (F45.8)

K31 OTHER DISEASES OF STOMACH AND DUODENUM

Includes: functional disorders of stomach

Excludes2: diabetic gastroparesis (E08.43, E09.43, E10.43, E11.43, E13.43)
diverticulum of duodenum (K57.00-K57.13)

- K31.0 Acute dilatation of stomach
  - Acute distention of stomach
- K31.1 Adult hypertrophic pyloric stenosis
  - Pyloric stenosis NOS
  - *Excludes1:* congenital or infantile pyloric stenosis (Q40.0)
- K31.3 Pylorospasm, NEC
  - *Excludes1:* congenital or infantile pylorospasm (Q40.0)
  - neurotic pylorospasm (F45.8)
  - psychogenic pylorospasm (F45.8)
- K31.5 Obstruction of duodenum
  - Constriction of duodenum
  - Duodenal ileus (chronic)
  - Stenosis of duodenum
  - Stricture of duodenum
  - Volvulus of duodenum
  - *Excludes 1:* congenital stenosis of duodenum (Q41.0)
- K31.6 Fistula of stomach and duodenum
  - Gastrocolic fistula
  - Gastrojejunocolic fistula
  - **Code also**, if applicable, disruption of internal operation (surgical) wound (T81.32-)
- K31.7 Polyp of stomach and duodenum
  - *Excludes1:* adenomatous polyp of stomach (D13.1)
- K31.8 Other specified diseases of stomach and duodenum
  - K31.83 Achlorhydria
  - K31.84 Gastroparesis
    - Gastroparalysis
    - **Code first** underlying disease, if known, such as:
      - anorexia nervosa (F50.0-)
      - diabetes mellitus (E08.43, E09.43, E10.43, E11.43, E13.43)
      - scleroderma (M34.-)
  - K31.89 Other diseases of stomach and duodenum
- K31.9 Disease of stomach and duodenum, unspecified
- K31.A Gastric intestinal metaplasia
  - K31.A0 Gastric intestinal metaplasia, unspecified
    - Gastric intestinal metaplasia indefinite for dysplasia
    - Gastric intestinal metaplasia NOS
  - K31.A1 Gastric intestinal metaplasia without dysplasia
    - K31.A11 Gastric intestinal metaplasia without dysplasia, involving the antrum
    - K31.A12 Gastric intestinal metaplasia without dysplasia, involving the body (corpus)
    - K31.A13 Gastric intestinal metaplasia without dysplasia, involving the fundus

K31.A14 Gastric intestinal metaplasia without dysplasia, involving the cardia

K31.A15 Gastric intestinal metaplasia without dysplasia, involving multiple sites

K31.A19 Gastric intestinal metaplasia without dysplasia, unspecified site

K31.A2 Gastric intestinal metaplasia with dysplasia

K31.A21 Gastric intestinal metaplasia with low grade dysplasia

K31.A22 Gastric intestinal metaplasia with high grade dysplasia

K31.A29 Gastric intestinal metaplasia with dysplasia, unspecified

(K35–K38) DISEASES OF APPENDIX

K35 ACUTE APPENDICITIS

K35.2 Acute appendicitis with generalized peritonitis

K35.20 Acute appendicitis with generalized peritonitis, without abscess

K35.200 Acute appendicitis with generalized peritonitis, without perforation or abscess

(Acute) appendicitis with generalized peritonitis without rupture or perforation of appendix NOS

K35.201 Acute appendicitis with generalized peritonitis, with perforation, without abscess

Appendicitis (acute) with generalized (diffuse) peritonitis following rupture or perforation of appendix NOS

K35.209 Acute appendicitis with generalized peritonitis, without abscess, unspecified as to perforation

(Acute) appendicitis with generalized peritonitis NOS

K35.21 Acute appendicitis with generalized peritonitis, with abscess

K35.210 Acute appendicitis with generalized peritonitis, without perforation, with abscess

(Acute) appendicitis with generalized peritonitis without rupture or perforation of appendix, with abscess

K35.211 Acute appendicitis with generalized peritonitis, with perforation and abscess

Appendicitis (acute) with generalized (diffuse) peritonitis following rupture or perforation of appendix, with abscess

K35.219 Acute appendicitis with generalized peritonitis, with abscess, unspecified as to perforation

(Acute) appendicitis with generalized peritonitis and abscess NOS

K35.3 Acute appendicitis with localized peritonitis

K35.30 Acute appendicitis with localized peritonitis, without perforation or gangrene

Acute appendicitis with localized peritonitis NOS

K35.31 Acute appendicitis with localized peritonitis and gangrene, without perforation

K35.32 Acute appendicitis with perforation, localized peritonitis, and gangrene, without abscess

(Acute) appendicitis with perforation NOS

Perforated appendix NOS

Ruptured appendix (with localized peritonitis) NOS

K35.33 Acute appendicitis with perforation, localized peritonitis, and gangrene, with abscess

(Acute) appendicitis with (peritoneal) abscess NOS

Ruptured appendix with localized peritonitis and abscess

K35.8 Other and unspecified acute appendicitis

K35.80 Unspecified acute appendicitis

Acute appendicitis NOS

Acute appendicitis without (localized) (generalized) peritonitis

K35.89 Other acute appendicitis

K35.890 Other acute appendicitis without perforation or gangrene

K35.891 Other acute appendicitis without perforation, with gangrene

K37 UNSPECIFIED APPENDICITIS

Excludes1: unspecified appendicitis with peritonitis (K35.2-, K35.3-)

(K40–K46) HERNIA

Note: Hernia with both gangrene and obstruction is classified to hernia with gangrene.

Includes: acquired hernia

congenital [except diaphragmatic or hiatus] hernia

recurrent hernia

K40 INGUINAL HERNIA

Includes: bubonocele

direct inguinal hernia

double inguinal hernia

indirect inguinal hernia

inguinal hernia NOS

oblique inguinal hernia

scrotal hernia

K40.0 Bilateral inguinal hernia, with obstruction, without gangrene

Inguinal hernia (bilateral) causing obstruction without gangrene

Incarcerated or Irreducible or Strangulated inguinal hernia (bilateral) without gangrene

K40.00 Bilateral inguinal hernia, with obstruction, without gangrene, not specified as recurrent

Bilateral inguinal hernia, with obstruction, without gangrene NOS

K40.01 Bilateral inguinal hernia, with obstruction, without gangrene, recurrent

K40.1 Bilateral inguinal hernia, with gangrene

K40.10 Bilateral inguinal hernia, with gangrene, not specified as recurrent

Bilateral inguinal hernia, with gangrene NOS

K40.11 Bilateral inguinal hernia, with gangrene, recurrent

K40.2 Bilateral inguinal hernia, without obstruction or gangrene

K40.20 Bilateral inguinal hernia, without obstruction or gangrene, not specified as recurrent

Bilateral inguinal hernia NOS

K40.21 Bilateral inguinal hernia, without obstruction or gangrene, recurrent

K40.3 Unilateral inguinal hernia, with obstruction, without gangrene

Inguinal hernia (unilateral) causing obstruction without gangrene

Incarcerated or Irreducible or Strangulated inguinal hernia (unilateral) without gangrene

K40.30 Unilateral inguinal hernia, with obstruction, without gangrene, not specified as recurrent

Inguinal hernia, with obstruction NOS

Unilateral inguinal hernia, with obstruction, without gangrene NOS

K40.31 Unilateral inguinal hernia, with obstruction, without gangrene, recurrent

K40.4 Unilateral inguinal hernia, with gangrene

K40.40 Unilateral inguinal hernia, with gangrene, not specified as recurrent

Inguinal hernia with gangrene NOS

Unilateral inguinal hernia with gangrene NOS

K40.41 Unilateral inguinal hernia, with gangrene, recurrent

K40.9 Unilateral inguinal hernia, without obstruction or gangrene

K40.90 Unilateral inguinal hernia, without obstruction or gangrene, not specified as recurrent

Inguinal hernia NOS

Unilateral inguinal hernia NOS

K40.91 Unilateral inguinal hernia, without obstruction or gangrene, recurrent

K42 UMBILICAL HERNIA

Includes: paraumbilical hernia

Excludes1: omphalocele (Q79.2)

K42.0 Umbilical hernia with obstruction, without gangrene
Umbilical hernia causing obstruction, without gangrene
Incarcerated or Irreducible or Strangulated umbilical hernia, without gangrene

K42.1 Umbilical hernia with gangrene
Gangrenous umbilical hernia

K42.9 Umbilical hernia without obstruction or gangrene
Umbilical hernia NOS

K43 VENTRAL HERNIA

K43.0 Incisional hernia with obstruction, without gangrene
Incisional hernia causing obstruction, without gangrene
Incarcerated or Irreducible or Strangulated incisional hernia, without gangrene

K43.1 Incisional hernia with gangrene
Gangrenous incisional hernia

K43.2 Incisional hernia without obstruction or gangrene
Incisional hernia NOS

K43.9 Ventral hernia without obstruction or gangrene
Epigastric hernia
Ventral hernia NOS

K44 DIAPHRAGMATIC HERNIA

Includes: hiatus hernia (esophageal) (sliding)
paraesophageal hernia
Excludes1: congenital diaphragmatic hernia (Q79.0)
congenital hiatus hernia (Q40.1)

K44.0 Diaphragmatic hernia with obstruction, without gangrene
Diaphragmatic hernia causing obstruction
Incarcerated or Irreducible or Strangulated diaphragmatic hernia

K44.1 Diaphragmatic hernia with gangrene
Gangrenous diaphragmatic hernia

K44.9 Diaphragmatic hernia without obstruction or gangrene
Diaphragmatic hernia NOS

K46 UNSPECIFIED ABDOMINAL HERNIA

Includes: enterocele
epiplocele
hernia NOS
interstitial hernia
intestinal hernia
intra-abdominal hernia
Excludes1: vaginal enterocele (N81.5)

K46.0 Unspecified abdominal hernia with obstruction, without gangrene
Unspecified abdominal hernia causing obstruction
Unspecified incarcerated abdominal hernia
Unspecified irreducible abdominal hernia
Unspecified strangulated abdominal hernia

K46.1 Unspecified abdominal hernia with gangrene
Any condition listed under K46 specified as gangrenous

K46.9 Unspecified abdominal hernia without obstruction or gangrene
Abdominal hernia NOS

(K50–K52) NONINFECTIVE ENTERITIS AND COLITIS

Includes: noninfective inflammatory bowel disease
Excludes1: irritable bowel syndrome (K58.-)
megacolon (K59.3-)

K50 CROHN'S DISEASE [REGIONAL ENTERITIS]

Includes: granulomatous enteritis
Use additional code to identify any associated fistulas, if applicable:
anal fistula (K60.3-)
anorectal fistula (K60.5-)
rectal fistula (K60.4-)
Use additional code to identify manifestations, such as: pyoderma gangrenosum (L88)
Excludes1: ulcerative colitis (K51.-)

K50.0 Crohn's disease of small intestine
Crohn's disease [regional enteritis] of duodenum or ileum or jejunum
Regional ileitis
Terminal ileitis
Excludes1: Crohn's disease of both small and large intestine (K50.8-)

K50.00 Crohn's disease of small intestine without complications

K50.01 Crohn's disease of small intestine with complications
- **K50.011** Crohn's disease of small intestine; with rectal bleeding
- **K50.012** with intestinal obstruction
- **K50.013** with fistula
- **K50.014** with abscess
- **K50.018** with other complication
- **K50.019** with unspecified complications

K50.1 Crohn's disease of large intestine
Crohn's disease [regional enteritis] of colon or large bowel or rectum
Granulomatous colitis
Regional colitis
Excludes1: Crohn's disease of both small and large intestine (K50.8)

K50.10 Crohn's disease of large intestine without complications

K50.11 Crohn's disease of large intestine with complications
- **K50.111** Crohn's disease of large intestine; with rectal bleeding
- **K50.112** with intestinal obstruction
- **K50.113** with fistula
- **K50.114** with abscess
- **K50.118** with other complication
- **K50.119** with unspecified complications

K50.8 Crohn's disease of both small and large intestine

K50.80 Crohn's disease of both small and large intestine without complications

K50.81 Crohn's disease of both small and large intestine with complications
- **K50.811** Crohn's disease of both small and large intestine; with rectal bleeding
- **K50.812** with intestinal obstruction
- **K50.813** with fistula
- **K50.814** with abscess
- **K50.818** with other complication
- **K50.819** with unspecified complications

K50.9 Crohn's disease, unspecified

K50.90 Crohn's disease, unspecified, without complications
Crohn's disease NOS
Regional enteritis NOS

K50.91 Crohn's disease, unspecified, with complications
- **K50.911** Crohn's disease, unspecified; with rectal bleeding
- **K50.912** with intestinal obstruction
- **K50.913** with fistula
- **K50.914** with abscess
- **K50.918** with other complication
- **K50.919** with unspecified complications

K51 ULCERATIVE COLITIS

Use additional code to identify manifestations, such as: pyoderma gangrenosum (L88)
Excludes1: Crohn's disease [regional enteritis] (K50.-)

K51.0 Ulcerative (chronic) pancolitis
Backwash ileitis

K51.00 Ulcerative (chronic) pancolitis without complications
Ulcerative (chronic) pancolitis NOS

K51.01 Ulcerative (chronic) pancolitis with complications
- **K51.011** Ulcerative (chronic) pancolitis; with rectal bleeding
- **K51.012** with intestinal obstruction
- **K51.013** with fistula
- **K51.014** with abscess
- **K51.018** with other complication
- **K51.019** with unspecified complications

K51.2 Ulcerative (chronic) proctitis

K51.20 Ulcerative (chronic) proctitis without complications
Ulcerative (chronic) proctitis NOS

K51.21 Ulcerative (chronic) proctitis with complications

6th **K51.211** Ulcerative (chronic) proctitis; with rectal bleeding

K51.212 with intestinal obstruction

K51.213 with fistula

K51.214 with abscess

K51.218 with other complication

K51.219 with unspecified complications

K51.3 Ulcerative (chronic) rectosigmoiditis

5th **K51.30** Ulcerative (chronic) rectosigmoiditis without complications
Ulcerative (chronic) rectosigmoiditis NOS

K51.31 Ulcerative (chronic) rectosigmoiditis with complications

6th **K51.311** Ulcerative (chronic) rectosigmoiditis; with rectal bleeding

K51.312 with intestinal obstruction

K51.313 with fistula

K51.314 with abscess

K51.318 with other complication

K51.319 with unspecified complications

K51.4 Inflammatory polyps of colon

5th *Excludes2:* adenomatous polyp of colon (D12.6)
polyposis of colon (D12.6)
polyps of colon NOS (K63.5)

K51.40 Inflammatory polyps of colon without complications
Inflammatory polyps of colon NOS

K51.41 Inflammatory polyps of colon with complications

6th **K51.411** Inflammatory polyps of colon; with rectal bleeding

K51.412 with intestinal obstruction

K51.413 with fistula

K51.414 with abscess

K51.418 with other complication

K51.419 with unspecified complications

K51.5 Left sided colitis

5th Left hemicolitis

K51.50 Left sided colitis without complications
Left sided colitis NOS

K51.51 Left sided colitis with complications

6th **K51.511** Left sided colitis; with rectal bleeding

K51.512 with intestinal obstruction

K51.513 with fistula

K51.514 with abscess

K51.518 with other complication

K51.519 with unspecified complications

K51.8 Other ulcerative colitis

5th **K51.80** Other ulcerative colitis without complications

K51.81 Other ulcerative colitis with complications

6th **K51.811** Other ulcerative colitis; with rectal bleeding

K51.812 with intestinal obstruction

K51.813 with fistula

K51.814 with abscess

K51.818 with other complication

K51.819 with unspecified complications

K51.9 Ulcerative colitis, unspecified

5th **K51.90** Ulcerative colitis, unspecified, without complications

K51.91 Ulcerative colitis, unspecified, with complications

6th **K51.911** Ulcerative colitis, unspecified; with rectal bleeding

K51.912 with intestinal obstruction

K51.913 with fistula

K51.914 with abscess

K51.918 with other complication

K51.919 with unspecified complications

K52 OTHER AND UNSPECIFIED NONINFECTIVE GASTROENTERITIS AND COLITIS

4th

K52.2 Allergic and dietetic gastroenteritis and colitis

5th Food hypersensitivity gastroenteritis or colitis
Use additional code to identify type of food allergy (Z91.01-, Z91.02-)
Excludes2: allergic eosinophilic colitis (K52.82)
allergic eosinophilic esophagitis (K20.0)
allergic eosinophilic gastritis (K52.81)
allergic eosinophilic gastroenteritis (K52.81)

K52.21 Food protein–induced enterocolitis syndrome (FPIES)
Use additional code for hypovolemic shock, if present (R57.1)

K52.22 Food protein–induced enteropathy

K52.29 Other allergic and dietetic gastroenteritis and colitis
Allergic proctocolitis
Food-induced eosinophilic proctocolitis
Food protein-induced proctocolitis
Food hypersensitivity gastroenteritis or colitis
Immediate gastrointestinal hypersensitivity
Milk protein-induced proctocolitis

K52.3 Indeterminate colitis
Colonic inflammatory bowel disease unclassified (IBDU)
Excludes1: unspecified colitis (K52.9)

K52.8 Other specified noninfective gastroenteritis and colitis

5th **K52.81** Eosinophilic gastritis or gastroenteritis
Eosinophilic enteritis
Excludes2: eosinophilic esophagitis (K20.0)

K52.82 Eosinophilic colitis
Excludes2: allergic proctocolitis (K52.29)
food-induced eosinophilic proctocolitis (K52.29)
food protein-induced enterocolitis syndrome (FPIES) (K52.21)
food protein-induced proctocolitis (K52.29)
milk protein-induced proctocolitis (K52.29)

K52.83 Microscopic colitis

6th **K52.831** Collagenous colitis

K52.832 Lymphocytic colitis

K52.838 Other microscopic colitis

K52.839 Microscopic colitis, unspecified

K52.89 Other specified noninfective gastroenteritis and colitis

K52.9 Noninfective gastroenteritis and colitis, unspecified
Colitis or Enteritis or Gastroenteritis NOS
Ileitis or Jejunitis or Sigmoiditis NOS
Excludes1: diarrhea NOS (R19.7)
functional diarrhea (K59.1)
infectious gastroenteritis and colitis NOS (A09)
neonatal diarrhea (noninfective) (P78.3)
psychogenic diarrhea (F45.8)

(K55–K64) OTHER DISEASES OF INTESTINES

K55 VASCULAR DISORDERS OF INTESTINES

4th **K55.0** Acute vascular disorders of intestine

5th *Excludes1:* necrotizing enterocolitis of newborn (P77.-)
Excludes2: angioectasia (angiodysplasia) duodenum (K31.81-)
Infarction of appendices epiploicae
Mesenteric (artery) (vein) embolism
Mesenteric (artery) (vein) infarction
Mesenteric (artery) (vein) thrombosis

K55.01 Ischemia of small intestines

6th **K55.011** Focal (segmental) acute (reversible) ischemia of small intestine

K55.012 Diffuse acute (reversible) ischemia of small intestine

K55.019 Acute (reversible) ischemia of small intestine, extent unspecified

K55.02 Infarction of small intestines

6th Gangrene or necrosis of small intestine

K55.021 Focal (segmental) acute infarction of small intestine

K55.022 Diffuse acute infarction of small intestine

4th 5th 6th 7th Additional Character Required ✓ 3-character code

●=New Code
▲=Revised Code

Excludes1—Not coded here, do not use together
Excludes2—Not included here

K55.029 Acute infarction of small intestine, extent unspecified

K55.03 Ischemia of small intestine

Acute fulminant ischemic colitis
Subacute ischemic colitis

K55.031 Focal (segmental) acute (reversible) ischemia of large intestine

K55.032 Diffuse acute (reversible) ischemia of large intestine

K55.039 Acute (reversible) ischemia of large intestine, extent unspecified

K55.04 Infarction of intestine, part unspecified

Gangrene or necrosis of large intestine

K55.041 Focal (segmental) acute infarction of large intestine

K55.042 Diffuse acute infarction of large intestine

K55.049 Acute infarction of large intestine, extent unspecified

K55.05 Ischemia of intestine, part unspecified

K55.051 Focal (segmental) acute (reversible) ischemia of intestine, part unspecified

K55.052 Diffuse acute (reversible) ischemia of intestine, part unspecified

K55.059 Acute (reversible) ischemia of intestine, part and extent unspecified

K55.06 Infarction of intestine, part unspecified

K55.061 Focal (segmental) acute infarction of intestine, part unspecified

K55.062 Diffuse acute infarction of intestine, part unspecified

K55.069 Acute infarction of intestine, part and extent unspecified

K55.1 Chronic vascular disorders of intestine

Chronic ischemic colitis
Chronic ischemic enteritis
Chronic ischemic enterocolitis
Ischemic stricture of intestine
Mesenteric atherosclerosis
Mesenteric vascular insufficiency

K55.3 Necrotizing enterocolitis

Excludes1: necrotizing enterocolitis of newborn (P77.-)
Excludes2: necrotizing enterocolitis due to Clostridium difficile (A04.7-)

K55.30 Necrotizing enterocolitis, unspecified
Necrotizing enterocolitis, NOS

K55.31 Stage 1 necrotizing enterocolitis
Necrotizing enterocolitis without pneumonia or perforation

K55.32 Stage 2 necrotizing enterocolitis
Necrotizing enterocolitis with pneumonia, without perforation

K55.33 Stage 3 necrotizing enterocolitis
Necrotizing enterocolitis with perforation
Necrotizing enterocolitis with pneumatosis and perforation

K55.9 Vascular disorder of intestine, unspecified

Ischemic colitis
Ischemic enteritis
Ischemic enterocolitis

K56 PARALYTIC ILEUS AND INTESTINAL OBSTRUCTION WITHOUT HERNIA

Excludes1: congenital stricture or stenosis of intestine (Q41–Q42)
cystic fibrosis with meconium ileus (E84.11)
ischemic stricture of intestine (K55.1)
meconium ileus NOS (P76.0)
neonatal intestinal obstructions classifiable to P76.-
obstruction of duodenum (K31.5)
postprocedural intestinal obstruction (K91.3-)

Excludes2: stenosis of anus or rectum (K62.4)

K56.0 Paralytic ileus

Paralysis of bowel, colon or intestine

Excludes1: gallstone ileus (K56.3)
ileus NOS (K56.7)
obstructive ileus NOS (K56.69-)

K56.1 Intussusception

Intussusception or invagination of bowel, colon, intestine or rectum

Excludes2: intussusception of appendix (K38.8)

K56.2 Volvulus

Strangulation of colon or intestine
Torsion or Twist of colon or intestine

Excludes2: volvulus of duodenum (K31.5)

K56.4 Other impaction of intestine

K56.41 Fecal impaction

Excludes1: constipation (K59.0-)
Excludes2: incomplete defecation (R15.0)

K56.49 Other impaction of intestine

K56.6 Other and unspecified intestinal obstruction

K56.60 Unspecified intestinal obstruction
Intestinal obstruction NOS

K56.600 Partial intestinal obstruction, unspecified as to cause
Incomplete intestinal obstruction, NOS

K56.601 Complete intestinal obstruction, unspecified as to cause

K56.609 Unspecified intestinal obstruction, unspecified as to partial versus complete obstruction
Intestinal obstruction NOS

K56.69 Other intestinal obstruction
Enterostenosis NOS
Obstructive ileus NOS
Occlusion or Stenosis or Stricture of colon or intestine NOS

Excludes1: intestinal obstruction due to specified condition-code to condition

K56.690 Other partial intestinal obstruction
Other incomplete intestinal obstruction

K56.691 Other complete intestinal obstruction

K56.699 Other intestinal obstruction unspecified as to partial versus complete obstruction
Other intestinal obstruction, NEC

K56.7 Ileus, unspecified

Excludes1: obstructive ileus (K56.69-)
Excludes2: intestinal obstruction with hernia (K40-K46)

K58 IRRITABLE BOWEL SYNDROME

Includes: irritable colon
spastic colon

K58.0 Irritable bowel syndrome with diarrhea

K58.1 Irritable bowel syndrome with constipation

K58.2 Mixed irritable bowel syndrome

K58.8 Other irritable bowel syndrome

▲ **K58.9** Irritable bowel syndrome, unspecified

K59 OTHER FUNCTIONAL INTESTINAL DISORDERS

Excludes1: change in bowel habit NOS (R19.4)
intestinal malabsorption (K90.-)
psychogenic intestinal disorders (F45.8)

Excludes2: functional disorders of stomach (K31.-)

K59.0 Constipation

Excludes1: fecal impaction (K56.41)
Excludes2: fecal impaction (K56.41)
incomplete defecation (R15.0)

K59.00 Constipation, unspecified

K59.01 Slow transit constipation

K59.02 Outlet dysfunction constipation

K59.03 Drug-induced constipation
Use additional code for adverse effect, if applicable, to identify drug (T36 –T50) with 5th or 6th character 5

K59.04 Chronic idiopathic constipation
Functional constipation

K59.09 Other constipation
Chronic constipation

K59.1 Functional diarrhea
Excludes1: diarrhea NOS (R19.7)
irritable bowel syndrome with diarrhea (K58.0)

K59.2 Neurogenic bowel, not elsewhere classified

K59.3 Megacolon, NEC
5th Dilatation of colon
Excludes1: congenital megacolon (aganglionic) (Q43.1)
megacolon (due to) (in) Chagas' disease (B57.32)
megacolon (due to) (in) Clostridium difficile (A04.7-)
megacolon (due to) (in) Hirschsprung's disease (Q43.1)

K59.31 Toxic megacolon
Code first (T51–T65) to identify toxic agent, if applicable

K59.39 Other megacolon
Megacolon NOS

K59.4 Anal spasm
Proctalgia fugax

K59.8 Other specified functional intestinal disorders

5th **K59.81 Ogilvie syndrome**
Acute colonic pseudo-obstruction (ACPO)

K59.89 Other specified functional intestinal disorders
Atony of colon
Pseudo-obstruction (acute) (chronic) of intestine

K59.9 Functional intestinal disorder, unspecified

K60 FISSURE AND FISTULA OF ANAL AND RECTAL REGIONS

4th *Excludes1:* fissure and fistula of anal and rectal regions with abscess or cellulitis (K61.-)
Excludes2: abscess or cellulitis of anal and rectal regions (K61.-)
anal sphincter tear (healed) (nontraumatic) (old) (K62.81)

K60.0 Acute anal fissure

K60.1 Chronic anal fissure

K60.2 Anal fissure, unspecified

K60.3 Anal fistula
5th **Code first**, if applicable:
Crohn's disease (K50.-)
ulcerative colitis (K51.-)
Excludes1: congenital fistula (Q43.6)

●**K60.30 Anal fistula, unspecified**
Anal fistula NOS

●**K60.31 Anal fistula, simple**
6th Low intersphincteric anal fistula
Superficial anal fistula

●**K60.311 Anal fistula, simple, initial**
Anal fistula, simple, new

●**K60.312 Anal fistula, simple, persistent**
Anal fistula, simple, chronic

●**K60.313 Anal fistula, simple, recurrent**
Anal fistula simple, occurring following complete healing

●**K60.319 Anal fistula, simple, unspecified**

●**K60.32 Anal fistula, complex**
6th Extrasphincteric anal fistula
High intersphincteric anal fistula
Suprasphincteric anal fistula
Transsphincteric anal fistula
Code also, if applicable:
perianal abscess (K61.0)
rectovaginal fistula (N82.3)
stenosis of anus and rectum (K62.4)

●**K60.321 Anal fistula, complex, initial**
Anal fistula, complex, new

●**K60.322 Anal fistula, complex, persistent**
Anal fistula, complex, chronic

●**K60.323 Anal fistula, complex, recurrent**
Anal fistula complex, occurring following complete healing

●**K60.329 Anal fistula, complex, unspecified**

K60.4 Rectal fistula
5th Fistula of rectum to skin
Code first, if applicable:
Crohn's disease (K50.-)
ulcerative colitis (K51.-)
Excludes1: rectovaginal fistula (N82.3)
vesicorectal fistula (N32.1)

●**K60.40 Rectal fistula, unspecified**
Rectal fistula NOS

●**K60.41 Rectal fistula, simple**
6th Low intersphincteric rectal fistula
Superficial rectal fistula

●**K60.411 Rectal fistula, simple, initial**
Rectal, fistula, simple, new

●**K60.412 Rectal fistula, simple, persistent**
Rectal fistula, simple, chronic

●**K60.413 Rectal fistula, simple, recurrent**
Rectal fistula, simple, occurring following complete healing

●**K60.419 Rectal fistula, simple, unspecified**

●**K60.42 Rectal fistula, complex**
6th Extrasphincteric rectal fistula
High intersphincteric rectal fistula
Suprasphincteric rectal fistula
Transsphincteric rectal fistula
Code also, if applicable:
perianal abscess (K61.0)
rectovaginal fistula (N82.3)
stenosis of anus and rectum (K62.4)

●**K60.421 Rectal fistula, complex, initial**
Rectal fistula, complex, new

●**K60.422 Rectal fistula, complex, persistent**
Rectal fistula, complex, chronic

●**K60.423 Rectal fistula, complex, recurrent**
Rectal fistula, complex, occurring following complete healing

●**K60.429 Rectal fistula, complex, unspecified**

K61 ABSCESS OF ANAL AND RECTAL REGIONS

4th *Includes:* abscess of anal and rectal regions
cellulitis of anal and rectal regions

K61.0 Anal abscess
Perianal abscess
Excludes2: intrasphincteric abscess (K61.4)

K61.1 Rectal abscess
Perirectal abscess
Excludes1: ischiorectal abscess (K61.39)

K61.2 Anorectal abscess

K61.3 Ischiorectal abscess
5th **K61.31 Horseshoe abscess**

K61.39 Other ischiorectal abscess
Abscess of ischiorectal fossa
Ischiorectal abscess, NOS

K61.4 Intrasphincteric abscess
Intersphincteric abscess

K61.5 Supralevator abscess

K62 OTHER DISEASES OF ANUS AND RECTUM

4th *Includes:* anal canal
Excludes2: colostomy and enterostomy malfunction (K94.0-, K94.1-)
fecal incontinence (R15.-)
hemorrhoids (K64.-)

K62.0 Anal polyp

K62.1 Rectal polyp
Excludes1: adenomatous polyp (D12.8)

K62.2 Anal prolapse
Prolapse of anal canal

K62.3 Rectal prolapse
Prolapse of rectal mucosa

K62.4 Stenosis of anus and rectum
Stricture of anus (sphincter)

K62.5 Hemorrhage of anus and rectum
Excludes1: gastrointestinal bleeding NOS (K92.2)
melena (K92.1)
neonatal rectal hemorrhage (P54.2)

K62.6 Ulcer of anus and rectum
Solitary ulcer of anus and rectum
Stercoral ulcer of anus and rectum

K62.8 Other specified diseases of anus and rectum

5th *Excludes2:* ulcerative proctitis (K51.2)

K62.81 Anal sphincter tear (healed) (nontraumatic) (old)
Tear of anus, nontraumatic
Use additional code for any associated fecal incontinence (R15.-)
Excludes2: anal fissure (K60.-)
anal sphincter tear (healed) (old) complicating delivery (O34.7-)
traumatic tear of anal sphincter (S31.831)

K62.82 Dysplasia of anus
Anal intraepithelial neoplasia I and II (AIN I and II) (histologically confirmed)
Dysplasia of anus NOS
Mild and moderate dysplasia of anus (histologically confirmed)
Excludes1: abnormal results from anal cytologic examination without histologic confirmation (R85.61-)
anal intraepithelial neoplasia III (D01.3)
carcinoma in situ of anus (D01.3)
HGSIL of anus (R85.613)
severe dysplasia of anus (D01.3)

K62.89 Other specified diseases of anus and rectum
Proctitis NOS
Use additional code for any associated fecal incontinence (R15.-)

K62.9 Disease of anus and rectum, unspecified

K63 OTHER DISEASES OF INTESTINE

4th

K63.0 Abscess of intestine
Excludes1: abscess of intestine with Crohn's disease (K50.014, K50.114, K50.814, K50.914)
abscess of intestine with diverticular disease (K57.0, K57.2, K57.4, K57.8)
abscess of intestine with ulcerative colitis (K51.014, K51.214, K51.314, K51.414, K51.514,K51.814, K51.914)
Excludes2: abscess of anal and rectal regions (K61.-)
abscess of appendix (K35.3-)

K63.2 Fistula of intestine
Code also, if applicable, disruption of internal operation (surgical) wound (T81.32-)

K63.3 Ulcer of intestine
Primary ulcer of small intestine
Excludes1: duodenal ulcer (K26.-)
gastrointestinal ulcer (K28.-)
gastrojejunal ulcer (K28.-)
jejunal ulcer (K28.-)
peptic ulcer, site unspecified (K27.-)
ulcer of intestine with perforation (K63.1)
ulcer of anus or rectum (K62.6)
ulcerative colitis (K51.-)

K63.5 Polyp of colon
Excludes2: adenomatous polyp of colon (D12.-)
inflammatory polyp of colon (K51.4-)
polyposis of colon (D12.6)

K63.8 Other specified diseases of intestine

5th **K63.81 Dieulafoy lesion of intestine**
Excludes2: Dieulafoy lesion of stomach and duodenum (K31.82)

K63.82 Intestinal microbial overgrowth

6th **K63.821 Small intestinal bacterial overgrowth**

7th **K63.8211 Small intestinal bacterial overgrowth, hydrogen-subtype**

K63.8212 Small intestinal bacterial overgrowth, hydrogen sulfide-subtype

K63.8219 Small intestinal bacterial overgrowth, unspecified

K63.822 Small intestinal fungal overgrowth

K63.829 Intestinal methanogen overgrowth, unspecified

K63.89 Other specified diseases of intestine

K63.9 Disease of intestine, unspecified

K64 HEMORRHOIDS AND PERIANAL VENOUS THROMBOSIS

4th *Includes:* piles
Excludes1: hemorrhoids complicating childbirth and the puerperium (O87.2)
hemorrhoids complicating pregnancy (O22.4)

K64.0 First degree hemorrhoids
Grade/stage I hemorrhoids
Hemorrhoids (bleeding) without prolapse outside of anal canal

K64.1 Second degree hemorrhoids
Grade/stage II hemorrhoids
Hemorrhoids (bleeding) that prolapse with straining, but retract spontaneously

K64.2 Third degree hemorrhoids
Grade/stage III hemorrhoids
Hemorrhoids (bleeding) that prolapse with straining and require manual replacement back inside anal canal

K64.3 Fourth degree hemorrhoids
Grade/stage IV hemorrhoids
Hemorrhoids (bleeding) with prolapsed tissue that cannot be manually replaced

K64.4 Residual hemorrhoidal skin tags
External hemorrhoids, NOS
Skin tags of anus

K64.5 Perianal venous thrombosis
External hemorrhoids with thrombosis
Perianal hematoma
Thrombosed hemorrhoids NOS

K64.8 Other hemorrhoids
Internal hemorrhoids, without mention of degree
Prolapsed hemorrhoids, degree not specified

K64.9 Unspecified hemorrhoids
Hemorrhoids (bleeding) NOS
Hemorrhoids (bleeding) without mention of degree

(K65–K68) DISEASES OF PERITONEUM AND RETROPERITONEUM

K65 PERITONITIS

4th **Use additional code** (B95–B97), to identify infectious agent, if known
Code also if applicable diverticular disease of intestine (K57.-)
Excludes1: acute appendicitis with generalized peritonitis (K35.2-)
aseptic peritonitis (T81.6)
benign paroxysmal peritonitis (E85.0)
chemical peritonitis (T81.6)
gonococcal peritonitis (A54.85)
neonatal peritonitis (P78.0–P78.1)
pelvic peritonitis, female (N73.3–N73.5)
periodic familial peritonitis (E85.0)
peritonitis due to talc or other foreign substance (T81.6)
peritonitis in chlamydia (A74.81) or in diphtheria (A36.89) or syphilis (late) (A52.74)
peritonitis in tuberculosis (A18.31)
peritonitis with or following appendicitis (K35.-)
retroperitoneal infections (K68.-)

K65.0 Generalized (acute) peritonitis
Pelvic peritonitis (acute), male
Subphrenic peritonitis (acute)
Suppurative peritonitis (acute)

K65.1 Peritoneal abscess
Abdominopelvic abscess
Abscess (of) omentum
Abscess (of) peritoneum
Mesenteric abscess
Retrocecal abscess
Subdiaphragmatic abscess
Subhepatic abscess
Subphrenic abscess

K65.2 **Spontaneous bacterial peritonitis**
Excludes1: bacterial peritonitis NOS (K65.9)

K65.8 **Other peritonitis**
Chronic proliferative peritonitis
Peritonitis due to urine

K65.9 **Peritonitis, unspecified**
Bacterial peritonitis NOS

K68 DISORDERS OF RETROPERITONEUM

K68.1 **Retroperitoneal abscess**
K68.19 **Other retroperitoneal abscess**

K68.2 **Retroperitoneal fibrosis**
Code also, if applicable, associated obstruction of ureter (N13.5)

K68.3 **Retroperitoneal hematoma**
Retroperitoneal hemorrhage

(K70–K77) DISEASES OF LIVER

Excludes1: jaundice NOS (R17)
Excludes2: hemochromatosis (E83.11-)
Reye's syndrome (G93.7)
viral hepatitis (B15–B19)
Wilson's disease (E83.01)

K73 CHRONIC HEPATITIS, NEC

Excludes1: alcoholic hepatitis (chronic) (K70.1-)
drug-induced hepatitis (chronic) (K71.-)
granulomatous hepatitis (chronic) NEC (K75.3)
reactive, nonspecific hepatitis (chronic) (K75.2)
viral hepatitis (chronic) (B15–B19)

K73.0 **Chronic persistent hepatitis, NEC**
K73.1 **Chronic lobular hepatitis, NEC**
K73.2 **Chronic active hepatitis, NEC**
K73.8 **Other chronic hepatitis, NEC**
K73.9 **Chronic hepatitis, unspecified**

K74 FIBROSIS AND CIRRHOSIS OF LIVER

Code also, if applicable, viral hepatitis (acute) (chronic) (B15-B19)
Excludes1: alcoholic cirrhosis (of liver) (K70.3)
alcoholic fibrosis of liver (K70.2)
cardiac sclerosis of liver (K76.1)
cirrhosis (of liver) with toxic liver disease (K71.7)
congenital cirrhosis (of liver) (P78.81)
pigmentary cirrhosis (of liver) (E83.110)

K74.5 **Biliary cirrhosis, unspecified**
K74.6 **Other and unspecified cirrhosis of liver**

K74.60 **Unspecified cirrhosis of liver**
Cirrhosis (of liver) NOS

K74.69 **Other cirrhosis of liver**
Cryptogenic cirrhosis (of liver)
Macronodular cirrhosis (of liver)
Micronodular cirrhosis (of liver)
Mixed type cirrhosis (of liver)
Portal cirrhosis (of liver)
Postnecrotic cirrhosis (of liver)

K75 OTHER INFLAMMATORY LIVER DISEASES

Excludes2: toxic liver disease (K71.-)

K75.2 **Nonspecific reactive hepatitis**
Excludes1: acute or subacute hepatitis (K72.0-)
chronic hepatitis NEC (K73.-)
viral hepatitis (B15-B19)

K75.3 **Granulomatous hepatitis, not elsewhere classified**
Excludes1: acute or subacute hepatitis (K72.0-)
chronic hepatitis NEC (K73.-)
viral hepatitis (B15-B19)

K75.9 **Inflammatory liver disease, unspecified**
Hepatitis NOS
Excludes1: acute or subacute hepatitis (K72.0-)
chronic hepatitis NEC (K73.-)
viral hepatitis (B15-B19)

K76 OTHER DISEASES OF LIVER

Excludes2: alcoholic liver disease (K70.-)
amyloid degeneration of liver (E85.-)
cystic disease of liver (congenital) (Q44.6)
hepatic vein thrombosis (I82.0)
hepatomegaly NOS (R16.0)
pigmentary cirrhosis (of liver) (E83.110)
portal vein thrombosis (I81)
toxic liver disease (K71.-)

K76.0 **Fatty (change of) liver, not elsewhere classified**
Nonalcoholic fatty liver disease (NAFLD)
Excludes1: nonalcoholic steatohepatitis (NASH) (K75.81)

K76.8 **Other specified diseases of liver**

K76.81 **Hepatopulmonary syndrome**
Code first underlying liver disease, such as:
alcoholic cirrhosis of liver (K70.3-)
cirrhosis of liver without mention of alcohol (K74.6-)

K76.82 **Hepatic encephalopathy**

K76.89 **Other specified diseases of liver**
Cyst (simple) of liver
Focal nodular hyperplasia of liver
Hepatoptosis

K76.9 **Liver disease, unspecified**

K77 LIVER DISORDERS IN DISEASES CLASSIFIED ELSEWHERE

Code first underlying disease, such as: amyloidosis (E85.-)
congenital syphilis (A50.0, A50.5)
congenital toxoplasmosis (P37.1)
infectious mononucleosis with liver disease (B27.0-B27.9 with .9)
schistosomiasis (B65.0–B65.9)

Excludes1: alcoholic hepatitis (K70.1-)
alcoholic liver disease (K70.-)
cytomegaloviral hepatitis (B25.1)
herpesviral [herpes simplex] hepatitis (B00.81)
mumps hepatitis (B26.81)
sarcoidosis with liver disease (D86.89)
secondary syphilis with liver disease (A51.45)
syphilis (late) with liver disease (A52.74)
toxoplasmosis (acquired) hepatitis (B58.1)
tuberculosis with liver disease (A18.83)

(K80–K87) DISORDERS OF GALLBLADDER, BILIARY TRACT AND PANCREAS

K80 CHOLELITHIASIS

Excludes1: retained cholelithiasis following cholecystectomy (K91.86)
Use additional code if applicable for associated gangrene of gallbladder (K82.A1), or perforation of gallbladder (K82.A2) for sub-categories K80.0-, K80.1-, K80.4-, K80.6-

K80.0 **Calculus of gallbladder with acute cholecystitis**
Any condition listed in K80.2 with acute cholecystitis

K80.00 **Calculus of gallbladder with acute cholecystitis without obstruction**

K80.01 **Calculus of gallbladder with acute cholecystitis with obstruction**

K80.1 **Calculus of gallbladder; with other cholecystitis**

K80.10 **with chronic cholecystitis without obstruction**
Cholelithiasis with cholecystitis NOS

K80.11 **with chronic cholecystitis with obstruction**

K80.12 **with acute and chronic cholecystitis without obstruction**

K80.13 **with acute and chronic cholecystitis with obstruction**

K80.18 **with other cholecystitis without obstruction**

K80.19 **with other cholecystitis with obstruction**

K80.2 **Calculus of gallbladder without cholecystitis**
Cholecystolithiasis with cholecystitis
Cholelithiasis (without cholecystitis)
Colic (recurrent) of gallbladder (without cholecystitis)
Gallstone (impacted) of cystic duct (without cholecystitis)
Gallstone (impacted) of gallbladder (without cholecystitis)

K80.20 Calculus of gallbladder without cholecystitis without obstruction

K80.21 Calculus of gallbladder without cholecystitis with obstruction

K80.5 Calculus of bile duct without cholangitis or cholecystitis

5th Choledocholithiasis (without cholangitis or cholecystitis)

Gallstone (impacted) of bile duct NOS (without cholangitis or cholecystitis)

Gallstone (impacted) of common duct (without cholangitis or cholecystitis)

Gallstone (impacted) of hepatic duct (without cholangitis or cholecystitis)

Hepatic cholelithiasis (without cholangitis or cholecystitis)

Hepatic colic (recurrent) (without cholangitis or cholecystitis)

K80.50 Calculus of bile duct without cholangitis or cholecystitis without obstruction

K80.51 Calculus of bile duct without cholangitis or cholecystitis with obstruction

K80.8 Other cholelithiasis

5th **K80.80** Other cholelithiasis without obstruction

K80.81 Other cholelithiasis with obstruction

K81 CHOLECYSTITIS

4th Use additional code if applicable for associated gangrene of gallbladder (K82.A1), or perforation of gallbladder (K82.A2)

Excludes1: cholecystitis with cholelithiasis (K80.-)

K81.0 Acute cholecystitis

Abscess of gallbladder

Angiocholecystitis

Emphysematous (acute) cholecystitis

Empyema of gallbladder

Gangrene of gallbladder

Gangrenous cholecystitis

Suppurative cholecystitis

K81.1 Chronic cholecystitis

K81.2 Acute cholecystitis with chronic cholecystitis

K81.9 Cholecystitis, unspecified

K82 OTHER DISEASES OF GALLBLADDER

4th *Excludes1:* nonvisualization of gallbladder (R93.2)

postcholecystectomy syndrome (K91.5)

K82.0 Obstruction of gallbladder

Occlusion of cystic duct or gallbladder without cholelithiasis

Stenosis of cystic duct or gallbladder without cholelithiasis

Stricture of cystic duct or gallbladder without cholelithiasis

Excludes1: obstruction of gallbladder with cholelithiasis (K80.-)

K82.3 Fistula of gallbladder

Code also, if applicable, disruption of internal operation (surgical) wound (T81.32-)

K82.8 Other specified diseases of gallbladder

Adhesions of cystic duct or gallbladder

Atrophy of cystic duct or gallbladder

Cyst of cystic duct or gallbladder

Dyskinesia of cystic duct or gallbladder

Hypertrophy of cystic duct or gallbladder

Nonfunctioning of cystic duct or gallbladder

Ulcer of cystic duct or gallbladder

K82.9 Disease of gallbladder, unspecified

K82.A Disorders of gallbladder in diseases classified elsewhere

5th Code first the type of cholecystitis (K81.-), or cholelithiasis with cholecystitis (K80.00-K80.19, K80.40-K80.47,K80.60-K80.67)

K82.A1 Gangrene of gallbladder in cholecystitis

K82.A2 Perforation of gallbladder in cholecystitis

K83 OTHER DISEASES OF BILIARY TRACT

4th *Excludes1:* postcholecystectomy syndrome (K91.5)

Excludes2: conditions involving the gallbladder (K81-K82)

conditions involving the cystic duct (K81-K82)

K83.1 Obstruction of bile duct

Occlusion of bile duct without cholelithiasis

Stenosis of bile duct without cholelithiasis

Stricture of bile duct without cholelithiasis

Excludes1: congenital obstruction of bile duct (Q44.3)

obstruction of bile duct with cholelithiasis (K80.-)

K83.8 Other specified diseases of biliary tract

Adhesions of biliary tract

Atrophy of biliary tract

Hypertrophy of biliary tract

Ulcer of biliary tract

K83.9 Disease of biliary tract, unspecified

K85 ACUTE PANCREATITIS

4th *Includes:* acute (recurrent) pancreatitis

subacute pancreatitis

K85.0 Idiopathic acute pancreatitis

5th **K85.00** Idiopathic acute pancreatitis without necrosis or infection

K85.01 Idiopathic acute pancreatitis with uninfected necrosis

K85.02 Idiopathic acute pancreatitis with infected necrosis

K85.8 Other acute pancreatitis

5th **K85.80** Other acute pancreatitis without necrosis or infection

K85.81 Other acute pancreatitis with uninfected necrosis

K85.82 Other acute pancreatitis with infected necrosis

K85.9 Acute pancreatitis, unspecified

5th Pancreatitis NOS

K85.90 Acute pancreatitis without necrosis or infection, unspecified

K85.91 Acute pancreatitis with uninfected necrosis, unspecified

K85.92 Acute pancreatitis with infected necrosis, unspecified

K86 OTHER DISEASES OF PANCREAS

4th *Excludes2:* fibrocystic disease of pancreas (E84.-)

islet cell tumor (of pancreas) (D13.7)

pancreatic steatorrhea (K90.3)

K86.2 Cyst of pancreas

K86.8 Other specified diseases of pancreas

5th **K86.81** Exocrine pancreatic insufficiency

K86.89 Other specified diseases of pancreas

Aseptic pancreatic necrosis, unrelated to acute pancreatitis

Atrophy of pancreas

Calculus of pancreas

Cirrhosis of pancreas

Fibrosis of pancreas

Pancreatic fat necrosis, unrelated to acute pancreatitis

Pancreatic infantilism

Pancreatic necrosis NOS, unrelated to acute pancreatitis

K86.9 Disease of pancreas, unspecified

(K90–K95) OTHER DISEASES OF THE DIGESTIVE SYSTEM

K90 INTESTINAL MALABSORPTION

4th *Excludes1:* intestinal malabsorption following gastrointestinal surgery (K91.2)

K90.0 Celiac disease

Celiac disease with steatorrhea

Celiac gluten-sensitive enteropathy

Nontropical sprue

Code also exocrine pancreatic insufficiency (K86.81)

Use additional code for *associated disorders including:*

dermatitis herpetiformis (L13.0)

gluten ataxia (G32.81)

K90.1 Tropical sprue

Sprue NOS

Tropical steatorrhea

K90.2 Blind loop syndrome, not elsewhere classified

Blind loop syndrome NOS

Excludes1: congenital blind loop syndrome (Q43.8)

postsurgical blind loop syndrome (K91.2)

K90.3 Pancreatic steatorrhea

K90.4 Other malabsorption due to intolerance

5th *Excludes2:* celiac gluten-sensitive enteropathy (K90.0)

lactose intolerance (E73.-)

K90.41 Non-celiac gluten sensitivity
Gluten sensitivity NOS
Non-celiac gluten sensitive enteropathy

K90.49 Malabsorption due to intolerance, NEC
Malabsorption due to intolerance to carbohydrate or fat or protein or starch

K90.8 Other intestinal malabsorption

K90.81 Whipple's disease

K90.82 Short bowel syndrome
Short gut syndrome

K90.821 Short bowel syndrome with colon in continuity
Short bowel syndrome with colonic continuity

K90.822 Short bowel syndrome without colon in continuity
Short bowel syndrome without colonic continuity

K90.829 Short bowel syndrome, unspecified

K90.83 Intestinal failure

K90.89 Other intestinal malabsorption

K90.9 Intestinal malabsorption, unspecified

K91 INTRAOPERATIVE AND POSTPROCEDURAL COMPLICATIONS AND DISORDERS OF DIGESTIVE SYSTEM, NEC

Excludes2: complications of artificial opening of digestive system (K94.-)
complications of bariatric procedures (K95.-)
gastrojejunal ulcer (K28.-)
postprocedural (radiation) retroperitoneal abscess (K68.11)
radiation colitis (K52.0)
radiation gastroenteritis (K52.0)
radiation proctitis (K62.7)

K91.2 Postsurgical malabsorption, NEC
Postsurgical blind loop syndrome
Excludes1: malabsorption osteomalacia in adults (M83.2)
malabsorption osteoporosis, postsurgical (M80.8-, M81.8)

K91.3 Postprocedural intestinal obstruction

K91.30 Postprocedural intestinal obstruction, unspecified as to partial versus complete
Postprocedural intestinal obstruction NOS

K91.31 Postprocedural partial intestinal obstruction
Postprocedural incomplete intestinal obstruction

K91.32 Postprocedural complete intestinal obstruction

K91.8 Other intraoperative and postprocedural complications and disorders of digestive system

K91.89 Other postprocedural complications and disorders of digestive system
Use additional code, if applicable, to further specify disorder
Excludes2: postprocedural retroperitoneal abscess (K68.11)

K92 OTHER DISEASES OF DIGESTIVE SYSTEM

Excludes1: neonatal gastrointestinal hemorrhage (P54.0–P54.3)

K92.0 Hematemesis

K92.1 Melena
Excludes1: occult blood in feces (R19.5)

K92.2 Gastrointestinal hemorrhage, unspecified
Gastric hemorrhage NOS
Intestinal hemorrhage NOS
Excludes1: acute hemorrhagic gastritis (K29.01)
hemorrhage of anus and rectum (K62.5)
angiodysplasia of stomach with hemorrhage (K31.811)
diverticular disease with hemorrhage (K57.-)
gastritis and duodenitis with hemorrhage (K29.-)
peptic ulcer with hemorrhage (K25–K28)

K92.8 Other specified diseases of the digestive system

K92.81 Gastrointestinal mucositis (ulcerative)
Code also type of associated therapy, such as:
antineoplastic and immunosuppressive drugs (T45.1X-)
radiological procedure and radiotherapy (Y84.2)
Excludes2: mucositis (ulcerative) of vagina and vulva (N76.81)
nasal mucositis (ulcerative) (J34.81)
oral mucositis (ulcerative) (K12.3-)

K92.89 Other specified diseases of the digestive system

K92.9 Disease of digestive system, unspecified

K94 COMPLICATIONS OF ARTIFICIAL OPENINGS OF THE DIGESTIVE SYSTEM

K94.0 Colostomy complications

K94.00 Colostomy complication, unspecified

K94.01 Colostomy hemorrhage

K94.02 Colostomy infection
Use additional code to specify type of infection, such as:
cellulitis of abdominal wall (L03.311)
sepsis (A40.-, A41.-)

K94.03 Colostomy malfunction
Mechanical complication of colostomy

K94.09 Other complications of colostomy

K94.2 Gastrostomy complications

K94.20 Gastrostomy complication, unspecified

K94.21 Gastrostomy hemorrhage

K94.22 Gastrostomy infection
Use additional code *to specify type of infection, such as:* sepsis (A40.-, A41.-)
cellulitis of abdominal wall (L03.311)

K94.23 Gastrostomy malfunction
Mechanical complication of gastrostomy

K94.29 Other complications of gastrostomy

Chapter 12. Diseases of the skin and subcutaneous tissue (L00–L99)

GUIDELINES

Pressure ulcer stages

See category L89.

Excludes2: certain conditions originating in the perinatal period (P04–P96)
certain infectious and parasitic diseases (A00–B99)
complications of pregnancy, childbirth and the puerperium (O00–O9A)
congenital malformations, deformations, and chromosomal abnormalities (Q00–Q99)
endocrine, nutritional and metabolic diseases (E00–E88)
lipomelanotic reticulosis (I89.8)
neoplasms (C00–D49)
symptoms, signs and abnormal clinical and laboratory findings, NEC (R00–R94)
systemic connective tissue disorders (M30–M36)
viral warts (B07.-)

(L00–L08) INFECTIONS OF THE SKIN AND SUBCUTANEOUS TISSUE

Use additional code (B95–B97) to identify infectious agent.

Excludes2: hordeolum (H00.0)
infective dermatitis (L30.3)
local infections of skin classified in Chapter 1
lupus panniculitis (L93.2)
panniculitis NOS (M79.3)
panniculitis of neck and back (M54.0-)
Perlèche NOS (K13.0)
Perlèche due to candidiasis (B37.0)
Perlèche due to riboflavin deficiency (E53.0)
pyogenic granuloma (L98.0)
relapsing panniculitis [Weber-Christian] (M35.6)
viral warts (B07.-)
zoster (B02.-)

L00 STAPHYLOCOCCAL SCALDED SKIN SYNDROME

✓ Ritter's disease

Use **additional code** to identify percentage of skin exfoliation (L49.-)

Excludes1: bullous impetigo (L01.03)
pemphigus neonatorum (L01.03)
toxic epidermal necrolysis [Lyell] (L51.2)

L01 IMPETIGO

Excludes1: impetigo herpetiformis (L40.1)

- **L01.0 Impetigo**
  - Impetigo contagiosa
  - Impetigo vulgaris
  - **L01.00 Impetigo, unspecified**
    - Impetigo NOS
  - **L01.01 Non-bullous impetigo**
  - **L01.02 Bockhart's impetigo**
    - Impetigo follicularis
    - Perifolliculitis NOS
    - Superficial pustular perifolliculitis
  - **L01.03 Bullous impetigo**
    - Impetigo neonatorum
    - Pemphigus neonatorum
  - **L01.09 Other impetigo**
    - Ulcerative impetigo
- **L01.1 Impetiginization of other dermatoses**

L02 CUTANEOUS ABSCESS, FURUNCLE AND CARBUNCLE

Use additional code to identify organism (B95–B96)

Excludes2: abscess of anus and rectal regions (K61.-)
abscess of female genital organs (external) (N76.4)
abscess of male genital organs (external) (N48.2, N49.-)

- **L02.0 Cutaneous abscess, furuncle and carbuncle of face**
  - **Excludes2:** abscess of ear, external (H60.0)
    - abscess of eyelid (H00.0)
    - abscess of head [any part, except face] (L02.8)
    - abscess of lacrimal gland (H04.0)
    - abscess of lacrimal passages (H04.3)
    - abscess of mouth (K12.2)
    - abscess of nose (J34.0)
    - abscess of orbit (H05.0)
    - submandibular abscess (K12.2)
  - **L02.01 Cutaneous abscess of face**
  - **L02.02 Furuncle of face**
    - Boil of face
    - Folliculitis of face
  - **L02.03 Carbuncle of face**

- **L02.1 Cutaneous abscess, furuncle and carbuncle of neck**
  - **L02.11 Cutaneous abscess of neck**
  - **L02.12 Furuncle of neck**
    - Boil of neck
    - Folliculitis of neck
  - **L02.13 Carbuncle of neck**

- **L02.2 Cutaneous abscess, furuncle and carbuncle of trunk**
  - **Excludes1:** non-newborn omphalitis (L08.82)
    - omphalitis of newborn (P38.-)
  - **Excludes2:** abscess of breast (N61.1)
    - abscess of buttocks (L02.3)
    - abscess of female external genital organs (N76.4)
    - abscess of male external genital organs (N48.2, N49.-)
    - abscess of hip (L02.4)
  - **L02.21 Cutaneous abscess of trunk**
    - **L02.211 Cutaneous abscess of; abdominal wall**
    - **L02.212 back [any part, except buttock]**
    - **L02.213 chest wall**
    - **L02.214 groin**
    - **L02.215 perineum**
    - **L02.216 umbilicus**
    - **L02.219 trunk, unspecified**
  - **L02.22 Furuncle of trunk**
    - Boil of trunk
    - Folliculitis of trunk
    - **L02.221 Furuncle of; abdominal wall**
    - **L02.222 back [any part, except buttock]**
    - **L02.223 chest wall**
    - **L02.224 groin**
    - **L02.225 perineum**
    - **L02.226 umbilicus**
    - **L02.229 trunk, unspecified**
  - **L02.23 Carbuncle of trunk**
    - **L02.231 Carbuncle of; abdominal wall**
    - **L02.232 back [any part, except buttock]**
    - **L02.233 chest wall**
    - **L02.234 groin**
    - **L02.235 perineum**
    - **L02.236 umbilicus**
    - **L02.239 trunk, unspecified**

- **L02.3 Cutaneous abscess, furuncle and carbuncle of buttock**
  - **Excludes1:** pilonidal cyst with abscess (L05.01)
  - **L02.31 Cutaneous abscess of buttock**
    - Cutaneous abscess of gluteal region
  - **L02.32 Furuncle of buttock**
    - Boil of buttock
    - Folliculitis of buttock
    - Furuncle of gluteal region
  - **L02.33 Carbuncle of buttock**
    - Carbuncle of gluteal region

- **L02.4 Cutaneous abscess, furuncle and carbuncle of limb**
  - **Excludes2:** Cutaneous abscess, furuncle and carbuncle of groin (L02.214, L02.224, L02.234)
    - Cutaneous abscess, furuncle and carbuncle of hand (L02.5-)
    - Cutaneous abscess, furuncle and carbuncle of foot (L02.6-)
  - **L02.41 Cutaneous abscess of; limb**
    - **L02.411 right axilla**
    - **L02.412 left axilla**
    - **L02.413 right upper limb**
    - **L02.414 left upper limb**
    - **L02.415 right lower limb**
    - **L02.416 left lower limb**

L02.42 Furuncle of; limb

6th Boil of limb

Folliculitis of limb

L02.421 right axilla

L02.422 left axilla

L02.423 right upper limb

L02.424 left upper limb

L02.425 right lower limb

L02.426 left lower limb

L02.43 Carbuncle of; limb

6th L02.431 right axilla

L02.432 left axilla

L02.433 right upper limb

L02.434 left upper limb

L02.435 right lower limb

L02.436 left lower limb

L02.5 Cutaneous abscess, furuncle and carbuncle of hand

5th **L02.51 Cutaneous abscess of; hand**

6th L02.511 right hand

L02.512 left hand

L02.52 Furuncle; hand

6th Boil of hand

Folliculitis of hand

L02.521 right hand

L02.522 left hand

L02.53 Carbuncle of; hand

6th L02.531 right hand

L02.532 left hand

L02.6 Cutaneous abscess, furuncle and carbuncle of foot

5th **L02.61 Cutaneous abscess of; foot**

6th L02.611 right foot

L02.612 left foot

L02.62 Furuncle of; foot

6th Boil of foot

Folliculitis of foot

L02.621 right foot

L02.622 left foot

L02.63 Carbuncle of; foot

6th L02.631 right foot

L02.632 left foot

L02.8 Cutaneous abscess, furuncle and carbuncle of other sites

5th **L02.81 Cutaneous abscess of; other sites**

6th L02.811 head [any part, except face]

L02.818 other sites

L02.82 Furuncle of; other sites

6th Boil of other sites

Folliculitis of other sites

L02.821 head [any part, except face]

L02.828 other sites

L02.83 Carbuncle of; other sites

6th L02.831 head [any part, except face]

L02.838 other sites

L02.9 Cutaneous abscess, furuncle and carbuncle, unspecified

5th **L02.91 Cutaneous abscess, unspecified**

L02.92 Furuncle, unspecified

Boil NOS

Furunculosis NOS

L02.93 Carbuncle, unspecified

L03 CELLULITIS AND ACUTE LYMPHANGITIS

4th *Excludes2:* cellulitis of anal and rectal region (K61.-)

cellulitis of external auditory canal (H60.1)

cellulitis of eyelid (H00.0)

cellulitis of female external genital organs (N76.4)

cellulitis of lacrimal apparatus (H04.3)

cellulitis of male external genital organs (N48.2, N49.-)

cellulitis of mouth (K12.2)

cellulitis of nose (J34.0)

eosinophilic cellulitis [Wells] (L98.3)

febrile neutrophilic dermatosis [Sweet] (L98.2)

lymphangitis (chronic) (subacute) (I89.1)

L03.0 Cellulitis and acute lymphangitis of finger and toe

5th Infection of nail

Onychia

Paronychia

Perionychia

L03.01 Cellulitis of; finger

6th Felon

Whitlow

Excludes1: herpetic whitlow (B00.89)

L03.011 right finger

L03.012 left finger

L03.02 Acute lymphangitis of; finger

6th Hangnail with lymphangitis of finger

L03.021 right finger

L03.022 left finger

L03.03 Cellulitis of; toe

6th L03.031 right toe

L03.032 left toe

L03.04 Acute lymphangitis of; toe

6th Hangnail with lymphangitis of toe

L03.041 right toe

L03.042 left toe

L03.1 Cellulitis and acute lymphangitis of other parts of limb

5th **L03.11 Cellulitis of other parts of limb**

6th *Excludes2:* cellulitis of fingers (L03.01-)

cellulitis of toes (L03.03-)

groin (L03.314)

L03.111 Cellulitis of; right axilla

L03.112 left axilla

L03.113 right upper limb

L03.114 left upper limb

L03.115 right lower limb

L03.116 left lower limb

L03.12 Acute lymphangitis of other parts of limb

6th *Excludes2:* acute lymphangitis of fingers (L03.2-)

acute lymphangitis of toes (L03.04-)

acute lymphangitis of groin (L03.324)

L03.121 Acute lymphangitis of; right axilla

L03.122 left axilla

L03.123 right upper limb

L03.124 left upper limb

L03.125 right lower limb

L03.126 left lower limb

L03.2 Cellulitis and acute lymphangitis of face and neck

5th **L03.21 Cellulitis and acute lymphangitis of face**

6th **L03.211 Cellulitis of face**

Excludes2: abscess of orbit (H05.01-)

cellulitis of ear (H60.1-)

cellulitis of eyelid (H00.0-)

cellulitis of head or scalp (L03.81)

cellulitis of lacrimal apparatus (H04.3)

cellulitis of lip (K13.0)

cellulitis of mouth (K12.2)

cellulitis of nose (internal) (J34.0)

cellulitis of orbit (H05.01-)

L03.212 Acute lymphangitis of face

L03.213 Periorbital cellulitis

Preseptal cellulitis

L03.22 Cellulitis and acute lymphangitis of neck

6th **L03.221 Cellulitis of neck**

L03.222 Acute lymphangitis of neck

L03.3 Cellulitis and acute lymphangitis of trunk

5th **L03.31 Cellulitis of trunk**

6th *Excludes2:* cellulitis of anal and rectal regions (K61.-)

cellulitis of breast NOS (N61.0)

cellulitis of female external genital organs (N76.4)

cellulitis of male external genital organs (N48.2, N49.-)

omphalitis of newborn (P38.-)

puerperal cellulitis of breast (O91.2)

L03.311 Cellulitis of; abdominal wall

Excludes2: cellulitis of umbilicus (L03.316)

cellulitis of groin (L03.314)

L03.312 back [any part except buttock]

L03.313 chest wall
L03.314 groin
L03.315 perineum
L03.316 umbilicus
L03.317 buttock
L03.319 trunk, unspecified

L03.32 Acute lymphangitis of; trunk

6th L03.321 abdominal wall
L03.322 back [any part except buttock]
L03.323 chest wall
L03.324 groin
L03.325 perineum
L03.326 umbilicus
L03.327 buttock
L03.329 trunk, unspecified

L03.8 Cellulitis and acute lymphangitis of other sites

5th L03.81 Cellulitis of; other sites

6th L03.811 head [any part, except face]
Cellulitis of scalp
Excludes2: cellulitis of face (L03.211)

L03.818 other sites

L03.89 Acute lymphangitis of; other sites

6th L03.891 head [any part, except face]
L03.898 other sites

L03.9 Cellulitis and acute lymphangitis, unspecified

5th L03.90 Cellulitis, unspecified
L03.91 Acute lymphangitis, unspecified
Excludes1: lymphangitis NOS (I89.1)

L04 ACUTE LYMPHADENITIS

4th *Includes:* abscess (acute) of lymph nodes, except mesenteric acute lymphadenitis, except mesenteric

Excludes1: chronic or subacute lymphadenitis, except mesenteric (I88.1)
enlarged lymph nodes (R59.-)
HIV disease resulting in generalized lymphadenopathy (B20)
lymphadenitis NOS (I88.9)
nonspecific mesenteric lymphadenitis (I88.0)

L04.0 Acute lymphadenitis of; face, head and neck
L04.1 trunk
L04.2 upper limb
Acute lymphadenitis of axilla or shoulder
L04.3 lower limb
Acute lymphadenitis of hip
Excludes2: acute lymphadenitis of groin (L04.1)
L04.8 other sites
L04.9 unspecified

L05 PILONIDAL CYST AND SINUS

4th L05.0 Pilonidal cyst and sinus with abscess

5th L05.01 Pilonidal cyst with abscess
Parasacral dimple with abscess
Excludes 2: congenital sacral dimple (Q82.6)
parasacral dimple (Q82.6)

L05.02 Pilonidal sinus with abscess

L05.9 Pilonidal cyst and sinus without abscess

5th L05.91 Pilonidal cyst without abscess
Parasacral or Pilonidal or Postanal dimple
Pilonidal cyst NOS
Excludes 2: congenital sacral dimple (Q82.6)
parasacral dimple (Q82.6)

L05.92 Pilonidal sinus without abscess
Coccygeal fistula
Coccygeal sinus without abscess
Pilonidal fistula

L08 OTHER LOCAL INFECTIONS OF SKIN AND SUBCUTANEOUS TISSUE

4th L08.0 Pyoderma
Dermatitis gangrenosa
Purulent or Septic or Suppurative dermatitis
Excludes1: pyoderma gangrenosum (L88)
pyoderma vegetans (L08.81)

L08.9 Local infection of the skin and subcutaneous tissue, unspecified

(L10–L14) BULLOUS DISORDERS

Excludes1: benign familial pemphigus [Hailey-Hailey] (Q82.8)
staphylococcal scalded skin syndrome (L00)
toxic epidermal necrolysis [Lyell] (L51.2)

(L20–L30) DERMATITIS AND ECZEMA

Note: In this block the terms dermatitis and eczema are used synonymously and interchangeably.

Excludes2: chronic (childhood) granulomatous disease (D71)
dermatitis gangrenosa (L08.0)
dermatitis herpetiformis (L13.0)
dry skin dermatitis (L85.3)
factitial dermatitis (L98.1)
perioral dermatitis (L71.0)
radiation-related disorders of the skin and subcutaneous tissue (L55–L59)
stasis dermatitis (I87.2)

L20 ATOPIC DERMATITIS

4th L20.0 Besnier's prurigo
L20.8 Other atopic dermatitis

5th *Excludes2:* circumscribed neurodermatitis (L28.0)

L20.81 Atopic neurodermatitis
Diffuse neurodermatitis
L20.82 Flexural eczema
L20.83 Infantile (acute) (chronic) eczema
L20.84 Intrinsic (allergic) eczema
L20.89 Other atopic dermatitis

L20.9 Atopic dermatitis, unspecified

L21 SEBORRHEIC DERMATITIS

4th *Excludes2:* infective dermatitis (L30.3)
seborrheic keratosis (L82.-)

L21.0 Seborrhea capitis
Cradle cap
L21.1 Seborrheic infantile dermatitis
L21.8 Other seborrheic dermatitis
L21.9 Seborrheic dermatitis, unspecified
Seborrhea NOS

L22 DIAPER DERMATITIS

✔ Diaper erythema
Diaper rash
Psoriasiform diaper rash

L23 ALLERGIC CONTACT DERMATITIS

4th *Excludes1:* allergy NOS (T78.40)
contact dermatitis NOS (L25.9)
dermatitis NOS (L30.9)

Excludes2: dermatitis due to substances taken internally (L27.-)
dermatitis of eyelid (H01.1-)
diaper dermatitis (L22)
eczema of external ear (H60.5-)
irritant contact dermatitis (L24.-)
perioral dermatitis (L71.0)
radiation-related disorders of the skin and subcutaneous tissue (L55–L59)

L23.0 Allergic contact dermatitis due to; metals
Allergic contact dermatitis due to chromium or nickel
L23.1 adhesives
L23.2 cosmetics
L23.3 drugs in contact with skin
Use additional code for adverse effect, if applicable, to identify drug (T36–T50 with fifth or sixth character 5)
Excludes2: dermatitis due to ingested drugs and medicaments (L27.0–L27.1)
L23.4 Allergic contact dermatitis due to; dyes
L23.5 other chemical products
Allergic contact dermatitis due to cement or to insecticide
L23.6 food in contact with the skin
Excludes2: dermatitis due to ingested food (L27.2)
L23.7 plants, except food
Excludes2: allergy NOS due to pollen (J30.1)

L23.8 Allergic contact dermatitis due to; other agents

- **L23.81** animal (cat) (dog) dander or hair
- **L23.89** other agents

L23.9 Allergic contact dermatitis, unspecified cause

Allergic contact eczema NOS

L24 IRRITANT CONTACT DERMATITIS

Excludes1: allergy NOS (T78.40)
contact dermatitis NOS (L25.9)
dermatitis NOS (L30.9)

Excludes2: allergic contact dermatitis (L23.-)
dermatitis due to substances taken internally (L27.-)
dermatitis of eyelid (H01.1-)
diaper dermatitis (L22)
eczema of external ear (H60.5-)
perioral dermatitis (L71.0)
radiation-related disorders of the skin and subcutaneous tissue (L55-L59)

L24.0 Irritant contact dermatitis due to detergents

L24.1 Irritant contact dermatitis due to oils and greases

L24.2 Irritant contact dermatitis due to solvents

Irritant contact dermatitis due to chlorocompound or cyclohexane or glycol or hydrocarbon or ketone

L24.3 Irritant contact dermatitis due to cosmetics

L24.4 Irritant contact dermatitis due to drugs in contact with skin

Use additional code for adverse effect, if applicable, to identify drug (T36-T50 with fifth or sixth character 5)

L24.5 Irritant contact dermatitis due to other chemical products

Irritant contact dermatitis due to cement
Irritant contact dermatitis due to insecticide
Irritant contact dermatitis due to plastic
Irritant contact dermatitis due to rubber

L24.8 Irritant contact dermatitis due to other agents

- **L24.81 Irritant contact dermatitis due to metals**
  Irritant contact dermatitis due to chromium
  Irritant contact dermatitis due to nickel
- **L24.89 Irritant contact dermatitis due to other agents**
  Irritant contact dermatitis due to dyes

L24.9 Irritant contact dermatitis, unspecified cause

Irritant contact eczema NOS

L24.A Irritant contact dermatitis due to friction or contact with body fluids

Excludes1: irritant contact dermatitis related to stoma or fistula (L24.B-)

Excludes2: erythema intertrigo (L30.4)

- **L24.A0 Irritant contact dermatitis due to friction or contact with body fluids, unspecified**
- **L24.A1 Irritant contact dermatitis due to saliva**
- **L24.A2 Irritant contact dermatitis due to fecal, urinary or dual incontinence**
  Excludes1: diaper dermatitis (L22)
- **L24.A9 Irritant contact dermatitis due to friction or contact with other specified body fluids**
  Irritant contact dermatitis related to endotracheal tube
  Wound fluids, exudate

L24.B Irritant contact dermatitis related to stoma or fistula

Use Additional code to identify any artificial opening status (Z93.-), if applicable, for contact dermatitis related to stoma secretions

- **L24.B0 Irritant contact dermatitis related to unspecified stoma or fistula**
  Irritant contact dermatitis related to fistula NOS
  Irritant contact dermatitis related to stoma NOS
- **L24.B1 Irritant contact dermatitis related to digestive stoma or fistula**
  Irritant contact dermatitis related to gastrostomy
  Irritant contact dermatitis related to jejunostomy
  Irritant contact dermatitis related to saliva or spit fistula
- **L24.B2 Irritant contact dermatitis related to respiratory stoma or fistula**
  Irritant contact dermatitis related to tracheostomy

- **L24.B3 Irritant contact dermatitis related to fecal or urinary stoma or fistula**
  Irritant contact dermatitis related to colostomy
  Irritant contact dermatitis related to enterocutaneous fistula
  Irritant contact dermatitis related to ileostomy

L25 UNSPECIFIED CONTACT DERMATITIS

Excludes1: allergic contact dermatitis (L23.-)
allergy NOS (T78.40)
dermatitis NOS (L30.9)
irritant contact dermatitis (L24.-)

Excludes2: dermatitis due to ingested substances (L27.-)
dermatitis of eyelid (H01.1-)
eczema of external ear (H60.5-)
perioral dermatitis (L71.0)
radiation-related disorders of the skin and subcutaneous tissue (L55-L59)

L25.0 Unspecified contact dermatitis due to cosmetics

L25.1 Unspecified contact dermatitis due to drugs in contact with skin

Use additional code for adverse effect, if applicable, to identify drug (T36-T50 with fifth or sixth character 5)

Excludes2: dermatitis due to ingested drugs and medicaments (L27.0-L27.1)

L25.2 Unspecified contact dermatitis due to dyes

L25.3 Unspecified contact dermatitis due to other chemical products

Unspecified contact dermatitis due to cement
Unspecified contact dermatitis due to insecticide

L25.4 Unspecified contact dermatitis due to food in contact with skin

Excludes2: dermatitis due to ingested food (L27.2)

L25.5 Unspecified contact dermatitis due to plants, except food

Excludes1: nettle rash (L50.9)

Excludes2: allergy NOS due to pollen (J30.1)

L25.8 Unspecified contact dermatitis due to other agents

L25.9 Unspecified contact dermatitis, unspecified cause

Contact dermatitis (occupational) NOS
Contact eczema (occupational) NOS

L26 EXFOLIATIVE DERMATITIS

Hebra's pityriasis

Excludes1: Ritter's disease (L00)

L27 DERMATITIS DUE TO SUBSTANCES TAKEN INTERNALLY

Excludes1: allergy NOS (T78.40)

Excludes2: adverse food reaction, except dermatitis (T78.0-T78.1)
contact dermatitis (L23-L25)
drug photoallergic response (L56.1)
drug phototoxic response (L56.0)
urticaria (L50.-)

L27.0 Generalized skin eruption due to drugs and medicaments taken internally

Use additional code for adverse effect, if applicable, to identify drug (T36-T50 with fifth or sixth character 5)

L27.1 Localized skin eruption due to drugs and medicaments taken internally

Use additional code for adverse effect, if applicable, to identify drug (T36-T50 with fifth or sixth character 5)

L27.2 Dermatitis due to ingested food

Excludes2: dermatitis due to food in contact with skin (L23.6, L24.6, L25.4)

L27.8 Dermatitis due to other substances taken internally

L27.9 Dermatitis due to unspecified substance taken internally

L28 LICHEN SIMPLEX CHRONICUS AND PRURIGO

L28.0 Lichen simplex chronicus

Circumscribed neurodermatitis
Lichen NOS

L28.1 Prurigo nodularis

L28.2 Other prurigo

Prurigo NOS
Prurigo Hebra
Prurigo mitis
Urticaria papulosa

L29 PRURITUS

Excludes1: neurotic excoriation (L98.1)
psychogenic pruritus (F45.8)

- **L29.0 Pruritus ani**
- **L29.1 Pruritus scroti**
- **L29.2 Pruritus vulvae**
- **L29.3 Anogenital pruritus, unspecified**
- **L29.8 Other pruritus**
  - **●L29.81 Cholestatic pruritus**
    - **Code also**, if applicable, type of liver disease
    - **Use additional code** for adverse effect, if applicable, to identify drug (T36–T50 with fifth or sixth character 5)
  - **●L29.89 Other pruritus**
- **L29.9 Pruritus, unspecified**
  - Itch NOS

L30 OTHER AND UNSPECIFIED DERMATITIS

Excludes2: contact dermatitis (L23–L25)

- dry skin dermatitis (L85.3)
- small plaque parapsoriasis (L41.3)
- stasis dermatitis (I83.1–.2)
- **L30.1 Dyshidrosis [pompholyx]**
- **L30.3 Infective dermatitis**
  - Infectious eczematoid dermatitis
- **L30.4 Erythema intertrigo**
- **L30.5 Pityriasis alba**
- **L30.8 Other specified dermatitis**
- **L30.9 Dermatitis, unspecified**
  - Eczema NOS

(L40–L45) PAPULOSQUAMOUS DISORDERS

L40 PSORIASIS

- **L40.5 Arthropathic psoriasis**
  - **L40.54 Psoriatic juvenile arthropathy**
- **L40.8 Other psoriasis**
  - Flexural psoriasis
- **L40.9 Psoriasis, unspecified**

L42 PITYRIASIS ROSEA

✓

L44 OTHER PAPULOSQUAMOUS DISORDERS

- **L44.0 Pityriasis rubra pilaris**
- **L44.1 Lichen nitidus**
- **L44.2 Lichen striatus**
- **L44.3 Lichen ruber moniliformis**
- **L44.4 Infantile papular acrodermatitis [Gianotti-Crosti]**
- **L44.8 Other specified papulosquamous disorders**
- **L44.9 Papulosquamous disorder, unspecified**

(L49–L54) URTICARIA AND ERYTHEMA

Excludes1: Lyme disease (A69.2-)
rosacea (L71.-)

L50 URTICARIA

Excludes1: allergic contact dermatitis (L23.-)
angioneurotic edema or giant urticarial or Quincke's edema (T78.3)
hereditary angio-edema (D84.1)
serum urticaria (T80.6-)
solar urticaria (L56.3)
urticaria neonatorum (P83.8)
urticaria papulosa (L28.2)
urticaria pigmentosa (D47.01)

- **L50.0 Allergic urticaria**
- **L50.1 Idiopathic urticaria**
- **L50.2 Urticaria due to cold and heat**
  - **Excludes2:** familial cold urticaria (M04.2)
- **L50.3 Dermatographic urticaria**
- **L50.4 Vibratory urticaria**
- **L50.5 Cholinergic urticaria**
- **L50.6 Contact urticaria**
- **L50.8 Other urticaria**
  - Chronic urticaria
  - Recurrent periodic urticaria
- **L50.9 Urticaria, unspecified**

L51 ERYTHEMA MULTIFORME

Use additional code for adverse effect, if applicable, to identify drug (T36–T50 with fifth or sixth character 5)

Use additional code to identify associated manifestations, such as:
arthropathy associated with dermatological disorders (M14.8-)
conjunctival edema (H11.42)
conjunctivitis (H10.22-)
corneal scars and opacities (H17.-)
corneal ulcer (H16.0-)
edema of eyelid (H02.84-)
inflammation of eyelid (H01.8)
keratoconjunctivitis sicca (H16.22-)
mechanical lagophthalmos (H02.22-)
stomatitis (K12.-)
symblepharon (H11.23-)

Use additional code to identify percentage of skin exfoliation (L49.-)

Excludes1: staphylococcal scalded skin syndrome (L00)
Ritter's disease (L00)

- **L51.0 Nonbullous erythema multiforme**
- **L51.1 Stevens-Johnson syndrome**
- **L51.2 Toxic epidermal necrolysis [Lyell]**
- **L51.3 Stevens-Johnson syndrome-toxic epidermal necrolysis overlap syndrome**
  - SJS-TEN overlap syndrome
- **L51.8 Other erythema multiforme**
- **L51.9 Erythema multiforme, unspecified**
  - Erythema iris
  - Erythema multiforme major NOS
  - Erythema multiforme minor NOS
  - Herpes iris

L52 ERYTHEMA NODOSUM

✓

Excludes1: tuberculous erythema nodosum (A18.4)

L53 OTHER ERYTHEMATOUS CONDITIONS

Excludes1: erythema ab igne (L59.0)
erythema due to external agents in contact with skin (L23-L25)
erythema intertrigo (L30.4)

- **L53.0 Toxic erythema**
  - **Code first** poisoning due to drug or toxin, if applicable (T36-T65 with fifth or sixth character 1-4)
  - **Use additional code** for adverse effect, if applicable, to identify drug (T36-T50 with fifth or sixth character 5)
  - **Excludes1:** neonatal erythema toxicum (P83.1)
- **L53.1 Erythema annulare centrifugum**
- **L53.2 Erythema marginatum**
- **L53.8 Other specified erythematous conditions**
- **L53.9 Erythematous condition, unspecified**
  - Erythema NOS
  - Erythroderma NOS

(L55–L59) RADIATION-RELATED DISORDERS OF THE SKIN AND SUBCUTANEOUS TISSUE

L55 SUNBURN

- **L55.0 Sunburn of first degree**
- **L55.1 Sunburn of second degree**
- **L55.2 Sunburn of third degree**
- **L55.9 Sunburn, unspecified**

L56 OTHER ACUTE SKIN CHANGES DUE TO ULTRAVIOLET RADIATION

Use additional code to identify the source of the ultraviolet radiation (W89, X32)

- **L56.0 Drug phototoxic response**
  - **Use additional code** for adverse effect, if applicable, to identify drug (T36-T50 with fifth or sixth character 5)
- **L56.1 Drug photoallergic response**
  - **Use additional code** for adverse effect, if applicable, to identify drug (T36-T50 with fifth or sixth character 5)
- **L56.3 Solar urticaria**
- **L56.8 Other specified acute skin changes due to ultraviolet radiation**
- **L56.9 Acute skin change due to ultraviolet radiation, unspecified**

(L60–L75) DISORDERS OF SKIN APPENDAGES

Excludes1: congenital malformations of integument (Q84.-)

L60 NAIL DISORDERS

Excludes2: clubbing of nails (R68.3)
onychia and paronychia (L03.0-)

- L60.0 Ingrowing nail
- L60.1 Onycholysis
- L60.3 Nail dystrophy
- L60.8 Other nail disorders
- L60.9 Nail disorder, unspecified

L65 OTHER NON-SCARRING HAIR LOSS

Use additional code for adverse effect, if applicable, to identify drug (T36–T50 with fifth or sixth character 5)

Excludes1: trichotillomania (F63.3)

- L65.8 Other specified non-scarring hair loss
- L65.9 Non-scarring hair loss, unspecified
Alopecia NOS

L68 HYPERTRICHOSIS

Includes: excess hair

Excludes1: congenital hypertrichosis (Q84.2)
persistent lanugo (Q84.2)

- L68.0 Hirsutism

L70 ACNE

Excludes2: acne keloid (L73.0)

- L70.0 Acne vulgaris
- L70.1 Acne conglobata
- L70.2 Acne varioliformis
Acne necrotica miliaris
- L70.3 Acne tropica
- L70.4 Infantile acne
- L70.5 Acné excoriée
Acné excoriée des jeunes filles
Picker's acne
- L70.8 Other acne
- L70.9 Acne, unspecified

L72 FOLLICULAR CYSTS OF SKIN AND SUBCUTANEOUS TISSUE

- L72.0 Epidermal cyst
- L72.1 Pilar and trichodermal cyst
  - L72.11 Pilar cyst
  - L72.12 Trichodermal cyst
Trichilemmal (proliferating) cyst
- L72.3 Sebaceous cyst
Excludes2: pilar cyst (L72.11)
trichilemmal (proliferating) cyst (L72.12)
- L72.8 Other follicular cysts of the skin and subcutaneous tissue
- L72.9 Follicular cyst of the skin and subcutaneous tissue, unspecified

L73 OTHER FOLLICULAR DISORDERS

- L73.0 Acne keloid
- L73.1 Pseudofolliculitis barbae
- L73.2 Hidradenitis suppurativa
- L73.8 Other specified follicular disorders
Sycosis barbae
- L73.9 Follicular disorder, unspecified

L74 ECCRINE SWEAT DISORDERS

Excludes2: generalized hyperhidrosis (R61)

- L74.0 Miliaria rubra
- L74.1 Miliaria crystallina
- L74.3 Miliaria, unspecified
- L74.5 Focal hyperhidrosis
  - L74.51 Primary focal hyperhidrosis
    - L74.510 Primary focal hyperhidrosis, axilla
    - L74.511 Primary focal hyperhidrosis, face
    - L74.512 Primary focal hyperhidrosis, palms
    - L74.513 Primary focal hyperhidrosis, soles
    - L74.519 Primary focal hyperhidrosis, unspecified
  - L74.52 Secondary focal hyperhidrosis
Frey's syndrome

(L76) INTRAOPERATIVE AND POSTPROCEDURAL COMPLICATIONS OF SKIN AND SUBCUTANEOUS TISSUE

(L80–L99) OTHER DISORDERS OF THE SKIN AND SUBCUTANEOUS TISSUE

L80 VITILIGO

Excludes2: vitiligo of eyelids (H02.73-)
vitiligo of vulva (N90.89)

L81 OTHER DISORDERS OF PIGMENTATION

Excludes1: birthmark NOS (Q82.5)
Peutz-Jeghers syndrome (Q85.8)

Excludes2: nevus — see Alphabetical Index

- L81.2 Freckles
- L81.3 Café au lait spots
- L81.4 Other melanin hyperpigmentation
Lentigo
- L81.6 Other disorders of diminished melanin formation
- L81.7 Pigmented purpuric dermatosis
Angioma serpiginosum
- L81.8 Other specified disorders of pigmentation
Iron pigmentation
Tattoo pigmentation
- L81.9 Disorder of pigmentation, unspecified

L82 SEBORRHEIC KERATOSIS

Includes: basal cell papilloma
dermatosis papulosa nigra
Leser-Trélat disease

Excludes2: seborrheic dermatitis (L21.-)

- L82.0 Inflamed seborrheic keratosis
- L82.1 Other seborrheic keratosis
Seborrheic keratosis NOS

L83 ACANTHOSIS NIGRICANS

Confluent and reticulated papillomatosis

L84 CORNS AND CALLOSITIES

Callus
Clavus

L85 OTHER EPIDERMAL THICKENING

Excludes2: hypertrophic disorders of the skin (L91.-)

- L85.0 Acquired ichthyosis
Excludes1: congenital ichthyosis (Q80.-)
- L85.1 Acquired keratosis [keratoderma] palmaris et plantaris
Excludes1: inherited keratosis palmaris et plantaris (Q82.8)
- L85.2 Keratosis punctata (palmaris et plantaris)
- L85.3 Xerosis cutis
Dry skin dermatitis
- L85.8 Other specified epidermal thickening
Cutaneous horn
- L85.9 Epidermal thickening, unspecified

L88 PYODERMA GANGRENOSUM

Phagedenic pyoderma

Excludes1: dermatitis gangrenosa (L08.0)

L89 PRESSURE ULCER

GUIDELINES

Pressure ulcer stages

Codes in category L89, Pressure ulcer, identify the site and stage of the pressure ulcer. The *ICD-10-CM* classifies pressure ulcer stages based on severity, which is designated by stages 1–4, deep tissue pressure injury, unspecified stage, and unstageable. Assign as many codes from category L89 as needed to identify all the pressure ulcers the patient has, if applicable. See *ICD-10-CM Official Guidelines for Coding and Reporting FY 2024* in front matter, "Documentation by Clinicians Other than the Patient's Provider," for pressure ulcer stage documentation by clinicians other than the patient's provider.

Unstageable pressure ulcers

Assignment of the code for unstageable pressure ulcer (L89.--0) should be based on the clinical documentation. These codes are used for pressure ulcers whose stage cannot be clinically determined (e.g., the ulcer is covered by eschar or has been treated with a skin or muscle graft). This code should not be confused with the codes for unspecified stage (L89.--9). When there is no documentation regarding the stage of the pressure ulcer, assign the appropriate code for unspecified stage (L89.--9).

If during an encounter, the stage of an unstageable pressure ulcer is revealed after debridement, assign only the code for the stage revealed following debridement.

Documented pressure ulcer stage

Assignment of the pressure ulcer stage code should be guided by clinical documentation of the stage or documentation of the terms found in the Alphabetic Index. For clinical terms describing the stage that are not found in the Alphabetic Index, and there is no documentation of the stage, the provider should be queried.

Patients admitted with pressure ulcers documented as healed

No code is assigned if the documentation states that the pressure ulcer is completely healed.

Patients admitted with pressure ulcers documented as healing

See the ICD-10-CM manual.

Patient admitted with pressure ulcer evolving into another stage during the admission

See the ICD-10-CM manual.

Pressure-induced deep tissue damage

For pressure-induced deep tissue damage or deep tissue pressure injury, assign only the appropriate code for pressure-induced deep tissue damage (L89.--6).

L89 PRESSURE ULCER

Includes: bed sore, decubitus ulcer, plaster ulcer, pressure area, pressure sore

Code first any associated gangrene (I96)

Excludes2: decubitus (trophic) ulcer of cervix (uteri) (N86) diabetic ulcers (E08.621, E08.622, E09.621, E09.622, E10.621, E10.622, E11.621, E11.622, E13.621, E13.622) non-pressure chronic ulcer of skin (L97.-) skin infections (L00–L08) varicose ulcer (I83.0, I83.2)

L89.0 Pressure ulcer of elbow

L89.01 Pressure ulcer of right elbow

Healing pressure ulcer of right elbow

L89.010 Pressure ulcer of right elbow; unstageable

L89.011 stage 1

L89.012 stage 2

L89.013 stage 3

L89.014 stage 4

L89.016 Pressure-induced deep tissue damage of right elbow

L89.019 unspecified stage

Healing pressure ulcer right of elbow NOS

L89.02 Pressure ulcer of left elbow

Healing pressure ulcer of left elbow

L89.020 Pressure ulcer of left elbow; unstageable

L89.021 stage 1

L89.022 stage 2

L89.023 stage 3

L89.024 stage 4

L89.026 Pressure-induced deep tissue damage of left elbow

L89.029 Pressure ulcer of left elbow, unspecified stage

Healing pressure ulcer of left of elbow NOS

L89.1 Pressure ulcer of back

L89.10 Pressure ulcer of unspecified part of back

Healing pressure ulcer of unspecified part of back

Pressure pre-ulcer skin changes limited to persistent focal edema, unspecified part of back

L89.100 Pressure ulcer of unspecified part of back; unstageable

L89.101 stage 1

L89.102 stage 2

L89.103 stage 3

L89.104 stage 4

L89.106 Pressure-induced deep tissue damage of unspecified part of back

L89.109 unspecified stage

Healing pressure ulcer of unspecified part of back NOS

L89.11 Pressure ulcer of right upper back

Pressure ulcer of right shoulder blade

Healing pressure ulcer of right upper back

L89.110 Pressure ulcer of right upper back; unstageable

L89.111 stage 1

L89.112 stage 2

L89.113 stage 3

L89.114 stage 4

L89.116 Pressure-induced deep tissue damage of right upper back

L89.119 unspecified stage

Healing pressure ulcer of right upper back NOS

L89.12 Pressure ulcer of left upper back

Healing pressure ulcer of left upper back,

Pressure ulcer of left shoulder blade

L89.120 Pressure ulcer of left upper back; unstageable

L89.121 stage 1

L89.122 stage 2

L89.123 stage 3

L89.124 stage 4

L89.126 Pressure-induced deep tissue damage of left upper back

L89.129 unspecified stage

Healing pressure ulcer of left upper back NOS

Healing pressure ulcer of left upper back, unspecified stage

L89.13 Pressure ulcer of right lower back

Healing pressure ulcer of right lower back

L89.130 Pressure ulcer of right lower back; unstageable

L89.131 stage 1

L89.132 stage 2

L89.133 stage 3

L89.134 stage 4

L89.136 Pressure-induced deep tissue damage of right lower back

L89.139 unspecified stage

Healing pressure ulcer of right lower back NOS

L89.14 Pressure ulcer of left lower back

Healing pressure ulcer of left lower back

L89.140 Pressure ulcer of left lower back; unstageable

L89.141 stage 1

L89.142 stage 2

L89.143 stage 3

L89.144 stage 4

L89.146 Pressure-induced deep tissue damage of left lower back

L89.149 unspecified stage
Healing pressure ulcer of left lower back NOS

L89.15 Pressure ulcer of sacral region

Healing pressure ulcer of sacral region,
Pressure ulcer of coccyx
Pressure ulcer of tailbone

L89.150 Pressure ulcer of sacral region; unstageable

L89.151 stage 1

L89.152 stage 2

L89.153 stage 3

L89.154 stage 4

L89.156 Pressure-induced deep tissue damage of sacral region

L89.159 unspecified stage
Healing pressure ulcer of sacral region NOS

L89.2 Pressure ulcer of hip

L89.21 Pressure ulcer of right hip
Healing pressure ulcer of right hip

L89.210 Pressure ulcer of right hip; unstageable

L89.211 stage 1

L89.212 stage 2

L89.213 stage 3

L89.214 stage 4

L89.216 Pressure-induced deep tissue damage of right hip

L89.219 unspecified stage
Healing pressure ulcer of right hip NOS

L89.22 Pressure ulcer of left hip
Healing pressure ulcer of left hip back

L89.220 Pressure ulcer of left hip; unstageable

L89.221 stage 1

L89.222 stage 2

L89.223 stage 3

L89.224 stage 4

L89.226 Pressure-induced deep tissue damage of left hip

L89.229 unspecified stage
Healing pressure ulcer of left hip NOS

L89.3 Pressure ulcer of buttock

L89.31 Pressure ulcer of right buttock
Healing pressure ulcer of right buttock

L89.310 Pressure ulcer of right buttock; unstageable

L89.311 stage 1

L89.312 stage 2

L89.313 stage 3

L89.314 stage 4

L89.316 Pressure-induced deep tissue damage of right buttock

L89.319 unspecified stage
Healing pressure ulcer of right buttock NOS

L89.32 Pressure ulcer of left buttock
Healing pressure ulcer of left buttock

L89.320 Pressure ulcer of left buttock; unstageable

L89.321 stage 1

L89.322 stage 2

L89.323 stage 3

L89.324 stage 4

L89.326 Pressure-induced deep tissue damage of left buttock

L89.329 Pressure ulcer of left buttock, unspecified stage
Healing pressure ulcer of left buttock NOS

L89.4 Pressure ulcer of contiguous site of back, buttock and hip
Healing pressure ulcer of contiguous site of back, buttock and hip

L89.40 Pressure ulcer of contiguous site of back, buttock and hip; unspecified stage
Healing pressure ulcer of contiguous site of back, buttock and hip NOS

L89.41 stage 1

L89.42 stage 2

L89.43 stage 3

L89.44 stage 4

L89.45 unstageable

L89.46 Pressure-induced deep tissue damage of contiguous site of back, buttock and hip

L89.5 Pressure ulcer of ankle

L89.51 Pressure ulcer of right ankle
Healing pressure ulcer of right ankle

L89.510 Pressure ulcer of right ankle; unstageable

L89.511 stage 1

L89.512 stage 2

L89.513 stage 3

L89.514 stage 4

L89.516 Pressure-induced deep tissue damage of right ankle

L89.519 unspecified stage
Healing pressure ulcer of right ankle NOS

L89.52 Pressure ulcer of left ankle
Healing pressure ulcer of left ankle

L89.520 Pressure ulcer of left ankle; unstageable

L89.521 stage 1
Pressure pre-ulcer skin changes limited to persistent focal edema, left ankle

L89.522 stage 2

L89.523 stage 3

L89.524 stage 4

L89.526 Pressure-induced deep tissue damage of left ankle

L89.529 unspecified stage
Healing pressure ulcer of left ankle NOS

L89.6 Pressure ulcer of heel

L89.61 Pressure ulcer of right heel
Healing pressure ulcer of right heel

L89.610 Pressure ulcer of right heel; unstageable

L89.611 stage 1

L89.612 stage 2

L89.613 stage 3

L89.614 stage 4

L89.616 Pressure-induced deep tissue damage of right heel

L89.619 unspecified stage
Healing pressure ulcer of right heel NOS

L89.62 Pressure ulcer of left heel
Healing pressure ulcer of left heel

L89.620 Pressure ulcer of left heel; unstageable

L89.621 stage 1

L89.622 stage 2

L89.623 stage 3

L89.624 stage 4

L89.626 Pressure-induced deep tissue damage of left heel

L89.629 unspecified stage
Healing pressure ulcer of left heel NOS

L89.8 Pressure ulcer of other site

L89.81 Pressure ulcer of head
Pressure ulcer of face
Healing pressure ulcer of head

L89.810 Pressure ulcer of head; unstageable

L89.811 stage 1

L89.812 stage 2

L89.813 stage 3

L89.814 stage 4

L89.816 Pressure-induced deep tissue damage of head

L89.819 unspecified stage
Healing pressure ulcer of head NOS

L89.89 Pressure ulcer of other site

Healing pressure ulcer of other site

L89.890 Pressure ulcer of other site; unstageable

L89.891 stage 1

L89.892 stage 2

L89.893 stage 3

L89.894 stage 4

L89.896 Pressure-induced deep tissue damage of other site

L89.899 unspecified stage

Healing pressure ulcer of other site NOS

L89.9 Pressure ulcer of unspecified site

Healing pressure ulcer of unspecified site

L89.90 Pressure ulcer of unspecified site; unspecified stage

L89.91 stage 1

L89.92 stage 2

L89.93 stage 3

L89.94 stage 4

L89.95 unstageable

L89.96 Pressure-induced deep tissue damage of unspecified site

L90 ATROPHIC DISORDERS OF SKIN

L90.5 Scar conditions and fibrosis of skin

Adherent scar (skin)

Cicatrix

Disfigurement of skin due to scar

Fibrosis of skin NOS

L91 HYPERTROPHIC DISORDERS OF SKIN

L91.0 Hypertrophic scar

Keloid

Keloid scar

Excludes2: acne keloid (L73.0)

scar NOS (L90.5)

L91.8 Other hypertrophic disorders of the skin

L91.9 Hypertrophic disorder of the skin, unspecified

L92 GRANULOMATOUS DISORDERS OF SKIN AND SUBCUTANEOUS TISSUE

Excludes2: actinic granuloma (L57.5)

L92.0 Granuloma annulare

Perforating granuloma annulare

L92.3 FB granuloma of the skin and subcutaneous tissue

Use additional code to identify the type of retained FB (Z18.-)

L92.9 Granulomatous disorder of the skin and subcutaneous tissue, unspecified

Excludes2: umbilical granuloma (P83.81)

L94 OTHER LOCALIZED CONNECTIVE TISSUE DISORDERS

Excludes1: systemic connective tissue disorders (M30–M36)

L94.2 Calcinosis cutis

L98 OTHER DISORDERS OF SKIN AND SUBCUTANEOUS TISSUE, NOT ELSEWHERE CLASSIFIED

L98.0 Pyogenic granuloma

Excludes2: pyogenic granuloma of gingiva (K06.8)

pyogenic granuloma of maxillary alveolar ridge (K04.5)

pyogenic granuloma of oral mucosa (K13.4)

L98.1 Factitial dermatitis

Neurotic excoriation

Excludes1: excoriation (skin-picking) disorder (F42.4)

L98.5 Mucinosis of the skin

Focal mucinosis

Lichen myxedematosus

Reticular erythematous mucinosis

Excludes1: focal oral mucinosis (K13.79)

myxedema (E03.9)

L98.7 Excessive and redundant skin and subcutaneous tissue

Loose or sagging skin following bariatric surgery weight loss

Loose or sagging skin following dietary weight loss

Loose or sagging skin, NOS

Excludes2: acquired excess or redundant skin of eyelid (H02.3-)

congenital excess or redundant skin of eyelid (Q10.3)

skin changes due to chronic exposure to nonionizing radiation (L57.-)

L98.8 Other specified disorders of the skin and subcutaneous tissue

L98.9 Disorder of the skin and subcutaneous tissue, unspecified

L99 OTHER DISORDERS OF SKIN AND SUBCUTANEOUS TISSUE IN DISEASES CLASSIFIED ELSEWHERE

Code first underlying disease, such as:

amyloidosis (E85.-)

Excludes1: skin disorders in diabetes (E08–E13 with .62-)

skin disorders in gonorrhea (A54.89)

skin disorders in syphilis (A51.31, A52.79)

Chapter 13. Diseases of the musculoskeletal system and connective tissue (M00–M99)

An "X" may be listed at the end of the code to indicate a placeholder digit(s). The X will be required in order to get to the 7th character, which indicates the type of encounter. Be sure to use all indicated placeholder digits prior to the appropriate 7th character digit.

GUIDELINES

Site and laterality

Most of the codes within Chapter 13 have site and laterality designations. The site represents the bone, joint or the muscle involved. For some conditions where more than one bone, joint or muscle is usually involved, such as osteoarthritis, there is a "multiple sites" code available. For categories where no multiple site code is provided and more than one bone, joint or muscle is involved, multiple codes should be used to indicate the different sites involved.

BONE VERSUS JOINT

For certain conditions, the bone may be affected at the upper or lower end. Though the portion of the bone affected may be at the joint, the site designation will be the bone, not the joint.

Acute traumatic versus chronic or recurrent musculoskeletal conditions

Many musculoskeletal conditions are a result of previous injury or trauma to a site, or are recurrent conditions. Bone, joint or muscle conditions that are the result of a healed injury are usually found in Chapter 13. Recurrent bone, joint or muscle conditions are also usually found in Chapter 13. Any current, acute injury should be coded to the appropriate injury code from Chapter 19. Chronic or recurrent conditions should generally be coded with a code from Chapter 13. If it is difficult to determine from the documentation in the record which code is best to describe a condition, query the provider.

Coding of Pathologic Fractures

See category M84.

Note: Use an external cause code following the code for the musculoskeletal condition, if applicable, to identify the cause of the musculoskeletal condition

Excludes2: arthropathic psoriasis (L40.5-)
certain conditions originating in the perinatal period (P04–P96)
certain infectious and parasitic diseases (A00–B99)
compartment syndrome (traumatic) (T79.A-)
complications of pregnancy, childbirth and the puerperium (O00–O9A)
congenital malformations, deformations, and chromosomal abnormalities (Q00–Q99)
endocrine, nutritional and metabolic diseases (E00–E88)
injury, poisoning and certain other consequences of external causes (S00–T88)
neoplasms (C00–D49)
symptoms, signs and abnormal clinical and laboratory findings, NEC (R00–R94)

(M00–M25) ARTHROPATHIES

Includes: disorders affecting predominantly peripheral (limb) joints

(M00–M02) INFECTIOUS ARTHROPATHIES

Note: This block comprises arthropathies due to microbiological agents. Distinction is made between the following types of etiological relationship:
a) a direct infection of joint, where organisms invade synovial tissue and microbial antigen is present in the joint;
b) indirect infection, which may be of two types: a reactive arthropathy, where microbial infection of the body is established but neither organisms nor antigens can be identified in the joint, and a postinfective arthropathy, where microbial antigen is present but recovery of an organism is inconstant and evidence of local multiplication is lacking.

M00 PYOGENIC ARTHRITIS

Excludes2: infection and inflammatory reaction due to internal joint prosthesis (T84.5-)

M00.0 Staphylococcal arthritis and polyarthritis

Use additional code (B95.61–B95.8) to identify bacterial agent

M00.00 Staphylococcal arthritis, unspecified joint

M00.01 Staphylococcal arthritis, shoulder

M00.011 Staphylococcal arthritis, right shoulder

M00.012 Staphylococcal arthritis, left shoulder

M00.02 Staphylococcal arthritis, elbow

M00.021 Staphylococcal arthritis, right elbow

M00.022 Staphylococcal arthritis, left elbow

M00.03 Staphylococcal arthritis, wrist

Staphylococcal arthritis of carpal bones

M00.031 Staphylococcal arthritis, right wrist

M00.032 Staphylococcal arthritis, left wrist

M00.04 Staphylococcal arthritis, hand

Staphylococcal arthritis of metacarpus and phalanges

M00.041 Staphylococcal arthritis, right hand

M00.042 Staphylococcal arthritis, left hand

M00.05 Staphylococcal arthritis, hip

M00.051 Staphylococcal arthritis, right hip

M00.052 Staphylococcal arthritis, left hip

M00.06 Staphylococcal arthritis, knee

M00.061 Staphylococcal arthritis, right knee

M00.062 Staphylococcal arthritis, left knee

M00.07 Staphylococcal arthritis, ankle and foot

Staphylococcal arthritis, tarsus, metatarsus and phalanges

M00.071 Staphylococcal arthritis, right ankle and foot

M00.072 Staphylococcal arthritis, left ankle and foot

M00.08 Staphylococcal arthritis, vertebrae

M00.09 Staphylococcal polyarthritis

M00.1 Pneumococcal arthritis and polyarthritis

M00.10 Pneumococcal arthritis, unspecified joint

M00.11 Pneumococcal arthritis, shoulder

M00.111 Pneumococcal arthritis, right shoulder

M00.112 Pneumococcal arthritis, left shoulder

M00.12 Pneumococcal arthritis, elbow

M00.121 Pneumococcal arthritis, right elbow

M00.122 Pneumococcal arthritis, left elbow

M00.13 Pneumococcal arthritis, wrist

Pneumococcal arthritis of carpal bones

M00.131 Pneumococcal arthritis, right wrist

M00.132 Pneumococcal arthritis, left wrist

M00.14 Pneumococcal arthritis, hand

Pneumococcal arthritis of metacarpus and phalanges

M00.141 Pneumococcal arthritis, right hand

M00.142 Pneumococcal arthritis, left hand

M00.15 Pneumococcal arthritis, hip

M00.151 Pneumococcal arthritis, right hip

M00.152 Pneumococcal arthritis, left hip

M00.16 Pneumococcal arthritis, knee

M00.161 Pneumococcal arthritis, right knee

M00.162 Pneumococcal arthritis, left knee

M00.17 Pneumococcal arthritis, ankle and foot

Pneumococcal arthritis, tarsus, metatarsus and phalanges

M00.171 Pneumococcal arthritis, right ankle and foot

M00.172 Pneumococcal arthritis, left ankle and foot

M00.18 Pneumococcal arthritis, vertebrae

M00.19 Pneumococcal polyarthritis

M00.2 Other streptococcal arthritis and polyarthritis

Use additional code (B95.0–B95.2, B95.4–B95.5) to identify bacterial agent

M00.20 Other streptococcal arthritis, unspecified joint

M00.21 Other streptococcal arthritis, shoulder

M00.211 Other streptococcal arthritis, right shoulder

M00.212 Other streptococcal arthritis, left shoulder

M00.22 Other streptococcal arthritis, elbow

M00.221 Other streptococcal arthritis, right elbow

M00.222 Other streptococcal arthritis, left elbow

M00.23 Other streptococcal arthritis, wrist

Other streptococcal arthritis of carpal bones

M00.231 Other streptococcal arthritis, right wrist

M00.232 Other streptococcal arthritis, left wrist

- **M00.24** Other streptococcal arthritis, hand
  - 6th — Other streptococcal arthritis metacarpus and phalanges
  - **M00.241** Other streptococcal arthritis, right hand
  - **M00.242** Other streptococcal arthritis, left hand
- **M00.25** Other streptococcal arthritis, hip
  - 6th
  - **M00.251** Other streptococcal arthritis, right hip
  - **M00.252** Other streptococcal arthritis, left hip
- **M00.26** Other streptococcal arthritis, knee
  - 6th
  - **M00.261** Other streptococcal arthritis, right knee
  - **M00.262** Other streptococcal arthritis, left knee
- **M00.27** Other streptococcal arthritis, ankle and foot
  - 6th — Other streptococcal arthritis, tarsus, metatarsus and phalanges
  - **M00.271** Other streptococcal arthritis, right ankle and foot
  - **M00.272** Other streptococcal arthritis, left ankle and foot
- **M00.28** Other streptococcal arthritis, vertebrae
- **M00.29** Other streptococcal polyarthritis
- **M00.8 Arthritis and polyarthritis due to other bacteria**
  - 5th — Use additional code (B96) to identify bacteria
  - **M00.80** Arthritis due to other bacteria, unspecified joint
  - **M00.81** Arthritis due to other bacteria, shoulder
    - 6th
    - **M00.811** Arthritis due to other bacteria, right shoulder
    - **M00.812** Arthritis due to other bacteria, left shoulder
  - **M00.82** Arthritis due to other bacteria, elbow
    - 6th
    - **M00.821** Arthritis due to other bacteria, right elbow
    - **M00.822** Arthritis due to other bacteria, left elbow
  - **M00.83** Arthritis due to other bacteria, wrist
    - 6th — Arthritis due to other bacteria, carpal bones
    - **M00.831** Arthritis due to other bacteria, right wrist
    - **M00.832** Arthritis due to other bacteria, left wrist
  - **M00.84** Arthritis due to other bacteria, hand
    - 6th — Arthritis due to other bacteria, metacarpus and phalanges
    - **M00.841** Arthritis due to other bacteria, right hand
    - **M00.842** Arthritis due to other bacteria, left hand
  - **M00.85** Arthritis due to other bacteria, hip
    - 6th
    - **M00.851** Arthritis due to other bacteria, right hip
    - **M00.852** Arthritis due to other bacteria, left hip
  - **M00.86** Arthritis due to other bacteria, knee
    - 6th
    - **M00.861** Arthritis due to other bacteria, right knee
    - **M00.862** Arthritis due to other bacteria, left knee
  - **M00.87** Arthritis due to other bacteria, ankle and foot
    - 6th — Arthritis due to other bacteria, tarsus, metatarsus, and phalanges
    - **M00.871** Arthritis due to other bacteria, right ankle and foot
    - **M00.872** Arthritis due to other bacteria, left ankle and foot
  - **M00.88** Arthritis due to other bacteria, vertebrae
  - **M00.89** Polyarthritis due to other bacteria
- **M00.9** Pyogenic arthritis, unspecified
  - Infective arthritis NOS
  - Autoinflammatory syndromes (M04)

M01 DIRECT INFECTIONS OF JOINT IN INFECTIOUS AND PARASITIC DISEASES CLASSIFIED ELSEWHERE

4th

Code first underlying disease, such as:
- leprosy [Hansen's disease] (A30.-)
- mycoses (B35-B49)
- O'nyong-nyong fever (A92.1)
- paratyphoid fever (A01.1-A01.4)

Excludes1: arthropathy in Lyme disease (A69.23)
- gonococcal arthritis (A54.42)
- meningococcal arthritis (A39.83)
- mumps arthritis (B26.85)
- postinfective arthropathy (M02.-)
- postmeningococcal arthritis (A39.84)
- reactive arthritis (M02.3)
- rubella arthritis (B06.82)

sarcoidosis arthritis (D86.86)
typhoid fever arthritis (A01.04)
tuberculosis arthritis (A18.01-A18.02)

- **M01.X Direct infection of joint in infectious and parasitic diseases classified elsewhere**
  - 5th
  - **M01.X0** Direct infection of unspecified joint in infectious and parasitic diseases classified elsewhere
  - **M01.X1** Direct infection of shoulder joint in infectious and parasitic diseases classified elsewhere
    - 6th
    - **M01.X11** Direct infection of right shoulder in infectious and parasitic diseases classified elsewhere
    - **M01.X12** Direct infection of left shoulder in infectious and parasitic diseases classified elsewhere
  - **M01.X2** Direct infection of elbow in infectious and parasitic diseases classified elsewhere
    - 6th
    - **M01.X21** Direct infection of right elbow in infectious and parasitic diseases classified elsewhere
    - **M01.X22** Direct infection of left elbow in infectious and parasitic diseases classified elsewhere
  - **M01.X3** Direct infection of wrist in infectious and parasitic diseases classified elsewhere
    - 6th — Direct infection of carpal bones in infectious and parasitic diseases classified elsewhere
    - **M01.X31** Direct infection of right wrist in infectious and parasitic diseases classified elsewhere
    - **M01.X32** Direct infection of left wrist in infectious and parasitic diseases classified elsewhere
  - **M01.X4** Direct infection of hand in infectious and parasitic diseases classified elsewhere
    - 6th — Direct infection of metacarpus and phalanges in infectious and parasitic diseases classified elsewhere
    - **M01.X41** Direct infection of right hand in infectious and parasitic diseases classified elsewhere
    - **M01.X42** Direct infection of left hand in infectious and parasitic diseases classified elsewhere
  - **M01.X5** Direct infection of hip in infectious and parasitic diseases classified elsewhere
    - 6th
    - **M01.X51** Direct infection of right hip in infectious and parasitic diseases classified elsewhere
    - **M01.X52** Direct infection of left hip in infectious and parasitic diseases classified elsewhere
  - **M01.X6** Direct infection of knee in infectious and parasitic diseases classified elsewhere
    - 6th
    - **M01.X61** Direct infection of right knee in infectious and parasitic diseases classified elsewhere
    - **M01.X62** Direct infection of left knee in infectious and parasitic diseases classified elsewhere
  - **M01.X7 Direct infection of ankle and foot in infectious and parasitic diseases classified elsewhere**
    - 6th — Direct infection of tarsus, metatarsus and phalanges in infectious and parasitic diseases classified elsewhere
    - **M01.X71** Direct infection of right ankle and foot in infectious and parasitic diseases classified elsewhere
    - **M01.X72** Direct infection of left ankle and foot in infectious and parasitic diseases classified elsewhere
  - **M01.X8** Direct infection of vertebrae in infectious and parasitic diseases classified elsewhere
  - **M01.X9** Direct infection of multiple joints in infectious and parasitic diseases classified elsewhere

(M04) AUTOINFLAMMATORY SYNDROMES

M04 AUTOINFLAMMATORY SYNDROMES

4th *Excludes2:* Crohn's disease (K50.-)

M04.1 Periodic fever syndromes

Familial Mediterranean fever

Hyperimmunoglobin D syndrome

Mevalonate kinase deficiency

Tumor necrosis factor receptor associated periodic syndrome [TRAPS]

M04.2 Cryopyrin-associated periodic syndromes

Chronic infantile neurological, cutaneous and articular syndrome [CINCA]

Familial cold autoinflammatory syndrome

Familial cold urticaria

Muckle-Wells syndrome

Neonatal onset multisystemic inflammatory disorder [NOMID]

M04.8 Other autoinflammatory syndromes

Blau syndrome

Deficiency of interleukin 1 receptor antagonist [DIRA]

Majeed syndrome

Periodic fever, aphthous stomatitis, pharyngitis, and adenopathy syndrome [PFAPA]

Pyogenic arthritis, pyoderma gangrenosum, and acne syndrome [PAPA]

M04.9 Autoinflammatory syndrome, unspecified

(M05–M14) INFLAMMATORY POLYARTHROPATHIES

M06 OTHER RHEUMATOID ARTHRITIS

4th **M06.9 Rheumatoid arthritis, unspecified**

M08 JUVENILE ARTHRITIS

4th Code also any associated underlying condition, such as: regional enteritis [Crohn's disease] (K50.-)

ulcerative colitis (K51.-)

Excludes1: arthropathy in Whipple's disease (M14.8)

Felty's syndrome (M05.0)

juvenile dermatomyositis (M33.0-)

psoriatic juvenile arthropathy (L40.54)

M08.0 Unspecified juvenile rheumatoid arthritis

5th Juvenile rheumatoid arthritis with or without rheumatoid factor

M08.00 Unspecified juvenile rheumatoid arthritis of unspecified site

M08.01 Unspecified juvenile rheumatoid arthritis, shoulder

6th **M08.011** right shoulder

M08.012 left shoulder

M08.02 Unspecified juvenile rheumatoid arthritis of elbow

6th **M08.021** right elbow

M08.022 left elbow

M08.03 Unspecified juvenile rheumatoid arthritis, wrist

6th **M08.031** right wrist

M08.032 left wrist

M08.04 Unspecified juvenile rheumatoid arthritis, hand

6th **M08.041** right hand

M08.042 left hand

M08.05 Unspecified juvenile rheumatoid arthritis, hip

6th **M08.051** right hip

M08.052 left hip

M08.06 Unspecified juvenile rheumatoid arthritis, knee

6th **M08.061** right knee

M08.062 left knee

M08.07 Unspecified juvenile rheumatoid arthritis, ankle and foot

6th **M08.071** right ankle and foot

M08.072 left ankle and foot

M08.08 Unspecified juvenile rheumatoid arthritis, vertebrae

M08.09 Unspecified juvenile rheumatoid arthritis, multiple sites

M08.0A Unspecified juvenile rheumatoid arthritis, other specified site

M08.1 Juvenile ankylosing spondylitis

Excludes1: ankylosing spondylitis in adults (M45.0-)

M08.2 Juvenile rheumatoid arthritis with systemic onset

5th Still's disease NOS

Excludes1: adult-onset Still's disease (M06.1-)

M08.20 Juvenile rheumatoid arthritis with systemic onset, unspecified site

M08.21 Juvenile rheumatoid arthritis with systemic onset, shoulder

6th **M08.211** right shoulder

M08.212 left shoulder

M08.22 Juvenile rheumatoid arthritis with systemic onset, elbow

6th **M08.221** right elbow

M08.222 left elbow

M08.23 Juvenile rheumatoid arthritis with systemic onset, wrist

6th **M08.231** right wrist

M08.232 left wrist

M08.24 Juvenile rheumatoid arthritis with systemic onset, hand

6th **M08.241** right hand

M08.242 left hand

M08.25 Juvenile rheumatoid arthritis with systemic onset, hip

6th **M08.251** right hip

M08.252 left hip

M08.26 Juvenile rheumatoid arthritis with systemic onset, knee

6th **M08.261** right knee

M08.262 left knee

M08.27 Juvenile rheumatoid arthritis with systemic onset, ankle and foot

6th **M08.271** right ankle and foot

M08.272 left ankle and foot

M08.28 Juvenile rheumatoid arthritis with systemic onset, vertebrae

M08.29 Juvenile rheumatoid arthritis with systemic onset, multiple sites

M08.2A Juvenile rheumatoid arthritis with systemic onset, other specified site

M08.3 Juvenile rheumatoid polyarthritis (seronegative)

M08.4 Pauciarticular juvenile rheumatoid arthritis

5th **M08.40** Pauciarticular juvenile rheumatoid arthritis, unspecified site

M08.41 Pauciarticular juvenile rheumatoid arthritis, shoulder

6th **M08.411** right shoulder

M08.412 left shoulder

M08.42 Pauciarticular juvenile rheumatoid arthritis, elbow

6th **M08.421** right elbow

M08.422 left elbow

M08.43 Pauciarticular juvenile rheumatoid arthritis, wrist

6th **M08.431** right wrist

M08.432 left wrist

M08.44 Pauciarticular juvenile rheumatoid arthritis, hand

6th **M08.441** right hand

M08.442 left hand

M08.45 Pauciarticular juvenile rheumatoid arthritis, hip

6th **M08.451** right hip

M08.452 left hip

M08.46 Pauciarticular juvenile rheumatoid arthritis, knee

6th **M08.461** right knee

M08.462 left knee

M08.47 Pauciarticular juvenile rheumatoid arthritis, ankle and foot

6th **M08.471** right ankle and foot

M08.472 left ankle and foot

M08.48 Pauciarticular juvenile rheumatoid arthritis, vertebrae

M08.4A Pauciarticular juvenile rheumatoid arthritis, other specified site

M08.8 Other juvenile arthritis

5th **M08.81** Other juvenile arthritis, shoulder

6th **M08.811** right shoulder

M08.812 left shoulder

M08.82 Other juvenile arthritis, elbow

6th M08.821 right elbow

M08.822 left elbow

M08.83 Other juvenile arthritis, wrist

6th M08.831 right wrist

M08.832 left wrist

M08.84 Other juvenile arthritis, hand

6th M08.841 right hand

M08.842 left hand

M08.85 Other juvenile arthritis, hip

6th M08.851 right hip

M08.852 left hip

M08.86 Other juvenile arthritis, knee

6th M08.861 right knee

M08.862 left knee

M08.87 Other juvenile arthritis, ankle and foot

6th M08.871 right ankle and foot

M08.872 left ankle and foot

M08.88 Other juvenile arthritis, other specified site

Other juvenile arthritis, vertebrae

M08.89 Other juvenile arthritis, multiple sites

M08.9 Juvenile arthritis, unspecified

5th *Excludes1:* juvenile rheumatoid arthritis, unspecified (M08.0-)

M08.90 Juvenile arthritis, unspecified, unspecified site

M08.91 Juvenile arthritis, unspecified, shoulder

6th M08.911 right shoulder

M08.912 left shoulder

M08.92 Juvenile arthritis, unspecified, elbow

6th M08.921 right elbow

M08.922 left elbow

M08.93 Juvenile arthritis, unspecified, wrist

6th M08.931 right wrist

M08.932 left wrist

M08.94 Juvenile arthritis, unspecified, hand

6th M08.941 right hand

M08.942 left hand

M08.95 Juvenile arthritis, unspecified, hip

6th M08.951 right hip

M08.952 left hip

M08.96 Juvenile arthritis, unspecified, knee

6th M08.961 right knee

M08.962 left knee

M08.97 Juvenile arthritis, unspecified, ankle and foot

6th M08.971 right ankle and foot

M08.972 left ankle and foot

M08.98 Juvenile arthritis, unspecified, vertebrae

M08.99 Juvenile arthritis, unspecified, multiple sites

M08.9A Juvenile arthritis, unspecified, other specified site

M10 GOUT

4th Acute gout

Gout attack

Gout flare

Podagra

Use additional code to identify:

Autonomic neuropathy in diseases classified elsewhere (G99.0)

Calculus of urinary tract in diseases classified elsewhere (N22)

Cardiomyopathy in diseases classified elsewhere (I43)

Disorders of external ear in diseases classified elsewhere (H61.1-, H62.8-)

Disorders of iris and ciliary body in diseases classified elsewhere (H22)

Glomerular disorders in diseases classified elsewhere (N08)

Excludes2: chronic gout (M1A.-)

M10.0 Idiopathic gout

5th Gouty bursitis

Primary gout

M10.01 Idiopathic gout, shoulder

6th M10.011 right shoulder

M10.012 left shoulder

M10.02 Idiopathic gout, elbow

6th M10.021 right elbow

M10.022 left elbow

M10.03 Idiopathic gout, wrist

6th M10.031 right wrist

M10.032 left wrist

M10.04 Idiopathic gout, hand

6th M10.041 right hand

M10.042 left hand

M10.05 Idiopathic gout, hip

6th M10.051 right hip

M10.052 left hip

M10.06 Idiopathic gout, knee

6th M10.061 right knee

M10.062 left knee

M10.07 Idiopathic gout, ankle and foot

6th M10.071 right ankle and foot

M10.072 left ankle and foot

M10.08 Idiopathic gout, vertebrae

M10.09 Idiopathic gout, multiple sites

M10.9 Gout, unspecified

Gout NOS

M12 OTHER AND UNSPECIFIED ARTHROPATHY

4th *Excludes1:* arthrosis (M15-M19)

cricoarytenoid arthropathy (J38.7)

M12.4 Intermittent hydrarthrosis

5th **M12.41** Intermittent hydrarthrosis, shoulder

6th M12.411 right shoulder

M12.412 left shoulder

M12.42 Intermittent hydrarthrosis, elbow

6th M12.421 right elbow

M12.422 left elbow

M12.43 Intermittent hydrarthrosis, wrist

6th M12.431 right wrist

M12.432 left wrist

M12.44 Intermittent hydrarthrosis, hand

6th M12.441 right hand

M12.442 left hand

M12.45 Intermittent hydrarthrosis, hip

6th M12.451 right hip

M12.452 left hip

M12.46 Intermittent hydrarthrosis, knee

6th M12.461 right knee

M12.462 left knee

M12.47 Intermittent hydrarthrosis, ankle and foot

6th M12.471 right ankle and foot

M12.472 left ankle and foot

M12.48 Intermittent hydrarthrosis, other site

M12.49 Intermittent hydrarthrosis, multiple sites

M12.5 Traumatic arthropathy

5th *Excludes1:* current injury — see Alphabetic Index

post-traumatic osteoarthritis of first carpometacarpal joint (M18.2-M18.3)

post-traumatic osteoarthritis of hip (M16.4-M16.5)

post-traumatic osteoarthritis of knee (M17.2-M17.3)

post-traumatic osteoarthritis NOS (M19.1-)

post-traumatic osteoarthritis of other single joints (M19.1-)

M12.50 Traumatic arthropathy, unspecified site

M12.51 Traumatic arthropathy, shoulder

6th M12.511 right shoulder

M12.512 left shoulder

M12.52 Traumatic arthropathy, elbow

6th M12.521 right elbow

M12.522 left elbow

M12.53 Traumatic arthropathy, wrist

6th M12.531 right wrist

M12.532 left wrist

M12.54 Traumatic arthropathy, hand

6th M12.541 right hand

M12.542 left hand

M12.55 Traumatic arthropathy, hip

6th M12.551 right hip

M12.552 left hip

M12.56 Traumatic arthropathy, knee

6th M12.561 right knee

M12.562 left knee

M12.57 Traumatic arthropathy, ankle and foot

6th M12.571 right ankle and foot

M12.572 left ankle and foot

M12.58 Traumatic arthropathy, other specified site

Traumatic arthropathy, vertebrae

M12.59 Traumatic arthropathy, multiple sites

M12.9 Arthropathy, unspecified

M14 ARTHROPATHIES IN OTHER DISEASES CLASSIFIED ELSEWHERE

4th

Excludes1: arthropathy in:
DM (E08-E13 with .61-)
hematological disorders (M36.2-M36.3)
hypersensitivity reactions (M36.4)
neoplastic disease (M36.1)
neurosyphillis (A52.16)
sarcoidosis (D86.86)
enteropathic arthropathies (M07.-)
juvenile psoriatic arthropathy (L40.54)
lipoid dermatoarthritis (E78.81)

M14.8 Arthropathies in other specified diseases classified elsewhere

5th **Code first:** underlying disease, such as:
amyloidosis (E85.-)
erythema multiforme (L51.-)
erythema nodosum (L52)
hemochromatosis (E83.11-)
hyperparathyroidism (E21.-)
hypothyroidism (E00-E03)
sickle-cell disorders (D57.-)
thyrotoxicosis [hyperthyroidism] (E05.-)
Whipple's disease (K90.81)

M14.80 Arthropathies in other specified diseases classified elsewhere, unspecified site

M14.81 Arthropathies in other specified diseases classified elsewhere; shoulder

6th

M14.811 right shoulder

M14.812 left shoulder

M14.82 Arthropathies in other specified diseases classified elsewhere; elbow

6th

M14.821 right elbow

M14.822 left elbow

M14.83 Arthropathies in other specified diseases classified elsewhere; wrist

6th

M14.831 right wrist

M14.832 left wrist

M14.84 Arthropathies in other specified diseases classified elsewhere; hand

6th

M14.841 right hand

M14.842 left hand

M14.85 Arthropathies in other specified diseases classified elsewhere; hip

6th

M14.851 right hip

M14.852 left hip

M14.86 Arthropathies in other specified diseases classified elsewhere; knee

6th

M14.861 right knee

M14.862 left knee

M14.87 Arthropathies in other specified diseases classified elsewhere; ankle and foot

6th

M14.871 right ankle and foot

M14.872 left ankle and foot

M14.88 Arthropathies in other specified diseases classified elsewhere, vertebrae

M14.89 Arthropathies in other specified diseases classified elsewhere, multiple sites

(M15-M19) OSTEOARTHRITIS

Excludes2: osteoarthritis of spine (M47.-)

(M20-M25) OTHER JOINT DISORDERS

Excludes2: joints of the spine (M40-M54)

M20 ACQUIRED DEFORMITIES OF FINGERS AND TOES

4th

Excludes1: acquired absence of fingers and toes (Z89.-)
congenital absence of fingers and toes (Q71.3-, Q72.3-)
congenital deformities and malformations of fingers and toes (Q66.-, Q68-Q70, Q74.-)

M20.0 Deformity of finger(s)

5th *Excludes1:* clubbing of fingers (R68.3)
palmar fascial fibromatosis [Dupuytren] (M72.0)
trigger finger (M65.3)

M20.00 Unspecified deformity of finger(s)

6th M20.001 Unspecified deformity of right finger(s)

M20.002 Unspecified deformity of left finger(s)

M20.01 Mallet finger

6th M20.011 Mallet finger of right finger(s)

M20.012 Mallet finger of left finger(s)

M20.09 Other deformity of finger(s)

6th M20.091 Other deformity of right finger(s)

M20.092 Other deformity of left finger(s)

M20.1 Hallux valgus (acquired)

5th *Excludes2:* bunion (M21.6-)

M20.11 Hallux valgus (acquired), right foot

M20.12 Hallux valgus (acquired), left foot

M20.5 Other deformities of toe(s) (acquired)

5th **M20.5X Other deformities of toe(s) (acquired)**

6th M20.5X1 right foot

M20.5X2 left foot

M20.6 Acquired deformities of toe(s), unspecified

5th M20.61 Acquired deformities of toe(s), unspecified, right foot

M20.62 Acquired deformities of toe(s), unspecified, left foot

M21 OTHER ACQUIRED DEFORMITIES OF LIMBS

4th

Excludes1: acquired absence of limb (Z89.-)
congenital absence of limbs (Q71-Q73)
congenital deformities and malformations of limbs (Q65-Q66, Q68-Q74)

Excludes2: acquired deformities of fingers or toes (M20.-)
coxa plana (M91.2)

M21.0 Valgus deformity, NEC

5th *Excludes1:* metatarsus valgus (Q66.6)
talipes calcaneovalgus (Q66.4-)

M21.06 Valgus deformity, NEC, knee

6th Genu valgum

Knock knee

M21.061 right knee

M21.062 left knee

M21.1 Varus deformity, NEC

5th *Excludes1:* metatarsus varus (Q66.22-)
tibia vara (M92.51-)

M21.16 Varus deformity, NEC, knee

6th Bow leg

Genu varum

M21.161 right knee

M21.162 left knee

M21.2 Flexion deformity

5th **M21.21 Flexion deformity, shoulder**

6th M21.211 right shoulder

M21.212 left shoulder

M21.22 Flexion deformity, elbow

6th M21.221 right elbow

M21.222 left elbow

M21.23 Flexion deformity, wrist

6th M21.231 right wrist

M21.232 left wrist

M21.24 Flexion deformity, finger joints

6th M21.241 right finger joints

M21.242 left finger joints

M21.25 Flexion deformity, hip

6th M21.251 right hip

M21.252 left hip

M21.26 Flexion deformity, knee

6th M21.261 right knee

M21.262 left knee

M21.27 Flexion deformity, ankle and toes

6th

	M21.271	right ankle and toes
	M21.272	left ankle and toes
M21.3	Wrist or foot drop (acquired)	
M21.33	Wrist drop (acquired)	
	M21.331	right wrist
	M21.332	left wrist
M21.37	Foot drop (acquired)	
	M21.371	right foot
	M21.372	left foot
M21.4	Flat foot [pes planus] (acquired)	
	Excludes1: congenital pes planus (Q66.5-)	
	M21.41	right foot
	M21.42	left foot
M21.6	Other acquired deformities of foot	
	Excludes2: deformities of toe (acquired) (M20.1-M20.6-)	
M21.61	Bunion	
	M21.611	right foot
	M21.612	left foot
M21.62	Bunionette	
	M21.621	right foot
	M21.622	left foot
M21.6X	Other acquired deformities of foot	
	M21.6X1	right foot
	M21.6X2	left foot
M21.8	Other specified acquired deformities of limbs	
	Excludes2: coxa plana (M91.2)	
M21.82	Other specified acquired deformities of upper arm	
	M21.821	right upper arm
	M21.822	left upper arm
M21.86	Other specified acquired deformities of lower leg	
	M21.861	right lower leg
	M21.862	left lower leg

M22 DISORDER OF PATELLA

Excludes2: traumatic dislocation of patella (S83.0-)

M22.0 Recurrent dislocation of patella

- M22.01 right knee
- M22.02 left knee

M22.1 Recurrent subluxation of patella

Incomplete dislocation of patella

- M22.11 right knee
- M22.12 left knee

M22.4 Chondromalacia patellae

- M22.41 right knee
- M22.42 left knee

M23 INTERNAL DERANGEMENT OF KNEE

Excludes1: ankylosis (M24.66)
deformity of knee (M21.-)
osteochondritis dissecans (M93.2)

Excludes2: current injury—see injury of knee and lower leg (S80-S89)
recurrent dislocation or subluxation of joints (M24.4)
recurrent dislocation or subluxation of patella (M22.0-M22.1)

M23.5 Chronic instability of knee

- M23.51 Chronic instability of knee, right knee
- M23.52 Chronic instability of knee, left knee

M23.8 Other internal derangements of knee

Laxity of ligament of knee
Snapping knee

M23.8X Other internal derangements of knee

- M23.8X1 right knee
- M23.8X2 left knee

M24 OTHER SPECIFIC JOINT DERANGEMENTS

Excludes1: current injury — see injury of joint by body region
Excludes2: ganglion (M67.4)
snapping knee (M23.8-)
TMJ disorders (M26.6-)

M24.5 Contracture of joint

Excludes1: contracture of muscle without contracture of joint (M62.4-)
contracture of tendon (sheath) without contracture of joint (M62.4-)
Dupuytren's contracture (M72.0)
Excludes2: acquired deformities of limbs (M20-M21)

M24.51 Contracture, shoulder

- M24.511 right shoulder
- M24.512 left shoulder

M24.52 Contracture, elbow

- M24.521 right elbow
- M24.522 left elbow

M24.53 Contracture, wrist

- M24.531 right wrist
- M24.532 left wrist

M24.54 Contracture, hand

- M24.541 right hand
- M24.542 left hand

M24.55 Contracture, hip

- M24.551 right hip
- M24.552 left hip

M24.56 Contracture, knee

- M24.561 right knee
- M24.562 left knee

M24.57 Contracture, ankle and foot

- M24.571 right ankle
- M24.572 left ankle
- M24.574 right foot
- M24.575 left foot

M24.59 Contracture, other specified joint

M24.8 Other specific joint derangements, NEC

Excludes2: iliotibial band syndrome (M76.3)

M24.81 Other specific joint derangements of shoulder, NEC

- M24.811 right shoulder, NEC
- M24.812 left shoulder, NEC

M24.82 Other specific joint derangements of elbow, NEC

- M24.821 right elbow, NEC
- M24.822 left elbow, NEC

M24.83 Other specific joint derangements of wrist, NEC

- M24.831 right wrist, NEC
- M24.832 left wrist, NEC

M24.84 Other specific joint derangements of hand, NEC

- M24.841 right hand, NEC
- M24.842 left hand, NEC

M24.85 Other specific joint derangements of hip, NEC

Irritable hip

- M24.851 right hip, NEC
- M24.852 left hip, NEC

M24.87 Other specific joint derangements of ankle and foot, NEC

- M24.871 right ankle, NEC
- M24.872 left ankle, NEC
- M24.874 right foot, NEC
- M24.875 left foot, NEC

M24.89 Other specific joint derangement of other specified joint, NEC

M24.9 Joint derangement, unspecified

M25 OTHER JOINT DISORDER, NEC

Excludes2: abnormality of gait and mobility (R26.-)
acquired deformities of limb (M20-M21)
calcification of bursa (M71.4-)
calcification of shoulder (joint) (M75.3)
calcification of tendon (M65.2-)
difficulty in walking (R26.2)
temporomandibular joint disorder (M26.6-)

M25.0 Hemarthrosis

Excludes1: current injury — see injury of joint by body region
hemophilic arthropathy (M36.2)

- M25.00 Hemarthrosis, unspecified joint

M25.01 Hemarthrosis, shoulder

- M25.011 right shoulder
- M25.012 left shoulder

M25.02 Hemarthrosis, elbow

- M25.021 right elbow
- M25.022 left elbow

M25.03 Hemarthrosis, wrist

- M25.031 right wrist
- M25.032 left wrist

M25.04 Hemarthrosis, hand
- 6th M25.041 right hand
- M25.042 left hand

M25.05 Hemarthrosis, hip
- 6th M25.051 right hip
- M25.052 left hip

M25.06 Hemarthrosis, knee
- 6th M25.061 right knee
- M25.062 left knee

M25.07 Hemarthrosis, ankle and foot
- 6th M25.071 right ankle
- M25.072 left ankle
- M25.074 right foot
- M25.075 left foot

M25.08 Hemarthrosis, other specified site
- Hemarthrosis, vertebrae

M25.2 Flail joint
- 5th

M25.21 Flail joint, shoulder
- 6th M25.211 right shoulder
- M25.212 left shoulder

M25.22 Flail joint, elbow
- 6th M25.221 right elbow
- M25.222 left elbow

M25.23 Flail joint, wrist
- 6th M25.231 right wrist
- M25.232 left wrist

M25.24 Flail joint, hand
- 6th M25.241 right hand
- M25.242 left hand

M25.25 Flail joint, hip
- 6th M25.251 right hip
- M25.252 left hip

M25.26 Flail joint, knee
- 6th M25.261 right knee
- M25.262 left knee

M25.27 Flail joint, ankle and foot
- 6th M25.271 right ankle and foot
- M25.272 left ankle and foot

M25.28 Flail joint, other site

M25.3 Other instability of joint
- 5th *Excludes1:* instability of joint secondary to old ligament injury (M24.2-)
- instability of joint secondary to removal of joint prosthesis (M96.8-)
- *Excludes2:* spinal instabilities (M53.2-)

M25.30 Other instability, unspecified joint

M25.31 Other instability, shoulder
- 6th M25.311 right shoulder
- M25.312 left shoulder

M25.32 Other instability, elbow
- 6th M25.321 right elbow
- M25.322 left elbow

M25.33 Other instability, wrist
- 6th M25.331 right wrist
- M25.332 left wrist

M25.34 Other instability, hand
- 6th M25.341 right hand
- M25.342 left hand

M25.35 Other instability, hip
- 6th M25.351 right hip
- M25.352 left hip

M25.36 Other instability, knee
- 6th M25.361 right knee
- M25.362 left knee

M25.37 Other instability, ankle and foot
- 6th M25.371 right ankle
- M25.372 left ankle
- M25.374 right foot
- M25.375 left foot

M25.39 Other instability, other specified joint

M25.4 Effusion of joint
- 5th *Excludes1:* hydrarthrosis in yaws (A66.6)
- intermittent hydrarthrosis (M12.4-)
- other infective (teno)synovitis (M65.1-)

M25.40 Effusion, unspecified joint

M25.41 Effusion, shoulder
- 6th M25.411 right shoulder
- M25.412 left shoulder

M25.42 Effusion, elbow
- 6th M25.421 right elbow
- M25.422 left elbow

M25.43 Effusion, wrist
- 6th M25.431 right wrist
- M25.432 left wrist

M25.44 Effusion, hand
- 6th M25.441 right hand
- M25.442 left hand

M25.45 Effusion, hip
- 6th M25.451 right hip
- M25.452 left hip

M25.46 Effusion, knee
- 6th M25.461 right knee
- M25.462 left knee

M25.47 Effusion, ankle and foot
- 6th M25.471 right ankle
- M25.472 left ankle
- M25.474 right foot
- M25.475 left foot

M25.48 Effusion, other site

M25.5 Pain in joint
- 5th *Excludes2:* pain in hand (M79.64-)
- pain in fingers (M79.64-)
- pain in foot (M79.67-)
- pain in limb (M79.6-)
- pain in toes (M79.67-)

M25.50 Pain in unspecified joint

M25.51 Pain in shoulder
- 6th M25.511 right shoulder
- M25.512 left shoulder

M25.52 Pain in elbow
- 6th M25.521 right elbow
- M25.522 left elbow

M25.53 Pain in wrist
- 6th M25.531 right wrist
- M25.532 left wrist

M25.54 Pain in hand joints
- 6th M25.541 right hand
- M25.542 left hand

M25.55 Pain in hip
- 6th M25.551 right hip
- M25.552 left hip

M25.56 Pain in knee
- 6th M25.561 right knee
- M25.562 left knee

M25.57 Pain in ankle and joints of foot
- 6th M25.571 Pain in right ankle and joints of right foot
- M25.572 Pain in left ankle and joints of left foot

M25.59 Pain in other specified joint

M25.6 Stiffness of joint, NEC
- 5th *Excludes1:* ankylosis of joint (M24.6-)
- contracture of joint (M24.5-)

M25.60 Stiffness of unspecified joint, NEC

M25.61 Stiffness of shoulder, NEC
- 6th M25.611 Stiffness of right shoulder, NEC
- M25.612 Stiffness of left shoulder, NEC

M25.62 Stiffness of elbow, NEC
- 6th M25.621 Stiffness of right elbow, NEC
- M25.622 Stiffness of left elbow, NEC

M25.63 Stiffness of wrist, NEC
- 6th M25.631 Stiffness of right wrist, NEC
- M25.632 Stiffness of left wrist, NEC

M25.64 Stiffness of hand, NEC
- 6th M25.641 Stiffness of right hand, NEC
- M25.642 Stiffness of left hand, NEC

M25.65 Stiffness of hip, NEC
- 6th M25.651 Stiffness of right hip, NEC
- M25.652 Stiffness of left hip, NEC

M25.66 Stiffness of knee, NEC
- M25.661 Stiffness of right knee, NEC
- M25.662 Stiffness of left knee, NEC

M25.67 Stiffness of ankle and foot, NEC
- M25.671 Stiffness of right ankle, NEC
- M25.672 Stiffness of left ankle, NEC
- M25.674 Stiffness of right foot, NEC
- M25.675 Stiffness of left foot, NEC

M25.69 Stiffness of other specified joint, NEC

M25.7 Osteophyte
- M25.70 Osteophyte, unspecified joint
- M25.71 Osteophyte, shoulder
  - M25.711 right shoulder
  - M25.712 left shoulder
- M25.72 Osteophyte, elbow
  - M25.721 right elbow
  - M25.722 left elbow
- M25.73 Osteophyte, wrist
  - M25.731 right wrist
  - M25.732 left wrist
- M25.74 Osteophyte, hand
  - M25.741 right hand
  - M25.742 left hand
- M25.75 Osteophyte, hip
  - M25.751 right hip
  - M25.752 left hip
- M25.76 Osteophyte, knee
  - M25.761 right knee
  - M25.762 left knee
- M25.77 Osteophyte, ankle and foot
  - M25.771 right ankle
  - M25.772 left ankle
  - M25.774 right foot
  - M25.775 left foot
- M25.78 Osteophyte, vertebrae

M25.9 Joint disorder, unspecified

(M26–M27) DENTOFACIAL ANOMALIES [INCLUDING MALOCCLUSION] AND OTHER DISORDERS OF JAW

Excludes1: hemifacial atrophy or hypertrophy (Q67.4)
unilateral condylar hyperplasia or hypoplasia (M27.8)

M26 DENTOFACIAL ANOMALIES [INCLUDING MALOCCLUSION]

M26.0 Major anomalies of jaw size
Excludes1: acromegaly (E22.0)
Robin's syndrome (Q87.0)
- M26.00 Unspecified anomaly of jaw size
- M26.04 Mandibular hypoplasia
- M26.09 Other specified anomalies of jaw size

M26.2 Anomalies of dental arch relationship
- M26.20 Unspecified anomaly of dental arch relationship
- M26.29 Other anomalies of dental arch relationship
  - Midline deviation of dental arch
  - Overbite (excessive) deep
  - Overbite (excessive) horizontal
  - Overbite (excessive) vertical
  - Posterior lingual occlusion of mandibular teeth

M26.4 Malocclusion, unspecified

M26.6 Temporomandibular joint disorders
Excludes2: current temporomandibular joint dislocation (S03.0)
current temporomandibular joint sprain (S03.4)
- M26.60 Temporomandibular joint disorder, unspecified
  - M26.601 Right temporomandibular joint disorder
  - M26.602 Left temporomandibular joint disorder
  - M26.603 Bilateral temporomandibular joint disorder
- M26.61 Adhesions and ankylosis of temporomandibular joint
  - M26.611 Adhesions and ankylosis of right temporomandibular joint
  - M26.612 Adhesions and ankylosis of left temporomandibular joint

- M26.613 Adhesions and ankylosis of bilateral temporomandibular joint
- M26.62 Arthralgia of temporomandibular joint
  - M26.621 Arthralgia of right temporomandibular joint
  - M26.622 Arthralgia of left temporomandibular joint
  - M26.623 Arthralgia of bilateral temporomandibular joint
- M26.63 Articular disc disorder of temporomandibular joint
  - M26.631 Articular disc disorder of right temporomandibular joint
  - M26.632 Articular disc disorder of left temporomandibular joint
  - M26.633 Articular disc disorder of bilateral temporomandibular joint

M26.69 Other specified disorders of temporomandibular joint

M27 OTHER DISEASES OF JAWS

M27.0 Developmental disorders of jaws
- Latent bone cyst of jaw
- Stafne's cyst
- Torus mandibularis
- Torus palatinus

M27.2 Inflammatory conditions of jaws
- Osteitis of jaw(s)
- Osteomyelitis (neonatal) jaw(s)
- Osteoradionecrosis jaw(s)
- Periostitis jaw(s)
- Sequestrum of jaw bone
- **Use additional code** (W88–W90, X39.0) to identify radiation, if radiation-induced

Excludes2: osteonecrosis of jaw due to drug (M87.180)

M27.4 Other and unspecified cysts of jaw
Excludes1: cysts of oral region (K09.-)
latent bone cyst of jaw (M27.0)
Stafne's cyst (M27.0)
- M27.40 Unspecified cyst of jaw
  - Cyst of jaw NOS
- M27.49 Other cysts of jaw
  - Aneurysmal cyst of jaw
  - Hemorrhagic cyst of jaw
  - Traumatic cyst of jaw

M27.8 Other specified diseases of jaws
- Cherubism
- Exostosis
- Fibrous dysplasia
- Unilateral condylar hyperplasia
- Unilateral condylar hypoplasia

Excludes1: jaw pain (R68.84)

(M30–M36) SYSTEMIC CONNECTIVE TISSUE DISORDERS

Includes: autoimmune disease NOS
collagen (vascular) disease NOS
systemic autoimmune disease
systemic collagen (vascular) disease

Excludes1: autoimmune disease, single organ or single cell type—code to relevant condition category

M30 POLYARTERITIS NODOSA AND RELATED CONDITIONS

Excludes1: microscopic polyarteritis (M31.7)

M30.2 Juvenile polyarteritis

M30.3 Mucocutaneous lymph node syndrome [Kawasaki]

M30.8 Other conditions related to polyarteritis nodosa
- Polyangiitis overlap syndrome

M31 OTHER NECROTIZING VASCULOPATHIES

M31.0 Hypersensitivity angiitis
- Goodpasture's syndrome

M31.1 Thrombotic microangiopathy
- M31.10 Thrombotic microangiopathy, unspecified
- M31.11 Hematopoietic stem cell transplantation-associated thrombotic microangiopathy [HSCT-TMA]
  - Transplant-associated thrombotic microangiopathy [TA-TMA]

Code first if applicable:
complications of bone marrow transplant (T86.0-)
complications of stem cell transplant (T86.5)

Use Additional code to identify specific organ dysfunction, such as:
acute kidney failure (N17.-)
acute respiratory distress syndrome (J80)
capillary leak syndrome (I78.8)
diffuse alveolar hemorrhage (R04.89)
encephalopathy (metabolic) (septic) (G93.41)
fluid overload, unspecified (E87.70)
graft versus host disease (D89.81-)
hemolytic uremic syndrome (D59.3)
hepatic failure (K72.-)
hepatic veno-occlusive disease (K76.5)
idiopathic interstitial pneumonia (J84.11-)
sinusoidal obstruction syndrome (K76.5)

- **M31.19** Other thrombotic microangiopathy
  - Thrombotic thrombocytopenic purpura
- **M31.3** Wegener's granulomatosis
  - Granulomatosis with polyangiitis
  - Necrotizing respiratory granulomatosis
  - **M31.30** Wegener's granulomatosis without renal involvement
    - Wegener's granulomatosis NOS
  - **M31.31** Wegener's granulomatosis with renal involvement
- **M31.4** Aortic arch syndrome [Takayasu]
- **M31.8** Other specified necrotizing vasculopathies
  - Hypocomplementemic vasculitis
  - Septic vasculitis
- **M31.9** Necrotizing vasculopathy, unspecified

M32 SLE

Excludes1: lupus erythematosus (discoid) (NOS) (L93.0)

- **M32.0** Drug-induced systemic lupus erythematosus
  - **Use additional code** for adverse effect, if applicable, to identify drug (T36–T50 with fifth or sixth character 5)
- **M32.1** SLE with organ or system involvement
  - **M32.10** SLE, organ or system involvement unspecified
  - **M32.11** Endocarditis in SLE
    - Libman-Sacks disease
  - **M32.12** Pericarditis in SLE
    - Lupus pericarditis
  - **M32.13** Lung involvement in SLE
    - Pleural effusion due to SLE
  - **M32.14** Glomerular disease in SLE
    - Lupus renal disease NOS
  - **M32.15** Tubulo-interstitial nephropathy in SLE
  - **M32.19** Other organ or system involvement in SLE
    - **Use additional** code(s) to identify organ or system involvement, such as encephalitis (G05.3)
- **M32.8** Other forms of SLE
- **M32.9** SLE, unspecified
  - SLE NOS
  - SLE NOS
  - SLE without organ involvement

M33 DERMATOPOLYMYOSITIS

- **M33.0** Juvenile dermatomyositis
  - **M33.00** Juvenile dermatomyositis, organ involvement unspecified
  - **M33.01** Juvenile dermatomyositis with respiratory involvement
  - **M33.02** Juvenile dermatomyositis with myopathy
  - **M33.03** Juvenile dermatomyositis without myopathy
  - **M33.09** Juvenile dermatomyositis with other organ involvement
- **M33.1** Other dermatomyositis
  - Adult dermatomyositis
  - **M33.10** Other dermatomyositis, organ involvement unspecified
  - **M33.11** Other dermatomyositis with respiratory involvement
  - **M33.12** Other dermatomyositis with myopathy
  - **M33.13** Other dermatomyositis without myopathy
    - Dermatomyositis NOS
  - **M33.19** Other dermatomyositis with other organ involvement

- **M33.9** Dermatopolymyositis, unspecified
  - **M33.90** Dermatopolymyositis, unspecified, organ involvement unspecified
  - **M33.91** Dermatopolymyositis, unspecified with respiratory involvement
  - **M33.92** Dermatopolymyositis, unspecified with myopathy
  - **M33.93** Dermatopolymyositis, unspecified without myopathy
  - **M33.99** Dermatopolymyositis, unspecified with other organ involvement

M35 OTHER SYSTEMIC INVOLVEMENT OF CONNECTIVE TISSUE

Excludes1: reactive perforating collagenosis (L87.1)

- **M35.7** Hypermobility syndrome
  - Familial ligamentous laxity
  - *Excludes1:* Ehlers-Danlos syndromes (Q79.6-)
    - ligamentous laxity, NOS (M24.2-)
- **M35.8** Other specified systemic involvement of connective tissue
  - **GUIDELINE**
  - See code U07.1 for details.
  - **M35.81** Multisystem inflammatory syndrome
    - MIS
    - MIS-C
    - **Use Additional** post COVID-19 condition (U09.9)
  - **M35.89** Other specified systemic involvement of connective tissue
- **M35.9** Systemic involvement of connective tissue, unspecified
  - Autoimmune disease (systemic) NOS
  - Collagen (vascular) disease NOS

M36 SYSTEMIC DISORDERS OF CONNECTIVE TISSUE IN DISEASES CLASSIFIED ELSEWHERE

Excludes2: arthropathies in diseases classified elsewhere (M14.-)

- **M36.0** Dermato(poly)myositis in neoplastic disease
  - **Code first** underlying neoplasm (C00-D49)
- **M36.1** Arthropathy in neoplastic disease
  - **Code first** underlying neoplasm, such as:
    - leukemia (C91-C95)
    - malignant histiocytosis (C96.A)
    - multiple myeloma (C90.0)
- **M36.2** Hemophilic arthropathy
  - Hemarthrosis in hemophilic arthropathy
  - **Code first:** underlying disease, such as: factor VIII deficiency (D66)
    - with vascular defect (D68.0)
    - factor IX deficiency (D67)
    - hemophilia (classical) (D66)
    - hemophilia B (D67)
    - hemophilia C (D68.1)
- **M36.3** Arthropathy in other blood disorders
- **M36.4** Arthropathy in hypersensitivity reactions classified elsewhere
  - **Code first** underlying disease, such as Henoch (-Schönlein)
    - purpura (D69.0)
    - serum sickness (T80.6-)
- **M36.8** Systemic disorders of connective tissue in other diseases classified elsewhere
  - **Code first** underlying disease, such as:
    - alkaptonuria (E70.29)
    - hypogammaglobulinemia (D80.-)
    - ochronosis (E70.29)

(M40–M43) DEFORMING DORSOPATHIES

M40 KYPHOSIS AND LORDOSIS

Code first underlying disease

Excludes1: congenital kyphosis and lordosis (Q76.4)
kyphoscoliosis (M41.-)
postprocedural kyphosis and lordosis (M96.-)

- **M40.2** Other and unspecified kyphosis
  - **M40.20** Unspecified kyphosis
    - **M40.202** cervical region
    - **M40.203** cervicothoracic region
    - **M40.204** thoracic region
    - **M40.205** thoracolumbar region
    - **M40.209** site unspecified

M40.29 Other kyphosis

	M40.292	cervical region
	M40.293	cervicothoracic region
	M40.294	thoracic region
	M40.295	thoracolumbar region
	M40.299	site unspecified

M40.4 Postural lordosis

Acquired lordosis

M40.40	site unspecified
M40.45	thoracolumbar region
M40.46	lumbar region
M40.47	lumbosacral region

M40.5 Lordosis, unspecified

M40.50	site unspecified
M40.55	thoracolumbar region
M40.56	lumbar region
M40.57	lumbosacral region

M41 SCOLIOSIS

Includes: kyphoscoliosis

Excludes1: congenital scoliosis NOS (Q67.5)
congenital scoliosis due to bony malformation (Q76.3)
postural congenital scoliosis (Q67.5)
kyphoscoliotic heart disease (I27.1)

Excludes2: postprocedural scoliosis (M96.89)
postradiation scoliosis (M96.5)

M41.0 Infantile idiopathic scoliosis

M41.00	site unspecified
M41.02	cervical region
M41.03	cervicothoracic region
M41.04	thoracic region
M41.05	thoracolumbar region
M41.06	lumbar region
M41.07	lumbosacral region
M41.08	sacral and sacrococcygeal region

M41.1 Juvenile and adolescent idiopathic scoliosis

M41.11 Juvenile idiopathic scoliosis

M41.112	cervical region
M41.113	cervicothoracic region
M41.114	thoracic region
M41.115	thoracolumbar region
M41.116	lumbar region
M41.117	lumbosacral region
M41.119	site unspecified

M41.12 Adolescent idiopathic scoliosis

M41.122	Adolescent idiopathic scoliosis, cervical region
M41.123	Adolescent idiopathic scoliosis, cervicothoracic region
M41.124	Adolescent idiopathic scoliosis, thoracic region
M41.125	Adolescent idiopathic scoliosis, thoracolumbar region
M41.126	Adolescent idiopathic scoliosis, lumbar region
M41.127	Adolescent idiopathic scoliosis, lumbosacral region
M41.129	Adolescent idiopathic scoliosis, site unspecified

M41.2 Other idiopathic scoliosis

M41.20	Other idiopathic scoliosis, site unspecified
M41.22	cervical region
M41.23	cervicothoracic region
M41.24	thoracic region
M41.25	thoracolumbar region
M41.26	lumbar region
M41.27	lumbosacral region

M41.9 Scoliosis, unspecified

M43 OTHER DEFORMING DORSOPATHIES

Excludes1: congenital spondylolysis and spondylolisthesis (Q76.2)
hemivertebra (Q76.3–Q76.4)
Klippel-Feil syndrome (Q76.1)
lumbarization and sacralization (Q76.4)
platyspondylisis (Q76.4)

spina bifida occulta (Q76.0)
spinal curvature in osteoporosis (M80.-)
spinal curvature in Paget's disease of bone [osteitis deformans] (M88.-)

M43.0 Spondylolysis

Excludes1: congenital spondylolysis (Q76.2)
spondylolisthesis (M43.1)

M43.00	Spondylolysis, site unspecified
M43.01	occipito-atlanto-axial region
M43.02	cervical region
M43.03	cervicothoracic region
M43.04	thoracic region
M43.05	thoracolumbar region
M43.06	lumbar region
M43.07	lumbosacral region
M43.08	sacral and sacrococcygeal region
M43.09	multiple sites in spine

M43.1 Spondylolisthesis

Excludes1: acute traumatic of lumbosacral region (S33.1)
acute traumatic of sites other than lumbosacral- code to
Fracture, vertebra, by region
congenital spondylolisthesis (Q76.2)

M43.10	Spondylolisthesis, site unspecified
M43.11	occipito-atlanto-axial region
M43.12	cervical region
M43.13	cervicothoracic region
M43.14	thoracic region
M43.15	thoracolumbar region
M43.16	lumbar region
M43.17	lumbosacral region
M43.18	sacral and sacrococcygeal region
M43.19	multiple sites in spine

M43.6 Torticollis

Excludes1: congenital (sternomastoid) torticollis (Q68.0)
current injury — see Injury, of spine, by body region
ocular torticollis (R29.891)
psychogenic torticollis (F45.8)
spasmodic torticollis (G24.3)
torticollis due to birth injury (P15.2)

(M45–M49) SPONDYLOPATHIES

M48 OTHER SPONDYLOPATHIES

M48.0 Spinal stenosis

Caudal stenosis

M48.00	Spinal stenosis, site unspecified
M48.01	Spinal stenosis, occipito-atlanto-axial region
M48.02	Spinal stenosis, cervical region
M48.03	Spinal stenosis, cervicothoracic region
M48.04	Spinal stenosis, thoracic region
M48.05	Spinal stenosis, thoracolumbar region
M48.06	Spinal stenosis, lumbar region
	M48.061 Spinal stenosis, lumbar region without neurogenic claudication
	Spinal stenosis, lumbar region NOS
	M48.062 Spinal stenosis, lumbar region with neurogenic claudication
M48.07	Spinal stenosis, lumbosacral region
M48.08	Spinal stenosis, sacral and sacrococcygeal region

(M50–M54) OTHER DORSOPATHIES

Excludes1: current injury — see injury of spine by body region
discitis NOS (M46.4-)

M53 OTHER AND UNSPECIFIED DORSOPATHIES, NOT ELSEWHERE CLASSIFIED

M53.3 Sacrococcygeal disorders, not elsewhere classified

Coccygodynia

M53.9 Dorsopathy, unspecified

M54 DORSALGIA

Excludes1: psychogenic dorsalgia (F45.41)

M54.2 Cervicalgia

Excludes1: cervicalgia due to intervertebral cervical disc disorder (M50.-)

M54.4 Lumbago with sciatica

5th *Excludes1:* intervertebral disc degeneration, lumbar region with discogenic back pain and lower extremitypain (M51.362) intervertebral disc degeneration, lumbosacral region with discogenic back pain and lowerextremity pain (M51.372) lumbago with sciatica due to intervertebral disc disorder (M51.1-)

- **M54.40 Lumbago with sciatica, unspecified side**
- **M54.41 Lumbago with sciatica, right side**
- **M54.42 Lumbago with sciatica, left side**

M54.5 Low back pain

5th *Excludes1:* intervertebral disc degeneration, lumbar region with discogenic back pain only (M51.360) intervertebral disc degeneration, lumbosacral region with discogenic back pain only (M51.370) low back strain (S39.012) lumbago due to intervertebral disc displacement (M51.2-) lumbago with sciatica (M54.4-)

- **M54.50 Low back pain, unspecified**
  - Loin pain
  - Lumbago NOS
- **M54.51 Vertebrogenic low back pain**
  - Low back vertebral endplate pain
- **M54.59 Other low back pain**

M54.9 Dorsalgia, unspecified

Backache NOS
Back pain NOS

(M60–M79) SOFT TISSUE DISORDERS

(M60–M63) DISORDERS OF MUSCLES

Excludes1: dermatopolymyositis (M33.-)
myopathy in amyloidosis (E85.-)
myopathy in polyarteritis nodosa (M30.0)
myopathy in rheumatoid arthritis (M05.32)
myopathy in scleroderma (M34.-)
myopathy in Sjögren's syndrome (M35.03)
myopathy in systemic lupus erythematosus (M32.-)
Excludes2: muscular dystrophies and myopathies (G71-G72)

M60 MYOSITIS

4th *Excludes2:* inclusion body myositis [IBM] (G72.41)

M60.0 Infective myositis

5th Tropical pyomyositis

Use additional code (B95–B97) to identify infectious agent

- **M60.00 Infective myositis, unspecified site**
  - 6th **M60.000** unspecified right arm
    - Infective myositis, right upper limb NOS
  - **M60.001** unspecified left arm
    - Infective myositis, left upper limb NOS
  - **M60.003** unspecified right leg
    - Infective myositis, right lower limb NOS
  - **M60.004** unspecified left leg
    - Infective myositis, left lower limb NOS
  - **M60.009** unspecified site
- **M60.01 Infective myositis, shoulder**
  - 6th **M60.011** right shoulder
  - **M60.012** left shoulder
- **M60.02 Infective myositis, upper arm**
  - 6th **M60.021** right upper arm
  - **M60.022** left upper arm
- **M60.03 Infective myositis, forearm**
  - 6th **M60.031** right forearm
  - **M60.032** left forearm
- **M60.04 Infective myositis, hand and fingers**
  - 6th **M60.041** right hand
  - **M60.042** left hand
  - **M60.044** right finger(s)
  - **M60.045** left finger(s)
- **M60.05 Infective myositis, thigh**
  - 6th **M60.051** right thigh
  - **M60.052** left thigh
- **M60.06 Infective myositis, lower leg**
  - 6th **M60.061** right lower leg
  - **M60.062** left lower leg
- **M60.07 Infective myositis, ankle, foot and toes**
  - 6th **M60.070** right ankle
  - **M60.071** left ankle
  - **M60.073** right foot
  - **M60.074** left foot
  - **M60.076** right toe(s)
  - **M60.077** left toe(s)
- **M60.08 Infective myositis, other site**
- **M60.09 Infective myositis, multiple sites**

M60.1 Interstitial myositis

- 5th **M60.10 Interstitial myositis of unspecified site**
- **M60.11 Interstitial myositis, shoulder**
  - 6th **M60.111** right shoulder
  - **M60.112** left shoulder
- **M60.12 Interstitial myositis, upper arm**
  - 6th **M60.121** right upper arm
  - **M60.122** left upper arm
- **M60.13 Interstitial myositis, forearm**
  - 6th **M60.131** right forearm
  - **M60.132** left forearm
- **M60.14 Interstitial myositis, hand**
  - 6th **M60.141** right hand
  - **M60.142** left hand
- **M60.15 Interstitial myositis, thigh**
  - 6th **M60.151** right thigh
  - **M60.152** left thigh
- **M60.16 Interstitial myositis, lower leg**
  - 6th **M60.161** right lower leg
  - **M60.162** left lower leg

M60.2 Foreign body granuloma of soft tissue, not elsewhere classified

5th Use additional code to identify the type of retained foreign body (Z18.-)

Excludes1: foreign body granuloma of skin and subcutaneous tissue (L92.3)

- **M60.21 Foreign body granuloma of soft tissue, NEC, shoulder**
  - 6th **M60.211** right shoulder
  - **M60.212** left shoulder
- **M60.22 Foreign body granuloma of soft tissue, NEC, upper arm**
  - 6th **M60.221** right upper arm
  - **M60.222** left upper arm
- **M60.23 Foreign body granuloma of soft tissue, NEC, forearm**
  - 6th **M60.231** right forearm
  - **M60.232** left forearm
- **M60.24 Foreign body granuloma of soft tissue, NEC, hand**
  - 6th **M60.241** right hand
  - **M60.242** left hand
- **M60.25 Foreign body granuloma of soft tissue, NEC, thigh**
  - 6th **M60.251** right thigh
  - **M60.252** left thigh
- **M60.26 Foreign body granuloma of soft tissue, NEC, lower leg**
  - 6th **M60.261** right lower leg
  - **M60.262** left lower leg
- **M60.27 Foreign body granuloma of soft tissue, NEC, ankle and foot**
  - 6th **M60.271** right ankle and foot
  - **M60.272** left ankle and foot
- **M60.28 Foreign body granuloma of soft tissue, NEC, other site**

M60.9 Myositis, unspecified

M62 OTHER DISORDERS OF MUSCLE

4th *Excludes1:* alcoholic myopathy (G72.1)
cramp and spasm (R25.2)
drug-induced myopathy (G72.0)
myalgia (M79.1-)
stiff-man syndrome (G25.82)
Excludes2: nontraumatic hematoma of muscle (M79.81)

M62.4 Contracture of muscle

Contracture of tendon (sheath)

Excludes1: contracture of joint (M24.5-)

- M62.40 Contracture of muscle, unspecified site
- M62.41 Contracture of muscle, shoulder
  - M62.411 right shoulder
  - M62.412 left shoulder
- M62.42 Contracture of muscle, upper arm
  - M62.421 right upper arm
  - M62.422 left upper arm
- M62.43 Contracture of muscle, forearm
  - M62.431 right forearm
  - M62.432 left forearm
- M62.44 Contracture of muscle, hand
  - M62.441 right hand
  - M62.442 left hand
- M62.45 Contracture of muscle, thigh
  - M62.451 right thigh
  - M62.452 left thigh
- M62.46 Contracture of muscle, lower leg
  - M62.461 right lower leg
  - M62.462 left lower leg
- M62.47 Contracture of muscle, ankle and foot
  - M62.471 right ankle and foot
  - M62.472 left ankle and foot
- M62.48 Contracture of muscle, other site
- M62.49 Contracture of muscle, multiple sites

M62.5 Muscle wasting and atrophy, not elsewhere classified

Disuse atrophy NEC

Excludes1: neuralgic amyotrophy (G54.5)
progressive muscular atrophy (G12.21) sarcopenia (M62.84)

Excludes2: pelvic muscle wasting (N81.84)

- M62.5A0 Muscle wasting and atrophy, not elsewhere classified, back, cervical
- M62.5A1 Muscle wasting and atrophy, not elsewhere classified, back, thoracic
- M62.5A2 Muscle wasting and atrophy, not elsewhere classified, back, lumbosacral

M62.8 Other specified disorders of muscle

Excludes2: nontraumatic hematoma of muscle (M79.81)

- M62.81 Muscle weakness (generalized)
  - *Excludes1:* muscle weakness in sarcopenia (M62.84)
- M62.82 Rhabdomyolysis
  - *Excludes1:* traumatic rhabdomyolysis (T79.6)
- M62.83 Muscle spasm
  - M62.830 Muscle spasm of back
  - M62.831 Muscle spasm of calf
    - Charley-horse
  - M62.838 Other muscle spasm
- •M62.85 Dysfunction of the multifidus muscles, lumbar region
- M62.89 Other specified disorders of muscle
  - Muscle (sheath) hernia

M62.9 Disorder of muscle, unspecified

(M65–M67) DISORDERS OF SYNOVIUM AND TENDON

M65 SYNOVITIS AND TENOSYNOVITIS

Excludes1: chronic crepitant synovitis of hand and wrist (M70.0-)
current injury — see injury of ligament or tendon by body region
soft tissue disorders related to use, overuse and pressure (M70.-)

- **M65.4** Radial styloid tenosynovitis [de Quervain]
- **M65.8** Other synovitis and tenosynovitis
  - M65.80 Other synovitis and tenosynovitis, unspecified site
  - M65.81 Other synovitis and tenosynovitis; shoulder
    - M65.811 right shoulder
    - M65.812 left shoulder
  - M65.82 Other synovitis and tenosynovitis; upper arm
    - M65.821 right upper arm
    - M65.822 left upper arm
  - M65.83 Other synovitis and tenosynovitis; forearm
    - M65.831 right forearm
    - M65.832 left forearm
  - M65.84 Other synovitis and tenosynovitis; hand

- M65.841 right hand
- M65.842 left hand
- M65.85 Other synovitis and tenosynovitis; thigh
  - M65.851 right thigh
  - M65.852 left thigh
- M65.86 Other synovitis and tenosynovitis; lower leg
  - M65.861 right lower leg
  - M65.862 left lower leg
- M65.87 Other synovitis and tenosynovitis; ankle and foot
  - M65.871 right ankle and foot
  - M65.872 left ankle and foot
- M65.88 Other synovitis and tenosynovitis, other site
- M65.89 Other synovitis and tenosynovitis, multiple sites

M65.9 Synovitis and tenosynovitis, unspecified

- •M65.90 Unspecified synovitis and tenosynovitis, unspecified site
- •M65.91 Unspecified synovitis and tenosynovitis, shoulder
  - •M65.911 right shoulder
  - •M65.912 left shoulder
  - M65.919 unspecified shoulder
- •M65.92 Unspecified synovitis and tenosynovitis, upper arm
  - •M65.921 right upper arm
  - •M65.922 left upper arm
  - •M65.929 unspecified upper arm
- •M65.93 Unspecified synovitis and tenosynovitis, forearm
  - •M65.931 right forearm
  - •M65.932 left forearm
  - •M65.939 unspecified forearm
- •M65.94 Unspecified synovitis and tenosynovitis, hand
  - •M65.941 right hand
  - •M65.942 left hand
  - •M65.949 unspecified hand
- •M65.95 Unspecified synovitis and tenosynovitis, thigh
  - •M65.951 right thigh
  - M65.952 left thigh
  - •M65.959 unspecified thigh
- •M65.96 Unspecified synovitis and tenosynovitis, lower leg
  - •M65.961 right lower leg
  - •M65.962 left lower leg
  - •M65.969 unspecified lower leg
- •M65.97 Unspecified synovitis and tenosynovitis, ankle and foot
  - •M65.971 right ankle and foot
  - •M65.972 left ankle and foot
  - •M65.979 unspecified ankle and foot
- •M65.98 Unspecified synovitis and tenosynovitis, other site
- •M65.99 Unspecified synovitis and tenosynovitis, multiple sites

M67 OTHER DISORDERS OF SYNOVIUM AND TENDON

Excludes1: palmar fascial fibromatosis [Dupuytren] (M72.0)
tendinitis NOS (M77.9-)
xanthomatosis localized to tendons (E78.2)

- **M67.0** Short Achilles tendon (acquired)
  - M67.01 right ankle
  - M67.02 left ankle
- **M67.4** Ganglion

Ganglion of joint or tendon (sheath)

Excludes1: ganglion in yaws (A66.6)

Excludes2: cyst of bursa (M71.2– M71.3)
cyst of synovium (M71.2–M71.3)

- M67.40 Ganglion, unspecified site
- M67.41 Ganglion, shoulder
  - M67.411 right shoulder
  - M67.412 left shoulder
- M67.42 Ganglion, elbow
  - M67.421 right elbow
  - M67.422 left elbow
- M67.43 Ganglion, wrist
  - M67.431 right wrist
  - M67.432 left wrist
- M67.44 Ganglion, hand
  - M67.441 right hand
  - M67.442 left hand

M67.45 Ganglion, hip

M67.451 right hip

M67.452 left hip

M67.46 Ganglion, knee

M67.461 right knee

M67.462 left knee

M67.47 Ganglion, ankle and foot

M67.471 right ankle and foot

M67.472 left ankle and foot

M67.48 Ganglion, other site

M67.49 Ganglion, multiple sites

(M70–M79) OTHER SOFT TISSUE DISORDERS

M70 SOFT TISSUE DISORDERS RELATED TO USE, OVERUSE AND PRESSURE

Includes: soft tissue disorders of occupational origin

Use additional external cause code to identify activity causing disorder (Y93.-)

Excludes1: bursitis NOS (M71.9-)

Excludes2: bursitis of shoulder (M75.5)

enthesopathies (M76-M77)

pressure ulcer (pressure area) (L89.-)

M70.3 Other bursitis of elbow

M70.31 right elbow

M70.32 left elbow

M70.6 Trochanteric bursitis

Trochanteric tendinitis

M70.61 right hip

M70.62 left hip

M70.7 Other bursitis of hip

Ischial bursitis

M70.71 right hip

M70.72 left hip

M71 OTHER BURSOPATHIES

Excludes1: bunion (M20.1)

bursitis related to use, overuse or pressure (M70.-)

enthesopathies (M76–M77)

M71.2 Synovial cyst of popliteal space [Baker]

Excludes1: synovial cyst of popliteal space with rupture (M66.0)

M71.21 right knee

M71.22 left knee

M71.5 Other bursitis, NEC

Excludes1: bursitis NOS (M71.9-)

Excludes2: bursitis of shoulder (M75.5)

bursitis of tibial collateral [Pellegrini-Stieda] (M76.4-)

M71.50 unspecified site

M71.52 elbow

M71.521 right elbow

M71.522 left elbow

M71.53 wrist

M71.531 right wrist

M71.532 left wrist

M71.54 hand

M71.541 right hand

M71.542 left hand

M71.55 hip

M71.551 right hip

M71.552 left hip

M71.56 knee

M71.561 right knee

M71.562 left knee

M71.57 ankle and foot

M71.571 right ankle and foot

M71.572 left ankle and foot

M71.58 other site

M71.9 Bursopathy, unspecified

Bursitis NOS

M72 FIBROBLASTIC DISORDERS

Excludes2: retroperitoneal fibromatosis (D48.3)

M72.6 Necrotizing fasciitis

Use additional code (B95.-, B96.-) to identify causative organism

M72.8 Other fibroblastic disorders

Abscess of fascia

Fasciitis NEC

Other infective fasciitis

Use additional code to (B95.-, B96.-) identify causative organism

Excludes1: diffuse (eosinophilic) fasciitis (M35.4)

necrotizing fasciitis (M72.6)

nodular fasciitis (M72.4)

perirenal fasciitis NOS (N13.5)

perirenal fasciitis with infection (N13.6)

plantar fasciitis (M72.2)

M72.9 Fibroblastic disorder, unspecified

Fasciitis NOS

Fibromatosis NOS

M75 SHOULDER LESIONS

M75.1 Rotator cuff tear or rupture, not specified as traumatic

Rotator cuff syndrome

Supraspinatus tear or rupture, not specified as traumatic

Supraspinatus syndrome

Excludes1: tear of rotator cuff, traumatic (S46.01-)

Excludes2: shoulder-hand syndrome (M89.0-)

M75.10 Unspecified rotator cuff tear or rupture, not specified as traumatic

M75.101 Unspecified rotator cuff tear or rupture of right shoulder, not specified as traumatic

M75.102 Unspecified rotator cuff tear or rupture of left shoulder, not specified as traumatic

M75.11 Incomplete rotator cuff tear or rupture not specified as traumatic

M75.111 Incomplete rotator cuff tear or rupture of right shoulder, not specified as traumatic

M75.112 Incomplete rotator cuff tear or rupture of left shoulder, not specified as traumatic

M75.12 Complete rotator cuff tear or rupture not specified as traumatic

M75.121 Complete rotator cuff tear or rupture of right shoulder, not specified as traumatic

M75.122 Complete rotator cuff tear or rupture of left shoulder, not specified as traumatic

M76 ENTHESOPATHIES, LOWER LIMB, EXCLUDING FOOT

Excludes2: bursitis due to use, overuse and pressure (M70.-)

enthesopathies of ankle and foot (M77.5-)

M76.0 Gluteal tendinitis

M76.01 right hip

M76.02 left hip

M76.1 Psoas tendinitis

M76.11 right hip

M76.12 left hip

M76.2 Iliac crest spur

M76.21 right hip

M76.22 left hip

M76.3 Iliotibial band syndrome

M76.31 right leg

M76.32 left leg

M76.4 Tibial collateral bursitis [Pellegrini-Stieda]

M76.41 right leg

M76.42 left leg

M76.6 Achilles tendinitis

Achilles bursitis

M76.61 right leg

M76.62 left leg

M76.7 Peroneal tendinitis

M76.71 right leg

M76.72 left leg

M76.8 Other specified enthesopathies of lower limb, excluding foot

M76.81 Anterior tibial syndrome

M76.811 right leg

M76.812 left leg

M76.82 Posterior tibial tendinitis

M76.821 right leg

M76.822 left leg

M76.89 Other specified enthesopathies of lower limb, excluding foot

M76.891 Other specified enthesopathies of right lower limb, excluding foot
M76.892 Other specified enthesopathies of left lower limb, excluding foot
M76.9 Unspecified enthesopathy, lower limb, excluding foot

M77 OTHER ENTHESOPATHIES

4th

Excludes1: bursitis NOS (M71.9-)
Excludes2: bursitis due to use, overuse and pressure (M70.-)
osteophyte (M25.7)
spinal enthesopathy (M46.0-)

M77.0 Medial epicondylitis

5th

M77.01 right elbow
M77.02 left elbow

M77.1 Lateral epicondylitis

5th

Tennis elbow
M77.11 right elbow
M77.12 left elbow

M77.5 Other enthesopathy of foot and ankle

5th

M77.51 Other enthesopathy of right foot and ankle
M77.52 Other enthesopathy of left foot and ankle

M77.8 Other enthesopathies, NEC

M77.9 Enthesopathy, unspecified
Bone spur NOS
Capsulitis NOS
Periarthritis NOS
Tendinitis NOS

M79 OTHER AND UNSPECIFIED SOFT TISSUE DISORDERS, NEC

4th

Excludes1: psychogenic rheumatism (F45.8)
soft tissue pain, psychogenic (F45.41)

M79.0 Rheumatism, unspecified
Excludes1: fibromyalgia (M79.7)
palindromic rheumatism (M12.3-)

M79.1 Myalgia

5th

Myofascial pain syndrome
Excludes1: fibromyalgia (M79.7)
myositis (M60.-)

M79.10 Myalgia, unspecified site
M79.11 Myalgia of mastication muscle
M79.12 Myalgia of auxiliary muscles, head and neck
M79.18 Myalgia, other site

M79.2 Neuralgia and neuritis, unspecified
Excludes1: brachial radiculitis NOS (M54.1)
lumbosacral radiculitis NOS (M54.1)
mononeuropathies (G56-G58)
radiculitis NOS (M54.1)
sciatica (M54.3-M54.4)

M79.5 Residual foreign body in soft tissue
Excludes1: foreign body granuloma of skin and subcutaneous tissue (L92.3)
foreign body granuloma of soft tissue (M60.2-)

M79.6 Pain in limb, hand, foot, fingers and toes

5th

Excludes2: pain in joint (M25.5-)

M79.60 Pain in limb, unspecified

6th

M79.601 Pain in right arm
Pain in right upper limb NOS
M79.602 Pain in left arm
Pain in left upper limb NOS
M79.604 Pain in right leg
Pain in right lower limb NOS
M79.605 Pain in left leg
Pain in left lower limb NOS

M79.62 Pain in upper arm

6th

Pain in axillary region
M79.621 Pain in right upper arm
M79.622 Pain in left upper arm

M79.63 Pain in forearm

6th

M79.631 Pain in right forearm
M79.632 Pain in left forearm

M79.64 Pain in hand and fingers

6th

M79.641 Pain in right hand
M79.642 Pain in left hand
M79.644 Pain in right finger(s)

M79.645 Pain in left finger(s)

M79.65 Pain in thigh

6th

M79.651 Pain in right thigh
M79.652 Pain in left thigh

M79.66 Pain in lower leg

6th

M79.661 Pain in right lower leg
M79.662 Pain in left lower leg

M79.67 Pain in foot and toes

6th

M79.671 Pain in right foot
M79.672 Pain in left foot
M79.674 Pain in right toe(s)
M79.675 Pain in left toe(s)

M79.8 Other specified soft tissue disorders

5th

M79.81 Nontraumatic hematoma of soft tissue
Nontraumatic hematoma of muscle
Nontraumatic seroma of muscle and soft tissue

M79.89 Other specified soft tissue disorders
Polyalgia

M79.9 Soft tissue disorder, unspecified

(M80–M94) OSTEOPATHIES AND CHONDROPATHIES

(M80–M85) DISORDERS OF BONE DENSITY AND STRUCTURE

M84 DISORDER OF CONTINUITY OF BONE

4th

GUIDELINES

Coding of Pathologic Fractures

7th character A is for use as long as the patient is receiving active treatment for the fracture. While the patient may be seen by a new or different provider over the course of treatment for a pathological fracture, assignment of the 7th character is based on whether the patient is undergoing active treatment and not whether the provider is seeing the patient for the first time. 7th character D is to be used for encounters after the patient has completed active treatment for the fracture and is receiving routine care for the fracture during the healing or recovery phase. The other 7th characters, listed under each subcategory in the Tabular List, are to be used for subsequent encounters for treatment of problems associated with the healing, such as malunions, nonunions, and sequelae.

Care for complications of surgical treatment for fracture repairs during the healing or recovery phase should be coded with the appropriate complication codes.

Excludes2: traumatic fracture of bone—see fracture, by site

M84.3 Stress fracture

5th

Fatigue fracture
March fracture
Stress fracture NOS
Stress reaction
Use additional external cause code(s) to identify the cause of the stress fracture
Excludes1: pathological fracture NOS (M84.4.-)
pathological fracture due to osteoporosis (M80.-)
traumatic fracture (S12.-, S22.-, S32.-, S42.-, S52.-, S62.-, S72.-, S82.-, S92.-)
Excludes2: personal history of (healed) stress (fatigue) fracture (Z87.312)
stress fracture of vertebra (M48.4-)

M84.3 requires a 7th character
A—initial encounter for fracture care
D—subsequent encounter with routine healing
G—subsequent encounter for fracture with delayed healing
K—subsequent encounter for fracture with nonunion
P—subsequent encounter for fracture with malunion
S—sequela

M84.30X- Stress fracture, unspecified site

7th

M84.31 Stress fracture, shoulder

6th

M84.311- Stress fracture, right shoulder

7th

M84.312- Stress fracture, left shoulder

7th

M84.32 Stress fracture, humerus

6th

M84.321- Stress fracture, right humerus

7th

M84.322- Stress fracture, left humerus

M84.33 Stress fracture, ulna and radius
M84.331- Stress fracture, right ulna
M84.332- Stress fracture, left ulna
M84.333- Stress fracture, right radius
M84.334- Stress fracture, left radius

M84.34 Stress fracture, hand and fingers
M84.341- Stress fracture, right hand
M84.342- Stress fracture, left hand
M84.344- Stress fracture, right finger(s)
M84.345- Stress fracture, left finger(s)

M84.35 Stress fracture, pelvis and femur
Stress fracture, hip
M84.350- Stress fracture, pelvis
M84.351- Stress fracture, right femur
M84.352- Stress fracture, left femur
M84.359- Stress fracture, hip, unspecified

M84.36 Stress fracture, tibia and fibula
M84.361- Stress fracture, right tibia
M84.362- Stress fracture, left tibia
M84.363- Stress fracture, right fibula
M84.364- Stress fracture, left fibula

M84.37 Stress fracture, ankle, foot and toes
M84.371- Stress fracture, right ankle
M84.372- Stress fracture, left ankle
M84.374- Stress fracture, right foot
M84.375- Stress fracture, left foot
M84.377- Stress fracture, right toe(s)
M84.378- Stress fracture, left toe(s)

M84.38X- Stress fracture, other site
Excludes2: stress fracture of vertebra (M48.4-)

M84.8 Other disorders of continuity of bone
M84.88 Other disorders of continuity of bone, other site

M85 OTHER DISORDERS OF BONE DENSITY AND STRUCTURE

Excludes1: osteogenesis imperfecta (Q78.0)
osteopetrosis (Q78.2)
osteopoikilosis (Q78.8)
polyostotic fibrous dysplasia (Q78.1)

M85.2 Hyperostosis of skull

M85.6 Other cyst of bone
Excludes1: cyst of jaw NEC (M27.4)
osteitis fibrosa cystica generalisata [von Recklinghausen's disease of bone] (E21.0)

M85.60 Other cyst of bone, unspecified site
M85.61 Other cyst of bone, shoulder
M85.611 right shoulder
M85.612 left shoulder
M85.62 Other cyst of bone, upper arm
M85.621 right upper arm

M85.622 left upper arm
M85.63 Other cyst of bone, forearm
M85.631 right forearm
M85.632 left forearm
M85.64 Other cyst of bone, hand
M85.641 right hand
M85.642 left hand
M85.65 Other cyst of bone, thigh
M85.651 right thigh
M85.652 left thigh
M85.66 Other cyst of bone, lower leg
M85.661 right lower leg
M85.662 left lower leg
M85.67 Other cyst of bone, ankle and foot
M85.671 right ankle and foot
M85.672 left ankle and foot
M85.68 Other cyst of bone, other site
M85.69 Other cyst of bone, multiple sites

(M86–M90) OTHER OSTEOPATHIES

Excludes1: postprocedural osteopathies (M96.-)

M86 OSTEOMYELITIS

Use additional code (B95–B97) to identify infectious agent
Use additional code to identify major osseous defect, if applicable (M89.7-)

Excludes1: osteomyelitis due to:
Echinococcus (B67.2)
gonococcus (A54.43)
Salmonella (A02.24)

Excludes2: osteomyelitis of:
orbit (H05.0-)
petrous bone (H70.2-)
vertebra (M46.2-)

M86.1 Other acute osteomyelitis

M86.10 Other acute osteomyelitis, unspecified site
M86.11 Other acute osteomyelitis, shoulder
M86.111 right shoulder
M86.112 left shoulder
M86.12 Other acute osteomyelitis, humerus
M86.121 right humerus
M86.122 left humerus
M86.13 Other acute osteomyelitis, radius and ulna
M86.131 right radius and ulna
M86.132 left radius and ulna
M86.14 Other acute osteomyelitis, hand
M86.141 right hand
M86.142 left hand
M86.15 Other acute osteomyelitis, femur
M86.151 right femur
M86.152 left femur
M86.16 Other acute osteomyelitis, tibia and fibula
M86.161 right tibia and fibula
M86.162 left tibia and fibula
M86.17 Other acute osteomyelitis, ankle and foot
M86.171 right ankle and foot
M86.172 left ankle and foot
M86.18 Other acute osteomyelitis, other site
M86.19 Other acute osteomyelitis, multiple sites

M86.9 Osteomyelitis, unspecified
Infection of bone NOS
Periostitis without osteomyelitis

M88 OSTEITIS DEFORMANS [PAGET'S DISEASE OF BONE]

Excludes1: osteitis deformans in neoplastic disease (M90.6)

M88.0 Osteitis deformans of skull
M88.1 Osteitis deformans of vertebrae
M88.8 Osteitis deformans of other bones
M88.81 Osteitis deformans of shoulder
M88.811 right shoulder
M88.812 left shoulder
M88.82 Osteitis deformans of upper arm
M88.821 right upper arm
M88.822 left upper arm

M88.83 Osteitis deformans of forearm
- M88.831 right forearm
- M88.832 left forearm

M88.84 Osteitis deformans of hand
- M88.841 right hand
- M88.842 left hand

M88.85 Osteitis deformans of thigh
- M88.851 right thigh
- M88.852 left thigh

M88.86 Osteitis deformans of lower leg
- M88.861 right lower leg
- M88.862 left lower leg

M88.87 Osteitis deformans of ankle and foot
- M88.871 right ankle and foot
- M88.872 left ankle and foot

M88.88 Osteitis deformans of other bones
- *Excludes2:* osteitis deformans of skull (M88.0)
- osteitis deformans of vertebrae (M88.1)

M88.89 Osteitis deformans of multiple sites

M88.9 Osteitis deformans of unspecified bone

M89 OTHER DISORDERS OF BONE

M89.1 Physeal arrest

Arrest of growth plate
Epiphyseal arrest
Growth plate arrest

M89.12 Physeal arrest, humerus

M89.121 Complete physeal arrest, right proximal humerus

M89.122 Complete physeal arrest, left proximal humerus

M89.123 Partial physeal arrest, right proximal humerus

M89.124 Partial physeal arrest, left proximal humerus

M89.125 Complete physeal arrest, right distal humerus

M89.126 Complete physeal arrest, left distal humerus

M89.127 Partial physeal arrest, right distal humerus

M89.128 Partial physeal arrest, left distal humerus

M89.129 Physeal arrest, humerus, unspecified

M89.13 Physeal arrest, forearm

M89.131 Complete physeal arrest, right distal radius

M89.132 Complete physeal arrest, left distal radius

M89.133 Partial physeal arrest, right distal radius

M89.134 Partial physeal arrest, left distal radius

M89.138 Other physeal arrest of forearm

M89.139 Physeal arrest, forearm, unspecified

M89.15 Physeal arrest, femur

M89.151 Complete physeal arrest, right proximal femur

M89.152 Complete physeal arrest, left proximal femur

M89.153 Partial physeal arrest, right proximal femur

M89.154 Partial physeal arrest, left proximal femur

M89.155 Complete physeal arrest, right distal femur

M89.156 Complete physeal arrest, left distal femur

M89.157 Partial physeal arrest, right distal femur

M89.158 Partial physeal arrest, left distal femur

M89.159 Physeal arrest, femur, unspecified

M89.16 Physeal arrest, lower leg

M89.160 Complete physeal arrest, right proximal tibia

M89.161 Complete physeal arrest, left proximal tibia

M89.162 Partial physeal arrest, right proximal tibia

M89.163 Partial physeal arrest, left proximal tibia

M89.164 Complete physeal arrest, right distal tibia

M89.165 Complete physeal arrest, left distal tibia

M89.166 Partial physeal arrest, right distal tibia

M89.167 Partial physeal arrest, left distal tibia

M89.168 Other physeal arrest of lower leg

M89.169 Physeal arrest, lower leg, unspecified

M89.18 Physeal arrest, other site

M90 OSTEOPATHIES IN DISEASES CLASSIFIED ELSEWHERE

Excludes1: osteochondritis, osteomyelitis, and osteopathy (in):
- cryptococcosis (B45.3)
- DM (E08–E13 with .69-)
- gonococcal (A54.43)
- neurogenic syphilis (A52.11)
- renal osteodystrophy (N25.0)
- salmonellosis (A02.24)
- secondary syphilis (A51.46)
- syphilis (late) (A52.77)

M90.5 Osteonecrosis in diseases classified elsewhere

Code first underlying disease, such as: caisson disease (T70.3) hemoglobinopathy (D50–D64)

M90.50 Osteonecrosis in diseases classified elsewhere, unspecified site

M90.51 Osteonecrosis in diseases classified elsewhere; shoulder
- M90.511 right shoulder
- M90.512 left shoulder

M90.52 Osteonecrosis in diseases classified elsewhere; upper arm
- M90.521 right upper arm
- M90.522 left upper arm

M90.53 Osteonecrosis in diseases classified elsewhere; forearm
- M90.531 right forearm
- M90.532 left forearm

M90.54 Osteonecrosis in diseases classified elsewhere; hand
- M90.541 right hand
- M90.542 left hand

M90.55 Osteonecrosis in diseases classified elsewhere; thigh
- M90.551 right thigh
- M90.552 left thigh

M90.56 Osteonecrosis in diseases classified elsewhere; lower leg
- M90.561 right lower leg
- M90.562 left lower leg

M90.57 Osteonecrosis in diseases classified elsewhere; ankle and foot
- M90.571 right ankle and foot
- M90.572 left ankle and foot

M90.58 Osteonecrosis in diseases classified elsewhere, other site

M90.59 Osteonecrosis in diseases classified elsewhere, multiple sites

M90.6 Osteitis deformans in neoplastic diseases

Osteitis deformans in malignant neoplasm of bone
Code first the neoplasm (C40.-, C41.-)
Excludes1: osteitis deformans [Paget's disease of bone] (M88.-)
Refer to the full *ICD-10-CM* manual for full codes

M90.8 Osteopathy in diseases classified elsewhere

Code first underlying disease, such as:
- rickets (E55.0)
- vitamin-D-resistant rickets (E83.31)

M90.80 Osteopathy in diseases classified elsewhere, unspecified site

(M91–M94) CHONDROPATHIES

Excludes1: postprocedural chondropathies (M96.-)

M91 JUVENILE OSTEOCHONDROSIS OF HIP AND PELVIS

Excludes1: slipped upper femoral epiphysis (nontraumatic) (M93.0)

M91.0 Juvenile osteochondrosis of pelvis
- Osteochondrosis (juvenile) of acetabulum
- Osteochondrosis (juvenile) of iliac crest [Buchanan]
- Osteochondrosis (juvenile) of ischiopubic synchondrosis [van Neck]
- Osteochondrosis (juvenile) of symphysis pubis [Pierson]

M91.1 Juvenile osteochondrosis of head of femur [Legg-Calvé-Perthes]

M91.11 Juvenile osteochondrosis of head of femur [Legg-Calvé-Perthes], right leg
M91.12 Juvenile osteochondrosis of head of femur [Legg-Calvé-Perthes], left leg
M91.2 Coxa plana
Hip deformity due to previous juvenile osteochondrosis
M91.21 Coxa plana, right hip
M91.22 Coxa plana, left hip
M91.3 Pseudocoxalgia
M91.31 Pseudocoxalgia, right hip
M91.32 Pseudocoxalgia, left hip
M91.4 Coxa magna
M91.41 Coxa magna, right hip
M91.42 Coxa magna, left hip
M91.8 Other juvenile osteochondrosis of hip and pelvis
Juvenile osteochondrosis after reduction of congenital dislocation of hip
M91.81 Other juvenile osteochondrosis of hip and pelvis, right leg
M91.82 Other juvenile osteochondrosis of hip and pelvis, left leg
M91.9 Juvenile osteochondrosis of hip and pelvis, unspecified
M91.91 Juvenile osteochondrosis of hip and pelvis, unspecified, right leg
M91.92 Juvenile osteochondrosis of hip and pelvis, unspecified, left leg

M92 OTHER JUVENILE OSTEOCHONDROSIS

M92.0 Juvenile osteochondrosis of humerus
Osteochondrosis (juvenile) of capitulum of humerus [Panner]
Osteochondrosis (juvenile) of head of humerus [Haas]
M92.01 right arm
M92.02 left arm

M92.1 Juvenile osteochondrosis of radius and ulna
Osteochondrosis (juvenile) of lower ulna [Burns]
Osteochondrosis (juvenile) of radial head [Brailsford]
M92.11 right arm
M92.12 left arm

M92.2 Juvenile osteochondrosis, hand
M92.20 Unspecified juvenile osteochondrosis; hand
M92.201 right hand
M92.202 left hand
M92.21 Osteochondrosis (juvenile) of carpal lunate [Kienböck];
M92.211 right hand
M92.212 left hand
M92.22 Osteochondrosis (juvenile) of metacarpal heads [Mauclaire];
M92.221 right hand
M92.222 left hand
M92.29 Other juvenile osteochondrosis; hand
M92.291 right hand
M92.292 left hand

M92.3 Other juvenile osteochondrosis; upper limb
M92.31 right upper limb
M92.32 left upper limb

M92.4 Juvenile osteochondrosis of patella;
Osteochondrosis (juvenile) of primary patellar center [Köhler]
Osteochondrosis (juvenile) of secondary patellar centre [Sinding Larsen]
M92.41 right knee
M92.42 left knee

M92.5 Juvenile osteochondrosis of tibia and fibula;
M92.50 Unspecified juvenile osteochondrosis of tibia and fibula
M92.501 right leg
M92.502 left leg
M92.503 bilateral leg
M92.51 Juvenile osteochondrosis of proximal tibia
Blount disease
Tibia vara
M92.511 right leg
M92.512 left leg
M92.513 bilateral

M92.52 Juvenile osteochondrosis of tibia tubercle
Osgood-Schlatter disease
M92.521 right leg
M92.522 left leg
M92.523 bilateral
M92.59 Other juvenile osteochondrosis of tibia and fibula
M92.591 right leg
M92.592 left leg
M92.593 bilateral

M92.6 Juvenile osteochondrosis of tarsus;
Osteochondrosis (juvenile) of calcaneum [Sever]
Osteochondrosis (juvenile) of os tibiale externum [Haglund]
Osteochondrosis (juvenile) of talus [Diaz]
Osteochondrosis (juvenile) of tarsal navicular [Köhler]
M92.61 right ankle
M92.62 left ankle

M92.7 Juvenile osteochondrosis of metatarsus;
Osteochondrosis (juvenile) of fifth metatarsus [Iselin]
Osteochondrosis (juvenile) of second metatarsus [Freiberg]
M92.71 right foot
M92.72 left foot

M92.8 Other specified juvenile osteochondrosis

M92.9 Juvenile osteochondrosis, unspecified
Juvenile apophysitis NOS
Juvenile epiphysitis NOS
Juvenile osteochondritis NOS
Juvenile osteochondrosis NOS

M93 OTHER OSTEOCHONDROPATHIES

Excludes2: osteochondrosis of spine (M42.-)

M93.0 Slipped upper femoral epiphysis (nontraumatic)
Use additional code for associated chondrolysis (M94.3)
M93.00 Unspecified slipped upper femoral epiphysis (nontraumatic);
M93.001 right hip
M93.002 left hip
M93.004 bilateral hips
M93.01 Acute slipped upper femoral epiphysis, stable (nontraumatic);
M93.011 right hip
M93.012 left hip
M93.014 bilateral hips
M93.02 Chronic slipped upper femoral epiphysis, stable (nontraumatic);
M93.021 right hip
M93.022 left hip
M93.024 bilateral hips
M93.03 Acute on chronic slipped upper femoral epiphysis, stable (nontraumatic);
M93.031 right hip
M93.032 left hip
M93.034 bilateral hips
M93.04 Acute slipped upper femoral epiphysis, unstable (nontraumatic);
M93.041 right hip
M93.042 left hip
M93.044 bilateral hips
M93.05 Acute on chronic slipped upper femoral epiphysis, unstable (nontraumatic);
M93.051 right hip
M93.052 left hip
M93.054 bilateral hips
M93.06 Acute slipped upper femoral epiphysis, unspecified stability (nontraumatic);
M93.061 right hip
M93.062 left hip
M93.064 bilateral hips
M93.07 Acute on chronic slipped upper femoral epiphysis, unspecified stability (nontraumatic);
M93.071 right hip
M93.072 left hip
M93.074 bilateral hips

M93.9 Osteochondropathy, unspecified

Apophysitis NOS
Epiphysitis NOS
Osteochondritis NOS
Osteochondrosis NOS
Refer to full *ICD-10-CM* manual for codes

M94 OTHER DISORDERS OF CARTILAGE

M94.0 Chondrocostal junction syndrome [Tietze]
Costochondritis

M94.2 Chondromalacia

M94.26 Chondromalacia, knee

M94.261 Chondromalacia, right knee

M94.262 Chondromalacia, left knee

M94.8 Other specified disorders of cartilage

M94.8X Other specified disorders of cartilage

M94.8X0	multiple sites
M94.8X1	shoulder
M94.8X2	upper arm
M94.8X3	forearm
M94.8X4	hand
M94.8X5	thigh
M94.8X6	lower leg
M94.8X7	ankle and foot
M94.8X8	other site
M94.8X9	unspecified sites

(M95) OTHER DISORDERS OF MUSCULOSKELETAL SYSTEM AND CONNECTIVE TISSUE

M95 OTHER ACQUIRED DEFORMITIES OF MUSCULOSKELETAL SYSTEM AND CONNECTIVE TISSUE

Excludes2: acquired absence of limbs and organs (Z89–Z90)
acquired deformities of limbs (M20–M21)
congenital malformations and deformations of the musculoskeletal system (Q65–Q79)
deforming dorsopathies (M40–M43)
dentofacial anomalies [including malocclusion] (M26.-)
postprocedural musculoskeletal disorders (M96.-)

M95.0 Acquired deformity of nose
Excludes2: deviated nasal septum (J34.2)

M95.2 Other acquired deformity of head

M95.3 Acquired deformity of neck

M95.4 Acquired deformity of chest and rib

M95.5 Acquired deformity of pelvis

M95.8 Other specified acquired deformities of musculoskeletal system

M95.9 Acquired deformity of musculoskeletal system, unspecified

M96 INTRAOPERATIVE AND POSTPROCEDURAL COMPLICATIONS AND DISORDERS OF MUSCULOSKELETAL SYSTEM, NOT ELSEWHERE CLASSIFIED

Excludes2: arthropathy following intestinal bypass (M02.0-)
complications of internal orthopedic prosthetic devices, implants and grafts (T84.-)
disorders associated with osteoporosis (M80)
periprosthetic fracture around internal prosthetic joint (M97.-)
presence of functional implants and other devices (Z96-Z97)

M96.A1 Fracture of sternum associated with chest compression and cardiopulmonary resuscitation

M96.A2 Fracture of one rib associated with chest compression and cardiopulmonary resuscitation

M96.A3 Multiple fractures of ribs associated with chest compression and cardiopulmonary resuscitation

M96.A4 Flail chest associated with chest compression and cardiopulmonary resuscitation

M96.A9 Other fracture associated with chest compression and cardiopulmonary resuscitation

Chapter 14. Diseases of the genitourinary system (N00–N99)

GUIDELINES

Chronic kidney disease

STAGES OF CKD
See category N18.

CKD AND KIDNEY TRANSPLANT STATUS
See category N18.

CKD WITH OTHER CONDITIONS
Patients with CKD may also suffer from other serious conditions, most commonly DM and hypertension (in adults). The sequencing of the CKD code in relationship to codes for other contributing conditions is based on the conventions in the Tabular List.

See Chapter 19 for CKD and kidney transplant complications.
Excludes2: certain conditions originating in the perinatal period (P04–P96)
certain infectious and parasitic diseases (A00–B99)
complications of pregnancy, childbirth and the puerperium (O00–O9A)
congenital malformations, deformations and chromosomal abnormalities (Q00–Q99)
endocrine, nutritional and metabolic diseases (E00–E88)
injury, poisoning and certain other consequences of external causes (S00–T88)
neoplasms (C00–D49)
symptoms, signs and abnormal clinical and laboratory findings, NEC (R00–R94)

(N00–N08) GLOMERULAR DISEASES

Code also any associated kidney failure (N17–N19).
Excludes1: hypertensive CKD (I12.-)

N00 ACUTE NEPHRITIC SYNDROME

Includes: acute glomerular disease
acute glomerulonephritis
acute nephritis
Excludes1: acute tubulo-interstitial nephritis (N10)
nephritic syndrome NOS (N05.-)

- **N00.0 Acute nephritic syndrome with; minor glomerular abnormality**
  Acute nephritic syndrome with minimal change lesion
- **N00.1 focal and segmental glomerular lesions**
  Acute nephritic syndrome with focal and segmental hyalinosis or with focal and segmental sclerosis or with focal glomerulonephritis
- **N00.2 diffuse membranous glomerulonephritis**
- **N00.3 diffuse mesangial proliferative glomerulonephritis**
- **N00.4 diffuse endocapillary proliferative glomerulonephritis**
- **N00.5 diffuse mesangiocapillary glomerulonephritis**
  Acute nephritic syndrome with MPGN, types 1 and 3, or NOS
  Excludes1: Acute nephritic syndrome with C3 glomerulonephritis or glomerulopathy (N00.A)
- **N00.6 dense deposit disease**
  Acute nephritic syndrome with C3 glomerulopathy with dense deposit disease
  Acute nephritic syndrome with MPGN, type 2
- **N00.7 diffuse crescentic glomerulonephritis**
  Acute nephritic syndrome with extracapillary glomerulonephritis
- **N00.8 other morphologic changes**
  Acute nephritic syndrome with proliferative glomerulonephritis NOS
- **N00.9 unspecified morphologic changes**
- **N00.A Acute nephritic syndrome with C3 glomerulonephritis**
  Acute nephritic syndrome with C3 glomerulopathy, NOS
  Excludes1: Acute nephritic syndrome (with C3 glomerulopathy) with dense deposit disease(N00.6)

N01 RAPIDLY PROGRESSIVE NEPHRITIC SYNDROME

Includes: rapidly progressive glomerular disease
rapidly progressive glomerulonephritis
rapidly progressive nephritis
Excludes1: nephritic syndrome NOS (N05.-)

- **N01.0 Rapidly progressive nephritic syndrome with; minor glomerular abnormality**
  Rapidly progressive nephritic syndrome with minimal change lesion
- **N01.1 focal and segmental glomerular lesions**
  Rapidly progressive nephritic syndrome with focal and segmental hyalinosis or with focal and segmental sclerosis or with focal glomerulonephritis
- **N01.2 diffuse membranous glomerulonephritis**
- **N01.3 diffuse mesangial proliferative glomerulonephritis**
- **N01.4 diffuse endocapillary proliferative glomerulonephritis**
- **N01.5 diffuse mesangiocapillary glomerulonephritis**
  Rapidly progressive nephritic syndrome with MPGN, types 1 and 3, or NOS
  Excludes1: Rapidly progressive nephritic syndrome with C3 glomerulonephritis or glomerulopathy (N01.A)
- **N01.6 dense deposit disease**
  Rapidly progressive nephritic syndrome with C3 glomerulopathy with dense deposit disease
  Rapidly progressive nephritic syndrome with MPGN, type 2
- **N01.7 diffuse crescentic glomerulonephritis**
  Rapidly progressive nephritic syndrome with extracapillary glomerulonephritis
- **N01.8 other morphologic changes**
  Rapidly progressive nephritic syndrome with proliferative glomerulonephritis NOS
- **N01.9 unspecified morphologic changes**
- **N01.A Rapidly progressive nephritic syndrome with C3 glomerulonephritis**
  Rapidly progressive nephritic syndrome with C3 glomerulopathy, NOS
  Excludes1: Rapidly progressive nephritic syndrome (with C3 glomerulopathy) with dense depositdisease (N01.6)

N02 RECURRENT AND PERSISTENT HEMATURIA

Excludes1: acute cystitis with hematuria (N30.01)
hematuria NOS (R31.9)
hematuria not associated with specified morphologic lesions (R31.-)

- **N02.B Recurrent and persistent immunoglobulin A nephropathy**
  - **N02.B1 Recurrent and persistent immunoglobulin A nephropathy with glomerular lesion**
  - **N02.B2 Recurrent and persistent immunoglobulin A nephropathy with focal and segmental glomerular lesion**
    Recurrent and persistent immunoglobulin A nephropathy with focal and segmental hyalinosis or sclerosis
  - **N02.B3 Recurrent and persistent immunoglobulin A nephropathy with diffuse membranoproliferative glomerulonephritis**
  - **N02.B4 Recurrent and persistent immunoglobulin A nephropathy with diffuse membranous glomerulonephritis**
  - **N02.B5 Recurrent and persistent immunoglobulin A nephropathy with diffuse mesangial proliferative glomerulonephritis**
  - **N02.B6 Recurrent and persistent immunoglobulin A nephropathy with diffuse mesangiocapillary glomerulonephritis**
  - **N02.B9 Other recurrent and persistent immunoglobulin A nephropathy**

N03 CHRONIC NEPHRITIC SYNDROME

Includes: chronic glomerular disease
chronic glomerulonephritis
chronic nephritis
Excludes1: chronic tubulo-interstitial nephritis (N11.-)
diffuse sclerosing glomerulonephritis (N05.8-)
nephritic syndrome NOS (N05.-)

- **N03.0 Chronic nephritic syndrome with; minor glomerular abnormality**
  Chronic nephritic syndrome with minimal change lesion
- **N03.1 focal and segmental glomerular lesions**
  Chronic nephritic syndrome with focal and segmental hyalinosis or with focal and segmental sclerosis or with focal glomerulonephritis
- **N03.2 diffuse membranous glomerulonephritis**
- **N03.3 diffuse mesangial proliferative glomerulonephritis**

N03.4 diffuse endocapillary proliferative glomerulonephritis

N03.5 diffuse mesangiocapillary glomerulonephritis

Chronic nephritic syndrome with MPGN, types 1 and 3, or NOS

Excludes1: Chronic nephritic syndrome with C3 glomerulonephritis or glomerulopathy (N03.A)

N03.6 dense deposit disease

Chronic nephritic syndrome with MPGN, type 2

N03.7 diffuse crescentic glomerulonephritis

Chronic nephritic syndrome with C3 glomerulopathy with dense deposit disease

Chronic nephritic syndrome with extracapillary glomerulonephritis

N03.8 other morphologic changes

Chronic nephritic syndrome with proliferative glomerulonephritis NOS

N03.9 unspecified morphologic changes

N03.A Chronic nephritic syndrome with C3 glomerulonephritis

Chronic nephritic syndrome with C3 glomerulopathy

Excludes1: Chronic nephritic syndrome (with C3 glomerulopathy) with dense deposit disease (N03.6)

N04 NEPHROTIC SYNDROME

Includes: congenital nephrotic syndrome lipoid nephrosis

N04.0 Nephrotic syndrome with; minor glomerular abnormality

Nephrotic syndrome with minimal change lesion

N04.1 focal and segmental glomerular lesions

Nephrotic syndrome with focal and segmental hyalinosis or with focal and segmental sclerosis or with focal glomerulonephritis

N04.2 diffuse membranous glomerulonephritis

N04.20 Nephrotic syndrome with diffuse membranous glomerulonephritis, unspecified

Membranous nephropathy NOS with nephrotic syndrome

N04.21 Primary membranous nephropathy with nephrotic syndrome

Idiopathic membranous nephropathy with nephrotic syndrome

N04.22 Secondary membranous nephropathy with nephrotic syndrome

Code first, if applicable, other disease or disorder or poisoning causing membranous nephropathy

Use additional code, if applicable, for adverse effect of drug causing membranous nephropathy

N04.29 Other nephrotic syndrome with diffuse membranous glomerulonephritis

N04.3 diffuse mesangial proliferative glomerulonephritis

N04.4 diffuse endocapillary proliferative glomerulonephritis

N04.5 diffuse mesangiocapillary glomerulonephritis

Nephrotic syndrome with MPGN, types 1 and 3, or NOS

Excludes1: Nephrotic syndrome with C3 glomerulonephritis or glomerulopathy (N04.A)

N04.6 dense deposit disease

Nephrotic syndrome with C3 glomerulopathy with dense deposit disease

Nephrotic syndrome with MPGN, type 2

N04.7 diffuse crescentic glomerulonephritis

Nephrotic syndrome with extracapillary glomerulonephritis

N04.8 other morphologic changes

Nephrotic syndrome with proliferative glomerulonephritis NOS

N04.9 unspecified morphologic changes

N04.A Nephrotic syndrome with C3 glomerulonephritis

Nephrotic syndrome with C3 glomerulopathy

Excludes1: Nephrotic syndrome (with C3 glomerulopathy) with dense deposit disease (N04.6)

N05 UNSPECIFIED NEPHRITIC SYNDROME

Includes: glomerular disease NOS glomerulonephritis NOS nephritis NOS nephropathy NOS and renal disease NOS with morphological lesion specified in .0-.8

Excludes1: nephropathy NOS with no stated morphological lesion (N28.9) renal disease NOS with no stated morphological lesion (N28.9) tubulo-interstitial nephritis NOS (N12)

N05.0 Unspecified nephritic syndrome with minor glomerular abnormality

Unspecified nephritic syndrome with minimal change lesion

N05.1 Unspecified nephritic syndrome with focal and segmental glomerular lesions

Unspecified nephritic syndrome with focal and segmental hyalinosis

Unspecified nephritic syndrome with focal and segmental sclerosis

Unspecified nephritic syndrome with focal glomerulonephritis

N05.2 Unspecified nephritic syndrome with diffuse membranous glomerulonephritis

N05.3 Unspecified nephritic syndrome with diffuse mesangial proliferative glomerulonephritis

N05.4 Unspecified nephritic syndrome with diffuse endocapillary proliferative glomerulonephritis

N05.5 Unspecified nephritic syndrome with diffuse mesangiocapillary glomerulonephritis

Unspecified nephritic syndrome with membranoproliferative glomerulonephritis, types 1 and 3, or NOS

Excludes1: Unspecified nephritic syndrome with C3 glomerulonephritis or glomerulopathy (N05.A)

N05.6 Unspecified nephritic syndrome with dense deposit disease

Unspecified nephritic syndrome with membranoproliferative glomerulonephritis, type 2

Unspecified nephritic syndrome with C3 glomerulopathy with dense deposit disease

N05.7 Unspecified nephritic syndrome with diffuse crescentic glomerulonephritis

Unspecified nephritic syndrome with extracapillary glomerulonephritis

N05.8 Unspecified nephritic syndrome with other morphologic changes

Unspecified nephritic syndrome with proliferative glomerulonephritis NOS

N05.9 Unspecified nephritic syndrome with unspecified morphologic changes

N05.A Unspecified nephritic syndrome with C3 glomerulonephritis

Unspecified nephritic syndrome with C3 glomerulopathy

Excludes1: Unspecified nephritic syndrome (with C3 glomerulopathy) with dense deposit disease (N05.6)

N06 ISOLATED PROTEINURIA WITH SPECIFIED MORPHOLOGICAL LESION

Excludes1: Proteinuria not associated with specific morphologic lesions (R80.0)

N06.2 Isolated proteinuria with diffuse membranous glomerulonephritis

N06.20 Isolated proteinuria with diffuse membranous glomerulonephritis, unspecified

Membranous nephropathy, NOS

Excludes1: membranous nephropathy NOS with nephrotic syndrome (N04.20)

N06.21 Primary membranous nephropathy with isolated proteinuria

Idiopathic membranous nephropathy (with isolated proteinuria)

Primary membranous nephropathy, NOS

Excludes1: primary membranous nephropathy with nephrotic syndrome (N04.21)

N06.22 Secondary membranous nephropathy with isolated proteinuria

Secondary membranous nephropathy, NOS

Code first, if applicable, other disease or disorder or poisoning causing membranous nephropathy

Use additional code, if applicable, for adverse effect of drug causing membranous nephropathy

Excludes1: secondary membranous nephropathy with nephrotic syndrome (N04.22)

N06.29 Other isolated proteinuria with diffuse membranous glomerulonephritis

CHAPTER 14. DISEASES OF THE GENITOURINARY SYSTEM (N00–N17.0)

N08 CULTURAL DISEASES IN GENITOURINARY SYSTEM

N08 GLOMERULAR DISORDERS IN DISEASES CLASSIFIED ELSEWHERE

Glomerulonephritis
Nephritis
Nephropathy

Code first underlying disease, such as:
- amyloidosis (E85.-)
- congenital syphilis (A50.5)
- cryoglobulinemia (A89.1)
- disseminated intravascular coagulation (D65)
- gout (M1A.-, M10.-)
- microscopic polyangiitis (M31.7)
- multiple myeloma (C90.0-)
- sepsis (A40.0-A41.9)
- sickle-cell disease (D57.0-D57.8)

Excludes1: glomerulonephritis, nephritis and nephropathy (in):
- antoglomerular basement membrane disease (M31.0)
- diabetes (E08-E13 with .21)
- gonococcal (A54.21)
- Goodpasture's syndrome (M31.0)
- hemolytic-uremic syndrome (D59.3)
- lupus (M32.14)
- mumps (B26.83)
- syphilis (A52.75)
- SLE (M32.14)
- Wegener's granulomatosis (M31.31)
- pyelonephritis in diseases classified elsewhere (N16)
- renal tubulo-interstitial disorders classified elsewhere (N16)

(N10–N16) RENAL TUBULO-INTERSTITIAL DISEASES

Includes: pyelonephritis
Excludes1: pyeloureteritis cystica (N28.85)

N10 ACUTE PYELONEPHRITIS
🔵 Acute infectious interstitial nephritis
Acute pyelitis
Hemoglobin nephrosis
Myoglobin nephrosis
Use additional code (B95-B97), to identify infectious agent.

N11 CHRONIC TUBULO-INTERSTITIAL NEPHRITIS
Includes: chronic infectious interstitial nephritis
- chronic pyelitis
- chronic pyelonephritis

Use additional code (B95-B97), to identify infectious agent

N11.9 Chronic tubulo-interstitial nephritis, unspecified
- Chronic interstitial nephritis NOS
- Chronic pyelitis NOS
- Chronic pyelonephritis NOS

N12 TUBULO-INTERSTITIAL NEPHRITIS, NOT SPECIFIED AS ACUTE OR CHRONIC
🔵 Interstitial nephritis NOS
Pyelitis NOS
Pyelonephritis NOS
Excludes1: calculous pyelonephritis (N20.9)

N13 OBSTRUCTIVE AND REFLUX UROPATHY
Excludes2: calculus of kidney and ureter without hydronephrosis (N20.-)
- congenital obstructive defects of renal pelvis and ureter (Q62.0-Q62.3)
- hydronephrosis with ureteropelvic junction obstruction (Q62.11)
- obstructive pyelonephritis (N11.1)

N13.0 Hydronephrosis with ureteropelvic junction obstruction
Hydronephrosis due to acquired occlusion ureteropelvic junction
Excludes2: hydronephrosis with ureteropelvic junction obstruction due to calculus (N13.2)

N13.1 Hydronephrosis with ureteral stricture, NEC
Excludes1: hydronephrosis with ureteral stricture with infection (N13.6)

N13.2 Hydronephrosis with renal and ureteral calculous obstruction
Excludes1: hydronephrosis with renal and ureteral calculous obstruction with infection (N13.6)

N13.3 Other and unspecified hydronephrosis
Excludes1: hydronephrosis with infection (N13.6)

N13.30 Unspecified hydronephrosis

N13.39 Other hydronephrosis

N13.5 Crossing vessel and stricture of ureter without hydronephrosis
Kinking and stricture of ureter without hydronephrosis
Excludes1: Crossing vessel and stricture of ureter without hydronephrosis with infection (N13.6)

N13.6 Pyonephrosis
Conditions in N13.0-N13.5 with infection
Obstructive uropathy with infection
Use additional code (B95-B97), to identify infectious agent.

N13.7 Vesicoureteral-reflux
Excludes1: reflux-associated pyelonephritis (N11.0)

N13.70 Vesicoureteral-reflux, unspecified
Vesicoureteral-reflux NOS

N13.71 Vesicoureteral-reflux without reflux nephropathy

N13.8 Other obstructive and reflux uropathy
Urinary tract obstruction due to specified cause
Code first, if applicable, any causal condition, such as:
- enlarged prostate (N40.1)

N13.9 Obstructive and reflux uropathy, unspecified
Urinary tract obstruction NOS

N14 DRUG- AND CHEMICAL-INDUCED TUBULO-INTERSTITIAL AND TUBULAR CONDITIONS
Code first poisoning due to drug or toxin, if applicable (T36-T65 with fifth or sixth character 1-4)
Use additional code for adverse effect, if applicable, to identify drug (T36-T50 with fifth or sixth character 5)

N14.0 Analgesic nephropathy

N16 RENAL TUBULO-INTERSTITIAL DISORDERS IN DISEASES CLASSIFIED ELSEWHERE
🔵 Pyelonephritis
Tubulo-interstitial nephritis
Code first underlying disease, such as:
- brucellosis (A23)
- cryoglobulinemia (D89.1)
- glycogen storage disease (E74.0-)
- leukemia (C91-C95)
- lymphoma (C81.0-C85.9, C96.0-C96.9)
- multiple myeloma (C90.0-)
- sepsis (A40.0-A41.9)
- Wilson's disease (E83.01)

Excludes1: diphtheritic pyelonephritis and tubulo-interstitial nephritis (A36.84)
- pyelonephritis and tubulo-interstitial nephritis in candidiasis (B37.49)
- in cystinosis (E72.04)
- in Salmonella infection (A02.25)
- in sarcoidosis (D86.84)
- in Sjögren syndrome (M35.04)
- in systemic lupus erythematosus (M32.15)
- in toxoplasmosis (B58.83)
- renal tubular degeneration in diabetes (E08-E13 with .29)
- syphilitic pyelonephritis and tubulo-interstitial nephritis (A52.75)

(N17–N19) ACUTE KIDNEY FAILURE AND CKD

Excludes2: congenital renal failure (P96.0)
- drug- and heavy-metal-induced tubulo-interstitial and tubular conditions (N14.-)
- extrarenal uremia (R39.2)
- hemolytic-uremic syndrome (D59.3)
- hepatorenal syndrome (K76.7)
- postpartum hepatorenal syndrome (O90.41)
- posttraumatic renal failure (T79.5)
- prerenal uremia (R39.2)
- renal failure complicating abortion or ectopic or molar pregnancy (O00-O07, O08.4)
- renal failure following labor and delivery (O90.41)
- renal failure postprocedural (N99.0)

N17 ACUTE KIDNEY FAILURE
Code also associated underlying condition
Excludes1: posttraumatic renal failure (T79.5)

N17.0 Acute kidney failure with tubular necrosis
- Acute tubular necrosis
- Renal tubular necrosis
- Tubular necrosis NOS

N17.1 Acute kidney failure with acute cortical necrosis
Acute cortical necrosis
Cortical necrosis NOS
Renal cortical necrosis

N17.2 Acute kidney failure with medullary necrosis
Medullary [papillary] necrosis NOS
Acute medullary [papillary] necrosis
Renal medullary [papillary] necrosis

N17.8 Other acute kidney failure

N17.9 Acute kidney failure, unspecified
Acute kidney injury (nontraumatic)
Excludes2: traumatic kidney injury (S37.0-)

N18 CHRONIC KIDNEY DISEASE (CKD)

GUIDELINES

Stages of CKD

The *ICD-10-CM* classifies CKD based on severity. The severity of CKD is designated by stages 1–5. Stage 2, code N18.2, equates to mild CKD; stage 3, codes N18.30–N18.32, equate to moderate CKD; and stage 4, code N18.4, equates to severe CKD. Code N18.6, ESRD, is assigned when the provider has documented ESRD.

If both a stage of CKD and ESRD are documented, assign code N18.6 only.

Chronic kidney disease and kidney transplant status

Patients who have undergone kidney transplant may still have some form of CKD because the kidney transplant may not fully restore kidney function. Therefore, the presence of CKD alone does not constitute a transplant complication. Assign the appropriate N18 code for the patient's stage of CKD and code Z94.0, Kidney transplant status. If a transplant complication such as failure or rejection or other transplant complication is documented, refer to code T86.1 for information on coding complications of a kidney transplant. If the documentation is unclear as to whether the patient has a complication of the transplant, query the provider.

Code first any associated diabetic CKD (E08.22, E09.22, E10.22, E11.22, E13.22)
hypertensive chronic kidney disease (I12.-, I13.-)

Use additional code to identify kidney transplant status, if applicable, (Z94.0)

N18.1 CKD stage 1

N18.2 CKD stage 2 (mild)

N18.3 CKD stage 3 (moderate)

N18.30 CKD, stage 3 unspecified

N18.31 CKD, stage 3a

N18.32 CKD, stage 3b

N18.4 CKD stage 4 (severe)

N18.5 CKD stage 5
Excludes1: CKD, stage 5 requiring chronic dialysis (N18.6)

N18.6 ESRD
CKD requiring chronic dialysis
Use additional code to identify dialysis status (Z99.2)

N18.9 CKD, unspecified
Chronic renal disease
Chronic renal failure NOS
Chronic renal insufficiency
Chronic uremia NOS

N19 UNSPECIFIED KIDNEY FAILURE

Uremia NOS
Excludes1: acute kidney failure (N17.-)
chronic kidney disease (N18.-)
chronic uremia (N18.9)
extrarenal uremia (R39.2)
prerenal uremia (R39.2)
renal insufficiency (acute) (N28.9)
uremia of newborn (P96.0)

(N20–N23) UROLITHIASIS

N20 CALCULUS OF KIDNEY AND URETER

Calculous pyelonephritis
Excludes1: nephrocalcinosis (E83.59)
that with hydronephrosis (N13.2)

N20.0 Calculus of kidney
Nephrolithiasis NOS
Renal calculus
Renal stone
Staghorn calculus
Stone in kidney

N20.1 Calculus of ureter
Ureteric stone
Calculus of the ureteropelvic junction

N20.2 Calculus of kidney with calculus of ureter

N20.9 Urinary calculus, unspecified

N21 CALCULUS OF LOWER URINARY TRACT

Includes: calculus of lower urinary tract with cystitis and urethritis

N21.0 Calculus in bladder
Calculus in diverticulum of bladder
Urinary bladder stone
Excludes2: staghorn calculus (N20.0)

N21.1 Calculus in urethra
Excludes2: calculus of prostate (N42.0)

N22 CALCULUS OF URINARY TRACT IN DISEASES CLASSIFIED ELSEWHERE

Code first underlying disease, such as:
gout (M1A.-, M10.-)
schistosomiasis (B65.0-B65.9)

N23 UNSPECIFIED RENAL COLIC

(N25–N29) OTHER DISORDERS OF KIDNEY AND URETER

Excludes2: disorders of kidney and ureter with urolithiasis (N20–N23)

N25 DISORDERS RESULTING FROM IMPAIRED RENAL TUBULAR FUNCTION

N25.0 Renal osteodystrophy
Azotemic osteodystrophy
Phosphate-losing tubular disorders
Renal rickets
Renal short stature
Excludes2: metabolic disorders classifiable to E70–E88

N25.1 Nephrogenic diabetes insipidus
Excludes1: diabetes insipidus NOS (E23.2)

N27 SMALL KIDNEY OF UNKNOWN CAUSE

Includes: oligonephronia

N27.0 Small kidney, unilateral

N27.1 Small kidney, bilateral

N28 OTHER DISORDERS OF KIDNEY AND URETER, NEC

N28.0 Ischemia and infarction of kidney
Renal artery embolism or obstruction or occlusion or thrombosis
Renal infarct
Excludes1: atherosclerosis of renal artery (extrarenal part) (I70.1)
congenital stenosis of renal artery (Q27.1)
Goldblatt's kidney (I70.1)

N28.1 Cyst of kidney, acquired
Cyst (multiple)(solitary) of kidney (acquired)
Excludes1: cystic kidney disease (congenital) (Q61.-)

N28.8 Other specified disorders of kidney and ureter
Excludes1: hydroureter (N13.4)
ureteric stricture with hydronephrosis (N13.1)
ureteric stricture without hydronephrosis (N13.5)

N28.85 Pyeloureteritis cystica

N28.89 Other specified disorders of kidney and ureter

N28.9 Disorder of kidney and ureter, unspecified
Nephropathy NOS
Renal disease (acute) NOS
Renal insufficiency (acute)
Excludes1: chronic renal insufficiency (N18.9)
unspecified nephritic syndrome (N05.-)

N29 OTHER DISORDERS OF KIDNEY AND URETER IN DISEASES CLASSIFIED ELSEWHERE

✓ **Code first** underlying disease, such as:
amyloidosis (E85.-)
nephrocalcinosis (E83.59)
schistosomiasis (B65.0-B65.9)
Excludes1: disorders of kidney and ureter in:
cystinosis (E72.0)
gonorrhea (A54.21)
syphilis (A52.75)
tuberculosis (A18.11)

(N30–N39) OTHER DISEASES OF THE URINARY SYSTEM

Excludes2: urinary infection (complicating): abortion or ectopic or molar pregnancy (O00–O07, O08.8)
pregnancy, childbirth and the puerperium (O23.-, O75.3, O86.2-)

N30 CYSTITIS

4th **Use additional code** to identify infectious agent (B95–B97)
Excludes1: prostatocystitis (N41.3)

N30.0 Acute cystitis
5th ***Excludes1:*** irradiation cystitis (N30.4-)
trigonitis (N30.3-)
- **N30.00 Acute cystitis without hematuria**
- **N30.01 Acute cystitis with hematuria**

N30.3 Trigonitis
5th Urethrotrigonitis
- **N30.30 Trigonitis without hematuria**
- **N30.31 Trigonitis with hematuria**

N30.4 Irradiation cystitis
5th
- **N30.40 Irradiation cystitis without hematuria**
- **N30.41 Irradiation cystitis with hematuria**

N30.8 Other cystitis
5th Abscess of bladder
- **N30.80 Other cystitis without hematuria**
- **N30.81 Other cystitis with hematuria**

N30.9 Cystitis, unspecified
5th
- **N30.90 Cystitis, unspecified without hematuria**
- **N30.91 Cystitis, unspecified with hematuria**

N31 NEUROMUSCULAR DYSFUNCTION OF BLADDER, NEC

4th **Use additional code** to identify any associated urinary incontinence (N39.3–N39.4-)
Excludes1: cord bladder NOS (G95.89)
neurogenic bladder due to cauda equina syndrome (G83.4)
neuromuscular dysfunction due to spinal cord lesion (G95.89)

N31.0 Uninhibited neuropathic bladder, NEC

N31.1 Reflex neuropathic bladder, NEC

N31.2 Flaccid neuropathic bladder, NEC
Atonic (motor) (sensory) neuropathic bladder
Autonomous neuropathic bladder
Nonreflex neuropathic bladder

N31.8 Other neuromuscular dysfunction of bladder

N31.9 Neuromuscular dysfunction of bladder, unspecified
Neurogenic bladder dysfunction NOS

N32 OTHER DISORDERS OF BLADDER

4th ***Excludes2:*** calculus of bladder (N21.0)
cystocele (N81.1-)
hernia or prolapse of bladder, female (N81.1-)

N32.0 Bladder-neck obstruction
Bladder-neck stenosis (acquired)
Excludes1: congenital bladder-neck obstruction (Q64.3-)

N32.1 Vesicointestinal fistula
Vesicorectal fistula

N32.2 Vesical fistula, NEC
Excludes1: fistula between bladder and female genital tract (N82.0–N82.1)

N32.3 Diverticulum of bladder
Excludes1: congenital diverticulum of bladder (Q64.6)
diverticulitis of bladder (N30.8-)

N32.8 Other specified disorders of bladder
5th

N32.81 Overactive bladder
Detrusor muscle hyperactivity
Excludes1: frequent urination due to specified bladder condition — code to condition

N32.89 Other specified disorders of bladder
Bladder hemorrhage
Bladder hypertrophy
Calcified bladder
Contracted bladder

N32.9 Bladder disorder, unspecified

N34 URETHRITIS AND URETHRAL SYNDROME

4th **Use additional code** (B95–B97), to identify infectious agent.
Excludes2: Reiter's disease (M02.3-)
urethritis in diseases with a predominantly sexual mode of transmission (A50–A64)
urethrotrigonitis (N30.3-)

N34.0 Urethral abscess
Abscess (of) Cowper's gland
Abscess (of) Littré's gland
Abscess (of) urethral (gland)
Periurethral abscess
Excludes1: urethral caruncle (N36.2)

N34.1 Nonspecific urethritis
Nongonococcal urethritis
Nonvenereal urethritis

N34.2 Other urethritis
Meatitis, urethral
Postmenopausal urethritis
Ulcer of urethra (meatus)
Urethritis NOS

N34.3 Urethral syndrome, unspecified

N35 URETHRAL STRICTURE

4th ***Excludes1:*** congenital urethral stricture (Q64.3-)
postprocedural urethral stricture (N99.1-)

N35.0 Post-traumatic urethral stricture
5th Urethral stricture due to injury
Excludes1: postprocedural urethral stricture (N99.1-)

- **N35.01 Post-traumatic urethral stricture, male**
  6th
  - **N35.010 Post-traumatic urethral stricture, male, meatal**
  - **N35.011 Post-traumatic bulbous urethral stricture**
  - **N35.012 Post-traumatic membranous urethral stricture**
  - **N35.013 Post-traumatic anterior urethral stricture**
  - **N35.014 Post-traumatic urethral stricture, male, unspecified**
  - **N35.016 Post-traumatic urethral stricture, male, overlapping sites**

- **N35.02 Post-traumatic urethral stricture, female**
  6th
  - **N35.021 Urethral stricture due to childbirth**
  - **N35.028 Other post-traumatic urethral stricture, female**

N35.1 Postinfective urethral stricture, NEC
5th ***Excludes1:*** urethral stricture associated with schistosomiasis (B65.-, N29)
gonococcal urethral stricture (A54.01)
syphilitic urethral stricture (A52.76)

- **N35.11 Postinfective urethral stricture, NEC, male**
  6th
  - **N35.111 Postinfective urethral stricture, NEC, male, meatal**
  - **N35.112 Postinfective bulbous urethral stricture, NEC, male**
  - **N35.113 Postinfective membranous urethral stricture, NEC, male**
  - **N35.114 Postinfective anterior urethral stricture, NEC, male**
  - **N35.116 Postinfective urethral stricture, NEC, male, overlapping sites**
  - **N35.119 Postinfective urethral stricture, NEC, male, unspecified**

- **N35.12 Postinfective urethral stricture, NEC, female**

N35.8 Other urethral stricture

5th *Excludes1:* postprocedural urethral stricture (N99.1-)

N35.81 Other urethral stricture, male

6th **N35.811 Other urethral stricture, male, meatal**

N35.812 Other bulbous urethral stricture, male

N35.813 Other membranous urethral stricture, male

N35.814 Other anterior urethral stricture, male

N35.816 Other urethral stricture, male, overlapping sites

N35.819 Other urethral stricture, male, unspecified site

N35.82 Other urethral stricture, female

N35.9 Urethral stricture, unspecified

5th **N35.91 Urethral stricture, unspecified, male**

6th **N35.911 Unspecified urethral stricture, male, meatal**

N35.912 Unspecified bulbous urethral stricture, male

N35.913 Unspecified membranous urethral stricture, male

N35.914 Unspecified anterior urethral stricture, male

N35.916 Unspecified urethral stricture, male, overlapping sites

N35.919 Unspecified urethral stricture, male, unspecified site

N35.92 Unspecified urethral stricture, female

N39 OTHER DISORDERS OF URINARY SYSTEM

4th *Excludes2:* hematuria NOS (R31.-)

recurrent or persistent hematuria (N02.-)

recurrent or persistent hematuria with specified morphological lesion (N02.-)

proteinuria NOS (R80.-)

N39.0 Urinary tract infection, site not specified

Use additional code (B95–B97), to identify infectious agent.

Excludes1: candidiasis of urinary tract (B37.4-)

neonatal urinary tract infection (P39.3)

pyonephrosis (N13.6)

pyuria (R82.81)

urinary tract infection of specified site, such as:

cystitis (N30.-)

urethritis (N34.-)

N39.4 Other specified urinary incontinence

5th Code also any associated overactive bladder (N32.81)

Excludes1: enuresis NOS (R32)

functional urinary incontinence (R39.81)

urinary incontinence associated with cognitive impairment (R39.81)

urinary incontinence NOS (R32)

urinary incontinence of nonorganic origin (F98.0)

N39.44 Nocturnal enuresis

Excludes2: nocturnal polyuria (R35.81)

N39.8 Other specified disorders of urinary system

N39.9 Disorder of urinary system, unspecified

(N40–N53) DISEASES OF MALE GENITAL ORGANS

N41 INFLAMMATORY DISEASES OF PROSTATE

4th Use additional code (B95–B97), to identify infectious agent.

N41.0 Acute prostatitis

N41.9 Inflammatory disease of prostate, unspecified

Prostatitis NOS

N43 HYDROCELE AND SPERMATOCELE

4th *Includes:* hydrocele of spermatic cord, testis or tunica vaginalis

Excludes1: congenital hydrocele (P83.5)

N43.0 Encysted hydrocele

N43.1 Infected hydrocele

Use additional code (B95–B97), to identify infectious agent

N43.2 Other hydrocele

N43.3 Hydrocele, unspecified

N43.4 Spermatocele of epididymis

5th Spermatic cyst

N43.40 Spermatocele of epididymis, unspecified

N43.41 Spermatocele of epididymis, single

N43.42 Spermatocele of epididymis, multiple

N44 NONINFLAMMATORY DISORDERS OF TESTIS

4th **N44.0 Torsion of testis**

5th **N44.00 Torsion of testis, unspecified**

N44.01 Extravaginal torsion of spermatic cord

N44.02 Intravaginal torsion of spermatic cord

Torsion of spermatic cord NOS

N44.03 Torsion of appendix testis

N44.04 Torsion of appendix epididymis

N44.1 Cyst of tunica albuginea testis

N44.2 Benign cyst of testis

N44.8 Other noninflammatory disorders of the testis

N45 ORCHITIS AND EPIDIDYMITIS

4th Use additional code (B95–B97), to identify infectious agent.

N45.1 Epididymitis

N45.2 Orchitis

N45.3 Epididymo-orchitis

N45.4 Abscess of epididymis or testis

N47 DISORDERS OF PREPUCE

4th **N47.0 Adherent prepuce, newborn**

N47.1 Phimosis

N47.2 Paraphimosis

N47.4 Benign cyst of prepuce

N47.5 Adhesions of prepuce and glans penis

N47.6 Balanoposthitis

N47.7 Other inflammatory diseases of prepuce

Use additional code (B95 – B97), to identify infectious agent.

N47.8 Other disorders of prepuce

Use additional code (B95–B97), to identify infectious agent.

Excludes1: balanitis (N48.1)

N48 OTHER DISORDERS OF PENIS

4th **N48.1 Balanitis**

Use additional code (B95–B97), to identify infectious agent

Excludes1: amebic balanitis (A06.8)

balanitis xerotica obliterans (N48.0)

candidal balanitis (B37.42)

gonococcal balanitis (A54.23)

herpesviral [herpes simplex] balanitis (A60.01)

N48.3 Priapism

5th Painful erection

Code first underlying cause

N48.30 Priapism, unspecified

N48.31 Priapism due to trauma

N48.32 Priapism due to disease classified elsewhere

N48.33 Priapism, drug-induced

N48.39 Other priapism

N48.8 Other specified disorders of penis

5th **N48.82 Acquired torsion of penis**

Acquired torsion of penis NOS

Excludes1: congenital torsion of penis (Q55.63)

N48.89 Other specified disorders of penis

N48.9 Disorder of penis, unspecified

N49 INFLAMMATORY DISORDERS OF MALE GENITAL ORGANS, NOT ELSEWHERE CLASSIFIED

4th Use additional code (B95–B97), to identify infectious agent.

Excludes1: inflammation of penis (N48.1, N48.2-)

orchitis and epididymitis (N45.-)

N49.0 Inflammatory disorders of seminal vesicle

Vesiculitis NOS

N50 OTHER AND UNSPECIFIED DISORDERS OF MALE GENITAL ORGANS

4th *Excludes2:* torsion of testis (N44.0-)

N50.0 Atrophy of testis

N50.8 Other specified disorders of male genital organs

5th **N50.81 Testicular pain**

6th **N50.811 Right testicular pain**

N50.812 Left testicular pain

N50.82 Scrotal pain

N50.89 Other specified disorders of the male genital organs
Atrophy or edema or hypertrophy or ulcer of scrotum, seminal vesicle, spermatic cord, tunica vaginalis and vas deferens
Chylocele, tunica vaginalis (nonfilarial) NOS
Urethroscrotal fistula
Stricture of spermatic cord, tunica vaginalis, and vas deferens

N50.9 Disorder of male genital organs, unspecified

(N60–N65) DISORDERS OF BREAST

Excludes1: disorders of breast associated with childbirth (O91–O92)

N60 BENIGN MAMMARY DYSPLASIA

4th *Includes:* fibrocystic mastopathy

N60.0 Solitary cyst of breast

5th Cyst of breast

- **N60.01 Solitary cyst of right breast**
- **N60.02 Solitary cyst of left breast**
- **N60.09 Solitary cyst of unspecified breast**

N61 INFLAMMATORY DISORDERS OF BREAST

4th *Excludes1:* inflammatory carcinoma of breast (C50.9) inflammatory disorder of breast associated with childbirth (O91.-) neonatal infective mastitis (P39.0) thrombophlebitis of breast [Mondor's disease] (I80.8)

N61.0 Mastitis without abscess
Infective mastitis (acute) (subacute) (nonpuerperal)
Mastitis (acute) (subacute) (nonpuerperal) NOS
Cellulitis (acute) (nonpuerperal) (subacute) of breast or nipple NOS

N61.1 Abscess of the breast and nipple
Abscess (acute) (chronic) (nonpuerperal) of areola or breast
Carbuncle of breast
Mastitis with abscess

N62 HYPERTROPHY OF BREAST

✓ Gynecomastia
Hypertrophy of breast NOS
Massive pubertal hypertrophy of breast
Excludes1: breast engorgement of newborn (P83.4) disproportion of reconstructed breast (N65.1)

N63 UNSPECIFIED LUMP IN BREAST

4th Nodule(s) NOS in breast

N63.0 Unspecified lump in unspecified breast

N63.1 Unspecified lump in the right breast

5th **N63.10 Unspecified lump in the right breast, unspecified quadrant**

- **N63.11** upper outer quadrant
- **N63.12** upper inner quadrant
- **N63.13** lower outer quadrant
- **N63.14** lower inner quadrant
- **N63.15** overlapping quadrants

N63.2 Unspecified lump in the left breast

5th **N63.20 Unspecified lump in the left breast, unspecified quadrant**

- **N63.21** upper outer quadrant
- **N63.22** upper inner quadrant
- **N63.23** lower outer quadrant
- **N63.24** lower inner quadrant
- **N63.25** overlapping quadrants

N63.3 Unspecified lump in axillary tail

5th **N63.31 Unspecified lump in axillary tail of the right breast**
N63.32 Unspecified lump in axillary tail of the left breast

N63.4 Unspecified lump in breast, subareolar

5th **N63.41 Unspecified lump in right breast, subareolar**
N63.42 Unspecified lump in left breast, subareolar

N64 OTHER DISORDERS OF BREAST

4th *Excludes2:* mechanical complication of breast prosthesis and implant (T85.4-)

N64.3 Galactorrhea not associated with childbirth

N64.4 Mastodynia

N64.5 Other signs and symptoms in breast

5th *Excludes2:* abnormal findings on diagnostic imaging of breast (R92.-)

- **N64.51 Induration of breast**
- **N64.52 Nipple discharge**
  Excludes1: abnormal findings in nipple discharge (R89.-)
- **N64.53 Retraction of nipple**
- **N64.59 Other signs and symptoms in breast**

N64.8 Other specified disorders of breast

5th **N64.89 Other specified disorders of breast**
Galactocele
Subinvolution of breast (postlactational)

(N70–N77) INFLAMMATORY DISEASES OF FEMALE PELVIC ORGANS

Excludes1: inflammatory diseases of female pelvic organs complicating: abortion or ectopic or molar pregnancy (O00–O07, O08.0) pregnancy, childbirth and the puerperium (O23.-, O75.3, O85, O86.-)

N70 SALPINGITIS AND OOPHORITIS

4th *Includes:* abscess (of) fallopian tube
abscess (of) ovary
pyosalpinx
salpingo-oophoritis
tubo-ovarian abscess
tubo-ovarian inflammatory disease

Use additional code (B95–B97), to identify infectious agent
Excludes1: gonococcal infection (A54.24) tuberculous infection (A18.17)

N70.0 Acute salpingitis and oophoritis

5th **N70.01 Acute salpingitis**
N70.02 Acute oophoritis
N70.03 Acute salpingitis and oophoritis

N70.1 Chronic salpingitis and oophoritis

5th Hydrosalpinx

- **N70.11 Chronic salpingitis**
- **N70.12 Chronic oophoritis**
- **N70.13 Chronic salpingitis and oophoritis**

N70.9 Salpingitis and oophoritis, unspecified

5th **N70.91 Salpingitis, unspecified**
N70.92 Oophoritis, unspecified
N70.93 Salpingitis and oophoritis, unspecified

N71 INFLAMMATORY DISEASE OF UTERUS, EXCEPT CERVIX

4th *Includes:* endo (myo) metritis
metritis
myometritis
pyometra
uterine abscess

Use additional code (B95 – B97), to identify infectious agent
Excludes1: hyperplastic endometritis (N85.0-) infection of uterus following delivery (O85, O86.-)

N71.0 Acute inflammatory disease of uterus

N71.9 Inflammatory disease of uterus, unspecified

N72 INFLAMMATORY DISEASE OF CERVIX UTERI

✓ *Includes:* cervicitis or endocervicitis or exocervicitis (all with or without erosion or ectropion)

Use additional code (B95–B97), to identify infectious agent
Excludes1: erosion and ectropion of cervix without cervicitis (N86)

N73 OTHER FEMALE PELVIC INFLAMMATORY DISEASES

4th **Use additional code** (B95–B97), to identify infectious agent.

N73.0 Acute parametritis and pelvic cellulitis
Abscess of broad ligament
Abscess of parametrium
Pelvic cellulitis, female

N73.1 Chronic parametritis and pelvic cellulitis
Any condition in N73.0 specified as chronic
Excludes1: tuberculous parametritis and pelvic cellulitis (A18.17)

N73.3 Female acute pelvic peritonitis

N73.4 Female chronic pelvic peritonitis
Excludes1: tuberculous pelvic (female) peritonitis (A18.17)

N73.5 Female pelvic peritonitis, unspecified

N73.6 Female pelvic peritoneal adhesions (postinfective)
Excludes2: postprocedural peritoneal adhesions (N99.4)

N73.8 Other specified female pelvic inflammatory diseases

N73.9 Female pelvic inflammatory disease, unspecified
Female pelvic infection or inflammation NOS

N75 DISEASES OF BARTHOLIN'S GLAND

N75.0 Cyst of Bartholin's gland

N75.1 Abscess of Bartholin's gland

N76 OTHER INFLAMMATION OF VAGINA AND VULVA

Use additional code (B95–B97), to identify infectious agent

Excludes2: vulvar vestibulitis (N94.810)

N76.0 Acute vaginitis
Acute vulvovaginitis

N76.1 Subacute and chronic vaginitis
Chronic vulvovaginitis
Subacute vulvovaginitis

N76.2 Acute vulvitis
Vulvitis NOS

N76.4 Abscess of vulva
Furuncle of vulva

N76.8 Other specified inflammation of vagina and vulva

N76.82 Fournier disease of vagina and vulva
Fournier gangrene of vagina and vulva
Code also, if applicable, diabetes mellitus (E08-E13 with .9)
Excludes1: gangrene in diabetes mellitus (E08-E13 with .52)

N76.89 Other specified inflammation of vagina and vulva

N77 VULVOVAGINAL ULCERATION AND INFLAMMATION IN DISEASES CLASSIFIED ELSEWHERE

N77.1 Vaginitis, vulvitis and vulvovaginitis in diseases classified elsewhere
Code first underlying disease, such as:
pinworm (B80)
Excludes1: candidal vulvovaginitis (B37.3)
chlamydial vulvovaginitis (A56.02)
gonococcal vulvovaginitis (A54.02)
herpesviral [herpes simplex] vulvovaginitis (A60.04)
trichomonal vulvovaginitis (A59.01)
tuberculous vulvovaginitis (A18.18)
vulvovaginitis in early syphilis (A51.0)
vulvovaginitis in late syphilis (A52.76)

(N80–N98) NONINFLAMMATORY DISORDERS OF FEMALE GENITAL TRACT

N83 NONINFLAMMATORY DISORDERS OF OVARY, FALLOPIAN TUBE AND BROAD LIGAMENT

Excludes2: hydrosalpinx (N70.1-)

N83.0 Follicular cyst of ovary
Cyst of graafian follicle
Hemorrhagic follicular cyst (of ovary)

N83.00 Follicular cyst of ovary, unspecified side

N83.01 Follicular cyst of right ovary

N83.02 Follicular cyst of left ovary

N83.1 Corpus luteum cyst
Hemorrhagic corpus luteum cyst

N83.10 Corpus luteum cyst of ovary, unspecified side

N83.11 Corpus luteum cyst of right ovary

N83.12 Corpus luteum cyst of left ovary

N83.2 Other and unspecified ovarian cysts
Excludes1: developmental ovarian cyst (Q50.1)
neoplastic ovarian cyst (D27.-)
polycystic ovarian syndrome (E28.2)
Stein-Leventhal syndrome (E28.2)

N83.20 Unspecified ovarian cysts

N83.201 Unspecified ovarian cyst, right side

N83.202 Unspecified ovarian cyst, left side

N83.209 Unspecified ovarian cyst, unspecified side

N83.29 Other ovarian cysts
Retention cyst of ovary
Simple cyst of ovary

N83.291 Other ovarian cyst, right side

N83.292 Other ovarian cyst, left side

N83.299 Other ovarian cyst, unspecified side

N83.4 Prolapse and hernia of ovary and fallopian tube

N83.40 Prolapse and hernia of ovary and fallopian tube, unspecified side
Prolapse and hernia of ovary and fallopian tube, NOS

N83.41 Prolapse and hernia of right ovary and fallopian tube

N83.42 Prolapse and hernia of left ovary and fallopian tube

N83.5 Torsion of ovary, ovarian pedicle and fallopian tube
Torsion of accessory tube

N83.51 Torsion of ovary and ovarian pedicle

N83.511 Torsion of right ovary and ovarian pedicle

N83.512 Torsion of left ovary and ovarian pedicle

N83.519 Torsion of ovary and ovarian pedicle, unspecified side
Torsion of ovary and ovarian pedicle, NOS

N83.53 Torsion of ovary, ovarian pedicle and fallopian tube

N83.8 Other noninflammatory disorders of ovary, fallopian tube and broad ligament
Broad ligament laceration syndrome [Allen-Masters]

N85 OTHER NONINFLAMMATORY DISORDERS OF UTERUS, EXCEPT CERVIX

Excludes1: endometriosis (N80.-)
inflammatory diseases of uterus (N71.-)
noninflammatory disorders of cervix, except malposition (N86–N88)
polyp of corpus uteri (N84.0)
uterine prolapse (N81.-)

N85.0 Endometrial hyperplasia

N85.00 Endometrial hyperplasia, unspecified
Hyperplasia (adenomatous) (cystic) (glandular) of endometrium
Hyperplastic endometritis

N85.8 Other specified noninflammatory disorders of uterus
Atrophy of uterus, acquired
Fibrosis of uterus NOS
[Prod: Add new text with new code bullet after N85.8]

N85.A Isthmocele
Isthmocele (non-pregnant state)
Code also any associated conditions such as:
abnormal uterine and vaginal bleeding, unspecified (N93.9)
female infertility of uterine origin (N97.2)
pelvic and perineal pain (R10.2)
Excludes1: maternal care for cesarean scar defect (isthmocele) (O34.22)

N86 EROSION AND ECTROPION OF CERVIX UTERI

Decubitus (trophic) ulcer of cervix
Eversion of cervix
Excludes1: erosion and ectropion of cervix with cervicitis (N72)

N88 OTHER NONINFLAMMATORY DISORDERS OF CERVIX UTERI

Excludes2: inflammatory disease of cervix (N72)
polyp of cervix (N84.1)

N88.1 Old laceration of cervix uteri
Adhesions of cervix
Excludes1: current obstetric trauma (O71.3)

N88.2 Stricture and stenosis of cervix uteri
Excludes1: stricture and stenosis of cervix uteri complicating labor (O65.5)

N89 OTHER NONINFLAMMATORY DISORDERS OF VAGINA

Excludes1: abnormal results from vaginal cytologic examination without histologic confirmation (R87.62-)
carcinoma in situ of vagina (D07.2)
HGSIL of vagina (R87.623)
inflammation of vagina (N76.-)
senile (atrophic) vaginitis (N95.2)
severe dysplasia of vagina (D07.2)
trichomonal leukorrhea (A59.00)
vaginal intraepithelial neoplasia [VAIN], grade III (D07.2)

N89.5 Stricture and atresia of vagina
Vaginal adhesions
Vaginal stenosis
Excludes1: congenital atresia or stricture (Q52.4)
postprocedural adhesions of vagina (N99.2)

N89.6 Tight hymenal ring
Rigid hymen
Tight introitus
Excludes1: imperforate hymen (Q52.3)

N89.7 Hematocolpos
Hematocolpos with hematometra or hematosalpinx

N89.8 Other specified noninflammatory disorders of vagina
Leukorrhea NOS
Old vaginal laceration
Pessary ulcer of vagina
Excludes1: current obstetric trauma (O70.-, O71.4, O71.7-O71.8)
old laceration involving muscles of pelvic floor (N81.8)

N89.9 Noninflammatory disorder of vagina, unspecified

N90 OTHER NONINFLAMMATORY DISORDERS OF VULVA AND PERINEUM

Excludes1: anogenital (venereal) warts (A63.0)
carcinoma in situ of vulva (D07.1)
condyloma acuminatum (A63.0)
current obstetric trauma (O70.-, O71.7-O71.8)
inflammation of vulva (N76.-)
severe dysplasia of vulva (D07.1)
vulvar intraepithelial neoplasm III [VIN III] (D07.1)

N90.0 Mild vulvar dysplasia
Vulvar intraepithelial neoplasia [VIN], grade I

N90.1 Moderate vulvar dysplasia
Vulvar intraepithelial neoplasia [VIN], grade II

N90.3 Dysplasia of vulva, unspecified

N90.4 Leukoplakia of vulva
Dystrophy of vulva
Kraurosis of vulva
Lichen sclerosus of external female genital organs

N90.5 Atrophy of vulva
Stenosis of vulva

N90.6 Hypertrophy of vulva

N90.60 Unspecified hypertrophy of vulva
Unspecified hypertrophy of labia

N90.61 Childhood asymmetric labium majus enlargement CALME

N90.69 Other specified hypertrophy of vulva
Other specified hypertrophy of labia

N90.7 Vulvar cyst

N90.8 Other specified noninflammatory disorders of vulva and perineum

N90.81 Female genital mutilation status
Female genital cutting status

N90.810 Female genital mutilation status, unspecified
Female genital cutting status, unspecified
Female genital mutilation status NOS

N90.811 Female genital mutilation Type I status
Clitorectomy status
Female genital cutting Type I status

N90.812 Female genital mutilation Type II status
Clitorectomy with excision of labia minora status

N90.813 Female genital mutilation Type III status
Female genital cutting Type III status
Infibulation status

N90.818 Other female genital mutilation status
Female genital cutting or mutilation Type IV status
Other female genital cutting status

N90.89 Other specified noninflammatory disorders of vulva and perineum
Adhesions of vulva
Hypertrophy of clitoris

N90.9 Noninflammatory disorder of vulva and perineum, unspecified

N91 ABSENT, SCANTY AND RARE MENSTRUATION

Excludes1: ovarian dysfunction (E28.-)

N91.0 Primary amenorrhea

N91.1 Secondary amenorrhea

N91.2 Amenorrhea, unspecified

N92 EXCESSIVE, FREQUENT AND IRREGULAR MENSTRUATION

Excludes1: postmenopausal bleeding (N95.0)
precocious puberty (menstruation) (E30.1)

N92.0 Excessive and frequent menstruation with regular cycle
Heavy periods NOS
Menorrhagia NOS
Polymenorrhea

N92.1 Excessive and frequent menstruation with irregular cycle
Irregular intermenstrual bleeding
Irregular, shortened intervals between menstrual bleeding
Menometrorrhagia
Metrorrhagia

N92.2 Excessive menstruation at puberty
Excessive bleeding associated with onset of menstrual periods
Pubertal menorrhagia
Puberty bleeding

N92.3 Ovulation bleeding
Regular intermenstrual bleeding

N92.5 Other specified irregular menstruation

N92.6 Irregular menstruation, unspecified
Irregular bleeding NOS
Irregular periods NOS
Excludes1: irregular menstruation with:
lengthened intervals or scanty bleeding (N91.3-N91.5)
shortened intervals or excessive bleeding (N92.1)

N93 OTHER ABNORMAL UTERINE AND VAGINAL BLEEDING

Excludes1: neonatal vaginal hemorrhage (P54.6)
precocious puberty (menstruation) (E30.1)
pseudomenses (P54.6)

N93.1 Pre-pubertal vaginal bleeding

N93.8 Other specified abnormal uterine and vaginal bleeding
Dysfunctional or functional uterine or vaginal bleeding NOS

N93.9 Abnormal uterine and vaginal bleeding, unspecified

N94 PAIN AND OTHER CONDITIONS ASSOCIATED WITH FEMALE GENITAL ORGANS AND MENSTRUAL CYCLE

N94.0 Mittelschmerz

N94.1 Dyspareunia
Excludes1: psychogenic dyspareunia (F52.6)

N94.10 Unspecified dyspareunia

N94.11 Superficial (introital) dyspareunia

N94.12 Deep dyspareunia

N94.19 Other specified dyspareunia

N94.2 Vaginismus
Excludes1: psychogenic vaginismus (F52.5)

N94.3 Premenstrual tension syndrome
Excludes 1: premenstrual dysphoric disorder (F32.81)
Code also associated menstrual migraine (G43.82-, G43.83-)

N94.4 Primary dysmenorrhea

N94.5 Secondary dysmenorrhea

N94.6 Dysmenorrhea, unspecified
Excludes1: psychogenic dysmenorrhea (F45.8)

N94.8 Other specified conditions associated with female genital organs and menstrual cycle

N94.81 Vulvodynia

N94.810 Vulvar vestibulitis

N94.818 Other vulvodynia

N94.819 Vulvodynia, unspecified
Vulvodynia NOS

N94.89 Other specified conditions associated with female genital organs and menstrual cycle

N94.9 Unspecified condition associated with female genital organs and menstrual cycle

N97 FEMALE INFERTILITY

Includes: inability to achieve a pregnancy
sterility, female NOS

Excludes2: female infertility associated with:
hypopituitarism (E23.0)
Stein-Leventhal syndrome (E28.2)
incompetence of cervix uteri (N88.3)

N97.0 Female infertility associated with anovulation

N97.1 Female infertility of tubal origin
Female infertility associated with congenital anomaly of tube
Female infertility due to tubal block
Female infertility due to tubal occlusion
Female infertility due to tubal stenosis

N97.9 Female infertility, unspecified

(N99) INTRAOPERATIVE AND POSTPROCEDURAL COMPLICATIONS AND DISORDERS OF GENITOURINARY SYSTEM, NEC

N99 INTRAOPERATIVE AND POSTPROCEDURAL COMPLICATIONS AND DISORDERS OF GENITOURINARY SYSTEM, NEC

Excludes2: irradiation cystitis (N30.4-)
postoophorectomy osteoporosis with current pathological fracture (M80.8-)
postoophorectomy osteoporosis without current pathological fracture (M81.8)

N99.0 Postprocedural (acute) (chronic) kidney failure
Use additional code to type of kidney disease

N99.1 Postprocedural urethral stricture
Postcatheterization urethral stricture

N99.11 Postprocedural urethral stricture, male

N99.110 Postprocedural urethral stricture, male, meatal

N99.111 Postprocedural bulbous urethral stricture, male

N99.112 Postprocedural membranous urethral stricture, male

N99.113 Postprocedural anterior bulbous urethral stricture, male

N99.114 Postprocedural urethral stricture, male, unspecified

N99.115 Postprocedural fossa navicularis urethral stricture

N99.116 Postprocedural urethral stricture, male, overlapping sites

N99.12 Postprocedural urethral stricture, female

N99.2 Postprocedural adhesions of vagina

N99.3 Prolapse of vaginal vault after hysterectomy

N99.4 Postprocedural pelvic peritoneal adhesions
Excludes2: pelvic peritoneal adhesions NOS (N73.6)
postinfective pelvic peritoneal adhesions (N73.6)

N99.5 Complications of stoma of urinary tract
Excludes2: mechanical complication of urinary catheter (T83.0-)

N99.51 Complication of cystostomy

N99.510 Cystostomy hemorrhage

N99.511 Cystostomy infection

N99.512 Cystostomy malfunction

N99.518 Other cystostomy complication

N99.52 Complication of incontinent external stoma of urinary tract

N99.520 Hemorrhage of incontinent external stoma of urinary tract

N99.521 Infection of incontinent external stoma of urinary tract

N99.522 Malfunction of incontinent external stoma of urinary tract

N99.523 Herniation of incontinent stoma of urinary tract

N99.524 Stenosis of incontinent stoma of urinary tract

N99.528 Other complication of incontinent external stoma of urinary tract

N99.53 Complication of continent stoma of urinary tract

N99.530 Hemorrhage of continent stoma of urinary tract

N99.531 Infection of continent stoma of urinary tract

N99.532 Malfunction of continent stoma of urinary tract

N99.533 Herniation of continent stoma of urinary tract

N99.534 Stenosis of continent stoma of urinary tract

N99.538 Other complication of continent stoma of urinary tract

N99.8 Other intraoperative and postprocedural complications and disorders of GI system

N99.81 Other intraoperative complications of GI system

N99.82 Postprocedural hemorrhage of a GI system organ or structure following a procedure

N99.820 Postprocedural hemorrhage of a GI system organ or structure following a GI system procedure

N99.821 Postprocedural hemorrhage of a GI system organ or structure following other procedure

N99.83 Residual ovary syndrome

N99.84 Postprocedural hematoma and seroma of a GI system organ or structure following a procedure

N99.840 Postprocedural hematoma of a GI system organ or structure following a GI system procedure

N99.841 Postprocedural hematoma of a GI system organ or structure following other procedure

N99.842 Postprocedural seroma of a GI system organ or structure following a GI system procedure

N99.843 Postprocedural seroma of a GI system organ or structure following other procedure

N99.89 Other postprocedural complications and disorders of GI system

Chapter 15. Pregnancy, childbirth and the puerperium (O00–O9A)

GUIDELINES

General Rules for Obstetric Cases

CODES FROM CHAPTER 15 AND SEQUENCING PRIORITY

Obstetric cases require codes from Chapter 15, codes in the range O00–O9A, Pregnancy, Childbirth, and the Puerperium. Chapter 15 codes have sequencing priority over codes from other chapters. Additional codes from other chapters may be used in conjunction with Chapter 15 codes to further specify conditions. Should the provider document that the pregnancy is incidental to the encounter, then code Z33.1, Pregnant state, incidental, should be used in place of any Chapter 15 codes. It is the provider's responsibility to state that the condition being treated is not affecting the pregnancy.

CHAPTER 15 CODES USED ONLY ON THE MATERNAL RECORD

Chapter 15 codes are to be used only on the maternal record, never on the record of the newborn.

FINAL CHARACTER FOR TRIMESTER

The majority of codes in Chapter 15 have a final character indicating the trimester of pregnancy. The timeframes for the trimesters are indicated at the beginning of the chapter. If trimester is not a component of a code, it is because the condition always occurs in a specific trimester, or the concept of trimester of pregnancy is not applicable. Certain codes have characters for only certain trimesters because the condition does not occur in all trimesters, but it may occur in more than just one.

Assignment of the final character for trimester should be based on the provider's documentation of the trimester (or number of weeks) for the current admission/ encounter. This applies to the assignment of trimester for pre-existing conditions as well as those that develop during or are due to the pregnancy. The provider's documentation of the number of weeks may be used to assign the appropriate code identifying the trimester.

Whenever delivery occurs during the current admission, and there is an "in childbirth" option for the obstetric complication being coded, the "in childbirth" code should be assigned. When the classification does not provide an obstetric code with an "in childbirth" option, it is appropriate to assign a code describing the current trimester.

SELECTION OF TRIMESTER FOR INPATIENT ADMISSIONS THAT ENCOMPASS MORE THAN ONE TRIMESTER

In instances when a patient is admitted to a hospital for complications of pregnancy during one trimester and remains in the hospital into a subsequent trimester, the trimester character for the antepartum complication code should be assigned on the basis of the trimester when the complication developed, not the trimester of the discharge. If the condition developed prior to the current admission/encounter or represents a pre-existing condition, the trimester character for the trimester at the time of the admission/encounter should be assigned.

UNSPECIFIED TRIMESTER

Each category that includes codes for trimester has a code for "unspecified trimester." The "unspecified trimester" code should rarely be used, such as when the documentation in the record is insufficient to determine the trimester and it is not possible to obtain clarification.

7TH CHARACTER FOR FETUS IDENTIFICATION

Where applicable, a 7th character is to be assigned for certain categories (O31, O32, O33.3–O33.6, O35, O36, O40, O41, O60.1, O60.2, O64, and O69) to identify the fetus for which the complication code applies.

Assign 7th character "0":

- For single gestations
- When the documentation in the record is insufficient to determine the fetus affected and it is not possible to obtain clarification.
- When it is not possible to clinically determine which fetus is affected.

Completed weeks of gestation

In *ICD-10-CM*, "completed" weeks of gestation refers to full weeks. For example, if the provider documents gestation at 39 weeks and 6 days, the code for 39 weeks of gestation should be assigned, as the patient has not yet reached 40 completed weeks.

Selection of OB Principal or First-listed Diagnosis

ROUTINE OUTPATIENT PRENATAL VISITS

Refer to the *ICD-10-CM* manual for complete guidelines.

SUPERVISION OF HIGH-RISK PREGNANCY

Codes from category O09, Supervision of high-risk pregnancy, are intended for use only during the prenatal period. For complications during the labor or delivery episode as a result of a high-risk pregnancy, assign the applicable complication codes from Chapter 15. If there are no complications during the labor or delivery episode, assign code O80, Encounter for full-term uncomplicated delivery.

For routine prenatal outpatient visits for patients with high-risk pregnancies, a code from category O09, Supervision of high-risk pregnancy, should be used as the first-listed diagnosis. Secondary chapter 15 codes may be used in conjunction with these codes if appropriate.

EPISODES WHEN NO DELIVERY OCCURS

Refer to the *ICD-10-CM* manual for complete guidelines.

WHEN A DELIVERY OCCURS

Refer to the *ICD-10-CM* manual for complete guidelines.

OUTCOME OF DELIVERY

A code from category Z37, Outcome of delivery, should be included on every maternal record when a delivery has occurred. These codes are not to be used on subsequent records or on the newborn record.

Pre-existing conditions versus conditions due to the pregnancy

Certain categories in Chapter 15 distinguish between conditions of the mother that existed prior to pregnancy (pre-existing) and those that are a direct result of pregnancy. When assigning codes from Chapter 15, it is important to assess if a condition was pre-existing prior to pregnancy or developed during or due to the pregnancy in order to assign the correct code.

Categories that do not distinguish between pre-existing and pregnancy-related conditions may be used for either. It is acceptable to use codes specifically for the puerperium with codes complicating pregnancy and childbirth if a condition arises postpartum during the delivery encounter.

Pre-existing hypertension in pregnancy

See category O10.
See Chapter 9, Hypertension.

Fetal Conditions Affecting the Management of the Mother

CODES FROM CATEGORIES O35 AND O36

See categories O35 and O36.

IN UTERO SURGERY

See category O35.

No code from Chapter 16, the perinatal codes, should be used on the mother's record to identify fetal conditions. Surgery performed in utero on a fetus is still to be coded as an obstetric encounter.

HIV Infection in Pregnancy, Childbirth and the Puerperium

During pregnancy, childbirth or the puerperium, a patient admitted because of an HIV-related illness should receive a principal diagnosis from subcategory O98.7-, HIV disease complicating pregnancy, childbirth and the puerperium, followed by the code(s) for the HIV-related illness(es).

Patients with asymptomatic HIV infection status admitted during pregnancy, childbirth, or the puerperium should receive codes of O98.7- and Z21, Asymptomatic HIV infection status.

DM in pregnancy

Diabetes mellitus is a significant complicating factor in pregnancy. Pregnant women who are diabetic should be assigned a code from category O24, DM in pregnancy, childbirth, and the puerperium, first, followed by the appropriate diabetes code(s) (E08–E13) from Chapter 4.

Long-term use of insulin

Code Z79.4, Long-term (current) use of insulin, should also be assigned if the DM is being treated with insulin.

Gestational (pregnancy induced) diabetes

Gestational (pregnancy induced) diabetes can occur during the second and third trimester of pregnancy in women who were not diabetic prior to pregnancy. Gestational diabetes can cause complications in the pregnancy similar to those of pre-existing DM. It also puts the woman at greater risk of developing diabetes after the pregnancy. Codes for gestational diabetes are in subcategory O24.4, Gestational DM. No other code from category O24, DM in pregnancy, childbirth, and the puerperium, should be used with a code from O24.4

The codes under subcategory O24.4 include diet controlled and insulin controlled. *If a patient with gestational diabetes is treated with both diet and insulin, only the code for insulin-controlled is required.*

Refer to the *ICD-10-CM* manual for complete guidelines.

Refer to the *ICD-10-CM* manual for guidelines for normal delivery (O80); peripartum and postpartum periods; sequela of complication of pregnancy, childbirth, and the puerperium (O94); sepsis and septic shock complicating abortion, pregnancy, childbirth and the puerperium; puerperal sepsis; termination of pregnancy and spontaneous abortion and alcohol, tobacco and *drug* use during pregnancy, childbirth and the puerperium.

Abuse in a pregnant patient

Refer to the *ICD-10-CM* manual for complete guidelines.

Refer to Chapter 19. Adult and child abuse, neglect and other maltreatment.

Note: CODES FROM THIS CHAPTER ARE FOR USE ONLY ON MATERNAL RECORDS, NEVER ON NEWBORN RECORDS.

Codes from this chapter are for use for conditions related to or aggravated by the pregnancy, childbirth, or by the puerperium (maternal causes or obstetric causes).

Use additional code from category Z3A, Weeks of gestation, to identify the specific week of the pregnancy, if known

Excludes1: supervision of normal pregnancy (Z34.-)

Excludes2: mental and behavioral disorders associated with the puerperium (F53) obstetrical tetanus (A34) postpartum necrosis of pituitary gland (E23.0) puerperal osteomalacia (M83.0)

(O00–O08) PREGNANCY WITH ABORTIVE OUTCOME

O00 ECTOPIC PREGNANCY

4th *Includes:* ruptured ectopic pregnancy

Use additional code from category O08 to identify any associated complication

O00.0 Abdominal pregnancy

5th *Excludes1:* maternal care for viable fetus in abdominal pregnancy (O36.7-)

- **O00.00** Abdominal pregnancy without intrauterine pregnancy
- **O00.01** Abdominal pregnancy with intrauterine pregnancy

O00.1 Tubal pregnancy

5th Fallopian pregnancy

Rupture of (fallopian) tube due to pregnancy

Tubal abortion

- **O00.10** Tubal pregnancy without intrauterine pregnancy
  - **6th** **O00.101** Right tubal pregnancy without intrauterine pregnancy
  - **O00.102** Left tubal pregnancy without intrauterine pregnancy
  - **O00.109** Unspecified tubal pregnancy without intrauterine pregnancy

O00.11 Tubal pregnancy with intrauterine pregnancy

- **6th** **O00.111** Right tubal pregnancy with intrauterine pregnancy
- **O00.112** Left tubal pregnancy with intrauterine pregnancy
- **O00.119** Unspecified tubal pregnancy with intrauterine pregnancy

O00.2 Ovarian pregnancy

- **5th** **O00.20** Ovarian pregnancy without intrauterine pregnancy
  - **6th** **O00.201** Right ovarian pregnancy without intrauterine pregnancy
  - **O00.202** Left ovarian pregnancy without intrauterine pregnancy
  - **O00.209** Unspecified ovarian pregnancy without intrauterine pregnancy
- **O00.21** Ovarian pregnancy with intrauterine pregnancy
  - **6th** **O00.211** Right ovarian pregnancy with intrauterine pregnancy
  - **O00.212** Left ovarian pregnancy without intrauterine pregnancy
  - **O00.219** Unspecified ovarian pregnancy with intrauterine pregnancy

O00.8 Other ectopic pregnancy

5th Cervical pregnancy

Cornual pregnancy

Intraligamentous pregnancy

Mural pregnancy

- **O00.80** Other ectopic pregnancy without intrauterine pregnancy
- **O00.81** Other ectopic pregnancy with intrauterine pregnancy

O00.9 Ectopic pregnancy, unspecified

- **5th** **O00.90** Unspecified ectopic pregnancy without intrauterine pregnancy
- **O00.91** Unspecified ectopic pregnancy with intrauterine pregnancy

O02 OTHER ABNORMAL PRODUCTS OF CONCEPTION

4th **Use additional code** from category O08 to identify any associated complication.

Excludes1: papyraceous fetus (O31.0-)

O02.1 Missed abortion

Early fetal death, before completion of 20 weeks of gestation, with retention of dead fetus

Excludes1: failed induced abortion (O07.-)

fetal death (intrauterine) (late) (O36.4)

missed abortion with blighted ovum (O02.0)

missed abortion with hydatidiform mole (O01.-)

missed abortion with nonhydatidiform (O02.0)

missed abortion with other abnormal products of conception (O02.8-)

missed delivery (O36.4)

stillbirth (P95)

O03 SPONTANEOUS ABORTION

4th **Note:** Incomplete abortion includes retained products of conception following spontaneous abortion

Includes: miscarriage

O03.4 Incomplete spontaneous abortion without complication

O03.9 Complete or unspecified spontaneous abortion without complication

Miscarriage NOS

Spontaneous abortion NOS

(O09) SUPERVISION OF HIGH RISK PREGNANCY

O09 SUPERVISION OF HIGH RISK PREGNANCY

4th **O09.6 Supervision of young primigravida and multigravida**

5th Supervision of pregnancy for a female <16 years old at expected date of delivery

O09.61- Supervision of young primigravida **6th**

O09.62- Supervision of young multigravida **6th**

(O10–O16) EDEMA, PROTEINURIA AND HYPERTENSIVE DISORDERS IN PREGNANCY, CHILDBIRTH AND THE PUERPERIUM

Category O10, Pre-existing hypertension complicating pregnancy, childbirth and the puerperium, includes codes for hypertensive heart and hypertensive CKD. When assigning one of the O10 codes that includes hypertensive heart disease or hypertensive CKD, it is necessary to add a secondary code from the appropriate hypertension category to specify the type of heart failure or CKD.

O10 PRE-EXISTING HYPERTENSION COMPLICATING PREGNANCY, CHILDBIRTH AND THE PUERPERIUM

4th

Includes: pre-existing hypertension with pre-existing proteinuria complicating pregnancy, childbirth and the puerperium

Excludes2: pre-existing hypertension with superimposed pre-eclampsia complicating pregnancy, childbirth and the puerperium (O11.-)

O10.0 Pre-existing essential hypertension complicating pregnancy, childbirth and the puerperium

5th

Any condition in I10 specified as a reason for obstetric care during pregnancy, childbirth or the puerperium

O10.01- Pre-existing essential hypertension complicating pregnancy

6th

O10.01 requires 6th character to identify trimester
1 first trimester
2 second trimester
3 third trimester
9 unspecified trimester

O10.02 Pre-existing essential hypertension complicating childbirth

O10.03 Pre-existing essential hypertension complicating the puerperium

O10.1 Pre-existing hypertensive heart disease complicating pregnancy, childbirth and the puerperium

5th

Any condition in I11 specified as a reason for obstetric care during pregnancy, childbirth or the puerperium

O10.1 and O10.4 require a 6th character
1 first trimester
2 second trimester
3 third trimester
9 unspecified trimester

Use additional code from I11 to identify the type of hypertensive heart disease

O10.11- Pre-existing hypertensive heart disease complicating pregnancy

6th

O10.4 Pre-existing secondary hypertension complicating pregnancy, childbirth and the puerperium

5th

Any condition in I15 specified as a reason for obstetric care during pregnancy, childbirth or the puerperium

Use additional code from I15 to identify the type of secondary hypertension

O10.41- Pre-existing secondary hypertension complicating pregnancy

6th

O11 PRE-EXISTING HYPERTENSION WITH PRE-ECLAMPSIA

4th

Includes: conditions in O10 complicated by pre-eclampsia pre-eclampsia superimposed pre-existing hypertension

Use additional code from O10 to identify the type of hypertension

O11.1 Pre-existing hypertension with pre-eclampsia, first trimester

O11.2 Pre-existing hypertension with pre-eclampsia, second trimester

O11.3 Pre-existing hypertension with pre-eclampsia, third trimester

O14 PRE-ECLAMPSIA

4th

Excludes1: pre-existing hypertension with pre-eclampsia (O11)

O14.0- Mild to moderate pre-eclampsia

5th

O14.1- Severe pre-eclampsia

5th

Excludes1: HELLP syndrome (O14.2-)

O14.2- HELLP syndrome

5th

Severe pre-eclampsia with hemolysis, elevated liver enzymes and low platelet count (HELLP)

O14.9- Unspecified pre-eclampsia

5th

O14 requires a 5th character
0 unspecified trimester
2 second trimester
3 third trimester
4 complicating childbirth
5 complicating the puerperium

(O20–O29) OTHER MATERNAL DISORDERS PREDOMINANTLY RELATED TO PREGNANCY

Excludes2: maternal care related to the fetus and amniotic cavity and possible delivery problems (O30–O48)
maternal diseases classifiable elsewhere but complicating pregnancy, labor and delivery, and the puerperium (O98–O99)

O20 HEMORRHAGE IN EARLY PREGNANCY

4th

Includes: hemorrhage before completion of 20 weeks gestation

Excludes1: pregnancy with abortive outcome (O00–O08)

O20.0 Threatened abortion

Hemorrhage specified as due to threatened abortion

O20.8 Other hemorrhage in early pregnancy

O20.9 Hemorrhage in early pregnancy, unspecified

O24 DM IN PREGNANCY, CHILDBIRTH, AND THE PUERPERIUM

4th

O24.0 Pre-existing type 1 DM

5th

Juvenile onset DM, in pregnancy, childbirth and the puerperium Ketosis-prone DM in pregnancy, childbirth and the puerperium

Use additional code from category E10 to further identify any manifestations

O24.01 and O24.11 require a 6th character
1 first trimester
2 second trimester
3 third trimester
9 unspecified trimester

O24.01- Pre-existing type 1 DM, in pregnancy

6th

O24.1 Pre-existing type 2 DM

5th

Insulin-resistant DM in pregnancy, childbirth and the puerperium

Use additional code (for):
from category E11 to further identify any manifestation
injectable non-insulin antidiabetic drugs (Z79.85)
long-term (current) use of insulin (Z79.4)

O24.11- Pre-existing type 2 DM, in pregnancy

6th

O24.12 Pre-existing type 2 diabetes mellitus, in childbirth

O24.13 Pre-existing type 2 diabetes mellitus, in the puerperium

O24.3 Unspecified pre-existing diabetes mellitus in pregnancy, childbirth and the puerperium

Use additional code (for):
from category E11 to further identify any manifestation
injectable non-insulin antidiabetic drugs (Z79.85)
long-term (current) use of insulin (Z79.4)

O24.31 Unspecified pre-existing diabetes mellitus in pregnancy

O24.311 first trimester

O24.312 second trimester

O24.313 third trimester

O24.319 unspecified trimester

O24.32 Unspecified pre-existing diabetes mellitus in childbirth

O24.33 Unspecified pre-existing diabetes mellitus in the puerperium

O24.4 Gestational DM

5th

DM arising in pregnancy
Gestational diabetes mellitus NOS

O24.41 Gestational DM in pregnancy

6th

O24.410 Gestational DM in pregnancy, diet controlled

O24.414 Gestational DM in pregnancy, insulin controlled

O24.415 Gestational DM in pregnancy, controlled by oral hypoglycemic drugs

Gestational diabetes mellitus in pregnancy, controlled by oral antidiabetic drugs

O24.8 Other pre-existing diabetes mellitus in pregnancy, childbirth, and the puerperium

Use additional code (for):
from categories E08, E09 and E13 to further identify any manifestation
injectable non-insulin antidiabetic drugs (Z79.85)
long-term (current) use of insulin (Z79.4)

O24.81 Other pre-existing diabetes mellitus in pregnancy
- O24.811 first trimester
- O24.812 second trimester
- O24.813 third trimester
- O24.819 unspecified trimester

O24.82 Other pre-existing diabetes mellitus in childbirth

O24.83 Other pre-existing diabetes mellitus in the puerperium

O24.9 Unspecified diabetes mellitus in pregnancy, childbirth and the puerperium

Use additional code (for):
- from categories E08, E09 and E13 to further identify any manifestation
- injectable non-insulin antidiabetic drugs (Z79.85)
- long-term (current) use of insulin (Z79.4)

- O24.91 Unspecified diabetes mellitus in pregnancy
  - O24.911 first trimester
  - O24.912 second trimester
  - O24.913 third trimester
  - O24.919 unspecified trimester
- O24.92 Unspecified diabetes mellitus in childbirth
- O24.93 Unspecified diabetes mellitus in the puerperium

O28 ABNORMAL FINDINGS ON ANTENATAL SCREENING OF MOTHER

Excludes1: diagnostic findings classified elsewhere—**see** Alphabetical Index

- O28.0 Abnormal hematological finding on antenatal screening of mother
- O28.1 Abnormal biochemical finding on antenatal screening of mother
- O28.2 Abnormal cytological finding on antenatal screening of mother
- O28.3 Abnormal ultrasonic finding on antenatal screening of mother
- O28.4 Abnormal radiological finding on antenatal screening of mother
- O28.5 Abnormal chromosomal and genetic finding on antenatal screening of mother
- O28.8 Other abnormal findings on antenatal screening of mother
- O28.9 Unspecified abnormal findings on antenatal screening of mother

(O30–O48) MATERNAL CARE RELATED TO THE FETUS AND AMNIOTIC CAVITY AND POSSIBLE DELIVERY PROBLEMS

O30 MULTIPLE GESTATION

Code **also** any complications specific to multiple gestation

O30.0 Twin pregnancy

- O30.00- Twin pregnancy, unspecified number of placenta and unspecified number of amniotic sacs
- O30.01- Twin pregnancy, monochorionic/monoamniotic Twin pregnancy, one placenta, one amniotic sac *Excludes1:* conjoined twins (O30.02-)

O30 requires a 6th character: 1 first trimester, 2 second trimester, 3 third trimester, 9 unspecified trimester

- O30.02- Conjoined twin pregnancy
- O30.03- Twin pregnancy, monochorionic/diamniotic Twin pregnancy, one placenta, two amniotic sacs
- O30.04- Twin pregnancy, dichorionic/diamniotic Twin pregnancy, two placentae, two amniotic sacs
- O30.09- Twin pregnancy, unable to determine number of placenta and number of amniotic sacs

O30.1 Triplet pregnancy;

- O30.10- unspecified number of placenta and unspecified number of amniotic sacs
- O30.11- with two or more monochorionic fetuses
- O30.12- with two or more monoamniotic fetuses
- O30.13- trichorionic/triamniotic
- O30.19- unable to determine number of placenta and number of amniotic sacs

O30.2 Quadruplet pregnancy;

- O30.20- unspecified number of placenta
- O30.21- with two or more monochorionic fetuses
- O30.22- with two or more monoamniotic fetuses
- O30.23- quadrachorionic/quadraamniotic
- O30.29- unable to determine number of placenta and number of amniotic sacs

O30.8 Other specified multiple gestation;

Multiple gestation pregnancy greater then quadruplets

- O30.80- unspecified number of placenta and unspecified number of amniotic sacs
- O30.81- with two or more monochorionic fetuses
- O30.82- with two or more monoamniotic fetuses
- O30.83- number of chorions and amnions are both equal to the number of fetuses Pentachorionic, penta-amniotic pregnancy (quintuplets) Hexachorionic, hexa-amniotic pregnancy (sextuplets) Heptachorionic, hepta-amniotic pregnancy (septuplets)
- O30.89- unable to determine number of placenta and number of amniotic sacs

O31 COMPLICATIONS SPECIFIC TO MULTIPLE GESTATION

Assign a 7th character to identify the fetus for which the complication code applies.

Assign 7th character "0" for either a single gestation or when the documentation is insufficient to determine the fetus affected and it is not possible to obtain clarification or when it is not possible to clinically determine which fetus is affected.

O31 requires a 7th character: 0 not applicable (ie, only one fetus) or unspecified, 1 fetus 1, 2 fetus 2, 3 fetus 3, 4 fetus 4, 5 fetus 5, 9 other fetus

Excludes2: delayed delivery of second twin, triplet, etc. (O63.2) malpresentation of one fetus or more (O32.9) placental transfusion syndromes (O43.0-)

Code **also** the appropriate code from category O30, Multiple gestation, when assigning a code from category O31 that has a 7th character of 1 through 9.

- O31.1 Continuing pregnancy after spontaneous abortion of one fetus or more;
  - O31.10X- unspecified trimester
  - O31.11X- first trimester
  - O31.12X- second trimester
  - O31.13X- third trimester

- O31.2 Continuing pregnancy after intrauterine death of one fetus or more;
  - O31.20X- unspecified trimester
  - O31.21X- first trimester
  - O31.22X- second trimester
  - O31.23X- third trimester

- O31.8 Other complications specific to multiple gestation
  - O31.8X Other complications specific to multiple gestation;
    - O31.8X1- first trimester
    - O31.8X2- second trimester
    - O31.8X3- third trimester

GUIDELINES

Codes from categories O35, Maternal care for known or suspected fetal abnormality and damage, and O36, Maternal care for other fetal problems, are assigned only when the fetal condition is actually responsible for modifying the management of the mother, i.e., by requiring diagnostic studies, additional observation, special care, or termination of pregnancy. The fact that the fetal condition exists does not justify assigning a code from this series to the mother's record.

O35 MATERNAL CARE FOR KNOWN OR SUSPECTED FETAL ABNORMALITY AND DAMAGE

Assign only when the fetal condition is actually responsible for modifying the management of the mother, ie, by requiring diagnostic studies, additional observation, special care, or termination of pregnancy. The fact that the fetal condition exists does not justify assigning a code from this series to the mother's record.

In cases when surgery is performed on the fetus, a diagnosis code from category O35, Maternal care for known or suspected fetal abnormality and damage, should be assigned identifying the fetal condition. Assign the appropriate procedure code for the procedure performed.

No code from Chapter 16, the perinatal codes, should be used on the mother's record to identify fetal conditions. Surgery performed in utero on a fetus is still to be coded as an obstetric encounter.

Assign a 7th character to identify the fetus for which the complication code applies.

Assign 7th character "0" for either a single gestation or when the documentation is insufficient to determine the fetus affected and it is not possible to obtain clarification or when it is not possible to clinically determine which fetus is affected.

Includes: the listed conditions in the fetus as a reason for hospitalization or other obstetric care to the mother, or for termination of pregnancy

Code also any associated maternal condition

Excludes1: encounter for suspected maternal and fetal conditions ruled out (Z03.7-)

Code also the appropriate code from category O30, Multiple gestation, when assigning a code from category O35 that has a 7th character of 1 through 9.

O35.0 Maternal care for (suspected) central nervous system malformation in fetus

Excludes2: chromosomal abnormality in fetus (O35.1-)

O35.00X- Maternal care for (suspected) central nervous system malformation or damage in fetus;

O35.01X- agenesis of the corpus callosum

O35.02X- anencephaly

O35.03X- choroid plexus cysts

O35.04X- encephalocele, not applicable or unspecified

O35.05X- holoprosencephaly, not applicable or unspecified

O35.06X- hydrocephaly

O35.07X- microcephaly

O35.08X- spina bifida

O35.09X- Maternal care for (suspected) other central nervous system malformation or damage in fetus

O35.1 Maternal care for (suspected) chromosomal abnormality in fetus;

O35.10X- unspecified

O35.11X- Trisomy 13

O35.12X- Trisomy 18

O35 requires a 7th character
0 not applicable (ie, only one fetus) or unspecified
1 fetus 1
2 fetus 2
3 fetus 3
4 fetus 4
5 fetus 5
9 other fetus

O35 requires a 7th character
0 not applicable (ie, only one fetus) or unspecified
1 fetus 1
2 fetus 2
3 fetus 3
4 fetus 4
5 fetus 5
9 other fetus

O35.13X- Trisomy 21

O35.14X- Turner Syndrome

O35.15X- sex chromosome abnormality

O35.19X- other chromosomal abnormality

O35.AXX- fetal facial anomalies

O35.BXX- fetal cardiac anomalies

O35.CXX- fetal abnormality and damage, fetal pulmonary anomalies

O35.DXX- fetal gastrointestinal anomalies

O35.EXX- fetal genitourinary anomalies

O35.FXX- fetal musculoskeletal anomalies of trunk

O35.GXX- fetal upper extremities anomalies

O35.HXX- fetal lower extremities anomalies

O35.2XX- Maternal care for (suspected) hereditary disease in fetus

Excludes2: chromosomal abnormality in fetus (O35.1)

O35.3XX- Maternal care for (suspected) damage to fetus from viral disease in mother

Maternal care for damage to fetus from maternal cytomegalovirus infection

Maternal care for damage to fetus from maternal rubella

O35.4XX- Maternal care for (suspected) damage to fetus from alcohol

O35.5XX- Maternal care for (suspected) damage to fetus by drugs

Maternal care for damage to fetus from drug addiction

O35.6XX- Maternal care for (suspected) damage to fetus by radiation

O35.7XX- Maternal care for (suspected) damage to fetus by other medical procedures

Maternal care for damage to fetus by amniocentesis

Maternal care for damage to fetus by biopsy procedures

Maternal care for damage to fetus by hematological investigation

Maternal care for damage to fetus by intrauterine contraceptive device

Maternal care for damage to fetus by intrauterine surgery

O35.8XX- Maternal care for other (suspected) fetal abnormality and damage

Maternal care for other (suspected) fetal abnormality and damage

Maternal care for damage to fetus from maternal listeriosis

Maternal care for damage to fetus from maternal toxoplasmosis

O35.9XX- Maternal care for (suspected) fetal abnormality and damage, unspecified

O36 MATERNAL CARE FOR OTHER FETAL PROBLEMS

Assign a 7th character to identify the fetus for which the complication code applies.

Assign 7th character "0" for either a single gestation or when the documentation is insufficient to determine the fetus affected and it is not possible to obtain clarification or when it is not possible to clinically determine which fetus is affected.

Includes: the listed conditions in the fetus as a reason for hospitalization or other obstetric care of the mother, or for termination of pregnancy

O36 requires a 7th character
0 not applicable (ie, only one fetus) or unspecified
1 fetus 1
2 fetus 2
3 fetus 3
4 fetus 4
5 fetus 5
9 other fetus

Excludes1: encounter for suspected maternal and fetal conditions ruled out (Z03.7-)
placental transfusion syndromes (O43.0-)

Excludes2: labor and delivery complicated by fetal stress (O77.-)

Code also the appropriate code from category O30, Multiple gestation, when assigning a code from category O36 that has a 7th character of 1 through 9.

O36.0 Maternal care for rhesus isoimmunization

5th Maternal care for Rh incompatibility (with hydrops fetalis)

O36.01 Maternal care for anti-D [Rh] antibodies;

6th **O36.011-** first trimester

7th

O36.012- second trimester

7th

O36.013- third trimester

7th

O36.09 Maternal care for other rhesus isoimmunization;

6th **O36.091-** first trimester

7th

O36.092- second trimester

7th

O36.093- third trimester

7th

O36.1 Maternal care for other isoimmunization

5th Maternal care for ABO isoimmunization

O36.11 Maternal care for Anti-A sensitization;

6th Maternal care for isoimmunization NOS (with hydrops fetalis)

O36.111- first trimester

7th

O36.112- second trimester

7th

O36.113- third trimester

7th

O36.19 Maternal care for other isoimmunization;

6th Maternal care for Anti-B sensitization

O36.191- first trimester

7th

O36.192- second trimester

7th

O36.193- third trimester

7th

O36.2 Maternal care for hydrops fetalis;

5th Maternal care for hydrops fetalis NOS
Maternal care for hydrops fetalis not associated with isoimmunization

Excludes1: hydrops fetalis associated with ABO isoimmunization (O36.1-)
hydrops fetalis associated with rhesus isoimmunization (O36.0-)

O36.21X- first trimester

7th

O36.22X- second trimester

7th

O36.23X- third trimester

7th

O36.4XX- Maternal care for intrauterine death

7th Maternal care for intrauterine fetal death NOS
Maternal care for intrauterine fetal death after completion of 20 weeks of gestation
Maternal care for late fetal death
Maternal care for missed delivery

Excludes1: missed abortion (O02.1)
stillbirth (P95)

O36.5 Maternal care for known or suspected poor fetal growth

5th **O36.51 Maternal care for known or suspected placental insufficiency;**

6th **O36.511-** first trimester

7th

O36.512- second trimester

7th

O36.513- third trimester

7th

O36.59 Maternal care for other known or suspected poor fetal growth;

6th Maternal care for known or suspected light-for-dates NOS
Maternal care for known or suspected small-for-dates NOS

O36.591- first trimester

7th

O36.592- second trimester

7th

O36.593- third trimester

7th

O36.6 Maternal care for excessive fetal growth;

5th Maternal care for known or suspected large-for-dates

O36.61X- first trimester

7th

O36.62X- second trimester

7th

O36.63X- third trimester

7th

O36.7 Maternal care for viable fetus in abdominal pregnancy;

5th **O36.71X-** first trimester

7th

O36.72X- second trimester

7th

O36.73X- third trimester

7th

O36.8 Maternal care for other specified fetal problems

5th **O36.80X-** Pregnancy with inconclusive fetal viability

7th Encounter to determine fetal viability of pregnancy

O36.81 Decreased fetal movements;

6th **O36.812-** second trimester

7th

O36.813- third trimester

7th

O36.82 Fetal anemia and thrombocytopenia;

6th **O36.821-** first trimester

7th

O36.822- second trimester

7th

O36.823- third trimester

7th

O36.83 Maternal care for abnormalities of the fetal heart rate or rhythm;

6th Maternal care for depressed fetal heart rate tones
Maternal care for fetal bradycardia
Maternal care for fetal heart rate abnormal variability
Maternal care for fetal heart rate decelerations
Maternal care for fetal heart rate irregularity
Maternal care for fetal tachycardia
Maternal care for non-reassuring fetal heart rate or rhythm

O36.831- first trimester

7th

O36.832- second trimester

7th

O36.833- third trimester

7th

O36.839- unspecified trimester

7th

O36.89 Maternal care for other specified fetal problems;

6th **O36.891-** first trimester

7th

O36.892- second trimester

7th

O36.893- third trimester

7th

4th 5th 6th 7th Additional Character Required ✓ 3-character code ●=New Code ▲=Revised Code *Excludes1*—Not coded here, do not use together *Excludes2*—Not included here

O40 POLYHYDRAMNIOS

4th Assign a 7th character to identify the fetus for which the complication code applies.

Assign 7th character "0" for either a single gestation or when the documentation is insufficient to determine the fetus affected and it is not possible to obtain clarification or when it is not possible to clinically determine which fetus is affected.

Includes: hydramnios

Excludes1: encounter for suspected maternal and fetal conditions ruled out (Z03.7-)

- **O40.1XX-** Polyhydramnios, first trimester **7th**
- **O40.2XX-** Polyhydramnios, second **7th** trimester
- **O40.3XX-** Polyhydramnios, third **7th** trimester
- **O40.9XX-** Polyhydramnios, unspecified trimester **7th**

O41 OTHER DISORDERS OF AMNIOTIC FLUID AND MEMBRANES

4th Assign a 7th character to identify the fetus for which the complication code applies.

Assign 7th character "0" for either a single gestation or when the documentation is insufficient to determine the fetus affected and it is not possible to obtain clarification or when it is not possible to clinically determine which fetus is affected.

Excludes1: encounter for suspected maternal and fetal conditions ruled out (Z03.7-)

Code also the appropriate code from category O30, Multiple gestation, when assigning a code from category O41 that has a 7th character of 1 through 9.

- **O41.01X-** Oligohydramnios, **7th** first trimester, not applicable or unspecified
- **O41.02X-** Oligohydramnios, **7th** second trimester, not applicable or unspecified
- **O41.03X-** Oligohydramnios, third **7th** trimester, not applicable or unspecified

O42 PREMATURE RUPTURE OF MEMBRANES

5th

- **O42.00** Premature rupture of membranes, onset of labor within 24 hours of rupture, unspecified weeks of gestation
- **O42.01** Preterm premature rupture of membranes, onset of **6th** labor within 24 hours of rupture Premature rupture of membranes before 37 completed weeks of gestation
  - **O42.011** Preterm premature rupture of membranes, onset of labor within 24 hours of rupture, first trimester
  - **O42.012** second trimester
  - **O42.013** third trimester
  - **O42.019** unspecified trimester
- **O42.02** Full-term premature rupture of membranes, onset of labor within 24 hours of rupture Premature rupture of membranes at or after 37 completed weeks of gestation, onset of labor within 24 hours of rupture
- **O42.1** Premature rupture of membranes, onset of labor more than **5th** 24 hours following rupture
  - **O42.10** Premature rupture of membranes, onset of labor more than 24 hours following rupture, unspecified weeks of gestation
  - **O42.11** Preterm premature rupture of membranes, onset of **6th** labor more than 24 hours following rupture Premature rupture of membranes before 37 completed weeks of gestation

- **O42.111** Preterm premature rupture of membranes, onset of labor more than 24 hours following rupture, first trimester
- **O42.112** second trimester
- **O42.113** third trimester
- **O42.119** unspecified trimester
- **O42.12** Full-term premature rupture of membranes, onset of labor more than 24 hours following rupture Premature rupture of membranes at or after 37 completed weeks of gestation, onset of labor more than 24 hours following rupture
- **O42.9** Premature rupture of membranes, unspecified as to length of **5th** time between rupture and onset of labor
  - **O42.90** Premature rupture of membranes, unspecified as to length of time between rupture and onset of labor, unspecified weeks of gestation
  - **O42.91** Preterm premature rupture of membranes, **6th** unspecified as to length of time between rupture and onset of labor Premature rupture of membranes before 37 completed weeks of gestation
    - **O42.911** Preterm premature rupture of membranes, unspecified as to length of time between rupture and onset of labor; first trimester
    - **O42.912** second trimester
    - **O42.913** third trimester
  - **O42.92** Full-term premature rupture of membranes, unspecified as to length of time between rupture and onset of labor Premature rupture of membranes at or after 37 completed weeks of gestation, unspecified as to length of time between rupture and onset of labor

O43 PLACENTAL DISORDERS

4th *Excludes2:* maternal care for poor fetal growth due to placental insufficiency (O36.5-) placenta previa (O44.-) placental polyp (O90.89) placentitis (O41.14-) premature separation of placenta [abruptio placentae] (O45.-)

- **O43.0** Placental transfusion syndromes
  - **5th**
  - **O43.01** Fetomaternal placental transfusion syndrome **6th** Maternofetal placental transfusion syndrome
    - **O43.011** Fetomaternal placental transfusion syndrome; first trimester
    - **O43.012** second trimester
    - **O43.013** third trimester
  - **O43.02** Fetus-to-fetus placental transfusion syndrome
    - **6th**
    - **O43.021** Fetus-to-fetus placental transfusion syndrome; first trimester
    - **O43.022** second trimester
    - **O43.023** third trimester

(O60–O77) COMPLICATIONS OF LABOR AND DELIVERY

O60 PRETERM LABOR

4th *Includes:* onset (spontaneous) of labor before 37 completed weeks of gestation

Excludes1: false labor (O47.0-) threatened labor NOS (O47.0-)

- **O60.0** Preterm labor without delivery, unspecified trimester
  - **5th**
  - **O60.02** Preterm labor without delivery, second trimester
  - **O60.03** Preterm labor without delivery, third trimester

O75 OTHER COMPLICATIONS OF LABOR AND DELIVERY, NOT ELSEWHERE CLASSIFIED

4th *Excludes2:* puerperal (postpartum) infection (O86.-) puerperal (postpartum) sepsis (O85)

- **O75.0** Maternal distress during labor and delivery
- **O75.1** Shock during or following labor and delivery Obstetric shock following labor and delivery
- **O75.2** Pyrexia during labor, not elsewhere classified
- **O75.3** Other infection during labor Sepsis during labor **Use additional code** (B95–B97), to identify infectious agent

O75.4 Other complications of obstetric surgery and procedures
Cardiac arrest following obstetric surgery or procedures
Cardiac failure following obstetric surgery or procedures
Cerebral anoxia following obstetric surgery or procedures
Pulmonary edema following obstetric surgery or procedures
Use additional code to identify specific complication
Excludes2: complications of anesthesia during labor and delivery (O74.-)
disruption of obstetrical (surgical) wound (O90.0-O90.1)
hematoma of obstetrical (surgical) wound (O90.2)
infection of obstetrical (surgical) wound (O86.0-)

O75.5 Delayed delivery after artificial rupture of membranes

O75.8 Other specified complications of labor and delivery

5th **O75.81 Maternal exhaustion complicating labor and delivery**

O75.82 Onset (spontaneous) of labor after 37 completed weeks of gestation but before 39 completed weeks gestation, with delivery by (planned) cesarean section
Delivery by (planned) cesarean section occurring after 37 completed weeks of gestation but before 39 completed weeks gestation due to (spontaneous) onset of labor
Code first to specify reason for planned cesarean section such as:
cephalopelvic disproportion (normally formed fetus) (O33.9)
previous cesarean delivery (O34.21-)

O75.89 Other specified complications of labor and delivery

O75.9 Complication of labor and delivery, unspecified

(O80-O82) ENCOUNTER FOR DELIVERY

(O85-O92) COMPLICATIONS PREDOMINANTLY RELATED TO THE PUERPERIUM

O92 OTHER DISORDERS OF BREAST AND DISORDERS OF LACTATION ASSOCIATED WITH PREGNANCY AND THE PUERPERIUM
4th

O92.0 Retracted nipple associated with pregnancy, the puerperium, and lactation
5th
O92.02 Retracted nipple associated with the puerperium
O92.03 Retracted nipple associated with lactation

O92.1 Cracked nipple associated with pregnancy, the puerperium, and lactation
5th
Fissure of nipple, gestational or puerperal
O92.12 Cracked nipple associated with the puerperium
O92.13 Cracked nipple associated with lactation

O92.2 Other and unspecified disorders of breast associated with pregnancy and the puerperium
5th
O92.20 Unspecified disorder of breast associated with pregnancy and the puerperium
O92.29 Other disorders of breast associated with pregnancy and the puerperium

O92.3 Agalactia
Primary agalactia
Excludes1: Elective agalactia (O92.5)
Secondary agalactia (O92.5)
Therapeutic agalactia (O92.5)

O92.4 Hypogalactia

O92.5 Suppressed lactation
Elective agalactia
Secondary agalactia
Therapeutic agalactia
Excludes1: primary agalactia (O92.3)

O92.6 Galactorrhea

O92.7 Other and unspecified disorders of lactation

5th **O92.70** Unspecified disorders of lactation

O92.79 Other disorders of lactation
Puerperal galactocele

(O94-O9A) OTHER OBSTETRIC CONDITIONS, NOT ELSEWHERE CLASSIFIED

Chapter 16. Certain conditions originating in the perinatal period (P00–P96)

GUIDELINES

For coding and reporting purposes the perinatal period is defined as before birth through the 28th day following birth. The following guidelines are provided for reporting purposes

General Perinatal Rules

Codes in this chapter are never for use on the maternal record. Codes from Chapter 15, the obstetric chapter, are never permitted on the newborn record. Chapter 16 codes may be used throughout the life of the patient if the condition is still present.

PRINCIPAL DIAGNOSIS FOR BIRTH RECORD

When coding the birth episode in a newborn record, assign a code from category Z38, Liveborn infants according to place of birth and type of delivery, as the principal diagnosis. A code from category Z38 is assigned only once, to a newborn at the time of birth. If a newborn is transferred to another institution, a code from category Z38 should not be used at the receiving hospital.

A code from category Z38 is used only on the newborn record, not on the mother's record.

USE OF CODES FROM OTHER CHAPTERS WITH CODES FROM CHAPTER 16

Codes from other chapters may be used with codes from Chapter 16 if the codes from the other chapters provide more specific detail. Codes for signs and symptoms may be assigned when a definitive diagnosis has not been established. If the reason for the encounter is a perinatal condition, the code from Chapter 16 should be sequenced first.

USE OF CHAPTER 16 CODES AFTER THE PERINATAL PERIOD

Should a condition originate in the perinatal period, and continue throughout the life of the patient, the perinatal code should continue to be used regardless of the patient's age.

BIRTH PROCESS OR COMMUNITY ACQUIRED CONDITIONS

If a newborn has a condition that may be either due to the birth process or community acquired and the documentation does not indicate which it is, the default is due to the birth process and the code from Chapter 16 should be used. If the condition is community-acquired, a code from Chapter 16 should not be assigned.

CODE ALL CLINICALLY SIGNIFICANT CONDITIONS

All clinically significant conditions noted on routine newborn examination should be coded. A condition is clinically significant if it requires:

- clinical evaluation; or
- therapeutic treatment; or
- diagnostic procedures; or
- extended length of hospital stay; or
- increased nursing care and/or monitoring; or
- has implications for future health care needs

Note: The perinatal guidelines listed above are the same as the general coding guidelines for "additional diagnoses," except for the final point regarding implications for future health care needs. Codes should be assigned for conditions that have been specified by the provider as having implications for future health care needs.

Observation and Evaluation of Newborns for Suspected Condition not Found

See category Z05.

Coding Additional Perinatal Diagnoses

ASSIGNING CODES FOR CONDITIONS THAT REQUIRE TREATMENT

Assign codes for conditions that require treatment or further investigation, prolong the length of stay, or require resource utilization.

CODES FOR CONDITIONS SPECIFIED AS HAVING IMPLICATIONS FOR FUTURE HEALTH CARE NEEDS

Assign codes for conditions that have been specified by the provider as having implications for future health care needs. Note: This guideline should not be used for adult patients.

Prematurity and Fetal Growth Retardation

See categories P05–P07.

LBW and Immaturity status

See category P07.

Bacterial Sepsis of Newborn

See category P36.

Stillbirth

See category P95.

COVID-19 Infection in Newborn

For a newborn that tests positive for COVID-19, assign code U07.1, COVID-19, and the appropriate codes for associated manifestation(s) in neonates/newborns in the absence of documentation indicating a specific type of transmission. For a newborn that tests positive for COVID-19 and the provider documents the condition was contracted in utero or during the birth process, assign codes P35.8, Other congenital viral diseases, and U07.1, COVID-19. When coding the birth episode in a newborn record, the appropriate code from category Z38, Liveborn infants according to place of birth and type of delivery, should be assigned as the principal diagnosis.

Note: Codes from this chapter are for use on newborn records only, never on maternal records

Includes: conditions that have their origin in the fetal or perinatal period (before birth through the first 28 days after birth) even if morbidity occurs later

Excludes2: congenital malformations, deformations and chromosomal abnormalities (Q00–Q99)
endocrine, nutritional and metabolic diseases (E00–E88)
injury, poisoning and certain other consequences of external causes (S00–T88)
neoplasms (C00–D49)
tetanus neonatorum (A33)

(P00–P04) NEWBORN AFFECTED BY MATERNAL FACTORS AND BY COMPLICATIONS OF PREGNANCY, LABOR, AND DELIVERY

Note: These codes are for use when the listed maternal conditions are specified as the cause of confirmed morbidity or potential morbidity which have their origin in the perinatal period (before birth through the first 28 days after birth). Codes from these categories are also for use for newborns who are suspected of having an abnormal condition resulting from exposure from the mother or the birth process.

P00 NEWBORN AFFECTED BY MATERNAL CONDITIONS THAT MAY BE UNRELATED TO PRESENT PREGNANCY

Code first any current condition in newborn

Excludes2: encounter for observation and evaluation of newborn for suspected diseases and conditions ruled out (Z05.-)
newborn affected by maternal complications of pregnancy (P01.-)
newborn affected by maternal endocrine and metabolic disorders (P70–P74)
newborn affected by noxious substances transmitted via placenta or breast milk (P04.-)

P00.0 Newborn affected by maternal hypertensive disorders
Newborn affected by maternal conditions classifiable to O10–O11, O13–O16

P00.1 Newborn affected by maternal renal and urinary tract diseases
Newborn affected by maternal conditions classifiable to N00–N39

P00.2 Newborn affected by maternal infectious and parasitic diseases
Newborn affected by maternal infectious disease classifiable to A00–B99, J09 and J10

Excludes2: infections specific to the perinatal period (P35–P39)
maternal genital tract or other localized infections (P00.8-)

P00.3 Newborn affected by other maternal circulatory and respiratory diseases
Newborn affected by maternal conditions classifiable to I00–I99, J00–J99, Q20–Q34 and not included in P00.0, P00.2

P00.4 Newborn affected by maternal nutritional disorders
Newborn affected by maternal disorders classifiable to E40–E64
Maternal malnutrition NOS

P00.5 Newborn affected by maternal injury
Newborn affected by maternal conditions classifiable to O9A.2-

P00.6 Newborn affected by surgical procedure on mother
Newborn affected by amniocentesis
Excludes1: cesarean delivery for present delivery (P03.4)
damage to placenta from amniocentesis, cesarean delivery or surgical induction (P02.1)
previous surgery to uterus or pelvic organs (P03.89)
Excludes2: newborn affected by complication of (fetal) intrauterine procedure (P96.5)

P00.7 Newborn affected by other medical procedures on mother, NEC
Newborn affected by radiation to mother
Excludes1: damage to placenta from amniocentesis, cesarean delivery or surgical induction (P02.1)
newborn affected by other complications of labor and delivery (P03.-)

P00.8 Newborn affected by other maternal conditions
- **P00.81 Newborn affected by periodontal disease in mother**
- **P00.82 Newborn affected by (positive) maternal group B streptococcus (GBS) colonization**
Contact with positive maternal group B streptococcus
- **P00.89 Newborn affected by other maternal conditions**
Newborn affected by conditions classifiable to T80–T88
Newborn affected by maternal genital tract or other localized infections
Newborn affected by maternal SLE
Use additional code to identify infectious agent, if known
Excludes 2: newborn affected by positive maternal group B streptococcus (GBS) colonization (P00.82)

P00.9 Newborn affected by unspecified maternal condition

P01 NEWBORN AFFECTED BY MATERNAL COMPLICATIONS OF PREGNANCY

Code first any current condition in newborn
Excludes2: encounter for observation of newborn for suspected diseases and conditions ruled out (Z05.-)

P01.0 Newborn affected by incompetent cervix

P01.1 Newborn affected by premature rupture of membranes

P01.2 Newborn affected by oligohydramnios
Excludes1: oligohydramnios due to premature rupture of membranes (P01.1)

P01.3 Newborn affected by polyhydramnios
Newborn affected by hydramnios

P01.4 Newborn affected by ectopic pregnancy
Newborn affected by abdominal pregnancy

P01.5 Newborn affected by multiple pregnancy
Newborn affected by triplet (pregnancy)
Newborn affected by twin (pregnancy)

P01.6 Newborn affected by maternal death

P01.7 Newborn affected by malpresentation before labor
Newborn affected by breech presentation before labor
Newborn affected by external version before labor
Newborn affected by face presentation before labor
Newborn affected by transverse lie before labor
Newborn affected by unstable lie before labor

P01.8 Newborn affected by other maternal complications of pregnancy

P01.9 Newborn affected by maternal complication of pregnancy, unspecified

P02 NEWBORN AFFECTED BY COMPLICATIONS OF PLACENTA, CORD AND MEMBRANES

Code first any current condition in newborn
Excludes2: encounter for observation of newborn for suspected diseases and conditions ruled out (Z05.-)

P02.0 Newborn affected by placenta previa

P02.1 Newborn affected by other forms of placental separation and hemorrhage
Newborn affected by abruptio placenta
Newborn affected by accidental hemorrhage
Newborn affected by antepartum hemorrhage
Newborn affected by damage to placenta from amniocentesis, cesarean delivery or surgical induction
Newborn affected by maternal blood loss
Newborn affected by premature separation of placenta

P02.2 Newborn affected by other and unspecified morphological and functional abnormalities of placenta
- **P02.20 Newborn affected by unspecified morphological and functional abnormalities of placenta**
- **P02.29 Newborn affected by other morphological and functional abnormalities of placenta**
Newborn affected by placental dysfunction
Newborn affected by placental infarction
Newborn affected by placental insufficiency

P02.3 Newborn affected by placental transfusion syndromes
Newborn affected by placental and cord abnormalities resulting in twin-to-twin or other transplacental transfusion

P02.4 Newborn affected by prolapsed cord

P02.5 Newborn affected by other compression of umbilical cord
Newborn affected by umbilical cord (tightly) around neck
Newborn affected by entanglement of umbilical cord
Newborn affected by knot in umbilical cord

P02.6 Newborn affected by other and unspecified conditions of umbilical cord
- **P02.60 Newborn affected by unspecified conditions of umbilical cord**
- **P02.69 Newborn affected by other conditions of umbilical cord**
Newborn affected by short umbilical cord
Newborn affected by vasa previa
Excludes1: newborn affected by single umbilical artery (Q27.0)

P02.7 Newborn affected by chorioamnionitis
- **P02.70 Newborn affected by fetal inflammatory response syndrome**
- **P02.78 Newborn affected by other conditions from chorioamnionitis**
Newborn affected by amnionitis
Newborn affected by membranitis
Newborn affected by placentitis

P02.8 Newborn affected by other abnormalities of membranes

P02.9 Newborn affected by abnormality of membranes, unspecified

P03 NEWBORN AFFECTED BY OTHER COMPLICATIONS OF LABOR AND DELIVERY

Code first any current condition in newborn
Excludes2: encounter for observation of newborn for suspected diseases and conditions ruled out (Z05.-)

P03.0 Newborn affected by breech delivery and extraction

P03.1 Newborn affected by other malpresentation, malposition and disproportion during labor and delivery
Newborn affected by contracted pelvis
Newborn affected by conditions classifiable to O64–O66
Newborn affected by persistent occipitoposterior
Newborn affected by transverse lie

P03.2 Newborn affected by forceps delivery

P03.3 Newborn affected by delivery by vacuum extractor [ventouse]

P03.4 Newborn affected by cesarean delivery

P03.5 Newborn affected by precipitate delivery
Newborn affected by rapid second stage

P03.6 Newborn affected by abnormal uterine contractions
Newborn affected by conditions classifiable to O62.-, except O62.3
Newborn affected by hypertonic labor
Newborn affected by uterine inertia

P03.8 Newborn affected by other specified complications of labor and delivery
- **P03.81 Newborn affected by abnormality in fetal (intrauterine) heart rate or rhythm**
Excludes1: neonatal cardiac dysrhythmia (P29.1-)

P03.810 Newborn affected by abnormality in fetal (intrauterine) heart rate or rhythm before the onset of labor

P03.811 Newborn affected by abnormality in fetal (intrauterine) heart rate or rhythm during labor

P03.819 Newborn affected by abnormality in fetal (intrauterine) heart rate or rhythm, unspecified as to time of onset

P03.82 Meconium passage during delivery

Excludes1: meconium aspiration (P24.00, P24.01) meconium staining (P96.83)

P03.89 Newborn affected by other specified complications of labor and delivery

Newborn affected by abnormality of maternal soft tissues

Newborn affected by conditions classifiable to O60–O75 and by procedures used in labor and delivery not included in P02.- and P03.0–P03.6

Newborn affected by induction of labor

P03.9 Newborn affected by complication of labor and delivery, unspecified

P04 NEWBORN AFFECTED BY NOXIOUS SUBSTANCES TRANSMITTED VIA PLACENTA OR BREAST MILK

Includes: nonteratogenic effects of substances transmitted via placenta Code **first** any current condition in newborn, if applicable

Excludes2: congenital malformations (Q00–Q99) encounter for observation of newborn for suspected diseases and conditions ruled out (Z05.-) neonatal jaundice from excessive hemolysis due to drugs or toxins transmitted from mother (P58.4) newborn in contact with and (suspected) exposures hazardous to health not transmitted via placenta or breast milk (Z77.-)

P04.0 Newborn affected by maternal anesthesia and analgesia in pregnancy, labor and delivery

Newborn affected by reactions and intoxications from maternal opiates and tranquilizers administered for procedures during pregnancy or labor and delivery

Excludes2: newborn affected by other maternal medication (P04.1-)

P04.1 Newborn affected by other maternal medication

Code **first**, if applicable, withdrawal symptoms from maternal use of drugs of addiction, if applicable (P96.1) withdrawal symptoms from therapeutic use of drugs in newborn (P96.2)

Excludes1: dysmorphism due to warfarin (Q86.2) fetal hydantoin syndrome (Q86.1)

Excludes2: maternal anesthesia and analgesia in pregnancy, labor and delivery (P04.0) maternal use of drugs of addiction (P04.4-)

P04.11 Newborn affected by maternal antineoplastic chemotherapy

P04.12 Newborn affected by maternal cytotoxic drugs

P04.13 Newborn affected by maternal use of anticonvulsants

P04.14 Newborn affected by maternal use of opiates

P04.15 Newborn affected by maternal use of antidepressants

P04.16 Newborn affected by maternal use of amphetamines

P04.17 Newborn affected by maternal use of sedative-hypnotics

P04.18 Newborn affected by other maternal medication

P04.19 Newborn affected by maternal use of unspecified medication

P04.1A Newborn affected by maternal use of anxiolytics

P04.2 Newborn affected by maternal use of tobacco

Newborn affected by exposure in utero to tobacco smoke

Excludes2: newborn exposure to environmental tobacco smoke (P96.81)

P04.3 Newborn affected by maternal use of alcohol

Excludes1: fetal alcohol syndrome (Q86.0)

P04.4 Newborn affected by maternal use of drugs of addiction

P04.40 Newborn affected by maternal use of unspecified drugs of addiction

P04.41 Newborn affected by maternal use of cocaine

P04.42 Newborn affected by maternal use of hallucinogens

Excludes2: newborn affected by other maternal medication (P04.1-)

P04.49 Newborn affected by maternal use of other drugs of addiction

Excludes2: newborn affected by maternal anesthesia and analgesia (P04.0) withdrawal symptoms from maternal use of drugs of addiction (P96.1)

P04.5 Newborn affected by maternal use of nutritional chemical substances

P04.6 Newborn affected by maternal exposure to environmental chemical substances

P04.8 Newborn affected by other maternal noxious substances

P04.81 Newborn affected by maternal use of cannabis

P04.89 Newborn affected by other maternal noxious substances

P04.9 Newborn affected by maternal noxious substance, unspecified

(P05–P08) DISORDERS OF NEWBORN RELATED TO LENGTH OF GESTATION AND FETAL GROWTH

GUIDELINES

Providers utilize different criteria in determining prematurity. A code for prematurity should not be assigned unless it is documented. Assignment of codes in categories P05, Disorders of newborn related to slow fetal growth and fetal malnutrition, and P07, Disorders of newborn related to short gestation and LBW, not elsewhere classified, should be based on the recorded birth weight and estimated gestational age. When both birth weight and gestational age are available, two codes from category P07 should be assigned, with the code for birth weight sequenced before the code for gestational age.

P05 DISORDERS OF NEWBORN RELATED TO SLOW FETAL GROWTH AND FETAL MALNUTRITION

P05.0 Newborn light for gestational age

Light-for-dates newborns are those who are smaller in size than normal for the gestational age, most commonly defined as weight below the 10th percentile but length above the 10th percentile for gestational age.

Newborn light-for-dates

P05.00 Newborn light for gestational age, unspecified weight

P05.01 Newborn light for gestational age, less than 500 g

P05.02 Newborn light for gestational age, 500–749 g

P05.03 Newborn light for gestational age, 750–999 g

P05.04 Newborn light for gestational age, 1000–1249 g

P05.05 Newborn light for gestational age, 1250–1499 g

P05.06 Newborn light for gestational age, 1500–1749 g

P05.07 Newborn light for gestational age, 1750–1999 g

P05.08 Newborn light for gestational age, 2000–2499 g

P05.09 Newborn light for gestational age, 2500 g and over

P05.1 Newborn small for gestational age

Small for gestational age newborns are those who are smaller in size than normal for the gestational age, most commonly defined as weight below the 10th percentile and length below the 10th percentile for the gestational age.

Newborn small-and-light-for-dates

Newborn small-for-dates

P05.10 Newborn small for gestational age, unspecified weight

P05.11 Newborn small for gestational age, less than 500 g

P05.12 Newborn small for gestational age, 500–749 g

P05.13 Newborn small for gestational age, 750–999 g

P05.14 Newborn small for gestational age, 1000–1249 g

P05.15 Newborn small for gestational age, 1250–1499 g

P05.16 Newborn small for gestational age, 1500–1749 g

P05.17 Newborn small for gestational age, 1750–1999 g

P05.18 Newborn small for gestational age, 2000–2499 g

P05.19 Newborn small for gestational age, other

Newborn small for gestational age, 2500 g and over

P05.2 Newborn affected by fetal (intrauterine) malnutrition not light or small for gestational age

Infant, not light or small for gestational age, showing signs of fetal malnutrition, such as dry, peeling skin and loss of subcutaneous tissue

Excludes1: newborn affected by fetal malnutrition with light for gestational age (P05.0-)
newborn affected by fetal malnutrition with small for gestational age (P05.1-)

P05.9 Newborn affected by slow intrauterine growth, unspecified
Newborn affected by fetal growth retardation NOS

P07 DISORDERS OF NEWBORN RELATED TO SHORT GESTATION AND LBW, NEC

GUIDELINES

Codes from category P07, Disorders of newborn related to short gestation and low birth weight, not elsewhere classified, are for use for a child or adult who was premature or had a low birth weight as a newborn and this is affecting the patient's current health status.

Note: When both birth weight and gestational age of the newborn are available, both should be coded with birth weight sequenced before gestational age

Includes: the listed conditions, without further specification, as the cause of morbidity or additional care, in newborn

P07.0 Extremely LBW newborn

Newborn birth weight 999 g or less

Excludes1: LBW due to slow fetal growth and fetal malnutrition (P05.-)

- **P07.00 Extremely LBW newborn, unspecified weight**
- **P07.01 Extremely LBW newborn, less than 500 g**
- **P07.02 Extremely LBW newborn, 500-749 g**
- **P07.03 Extremely LBW newborn, 750-999 g**

P07.1 Other LBW newborn

Newborn birth weight 1000-2499 g.

Excludes1: LBW due to slow fetal growth and fetal malnutrition (P05.-)

- **P07.10 Other LBW newborn, unspecified weight**
- **P07.14 Other LBW newborn, 1000-1249 g**
- **P07.15 Other LBW newborn, 1250-1499 g**
- **P07.16 Other LBW newborn, 1500-1749 g**
- **P07.17 Other LBW newborn, 1750-1999 g**
- **P07.18 Other LBW newborn, 2000-2499 g**

P07.2 Extreme immaturity of newborn

Less than 28 completed weeks (less than 196 completed days) of gestation.

- **P07.20 Extreme immaturity of newborn; unspecified weeks of gestation**
  Gestational age less than 28 completed weeks NOS
- **P07.21 gestational age less than 23 completed weeks**
  gestational age less than 23 weeks, 0 days
- **P07.22 gestational age 23 completed weeks**
  gestational age 23 weeks, 0 days through 23 weeks, 6 days
- **P07.23 gestational age 24 completed weeks**
  gestational age 24 weeks, 0 days through 24 weeks, 6 days
- **P07.24 gestational age 25 completed weeks**
  gestational age 25 weeks, 0 days through 25 weeks, 6 days
- **P07.25 gestational age 26 completed weeks**
  gestational age 26 weeks, 0 days through 26 weeks, 6 days
- **P07.26 gestational age 27 completed weeks**
  gestational age 27 weeks, 0 days through 27 weeks, 6 days

P07.3 Preterm [premature] newborn [other]

28 completed weeks or more but less than 37 completed weeks (196 completed days but less than 259 completed days) of gestation.

Prematurity NOS

- **P07.30 Preterm newborn, unspecified weeks of gestation**

- **P07.31 Preterm newborn, gestational age 28 completed weeks**
  Preterm newborn, gestational age 28 weeks, 0 days through 28 weeks, 6 days

- **P07.32 Preterm newborn, gestational age 29 completed weeks**
  Preterm newborn, gestational age 29 weeks, 0 days through 29 weeks, 6 days

- **P07.33 Preterm newborn, gestational age 30 completed weeks**
  Preterm newborn, gestational age 30 weeks, 0 days through 30 weeks, 6 days

- **P07.34 Preterm newborn, gestational age 31 completed weeks**
  Preterm newborn, gestational age 31 weeks, 0 days through 31 weeks, 6 days

- **P07.35 Preterm newborn, gestational age 32 completed weeks**
  Preterm newborn, gestational age 32 weeks, 0 days through 32 weeks, 6 days

- **P07.36 Preterm newborn, gestational age 33 completed weeks**
  Preterm newborn, gestational age 33 weeks, 0 days through 33 weeks, 6 days

- **P07.37 Preterm newborn, gestational age 34 completed weeks**
  Preterm newborn, gestational age 34 weeks, 0 days through 34 weeks, 6 days

- **P07.38 Preterm newborn, gestational age 35 completed weeks**
  Preterm newborn, gestational age 35 weeks, 0 days through 35 weeks, 6 days

- **P07.39 Preterm newborn, gestational age 36 completed weeks**
  Preterm newborn, gestational age 36 weeks, 0 days through 36 weeks, 6 days

P08 DISORDERS OF NEWBORN RELATED TO LONG GESTATION AND HIGH BIRTH WEIGHT

Note: When both birth weight and gestational age of the newborn are available, priority of assignment should be given to birth weight

Includes: the listed conditions, without further specification, as causes of morbidity or additional care, in newborn

P08.0 Exceptionally large newborn baby

Usually implies a birth weight of 4500 g. or more

Excludes1: syndrome of infant of diabetic mother (P70.1) syndrome of infant of mother with gestational diabetes (P70.0)

P08.1 Other heavy for gestational age newborn

Other newborn heavy- or large-for-dates regardless of period of gestation

Usually implies a birth weight of 4000 g. to 4499 g.

Excludes1: newborn with a birth weight of 4500 or more (P08.0) syndrome of infant of diabetic mother (P70.1) syndrome of infant of mother with gestational diabetes (P70.0).

P08.2 Late newborn, not heavy for gestational age

- **P08.21 Post-term newborn**
  Newborn with gestation period over 40 completed weeks to 42 completed weeks
- **P08.22 Prolonged gestation of newborn**
  Newborn with gestation period over 42 completed weeks (294 days or more), not heavy- or large-for-dates. Postmaturity NOS

(P09) ABNORMAL FINDINGS ON NEONATAL SCREENING

P09 ABNORMAL FINDINGS ON NEONATAL SCREENING

Includes: Abnormal findings on state mandated newborn screens Failed newborn screening

P09.1 Abnormal findings on neonatal screening for inborn errors of metabolism

Abnormal findings on neonatal screening for congenital adrenal hyperplasia

Abnormal findings on neonatal screening for hypothyroidism screen

P09.2 Abnormal findings on neonatal screening for congenital endocrine disease

P09.3 Abnormal findings on neonatal screening for congenital hematologic disorders
Abnormal findings for hemoglobinopathy screening
Abnormal findings on red cell membrane defects screen
Abnormal findings on sickle cell screen

P09.4 Abnormal findings on neonatal screening for cystic fibrosis

P09.5 Abnormal findings on neonatal screening for critical congenital heart disease
Neonatal congenital heart disease screening failure

P09.6 Abnormal findings on neonatal screening for neonatal hearing loss
Excludes2: Encounter for hearing examination following failed hearing screening (Z01.110)

P09.8 Other abnormal findings on neonatal screening

P09.9 Abnormal findings on neonatal screening, unspecified

(P10–P15) BIRTH TRAUMA

P10 INTRACRANIAL LACERATION AND HEMORRHAGE DUE TO BIRTH INJURY

Excludes1: intracranial hemorrhage of newborn NOS (P52.9)
intracranial hemorrhage of newborn due to anoxia or hypoxia (P52.-)
nontraumatic intracranial hemorrhage of newborn (P52.-)

P10.0 Subdural hemorrhage due to birth injury
Subdural hematoma (localized) due to birth injury

P10.1 Cerebral hemorrhage due to birth injury

P10.2 Intraventricular hemorrhage due to birth injury

P10.3 Subarachnoid hemorrhage due to birth injury

P10.4 Tentorial tear due to birth injury

P10.8 Other intracranial lacerations and hemorrhages due to birth injury

P10.9 Unspecified intracranial laceration and hemorrhage due to birth injury
Excludes1: subdural hemorrhage accompanying tentorial tear (P10.4)

P11 OTHER BIRTH INJURIES TO CENTRAL NERVOUS SYSTEM

P11.0 Cerebral edema due to birth injury

P11.1 Other specified brain damage due to birth injury

P11.2 Unspecified brain damage due to birth injury

P11.3 Birth injury to facial nerve
Facial palsy due to birth injury

P11.4 Birth injury to other cranial nerves

P11.5 Birth injury to spine and spinal cord
Fracture of spine due to birth injury

P11.9 Birth injury to central nervous system, unspecified

P12 BIRTH INJURY TO SCALP

P12.0 Cephalhematoma due to birth injury

P12.1 Chignon (from vacuum extraction) due to birth injury

P12.2 Epicranial subaponeurotic hemorrhage due to birth injury
Subgaleal hemorrhage

P12.3 Bruising of scalp due to birth injury

P12.4 Injury of scalp of newborn due to monitoring equipment
Sampling incision of scalp of newborn
Scalp clip (electrode) injury of newborn

P12.8 Other birth injuries to scalp

P12.81 Caput succedaneum

P12.89 Other birth injuries to scalp

P12.9 Birth injury to scalp, unspecified

P13 BIRTH INJURY TO SKELETON

Excludes2: birth injury to spine (P11.5)

P13.0 Fracture of skull due to birth injury

P13.1 Other birth injuries to skull
Excludes1: cephalhematoma (P12.0)

P13.2 Birth injury to femur

P13.3 Birth injury to other long bones

P13.4 Fracture of clavicle due to birth injury

P13.8 Birth injuries to other parts of skeleton

P13.9 Birth injury to skeleton, unspecified

P14 BIRTH INJURY TO PERIPHERAL NERVOUS SYSTEM

P14.0 Erb's paralysis due to birth injury

P14.1 Klumpke's paralysis due to birth injury

P14.2 Phrenic nerve paralysis due to birth injury

P14.3 Other brachial plexus birth injuries

P14.8 Birth injuries to other parts of peripheral nervous system

P14.9 Birth injury to peripheral nervous system, unspecified

P15 OTHER BIRTH INJURIES

P15.0 Birth injury to liver
Rupture of liver due to birth injury

P15.1 Birth injury to spleen
Rupture of spleen due to birth injury

P15.2 Sternomastoid injury due to birth injury

P15.3 Birth injury to eye
Subconjunctival hemorrhage due to birth injury
Traumatic glaucoma due to birth injury

P15.4 Birth injury to face
Facial congestion due to birth injury

P15.5 Birth injury to external genitalia

P15.6 Subcutaneous fat necrosis due to birth injury

P15.8 Other specified birth injuries

P15.9 Birth injury, unspecified

(P19–P29) RESPIRATORY AND CARDIOVASCULAR DISORDERS SPECIFIC TO THE PERINATAL PERIOD

P19 METABOLIC ACIDEMIA IN NEWBORN

Includes: metabolic acidemia in newborn

P19.0 Metabolic acidemia in newborn first noted before onset of labor

P19.1 Metabolic acidemia in newborn first noted during labor

P19.2 Metabolic acidemia noted at birth

P19.9 Metabolic acidemia in newborn, unspecified

P22 RESPIRATORY DISTRESS OF NEWBORN

P22.0 Respiratory distress syndrome of newborn
Cardiorespiratory distress syndrome of newborn
Hyaline membrane disease
Idiopathic respiratory distress syndrome [IRDS or RDS] of newborn
Pulmonary hypoperfusion syndrome
Respiratory distress syndrome, type I
Excludes2: respiratory arrest of newborn (P28.81)
respiratory failure of newborn NOS (P28.5)

P22.1 Transient tachypnea of newborn
Idiopathic tachypnea of newborn
Respiratory distress syndrome, type II
Wet lung syndrome
Excludes1: respiratory arrest of newborn (P28.81)
respiratory failure of newborn NOS (P28.5)

P22.8 Other respiratory distress of newborn

P22.9 Respiratory distress of newborn, unspecified
Excludes1: respiratory arrest of newborn (P28.81)
respiratory failure of newborn NOS (P28.5)

P23 CONGENITAL PNEUMONIA

Includes: infective pneumonia acquired in utero or during birth
Excludes1: neonatal pneumonia resulting from aspiration (P24.-)

P23.0 Congenital pneumonia; due to viral agent
Use additional code (B97) to identify organism
Excludes1: congenital rubella pneumonitis (P35.0)

P23.1 due to Chlamydia

P23.2 due to Staphylococcus

P23.3 due to Streptococcus, group B

P23.4 due to E. coli

P23.5 due to Pseudomonas

P23.6 due to other bacterial agents
due to H. influenzae
due to K. pneumoniae
due to Mycoplasma
due to Streptococcus, except group B
Use additional code (B95–B96) to identify organism

P23.8 due to other organisms

P23.9 unspecified

P24 NEONATAL ASPIRATION

Includes: aspiration in utero and during delivery

P24.0 Meconium aspiration

Excludes1: meconium passage (without aspiration) during delivery (P03.82)

meconium staining (P96.83)

P24.00 Meconium aspiration without respiratory symptoms

Meconium aspiration NOS

P24.01 Meconium aspiration with respiratory symptoms

Meconium aspiration pneumonia

Meconium aspiration pneumonitis

Meconium aspiration syndrome NOS

Use additional code to identify any secondary pulmonary hypertension, if applicable (I27.2-)

P24.1 Neonatal aspiration of (clear) amniotic fluid and mucus

Neonatal aspiration of liquor (amnii)

P24.10 Neonatal aspiration of (clear) amniotic fluid and mucus; without respiratory symptoms

Neonatal aspiration of amniotic fluid and mucus NOS

P24.11 with respiratory symptoms

with pneumonia

with pneumonitis

Use additional code to identify any secondary pulmonary hypertension, if applicable (I27.2-)

P24.2 Neonatal aspiration of blood;

P24.20 without respiratory symptoms

Neonatal aspiration of blood NOS

P24.21 with respiratory symptoms

with pneumonia

with pneumonitis

Use additional code to identify any secondary pulmonary hypertension, if applicable (I27.2-)

P24.3 Neonatal aspiration of milk and regurgitated food

Neonatal aspiration of stomach contents

P24.30 Neonatal aspiration of milk and regurgitated food; without respiratory symptoms

Neonatal aspiration of milk and regurgitated food NOS

P24.31 with respiratory symptoms

Use additional code to identify any secondary pulmonary hypertension, if applicable (I27.2-)

P24.8 Other neonatal aspiration;

P24.80 without respiratory symptoms

Neonatal aspiration NEC

P24.81 with respiratory symptoms

Neonatal aspiration pneumonia NEC

Neonatal aspiration with pneumonitis NEC

Neonatal aspiration with pneumonia NOS

Neonatal aspiration with pneumonitis NOS

Use additional code to identify any secondary pulmonary hypertension, if applicable (I27.2-)

P24.9 Neonatal aspiration, unspecified

P25 INTERSTITIAL EMPHYSEMA AND RELATED CONDITIONS ORIGINATING IN THE PERINATAL PERIOD

Do not report codes from P25 that do not originate in the perinatal period.

P25.0 Interstitial emphysema originating in the perinatal period

P25.1 Pneumothorax originating in the perinatal period

P25.2 Pneumomediastinum originating in the perinatal period

P25.3 Pneumopericardium originating in the perinatal period

P25.8 Other conditions related to interstitial emphysema originating in the perinatal period

P26 PULMONARY HEMORRHAGE ORIGINATING IN THE PERINATAL PERIOD

Do not report codes from P26 that do not originate in the perinatal period

Excludes1: acute idiopathic hemorrhage in infants over 28 days old (R04.81)

P26.0 Tracheobronchial hemorrhage

P26.1 Massive pulmonary hemorrhage

P26.8 Other pulmonary hemorrhages

P26.9 Unspecified pulmonary hemorrhage

P27 CHRONIC RESPIRATORY DISEASE ORIGINATING IN THE PERINATAL PERIOD

Do not report codes from P27 that do not originate in the perinatal period

Excludes2: respiratory distress of newborn (P22.0–P22.9)

P27.0 Wilson-Mikity syndrome

Pulmonary dysmaturity

P27.1 Bronchopulmonary dysplasia

P27.8 Other chronic respiratory diseases

Congenital pulmonary fibrosis

Ventilator lung in newborn

P27.9 Unspecified chronic respiratory disease

P28 OTHER RESPIRATORY CONDITIONS ORIGINATING IN THE PERINATAL PERIOD

Excludes1: congenital malformations of the respiratory system (Q30–Q34)

P28.0 Primary atelectasis of newborn

Primary failure to expand terminal respiratory units

Pulmonary hypoplasia associated with short gestation

Pulmonary immaturity NOS

P28.1 Other and unspecified atelectasis of newborn

P28.10 Unspecified atelectasis of newborn

Atelectasis of newborn NOS

P28.11 Resorption atelectasis without respiratory distress syndrome

Excludes1: resorption atelectasis with respiratory distress syndrome (P22.0)

P28.19 Other atelectasis of newborn

Partial atelectasis of newborn

Secondary atelectasis of newborn

P28.2 Cyanotic attacks of newborn

Excludes1: apnea of newborn (P28.3–P28.4)

P28.3 Primary sleep apnea of newborn

Central sleep apnea of newborn

Obstructive sleep apnea of newborn

Sleep apnea of newborn NOS

P28.30 Primary sleep apnea of newborn, unspecified

P28.31 Primary central sleep apnea of newborn

P28.32 Primary obstructive sleep apnea of newborn

P28.33 Primary mixed sleep apnea of newborn

P28.39 Other primary sleep apnea of newborn

P28.4 Other apnea of newborn

Apnea of prematurity

Obstructive apnea of newborn

Excludes1: obstructive sleep apnea of newborn (P28.3)

P28.40 Unspecified apnea of newborn

P28.41 Central neonatal apnea of newborn

P28.42 Obstructive apnea of newborn

P28.43 Mixed neonatal apnea of newborn

P28.49 Other apnea of newborn

P28.5 Respiratory failure of newborn

Excludes2: respiratory arrest of newborn (P28.81)

respiratory distress of newborn (P22.0)

P28.8 Other specified respiratory conditions of newborn

P28.81 Respiratory arrest of newborn

P28.89 Other specified respiratory conditions of newborn

Congenital laryngeal stridor

Sniffles in newborn

Snuffles in newborn

Excludes1: early congenital syphilitic rhinitis (A50.05)

P28.9 Respiratory condition of newborn, unspecified

Respiratory depression in newborn

P29 CARDIOVASCULAR DISORDERS ORIGINATING IN THE PERINATAL PERIOD

Excludes2: congenital malformations of the circulatory system (Q20–Q28)

P29.0 Neonatal cardiac failure

Code also associated underlying condition

P29.1 Neonatal cardiac dysrhythmia

P29.11 Neonatal tachycardia

P29.12 Neonatal bradycardia

P29.2 Neonatal hypertension

P29.3 Persistent fetal circulation

P29.30 Pulmonary hypertension of newborn

Persistent pulmonary hypertension of newborn

P29.38 Other persistent fetal circulation
Delayed closure of ductus arteriosus

P29.4 Transient myocardial ischemia in newborn

P29.8 Other cardiovascular disorders originating in the perinatal period

P29.81 Cardiac arrest of newborn

P29.89 Other cardiovascular disorders originating in the perinatal period

P29.9 Cardiovascular disorder originating in the perinatal period, unspecified

(P35–P39) INFECTIONS SPECIFIC TO THE PERINATAL PERIOD

Infections acquired in utero, during birth via the umbilicus, or during the first 28 days after birth

Excludes2: asymptomatic HIV infection status (Z21)
congenital gonococcal infection (A54.-)
congenital pneumonia (P23.-)
congenital syphilis (A50.-)
HIV disease (B20)
infant botulism (A48.51)
infectious diseases not specific to the perinatal period (A00–B99, J09, J10.-)
intestinal infectious disease (A00–A09)
laboratory evidence of HIV (R75)
tetanus neonatorum (A33)

P35 CONGENITAL VIRAL DISEASES

Includes: infections acquired in utero or during birth

P35.0 Congenital rubella syndrome
Congenital rubella pneumonitis

P35.1 Congenital cytomegalovirus infection

P35.2 Congenital herpesviral [herpes simplex] infection

P35.3 Congenital viral hepatitis

P35.4 Congenital Zika virus disease
Use additional code to identify manifestations of congenital Zika virus disease

P35.8 Other congenital viral diseases
Congenital varicella [chickenpox]

P35.9 Congenital viral disease, unspecified

P36 BACTERIAL SEPSIS OF NEWBORN

GUIDELINES

Category P36, Bacterial sepsis of newborn, includes congenital sepsis. If a perinate is documented as having sepsis without documentation of congenital or community acquired, the default is congenital and a code from category P36 should be assigned. If the P36 code includes the causal organism, an additional code from category B95, Streptococcus, Staphylococcus, and Enterococcus as the cause of diseases classified elsewhere, or B96, Other bacterial agents as the cause of diseases classified elsewhere, should not be assigned. If the P36 code does not include the causal organism, assign an additional code from category B96. If applicable, use additional codes to identify severe sepsis (R65.2-) and any associated acute organ dysfunction.

Includes: congenital sepsis

Use additional code(s), if applicable, to identify severe sepsis (R65.2-) and associated acute organ dysfunction(s)

P36.0 Sepsis of newborn due to Streptococcus, group B

P36.1 Sepsis of newborn due to other and unspecified streptococci

P36.10 Sepsis of newborn due to unspecified streptococci

P36.19 Sepsis of newborn due to other streptococci

P36.2 Sepsis of newborn due to Staphylococcus aureus

P36.3 Sepsis of newborn due to other and unspecified staphylococci

P36.30 Sepsis of newborn due to unspecified staphylococci

P36.39 Sepsis of newborn due to other staphylococci

P36.4 Sepsis of newborn due to E. coli

P36.5 Sepsis of newborn due to anaerobes

P36.8 Other bacterial sepsis of newborn
Use additional code from category B96 to identify organism

P36.9 Bacterial sepsis of newborn, unspecified

P37 OTHER CONGENITAL INFECTIOUS AND PARASITIC DISEASES

Excludes2: congenital syphilis (A50.-)
infectious neonatal diarrhea (A00–A09)
necrotizing enterocolitis in newborn (P77.-)
noninfectious neonatal diarrhea (P78.3)
ophthalmia neonatorum due to gonococcus (A54.31)
tetanus neonatorum (A33)

P37.0 Congenital tuberculosis

P37.1 Congenital toxoplasmosis
Hydrocephalus due to congenital toxoplasmosis

P37.2 Neonatal (disseminated) listeriosis

P37.3 Congenital falciparum malaria

P37.4 Other congenital malaria

P37.5 Neonatal candidiasis

P37.8 Other specified congenital infectious and parasitic diseases

P37.9 Congenital infectious or parasitic disease, unspecified

P38 OMPHALITIS OF NEWBORN

Excludes1: omphalitis not of newborn (L08.82)
tetanus omphalitis (A33)
umbilical hemorrhage of newborn (P51.-)

P38.1 Omphalitis with mild hemorrhage

P38.9 Omphalitis without hemorrhage
Omphalitis of newborn NOS

P39 OTHER INFECTIONS SPECIFIC TO THE PERINATAL PERIOD

Use additional code to identify organism or specific infection

P39.0 Neonatal infective mastitis
Excludes1: breast engorgement of newborn (P83.4)
noninfective mastitis of newborn (P83.4)

P39.1 Neonatal conjunctivitis and dacryocystitis
Neonatal chlamydial conjunctivitis
Ophthalmia neonatorum NOS
Excludes1: gonococcal conjunctivitis (A54.31)

P39.2 Intra-amniotic infection affecting newborn, NEC

P39.3 Neonatal urinary tract infection

P39.4 Neonatal skin infection
Neonatal pyoderma
Excludes1: pemphigus neonatorum (L00)
staphylococcal scalded skin syndrome (L00)

P39.8 Other specified infections specific to the perinatal period

P39.9 Infection specific to the perinatal period, unspecified

(P50–P61) HEMORRHAGIC AND HEMATOLOGICAL DISORDERS OF NEWBORN

Excludes1: congenital stenosis and stricture of bile ducts (Q44.3)
Crigler-Najjar syndrome (E80.5)
Dubin-Johnson syndrome (E80.6)
Gilbert syndrome (E80.4)
hereditary hemolytic anemias (D55–D58)

P50 NEWBORN AFFECTED BY INTRAUTERINE (FETAL) BLOOD LOSS

Excludes1: congenital anemia from intrauterine (fetal) blood loss (P61.3)

P50.0 Newborn affected by intrauterine (fetal) blood loss from vasa previa

P50.1 Newborn affected by intrauterine (fetal) blood loss from ruptured cord

P50.2 Newborn affected by intrauterine (fetal) blood loss from placenta

P50.3 Newborn affected by hemorrhage into co-twin

P50.4 Newborn affected by hemorrhage into maternal circulation

P50.5 Newborn affected by intrauterine (fetal) blood loss from cut end of co-twin's cord

P50.8 Newborn affected by other intrauterine (fetal) blood loss

P50.9 Newborn affected by intrauterine (fetal) blood loss, unspecified
Newborn affected by fetal hemorrhage NOS

P51 UMBILICAL HEMORRHAGE OF NEWBORN

Excludes1: omphalitis with mild hemorrhage (P38.1)
umbilical hemorrhage from cut end of co-twins cord (P50.5)

- P51.0 Massive umbilical hemorrhage of newborn
- P51.8 Other umbilical hemorrhages of newborn
  - Slipped umbilical ligature NOS
- P51.9 Umbilical hemorrhage of newborn, unspecified

P52 INTRACRANIAL NONTRAUMATIC HEMORRHAGE OF NEWBORN

Includes: intracranial hemorrhage due to anoxia or hypoxia
Excludes1: intracranial hemorrhage due to birth injury (P10.-)
intracranial hemorrhage due to other injury (S06.-)

- P52.0 Intraventricular (nontraumatic) hemorrhage, grade 1, of newborn
  - Subependymal hemorrhage (without intraventricular extension)
  - Bleeding into germinal matrix
- P52.1 Intraventricular (nontraumatic) hemorrhage, grade 2, of newborn
  - Subependymal hemorrhage with intraventricular extension
  - Bleeding into ventricle
- P52.2 Intraventricular (nontraumatic) hemorrhage, grade 3 and grade 4, of newborn
  - P52.21 Intraventricular (nontraumatic) hemorrhage, grade 3, of newborn
    - Subependymal hemorrhage with intraventricular extension with enlargement of ventricle
  - P52.22 Intraventricular (nontraumatic) hemorrhage, grade 4, of newborn
    - Bleeding into cerebral cortex
    - Subependymal hemorrhage with intracerebral extension
- P52.3 Unspecified intraventricular (nontraumatic) hemorrhage of newborn
- P52.4 Intracerebral (nontraumatic) hemorrhage of newborn
- P52.5 Subarachnoid (nontraumatic) hemorrhage of newborn
- P52.6 Cerebellar (nontraumatic) and posterior fossa hemorrhage of newborn
- P52.8 Other intracranial (nontraumatic) hemorrhages of newborn
- P52.9 Intracranial (nontraumatic) hemorrhage of newborn, unspecified

P53 HEMORRHAGIC DISEASE OF NEWBORN

Vitamin K deficiency of newborn

P54 OTHER NEONATAL HEMORRHAGES

Excludes1: newborn affected by (intrauterine) blood loss (P50.-)
pulmonary hemorrhage originating in the perinatal period (P26.-)

- P54.0 Neonatal hematemesis
  - *Excludes1:* neonatal hematemesis due to swallowed maternal blood (P78.2)
- P54.1 Neonatal melena
  - *Excludes1:* neonatal melena due to swallowed maternal blood (P78.2)
- P54.2 Neonatal rectal hemorrhage
- P54.3 Other neonatal gastrointestinal hemorrhage
- P54.4 Neonatal adrenal hemorrhage
- P54.5 Neonatal cutaneous hemorrhage
  - Neonatal bruising
  - Neonatal ecchymoses
  - Neonatal petechiae
  - Neonatal superficial hematomata
  - *Excludes2:* bruising of scalp due to birth injury (P12.3)
  cephalhematoma due to birth injury (P12.0)
- P54.6 Neonatal vaginal hemorrhage
  - Neonatal pseudomenses
- P54.8 Other specified neonatal hemorrhages
- P54.9 Neonatal hemorrhage, unspecified

P55 HEMOLYTIC DISEASE OF NEWBORN

- P55.0 Rh isoimmunization of newborn
- P55.1 ABO isoimmunization of newborn
- P55.8 Other hemolytic diseases of newborn
- P55.9 Hemolytic disease of newborn, unspecified

P56 HYDROPS FETALIS DUE TO HEMOLYTIC DISEASE

Excludes1: hydrops fetalis NOS (P83.2)

- P56.0 Hydrops fetalis due to isoimmunization
- P56.9 Hydrops fetalis due to other and unspecified hemolytic disease
  - P56.90 Hydrops fetalis due to unspecified hemolytic disease
  - P56.99 Hydrops fetalis due to other hemolytic disease

P57 KERNICTERUS

- P57.0 Kernicterus due to isoimmunization
- P57.8 Other specified kernicterus
  - *Excludes1:* Crigler-Najjar syndrome (E80.5)
- P57.9 Kernicterus, unspecified

P59 NEONATAL JAUNDICE FROM OTHER AND UNSPECIFIED CAUSES

Excludes1: jaundice due to inborn errors of metabolism (E70–E88)
kernicterus (P57.-)

- P59.0 Neonatal jaundice associated with preterm delivery
  - Hyperbilirubinemia of prematurity
  - Jaundice due to delayed conjugation associated with preterm delivery
- P59.1 Inspissated bile syndrome
- P59.2 Neonatal jaundice from other and unspecified hepatocellular damage
  - *Excludes1:* congenital viral hepatitis (P35.3)
  - P59.20 Neonatal jaundice from unspecified hepatocellular damage
  - P59.29 Neonatal jaundice from other hepatocellular damage
    - Neonatal giant cell hepatitis
    - Neonatal (idiopathic) hepatitis
- P59.3 Neonatal jaundice from breast milk inhibitor
- P59.8 Neonatal jaundice from other specified causes
- P59.9 Neonatal jaundice, unspecified
  - Neonatal physiological jaundice (intense)(prolonged) NOS

P60 DISSEMINATED INTRAVASCULAR COAGULATION OF NEWBORN

Defibrination syndrome of newborn

P61 OTHER PERINATAL HEMATOLOGICAL DISORDERS

Excludes1: transient hypogammaglobulinemia of infancy (D80.7)

- P61.0 Transient neonatal thrombocytopenia
  - Neonatal thrombocytopenia due to exchange transfusion
  - Neonatal thrombocytopenia due to idiopathic maternal thrombocytopenia
  - Neonatal thrombocytopenia due to isoimmunization
- P61.1 Polycythemia neonatorum
- P61.2 Anemia of prematurity
- P61.3 Congenital anemia from fetal blood loss
- P61.4 Other congenital anemias, NEC
  - Congenital anemia NOS
- P61.5 Transient neonatal neutropenia
  - *Excludes1:* congenital neutropenia (nontransient) (D70.0)
- P61.6 Other transient neonatal disorders of coagulation
- P61.8 Other specified perinatal hematological disorders
- P61.9 Perinatal hematological disorder, unspecified

(P70–P74) TRANSITORY ENDOCRINE AND METABOLIC DISORDERS SPECIFIC TO NEWBORN

Includes: transitory endocrine and metabolic disturbances caused by the infant's response to maternal endocrine and metabolic factors, or its adjustment to extrauterine environment

P70 TRANSITORY DISORDERS OF CARBOHYDRATE METABOLISM SPECIFIC TO NEWBORN

- P70.0 Syndrome of infant of mother with gestational diabetes
  - Newborn (with hypoglycemia) affected by maternal gestational diabetes
  - *Excludes1:* newborn (with hypoglycemia) affected by maternal (pre-existing) DM (P70.1)
  syndrome of infant of a diabetic mother (P70.1)

P70.1 Syndrome of infant of a diabetic mother
Newborn (with hypoglycemia) affected by maternal (pre-existing) DM

Excludes1: newborn (with hypoglycemia) affected by maternal gestational diabetes (P70.0)
syndrome of infant of mother with gestational diabetes (P70.0)

P70.2 Neonatal DM

P70.3 Iatrogenic neonatal hypoglycemia

P70.4 Other neonatal hypoglycemia
Transitory neonatal hypoglycemia

P70.8 Other transitory disorders of carbohydrate metabolism of newborn

P71 TRANSITORY NEONATAL DISORDERS OF CALCIUM AND MAGNESIUM METABOLISM

P71.0 Cow's milk hypocalcemia in newborn

P71.1 Other neonatal hypocalcemia
Excludes1: neonatal hypoparathyroidism (P71.4)

P71.3 Neonatal tetany without calcium or magnesium deficiency
Neonatal tetany NOS

P71.4 Transitory neonatal hypoparathyroidism

P71.8 Other transitory neonatal disorders of calcium and magnesium metabolism

P71.9 Transitory neonatal disorder of calcium and magnesium metabolism, unspecified

P72 OTHER TRANSITORY NEONATAL ENDOCRINE DISORDERS

Excludes1: congenital hypothyroidism with or without goiter (E03.0-E03.1)
dyshormogenetic goiter (E07.1)
dyshormonogenetic goiter (E07.1)
Pendred's syndrome (E07.1)

P72.0 Neonatal goiter, not elsewhere classified
Transitory congenital goiter with normal functioning

P72.1 Transitory neonatal hyperthyroidism
Neonatal thyrotoxicosis

P72.2 Other transitory neonatal disorders of thyroid function, not elsewhere classified
Transitory neonatal hypothyroidism

P72.8 Other specified transitory neonatal endocrine disorders

P72.9 Transitory neonatal endocrine disorder, unspecified

P74 OTHER TRANSITORY NEONATAL ELECTROLYTE AND METABOLIC DISTURBANCES

P74.0 Late metabolic acidosis of newborn
Excludes1: (fetal) metabolic acidosis of newborn (P19)

P74.1 Dehydration of newborn

P74.2 Disturbances of sodium balance of newborn
- **P74.21 Hypernatremia of newborn**
- **P74.22 Hyponatremia of newborn**

P74.3 Disturbances of potassium balance of newborn
- **P74.31 Hyperkalemia of newborn**
- **P74.32 Hypokalemia of newborn**

P74.4 Other transitory electrolyte disturbances of newborn
- **P74.41 Alkalosis of newborn**
- **P74.42 Disturbances of chlorine balance of newborn**
  - **P74.421 Hyperchloremia of newborn**
    Hyperchloremic metabolic acidosis
    Excludes2: late metabolic acidosis of the newborn (P47.0)
  - **P74.422 Hypochloremia of newborn**
- **P74.49 Other transitory electrolyte disturbance of newborn**

P74.5 Transitory tyrosinemia of newborn

P74.6 Transitory hyperammonemia of newborn

P74.8 Other transitory metabolic disturbances of newborn
Amino-acid metabolic disorders described as transitory

P74.9 Transitory metabolic disturbance of newborn, unspecified

(P76–P78) DIGESTIVE SYSTEM DISORDERS OF NEWBORN

P76 OTHER INTESTINAL OBSTRUCTION OF NEWBORN

P76.0 Meconium plug syndrome
Meconium ileus NOS
Excludes1: meconium ileus in cystic fibrosis (E84.11)

P76.1 Transitory ileus of newborn
Excludes1: Hirschsprung's disease (Q43.1)

P76.2 Intestinal obstruction due to inspissated milk

P76.8 Other specified intestinal obstruction of newborn
Excludes1: intestinal obstruction classifiable to K56.-

P76.9 Intestinal obstruction of newborn, unspecified

P77 NECROTIZING ENTEROCOLITIS OF NEWBORN

P77.1 Stage 1 necrotizing enterocolitis in newborn
Necrotizing enterocolitis without pneumatosis, without perforation

P77.2 Stage 2 necrotizing enterocolitis in newborn
Necrotizing enterocolitis with pneumatosis, without perforation

For necrotizing enterocolitis that begins after the 28th day, see the alphabetic index for the appropriate reference (eg, necrotizing enterocolitis due to *C. difficile* A04.7).

P77.3 Stage 3 necrotizing enterocolitis in newborn
Necrotizing enterocolitis with perforation
Necrotizing enterocolitis with pneumatosis and perforation

P77.9 Necrotizing enterocolitis in newborn, unspecified
Necrotizing enterocolitis in newborn, NOS

P78 OTHER PERINATAL DIGESTIVE SYSTEM DISORDERS

Excludes1: cystic fibrosis (E84.0–E84.9)
neonatal gastrointestinal hemorrhages (P54.0–P54.3)

P78.0 Perinatal intestinal perforation
Meconium peritonitis

P78.1 Other neonatal peritonitis
Neonatal peritonitis NOS

P78.2 Neonatal hematemesis and melena due to swallowed maternal blood

P78.3 Noninfective neonatal diarrhea
Neonatal diarrhea NOS

P78.8 Other specified perinatal digestive system disorders
- **P78.81 Congenital cirrhosis (of liver)**
- **P78.82 Peptic ulcer of newborn**
- **P78.83 Newborn esophageal reflux**
  Neonatal esophageal reflux
- **P78.84 Gestational alloimmune liver disease**
  GALD
  Neonatal hemochromatosis
  Excludes 1: hemochromatosis (E83.11-)
- **P78.89 Other specified perinatal digestive system disorders**

P78.9 Perinatal digestive system disorder, unspecified

(P80–P83) CONDITIONS INVOLVING THE INTEGUMENT AND TEMPERATURE REGULATION OF NEWBORN

P80 HYPOTHERMIA OF NEWBORN

P80.0 Cold injury syndrome
Severe and usually chronic hypothermia associated with a pink flushed appearance, edema and neurological and biochemical abnormalities.
Excludes1: mild hypothermia of newborn (P80.8)

P80.8 Other hypothermia of newborn
Mild hypothermia of newborn

P80.9 Hypothermia of newborn, unspecified

P81 OTHER DISTURBANCES OF TEMPERATURE REGULATION OF NEWBORN

P81.0 Environmental hyperthermia of newborn

P81.8 Other specified disturbances of temperature regulation of newborn

P81.9 Disturbance of temperature regulation of newborn, unspecified
Fever of newborn NOS

P83 OTHER CONDITIONS OF INTEGUMENT SPECIFIC TO NEWBORN

Excludes1: congenital malformations of skin and integument (Q80–Q84)
hydrops fetalis due to hemolytic disease (P56.-)
neonatal skin infection (P39.4)
staphylococcal scalded skin syndrome (L00)

Excludes2: cradle cap (L21.0)
diaper [napkin] dermatitis (L22)

P83.0 Sclerema neonatorum

P83.1 Neonatal erythema toxicum

P83.2 Hydrops fetalis not due to hemolytic disease
Hydrops fetalis NOS

P83.3 Other and unspecified edema specific to newborn
- **P83.30 Unspecified edema specific to newborn**
- **P83.39 Other edema specific to newborn**

P83.4 Breast engorgement of newborn
Noninfective mastitis of newborn

P83.5 Congenital hydrocele

P83.6 Umbilical polyp of newborn

P83.8 Other specified conditions of integument specific to newborn
- **P83.81 Umbilical granuloma**
  Excludes2: Granulomatous disorder of the skin and subcutaneous tissue, unspecified (L92.9)
- **P83.88 Other specified conditions of integument specific to newborn**
  Bronze baby syndrome
  Neonatal scleroderma
  Urticaria neonatorum

P83.9 Condition of the integument specific to newborn, unspecified

(P84) OTHER PROBLEMS WITH NEWBORN

P84 OTHER PROBLEMS WITH NEWBORN
✓
Acidemia of newborn
Acidosis of newborn
Anoxia of newborn NOS
Asphyxia of newborn NOS
Hypercapnia of newborn
Hypoxemia of newborn
Hypoxia of newborn NOS
Mixed metabolic and respiratory acidosis of newborn
Excludes1: intracranial hemorrhage due to anoxia or hypoxia (P52.-)
hypoxic ischemic encephalopathy [HIE] (P91.6-)
late metabolic acidosis of newborn (P74.0)

(P90–P96) OTHER DISORDERS ORIGINATING IN THE PERINATAL PERIOD

P90 CONVULSIONS OF NEWBORN
✓
Excludes1: benign myoclonic epilepsy in infancy (G40.3-)
benign neonatal convulsions (familial) (G40.3-)

P91 OTHER DISTURBANCES OF CEREBRAL STATUS OF NEWBORN

P91.0 Neonatal cerebral ischemia
Excludes1: Neonatal cerebral infarction (P91.82-)

P91.1 Acquired periventricular cysts of newborn

P91.2 Neonatal cerebral leukomalacia
Periventricular leukomalacia

P91.3 Neonatal cerebral irritability

P91.4 Neonatal cerebral depression

P91.5 Neonatal coma

P91.6 Hypoxic ischemic encephalopathy [HIE]
Excludes1: Neonatal cerebral depression (P91.4)
Neonatal cerebral irritability (P91.3)
Neonatal coma (P91.5)

- **P91.60 HIE, unspecified**
- **P91.61 Mild HIE**
- **P91.62 Moderate HIE**
- **P91.63 Severe HIE**

P91.8 Other specified disturbances of cerebral status of newborn
- **P91.81 Neonatal encephalopathy**
  - **P91.811 Neonatal encephalopathy in diseases classified elsewhere**
    Code first underlying condition, if known, such as:
    congenital cirrhosis (of liver) (P78.81)
    intracranial nontraumatic hemorrhage of newborn (P52.-)
    kernicterus (P57.-)
  - **P91.819 Neonatal encephalopathy, unspecified**

P91.82 Neonatal cerebral infarction
Neonatal stroke
Perinatal arterial ischemic stroke
Perinatal cerebral infarction
Excludes1: cerebral infarction (I63.-)
Excludes2: intracranial hemorrhage of newborn (P52.-)

- **P91.821 Neonatal cerebral infarction, right side of brain**
- **P91.822 Neonatal cerebral infarction, left side of brain**
- **P91.823 Neonatal cerebral infarction, bilateral**
- **P91.829 Neonatal cerebral infarction, unspecified side**

P91.88 Other specified disturbances of cerebral status of newborn

P91.9 Disturbance of cerebral status of newborn, unspecified

P92 FEEDING PROBLEMS OF NEWBORN
Excludes1: eating disorders (F50.-)
Excludes2: feeding problems in child over 28 days old (R63.3-)

P92.0 Vomiting of newborn
Excludes1: vomiting of child over 28 days old (R11.-)

Note: Report a code from P92 after 28 days of life if the feeding problem began within the first 28 days of life

- **P92.01 Bilious vomiting of newborn**
  Excludes1: bilious vomiting in child over 28 days old (R11.14)
- **P92.09 Other vomiting of newborn**
  Excludes1: regurgitation of food in newborn (P92.1)

P92.1 Regurgitation and rumination of newborn

P92.2 Slow feeding of newborn

P92.3 Underfeeding of newborn

P92.4 Overfeeding of newborn

P92.5 Neonatal difficulty in feeding at breast

P92.6 Failure to thrive in newborn
Excludes1: failure to thrive in child over 28 days old (R62.51)

P92.8 Other feeding problems of newborn

P92.9 Feeding problem of newborn, unspecified

P93 REACTIONS AND INTOXICATIONS DUE TO DRUGS ADMINISTERED TO NEWBORN
Includes: reactions and intoxications due to drugs administered to fetus affecting newborn
Excludes1: jaundice due to drugs or toxins transmitted from mother or given to newborn (P58.4-)
reactions and intoxications from maternal opiates, tranquilizers and other medication (P04.0-P04.1, P04.4-)
withdrawal symptoms from maternal use of drugs of addiction (P96.1)
withdrawal symptoms from therapeutic use of drugs in newborn (P96.2)

P93.0 Grey baby syndrome

P93.8 Other reactions and intoxications due to drugs administered to newborn
Use additional code for adverse effect, if applicable, to identify drug (T36-T50 with fifth or sixth character 5)

P94 DISORDERS OF MUSCLE TONE OF NEWBORN

P94.0 Transient neonatal myasthenia gravis
myasthenia gravis (G70.0)

P94.1 Congenital hypertonia

P94.2 Congenital hypotonia
Floppy baby syndrome, unspecified

P94.8 Other disorders of muscle tone of newborn

P94.9 Disorder of muscle tone of newborn, unspecified

P95 STILLBIRTH
✓

GUIDELINES

Code P95, Stillbirth, is only for use in institutions that maintain separate records for stillbirths. No other code should be used with P95. Code P95 should not be used on the mother's record.

Deadborn fetus NOS
Fetal death of unspecified cause
Stillbirth NOS

Excludes1: maternal care for intrauterine death (O36.4)
missed abortion (O02.1)
outcome of delivery, stillbirth (Z37.1, Z37.3, Z37.4, Z37.7)
Code P95, Stillbirth, is only for use in institutions that maintain separate records for stillbirths. No other code should be used with P95. Code P95 should not be used on the mother's record.

P96 OTHER CONDITIONS ORIGINATING IN THE PERINATAL PERIOD

- **P96.0 Congenital renal failure**
  Uremia of newborn
- **P96.1 Neonatal withdrawal symptoms from maternal use of drugs of addiction**
  Drug withdrawal syndrome in infant of dependent mother
  Neonatal abstinence syndrome
  Excludes1: reactions and intoxications from maternal opiates and tranquilizers administered during labor and delivery (P04.0)
- **P96.2 Withdrawal symptoms from therapeutic use of drugs in newborn**
- **P96.3 Wide cranial sutures of newborn**
  Neonatal craniotabes
- **P96.5 Complication to newborn due to (fetal) intrauterine procedure**
  newborn affected by amniocentesis (P00.6)
- **P96.8 Other specified conditions originating in the perinatal period**
  - **P96.81 Exposure to (parental) (environmental) tobacco smoke in the perinatal period**
    Excludes2: newborn affected by in utero exposure to tobacco (P04.2)
    exposure to environmental tobacco smoke after the perinatal period (Z77.22)
  - **P96.82 Delayed separation of umbilical cord**
  - **P96.83 Meconium staining**
    Excludes1: meconium aspiration (P24.00, P24.01)
    meconium passage during delivery (P03.82)
  - **P96.89 Other specified conditions originating in the perinatal period**
    Use additional code to specify condition
- **P96.9 Condition originating in the perinatal period, unspecified**
  Congenital debility NOS

Chapter 17. Congenital malformations, deformations and chromosomal abnormalities (Q00–Q99)

GUIDELINES

Assign an appropriate code(s) from categories Q00–Q99, Congenital malformations, deformations, and chromosomal abnormalities when a malformation/deformation or chromosomal abnormality is documented. A malformation/deformation or chromosomal abnormality may be the principal/first-listed diagnosis on a record or a secondary diagnosis.

When a malformation/deformation or chromosomal abnormality does not have a unique code assignment, assign additional code(s) for any manifestations that may be present.

When the code assignment specifically identifies the malformation/deformation or chromosomal abnormality, manifestations that are an inherent component of the anomaly should not be coded separately. Additional codes should be assigned for manifestations that are not an inherent component.

Codes from Chapter 17 may be used throughout the life of the patient. If a congenital malformation or deformity has been corrected, a personal history code should be used to identify the history of the malformation or deformity. Although present at birth, a malformation/deformation or chromosomal abnormality may not be identified until later in life. Whenever the condition is diagnosed by the provider, it is appropriate to assign a code from codes Q00–Q99. For the birth admission, the appropriate code from category Z38, Liveborn infants, according to place of birth and type of delivery, should be sequenced as the principal diagnosis, followed by any congenital anomaly codes, Q00–Q99.

Note: Codes from this chapter are not for use on maternal records

Excludes2: inborn errors of metabolism (E70–E88)

(Q00–Q07) CONGENITAL MALFORMATIONS OF THE NERVOUS SYSTEM

Q00 ANENCEPHALY AND SIMILAR MALFORMATIONS

Q00.0 Anencephaly
Acephaly
Acrania
Amyelencephaly
Hemianencephaly
Hemicephaly

Q00.1 Craniorachischisis

Q00.2 Iniencephaly

Q01 ENCEPHALOCELE

Includes: Arnold-Chiari syndrome, type III
encephalocystocele
encephalomyelocele
hydroencephalocele
hydromeningocele, cranial
meningocele, cerebral
meningoencephalocele

Excludes1: Meckel-Gruber syndrome (Q61.9)

Q01.0 Frontal encephalocele

Q01.1 Nasofrontal encephalocele

Q01.2 Occipital encephalocele

Q01.8 Encephalocele of other sites

Q01.9 Encephalocele, unspecified

Q02 MICROCEPHALY

Includes: hydromicrocephaly
micrencephalon

Code first, if applicable, to identify congenital Zika virus disease

Excludes1: Meckel-Gruber syndrome (Q61.9)

Q03 CONGENITAL HYDROCEPHALUS

Includes: hydrocephalus in newborn

Excludes1: Arnold-Chiari syndrome, type II (Q07.0-)
acquired hydrocephalus (G91.-)
hydrocephalus due to congenital toxoplasmosis (P37.1)
hydrocephalus with spina bifida (Q05.0–Q05.4)

Q03.0 Malformations of aqueduct of Sylvius
Anomaly of aqueduct of Sylvius
Obstruction of aqueduct of Sylvius, congenital
Stenosis of aqueduct of Sylvius

Q03.1 Atresia of foramina of Magendie and Luschka
Dandy-Walker syndrome

Q03.8 Other congenital hydrocephalus

Q03.9 Congenital hydrocephalus, unspecified

Q04 OTHER CONGENITAL MALFORMATIONS OF BRAIN

Excludes1: cyclopia (Q87.0)
macrocephaly (Q75.3)

Q04.0 Congenital malformations of corpus callosum
Agenesis of corpus callosum

Q04.3 Other reduction deformities of brain
Absence of part of brain
Agenesis of part of brain
Agyria
Aplasia of part of brain
Hydranencephaly
Hypoplasia of part of brain
Lissencephaly
Microgyria
Pachygyria

Excludes1: congenital malformations of corpus callosum (Q04.0)

Q04.6 Congenital cerebral cysts
Porencephaly
Schizencephaly

Excludes1: acquired porencephalic cyst (G93.0)

Q04.8 Other specified congenital malformations of brain
Arnold-Chiari syndrome, type IV
Macrogyria

Q04.9 Congenital malformation of brain, unspecified
Congenital anomaly NOS of brain
Congenital deformity NOS of brain
Congenital disease or lesion NOS of brain
Multiple anomalies NOS of brain, congenital

Q05 SPINA BIFIDA

Includes: hydromeningocele (spinal)
meningocele (spinal)
meningomyelocele
myelocele
myelomeningocele
rachischisis
spina bifida (aperta) (cystica)
syringomyelocele

Use additional code for any associated paraplegia (paraparesis) (G82.2-)

Excludes1: Arnold-Chiari syndrome, type II (Q07.0-)
spina bifida occulta (Q76.0)

Q05.0 Cervical spina bifida with hydrocephalus

Q05.1 Thoracic spina bifida with hydrocephalus
Dorsal spina bifida with hydrocephalus
Thoracolumbar spina bifida with hydrocephalus

Q05.2 Lumbar spina bifida with hydrocephalus
Lumbosacral spina bifida with hydrocephalus

Q05.3 Sacral spina bifida with hydrocephalus

Q05.4 Unspecified spina bifida with hydrocephalus

Q05.5 Cervical spina bifida without hydrocephalus

Q05.6 Thoracic spina bifida without hydrocephalus
Dorsal spina bifida NOS
Thoracolumbar spina bifida NOS

Q05.7 Lumbar spina bifida without hydrocephalus
Lumbosacral spina bifida NOS

Q05.8 Sacral spina bifida without hydrocephalus

Q05.9 Spina bifida, unspecified

Q06 OTHER CONGENITAL MALFORMATIONS OF SPINAL CORD

Q06.0 Amyelia

Q06.1 Hypoplasia and dysplasia of spinal cord
Atelomyelia
Myelatelia
Myelodysplasia of spinal cord

Q06.2 Diastematomyelia

Q06.3 Other congenital cauda equina malformations

Q06.4 Hydromyelia
Hydrorachis

Q06.8 Other specified congenital malformations of spinal cord

Q06.9 Congenital malformation of spinal cord, unspecified
Congenital anomaly NOS of spinal cord
Congenital deformity NOS of spinal cord
Congenital disease or lesion NOS of spinal cord

Q07 OTHER CONGENITAL MALFORMATIONS OF NERVOUS SYSTEM

Excludes2: congenital central alveolar hypoventilation syndrome (G47.35)
familial dysautonomia [Riley-Day] (G90.1)
neurofibromatosis (nonmalignant) (Q85.0-)

Q07.0 Arnold-Chiari syndrome
Arnold-Chiari syndrome, type II
Excludes1: Arnold-Chiari syndrome, type III (Q01.-)
Arnold-Chiari syndrome, type IV (Q04.8)
- **Q07.00** without spina bifida or hydrocephalus
- **Q07.01** with spina bifida
- **Q07.02** with hydrocephalus
- **Q07.03** with spina bifida and hydrocephalus

Q07.8 Other specified congenital malformations of nervous system
Agenesis of nerve
Displacement of brachial plexus
Jaw-winking syndrome
Marcus Gunn's syndrome

Q07.9 Congenital malformation of nervous system, unspecified
Congenital anomaly NOS of nervous system
Congenital deformity NOS of nervous system
Congenital disease or lesion NOS of nervous system

(Q10–Q18) CONGENITAL MALFORMATIONS OF EYE, EAR, FACE AND NECK

Excludes2: cleft lip and cleft palate (Q35–Q37)
congenital malformation of cervical spine (Q05.0, Q05.5, Q67.5, Q76.0–Q76.4)
congenital malformation of larynx (Q31.-)
congenital malformation of lip NEC (Q38.0)
congenital malformation of nose (Q30.-)
congenital malformation of parathyroid gland (Q89.2)
congenital malformation of thyroid gland (Q89.2)

Q10 CONGENITAL MALFORMATIONS OF EYELID, LACRIMAL APPARATUS AND ORBIT

Excludes1: cryptophthalmos NOS (Q11.2)
cryptophthalmos syndrome (Q87.0)

Q10.0 Congenital ptosis
Q10.1 Congenital ectropion
Q10.2 Congenital entropion
Q10.3 Other congenital malformations of eyelid
Ablepharon
Blepharophimosis, congenital
Coloboma of eyelid
Congenital absence or agenesis of cilia
Congenital absence or agenesis of eyelid
Congenital accessory eyelid
Congenital accessory eye muscle
Congenital malformation of eyelid NOS
Q10.4 Absence and agenesis of lacrimal apparatus
Congenital absence of punctum lacrimale
Q10.5 Congenital stenosis and stricture of lacrimal duct
Q10.6 Other congenital malformations of lacrimal apparatus
Congenital malformation of lacrimal apparatus NOS
Q10.7 Congenital malformation of orbit

Q11 ANOPHTHALMOS, MICROPHTHALMOS AND MACROPHTHALMOS

Q11.0 Cystic eyeball
Q11.1 Other anophthalmos
Anophthalmos NOS
Agenesis of eye
Aplasia of eye
Q11.2 Microphthalmos
Cryptophthalmos NOS
Dysplasia of eye
Hypoplasia of eye
Rudimentary eye
Excludes1: cryptophthalmos syndrome (Q87.0)

Q11.3 Macrophthalmos
Excludes1: macrophthalmos in congenital glaucoma (Q15.0)

Q12 CONGENITAL LENS MALFORMATIONS

Q12.0 Congenital cataract
Q12.1 Congenital displaced lens
Q12.2 Coloboma of lens
Q12.3 Congenital aphakia
Q12.4 Spherophakia
Q12.8 Other congenital lens malformations
Microphakia
Q12.9 Congenital lens malformation, unspecified

Q13 CONGENITAL MALFORMATIONS OF ANTERIOR SEGMENT OF EYE

Q13.0 Coloboma of iris
Coloboma NOS
Q13.1 Absence of iris
Aniridia
Use additional code for associated glaucoma (H42)
Q13.2 Other congenital malformations of iris
Anisocoria, congenital
Atresia of pupil
Congenital malformation of iris NOS
Corectopia
Q13.3 Congenital corneal opacity
Q13.4 Other congenital corneal malformations
Congenital malformation of cornea NOS
Microcornea
Peter's anomaly
Q13.5 Blue sclera
Q13.8 Other congenital malformations of anterior segment of eye
- **Q13.81** Rieger anomaly
Axenfeld-Rieger syndrome
Code also any other associated congenital malformations such as cardiac defects
Use additional code for associated glaucoma (H42)
- **Q13.89** Other congenital malformations of anterior segment of eye

Q13.9 Congenital malformation of anterior segment of eye, unspecified

Q14 CONGENITAL MALFORMATIONS OF POSTERIOR SEGMENT OF EYE

Excludes2: optic nerve hypoplasia (H47.03-)

Q14.0 Congenital malformation of vitreous humor
Congenital vitreous opacity
Q14.1 Congenital malformation of retina
Congenital retinal aneurysm
Q14.2 Congenital malformation of optic disc
Coloboma of optic disc
Q14.3 Congenital malformation of choroid
Q14.8 Other congenital malformations of posterior segment of eye
Coloboma of the fundus
Q14.9 Congenital malformation of posterior segment of eye, unspecified

Q15 OTHER CONGENITAL MALFORMATIONS OF EYE

Excludes1: congenital nystagmus (H55.01)
ocular albinism (E70.31-)
optic nerve hypoplasia (H47.03-)
retinitis pigmentosa (H35.52)

Q15.0 Congenital glaucoma
Axenfeld's anomaly
Buphthalmos
Glaucoma of childhood
Glaucoma of newborn
Hydrophthalmos
Keratoglobus, congenital, with glaucoma
Macrocornea with glaucoma
Macrophthalmos in congenital glaucoma
Megalocornea with glaucoma
Q15.8 Other specified congenital malformations of eye
Q15.9 Congenital malformation of eye, unspecified
Congenital anomaly of eye
Congenital deformity of eye

Q16 CONGENITAL MALFORMATIONS OF EAR CAUSING IMPAIRMENT OF HEARING

Excludes1: congenital deafness (H90.-)

- **Q16.0 Congenital absence of (ear) auricle**
- **Q16.1 Congenital absence, atresia and stricture of auditory canal (external)**
  - Congenital atresia or stricture of osseous meatus
- **Q16.2 Absence of eustachian tube**
- **Q16.3 Congenital malformation of ear ossicles**
  - Congenital fusion of ear ossicles
- **Q16.4 Other congenital malformations of middle ear**
  - Congenital malformation of middle ear NOS
- **Q16.5 Congenital malformation of inner ear**
  - Congenital anomaly of membranous labyrinth
  - Congenital anomaly of organ of Corti
- **Q16.9 Congenital malformation of ear causing impairment of hearing, unspecified**
  - Congenital absence of ear NOS

Q17 OTHER CONGENITAL MALFORMATIONS OF EAR

Excludes1: congenital malformations of ear with impairment of hearing (Q16.0–Q16.9)
preauricular sinus (Q18.1)

- **Q17.0 Accessory auricle**
  - Accessory tragus
  - Polyotia
  - Preauricular appendage or tag
  - Supernumerary ear
  - Supernumerary lobule
- **Q17.1 Macrotia**
- **Q17.2 Microtia**
- **Q17.3 Other misshapen ear**
  - Pointed ear
- **Q17.4 Misplaced ear**
  - Low-set ears
  - *Excludes1:* cervical auricle (Q18.2)
- **Q17.5 Prominent ear**
  - Bat ear
- **Q17.8 Other specified congenital malformations of ear**
  - Congenital absence of lobe of ear
- **Q17.9 Congenital malformation of ear, unspecified**
  - Congenital anomaly of ear NOS

Q18 OTHER CONGENITAL MALFORMATIONS OF FACE AND NECK

Excludes1: cleft lip and cleft palate (Q35-Q37)
conditions classified to Q67.0-Q67.4
congenital malformations of skull and face bones (Q75.-)
cyclopia (Q87.0)
dentofacial anomalies [including malocclusion] (M26.-)
malformation syndromes affecting facial appearance (Q87.0)
persistent thyroglossal duct (Q89.2)

- **Q18.0 Sinus, fistula and cyst of branchial cleft**
  - Branchial vestige
- **Q18.1 Preauricular sinus and cyst**
  - Fistula of auricle, congenital
  - Cervicoaural fistula
- **Q18.2 Other branchial cleft malformations**
  - Branchial cleft malformation NOS
  - Cervical auricle
  - Otocephaly
- **Q18.6 Macrocheilia**
  - Hypertrophy of lip, congenital
- **Q18.8 Other specified congenital malformations of face and neck**
  - Medial cyst of face and neck
  - Medial fistula of face and neck
  - Medial sinus of face and neck
- **Q18.9 Congenital malformation of face and neck, unspecified**
  - Congenital anomaly NOS of face and neck

(Q20–Q28) CONGENITAL MALFORMATIONS OF THE CIRCULATORY SYSTEM

Q20 CONGENITAL MALFORMATIONS OF CARDIAC CHAMBERS AND CONNECTIONS

Excludes1: dextrocardia with situs inversus (Q89.3)
mirror-image atrial arrangement with situs inversus (Q89.3)

- **Q20.0 Common arterial trunk**
  - Persistent truncus arteriosus
  - *Excludes1:* aortic septal defect (Q21.4)
- **Q20.3 Discordant ventriculoarterial connection**
  - Dextrotransposition of aorta
  - Transposition of great vessels (complete)
- **Q20.8 Other congenital malformations of cardiac chambers and connections**
  - Cor binoculare

Q21 CONGENITAL MALFORMATIONS OF CARDIAC SEPTA

Excludes1: acquired cardiac septal defect (I51.0)

- **Q21.0 Ventricular septal defect**
  - Roger's disease
- **Q21.1 Atrial septal defect;**
  - *Excludes2:* ostium primum atrial septal defect (type I) (Q21.20)
  - **Q21.10 unspecified**
  - **Q21.11 secundum**
    - Fenestrated atrial septum
    - Patent or persistent ostium secundum defect (type II)
  - **Q21.12 patent foramen ovale**
    - Persistent foramen ovale
  - **Q21.13 coronary sinus**
    - Coronary sinus defect
    - Unroofed coronary sinus
  - **Q21.14 superior sinus venosus**
    - Superior vena cava type atrial septal defect
  - **Q21.15 inferior sinus venosus**
    - Inferior vena cava type atrial septal defect
  - **Q21.16 sinus venosus, unspecified**
    - Sinus venosus defect, NOS
  - **Q21.19 other specified**
    - Common atrium
    - Other specified atrial septal abnormality
- **Q21.2 Atrioventricular septal defect;**
  - Common atrioventricular canal
  - Endocardial cushion defect
  - Ostium primum atrial septal defect (type I)
  - **Q21.20 unspecified as to partial or complete**
  - **Q21.21 partial**
  - **Q21.22 transitional**
  - **Q21.23 complete**
- **Q21.3 Tetralogy of Fallot**
  - Ventricular septal defect with pulmonary stenosis or atresia, dextroposition of aorta and hypertrophy of right ventricle
- **Q21.8 Other congenital malformations of cardiac septa**
  - Eisenmenger's defect
  - Pentalogy of Fallot
  - **Code also** Eisenmenger's complex or syndrome (I27.83)
- **Q21.9 Congenital malformation of cardiac septum, unspecified**
  - Septal (heart) defect NOS

Q22 CONGENITAL MALFORMATIONS OF PULMONARY AND TRICUSPID VALVES

- **Q22.0 Pulmonary valve atresia**
- **Q22.1 Congenital pulmonary valve stenosis**
- **Q22.2 Congenital pulmonary valve insufficiency**
  - Congenital pulmonary valve regurgitation
- **Q22.3 Other congenital malformations of pulmonary valve**
  - Congenital malformation of pulmonary valve NOS
  - Supernumerary cusps of pulmonary valve
- **Q22.4 Congenital tricuspid stenosis**
  - Congenital tricuspid atresia
- **Q22.5 Ebstein's anomaly**
- **Q22.6 Hypoplastic right heart syndrome**
- **Q22.8 Other congenital malformations of tricuspid valve**
- **Q22.9 Congenital malformation of tricuspid valve, unspecified**

Q23 CONGENITAL MALFORMATIONS OF AORTIC AND MITRAL VALVES

4th

Q23.0 Congenital stenosis of aortic valve
Congenital aortic atresia
Congenital aortic stenosis NOS
Excludes1: congenital stenosis of aortic valve in hypoplastic left heart syndrome (Q23.4)
congenital subaortic stenosis (Q24.4)
supravalvular aortic stenosis (congenital) (Q25.3)

Q23.1 Congenital insufficiency of aortic valve
Congenital aortic insufficiency

Q23.2 Congenital mitral stenosis
Congenital mitral atresia

Q23.3 Congenital mitral insufficiency

Q23.4 Hypoplastic left heart syndrome

Q23.8 Other congenital malformations of aortic and mitral valves

5th •**Q23.81 Bicuspid aortic valve**
Congenital bicuspid aortic valve
Unicuspid (congenital) aortic valve (at birth)
Code also, if applicable, acquired aortic valve disorders, such as:
aortic (valve) insufficiency (nonrheumatic) (I35.1)
aortic (valve) stenosis (nonrheumatic) (I35.0)
aortic (valve) stenosis with insufficiency (nonrheumatic) (I35.2)

•**Q23.82 Congenital mitral valve cleft leaflet**
Cleft mitral valve leaflet at birth

•**Q23.88 Other congenital malformations of aortic and mitral valves**

Q23.9 Congenital malformation of aortic and mitral valves, unspecified

Q24 OTHER CONGENITAL MALFORMATIONS OF HEART

4th

Excludes1: endocardial fibroelastosis (I42.4)

Q24.0 Dextrocardia
Excludes1: dextrocardia with situs inversus (Q89.3)
isomerism of atrial appendages (with asplenia or polysplenia) (Q20.6)
mirror-image atrial arrangement with situs inversus (Q89.3)

Q24.1 Levocardia

Q24.3 Pulmonary infundibular stenosis
Subvalvular pulmonic stenosis

Q24.4 Congenital subaortic stenosis

Q24.6 Congenital heart block

Q24.8 Other specified congenital malformations of heart
Congenital diverticulum of left ventricle
Congenital malformation of myocardium
Congenital malformation of pericardium
Malposition of heart
Uhl's disease

Q24.9 Congenital malformation of heart, unspecified
Congenital anomaly of heart
Congenital disease of heart

Q25 CONGENITAL MALFORMATIONS OF GREAT ARTERIES

4th

Q25.0 Patent ductus arteriosus
Patent ductus Botallo
Persistent ductus arteriosus

Q25.1 Coarctation of aorta
Coarctation of aorta (preductal) (postductal)
Stenosis of aorta

Q25.2 Atresia of aorta

5th Q25.21 **Interruption of aortic arch**
Atresia of aortic arch

Q25.29 **Other atresia of aorta**
Atresia of aorta

Q25.3 Supravalvular aortic stenosis
Excludes1: congenital aortic stenosis NOS (Q23.0)
congenital stenosis of aortic valve (Q23.0)

Q25.4 Other congenital malformations of aorta

5th Q25.40 **Congenital malformation of aorta unspecified**

Q25.41 **Absence and aplasia of aorta**

Q25.42 **Hypoplasia of aorta**

Q25.43 **Congenital aneurysm of aorta**
Congenital aneurysm of aortic root
Congenital aneurysm of aortic sinus

Q25.44 Congenital dilation of aorta

Q25.45 Double aortic arch
Vascular ring of aorta

Q25.46 Tortuous aortic arch
Persistent convolutions of aortic arch

Q25.47 Right aortic arch
Persistent right aortic arch

Q25.48 Anomalous origin of subclavian artery

Q25.49 Other congenital malformations of aorta
Aortic arch
Bovine arch

Q25.5 Atresia of pulmonary artery

Q25.6 Stenosis of pulmonary artery
Supravalvular pulmonary stenosis

Q25.7 Other congenital malformations of pulmonary artery

5th Q25.71 **Coarctation of pulmonary artery**

Q25.72 **Congenital pulmonary arteriovenous malformation**
Congenital pulmonary arteriovenous aneurysm

Q25.79 Other congenital malformations of pulmonary artery
Aberrant pulmonary artery
Agenesis of pulmonary artery
Congenital aneurysm of pulmonary artery
Congenital anomaly of pulmonary artery
Hypoplasia of pulmonary artery

Q25.9 Congenital malformation of great arteries, unspecified

Q26 CONGENITAL MALFORMATIONS OF GREAT VEINS

4th

Q26.2 Total anomalous pulmonary venous connection
TAPVR, subdiaphragmatic
TAPVR, supradiaphragmatic

Q26.3 Partial anomalous pulmonary venous connection
Partial anomalous pulmonary venous return

Q26.4 Anomalous pulmonary venous connection, unspecified

Q26.8 Other congenital malformations of great veins
Absence of vena cava (inferior) (superior)
Azygos continuation of inferior vena cava
Persistent left posterior cardinal vein
Scimitar syndrome

Q26.9 Congenital malformation of great vein, unspecified
Congenital anomaly of vena cava (inferior) (superior) NOS

Q27 OTHER CONGENITAL MALFORMATIONS OF PERIPHERAL VASCULAR SYSTEM

4th

Excludes2: anomalies of cerebral and precerebral vessels (Q28.0–Q28.3)
anomalies of coronary vessels (Q24.5)
anomalies of pulmonary artery (Q25.5–Q25.7)
congenital retinal aneurysm (Q14.1)
hemangioma and lymphangioma (D18.-)

Q27.0 Congenital absence and hypoplasia of umbilical artery
Single umbilical artery

Q27.3 Arteriovenous malformation (peripheral)

5th Arteriovenous aneurysm
Excludes1: acquired arteriovenous aneurysm (I77.0)
Excludes2: arteriovenous malformation of cerebral vessels (Q28.2)
arteriovenous malformation of precerebral vessels (Q28.0)

Q27.30 **Arteriovenous malformation, site unspecified**

Q27.31 **Arteriovenous malformation of vessel of upper limb**

Q27.32 **Arteriovenous malformation of vessel of lower limb**

Q27.33 **Arteriovenous malformation of digestive system vessel**

Q27.34 **Arteriovenous malformation of renal vessel**

Q27.39 **Arteriovenous malformation, other site**

Q27.8 Other specified congenital malformations of peripheral vascular system
Absence of peripheral vascular system
Atresia of peripheral vascular system
Congenital aneurysm (peripheral)
Congenital stricture, artery
Congenital varix
Excludes 1: arteriovenous malformation (Q27.3-)

Q27.9 Congenital malformation of peripheral vascular system, unspecified
Anomaly of artery or vein NOS

Q28 OTHER CONGENITAL MALFORMATIONS OF CIRCULATORY SYSTEM

Excludes1: congenital aneurysm NOS (Q27.8)
congenital coronary aneurysm (Q24.5)
ruptured cerebral arteriovenous malformation (I60.8)
ruptured malformation of precerebral vessels (I72.0)

Excludes2: congenital peripheral aneurysm (Q27.8)
congenital pulmonary aneurysm (Q25.79)
congenital retinal aneurysm (Q14.1)

Q28.2 Arteriovenous malformation of cerebral vessels
Arteriovenous malformation of brain NOS
Congenital arteriovenous cerebral aneurysm (nonruptured)

Q28.3 Other malformations of cerebral vessels
Congenital cerebral aneurysm (nonruptured)
Congenital malformation of cerebral vessels NOS
Developmental venous anomaly

Q28.8 Other specified congenital malformations of circulatory system
Congenital aneurysm, specified site NEC
Spinal vessel anomaly

(Q30–Q34) CONGENITAL MALFORMATIONS OF THE RESPIRATORY SYSTEM

Q30 CONGENITAL MALFORMATIONS OF NOSE

Excludes1: congenital deviation of nasal septum (Q67.4)

Q30.0 Choanal atresia
Atresia of nares (anterior) (posterior)
Congenital stenosis of nares (anterior) (posterior)

Q30.3 Congenital perforated nasal septum

Q30.8 Other congenital malformations of nose
Accessory nose
Congenital anomaly of nasal sinus wall

Q30.9 Congenital malformation of nose, unspecified

Q31 CONGENITAL MALFORMATIONS OF LARYNX

Excludes1: congenital laryngeal stridor NOS (P28.89)

Q31.2 Laryngeal hypoplasia

Q31.5 Congenital laryngomalacia

Q31.8 Other congenital malformations of larynx
Absence of larynx
Agenesis of larynx
Atresia of larynx
Congenital cleft thyroid cartilage
Congenital fissure of epiglottis
Congenital stenosis of larynx NEC
Posterior cleft of cricoid cartilage

Q32 CONGENITAL MALFORMATIONS OF TRACHEA AND BRONCHUS

Excludes1: congenital bronchiectasis (Q33.4)

Q32.0 Congenital tracheomalacia

Q32.4 Other congenital malformations of bronchus
Absence of bronchus
Agenesis of bronchus
Atresia of bronchus
Congenital diverticulum of bronchus
Congenital malformation of bronchus NOS

Q33 CONGENITAL MALFORMATIONS OF LUNG

Excludes1: pulmonary hypoplasia associated with short gestation (P28.0)

Q33.6 Congenital hypoplasia and dysplasia of lung

Q33.9 Congenital malformation of lung, unspecified

Q34 OTHER CONGENITAL MALFORMATIONS OF RESPIRATORY SYSTEM

Excludes2: congenital central alveolar hypoventilation syndrome (G47.35)

Q34.8 Other specified congenital malformations of respiratory system
Atresia of nasopharynx

Q34.9 Congenital malformation of respiratory system, unspecified
Congenital absence of respiratory system
Congenital anomaly of respiratory system NOS

(Q35–Q37) CLEFT LIP AND CLEFT PALATE

Use **additional code** to identify associated malformation of the nose (Q30.2)

Excludes2: Robin's syndrome (Q87.0)

Q35 CLEFT PALATE

Includes: fissure of palate
palatoschisis

Excludes1: cleft palate with cleft lip (Q37.-)

Q35.1 Cleft hard palate

Q35.3 Cleft soft palate

Q35.5 Cleft hard palate with cleft soft palate

Q35.7 Cleft uvula

Q35.9 Cleft palate, unspecified
Cleft palate NOS

Q36 CLEFT LIP

Includes: cheiloschisis
congenital fissure of lip
harelip
labium leporinum

Excludes1: cleft lip with cleft palate (Q37.-)

Q36.0 Cleft lip, bilateral

Q36.1 Cleft lip, median

Q36.9 Cleft lip, unilateral
Cleft lip NOS

Q37 CLEFT PALATE WITH CLEFT LIP

Includes: cheilopalatoschisis

Q37.0 Cleft hard palate with bilateral cleft lip

Q37.1 Cleft hard palate with unilateral cleft lip
Cleft hard palate with cleft lip NOS

Q37.2 Cleft soft palate with bilateral cleft lip

Q37.3 Cleft soft palate with unilateral cleft lip
Cleft soft palate with cleft lip NOS

Q37.4 Cleft hard and soft palate with bilateral cleft lip

Q37.5 Cleft hard and soft palate with unilateral cleft lip
Cleft hard and soft palate with cleft lip NOS

Q37.8 Unspecified cleft palate with bilateral cleft lip

Q37.9 Unspecified cleft palate with unilateral cleft lip

(Q38–Q45) OTHER CONGENITAL MALFORMATIONS OF THE DIGESTIVE SYSTEM

Q38 OTHER CONGENITAL MALFORMATIONS OF TONGUE, MOUTH AND PHARYNX

Excludes1: dentofacial anomalies (M26.-)
macrostomia (Q18.4)
microstomia (Q18.5)

Q38.0 Congenital malformations of lips, not elsewhere classified
Congenital fistula of lip
Congenital malformation of lip NOS
Van der Woude's syndrome
Excludes1: cleft lip (Q36.-)
cleft lip with cleft palate (Q37.-)
macrocheilia (Q18.6)
microcheilia (Q18.7)

Q38.1 Ankyloglossia
Tongue tie

Q38.2 Macroglossia
Congenital hypertrophy of tongue

Q38.3 Other congenital malformations of tongue
Aglossia
Bifid tongue
Congenital adhesion of tongue
Congenital fissure of tongue
Congenital malformation of tongue NOS
Double tongue
Hypoglossia
Hypoplasia of tongue
Microglossia

CHAPTER 17. CONGENITAL MALFORMATIONS, DEFORMATIONS AND CHROMOSOMAL ABNORMALITIES (Q00–Q99)

(Q38.5–Q45)

Q38.5 Congenital malformations of palate, not elsewhere classified
Congenital absence of uvula
Congenital malformation of palate NOS
Congenital high arched palate
Excludes1: cleft palate (Q35.-)
cleft palate with cleft lip (Q37.-)

Q38.6 Other congenital malformations of mouth
Congenital malformation of mouth NOS

Q38.8 Other congenital malformations of pharynx
Congenital malformation of pharynx NOS
Imperforate pharynx

Q39 CONGENITAL MALFORMATIONS OF ESOPHAGUS
4th

Q39.0 Atresia of esophagus without fistula
Atresia of esophagus NOS

Q39.1 Atresia of esophagus with tracheo-esophageal fistula
Atresia of esophagus with broncho-esophageal fistula

Q39.2 Congenital tracheo-esophageal fistula without atresia
Congenital tracheo-esophageal fistula NOS

Q39.5 Congenital dilatation of esophagus
Congenital cardiospasm

Q40 OTHER CONGENITAL MALFORMATIONS OF UPPER ALIMENTARY TRACT
4th

Q40.0 Congenital hypertrophic pyloric stenosis
Congenital or infantile constriction or hypertrophy or spasm
Congenital or infantile stenosis
Congenital or infantile stricture or stricture

Q40.1 Congenital hiatus hernia
Congenital displacement of cardia through esophageal hiatus
Excludes1: congenital diaphragmatic hernia (Q79.0)

Q40.2 Other specified congenital malformations of stomach
Congenital displacement of stomach
Congenital diverticulum of stomach
Congenital hourglass stomach
Congenital duplication of stomach
Megalogastria
Microgastria

Q40.8 Other specified congenital malformations of upper alimentary tract

Q40.9 Congenital malformation of upper alimentary tract, unspecified
Congenital anomaly of upper alimentary tract
Congenital deformity of upper alimentary tract

Q41 CONGENITAL ABSENCE, ATRESIA AND STENOSIS OF SMALL INTESTINE
4th

Includes: congenital obstruction, occlusion or stricture of small intestine or intestine NOS
Excludes1: cystic fibrosis with intestinal manifestation (E84.11)
meconium ileus NOS (without cystic fibrosis) (P76.0)

Q41.0 Congenital absence, atresia and stenosis of duodenum

Q41.1 Congenital absence, atresia and stenosis of jejunum
Apple peel syndrome
Imperforate jejunum

Q41.2 Congenital absence, atresia and stenosis of ileum

Q41.8 Congenital absence, atresia and stenosis of other specified parts of small intestine

Q41.9 Congenital absence, atresia and stenosis of small intestine, part unspecified
Congenital absence, atresia and stenosis of intestine NOS

Q42 CONGENITAL ABSENCE, ATRESIA AND STENOSIS OF LARGE INTESTINE
4th

Includes: congenital obstruction, occlusion and stricture of large intestine

Q42.0 Congenital absence, atresia and stenosis of rectum with fistula

Q42.1 Congenital absence, atresia and stenosis of rectum without fistula
Imperforate rectum

Q42.2 Congenital absence, atresia and stenosis of anus with fistula

Q42.3 Congenital absence, atresia and stenosis of anus without fistula
Imperforate anus

Q42.8 Congenital absence, atresia and stenosis of other parts of large intestine

Q42.9 Congenital absence, atresia and stenosis of large intestine, part unspecified

Q43 OTHER CONGENITAL MALFORMATIONS OF INTESTINE
4th

Q43.0 Meckel's diverticulum (displaced) (hypertrophic)
Persistent omphalomesenteric duct
Persistent vitelline duct

Q43.1 Hirschsprung's disease
Aganglionosis
Congenital (aganglionic) megacolon

Q43.2 Other congenital functional disorders of colon
Congenital dilatation of colon

Q43.3 Congenital malformations of intestinal fixation
Congenital omental, anomalous adhesions [bands]
Congenital peritoneal adhesions [bands]
Incomplete rotation of cecum and colon
Insufficient rotation of cecum and colon
Jackson's membrane
Malrotation of colon
Rotation failure of cecum and colon
Universal mesentery

Q43.6 Congenital fistula of rectum and anus
Excludes1: congenital fistula of anus with absence, atresia and stenosis (Q42.2)
congenital fistula of rectum with absence, atresia and stenosis (Q42.0)
congenital rectovaginal fistula (Q52.2)
congenital urethrorectal fistula (Q64.73)
pilonidal fistula or sinus (L05.-)

Q43.8 Other specified congenital malformations of intestine
Congenital blind loop syndrome
Congenital diverticulitis, colon
Congenital diverticulum, intestine
Dolichocolon
Megaloappendix
Megaloduodenum
Microcolon
Transposition of appendix
Transposition of colon
Transposition of intestine

Q43.9 Congenital malformation of intestine, unspecified

Q44 CONGENITAL MALFORMATIONS OF GALLBLADDER, BILE DUCTS AND LIVER
4th

Q44.0 Agenesis, aplasia and hypoplasia of gallbladder
Congenital absence of gallbladder

Q44.1 Other congenital malformations of gallbladder
Congenital malformation of gallbladder NOS
Intrahepatic gallbladder

Q44.2 Atresia of bile ducts

Q44.3 Congenital stenosis and stricture of bile ducts

Q44.4 Choledochal cyst

Q44.5 Other congenital malformations of bile ducts
Accessory hepatic duct
Biliary duct duplication
Congenital malformation of bile duct NOS
Cystic duct duplication

Q44.7 Other congenital malformations of liver
5th Code also, if applicable, associated malformations affecting other systems

Q44.70 Other congenital malformation of liver, unspecified
Congenital malformation of liver, NOS

Q44.71 Alagille syndrome
Alagille-Watson syndrome

Q44.79 Other congenital malformations of liver
Accessory liver
Congenital absence of liver
Congenital hepatomegaly

Q45 OTHER CONGENITAL MALFORMATIONS OF DIGESTIVE SYSTEM
4th

Excludes2: congenital diaphragmatic hernia (Q79.0)
congenital hiatus hernia (Q40.1)

4th	5th	6th	7th	Additional Character Required	✔	3-character code

*=New Code
▲=Revised Code

Excludes1—Not coded here, do not use together
Excludes2—Not included here

Q45.8 Other specified congenital malformations of digestive system
Absence (complete) (partial) of alimentary tract NOS
Duplication of digestive system
Malposition, congenital of digestive system

Q45.9 Congenital malformation of digestive system, unspecified
Congenital anomaly of digestive system
Congenital deformity of digestive system

(Q50–Q56) CONGENITAL MALFORMATIONS OF GENITAL ORGANS

Excludes1: androgen insensitivity syndrome (E34.5-)
syndromes associated with anomalies in the number and form of chromosomes (Q90–Q99)

Q50 CONGENITAL MALFORMATIONS OF OVARIES, FALLOPIAN TUBES AND BROAD LIGAMENTS

- Q50.0 Congenital absence of ovary
  - *Excludes1:* Turner's syndrome (Q96.-)
  - Q50.01 Congenital absence of ovary, unilateral
  - Q50.02 Congenital absence of ovary, bilateral
- Q50.1 Developmental ovarian cyst
- Q50.2 Congenital torsion of ovary
- Q50.3 Other congenital malformations of ovary
  - Q50.31 Accessory ovary
  - Q50.32 Ovarian streak
    - 46, XX with streak gonads
  - Q50.39 Other congenital malformation of ovary
    - Congenital malformation of ovary NOS
- Q50.4 Embryonic cyst of fallopian tube
  - Fimbrial cyst
- Q50.5 Embryonic cyst of broad ligament
  - Epoophoron cyst
  - Parovarian cyst
- Q50.6 Other congenital malformations of fallopian tube and broad ligament
  - Absence of fallopian tube and broad ligament
  - Accessory fallopian tube and broad ligament
  - Atresia of fallopian tube and broad ligament
  - Congenital malformation of fallopian tube or broad ligament NOS

Q51 CONGENITAL MALFORMATIONS OF UTERUS AND CERVIX

- Q51.0 Agenesis and aplasia of uterus
  - Congenital absence of uterus
- Q51.1 Doubling of uterus with doubling of cervix and vagina
  - Q51.10 Doubling of uterus with doubling of cervix and vagina without obstruction
    - Doubling of uterus with doubling of cervix and vagina NOS
  - Q51.11 Doubling of uterus with doubling of cervix and vagina with obstruction
- Q51.2 Other doubling of uterus
  - Doubling of uterus NOS
  - Septate uterus
  - Q51.21 Complete doubling of uterus
    - Complete septate uterus
  - Q51.22 Partial doubling of uterus
    - Partial septate uterus
  - Q51.28 Other and unspecified doubling of uterus
    - Septate uterus NOS
- Q51.3 Bicornate uterus
  - Bicornate uterus, complete or partial
- Q51.4 Unicornate uterus
  - Unicornate uterus with or without a separate uterine horn
  - Uterus with only one functioning horn
- Q51.5 Agenesis and aplasia of cervix
  - Congenital absence of cervix
- Q51.6 Embryonic cyst of cervix
- Q51.7 Congenital fistulae between uterus and digestive and urinary tracts
- Q51.8 Other congenital malformations of uterus and cervix
  - Q51.81 Other congenital malformations of uterus
    - Q51.810 Arcuate uterus
      - Arcuatus uterus
    - Q51.811 Hypoplasia of uterus
    - Q51.818 Other congenital malformations of uterus
      - Müllerian anomaly of uterus NEC
  - Q51.82 Other congenital malformations of cervix
    - Q51.820 Cervical duplication
    - Q51.821 Hypoplasia of cervix
    - Q51.828 Other congenital malformations of cervix
- Q51.9 Congenital malformation of uterus and cervix, unspecified

Q52 OTHER CONGENITAL MALFORMATIONS OF FEMALE GENITALIA

- Q52.0 Congenital absence of vagina
  - Vaginal agenesis, total or partial
- Q52.1 Doubling of vagina
  - *Excludes1:* doubling of vagina with doubling of uterus and cervix (Q51.1-)
  - Q52.10 Doubling of vagina, unspecified
    - Septate vagina NOS
  - Q52.11 Transverse vaginal septum
  - Q52.12 Longitudinal vaginal septum
    - Q52.120 Longitudinal vaginal septum, nonobstructing
    - Q52.121 Longitudinal vaginal septum, obstructing, right side
    - Q52.122 Longitudinal vaginal septum, obstructing, left side
    - Q52.123 Longitudinal vaginal septum, microperforate, right side
    - Q52.124 Longitudinal vaginal septum, microperforate, left side
    - Q52.129 Other and unspecified longitudinal vaginal septum
- Q52.2 Congenital rectovaginal fistula
  - *Excludes1:* cloaca (Q43.7)
- Q52.4 Other congenital malformations of vagina
  - Canal of Nuck cyst, congenital
  - Congenital malformation of vagina NOS
  - Embryonic vaginal cyst
  - Gartner's duct cyst
- Q52.5 Fusion of labia
- Q52.6 Congenital malformation of clitoris
- Q52.7 Other and unspecified congenital malformations of vulva
  - Q52.70 Unspecified congenital malformations of vulva
    - Congenital malformation of vulva NOS
  - Q52.71 Congenital absence of vulva
  - Q52.79 Other congenital malformations of vulva
    - Congenital cyst of vulva
- Q52.3 Imperforate hymen
- Q52.8 Other specified congenital malformations of female genitalia
- Q52.9 Congenital malformation of female genitalia, unspecified

Q53 UNDESCENDED AND ECTOPIC TESTICLE

- Q53.0 Ectopic testis
  - Q53.00 Ectopic testis, unspecified
  - Q53.01 Ectopic testis, unilateral
  - Q53.02 Ectopic testes, bilateral
- Q53.1 Undescended testicle, unilateral
  - Q53.10 Unspecified undescended testicle, unilateral
  - Q53.11 Abdominal testis, unilateral
    - Q53.111 Unilateral intraabdominal testis
    - Q53.112 Unilateral inguinal testis
  - Q53.12 Ectopic perineal testis, unilateral
  - Q53.13 Unilateral high scrotal testis
- Q53.2 Undescended testicle, bilateral
  - Q53.20 Undescended testicle, unspecified, bilateral
  - Q53.21 Abdominal testis, bilateral
    - Q53.211 Bilateral intraabdominal testes
    - Q53.212 Bilateral inguinal testes
  - Q53.22 Ectopic perineal testis, bilateral
  - Q53.23 Bilateral high scrotal testes
- Q53.9 Undescended testicle, unspecified
  - Cryptorchism NOS

Q54 HYPOSPADIAS

Excludes1: epispadias (Q64.0)

- Q54.0 Hypospadias, balanic
  - Hypospadias, coronal
  - Hypospadias, glandular
- Q54.1 Hypospadias, penile
- Q54.2 Hypospadias, penoscrotal
- Q54.3 Hypospadias, perineal
- Q54.4 Congenital chordee
  - Chordee without hypospadias
- Q54.8 Other hypospadias
  - Hypospadias with intersex state
- Q54.9 Hypospadias, unspecified

Q55 OTHER CONGENITAL MALFORMATIONS OF MALE GENITAL ORGANS

Excludes1: congenital hydrocele (P83.5)

hypospadias (Q54.-)

- Q55.0 Absence and aplasia of testis
  - Monorchism
- Q55.1 Hypoplasia of testis and scrotum
  - Fusion of testes
- Q55.2 Other and unspecified congenital malformations of testis and scrotum
  - Q55.20 Unspecified congenital malformations of testis and scrotum
    - Congenital malformation of testis or scrotum NOS
  - Q55.21 Polyorchism
  - Q55.22 Retractile testis
  - Q55.23 Scrotal transposition
  - Q55.29 Other congenital malformations of testis and scrotum
- Q55.4 Other congenital malformations of vas deferens, epididymis, seminal vesicles and prostate
  - Absence or aplasia of prostate
  - Absence or aplasia of spermatic cord
  - Congenital malformation of vas deferens, epididymis, seminal vesicles or prostate NOS
- Q55.5 Congenital absence and aplasia of penis
- Q55.6 Other congenital malformations of penis
  - Q55.61 Curvature of penis (lateral)
  - Q55.62 Hypoplasia of penis
    - Micropenis
  - Q55.63 Congenital torsion of penis
    - *Excludes1:* acquired torsion of penis (N48.82)
  - Q55.64 Hidden penis
    - Buried penis
    - Concealed penis
    - *Excludes1:* acquired buried penis (N48.83)
  - Q55.69 Other congenital malformation of penis
    - Congenital malformation of penis NOS
- Q55.8 Other specified congenital malformations of male genital organs
- Q55.9 Congenital malformation of male genital organ, unspecified
  - Congenital anomaly of male genital organ
  - Congenital deformity of male genital organ

Q56 INDETERMINATE SEX AND PSEUDOHERMAPHRODITISM

Excludes1: 46, XX true hermaphrodite (Q99.1)

androgen insensitivity syndrome (E34.5-)

chimera 46, XX/46, XY true hermaphrodite (Q99.0)

female pseudohermaphroditism with adrenocortical disorder (E25.-)

pseudohermaphroditism with specified chromosomal anomaly (Q96–Q99)

pure gonadal dysgenesis (Q99.1)

- Q56.1 Male pseudohermaphroditism, not elsewhere classified
  - 46, XY with streak gonads
  - Male pseudohermaphroditism NOS
- Q56.2 Female pseudohermaphroditism, not elsewhere classified
  - Female pseudohermaphroditism NOS
- Q56.3 Pseudohermaphroditism, unspecified
- Q56.4 Indeterminate sex, unspecified
  - Ambiguous genitalia

(Q60–Q64) CONGENITAL MALFORMATIONS OF THE URINARY SYSTEM

Q60 RENAL AGENESIS AND OTHER REDUCTION DEFECTS OF KIDNEY

Includes: congenital absence of kidney

congenital atrophy of kidney

infantile atrophy of kidney

- Q60.0 Renal agenesis, unilateral
- Q60.1 Renal agenesis, bilateral
- Q60.3 Renal hypoplasia, unilateral
- Q60.4 Renal hypoplasia, bilateral
- Q60.6 Potter's syndrome

Q61 CYSTIC KIDNEY DISEASE

Excludes1: acquired cyst of kidney (N28.1)

Potter's syndrome (Q60.6)

- Q61.0 Congenital renal cyst
  - Q61.00 Congenital renal cyst, unspecified
    - Cyst of kidney NOS (congenital)
  - Q61.01 Congenital single renal cyst
  - Q61.02 Congenital multiple renal cysts
- Q61.1 Polycystic kidney, infantile type
  - Polycystic kidney, autosomal recessive
  - Q61.11 Cystic dilatation of collecting ducts
  - Q61.19 Other polycystic kidney, infantile type
- Q61.2 Polycystic kidney, adult type
  - Polycystic kidney, autosomal dominant
- Q61.3 Polycystic kidney, unspecified
- Q61.4 Renal dysplasia
  - Multicystic dysplastic kidney
  - Multicystic kidney (development)
  - Multicystic kidney disease
  - Multicystic renal dysplasia
  - *Excludes1:* polycystic kidney disease (Q61.11–Q61.3)
- Q61.5 Medullary cystic kidney
  - Nephronophthisis
  - Sponge kidney NOS
- Q61.8 Other cystic kidney diseases
  - Fibrocystic kidney
  - Fibrocystic renal degeneration or disease
- Q61.9 Cystic kidney disease, unspecified
  - Meckel-Gruber syndrome

Q62 CONGENITAL OBSTRUCTIVE DEFECTS OF RENAL PELVIS AND CONGENITAL MALFORMATIONS OF URETER

- Q62.0 Congenital hydronephrosis
- Q62.1 Congenital occlusion of ureter
  - Atresia and stenosis of ureter
  - Q62.10 Congenital occlusion of ureter, unspecified
  - Q62.11 Congenital occlusion of ureteropelvic junction
  - Q62.12 Congenital occlusion of ureterovesical orifice
- Q62.3 Other obstructive defects of renal pelvis and ureter
  - Q62.31 Congenital ureterocele, orthotopic
  - Q62.32 Cecoureterocele
    - Ectopic ureterocele
  - Q62.39 Other obstructive defects of renal pelvis and ureter
    - Ureteropelvic junction obstruction NOS
- Q62.8 Other congenital malformations of ureter
  - Anomaly of ureter NOS

Q63 OTHER CONGENITAL MALFORMATIONS OF KIDNEY

Excludes1: congenital nephrotic syndrome (N04.-)

- Q63.0 Accessory kidney
- Q63.1 Lobulated, fused and horseshoe kidney
- Q63.2 Ectopic kidney
  - Congenital displaced kidney
  - Malrotation of kidney
- Q63.3 Hyperplastic and giant kidney
  - Compensatory hypertrophy of kidney
- Q63.8 Other specified congenital malformations of kidney
  - Congenital renal calculi
- Q63.9 Congenital malformation of kidney, unspecified

Q64 OTHER CONGENITAL MALFORMATIONS OF URINARY SYSTEM

- Q64.0 Epispadias
  - *Excludes1:* hypospadias (Q54.-)
- Q64.1 Exstrophy of urinary bladder
  - Q64.10 Exstrophy of urinary bladder, unspecified
    - Ectopia vesicae
  - Q64.11 Supravesical fissure of urinary bladder
  - Q64.12 Cloacal exstrophy of urinary bladder
  - Q64.19 Other exstrophy of urinary bladder
    - Extroversion of bladder
- Q64.2 Congenital posterior urethral valves
- Q64.3 Other atresia and stenosis of urethra and bladder neck
  - Q64.31 Congenital bladder neck obstruction
    - Congenital obstruction of vesicourethral orifice
  - Q64.39 Other atresia and stenosis of urethra and bladder neck
    - Atresia and stenosis of urethra and bladder neck NOS
- Q64.4 Malformation of urachus
  - Cyst of urachus
  - Patent urachus
  - Prolapse of urachus
- Q64.5 Congenital absence of bladder and urethra
- Q64.6 Congenital diverticulum of bladder
- Q64.7 Other and unspecified congenital malformations of bladder and urethra
  - *Excludes1:* congenital prolapse of bladder (mucosa) (Q79.4)
  - Q64.70 Unspecified congenital malformation of bladder and urethra
    - Malformation of bladder or urethra NOS
  - Q64.79 Other congenital malformations of bladder and urethra
- Q64.9 Congenital malformation of urinary system, unspecified
  - Congenital anomaly NOS of urinary system
  - Congenital deformity NOS of urinary system

(Q65–Q79) CONGENITAL MALFORMATIONS AND DEFORMATIONS OF THE MUSCULOSKELETAL SYSTEM

Q65 CONGENITAL DEFORMITIES OF HIP

Excludes1: clicking hip (R29.4)

- Q65.0 Congenital dislocation of hip, unilateral
  - Q65.00 Congenital dislocation of unspecified hip, unilateral
  - Q65.01 Congenital dislocation of right hip, unilateral
  - Q65.02 Congenital dislocation of left hip, unilateral
- Q65.1 Congenital dislocation of hip, bilateral
- Q65.2 Congenital dislocation of hip, unspecified
- Q65.3 Congenital partial dislocation of hip, unilateral
  - Q65.30 Congenital partial dislocation of unspecified hip, unilateral
  - Q65.31 Congenital partial dislocation of right hip, unilateral
  - Q65.32 Congenital partial dislocation of left hip, unilateral
- Q65.4 Congenital partial dislocation of hip, bilateral
- Q65.5 Congenital partial dislocation of hip, unspecified
- Q65.6 Congenital unstable hip
  - Congenital dislocatable hip
- Q65.8 Other congenital deformities of hip
  - Q65.81 Congenital coxa valga
  - Q65.82 Congenital coxa vara
  - Q65.89 Other specified congenital deformities of hip
    - Anteversion of femoral neck
    - Congenital acetabular dysplasia

Q66 CONGENITAL DEFORMITIES OF FEET

Excludes1: reduction defects of feet (Q72.-)
valgus deformities (acquired) (M21.0-)
varus deformities (acquired) (M21.1-)

- Q66.0 Congenital talipes equinovarus
  - Q66.01 Congenital talipes equinovarus, right foot
  - Q66.02 Congenital talipes equinovarus, left foot
- Q66.1 Congenital talipes calcaneovarus
  - Q66.11 Congenital talipes calcaneovarus, right foot
  - Q66.12 Congenital talipes calcaneovarus, left foot
- Q66.2 Congenital metatarsus deformities
  - Q66.21 Congenital metatarsus primus varus
    - Q66.211 Congenital metatarsus primus varus, right foot
    - Q66.212 Congenital metatarsus primus varus, left foot
  - Q66.22 Congenital metatarsus adductus
    - Congenital metatarsus varus
    - Q66.221 Congenital metatarsus adductus, right foot
    - Q66.222 Congenital metatarsus adductus, left foot
- Q66.3 Other congenital varus deformities of feet
  - Hallux varus, congenital
  - Q66.31 Other congenital varus deformities of feet, right foot
  - Q66.32 Other congenital varus deformities of feet, left foot
- Q66.4 Congenital talipes calcaneovalgus
  - Q66.41 Congenital talipes calcaneovalgus, right foot
  - Q66.42 Congenital talipes calcaneovalgus, left foot
- Q66.5 Congenital pes planus
  - Congenital flat foot
  - Congenital rigid flat foot
  - Congenital spastic (everted) flat foot
  - *Excludes1:* pes planus, acquired (M21.4)
  - Q66.50 Congenital pes planus, unspecified foot
  - Q66.51 Congenital pes planus, right foot
  - Q66.52 Congenital pes planus, left foot
- Q66.6 Other congenital valgus deformities of feet
  - Congenital metatarsus valgus
- Q66.7 Congenital pes cavus
  - Q66.71 Congenital pes cavus, right foot
  - Q66.72 Congenital pes cavus, left foot
- Q66.8 Other congenital deformities of feet
  - Q66.80 Congenital vertical talus deformity, unspecified foot
  - Q66.81 Congenital vertical talus deformity, right foot
  - Q66.82 Congenital vertical talus deformity, left foot
  - Q66.89 Other specified congenital deformities of feet
    - Congenital asymmetric talipes
    - Congenital clubfoot NOS
    - Congenital talipes NOS
    - Congenital tarsal coalition
    - Hammer toe, congenital
- Q66.9 Congenital deformity of feet, unspecified
  - Q66.91 Congenital deformity of feet, unspecified, right foot
  - Q66.92 Congenital deformity of feet, unspecified, left foot

Q67 CONGENITAL MUSCULOSKELETAL DEFORMITIES OF HEAD, FACE, SPINE AND CHEST

Excludes1: congenital malformation syndromes classified to Q87.-
Potter's syndrome (Q60.6)

- Q67.0 Congenital facial asymmetry
- Q67.1 Congenital compression facies
- Q67.2 Dolichocephaly
  - *Excludes1:* sagittal craniosynostosis (Q75.01)
- Q67.3 Plagiocephaly
  - *Excludes1:* coronal craniosynostosis (Q75.02-)
  - lambdoid craniosynostosis (Q75.04-)
- Q67.4 Other congenital deformities of skull, face and jaw
  - Congenital depressions in skull
  - Congenital hemifacial atrophy or hypertrophy
  - Deviation of nasal septum, congenital
  - Squashed or bent nose, congenital
  - *Excludes1:* dentofacial anomalies [including malocclusion] (M26.-)
  - syphilitic saddle nose (A50.5)
- Q67.5 Congenital deformity of spine
  - Congenital postural scoliosis
  - Congenital scoliosis NOS
  - *Excludes1:* infantile idiopathic scoliosis (M41.0)
  - scoliosis due to congenital bony malformation (Q76.3)
- Q67.6 Pectus excavatum
  - Congenital funnel chest
- Q67.7 Pectus carinatum
  - Congenital pigeon chest
- Q67.8 Other congenital deformities of chest
  - Congenital deformity of chest wall NOS

Q68 OTHER CONGENITAL MUSCULOSKELETAL DEFORMITIES

Excludes1: reduction defects of limb(s) (Q71-Q73)

Excludes2: congenital myotonic chondrodystrophy (G71.13)

- **Q68.0** Congenital deformity of sternocleidomastoid muscle
  - Congenital contracture of sternocleidomastoid (muscle)
  - Congenital (sternomastoid) torticollis
  - Sternomastoid tumor (congenital)
- **Q68.1** Congenital deformity of finger(s) and hand
  - Congenital clubfinger
  - Spade-like hand (congenital)
- **Q68.2** Congenital deformity of knee
  - Congenital dislocation of knee
  - Congenital genu recurvatum
- **Q68.5** Congenital bowing of long bones of leg, unspecified
- **Q68.8** Other specified congenital musculoskeletal deformities
  - Congenital deformity of clavicle or scapula
  - Congenital deformity of elbow or forearm or wrist
  - Congenital dislocation of elbow or shoulder or wrist

Q69 POLYDACTYLY

- **Q69.0** Accessory finger(s)
- **Q69.1** Accessory thumb(s)
- **Q69.2** Accessory toe(s)
  - Accessory hallux
- **Q69.9** Polydactyly, unspecified
  - Supernumerary digit(s) NOS

Q70 SYNDACTYLY

- **Q70.0** Fused fingers
  - Complex syndactyly of fingers with synostosis
  - Q70.00 Fused fingers, unspecified hand
  - Q70.01 Fused fingers, right hand
  - Q70.02 Fused fingers, left hand
  - Q70.03 Fused fingers, bilateral
- **Q70.1** Webbed fingers
  - Simple syndactyly of fingers without synostosis
  - Q70.10 Webbed fingers, unspecified hand
  - Q70.11 Webbed fingers, right hand
  - Q70.12 Webbed fingers, left hand
  - Q70.13 Webbed fingers, bilateral
- **Q70.2** Fused toes
  - Complex syndactyly of toes with synostosis
  - Q70.20 Fused toes, unspecified foot
  - Q70.21 Fused toes, right foot
  - Q70.22 Fused toes, left foot
  - Q70.23 Fused toes, bilateral
- **Q70.3** Webbed toes
  - Simple syndactyly of toes without synostosis
  - Q70.30 Webbed toes, unspecified foot
  - Q70.31 Webbed toes, right foot
  - Q70.32 Webbed toes, left foot
  - Q70.33 Webbed toes, bilateral
- **Q70.4** Polysyndactyly, unspecified
  - *Excludes1:* specified syndactyly of hand and feet—code to specified conditions (Q70.0-Q70.3-)
- **Q70.9** Syndactyly, unspecified
  - Symphalangy NOS

Q71 REDUCTION DEFECTS OF UPPER LIMB

- **Q71.4** Longitudinal reduction defect of radius
  - Clubhand (congenital)
  - Radial clubhand
  - Q71.41 Longitudinal reduction defect of right radius
  - Q71.42 Longitudinal reduction defect of left radius
  - Q71.43 Longitudinal reduction defect of radius, bilateral
- **Q71.5** Longitudinal reduction defect of ulna
  - Q71.51 Longitudinal reduction defect of right ulna
  - Q71.52 Longitudinal reduction defect of left ulna
  - Q71.53 Longitudinal reduction defect of ulna, bilateral
- **Q71.6** Lobster-claw hand
  - Q71.61 Lobster-claw right hand
  - Q71.62 Lobster-claw left hand
  - Q71.63 Lobster-claw hand, bilateral

- **Q71.8** Other reduction defects of upper limb
  - Q71.81 Congenital shortening of upper limb
    - Q71.811 Congenital shortening of right upper limb
    - Q71.812 Congenital shortening of left upper limb
    - Q71.813 Congenital shortening of upper limb, bilateral
  - Q71.89 Other reduction defects of upper limb
    - Q71.891 Other reduction defects of right upper limb
    - Q71.892 Other reduction defects of left upper limb
    - Q71.893 Other reduction defects of upper limb, bilateral
- **Q71.9** Unspecified reduction defect of upper limb
  - Q71.91 Unspecified reduction defect of right upper limb
  - Q71.92 Unspecified reduction defect of left upper limb
  - Q71.93 Unspecified reduction defect of upper limb, bilateral

Q72 REDUCTION DEFECTS OF LOWER LIMB

- **Q72.4** Longitudinal reduction defect of femur
  - Proximal femoral focal deficiency
  - Q72.41 Longitudinal reduction defect of right femur
  - Q72.42 Longitudinal reduction defect of left femur
  - Q72.43 Longitudinal reduction defect of femur, bilateral
- **Q72.5** Longitudinal reduction defect of tibia
  - Q72.51 Longitudinal reduction defect of right tibia
  - Q72.52 Longitudinal reduction defect of left tibia
  - Q72.53 Longitudinal reduction defect of tibia, bilateral
- **Q72.6** Longitudinal reduction defect of fibula
  - Q72.61 Longitudinal reduction defect of right fibula
  - Q72.62 Longitudinal reduction defect of left fibula
  - Q72.63 Longitudinal reduction defect of fibula, bilateral
- **Q72.7** Split foot
  - Q72.71 Split foot, right lower limb
  - Q72.72 Split foot, left lower limb
  - Q72.73 Split foot, bilateral
- **Q72.8** Other reduction defects of lower limb
  - Q72.81 Congenital shortening of lower limb
    - Q72.811 Congenital shortening of right lower limb
    - Q72.812 Congenital shortening of left lower limb
    - Q72.813 Congenital shortening of lower limb, bilateral
  - Q72.89 Other reduction defects of lower limb
    - Q72.891 Other reduction defects of right lower limb
    - Q72.892 Other reduction defects of left lower limb
    - Q72.893 Other reduction defects of lower limb, bilateral
- **Q72.9** Unspecified reduction defect of lower limb
  - Q72.91 Unspecified reduction defect of right lower limb
  - Q72.92 Unspecified reduction defect of left lower limb
  - Q72.93 Unspecified reduction defect of lower limb, bilateral

Q74 OTHER CONGENITAL MALFORMATIONS OF LIMB(S)

Excludes1: polydactyly (Q69.-)
reduction defect of limb (Q71-Q73)
syndactyly (Q70.-)

- **Q74.0** Other congenital malformations of upper limb(s), including shoulder girdle
  - Accessory carpal bones
  - Cleidocranial dysostosis
  - Congenital pseudarthrosis of clavicle
  - Macrodactylia (fingers)
  - Madelung's deformity
  - Radioulnar synostosis
  - Sprengel's deformity
  - Triphalangeal thumb
- **Q74.1** Congenital malformation of knee
  - Congenital absence of patella
  - Congenital dislocation of patella
  - Congenital genu valgum
  - Congenital genu varum
  - Rudimentary patella
  - *Excludes1:* congenital dislocation of knee (Q68.2)
  congenital genu recurvatum (Q68.2)
  nail patella syndrome (Q87.2)

- **Q74.2 Other congenital malformations of lower limb(s), including pelvic girdle**
  - Congenital fusion of sacroiliac joint
  - Congenital malformation of ankle joint
  - Congenital malformation of sacroiliac joint
  - *Excludes1:* anteversion of femur (neck) (Q65.89)
- **Q74.3 Arthrogryposis multiplex congenita**
- **Q74.8 Other specified congenital malformations of limb(s)**
- **Q74.9 Unspecified congenital malformation of limb(s)**
  - Congenital anomaly of limb(s) NOS

Q75 OTHER CONGENITAL MALFORMATIONS OF SKULL AND FACE BONES

4th

Excludes1: congenital malformation of face NOS (Q18.-)
congenital malformation syndromes classified to Q87.-
dentofacial anomalies [including malocclusion] (M26.-)
musculoskeletal deformities of head and face (Q67.0–Q67.4)
skull defects associated with congenital anomalies of brain such as:
  anencephaly (Q00.0)
  encephalocele (Q01.-)
  hydrocephalus (Q03.-)
  microcephaly (Q02)

- **Q75.0 Craniosynostosis**
  - **5th** **Q75.00 Craniosynostosis unspecified**
    - **6th** Craniosynostosis NOS
    - **Q75.001 Craniosynostosis unspecified, unilateral**
    - **Q75.002 Craniosynostosis unspecified, bilateral**
    - **Q75.009 Craniosynostosis unspecified**
      - Imperfect fusion of skull
  - **Q75.01 Sagittal craniosynostosis**
    - Non-deformational dolichocephaly
    - Non-deformational scaphocephaly
    - *Excludes1:* plagiocephaly (Q67.3)
  - **Q75.02 Coronal craniosynostosis**
    - **6th** Non-deformational anterior plagiocephaly
    - *Excludes1:* dolichocephaly (Q67.2)
    - **Q75.021 Coronal craniosynostosis unilateral**
      - Non-deformational anterior plagiocephaly
    - **Q75.022 Coronal craniosynostosis bilateral**
      - Non-deformational brachycephaly
    - **Q75.029 Coronal craniosynostosis unspecified**
  - **Q75.03 Metopic craniosynostosis**
  - **Q75.04 Lambdoid craniosynostosis**
    - **6th** Non-deformational posterior plagiocephaly
    - *Excludes1:* dolichocephaly (Q67.2)
    - **Q75.041 Lambdoid craniosynostosis, unilateral**
    - **Q75.042 Lambdoid craniosynostosis, bilateral**
    - **Q75.049 Lambdoid craniosynostosis, unspecified**
  - **Q75.05 Multi-suture craniosynostosis**
    - **6th** **Q75.051 Cloverleaf skull**
      - Kleeblattschaedel skull
    - **Q75.052 Pansynostosis**
    - **Q75.058 Other multi-suture craniosynostosis**
  - **Q75.08 Other single-suture craniosynostosis**
- **Q75.1 Craniofacial dysostosis**
  - Crouzon's disease
- **Q75.2 Hypertelorism**
- **Q75.3 Macrocephaly**
- **Q75.4 Mandibulofacial dysostosis**
  - Franceschetti syndrome
  - Treacher Collins syndrome
- **Q75.5 Oculomandibular dysostosis**
- **Q75.8 Other specified congenital malformations of skull and face bones**
  - Absence of skull bone, congenital
  - Congenital deformity of forehead
  - Platybasia
- **Q75.9 Congenital malformation of skull and face bones, unspecified**
  - Congenital anomaly of face bones NOS
  - Congenital anomaly of skull NOS

Q76 CONGENITAL MALFORMATIONS OF SPINE AND BONY THORAX

4th

Excludes1: congenital musculoskeletal deformities of spine and chest (Q67.5–Q67.8)

- **Q76.0 Spina bifida occulta**
  - *Excludes1:* meningocele (spinal) (Q05.-)
  - spina bifida (aperta) (cystica) (Q05.-)
- **Q76.2 Congenital spondylolisthesis**
  - Congenital spondylolysis
  - *Excludes1:* spondylolisthesis (acquired) (M43.1-)
  - spondylolysis (acquired) (M43.0-)
- **Q76.3 Congenital scoliosis due to congenital bony malformation**
  - Hemivertebra fusion or failure of segmentation with scoliosis
- **Q76.4 Other congenital malformations of spine, not associated with scoliosis**
  - **5th**
  - **Q76.42 Congenital lordosis**
    - **5th**
    - **Q76.425 Congenital lordosis, thoracolumbar region**
    - **Q76.426 Congenital lordosis, lumbar region**
    - **Q76.427 Congenital lordosis, lumbosacral region**
    - **Q76.428 Congenital lordosis, sacral and sacrococcygeal region**
    - **Q76.429 Congenital lordosis, unspecified region**
  - **Q76.49 Other congenital malformations of spine, not associated with scoliosis**
    - Congenital absence of vertebra NOS
    - Congenital fusion of spine NOS
    - Congenital malformation of lumbosacral (joint) (region) NOS
    - Congenital malformation of spine NOS
    - Hemivertebra NOS
    - Malformation of spine NOS
    - Platyspondylisis NOS
    - Supernumerary vertebra NOS

Q77 OSTEOCHONDRODYSPLASIA WITH DEFECTS OF GROWTH OF TUBULAR BONES AND SPINE

4th

Excludes1: mucopolysaccharidosis (E76.0-E76.3)

Excludes2: congenital myotonic chondrodystrophy (G71.13)

- **Q77.0 Achondrogenesis**
  - Hypochondrogenesis
- **Q77.1 Thanatophoric short stature**
- **Q77.2 Short rib syndrome**
  - Asphyxiating thoracic dysplasia [Jeune]
- **Q77.3 Chondrodysplasia punctata**
  - *Excludes1:* Rhizomelic chondrodysplasia punctata (E71.43)
- **Q77.4 Achondroplasia**
  - Hypochondroplasia
  - Osteosclerosis congenita
- **Q77.5 Diastrophic dysplasia**
- **Q77.6 Chondroectodermal dysplasia**
  - Ellis-van Creveld syndrome
- **Q77.7 Spondyloepiphyseal dysplasia**
- **Q77.8 Other osteochondrodysplasia with defects of growth of tubular bones and spine**
- **Q77.9 Osteochondrodysplasia with defects of growth of tubular bones and spine, unspecified**

Q78 OTHER OSTEOCHONDRODYSPLASIAS

4th

Excludes2: congenital myotonic chondrodystrophy (G71.13)

- **Q78.0 Osteogenesis imperfecta**
  - Fragilitas ossium
  - Osteopsathyrosis
- **Q78.2 Osteopetrosis**
  - Albers-Schönberg syndrome
  - Osteosclerosis NOS
- **Q78.4 Enchondromatosis**
  - Maffucci's syndrome
  - Ollier's disease
- **Q78.8 Other specified osteochondrodysplasias**
  - Osteopoikilosis
- **Q78.9 Osteochondrodysplasia, unspecified**
  - Chondrodystrophy NOS
  - Osteodystrophy NOS

Q79 CONGENITAL MALFORMATIONS OF MUSCULOSKELETAL SYSTEM, NEC

4th

Excludes2: congenital (sternomastoid) torticollis (Q68.0)

- **Q79.0 Congenital diaphragmatic hernia**
  - *Excludes1:* congenital hiatus hernia (Q40.1)

4th **5th** **6th** **7th** Additional Character Required ✓ 3-character code

●=New Code *Excludes1*—Not coded here, do not use together
▲=Revised Code *Excludes2*—Not included here

Q79.1 Other congenital malformations of diaphragm
Absence of diaphragm
Congenital malformation of diaphragm NOS
Eventration of diaphragm

Q79.2 Exomphalos
Omphalocele
Excludes1: umbilical hernia (K42.-)

Q79.3 Gastroschisis

Q79.4 Prune belly syndrome
Congenital prolapse of bladder mucosa
Eagle-Barrett syndrome

Q79.5 Other congenital malformations of abdominal wall
Excludes1: umbilical hernia (K42.-)

Q79.51 Congenital hernia of bladder

Q79.59 Other congenital malformations of abdominal wall

Q79.6 Ehlers-Danlos syndromes

Q79.60 Ehlers-Danlos syndrome, unspecified

Q79.61 Classical Ehlers-Danlos syndrome
Classical EDS (cEDS)

Q79.62 Hypermobile Ehlers-Danlos syndrome
Hypermobile EDS (hEDS)

Q79.63 Vascular Ehlers-Danlos syndrome
Vascular EDS (vEDS)

Q79.69 Other Ehlers-Danlos syndromes

Q79.8 Other congenital malformations of musculoskeletal system
Absence of muscle
Absence of tendon
Accessory muscle
Amyotrophia congenita
Congenital constricting bands
Congenital shortening of tendon
Poland syndrome

Q79.9 Congenital malformation of musculoskeletal system, unspecified
Congenital anomaly of musculoskeletal system NOS
Congenital deformity of musculoskeletal system NOS

(Q80–Q89) OTHER CONGENITAL MALFORMATIONS

Q80 CONGENITAL ICHTHYOSIS
Excludes1: Refsum's disease (G60.1)

Q80.0 Ichthyosis vulgaris

Q80.1 X-linked ichthyosis

Q80.2 Lamellar ichthyosis
Collodion baby

Q80.3 Congenital bullous ichthyosiform erythroderma

Q80.4 Harlequin fetus

Q80.8 Other congenital ichthyosis

Q80.9 Congenital ichthyosis, unspecified

Q81 EPIDERMOLYSIS BULLOSA

Q81.0 Epidermolysis bullosa simplex
Excludes1: Cockayne's syndrome (Q87.19)

Q81.1 Epidermolysis bullosa letalis
Herlitz' syndrome

Q81.2 Epidermolysis bullosa dystrophica

Q81.8 Other epidermolysis bullosa

Q81.9 Epidermolysis bullosa, unspecified

Q82 OTHER CONGENITAL MALFORMATIONS OF SKIN
Excludes1: acrodermatitis enteropathica (E83.2)
congenital erythropoietic porphyria (E80.0)
pilonidal cyst or sinus (L05.-)
Sturge-Weber (-Dimitri) syndrome (Q85.8)

Q82.0 Hereditary lymphedema

Q82.1 Xeroderma pigmentosum

Q82.2 Congenital cutaneous mastocytosis
Congenital diffuse cutaneous mastocytosis
Congenital maculopapular cutaneous mastocytosis
Congenital urticaria pigmentosa

Excludes1: cutaneous mastocytosis NOS (D47.01)
diffuse cutaneous mastocytosis (with onset after newborn period) (D47.01)
malignant mastocytosis (C96.2-)
systemic mastocytosis (D47.02)
urticaria pigmentosa (non-congenital) (with onset after newborn period) (D47.01)

Q82.3 Incontinentia pigmenti

Q82.4 Ectodermal dysplasia (anhidrotic)
Excludes1: Ellis-van Creveld syndrome (Q77.6)

Q82.5 Congenital non-neoplastic nevus
Birthmark NOS
Flammeus nevus
Portwine nevus
Sanguineous nevus
Strawberry nevus
Vascular nevus NOS
Verrucous nevus
Excludes2: Café au lait spots (L81.3)
lentigo (L81.4)
nevus NOS (D22.-)
araneus nevus (I78.1)
melanocytic nevus (D22.-)
pigmented nevus (D22.-)
spider nevus (I78.1)
stellar nevus (I78.1)

Q82.6 Congenital sacral dimple
Parasacral dimple
Excludes2: pilonidal cyst with abscess (L05.01)
pilonidal cyst without abscess (L05.91)

Q82.8 Other specified congenital malformations of skin
Abnormal palmar creases
Accessory skin tags
Benign familial pemphigus [Hailey-Hailey]
Congenital poikiloderma
Cutis laxa (hyperelastica)
Dermatoglyphic anomalies
Inherited keratosis palmaris et plantaris
Keratosis follicularis [Darier-White]
Excludes1: Ehlers-Danlos syndromes (Q79.6-).

Q82.9 Congenital malformation of skin, unspecified

Q83 CONGENITAL MALFORMATIONS OF BREAST
Excludes2: absence of pectoral muscle (Q79.8)
hypoplasia of breast (N64.82)
micromastia (N64.82)

Q83.0 Congenital absence of breast with absent nipple

Q83.3 Accessory nipple
Supernumerary nipple

Q83.8 Other congenital malformations of breast

Q84 OTHER CONGENITAL MALFORMATIONS OF INTEGUMENT

Q84.2 Other congenital malformations of hair
Congenital hypertrichosis
Congenital malformation of hair NOS
Persistent lanugo

Q84.3 Anonychia
Excludes1: nail patella syndrome (Q87.2)

Q84.4 Congenital leukonychia

Q84.6 Other congenital malformations of nails
Congenital clubnail
Congenital koilonychia
Congenital malformation of nail NOS

Q84.8 Other specified congenital malformations of integument
Aplasia cutis congenita

Q84.9 Congenital malformation of integument, unspecified
Congenital anomaly of integument NOS
Congenital deformity of integument NOS

Q85 PHAKOMATOSES, NES
Excludes1: ataxia telangiectasia [Louis-Bar] (G11.3)
familial dysautonomia [Riley-Day] (G90.1)

Q85.0 Neurofibromatosis (nonmalignant)

Q85.00 Neurofibromatosis, unspecified

Q85.01 Neurofibromatosis, type 1
Von Recklinghausen disease
Q85.02 Neurofibromatosis, type 2
Acoustic neurofibromatosis
Q85.03 Schwannomatosis
Q85.09 Other neurofibromatosis
Q85.1 Tuberous sclerosis
Bourneville's disease
Epiloia
Q85.8 Other phakomatoses, NEC
Peutz-Jeghers syndrome
Sturge-Weber (-Dimitri) syndrome
von Hippel-Lindau syndrome
Excludes1: Meckel-Gruber syndrome (Q61.9)
Q85.81 **PTEN hamartoma tumor syndrome**
PHTS
PTEN related Cowden syndrome
Code also, if applicable, genetic susceptibility to malignant neoplasm (Z15.0-)
Q85.82 Other Cowden syndrome
Q85.83 Von Hippel-Lindau syndrome
Code also manifestations
Q85.89 Other phakomatoses, not elsewhere classified
Peutz-Jeghers syndrome
Sturge-Weber(-Dimitri) syndrome
Q85.9 Phakomatosis, unspecified
Hamartosis NOS

Q86 CONGENITAL MALFORMATION SYNDROMES DUE TO KNOWN EXOGENOUS CAUSES, NEC

Excludes2: iodine-deficiency-related hypothyroidism (E00-E02)
nonteratogenic effects of substances transmitted via placenta or breast milk (P04.-)

Q86.0 Fetal alcohol syndrome (dysmorphic)

Q87 OTHER SPECIFIED CONGENITAL MALFORMATION SYNDROMES AFFECTING MULTIPLE SYSTEMS

Use additional code(s) to identify all associated manifestations

Q87.0 Congenital malformation syndromes predominantly affecting facial appearance
Acrocephalopolysyndactyly
Acrocephalosyndactyly [Apert]
Cryptophthalmos syndrome
Cyclopia
Goldenhar syndrome
Moebius syndrome
Oro-facial-digital syndrome
Robin syndrome
Whistling face

Q87.1 Congenital malformation syndromes predominantly associated with short stature
Excludes1: Ellis-van Creveld syndrome (Q77.6)
Smith-Lemli-Opitz syndrome (E78.72)
Q87.11 Prader-Willi syndrome
Q87.19 Other congenital malformation syndromes predominantly associated with short stature
Aarskog syndrome
Cockayne syndrome
De Lange syndrome
Dubowitz syndrome
Noonan syndrome
Robinow-Silverman-Smith syndrome
Russell-Silver syndrome
Seckel syndrome

Q87.2 Congenital malformation syndromes predominantly involving limbs
Holt-Oram syndrome
Klippel-Trenaunay-Weber syndrome
Nail patella syndrome
Rubinstein-Taybi syndrome
Sirenomelia syndrome
TAR syndrome
VATER syndrome

Q87.3 Congenital malformation syndromes involving early overgrowth
Beckwith-Wiedemann syndrome
Sotos syndrome
Weaver syndrome

Q87.4 Marfan syndrome
Q87.40 Marfan syndrome, unspecified
Q87.41 Marfan syndrome with cardiovascular manifestations
Q87.410 Marfan syndrome with aortic dilation
Q87.418 Marfan syndrome with other cardiovascular manifestations
Q87.42 Marfan syndrome with ocular manifestations
Q87.43 Marfan syndrome with skeletal manifestation

Q87.8 Other specified congenital malformation syndromes, NEC
Excludes1: Zellweger syndrome (E71.510)
Q87.81 Alport syndrome
Use additional code to identify stage of CKD (N18.1-N18.6)
Q87.82 Arterial tortuosity syndrome
Q87.83 Bardet-Biedl syndrome
Q87.84 Laurence-Moon syndrome
Q87.85 MED13L syndrome
Asadollahi-Rauch syndrome
Mediator complex subunit 13L syndrome
Code also, if applicable, any associated manifestations such as:
autism spectrum disorder (F84.0-)
congenital malformations of cardiac septa (Q21.-)
epilepsy and recurrent seizures (G40.-)
intellectual disability (F70-F79)
●**Q87.86** Kleefstra syndrome
Q87.89 Other specified congenital malformation syndromes, not elsewhere classified

Q89 OTHER CONGENITAL MALFORMATIONS, NEC

Q89.0 Congenital absence and malformations of spleen
Excludes1: isomerism of atrial appendages (with asplenia or polysplenia) (Q20.6)
Q89.01 Asplenia (congenital)
Q89.09 Congenital malformations of spleen
Congenital splenomegaly

Q89.1 Congenital malformations of adrenal gland
Excludes1: adrenogenital disorders (E25.-)
congenital adrenal hyperplasia (E25.0)

Q89.2 Congenital malformations of other endocrine glands
Congenital malformation of parathyroid or thyroid gland
Persistent thyroglossal duct
Thyroglossal cyst
Excludes1: congenital goiter (E03.0)
congenital hypothyroidism (E03.1)

Q89.3 Situs inversus
Dextrocardia with situs inversus
Mirror-image atrial arrangement with situs inversus
Situs inversus or transversus abdominalis
Situs inversus or transversus thoracis
Transposition of abdominal viscera
Transposition of thoracic viscera
Excludes1: dextrocardia NOS (Q24.0)

Q89.7 Multiple congenital malformations, NEC
Multiple congenital anomalies NOS
Multiple congenital deformities NOS
Excludes1: congenital malformation syndromes affecting multiple systems (Q87.-)

Q89.8 Other specified congenital malformations
Use additional code(s) to identify all associated manifestations

Q89.9 Congenital malformation, unspecified
Congenital anomaly NOS
Congenital deformity NOS

(Q90–Q99) CHROMOSOMAL ABNORMALITIES, NEC

Excludes2: mitochondrial metabolic disorders (E88.4-)

Q90 DOWN SYNDROME

Code also associated physical condition(s), such as atrioventricular septal defect (Q21.2-)

Use additional code(s) to identify any associated degree of intellectual disabilities (F70–F79)

- Q90.0 Trisomy 21, nonmosaicism (meiotic nondisjunction)
- Q90.1 Trisomy 21, mosaicism (mitotic nondisjunction)
- Q90.2 Trisomy 21, translocation
- Q90.9 Down syndrome, unspecified
  - Trisomy 21 NOS

Q91 TRISOMY 18 AND TRISOMY 13

- Q91.0 Trisomy 18, nonmosaicism (meiotic nondisjunction)
- Q91.1 Trisomy 18, mosaicism (mitotic nondisjunction)
- Q91.2 Trisomy 18, translocation
- Q91.3 Trisomy 18, unspecified
- Q91.4 Trisomy 13, nonmosaicism (meiotic nondisjunction)
- Q91.5 Trisomy 13, mosaicism (mitotic nondisjunction)
- Q91.6 Trisomy 13, translocation
- Q91.7 Trisomy 13, unspecified

Q92 OTHER TRISOMIES AND PARTIAL TRISOMIES OF THE AUTOSOMES, NOT ELSEWHERE CLASSIFIED

Includes: unbalanced translocations and insertions

Excludes1: trisomies of chromosomes 13, 18, 21 (Q90-Q91)

- Q92.9 Trisomy and partial trisomy of autosomes, unspecified

Q93 MONOSOMIES AND DELETIONS FROM THE AUTOSOMES, NEC

- Q93.0 Whole chromosome monosomy, nonmosaicism (meiotic nondisjunction)
- Q93.1 Whole chromosome monosomy, mosaicism (mitotic nondisjunction)
- Q93.2 Chromosome replaced with ring, dicentric or isochromosome
- Q93.3 Deletion of short arm of chromosome 4
  - Wolff-Hirschhorn syndrome
- Q93.4 Deletion of short arm of chromosome 5
  - Cri-du-chat syndrome
- Q93.5 Other deletions of part of a chromosome
  - Q93.51 Angelman syndrome
  - Q93.52 Phelan-McDermid syndrome
    - 22q13.3 deletion syndrome
    - **Use additional** code(s) to identify any associated conditions, such as:
    - autism spectrum disorder (F84.0)
    - degree of intellectual disabilities (F70-F79)
    - epilepsy and recurrent seizures (G40.-)
    - lymphedema (I89.0)
  - Q93.59 Other deletions of part of a chromosome
- Q93.7 Deletions with other complex rearrangements
  - Deletions due to unbalanced translocations, inversions and insertions
  - **Code also any associated** duplications due to unbalanced translocations, inversions and insertions (Q92.5)
- Q93.8 Other deletions from the autosomes
  - Q93.81 Velo-cardio-facial syndrome
    - Deletion 22q11.2
  - Q93.82 Williams syndrome
  - Q93.88 Other microdeletions
    - Miller-Dieker syndrome
    - Smith-Magenis syndrome
  - Q93.89 Other deletions from the autosomes
    - Deletions identified by fluorescence in situ hybridization (FISH)
    - Deletions identified by in situ hybridization (ISH)
    - Deletions seen only at prometaphase
- Q93.9 Deletion from autosomes, unspecified

Q95 BALANCED REARRANGEMENTS AND STRUCTURAL MARKERS, NOT ELSEWHERE CLASSIFIED

Includes: Robertsonian and balanced reciprocal translocations and insertions

- Q95.0 Balanced translocation and insertion in normal individual
- Q95.9 Balanced rearrangement and structural marker, unspecified

Q96 TURNER'S SYNDROME

Excludes1: Noonan syndrome (Q87.19)

- Q96.0 Karyotype 45, X
- Q96.1 Karyotype 46, X iso (Xq)
  - Karyotype 46, isochromosome Xq
- Q96.2 Karyotype 46, X with abnormal sex chromosome, except iso (Xq)
  - Karyotype 46, X with abnormal sex chromosome, except isochromosome Xq
- Q96.3 Mosaicism, 45, X/46, XX or XY
- Q96.4 Mosaicism, 45, X/other cell line(s) with abnormal sex chromosome
- Q96.8 Other variants of Turner's syndrome
- Q96.9 Turner's syndrome, unspecified

Q97 OTHER SEX CHROMOSOME ABNORMALITIES, FEMALE PHENOTYPE, NEC

Excludes1: Turner's syndrome (Q96.-)

- Q97.0 Karyotype 47, XXX
- Q97.2 Mosaicism, lines with various numbers of X chromosomes
- Q97.8 Other specified sex chromosome abnormalities, female phenotype
- Q97.9 Sex chromosome abnormality, female phenotype, unspecified

Q98 OTHER SEX CHROMOSOME ABNORMALITIES, MALE PHENOTYPE, NEC

- Q98.3 Other male with 46, XX karyotype
- Q98.4 Klinefelter syndrome, unspecified
- Q98.5 Karyotype 47, XYY
- Q98.7 Male with sex chromosome mosaicism
- Q98.9 Sex chromosome abnormality, male phenotype, unspecified

Q99 OTHER CHROMOSOME ABNORMALITIES, NEC

- Q99.1 46, XX true hermaphrodite
  - 46, XX with streak gonads
  - 46, XY with streak gonads
  - Pure gonadal dysgenesis
- Q99.2 Fragile X chromosome
  - Fragile X syndrome
- Q99.8 Other specified chromosome abnormalities
- Q99.9 Chromosomal abnormality, unspecified

Chapter 18. Symptoms, signs, and abnormal clinical and laboratory findings, not elsewhere classified (R00–R99)

GUIDELINES

Chapter 18 includes symptoms, signs, abnormal results of clinical or other investigative procedures, and ill-defined conditions regarding which no diagnosis classifiable elsewhere is recorded. Signs and symptoms that point to a specific diagnosis have been assigned to a category in other chapters of the classification.

Use of symptom codes

Codes that describe symptoms and signs are acceptable for reporting purposes when a related definitive diagnosis has not been established (confirmed) by the provider.

Use of a symptom code with a definitive diagnosis code

Codes for signs and symptoms may be reported in addition to a related definitive diagnosis when the sign or symptom is not routinely associated with that diagnosis, such as the various signs and symptoms associated with complex syndromes. The definitive diagnosis code should be sequenced before the symptom code.

Signs or symptoms that are associated routinely with a disease process should not be assigned as additional codes, unless otherwise instructed by the classification.

Combination codes that include symptoms

ICD-10-CM contains a number of combination codes that identify both the definitive diagnosis and common symptoms of that diagnosis. When using one of these combination codes, an additional code should not be assigned for the symptom.

Repeated falls

Refer to the ICD-10-CM manual.

Coma

See code R40.2.

SIRS due to Non-Infectious Process

See codes R65.10-R65.11.

Death NOS

See category R99.

Note: This chapter includes symptoms, signs, abnormal results of clinical or other investigative procedures, and ill-defined conditions regarding which no diagnosis classifiable elsewhere is recorded.

Signs and symptoms that point rather definitely to a given diagnosis have been assigned to a category in other chapters of the classification. In general, categories in this chapter include the less well-defined conditions and symptoms that, without the necessary study of the case to establish a final diagnosis, point perhaps equally to two or more diseases or to two or more systems of the body. Practically all categories in the chapter could be designated 'not otherwise specified,' 'unknown etiology' or 'transient'. The Alphabetical Index should be consulted to determine which symptoms and signs are to be allocated here and which to other chapters. The residual subcategories, numbered .8, are generally provided for other relevant symptoms that cannot be allocated elsewhere in the classification.

The conditions and signs or symptoms included in categories R00–R94 consist of:

a) cases for which no more specific diagnosis can be made even after all the facts bearing on the case have been investigated;
b) signs or symptoms existing at the time of initial encounter that proved to be transient and whose causes could not be determined;
c) provisional diagnosis in a patient who failed to return for further investigation or care;
d) cases referred elsewhere for investigation or treatment before the diagnosis was made;
e) cases in which a more precise diagnosis was not available for any other reason;
f) certain symptoms, for which supplementary information is provided, that represent important problems in medical care in their own right.

Excludes2: abnormal findings on antenatal screening of mother (O28.-)
certain conditions originating in the perinatal period (P04–P96)
signs and symptoms classified in the body system chapters signs and symptoms of breast (N63, N64.5)

(R00–R09) SYMPTOMS AND SIGNS INVOLVING THE CIRCULATORY AND RESPIRATORY SYSTEMS

R00 ABNORMALITIES OF HEART BEAT

Excludes1: abnormalities originating in the perinatal period (P29.1-)
Excludes 2: specified arrhythmias (I47–I49)

R00.0 Tachycardia, unspecified
Rapid heart beat
Sinoauricular tachycardia NOS
Sinus [sinusal] tachycardia NOS
Excludes1: inappropriate sinus tachycardia, so stated (I47.11)
neonatal tachycardia (P29.11)
paroxysmal tachycardia (I47.-)

R00.1 Bradycardia, unspecified
Sinoatrial bradycardia
Sinus bradycardia
Slow heart beat
Vagal bradycardia
Use additional code for adverse effect, if applicable, to identify drug (T36–T50 with fifth or sixth character 5)
Excludes1: neonatal bradycardia (P29.12)

R00.2 Palpitations
Awareness of heart beat

R00.8 Other abnormalities of heart beat

R00.9 Unspecified abnormalities of heart beat

R01 CARDIAC MURMURS AND OTHER CARDIAC SOUNDS

Excludes1: cardiac murmurs and sounds originating in the perinatal period (P29.8)

R01.0 Benign and innocent cardiac murmurs
Functional cardiac murmur

R01.1 Cardiac murmur, unspecified
Cardiac bruit NOS
Heart murmur NOS
Systolic murmur NOS

R01.2 Other cardiac sounds
Cardiac dullness, increased or decreased
Precordial friction

R03 ABNORMAL BLOOD-PRESSURE READING, WITHOUT DIAGNOSIS

R03.0 Elevated blood-pressure reading, without diagnosis of hypertension
Note: This category is to be used to record an episode of elevated blood pressure in a patient in whom no formal diagnosis of hypertension has been made, or as an isolated incidental finding.

R03.1 Nonspecific low blood-pressure reading
Excludes1: hypotension (I95.-)
maternal hypotension syndrome (O26.5-)
neurogenic orthostatic hypotension (G90.3)

R04 HEMORRHAGE FROM RESPIRATORY PASSAGES

R04.0 Epistaxis
Hemorrhage from nose
Nosebleed

R04.2 Hemoptysis
Blood-stained sputum
Cough with hemorrhage

R04.8 Hemorrhage from other sites in respiratory passages

R04.81 Acute idiopathic pulmonary hemorrhage in infants
AIPHI
Acute idiopathic hemorrhage in infants over 28 days old
Excludes1: perinatal pulmonary hemorrhage (P26.-)
von Willebrand's disease (D68.0)

R04.89 Hemorrhage from other sites in respiratory passages
Pulmonary hemorrhage NOS

R04.9 Hemorrhage from respiratory passages, unspecified

R05 COUGH

4th

Excludes1: paroxysmal cough due to Bordetella pertussis (A37.0-)
smoker's cough (J41.0)

Excludes2: cough with hemorrhage (R04.2)

R05.1 Acute cough

R05.2 Subacute cough

R05.3 Chronic cough
Persistent cough
Refractory cough
Unexplained cough

R05.4 Cough syncope
Code first syncope and collapse (R55)

R05.8 Other specified cough

R05.9 Cough, unspecified

R06 ABNORMALITIES OF BREATHING

4th

Excludes1: acute respiratory distress syndrome (J80)
respiratory arrest (R09.2)
respiratory arrest of newborn (P28.81)
respiratory distress syndrome of newborn (P22.-)
respiratory failure (J96.-)
respiratory failure of newborn (P28.5)

R06.0 Dyspnea

5th

Excludes1: tachypnea NOS (R06.82)
transient tachypnea of newborn (P22.1)

R06.00 Dyspnea, unspecified

R06.01 Orthopnea

R06.02 Shortness of breath

R06.03 Acute respiratory distress

R06.1 Stridor

Excludes1: congenital laryngeal stridor (P28.89)
laryngismus (stridulus) (J38.5)

R06.2 Wheezing

Excludes1: Asthma (J45.-)

R06.3 Periodic breathing
Cheyne-Stokes breathing

R06.4 Hyperventilation

Excludes1: psychogenic hyperventilation (F45.8)

R06.5 Mouth breathing

Excludes2: dry mouth NOS (R68.2)

R06.6 Hiccough

Excludes1: psychogenic hiccough (F45.8)

R06.7 Sneezing

R06.8 Other abnormalities of breathing

5th

R06.81 Apnea, NEC
Apnea NOS
Excludes1: apnea (of) newborn (P28.4)
sleep apnea (G47.3-)
sleep apnea of newborn (primary) (P28.3)

R06.82 Tachypnea, NEC
Tachypnea NOS
Excludes1: transitory tachypnea of newborn (P22.1)

R06.83 Snoring

R06.89 Other abnormalities of breathing
Breath-holding (spells)
Sighing
Hypercapnia

R07 PAIN IN THROAT AND CHEST

4th

Excludes1: epidemic myalgia (B33.0)

Excludes2: jaw pain R68.84
pain in breast (N64.4)

R07.0 Pain in throat

Excludes1: chronic sore throat (J31.2)
sore throat (acute) NOS (J02.9)

Excludes2: dysphagia (R13.1-)
pain in neck (M54.2)

R07.1 Chest pain on breathing
Painful respiration

R07.8 Other chest pain

5th

R07.81 Pleurodynia
Pleurodynia NOS
Excludes1: epidemic pleurodynia (B33.0)

R07.82 Intercostal pain

R07.89 Other chest pain
Anterior chest-wall pain NOS

R07.9 Chest pain, unspecified

R09 OTHER SYMPTOMS AND SIGNS INVOLVING THE CIRCULATORY AND RESPIRATORY SYSTEM

4th

Excludes1: acute respiratory distress syndrome (J80)
respiratory arrest of newborn (P28.81)
respiratory distress syndrome of newborn (P22.0)
respiratory failure (J96.-)
respiratory failure of newborn (P28.5)

R09.0 Asphyxia and hypoxemia

5th

Excludes1: asphyxia due to carbon monoxide (T58.-)
asphyxia due to FB in respiratory tract (T17.-)
birth (intrauterine) asphyxia (P84)
hyperventilation (R06.4)
traumatic asphyxia (T71.-)

Excludes 2: hypercapnia (R06.89)

R09.01 Asphyxia

R09.02 Hypoxemia

R09.1 Pleurisy

Excludes1: pleurisy with effusion (J90)

R09.2 Respiratory arrest
Cardiorespiratory failure
Excludes1: cardiac arrest (I46.-)
respiratory arrest of newborn (P28.81)
respiratory distress of newborn (P22.0)
respiratory failure (J96.-)
respiratory failure of newborn (P28.5)
respiratory insufficiency (R06.89)
respiratory insufficiency of newborn (P28.5)

R09.3 Abnormal sputum
Abnormal amount of sputum
Abnormal color of sputum
Abnormal odor of sputum
Excessive sputum
Excludes1: blood-stained sputum (R04.2)

R09.8 Other specified symptoms and signs involving the circulatory and respiratory systems

5th

R09.81 Nasal congestion

R09.82 Postnasal drip

R09.89 Other specified symptoms and signs involving the circulatory and respiratory systems
Bruit (arterial)
Abnormal chest percussion
Friction sounds in chest
Chest tympany
Choking sensation
Rales
Weak pulse
Excludes2: FB in throat (T17.2-)
wheezing (R06.2)

R09.A Foreign body sensation of the circulatory and respiratory system

5th

R09.A0 Foreign body sensation, unspecified

R09.A1 Foreign body sensation, nose

R09.A2 Foreign body sensation, throat
Foreign body sensation globus

R09.A9 Foreign body sensation, other site

(R10–R19) SYMPTOMS AND SIGNS INVOLVING THE DIGESTIVE SYSTEM AND ABDOMEN

Excludes2: congenital or infantile pylorospasm (Q40.0)
gastrointestinal hemorrhage (K92.0–K92.2)
intestinal obstruction (K56.-)
newborn gastrointestinal hemorrhage (P54.0–P54.3)
newborn intestinal obstruction (P76.-)
pylorospasm (K31.3)
signs and symptoms involving the urinary system (R30–R39)
symptoms referable to female genital organs (N94.-)
symptoms referable to male genital organs male (N48–N50)

R10 ABDOMINAL AND PELVIC PAIN

Excludes1: renal colic (N23)

Excludes2: dorsalgia (M54.-)

flatulence and related conditions (R14.-)

R10.0 Acute abdomen

Severe abdominal pain (generalized) (with abdominal rigidity)

Excludes1: abdominal rigidity NOS (R19.3)

generalized abdominal pain NOS (R10.84)

localized abdominal pain (R10.1-R10.3-)

R10.1 Pain localized to upper abdomen

R10.10 Upper abdominal pain, unspecified

R10.11 RUQ pain

R10.12 LUQ pain

R10.13 Epigastric pain

Dyspepsia

Excludes1: functional dyspepsia (K30)

R10.2 Pelvic and perineal pain

Excludes1: vulvodynia (N94.81)

R10.3 Pain localized to other parts of lower abdomen

R10.30 Lower abdominal pain, unspecified

R10.31 RLQ pain

R10.32 LLQ pain

R10.33 Periumbilical pain

R10.8 Other abdominal pain

R10.81 Abdominal tenderness

Abdominal tenderness NOS

R10.811 RUQ abdominal tenderness

R10.812 LUQ abdominal tenderness

R10.813 RLQ abdominal tenderness

R10.814 LLQ abdominal tenderness

R10.815 Periumbilic abdominal tenderness

R10.816 Epigastric abdominal tenderness

R10.817 Generalized abdominal tenderness

R10.819 Abdominal tenderness, unspecified site

R10.82 Rebound abdominal tenderness

R10.821 RUQ rebound abdominal tenderness

R10.822 LUQ rebound abdominal tenderness

R10.823 RLQ rebound abdominal tenderness

R10.824 LLQ rebound abdominal tenderness

R10.825 Periumbilic rebound abdominal tenderness

R10.826 Epigastric rebound abdominal tenderness

R10.827 Generalized rebound abdominal tenderness

R10.829 Rebound abdominal tenderness, unspecified site

R10.83 Colic

Colic NOS

Infantile colic

Excludes1: colic in adult and child over 12 months old (R10.84)

R10.84 Generalized abdominal pain

Excludes1: generalized abdominal pain associated with acute abdomen (R10.0)

R10.9 Unspecified abdominal pain

R11 NAUSEA AND VOMITING

Excludes1: cyclical vomiting associated with migraine (G43.A-)

excessive vomiting in pregnancy (O21.-)

hematemesis (K92.0)

neonatal hematemesis (P54.0)

newborn vomiting (P92.0-)

psychogenic vomiting (F50.89)

vomiting associated with bulimia nervosa (F50.2-)

vomiting following gastrointestinal surgery (K91.0)

R11.0 Nausea

Nausea NOS

Nausea without vomiting

R11.1 Vomiting

R11.10 Vomiting, unspecified

Vomiting NOS

R11.11 Vomiting without nausea

R11.12 Projectile vomiting

R11.13 Vomiting of fecal matter

R11.14 Bilious vomiting

Bilious emesis

R11.15 Cyclical vomiting syndrome unrelated to migraine

Cyclic vomiting syndrome NOS

Persistent vomiting

Excludes1: cyclical vomiting in migraine (G43.A-)

Excludes2: bulimia nervosa (F50.20)

diabetes mellitus due to underlying condition (E08.-)

R11.2 Nausea with vomiting, unspecified

Persistent nausea with vomiting NOS

R12 HEARTBURN

Excludes1: dyspepsia NOS (R10.13)

functional dyspepsia (K30)

R13 APHAGIA AND DYSPHAGIA

R13.0 Aphagia

Inability to swallow

Excludes1: psychogenic aphagia (F50.9)

R13.1 Dysphagia

Code first, if applicable, dysphagia following cerebrovascular disease (I69. with final characters -91)

Excludes1: psychogenic dysphagia (F45.8)

R13.10 Dysphagia, unspecified

Difficulty in swallowing NOS

R13.11 Dysphagia, oral phase

R13.12 Dysphagia, oropharyngeal phase

R13.13 Dysphagia, pharyngeal phase

R13.14 Dysphagia, pharyngoesophageal phase

R13.19 Other dysphagia

Cervical dysphagia

Neurogenic dysphagia

R14 FLATULENCE AND RELATED CONDITIONS

Excludes1: psychogenic aerophagy (F45.8)

R14.0 Abdominal distension (gaseous)

Bloating

Tympanites (abdominal) (intestinal)

R14.1 Gas pain

R14.2 Eructation

R14.3 Flatulence

R15 FECAL INCONTINENCE

Includes: encopresis NOS

Excludes1: fecal incontinence of nonorganic origin (F98.1)

R15.0 Incomplete defecation

Excludes1: constipation (K59.0-)

fecal impaction (K56.41)

R15.1 Fecal smearing

Fecal soiling

R15.2 Fecal urgency

R15.9 Full incontinence of feces

Fecal incontinence NOS

R16 HEPATOMEGALY AND SPLENOMEGALY, NEC

R16.0 Hepatomegaly, NEC

Hepatomegaly NOS

R16.1 Splenomegaly, NEC

Splenomegaly NOS

R16.2 Hepatomegaly with splenomegaly, NEC

Hepatosplenomegaly NOS

R17 UNSPECIFIED JAUNDICE

Excludes1: neonatal jaundice (P55, P57–P59)

R18 ASCITES

Includes: fluid in peritoneal cavity

Excludes1: ascites in alcoholic cirrhosis (K70.31)

ascites in alcoholic hepatitis (K70.11)

ascites in toxic liver disease with chronic active hepatitis (K71.51)

R18.0 Malignant ascites

Code first malignancy, such as: malignant neoplasm of ovary (C56.-)

secondary malignant neoplasm of retroperitoneum and peritoneum (C78.6)

R18.8 Other ascites
Ascites NOS
Peritoneal effusion (chronic)

R19 OTHER SYMPTOMS AND SIGNS INVOLVING THE DIGESTIVE SYSTEM AND ABDOMEN

4th

Excludes1: acute abdomen (R10.0)

R19.0 Intra-abdominal and pelvic swelling, mass and lump

5th *Excludes1:* abdominal distension (gaseous) (R14.-)
ascites (R18.-)

R19.00 Intra-abdominal and pelvic swelling, mass and lump, unspecified site

R19.01 RUQ abdominal swelling, mass and lump

R19.02 LUQ abdominal swelling, mass and lump

R19.03 RLQ abdominal swelling, mass and lump

R19.04 LLQ abdominal swelling, mass and lump

R19.05 Periumbiltic swelling, mass or lump
Diffuse or generalized umbilical swelling or mass

R19.06 Epigastric swelling, mass or lump

R19.07 Generalized intra-abdominal and pelvic swelling, mass and lump
Diffuse or generalized intra-abdominal swelling or mass NOS
Diffuse or generalized pelvic swelling or mass NOS

R19.09 Other intra-abdominal and pelvic swelling, mass and lump

R19.1 Abnormal bowel sounds

5th

R19.11 Absent bowel sounds

R19.12 Hyperactive bowel sounds

R19.15 Other abnormal bowel sounds
Abnormal bowel sounds NOS

R19.2 Visible peristalsis
Hyperperistalsis

R19.3 Abdominal rigidity

5th *Excludes1:* abdominal rigidity with severe abdominal pain (R10.0)

R19.30 Abdominal rigidity, unspecified site

R19.31 RUQ abdominal rigidity

R19.32 LUQ abdominal rigidity

R19.33 RLQ abdominal rigidity

R19.34 LLQ abdominal rigidity

R19.35 Periumbiltic abdominal rigidity

R19.36 Epigastric abdominal rigidity

R19.37 Generalized abdominal rigidity

R19.4 Change in bowel habit
Excludes1: constipation (K59.0-)
functional diarrhea (K59.1)

R19.5 Other fecal abnormalities
Abnormal stool color
Bulky stools
Mucus in stools
Occult blood in feces
Occult blood in stools
Excludes1: melena (K92.1)
neonatal melena (P54.1)

R19.6 Halitosis

R19.7 Diarrhea, unspecified
Diarrhea NOS
Excludes1: functional diarrhea (K59.1)
neonatal diarrhea (P78.3)
psychogenic diarrhea (F45.8)

R19.8 Other specified symptoms and signs involving the digestive system and abdomen

(R20–R23) SYMPTOMS AND SIGNS INVOLVING THE SKIN AND SUBCUTANEOUS TISSUE

Excludes2: symptoms relating to breast (N64.4–N64.5)

R20 DISTURBANCES OF SKIN SENSATION

4th *Excludes1:* dissociative anesthesia and sensory loss (F44.6)
psychogenic disturbances (F45.8)

R20.0 Anesthesia of skin

R20.1 Hypoesthesia of skin

R20.2 Paresthesia of skin
Formication
Pins and needles
Tingling skin
Excludes1: acroparesthesia (I73.8)

R20.3 Hyperesthesia

R20.8 Other disturbances of skin sensation

R20.9 Unspecified disturbances of skin sensation

R21 RASH AND OTHER NONSPECIFIC SKIN ERUPTION

✔ *Includes:* rash NOS
Excludes1: specified type of rash — code to condition
vesicular eruption (R23.8)

R22 LOCALIZED SWELLING, MASS AND LUMP OF SKIN AND SUBCUTANEOUS TISSUE

4th

Includes: subcutaneous nodules (localized)(superficial)
Excludes1: abnormal findings on diagnostic imaging (R90–R93)
edema (R60.-)
enlarged lymph nodes (R59.-)
localized adiposity (E65)
swelling of joint (M25.4-)

R22.0 Localized swelling, mass and lump; head

R22.1 neck

R22.2 trunk
Excludes1: intra-abdominal or pelvic mass and lump (R19.0-)
intra-abdominal or pelvic swelling (R19.0-)
Excludes2: breast mass and lump (N63)

R22.3 Localized swelling, mass and lump, upper limb

5th

R22.31 Localized swelling, mass and lump; right upper limb

R22.32 left upper limb

R22.33 upper limb, bilateral

R22.4 Localized swelling, mass and lump, lower limb

5th

R22.41 Localized swelling, mass and lump; right lower limb

R22.42 left lower limb

R22.43 lower limb, bilateral

R22.9 Localized swelling, mass and lump, unspecified

R23 OTHER SKIN CHANGES

4th

R23.0 Cyanosis
Excludes1: acrocyanosis (I73.8)
cyanotic attacks of newborn (P28.2)

R23.1 Pallor
Clammy skin

R23.2 Flushing
Excessive blushing
Code first, if applicable, menopausal and female climacteric states (N95.1)

R23.3 Spontaneous ecchymoses
Petechiae
Excludes1: ecchymoses of newborn (P54.5)
purpura (D69.-)

R23.8 Other skin changes

R23.9 Unspecified skin changes

(R25–R29) SYMPTOMS AND SIGNS INVOLVING THE NERVOUS AND MUSCULOSKELETAL SYSTEMS

R25 ABNORMAL INVOLUNTARY MOVEMENTS

4th *Excludes1:* specific movement disorders (G20–G26)
stereotyped movement disorders (F98.4)
tic disorders (F95.-)

R25.0 Abnormal head movements

R25.1 Tremor, unspecified
Excludes1: chorea NOS (G25.5)
essential tremor (G25.0)
hysterical tremor (F44.4)
intention tremor (G25.2)

R25.2 Cramp and spasm
Excludes2: carpopedal spasm (R29.0)
charley-horse (M62.831)
infantile spasms (G40.4-)
muscle spasm of back (M62.830)
muscle spasm of calf (M62.831)

R25.8 Other abnormal involuntary movements
R25.9 Unspecified abnormal involuntary movements

R26 ABNORMALITIES OF GAIT AND MOBILITY

Excludes1: ataxia NOS (R27.0)
hereditary ataxia (G11.-)
locomotor (syphilitic) ataxia (A52.11)
immobility syndrome (paraplegic) (M62.3)

R26.0 Ataxic gait
Staggering gait

R26.1 Paralytic gait
Spastic gait

R26.2 Difficulty in walking, NEC
Excludes1: falling (R29.6)
unsteadiness on feet (R26.81)

R26.8 Other abnormalities of gait and mobility
R26.81 Unsteadiness on feet
R26.89 Other abnormalities of gait and mobility

R26.9 Unspecified abnormalities of gait and mobility

R27 OTHER LACK OF COORDINATION

Excludes1: ataxic gait (R26.0)
hereditary ataxia (G11.-)
vertigo NOS (R42)

R27.0 Ataxia, unspecified
Excludes1: ataxia following cerebrovascular disease (I69. with final characters -93)

R27.8 Other lack of coordination

R27.9 Unspecified lack of coordination

R29 OTHER SYMPTOMS AND SIGNS INVOLVING THE NERVOUS AND MUSCULOSKELETAL SYSTEMS

R29.0 Tetany
Carpopedal spasm
Excludes1: hysterical tetany (F44.5)
neonatal tetany (P71.3)
parathyroid tetany (E20.9)
post-thyroidectomy tetany (E89.2)

R29.1 Meningismus

R29.2 Abnormal reflex
Excludes2: abnormal pupillary reflex (H57.0)
hyperactive gag reflex (J39.2)
vasovagal reaction or syncope (R55)

R29.3 Abnormal posture

R29.4 Clicking hip
Excludes1: congenital deformities of hip (Q65.-)

R29.8 Other symptoms and signs involving the nervous and musculoskeletal systems

R29.81 Other symptoms and signs involving the nervous system

R29.810 Facial weakness
Facial droop

R29.818 Other symptoms and signs involving the nervous system

R29.89 Other symptoms and signs involving the musculoskeletal system
Excludes2: pain in limb (M79.6-)

R29.891 Ocular torticollis
Excludes1: congenital (sternomastoid) torticollis Q68.0
psychogenic torticollis (F45.8)
spasmodic torticollis (G24.3)
torticollis due to birth injury (P15.8)
torticollis NOS M43.6

R29.898 Other symptoms and signs involving the musculoskeletal system

R29.9 Unspecified symptoms and signs involving the; nervous and musculoskeletal systems

R29.90 Nervous system
R29.91 Musculoskeletal system

(R30–R39) SYMPTOMS AND SIGNS INVOLVING THE GENITOURINARY SYSTEM

R30 PAIN ASSOCIATED WITH MICTURITION

Excludes1: psychogenic pain associated with micturition (F45.8)

R30.0 Dysuria
Strangury

R30.9 Painful micturition, unspecified
Painful urination NOS

R31 HEMATURIA

Excludes1: hematuria included with underlying conditions, such as:
acute cystitis with hematuria (N30.01)
recurrent and persistent hematuria in glomerular diseases (N02.-)

R31.0 Gross hematuria

R31.1 Benign essential microscopic hematuria

R31.2 Other microscopic hematuria

R31.21 Asymptomatic microscopic hematuria
R31.29 Other microscopic hematuria

R31.9 Hematuria, unspecified

R32 UNSPECIFIED URINARY INCONTINENCE

Enuresis NOS
Excludes1: functional urinary incontinence (R39.81)
nonorganic enuresis (F98.0)
stress incontinence and other specified urinary incontinence (N39.3–N39.4-)
urinary incontinence associated with cognitive impairment (R39.81)

R33 RETENTION OF URINE

Excludes1: psychogenic retention of urine (F45.8)

R33.8 Other retention of urine
Code first, if applicable, any causal condition, such as: enlarged prostate (N40.1)

R33.9 Retention of urine, unspecified

R34 ANURIA AND OLIGURIA

Excludes1: anuria and oliguria complicating abortion or ectopic or molar pregnancy (O00–O07, O08.4)
anuria and oliguria complicating pregnancy (O26.83-)
anuria and oliguria complicating the puerperium (O90.49)

R35 POLYURIA

Code first, if applicable, any causal condition, such as: enlarged prostate (N40.1)
Excludes1: psychogenic polyuria (F45.8)

R35.0 Frequency of micturition

R35.1 Nocturia

R35.8 Other polyuria

R35.81 Nocturnal polyuria
Excludes2: nocturnal enuresis (N39.44)

R35.89 Other polyuria
Polyuria NOS

R36 URETHRAL DISCHARGE

R36.0 Urethral discharge without blood

R36.1 Hematospermia

R36.9 Urethral discharge, unspecified
Penile discharge NOS
Urethrorrhea

R37 SEXUAL DYSFUNCTION, UNSPECIFIED

R39 OTHER AND UNSPECIFIED SYMPTOMS AND SIGNS INVOLVING THE GENITOURINARY SYSTEM

R39.0 Extravasation of urine

R39.1 Other difficulties with micturition
Code first, if applicable, any causal condition, such as: enlarged prostate (N40.1)

R39.11 Hesitancy of micturition
R39.12 Poor urinary stream
Weak urinary steam
R39.13 Splitting of urinary stream
R39.14 Feeling of incomplete bladder emptying
R39.15 Urgency of urination
Excludes1: urge incontinence (N39.41, N39.46)

R39.16 Straining to void
R39.19 Other difficulties with micturition
- **R39.191** Need to immediately re-void
- **R39.192** Position dependent micturition
- **R39.198** Other difficulties with micturition

R39.8 Other symptoms and signs involving the genitourinary system
- **R39.81** Functional urinary incontinence
- **R39.82** Chronic bladder pain
- **R39.83** Unilateral non-palpable testicle
- **R39.84** Bilateral non-palpable testicles
- **R39.89** Other symptoms and signs involving the genitourinary system

R39.9 Unspecified symptoms and signs involving the genitourinary system

(R40–R46) SYMPTOMS AND SIGNS INVOLVING COGNITION, PERCEPTION, EMOTIONAL STATE AND BEHAVIOR

Excludes2: symptoms and signs constituting part of a pattern of mental disorder (F01–F99)

R40 SOMNOLENCE, STUPOR AND COMA

Excludes1: neonatal coma (P91.5)
somnolence, stupor and coma in diabetes (E08–E13)
somnolence, stupor and coma in hepatic failure (K72.-)
somnolence, stupor and coma in hypoglycemia (nondiabetic) (E15)

R40.0 Somnolence
Drowsiness
Excludes1: coma (R40.2-)

R40.1 Stupor
Catatonic stupor
Semicoma
Excludes1: catatonic schizophrenia (F20.2)
coma (R40.2-)
depressive stupor (F31–F33)
dissociative stupor (F44.2)
manic stupor (F30.2)

R40.2 Coma

GUIDELINES

Code R40.20, Unspecified coma, **should** be assigned **when the underlying cause of the coma is not known, or the cause is a traumatic brain injury and the coma scale is not documented in the medical record.**

Do not report codes for unspecified coma, individual or total Glasgow coma scale scores for a patient with a medically induced coma or a sedated patient.

Coma Scale
The coma scale codes R40.21- to R40.24- can be used in conjunction with traumatic brain injury codes. These codes **cannot be used with code R40.2A, Nontraumatic coma due to underlying condition. They** are primarily for use by trauma registries, but they may be used in any setting where this information is collected. The coma scale codes should be sequenced after the diagnosis code(s).

These codes, one from each subcategory, are needed to complete the scale. The 7th character indicates when the scale was recorded. The 7th character should match for all three codes.

At a minimum, report the initial score documented on presentation at your facility. This may be a score from the emergency medicine technician (EMT) or in the emergency department. If desired, a facility may choose to capture multiple coma scale scores.

Assign code R40.24, Glasgow coma scale, total score, when only the total score is documented in the medical record and not the individual score(s). **If multiple coma scores are captured within the first 24 hours after hospital admission, assign only the code for the score at the time of admission. ICD-10-CM does not classify coma scores that are reported after admission but less than 24 hours later.**

See *ICD-10-CM* Official Guidelines for Coding and Reporting FY 2024 in front matter, "Documentation by Clinicians Other than the Patient's Provider," for coma scale documentation by clinicians other than the patient's provider.

Code **first** any associated: fracture of skull (S02.-)
intracranial injury (S06.-)

Note: One code from each subcategory R40.21–R40.23 is required to complete the coma scale

R40.20 Unspecified coma
Coma NOS
Unconsciousness NOS

R40.21 Coma scale, eyes open

R40.21 requires a 7th character:
0–unspecified time
1–in the field [EMT/ambulance]
2–at arrival to ED
3–at hospital admission
4–24 hours or more after hospital admission

- **R40.211-** Coma scale, eyes open, never
Coma scale eye opening score of 1
- **R40.212-** Coma scale, eyes open, to pain
Coma scale eye opening score of 2
- **R40.213-** Coma scale, eyes open, to sound
Coma scale eye opening score of 3
- **R40.214-** Coma scale, eyes open, spontaneous
Coma scale eye opening score of 4

R40.22 Coma scale, best verbal response

R40.22 requires a 7th character:
0–unspecified time
1–in the field [EMT/ambulance]
2–at arrival to ED
3–at hospital admission
4–24 hours or more after hospital admission

- **R40.221-** Coma scale, best verbal response, none
Coma scale verbal score of 1
- **R40.222-** Coma scale, best verbal response, incomprehensible words
Coma scale verbal score of 2
Incomprehensible sounds (2–5 years of age)
Moans/grunts to pain; restless (<2 years old)
- **R40.223-** Coma scale, best verbal response, inappropriate words
Coma scale verbal score of 3
Inappropriate crying or screaming (< 2 years of age)
Screaming (2–5 years of age)
- **R40.224-** Coma scale, best verbal response, confused conversation
Coma scale verbal score of 4
Inappropriate words (2–5 years of age)
Irritable cries (< 2 years of age)
- **R40.225-** Coma scale, best verbal response, oriented
Coma scale verbal score of 5
Cooing or babbling or crying appropriately (< 2 years of age)
Uses appropriate words (2–5 years of age)

R40.23 Coma scale, best motor response

R40.23 requires a 7th character:
0–unspecified time
1–in the field [EMT/ambulance]
2–at arrival to ED
3–at hospital admission
4–24 hours or more after hospital admission

- **R40.231-** Coma scale, best motor response, none
Coma scale motor score of 1
- **R40.232-** Coma scale, best motor response, extension
Coma scale motor score of 2
Abnormal extensor posturing to pain or noxious stimuli (< 2 years of age)
Extensor posturing to pain or noxious stimuli (2–5 years of age)
- **R40.233-** Coma scale, best motor response, abnormal
Coma scale motor score of 3
Abnormal flexure posturing to pain or noxious stimuli (0–5 years of age)
Flexion/decorticate posturing (< 2 years of age)

R40.234- Coma scale, best motor response, flexion withdrawal
Coma scale motor score of 4
Withdraws from pain or noxious stimuli (0-5 years of age)

R40.235- Coma scale, best motor response, localizes pain
Coma scale motor score of 5
Localizes pain (2-5 years of age)
Withdraws to touch (< 2 years of age)

R40.236- Coma scale, best motor response, obeys commands
Coma scale motor score of 6
Normal or spontaneous movement (< 2 years of age)
Obeys commands (2-5 years of age)

R40.24 Glasgow coma scale, total score
Note: Assign a code from subcategory R40.24, when only the total coma score is documented

R40.241- Glasgow coma scale score 13-15

R40.242- Glasgow coma scale score 9-12

R40.243- Glasgow coma scale score 3-8

R40.244- Other coma, without documented Glasgow coma scale score, or with partial score reported

R40.2A Nontraumatic coma due to underlying condition
Secondary coma
Code first underlying condition

R40.3 Persistent vegetative state

R41 OTHER SYMPTOMS AND SIGNS INVOLVING COGNITIVE FUNCTIONS AND AWARENESS

Excludes1: dissociative [conversion] disorders (F44.-)
mild cognitive impairment of uncertain or unknown etiology (G31.84)

R41.0 Disorientation, unspecified
Confusion NOS
Delirium NOS
Excludes1: delirium due to known physiological condition (F05)

R41.8 Other symptoms and signs involving cognitive functions and awareness

R41.81 Age-related cognitive decline
Senility NOS

R41.82 Altered mental status, unspecified
Change in mental status NOS
Excludes1: altered level of consciousness (R40.-)
altered mental status due to known condition—code to condition
delirium NOS (R41.0)

R41.83 Borderline intellectual functioning
IQ level 71 to 84
Excludes1: intellectual disabilities (F70-F79)

R41.84 Other specified cognitive deficit
Code first the underlying condition, if known, such as:
schizophrenia (F20.-)
Excludes1: cognitive deficits as sequelae of cerebrovascular disease (I69.01-, I69.11-, I69.21-, I69.31-, I69.81-, I69.91-)

R41.840 Attention and concentration deficit
Excludes1: attention-deficit hyperactivity disorders (F90.-)

R41.841 Cognitive communication deficit

R41.842 Visuospatial deficit

R41.843 Psychomotor deficit

R41.844 Frontal lobe and executive function deficit

●**R41.85 Anosognosia**

R41.89 Other symptoms and signs involving cognitive functions and awareness

R41.9 Unspecified symptoms and signs involving cognitive functions and awareness
Unspecified neurocognitive disorder

R42 DIZZINESS AND GIDDINESS

Light-headedness
Vertigo NOS
Excludes1: vertiginous syndromes (H81.-)
vertigo from infrasound (T75.23)

R43 DISTURBANCES OF SMELL AND TASTE

R43.0 Anosmia

R43.1 Parosmia

R43.2 Parageusia

R43.8 Other disturbances of smell and taste
Mixed disturbance of smell and taste

R43.9 Unspecified disturbances of smell and taste

R44 OTHER SYMPTOMS AND SIGNS INVOLVING GENERAL SENSATIONS AND PERCEPTIONS

Excludes1: alcoholic hallucinations (F10.151, F10.251, F10.951)
hallucinations in drug psychosis (F11-F19 with fifth to sixth characters 51)
hallucinations in mood disorders with psychotic symptoms (F30.2, F31.5, F32.3, F33.3)
hallucinations in schizophrenia, schizotypal and delusional disorders (F20-F29)
Excludes2: disturbances of skin sensation (R20.-)

R44.0 Auditory hallucinations

R44.1 Visual hallucinations

R44.2 Other hallucinations

R44.3 Hallucinations, unspecified

R44.8 Other symptoms and signs involving general sensations and perceptions

R44.9 Unspecified symptoms and signs involving general sensations and perceptions

R45 SYMPTOMS AND SIGNS INVOLVING EMOTIONAL STATE

R45.0 Nervousness
Nervous tension

R45.1 Restlessness and agitation

R45.2 Unhappiness

R45.3 Demoralization and apathy
Excludes1: anhedonia (R45.84)

R45.4 Irritability and anger

R45.5 Hostility

R45.6 Violent behavior

R45.7 State of emotional shock and stress, unspecified

R45.8 Other symptoms and signs involving emotional state

R45.81 Low self-esteem

R45.82 Worries

R45.83 Excessive crying of child, adolescent or adult
Excludes1: excessive crying of infant (baby) R68.11

R45.84 Anhedonia

R45.85 Homicidal and suicidal ideations
Excludes1: suicide attempt (T14.91)

R45.850 Homicidal ideations

R45.851 Suicidal ideations

R45.86 Emotional lability

R45.87 Impulsiveness

R45.88 Nonsuicidal self-harm
Nonsuicidal self-injury
Nonsuicidal self-mutilation
Self-inflicted injury without suicidal intent
Code also injury, if known

R45.89 Other symptoms and signs involving emotional state
Flat affect
Loneliness

R46 SYMPTOMS AND SIGNS INVOLVING APPEARANCE AND BEHAVIOR

4th

Excludes1: appearance and behavior in schizophrenia, schizotypal and delusional disorders (F20–F29)
mental and behavioral disorders (F01– F99)

- **R46.0** Very low level of personal hygiene
- **R46.1** Bizarre personal appearance
- **R46.2** Strange and inexplicable behavior
- **R46.3** Overactivity
- **R46.4** Slowness and poor responsiveness
  - **Excludes 1:** stupor (R40.1)
- **R46.5** Suspiciousness and marked evasiveness
- **R46.6** Undue concern and preoccupation with stressful events
- **R46.7** Verbosity and circumstantial detail obscuring reason for contact
- **R46.8** Other symptoms and signs involving appearance and behavior
  - 5th
  - **R46.81** Obsessive-compulsive behavior
    - obsessive-compulsive disorder (F42.-)
  - **R46.89** Other symptoms and signs involving appearance and behavior

(R47–R49) SYMPTOMS AND SIGNS INVOLVING SPEECH AND VOICE

R47 SPEECH DISTURBANCES, NEC

4th

Excludes1: autism (F84.0)
cluttering (F80.81)
specific developmental disorders of speech and language (F80.-)
stuttering (F80.81)

- **R47.1** Dysarthria and anarthria
  - **Excludes1:** dysarthria following cerebrovascular disease (I69. with final characters -22)
- **R47.8** Other speech disturbances
  - 5th
  - **Excludes1:** dysarthria following cerebrovascular disease (I69. with final characters -28)
  - **R47.81** Slurred speech
  - **R47.82** Fluency disorder in conditions classified elsewhere
    - Stuttering in conditions classified elsewhere
    - **Code first** underlying disease or condition, such as:
    - Parkinson's disease (G20.-)
    - **Excludes1:** adult onset fluency disorder (F98.5)
    - childhood onset fluency disorder (F80.81)
    - fluency disorder (stuttering) following cerebrovascular disease (I69. with final characters -23)
  - **R47.89** Other speech disturbances
- **R47.9** Unspecified speech disturbances

R48 DYSLEXIA AND OTHER SYMBOLIC DYSFUNCTIONS, NEC

4th

Excludes1: specific developmental disorders of scholastic skills (F81.-)

- **R48.0** Dyslexia and alexia
- **R48.1** Agnosia
  - Astereognosia (astereognosis)
  - Autotopagnosia
  - **Excludes1:** visual object agnosia (R48.3)
- **R48.8** Other symbolic dysfunctions
  - Acalculia
  - Agraphia
- **R48.9** Unspecified symbolic dysfunctions

R49 VOICE AND RESONANCE DISORDERS

4th

Excludes1: psychogenic voice and resonance disorders (F44.4)

- **R49.0** Dysphonia
  - Hoarseness
- **R49.1** Aphonia
  - Loss of voice
- **R49.2** Hypernasality and hyponasality
  - 5th
  - **R49.21** Hypernasality
  - **R49.22** Hyponasality
- **R49.8** Other voice and resonance disorders
- **R49.9** Unspecified voice and resonance disorder
  - Change in voice NOS
  - Resonance disorder NOS

(R50–R69) GENERAL SYMPTOMS AND SIGNS

R50 FEVER OF OTHER AND UNKNOWN ORIGIN

4th

Excludes1: chills without fever (R68.83)
febrile convulsions (R56.0-)
fever of unknown origin during labor (O75.2)
fever of unknown origin in newborn (P81.9)
hypothermia due to illness (R68.0)
malignant hyperthermia due to anesthesia (T88.3)
puerperal pyrexia NOS (O86.4)

- **R50.2** Drug-induced fever
  - **Use additional code** for adverse effect, if applicable, to identify drug (T36–T50 with fifth or sixth character 5)
  - **Excludes1:** postvaccination (postimmunization) fever (R50.83)
- **R50.8** Other specified fever
  - 5th
  - **R50.81** Fever presenting with conditions classified elsewhere
    - **Code first** underlying condition when associated fever is present, such as with: leukemia (C91–C95)
    - neutropenia (D70.-)
    - sickle-cell disease (D57.-)

- **R50.82** Postprocedural fever
  - **Excludes1:**
  - postprocedural infection (T81.4-)
  - posttransfusion fever (R50.84)
  - postvaccination (postimmunization) fever (R50.83)
- **R50.83** Postvaccination fever
  - Postimmunization fever
- **R50.84** Febrile nonhemolytic transfusion reaction
  - FNHTR
  - Posttransfusion fever
- **R50.9** Fever, unspecified
  - Fever NOS
  - Fever of unknown origin [FUO]
  - Fever with chills
  - Fever with rigors
  - Hyperpyrexia NOS
  - Persistent fever

R51 HEADACHE

4th

Excludes2: atypical face pain (G50.1)
migraine and other headache syndromes (G43–G44)
trigeminal neuralgia (G50.0)

- **R51.0** Headache with orthostatic component, NEC
  - Headache with positional component, NEC
- **R51.9** Headache, unspecified
  - Facial pain NOS

R52 PAIN, UNSPECIFIED

✓

Acute pain NOS
Generalized pain NOS
Pain NOS

Excludes1: acute and chronic pain, NEC (G89.-)
localized pain, unspecified type — code to pain by site, such as:
abdomen pain (R10.-)
back pain (M54.9)
breast pain (N64.4)
chest pain (R07.1–R07.9)
ear pain (H92.0-)
eye pain (H57.1)
headache (R51.9)
joint pain (M25.5-)
limb pain (M79.6-)
lumbar region pain (M54.5-)
pelvic and perineal pain (R10.2)
shoulder pain (M25.51-)
spine pain (M54.-)
throat pain (R07.0)
tongue pain (K14.6)
tooth pain (K08.8)
renal colic (N23)
pain disorders exclusively related to psychological factors (F45.41)

R53 MALAISE AND FATIGUE

R53.1 Weakness
Asthenia NOS
Excludes1: muscle weakness (M62.81)
sarcopenia (M62.84)

R53.8 Other malaise and fatigue

5th *Excludes1:* combat exhaustion and fatigue (F43.0)
congenital debility (P96.9)
exhaustion and fatigue due to excessive exertion (T73.3)
exhaustion and fatigue due to exposure (T73.2)
exhaustion and fatigue due to heat (T67.-)
exhaustion and fatigue due to recurrent depressive episode (F33)

R53.81 Other malaise
Chronic debility
Debility NOS
General physical deterioration
Malaise NOS
Nervous debility
Excludes1: age-related physical debility (R54)

R53.82 Chronic fatigue, unspecified
Excludes1: chronic fatigue syndrome (G93.32)
myalgic encephalomyelitis (G93.32)
other post infection and related fatigue syndromes (G93.39)
postviral fatigue syndrome (G93.31)

R53.83 Other fatigue
Fatigue NOS
Lack of energy
Lethargy
Tiredness
Excludes 2: exhaustion and fatigue due to depressive episode (F32.-)

R55 SYNCOPE AND COLLAPSE

✔ Blackout
Fainting
Vasovagal attack
Excludes1: cardiogenic shock (R57.0)
carotid sinus syncope (G90.01)
heat syncope (T67.1)
neurocirculatory asthenia (F45.8)
neurogenic orthostatic hypotension (G90.3)
orthostatic hypotension (I95.1)
postprocedural shock (T81.1-)
psychogenic syncope (F48.8)
shock NOS (R57.9)
shock complicating or following abortion or ectopic or molar pregnancy (O00-O07, O08.3)
Stokes-Adams attack (I45.9)
unconsciousness NOS (R40.2-)

R56 CONVULSIONS, NEC

4th *Excludes1:* dissociative convulsions and seizures (F44.5)
epileptic convulsions and seizures (G40.-)
newborn convulsions and seizures (P90)

R56.0 Febrile convulsions

5th **R56.00 Simple febrile convulsions**
Febrile convulsion NOS
Febrile seizure NOS

R56.01 Complex febrile convulsions
Atypical febrile seizure
Complex febrile seizure
Complicated febrile seizure
Excludes1: status epilepticus (G40.901)

R56.1 Post traumatic seizures
Excludes1: post traumatic epilepsy (G40.-)

R56.9 Unspecified convulsions
Convulsion disorder
Fit NOS
Recurrent convulsions
Seizure(s) (convulsive) NOS

R57 SHOCK, NEC

4th *Excludes1:* anaphylactic shock NOS (T78.2)
anaphylactic reaction or shock due to adverse food reaction (T78.0-)
anaphylactic shock due to adverse effect of correct drug or medicament properly administered (T88.6)
anaphylactic shock due to serum (T80.5-)
shock due to anesthetic (T88.3)
electric shock (T75.4)
obstetric shock (O75.1)
postprocedural shock (T81.1-)
psychic shock (F43.0)
shock complicating or following ectopic or molar pregnancy (O00-O07, O08.3)
shock due to anesthesia (T88.2)
shock due to lightning (T75.01)
traumatic shock (T79.4)
toxic shock syndrome (A48.3)

R57.0 Cardiogenic shock
Excludes 2: septic shock (R65.21)

R57.1 Hypovolemic shock

R57.8 Other shock

R57.9 Shock, unspecified
Failure of peripheral circulation NOS

R58 HEMORRHAGE, NEC

✔ Hemorrhage NOS
Excludes1: hemorrhage included with underlying conditions, such as:
acute duodenal ulcer with hemorrhage (K26.0)
acute gastritis with bleeding (K29.01)
ulcerative enterocolitis with rectal bleeding (K51.01)

R59 ENLARGED LYMPH NODES

4th *Includes:* swollen glands
Excludes1: lymphadenitis NOS (I88.9)
acute lymphadenitis (L04.-)
chronic lymphadenitis (I88.1)
mesenteric (acute) (chronic) lymphadenitis (I88.0)

R59.0 Localized enlarged lymph nodes

R59.1 Generalized enlarged lymph nodes
Lymphadenopathy NOS

R59.9 Enlarged lymph nodes, unspecified

R60 EDEMA, NEC

4th *Excludes1:* angioneurotic edema (T78.3)
ascites (R18.-)
cerebral edema (G93.6)
cerebral edema due to birth injury (P11.0)
edema of larynx (J38.4)
edema of nasopharynx (J39.2)
edema of pharynx (J39.2)
gestational edema (O12.0-)
hereditary edema (Q82.0)
hydrops fetalis NOS (P83.2)
hydrothorax (J94.8)
hydrops fetalis NOS (P83.2)
newborn edema (P83.3)
pulmonary edema (J81.-)

R60.0 Localized edema

R60.1 Generalized edema
Excludes 2: nutritional edema (E40-E46)

R60.9 Edema, unspecified
Fluid retention NOS

R61 GENERALIZED HYPERHIDROSIS

✔ Excessive sweating
Night sweats
Secondary hyperhidrosis
Code first, if applicable, menopausal and female climacteric states (N95.1)
Excludes1: focal (primary) (secondary) hyperhidrosis (L74.5-)
Frey's syndrome (L74.52)
localized (primary) (secondary) hyperhidrosis (L74.5-)

R62 LACK OF EXPECTED NORMAL PHYSIOLOGICAL DEVELOPMENT IN CHILDHOOD AND ADULTS

4th *Excludes1:* delayed puberty (E30.0)
gonadal dysgenesis (Q99.1)
hypopituitarism (E23.0)

R62.0 Delayed milestone in childhood

Delayed attainment of expected physiological developmental stage
Late talker
Late walker

R62.5 Other and unspecified lack of expected normal physiological development in childhood

Excludes1: HIV disease resulting in failure to thrive (B20)
physical retardation due to malnutrition (E45)

R62.50 Unspecified lack of expected normal physiological development in childhood
Infantilism NOS

R62.51 Failure to thrive (child)
Failure to gain weight
Excludes1: failure to thrive in child under 28 days old (P92.6)

R62.52 Short stature (child)
Lack of growth
Physical retardation
Short stature NOS
Excludes1: short stature due to endocrine disorder (E34.3)

R62.59 Other lack of expected normal physiological development in childhood

R63 SYMPTOMS AND SIGNS CONCERNING FOOD AND FLUID INTAKE

Excludes1: bulimia NOS (F50.2-)

R63.0 Anorexia
Loss of appetite
Excludes1: anorexia nervosa (F50.0-)
loss of appetite of nonorganic origin (F50.89)

R63.1 Polydipsia
Excessive thirst

R63.2 Polyphagia
Excessive eating
Hyperalimentation NOS

R63.3 Feeding difficulties
Excludes2: eating disorders (F50.-)
feeding problems of newborn (P92.-)
infant feeding disorder of nonorganic origin (F98.2-)

R63.30 Feeding difficulties, unspecified

R63.31 Pediatric feeding disorder, acute
Pediatric feeding dysfunction, acute
Code also, if applicable, associated conditions such as:
aspiration pneumonia (J69.0)
dysphagia (R13.1-)
gastro-esophageal reflux disease (K21.-)
malnutrition (E40-E46)

R63.32 Pediatric feeding disorder, chronic
Pediatric feeding dysfunction, chronic
Code also, if applicable, associated conditions such as:
aspiration pneumonia (J69.0)
dysphagia (R13.1-)
gastro-esophageal reflux disease (K21.-)
malnutrition (E40-E46)

R63.39 Other feeding difficulties
Feeding problem (elderly) (infant) NOS
Picky eater

R63.4 Abnormal weight loss

R63.5 Abnormal weight gain
Excludes1: excessive weight gain in pregnancy (O26.0-)
obesity (E66.-)

R63.6 Underweight
Use additional code to identify body mass index (BMI), if known (Z68.-)
Excludes1: abnormal weight loss (R63.4)
anorexia nervosa (F50.0-)
malnutrition (E40–E46)

R63.8 Other symptoms and signs concerning food and fluid intake

R64 CACHEXIA

Excludes1: abnormal weight loss (R63.4)
cachexia due to underlying condition (E88.A)
nutritional marasmus (E41)

R65 SYMPTOMS AND SIGNS SPECIFICALLY ASSOCIATED WITH SYSTEMIC INFLAMMATION AND INFECTION

R65.1 SIRS of non-infectious origin

GUIDELINE

The SIRS can develop as a result of certain non-infectious disease processes, such as trauma, malignant neoplasm, or pancreatitis. When SIRS is documented with a noninfectious condition, and no subsequent infection is documented, the code for the underlying condition, such as an injury, should be assigned, followed by code R65.10 or code R65.11, SIRS of non-infectious origin with acute organ dysfunction. If an associated acute organ dysfunction is documented, the appropriate code(s) for the specific type of organ dysfunction(s) should be assigned in addition to code R65.11. If acute organ dysfunction is documented, but it cannot be determined if the acute organ dysfunction is associated with SIRS or due to another condition (e.g., directly due to the trauma), the provider should be queried.
Code first underlying condition, such as: heatstroke (T67.0-)
injury and trauma (S00–T88)
Excludes1: sepsis- code to infection
severe sepsis (R65.2)

R65.10 SIRS of non-infectious origin without acute organ dysfunction
SIRS NOS

R65.11 SIRS of non-infectious origin with acute organ dysfunction
Use additional code to identify specific acute organ dysfunction, such as:
acute kidney failure (N17.-)
cute respiratory failure (J96.0-)
critical illness myopathy (G72.81)
critical illness polyneuropathy (G62.81)
disseminated intravascular coagulopathy [DIC] (D65)
encephalopathy (metabolic) (septic) (G93.41)
hepatic failure (K72.0-)

R65.2 Severe sepsis
Infection with associated acute organ dysfunction
Sepsis with acute organ dysfunction
Sepsis with multiple organ dysfunction
SIRS due to infectious process with acute organ dysfunction
Code first underlying infection, such as: infection following a procedure (T81.4-)
infections following infusion, transfusion and therapeutic injection (T80.2-)
puerperal sepsis (O85)
sepsis following complete or unspecified spontaneous abortion (O03.87)
sepsis following ectopic and molar pregnancy (O08.82)
sepsis following incomplete spontaneous abortion (O03.37)
sepsis following (induced) termination of pregnancy (O04.87)
sepsis NOS (A41.9)
Use additional code to identify specific acute organ dysfunction, such as:
acute kidney failure (N17.-)
acute respiratory failure (J96.0-)
critical illness myopathy (G72.81)
critical illness polyneuropathy (G62.81)
disseminated intravascular coagulopathy [DIC] (D65)
encephalopathy (metabolic) (septic) (G93.41)
hepatic failure (K72.0-)

R65.20 Severe sepsis without septic shock
Severe sepsis NOS

R65.21 Severe sepsis with septic shock

R68 OTHER GENERAL SYMPTOMS AND SIGNS

R68.0 Hypothermia, not associated with low environmental temperature
Excludes1: hypothermia NOS (accidental) (T68)
hypothermia due to anesthesia (T88.51)
hypothermia due to low environmental temperature (T68)
newborn hypothermia (P80.-)

R68.1 Nonspecific symptoms peculiar to infancy

5th *Excludes1:* colic, infantile (R10.83)
neonatal cerebral irritability (P91.3)
teething syndrome (K00.7)

R68.11 Excessive crying of infant (baby)
Excludes1: excessive crying of child, adolescent, or adult (R45.83)

R68.12 Fussy infant (baby)
Irritable infant

R68.13 Apparent life threatening event in infant (ALTE)
Apparent life threatening event in newborn
Brief resolved unexplained event (BRUE)
Code first confirmed diagnosis, if known
Use additional code(s) for associated signs and symptoms if no confirmed diagnosis established, or if signs and symptoms are not associated routinely with confirmed diagnosis, or provide additional information for cause of ALTE

R68.19 Other nonspecific symptoms peculiar to infancy

R68.2 Dry mouth, unspecified
Excludes1: dry mouth due to dehydration (E86.0)
dry mouth due to Sjögren syndrome (M35.0-)
Excludes2: salivary gland hyposecretion (K11.7)

R68.3 Clubbing of fingers
Clubbing of nails
Excludes1: congenital club finger (Q68.1)

R68.8 Other general symptoms and signs

5th **R68.81 Early satiety**

R68.83 Chills (without fever)
Chills NOS
Excludes1: chills with fever (R50.9)

R68.84 Jaw pain
Mandibular pain
Maxilla pain
Excludes1: temporomandibular joint arthralgia (M26.62-)

R68.89 Other general symptoms and signs

R69 ILLNESS, UNSPECIFIED

✓ Unknown and unspecified cases of morbidity

(R70–R79) ABNORMAL FINDINGS ON EXAMINATION OF BLOOD, WITHOUT DIAGNOSIS

Excludes2: abnormalities (of) (on):
abnormal findings on antenatal screening of mother (O28.-)
coagulation hemorrhagic disorders (D65–D68)
lipids (E78.-)
platelets and thrombocytes (D69.-)
white blood cells classified elsewhere (D70–D72)
diagnostic abnormal findings classified elsewhere—see Alphabetical Index
hemorrhagic and hematological disorders of newborn (P50–P61)

R70 ELEVATED ERYTHROCYTE SEDIMENTATION RATE AND ABNORMALITY OF PLASMA VISCOSITY

4th

R70.0 Elevated erythrocyte sedimentation rate

R70.1 Abnormal plasma viscosity

R71 ABNORMALITY OF RED BLOOD CELLS

4th *Excludes1:* anemias (D50–D64)
anemia of premature infant (P61.2)
benign (familial) polycythemia (D75.0)
congenital anemias (P61.2–P61.4)
newborn anemia due to isoimmunization (P55.-)
polycythemia neonatorum (P61.1)
polycythemia NOS (D75.1)
polycythemia vera (D45)
secondary polycythemia (D75.1)

R71.0 Precipitous drop in hematocrit
Drop (precipitous) in hemoglobin
Drop in hematocrit

R71.8 Other abnormality of red blood cells
Abnormal red-cell morphology NOS
Abnormal red-cell volume NOS
Anisocytosis
Poikilocytosis

R73 ELEVATED BLOOD GLUCOSE LEVEL

4th *Excludes1:* DM (E08–E13)
DM in pregnancy, childbirth and the puerperium (O24.-)
neonatal disorders (P70.0–P70.2)
postsurgical hypoinsulinemia (E89.1)

R73.0 Abnormal glucose

5th *Excludes1:* abnormal glucose in pregnancy (O99.81-)
diabetes mellitus (E08-E13)
dysmetabolic syndrome X (E88.81-)
gestational diabetes (O24.4-)
glycosuria (R81)
hypoglycemia (E16.2)
type 1 diabetes mellitus, presymptomatic (E10.A-)

R73.01 Impaired fasting glucose
Elevated fasting glucose

R73.02 Impaired glucose tolerance (oral)
Elevated glucose tolerance

R73.03 Prediabetes
Latent diabetes

R73.09 Other abnormal glucose

Abnormal glucose NOS
Abnormal non-fasting glucose tolerance

R73.9 Hyperglycemia, unspecified

R74 ABNORMAL SERUM ENZYME LEVELS

4th

R74.0 Nonspecific elevation of levels of transaminase and lactic acid dehydrogenase [LDH]

5th **R74.01 Elevation of levels of liver transaminase levels**
Elevation of levels of alanine transaminase (ALT)
Elevation of levels of aspartate transaminase (AST)

R74.02 Elevation of levels of lactic acid dehydrogenase [LDH]

R74.8 Abnormal levels of other serum enzymes
Abnormal level of acid phosphatase
Abnormal level of alkaline phosphatase
Abnormal level of amylase
Abnormal level of lipase [triacylglycerol lipase]

R74.9 Abnormal serum enzyme level, unspecified

R75 INCONCLUSIVE LABORATORY EVIDENCE OF HIV

✓

GUIDELINES

Patients with inconclusive HIV serology, but no definitive diagnosis or manifestations of the illness, may be assigned code R75, Inconclusive laboratory evidence of HIV.
Nonconclusive HIV-test finding in infants
Excludes1: asymptomatic HIV infection status (Z21)
HIV disease (B20)

R76 OTHER ABNORMAL IMMUNOLOGICAL FINDINGS IN SERUM

4th

R76.0 Raised antibody titer
Excludes1: isoimmunization in pregnancy (O36.0–O36.1)
isoimmunization affecting newborn (P55.-)

R76.1 Nonspecific reaction to test for tuberculosis

5th **R76.11 Nonspecific reaction to tuberculin skin test without active tuberculosis**
Abnormal result of Mantoux test
PPD positive
Tuberculin (skin test) positive
Tuberculin (skin test) reactor
Excludes1: nonspecific reaction to cell mediated immunity measurement of gamma interferon antigen response without active tuberculosis (R76.12)

R76.12 Nonspecific reaction to cell mediated immunity measurement of gamma interferon antigen response without active tuberculosis
Nonspecific reaction to QFT without active tuberculosis
Excludes1: nonspecific reaction to tuberculin skin test without active tuberculosis (R76.11)
positive tuberculin skin test (R76.11)

R76.8 Other specified abnormal immunological findings in serum
Raised level of immunoglobulins NOS

R76.9 Abnormal immunological finding in serum, unspecified

4th 5th 6th 7th Additional Character Required ✓ 3-character code

●=New Code *Excludes1*—Not coded here, do not use together
▲=Revised Code *Excludes2*—Not included here

R77 OTHER ABNORMALITIES OF PLASMA PROTEINS

4th

Excludes1: disorders of plasma-protein metabolism (E88.0-)

- R77.1 Abnormality of globulin
  - Hyperglobulinemia NOS
- R77.8 Other specified abnormalities of plasma proteins
- R77.9 Abnormality of plasma protein, unspecified

R78 FINDINGS OF DRUGS AND OTHER SUBSTANCES, NOT NORMALLY FOUND IN BLOOD

4th

Use additional code to identify the any retained FB, if applicable (Z18.-)

Excludes2: mental or behavioral disorders due to psychoactive substance use (F10–F19)

- R78.0 Finding of alcohol in blood
  - Use additional external cause code (Y90.-), for detail regarding alcohol level
- R78.1 Finding of opiate drug in blood
- R78.2 Finding of cocaine in blood
- R78.3 Finding of hallucinogen in blood
- R78.4 Finding of other drugs of addictive potential in blood
- R78.5 Finding of other psychotropic drug in blood
- R78.6 Finding of steroid agent in blood
- R78.7 Finding of abnormal level of heavy metals in blood
  - 5th R78.71 Abnormal lead level in blood
    - *Excludes1:* lead poisoning (T56.0-)
  - R78.79 Finding of abnormal level of heavy metals in blood
- R78.8 Finding of other specified substances, not normally found in blood
  - 5th
  - R78.81 Bacteremia
    - *Excludes1:* sepsis-code to specified infection
  - R78.89 Finding of other specified substances, not normally found in blood
    - Finding of abnormal level of lithium in blood
- R78.9 Finding of unspecified substance, not normally found in blood

R79 OTHER ABNORMAL FINDINGS OF BLOOD CHEMISTRY

4th

Use additional code to identify any retained FB, if applicable (Z18.-)

Excludes1: asymptomatic hyperuricemia (E79.0)
hyperglycemia NOS (R73.9)
hypoglycemia NOS (E16.2)
neonatal hypoglycemia (P70.3–P70.4)
specific findings indicating disorder of amino-acid metabolism (E70–E72)
specific findings indicating disorder of carbohydrate metabolism (E73–E74)
specific findings indicating disorder of lipid metabolism (E75.-)

- R79.1 **Abnormal coagulation profile**
  - Abnormal or prolonged bleeding time
  - Abnormal or prolonged coagulation time
  - Abnormal or prolonged partial thromboplastin time [PTT]
  - Abnormal or prolonged prothrombin time [PT]
  - *Excludes1:* coagulation defects (D68.-)
  - *Excludes2:* abnormality of fluid, electrolyte or acid-base balance (E86–E87)
- R79.8 Other specified abnormal findings of blood chemistry
  - 5th
  - R79.81 **Abnormal blood-gas level**
  - R79.82 **Elevated C-reactive protein (CRP)**
  - R79.83 **Abnormal findings of blood amino-acid level**
    - Homocysteinemia
    - *Excludes1:* disorders of amino-acid metabolism (E70–E72)
  - R79.89 Other specified abnormal findings of blood chemistry
- R79.9 Abnormal finding of blood chemistry, unspecified

(R80–R82) ABNORMAL FINDINGS ON EXAMINATION OF URINE, WITHOUT DIAGNOSIS

Excludes1: abnormal findings on antenatal screening of mother (O28.-)
diagnostic abnormal findings classified elsewhere—see Alphabetical Index
specific findings indicating disorder of amino-acid metabolism (E70–E72)
specific findings indicating disorder of carbohydrate metabolism (E73–E74)

R80 PROTEINURIA

4th

Excludes1: gestational proteinuria (O12.1-)

- R80.0 Isolated proteinuria
  - Idiopathic proteinuria
  - *Excludes1:* isolated proteinuria with specific morphological lesion (N06.-)
- R80.1 Persistent proteinuria, unspecified
- R80.2 Orthostatic proteinuria, unspecified
  - Postural proteinuria
- R80.3 Bence Jones proteinuria
- R80.8 Other proteinuria
- R80.9 Proteinuria, unspecified
  - Albuminuria NOS

R81 GLYCOSURIA

✓

Excludes1: renal glycosuria (E74.818)

R82 OTHER AND UNSPECIFIED ABNORMAL FINDINGS IN URINE

4th

Includes: chromoabnormalities in urine

Use additional code to identify any retained FB, if applicable (Z18.-)

Excludes2: hematuria (R31.-)

- R82.0 Chyluria
  - *Excludes1:* filarial chyluria (B74.-)
- R82.1 Myoglobinuria
- R82.2 Biliuria
- R82.3 Hemoglobinuria
  - *Excludes1:* hemoglobinuria due to hemolysis from external causes NEC (D59.6)
  - hemoglobinuria due to paroxysmal nocturnal [Marchiafava-Micheli] (D59.5)
- R82.7 Abnormal findings on microbiological examination of urine
  - 5th *Excludes1:* colonization status (Z22.-)
  - R82.71 Bacteriuria
  - R82.79 Other abnormal findings on microbiological examination of urine
- R82.8 Abnormal findings on cytological and histological examination of urine
  - 5th
  - R82.81 Pyuria
    - sterile pyuria
  - R82.89 Other abnormal findings on cytological and histological examination of urine
- R82.9 Other and unspecified abnormal findings in urine
  - 5th
  - R82.90 Unspecified abnormal findings in urine
  - R82.91 Other chromoabnormalities of urine
    - Chromoconversion (dipstick)
    - Idiopathic dipstick converts positive for blood with no cellular forms in sediment
    - *Excludes1:* hemoglobinuria (R82.3)
    - myoglobinuria (R82.1)
  - R82.99 Other abnormal findings in urine
    - 6th
    - R82.991 Hypocitraturia
    - R82.992 Hyperoxaluria
      - *Excludes1:* primary hyperoxaluria (E72.53)
    - R82.993 Hyperuricosuria
    - R82.994 Hypercalciuria
      - Idiopathic hypercalciuria
    - R82.998 Other abnormal findings in urine
      - Cells and casts in urine
      - Crystalluria
      - Melanuria

(R83–R89) ABNORMAL FINDINGS ON EXAMINATION OF OTHER BODY FLUIDS, SUBSTANCES AND TISSUES, WITHOUT DIAGNOSIS

Excludes1: abnormal findings on antenatal screening of mother (O28.-)
diagnostic abnormal findings classified elsewhere — see Alphabetical Index

Excludes2: abnormal findings on examination of blood, without diagnosis (R70–R79)
abnormal findings on examination of urine, without diagnosis (R80–R82)
abnormal tumor markers (R97.-)

R83 ABNORMAL FINDINGS IN CEREBROSPINAL FLUID

R83.3 Abnormal level of substances chiefly nonmedicinal as to source in cerebrospinal fluid

R83.4 Abnormal immunological findings in cerebrospinal fluid

R83.5 Abnormal microbiological findings in cerebrospinal fluid

Positive culture findings in cerebrospinal fluid

Excludes1: colonization status (Z22.-)

R83.6 Abnormal cytological findings in cerebrospinal fluid

R83.8 Other abnormal findings in cerebrospinal fluid

Abnormal chromosomal findings in cerebrospinal fluid

R83.9 Unspecified abnormal finding in cerebrospinal fluid

R84 ABNORMAL FINDINGS IN SPECIMENS FROM RESPIRATORY ORGANS AND THORAX

Includes: abnormal findings in bronchial washings
abnormal findings in nasal secretions
abnormal findings in pleural fluid
abnormal findings in sputum
abnormal findings in throat scrapings

Excludes1: blood-stained sputum (R04.2)

R84.3 Abnormal level of substances chiefly nonmedicinal as to source in specimens from respiratory organs and thorax

R84.4 Abnormal immunological findings in specimens from respiratory organs and thorax

R84.5 Abnormal microbiological findings in specimens from respiratory organs and thorax

Positive culture findings in specimens from respiratory organs and thorax

Excludes1: colonization status (Z22.-)

R84.6 Abnormal cytological findings in specimens from respiratory organs and thorax

R89 ABNORMAL FINDINGS IN SPECIMENS FROM OTHER ORGANS, SYSTEMS AND TISSUES

Includes: abnormal findings in nipple discharge
abnormal findings in synovial fluid
abnormal findings in wound secretions

R89.0 Abnormal level of enzymes in specimens from other organs, systems and tissues

R89.1 Abnormal level of hormones in specimens from other organs, systems and tissues

R89.2 Abnormal level of other drugs, medicaments and biological substances in specimens from other organs, systems and tissues

R89.3 Abnormal level of substances chiefly nonmedicinal as to source in specimens from other organs, systems and tissues

R89.4 Abnormal immunological findings in specimens from other organs, systems and tissues

R89.5 Abnormal microbiological findings in specimens from other organs, systems and tissues

Positive culture findings in specimens from other organs, systems and tissues

Excludes1: colonization status (Z22.-)

R89.6 Abnormal cytological findings in specimens from other organs, systems and tissues

R89.7 Abnormal histological findings in specimens from other organs, systems and tissues

R89.8 Other abnormal findings in specimens from other organs, systems and tissues

Abnormal chromosomal findings in specimens from other organs, systems and tissues

R89.9 Unspecified abnormal finding in specimens from other organs, systems and tissues

(R90–R94) ABNORMAL FINDINGS ON DIAGNOSTIC IMAGING AND IN FUNCTION STUDIES, WITHOUT DIAGNOSIS

Includes: nonspecific abnormal findings on diagnostic imaging by CAT scan
nonspecific abnormal findings on diagnostic imaging by MRI [NMR] or PET scan
nonspecific abnormal findings on diagnostic imaging by thermography
nonspecific abnormal findings on diagnostic imaging by ultrasound [echogram]
nonspecific abnormal findings on diagnostic imaging by X-ray examination

Excludes1: abnormal findings on antenatal screening of mother (O28.-)
diagnostic abnormal findings classified elsewhere — **see Alphabetical Index**

R91 ABNORMAL FINDINGS ON DIAGNOSTIC IMAGING OF LUNG

R91.1 Solitary pulmonary nodule

Coin lesion lung

Solitary pulmonary nodule, subsegmental branch of the bronchial tree

R91.8 Other nonspecific abnormal finding of lung field

Lung mass NOS found on diagnostic imaging of lung

Pulmonary infiltrate NOS

Shadow, lung

R93 ABNORMAL FINDINGS ON DIAGNOSTIC IMAGING OF OTHER BODY STRUCTURES

R93.0 Abnormal findings on diagnostic imaging of skull and head, NEC

Excludes1: intracranial space-occupying lesion found on diagnostic imaging (R90.0)

R93.1 Abnormal findings on diagnostic imaging of heart and coronary circulation

Abnormal echocardiogram NOS

Abnormal heart shadow

R93.2 Abnormal findings on diagnostic imaging of liver and biliary tract

Nonvisualization of gallbladder

R93.3 Abnormal findings on diagnostic imaging of other parts of digestive tract

R93.4 Abnormal findings on diagnostic imaging of urinary organs

Excludes2: hypertrophy of kidney (N28.81)

R93.41 Abnormal radiologic findings on diagnostic imaging of renal pelvis, ureter, or bladder

Filling defect of bladder found on diagnostic imaging

Filling defect of renal pelvis found on diagnostic imaging

Filling defect of ureter found on diagnostic imaging

R93.42 Abnormal radiologic findings on diagnostic imaging of kidney

R93.421 right kidney

R93.422 left kidney

R93.429 unspecified kidney

R93.49 Abnormal radiologic findings on diagnostic imaging of other urinary organs

R93.5 Abnormal findings on diagnostic imaging of other abdominal regions, including retroperitoneum

R93.6 Abnormal findings on diagnostic imaging of limbs

Excludes2: abnormal finding in skin and subcutaneous tissue (R93.8-)

R93.7 Abnormal findings on diagnostic imaging of other parts of musculoskeletal system

Excludes2: abnormal findings on diagnostic imaging of skull (R93.0)

R93.8 Abnormal findings on diagnostic imaging of other specified body structures

R93.81 Abnormal radiologic findings on diagnostic imaging of testicles

R93.811 Abnormal radiologic findings on diagnostic imaging of right testicle

R93.812 Abnormal radiologic findings on diagnostic imaging of left testicle

R93.813 Abnormal radiologic findings on diagnostic imaging of testicles, bilateral

R93.819 Abnormal radiologic findings on diagnostic imaging of unspecified testicle

R93.89 Abnormal findings on diagnostic imaging of other specified body structures

Abnormal finding by radioisotope localization of placenta

Abnormal radiological finding in skin and subcutaneous tissue

Mediastinal shift

R94 ABNORMAL RESULTS OF FUNCTION STUDIES

Includes: abnormal results of radionuclide [radioisotope] uptake studies
abnormal results of scintigraphy

R94.0 Abnormal results of function studies of central nervous system

R94.01 Abnormal electroencephalogram [EEG]

R94.02 Abnormal brain scan

R94.09 Abnormal results of other function studies of central nervous system

R94.1 Abnormal results of function studies of peripheral nervous system and special senses

R94.11 Abnormal results of function studies of eye

R94.110 Abnormal electro-oculogram [EOG]

R94.111 Abnormal electroretinogram[ERG] Abnormal retinal function study

R94.112 Abnormal visually evoked potential [VEP]

R94.113 Abnormal oculomotor study

R94.118 Abnormal results of other function studies of eye

R94.12 Abnormal results of function studies of ear and other special senses

R94.120 Abnormal auditory function study

R94.121 Abnormal vestibular function study

R94.128 Abnormal results of other function studies of ear and other special senses

R94.13 Abnormal results of function studies of peripheral nervous system

R94.130 Abnormal response to nerve stimulation, unspecified

R94.131 Abnormal electromyogram [EMG] *Excludes1:* electromyogram of eye (R94.113)

R94.138 Abnormal results of other function studies of peripheral nervous system

R94.2 Abnormal results of pulmonary function studies Reduced ventilatory capacity Reduced vital capacity

R94.3 Abnormal results of cardiovascular function studies

R94.30 Abnormal result of cardiovascular function study, unspecified

R94.31 Abnormal electrocardiogram [ECG] [EKG] *Excludes1:* long QT syndrome (I45.81)

R94.39 Abnormal result of other cardiovascular function study Abnormal electrophysiological intracardiac studies Abnormal phonocardiogram Abnormal vectorcardiogram

R94.4 Abnormal results of kidney function studies Abnormal renal function test

R94.5 Abnormal results of liver function studies

R94.6 Abnormal results of thyroid function studies

R94.7 Abnormal results of other endocrine function studies *Excludes2:* abnormal glucose (R73.0-)

R94.8 Abnormal results of function studies of other organs and systems Abnormal basal metabolic rate [BMR] Abnormal bladder function test Abnormal splenic function test

(R97) ABNORMAL TUMOR MARKERS

R97 ABNORMAL TUMOR MARKERS

Elevated tumor associated antigens [TAA] Elevated tumor specific antigens [TSA]

R97.0 Elevated carcinoembryonic antigen [CEA]

R97.1 Elevated cancer antigen 125 [CA 125]

R97.8 Other abnormal tumor markers

(R99) ILL-DEFINED AND UNKNOWN CAUSE OF MORTALITY

R99 ILL-DEFINED AND UNKNOWN CAUSE OF MORTALITY

Code R99, Ill-defined and unknown cause of mortality, is only for use in the very limited circumstance when a patient who has already died is brought into an emergency department or other healthcare facility and is pronounced dead upon arrival. It does not represent the discharge disposition of death.

Death (unexplained) NOS

Unspecified cause of mortality

Chapter 19. Injury, poisoning and certain other consequences of external causes (S00–T88)

GUIDELINES

Application of 7th Characters in Chapter 19

Most categories in Chapter 19 have a 7th character requirement for each applicable code. Most categories in this chapter have three 7th character values (with the exception of fractures): A, initial encounter, D, subsequent encounter and S, sequela. Categories for traumatic fractures have additional 7th character values. While the patient may be seen by a new or different provider over the course of treatment for an injury, assignment of the 7th character is based on whether the patient is undergoing active treatment and not whether the provider is seeing the patient for the first time.

For complication codes, active treatment refers to treatment for the condition described by the code, even though it may be related to an earlier precipitating problem. For example, code T84.50XA, Infection and inflammatory reaction due to unspecified internal joint prosthesis, initial encounter, is used when active treatment is provided for the infection, even though the condition relates to the prosthetic device, implant or graft that was placed at a previous encounter.

7th character "A," initial encounter, is used while the patient is receiving active treatment for the condition.

7th character "D," subsequent encounter, is used for encounters after the patient has received active treatment of the condition and is receiving routine care for the condition during the healing or recovery phase.

The aftercare Z codes should not be used for aftercare for conditions such as injuries or poisonings, where 7th characters are provided to identify subsequent care. For example, for aftercare of an injury, assign the acute injury code with the 7th character "D" (subsequent encounter).

7th character "S," sequela, is for use for complications or conditions that arise as a direct result of a condition, such as scar formation after a burn. The scars are sequelae of the burn. When using 7th character "S," it is necessary to use both the injury code that precipitated the sequela and the code for the sequela itself. The "S" is added only to the injury code, not the sequela code. The 7th character "S" identifies the injury responsible for the sequela. The specific type of sequela (eg, scar) is sequenced first, followed by the injury code.

Coding of Injuries

When coding injuries, assign separate codes for each injury unless a combination code is provided, in which case the combination code is assigned. Codes from category T07, Unspecified multiple injuries should not be assigned in the inpatient setting unless information for a more specific code is not available. Traumatic injury codes (S00–T14.9) are not to be used for normal, healing surgical wounds or to identify complications of surgical wounds.

The code for the most serious injury, as determined by the provider and the focus of treatment, is sequenced first.

SUPERFICIAL INJURIES

Superficial injuries such as abrasions or contusions are not coded when associated with more severe injuries of the same site.

PRIMARY INJURY WITH DAMAGE TO NERVES/BLOOD VESSELS

When a primary injury results in minor damage to peripheral nerves or blood vessels, the primary injury is sequenced first with additional code(s) for injuries to nerves and spinal cord (such as category S04), and/or injury to blood vessels (such as category S15). When the primary injury is to the blood vessels or nerves, that injury should be sequenced first.

IATROGENIC INJURIES

Injury codes from Chapter 19 should not be assigned for injuries that occur during, or as a result of, a medical intervention. Assign the appropriate complication code(s).

Coding of Traumatic Fractures

The principles of multiple coding of injuries should be followed in coding fractures. Fractures of specified sites are coded individually by site in accordance with both the provisions within categories S02, S12, S22, S32, S42, S49, S52, S59, S62, S72, S79, S82, S89, S92 and the level of detail furnished by medical record content.

A fracture not indicated as open or closed should be coded to closed. A fracture not indicated whether displaced or not displaced should be coded to displaced.

More specific guidelines are as follows:

INITIAL VS. SUBSEQUENT ENCOUNTER FOR FRACTURES

Traumatic fractures are coded using the appropriate 7th character for initial encounter (A, B, C) for each encounter where the patient is receiving active

treatment for the fracture. The appropriate 7th character for initial encounter should also be assigned for a patient who delayed seeking treatment for the fracture or nonunion.

Fractures are coded using the appropriate 7th character for subsequent care for encounters after the patient has completed active treatment of the fracture and is receiving routine care for the fracture during the healing or recovery phase.

Care for complications of surgical treatment for fracture repairs during the healing or recovery phase should be coded with the appropriate complication codes.

Care of complications of fractures, such as malunion and nonunion, should be reported with the appropriate 7th character for subsequent care with nonunion (K, M, N,) or subsequent care with malunion (P, Q, R).

Malunion/nonunion: The appropriate 7th character for initial encounter should also be assigned for a patient who delayed seeking treatment for the fracture or nonunion.

The open fracture designations in the assignment of the 7th character for fractures of the forearm, femur and lower leg, including ankle are based on the Gustilo open fracture classification. When the Gustilo classification type is not specified for an open fracture, the 7th character for open fracture type I or II should be assigned (B, E, H, M, Q).

A code from category M80, not a traumatic fracture code, should be used for any patient with known osteoporosis who suffers a fracture, even if the patient had a minor fall or trauma, if that fall or trauma would not usually break a normal, healthy bone.

The aftercare Z codes should not be used for aftercare for traumatic fractures. For aftercare of a traumatic fracture, assign the acute fracture code with the appropriate 7th character.

MULTIPLE FRACTURES SEQUENCING

Multiple fractures are sequenced in accordance with the severity of the fracture.

PHYSEAL FRACTURES

For physeal fractures, assign only the code identifying the type of physeal fracture. Do not assign a separate code to identify the specific bone that is fractured.

Coding of Burns and Corrosions

See category T20.

Adverse Effects, Poisoning, Underdosing and Toxic Effects

See category T36.

Adult and Child Abuse, Neglect and Other Maltreatment

See category T74.

Complications of care

GENERAL GUIDELINES FOR COMPLICATIONS OF CARE

Documentation of Complications of Care
See *ICD-10-CM* Official Guidelines for Coding and Reporting FY 2024 in front matter, "Documentation of Complications of Care."

PAIN DUE TO MEDICAL DEVICES

Pain associated with devices, implants or grafts left in a surgical site (for example painful hip prosthesis) is assigned to the appropriate code(s) found in Chapter 19, Injury, poisoning, and certain other consequences of external causes. Specific codes for pain due to medical devices are found in the T code section of the *ICD-10-CM*. **Use additional code(s)** from category G89 to identify acute or chronic pain due to presence of the device, implant or graft (G89.18 or G89.28).

TRANSPLANT COMPLICATIONS

Transplant complications other than kidney
See category T86.

Kidney transplant complications
See code T86.1.

COMPLICATION CODES THAT INCLUDE THE EXTERNAL CAUSE

As with certain other T codes, some of the complications of care codes have the external cause included in the code. The code includes the nature of the complication as well as the type of procedure that caused the complication. No external cause code indicating the type of procedure is necessary for these codes.

COMPLICATIONS OF CARE CODES WITHIN THE BODY SYSTEM CHAPTERS

Intraoperative and postprocedural complication codes are found within the body system chapters with codes specific to the organs and structures of that body system. These codes should be sequenced first, followed by a code(s) for the specific complication, if applicable.

Complication codes from the body system chapters should be assigned for intraoperative and postprocedural complications (e.g., the appropriate complication code from chapter 9 would be assigned for a vascular intraoperative or postprocedural complication) unless the complication is specifically indexed to a T code in chapter 19.

Note: Use secondary code(s) from Chapter 20, External causes of morbidity, to indicate cause of injury. Codes within the T section that include the external cause do not require an additional external cause code

Use additional code to identify any retained FB, if applicable (Z18.-)

Excludes1: birth trauma (P10–P15)
obstetric trauma (O70–O71)

Note: The chapter uses the S-section for coding different types of injuries related to single body regions and the T-section to cover injuries to unspecified body regions as well as poisoning and certain other consequences of external causes.

(S00–S09) INJURIES TO THE HEAD

Includes: Injuries of ear
injuries of eye
injuries of face [any part]
injuries of gum
injuries of jaw
injuries of oral cavity
injuries of palate
injuries of periocular area
injuries of scalp
injuries of temporomandibular joint area
injuries of tongue
injuries of tooth

Code also for any associated infection

Excludes2: burns and corrosions (T20–T32)
effects of FB in ear (T16)
effects of FB in larynx (T17.3)
effects of FB in mouth NOS (T18.0)
effects of FB in nose (T17.0–T17.1)
effects of FB in pharynx (T17.2)
effects of FB on external eye (T15.-)
frostbite (T33–T34)
insect bite or sting, venomous (T63.4)

S00 SUPERFICIAL INJURY OF HEAD

Excludes1: diffuse cerebral contusion (S06.2-)
focal cerebral contusion (S06.3-)
injury of eye and orbit (S05.-)
open wound of head (S01.-)

S00.0 Superficial injury of scalp

S00.00X- Unspecified superficial injury of scalp

S00.01X- Abrasion of scalp

S00.02X- Blister (nonthermal) of scalp

S00.03X- Contusion of scalp
Bruise of scalp
Hematoma of scalp

S00.04X- External constriction of part of scalp

S00.05X- Superficial FB of scalp
Splinter in the scalp

S00.06X- Insect bite (nonvenomous) of scalp

S00.07X- Other superficial bite of scalp
Excludes1: open bite of scalp (S01.05)

S00.1 Contusion of eyelid and periocular area
Black eye
Excludes2: contusion of eyeball and orbital tissues (S05.1-)

S00.10X- Contusion of unspecified eyelid and periocular area

S00.11X- Contusion of right eyelid and periocular area

S00.12X- Contusion of left eyelid and periocular area

S00.2 Other and unspecified superficial injuries of eyelid and periocular area
Excludes2: superficial injury of conjunctiva and cornea (S05.0-)

S00.20 Unspecified superficial injury of eyelid and periocular area

S00.201- Unspecified superficial injury of right eyelid and periocular area

S00.202- Unspecified superficial injury of left eyelid and periocular area

S00.21 Abrasion of eyelid and periocular area

S00.211- Abrasion of right eyelid and periocular area

S00.212- Abrasion of left eyelid and periocular area

S00.22 Blister (nonthermal) of eyelid and periocular area

S00.221- Blister (nonthermal) of right eyelid and periocular area

S00.222- Blister (nonthermal) of left eyelid and periocular area

S00.24 External constriction of eyelid and periocular area

S00.241- External constriction of right eyelid and periocular area

S00.242- External constriction of left eyelid and periocular area

S00.25 Superficial FB of eyelid and periocular area
Splinter of eyelid and periocular area
Excludes2: retained FB in eyelid (H02.81-)

S00.251- Superficial FB of right eyelid and periocular area

S00.252- Superficial FB of left eyelid and periocular area

S00.26 Insect bite (nonvenomous) of eyelid and periocular area

S00.261- Insect bite (nonvenomous) of right eyelid and periocular area

S00.262- Insect bite (nonvenomous) of left eyelid and periocular area

S00.27 Other superficial bite of eyelid and periocular area
Excludes1: open bite of eyelid and periocular area (S01.15)

S00.271- Other superficial bite of right eyelid and periocular area

S00.272- Other superficial bite of left eyelid and periocular area

S00.3 Superficial injury of nose

S00.30X- Unspecified superficial injury of nose

S00.31X- Abrasion of nose

S00.32X- Blister (nonthermal) of nose

S00.33X- Contusion of nose
Bruise of nose
Hematoma of nose

S00.34X- External constriction of nose

S00.35X- Superficial FB of nose
Splinter in the nose

S00.36X- Insect bite (nonvenomous) of nose

S00.37X- Other superficial bite of nose
Excludes1: open bite of nose (S01.25)

S00.4 Superficial injury of ear

S00 requires a 7th character
A—initial encounter
D—subsequent encounter
S—sequela

5th **S00.40 Unspecified superficial injury of ear**

6th S00.401- Unspecified superficial injury of right ear

7th

S00.402- Unspecified superficial injury of left ear

S00.41 Abrasion of ear

6th S00.411- Abrasion of right ear

7th

S00.412- Abrasion of left ear

7th

S00.42 Blister (nonthermal) of ear

6th S00.421- Blister (nonthermal) of right ear

7th

S00.422- Blister (nonthermal) of left ear

7th

S00.43 Contusion of ear

6th Bruise of ear
Hematoma of ear

S00.431- Contusion of right ear

7th

S00.432- Contusion of left ear

7th

S00.44 External constriction of ear

6th S00.441- External constriction of right ear

7th

S00.442- External constriction of left ear

7th

S00.45 Superficial FB of ear

6th Splinter in the ear

S00.451- Superficial FB of right ear

7th

S00.452- Superficial FB of left ear

7th

S00.46 Insect bite (nonvenomous) of ear

6th S00.461- Insect bite (nonvenomous) of right ear

7th

S00.462- Insect bite (nonvenomous) of left ear

7th

S00.47 Other superficial bite of ear

6th *Excludes1:* open bite of ear (S01.35)

S00.471- Other superficial bite of right ear

7th

S00.472- Other superficial bite of left ear

7th

S00.5 Superficial injury of lip and oral cavity

5th **S00.50 Unspecified superficial injury of lip and oral cavity**

6th S00.501- Unspecified superficial injury of lip

7th

S00.502- Unspecified superficial injury of oral cavity

7th

S00.51 Abrasion of lip and oral cavity

6th S00.511- Abrasion of lip

7th

S00.512- Abrasion of oral cavity

7th

S00.52 Blister (nonthermal) of lip and oral cavity

6th S00.521- Blister (nonthermal) of lip

7th

S00.522- Blister (nonthermal) of oral cavity

7th

S00.53 Contusion of lip and oral cavity

6th S00.531- Contusion of lip

7th Bruise of lip
Hematoma of lip

S00.532- Contusion of oral cavity

7th Bruise of oral cavity
Hematoma of oral cavity

S00.54 External constriction of lip and oral cavity

6th S00.541- External constriction of lip

7th

S00.542- External constriction of oral cavity

7th

S00.55 Superficial FB of lip and oral cavity

6th S00.551- Superficial FB of lip

7th Splinter of lip and oral cavity

S00.552- Superficial FB of oral cavity

7th Splinter of lip and oral cavity

S00.56 Insect bite (nonvenomous) of lip and oral cavity

6th S00.561- Insect bite (nonvenomous) of lip

7th

S00.562- Insect bite (nonvenomous) of oral cavity

7th

S00.57 Other superficial bite of lip and oral cavity

6th S00.571- Other superficial bite of lip

7th *Excludes1:* open bite of lip (S01.551)

S00.572- Other superficial bite of oral cavity

7th *Excludes1:* open bite of oral cavity (S01.552)

S00.8 Superficial injury of other parts of head

5th Superficial injuries of face [any part]

S00.80X- Unspecified superficial injury of other part of head

7th

S00.81X- Abrasion of other part of head

7th

S00.82X- Blister (nonthermal) of other part of head

7th

S00.83X- Contusion of other part of head

7th Bruise of other part of head
Hematoma of other part of head

S00.84X- External constriction of other part of head

7th

S00.85X- Superficial FB of other part of head

7th *Splinter in other part of head*

S00.86X- Insect bite (nonvenomous) of other part of head

7th

S00.87X- Other superficial bite of other part of head

7th *Excludes1:* open bite of other part of head (S01.85)

S00.9 Superficial injury of unspecified part of head

5th **S00.90X- Unspecified superficial injury of unspecified part of head**

7th

S00.91X- Abrasion of unspecified part of head

7th

S00.92X- Blister (nonthermal) of unspecified part of head

7th

S00.93X- Contusion of unspecified part of head

7th Bruise of head
Hematoma of head

S00.94X- External constriction of unspecified part of head

7th

S00.95X- Superficial FB of unspecified part of head

7th Splinter of head

S00.96X- Insect bite (nonvenomous) of unspecified part of head

7th

S00.97X- Other superficial bite of unspecified part of head

7th *Excludes1:* open bite of head (S01.95)

S01 OPEN WOUND OF HEAD

4th Code also any associated:
injury of cranial nerve (S04.-)
injury of muscle and tendon of head (S09.1-)
intracranial injury (S06.-)
wound infection

S01 requires a 7th character
A—initial encounter
D—subsequent encounter
S—sequela

Excludes1: open skull fracture (S02.- with 7th character)

Excludes2: injury of eye and orbit (S05.-)
traumatic amputation of part of head (S08.-)

S01.0 Open wound of scalp

5th *Excludes1:* avulsion of scalp (S08.0-)

S01.01X- Laceration without FB of scalp

7th

S01.02X- Laceration with FB of scalp

7th

S01.03X- Puncture wound without FB of scalp

7th

S01.04X- Puncture wound with FB of scalp

7th

S01.05X- Open bite of scalp
7th Bite of scalp NOS
Excludes1: superficial bite of scalp (S00.06, S00.07-)

S01.1 Open wound of eyelid and periocular area
5th Open wound of eyelid and periocular area with or without involvement of lacrimal passages
S01.11 Laceration without FB of eyelid and periocular area
6th S01.111- Laceration without FB of right eyelid and
7th periocular area
S01.112- Laceration without FB of left eyelid and
7th periocular area
S01.12 Laceration with FB of eyelid and periocular area
6th S01.121- Laceration with FB of right eyelid and
7th periocular area
S01.122- Laceration with FB of left eyelid and
7th periocular area
S01.13 Puncture wound without FB of eyelid and periocular
6th area
S01.131- Puncture wound without FB of right eyelid
7th and periocular area
S01.132- Puncture wound without FB of left eyelid
7th and periocular area
S01.14 Puncture wound with FB of eyelid and periocular
6th area
S01.141- Puncture wound with FB of right eyelid
7th and periocular area
S01.142- Puncture wound with FB of left eyelid and
7th periocular area
S01.15 Open bite of eyelid and periocular area
6th Bite of eyelid and periocular area NOS
Excludes1: superficial bite of eyelid and periocular area (S00.26, S00.27)
S01.151- Open bite of right eyelid and periocular
7th area
S01.152- Open bite of left eyelid and periocular area
7th

S01.2 Open wound of nose
5th **S01.21X-** Laceration without FB of nose
7th
S01.22X- Laceration with FB of nose
7th
S01.23X- Puncture wound without FB of nose
7th
S01.24X- Puncture wound with FB of nose
7th
S01.25X- Open bite of nose
7th Bite of nose NOS
Excludes1: superficial bite of nose (S00.36, S00.37)

S01.3 Open wound of ear
5th **S01.31** Laceration without FB of ear
6th S01.311- Laceration without FB of right ear
7th
S01.312- Laceration without FB of left ear
7th
S01.32 Laceration with FB of ear
6th S01.321- Laceration with FB of right ear
7th
S01.322- Laceration with FB of left ear
7th
S01.33 Puncture wound without FB of ear
6th S01.331- Puncture wound without FB of right ear
7th
S01.332- Puncture wound without FB of left ear
7th
S01.34 Puncture wound with FB of ear
6th S01.341- Puncture wound with FB of right ear
7th
S01.342- Puncture wound with FB of left ear
7th
S01.35 Open bite of ear
6th Bite of ear NOS
Excludes1: superficial bite of ear (S00.46, S00.47)

S01.351- Open bite of right ear
7th
S01.352- Open bite of left ear
7th

S01.4 Open wound of cheek and temporomandibular area
5th **S01.41** Laceration without FB of cheek and
6th temporomandibular area
S01.411- Laceration without FB of right cheek and
7th temporomandibular area
S01.412- Laceration without FB of left cheek and
7th temporomandibular area
S01.42 Laceration with FB of cheek and temporomandibular
6th area
S01.421- Laceration with FB of right cheek and
7th temporomandibular area
S01.422- Laceration with FB of left cheek and
7th temporomandibular area
S01.43 Puncture wound without FB of cheek and
6th temporomandibular area
S01.431- Puncture wound without FB of right cheek
7th and temporomandibular area
S01.432- Puncture wound without FB of left cheek
7th and temporomandibular area
S01.44 Puncture wound with FB of cheek and
6th temporomandibular area
S01.441- Puncture wound with FB of right cheek
7th and temporomandibular area
S01.442- Puncture wound with FB of left cheek and
7th temporomandibular area
S01.45 Open bite of cheek and temporomandibular area
6th Bite of cheek and temporomandibular area NOS
Excludes2: superficial bite of cheek and temporomandibular area (S00.86, S00.87)
S01.451- Open bite of right cheek and
7th temporomandibular area
S01.452- Open bite of left cheek and
7th temporomandibular area

S01.5 Open wound of lip and oral cavity
5th *Excludes2:* tooth dislocation (S03.2)
tooth fracture (S02.5)
S01.51 Laceration of lip and oral cavity without FB
6th **S01.511-** Laceration without FB of lip
7th
S01.512- Laceration without FB of oral cavity
7th
S01.52 Laceration of lip and oral cavity with FB
6th **S01.521-** Laceration with FB of lip
7th
S01.522- Laceration with FB of oral cavity
7th
S01.53 Puncture wound of lip and oral cavity without FB
6th **S01.531-** Puncture wound without FB of lip
7th
S01.532- Puncture wound without FB of oral cavity
7th
S01.54 Puncture wound of lip and oral cavity with FB
6th **S01.541-** Puncture wound with FB of lip
7th
S01.542- Puncture wound with FB of oral cavity
7th
S01.55 Open bite of lip and oral cavity
6th **S01.551-** Open bite of lip
7th Bite of lip NOS
Excludes1: superficial bite of lip (S00.571)
S01.552- Open bite of oral cavity
7th Bite of oral cavity NOS
Excludes1: superficial bite of oral cavity (S00.572)

S01.8 Open wound of other parts of head
5th **S01.81X-** Laceration without FB of other part of head
7th
S01.82X- Laceration with FB of other part of head
7th

S01.83X- Puncture wound without FB of other part of head

7th

S01.84X- Puncture wound with FB of other part of head

7th

S01.85X- Open bite of other part of head

7th Bite of other part of head NOS

Excludes1: superficial bite of other part of head (S00.87)

S01.9 Open wound of unspecified part of head

5th **S01.90X-** Unspecified open wound of unspecified part of head

7th

S01.91X- Laceration without FB of unspecified part of head

7th

S01.92X- Laceration with FB of unspecified part of head

7th

S01.93X- Puncture wound without FB of unspecified part of head

7th

S01.94X- Puncture wound with FB of unspecified part of head

7th

S01.95X- Open bite of unspecified part of head

7th Bite of head NOS

Excludes1: superficial bite of head NOS (S00.97)

S02 **FRACTURE OF SKULL AND FACIAL BONES**

4th

Note: A fracture not indicated as open or closed should be coded to closed

Code also any associated intracranial injury (S06.-)

S02.0 Fracture of vault of skull

Fracture of frontal bone

Fracture of parietal bone

S02.1 Fracture of base of skull,

5th *Excludes2:* lateral orbital wall (S02.84-)

medial orbital wall (S02.83-)

orbital floor (S02.3-)

S02.10 Unspecified fracture of base of skull

6th **S02.101-** right side

7th

S02.102- left side

7th

S02.109- unspecified side

7th

S02.11 Fracture of occiput

6th **S02.111-** Type II occipital condyle fracture, unspecified side

7th

S02.112- Type III occipital condyle fracture, unspecified side

7th

S02.113- Unspecified occipital condyle fracture

7th

S02.118- Other fracture of occiput, unspecified side

7th

S02.119- Unspecified fracture of occiput

7th

S02.11A- Type I occipital condyle fracture, right side

7th

S02.11B- Type I occipital condyle fracture, left side

7th

S02.11C- Type II occipital condyle fracture, right side

7th

S02.11D- Type II occipital condyle fracture, left side

7th

S02.11E- Type III occipital condyle fracture, right side

7th

S02.11F- Type III occipital condyle fracture, left side

7th

S02.11G- Other fracture of occiput, right side

7th

S02.11H- Other fracture of occiput, left side

7th

S02.12 Fracture of orbital roof,

6th

S02.121- right side, closed fracture

7th

S02.122- left side, closed fracture

7th

S02.129- unspecified side, closed fracture

7th

S02.19X- Other fracture of base of skull

7th Fracture of anterior fossa of base of skull

Fracture of ethmoid or frontal sinus

Fracture of middle fossa of base of skull

Fracture of orbital roof

Fracture of posterior fossa of base of skull

Fracture of sphenoid

Fracture of temporal bone

S02.2XX- Fracture of nasal bones

7th

S02.3 Fracture of orbital floor,

5th Fracture of inferior orbital wall

Excludes1: orbit NOS (S02.85)

Excludes2: lateral orbital wall (S02.84-)

medial orbital wall (S02.83-)

orbital roof (S02.1-)

S02.30X- unspecified side

7th *Excludes1:* orbit NOS (S02.85)

Excludes2: orbital roof (S02.1-)

S02.31X- right side

7th *Excludes1:* orbit NOS (S02.8)

Excludes2: orbital roof (S02.1-)

S02.32X- left side

7th *Excludes1:* orbit NOS (S02.8)

Excludes2: orbital roof (S02.1-)

S02.4 Fracture of malar, maxillary and zygoma bones,

5th Fracture of superior maxilla

Fracture of upper jaw (bone)

Fracture of zygomatic process of temporal bone

S02.40 unspecified

6th **S02.400-** Malar fracture, unspecified side

7th

S02.401- Maxillary fracture, unspecified side

7th

S02.402- Zygomatic fracture, unspecified side

7th

S02.40A- Malar fracture, right side

7th

S02.40B- Malar fracture, left side

7th

S02.40C- Maxillary fracture, right side

7th

S02.40D- Maxillary fracture, left side

7th

S02.40E- Zygomatic fracture, right side

7th

S02.40F- Zygomatic fracture, left side

7th

S02.5XX- Fracture of tooth (traumatic)

7th Broken tooth

Excludes1: cracked tooth (nontraumatic) (K03.81)

S02.6 Fracture of mandible

5th Fracture of lower jaw (bone)

S02.60 Fracture of mandible, unspecified

6th **S02.600-** Fracture of unspecified part of body of mandible, unspecified side

7th

S02.601- Fracture of unspecified part of body of right mandible

7th

S02.602- Fracture of unspecified part of body of left mandible

7th

S02.609- Fracture of mandible, unspecified

7th

S02.61 Fracture of condylar process of mandible

6th **S02.610-** Fracture of condylar process of mandible, unspecified side

7th

S02.611- Fracture of condylar process of right mandible

7th

(S02.612–S04.52X)

S02.612- Fracture of condylar process of left mandible

S02.62 Fracture of subcondylar process of mandible

S02.620- Fracture of subcondylar process of mandible, unspecified side

S02.621- Fracture of subcondylar process of right mandible

S02.622- Fracture of subcondylar process of left mandible

S02.63 Fracture of coronoid process of mandible

S02.630- Fracture of process of mandible, unspecified side

S02.631- Fracture of subcondylar process of right mandible

S02.632- Fracture of subcondylar process of left mandible

S02.64 Fracture of ramus of mandible

S02.640- Fracture of ramus of mandible, unspecified side

S02.641- Fracture of ramus of right mandible

S02.642- Fracture of ramus of left mandible

S02.65 Fracture of angle of mandible

S02.650- Fracture of angle of mandible, unspecified side

S02.651- Fracture of angle of right mandible

S02.652- Fracture of angle of left mandible

S02.66X- Fracture of symphysis of mandible

S02.67 Fracture of alveolus of mandible

S02.670- Fracture of alveolus of mandible, unspecified side

S02.671- Fracture of alveolus of right mandible

S02.672- Fracture of alveolus of left mandible

S02.69X- Fracture of mandible of other specified site

S02.8 Fractures of other specified skull and facial bones, Fracture of palate

Excludes2: fracture of orbital floor (S02.3-) fracture of orbital roof (S02.12-)

S02.80X- unspecified side

S02.81X- right side

S02.82X- left side

S02.83 Fracture of medial orbital wall, *Excludes2:* orbital floor (S02.3-) orbital roof (S02.12-)

S02.831- right side, closed fracture

S02.832- left side, closed fracture

S02.839- unspecified side, closed fracture

S02.84 Fracture of lateral orbital wall, *Excludes2:* orbital floor (S02.3-) orbital roof (S02.12-)

S02.841- right side, closed fracture

S02.842- left side, closed fracture

S02.849- unspecified side, closed fracture

S02.85X- Fracture of orbit, unspecified Fracture of orbit NOS Fracture of orbit wall NOS *Excludes1:* lateral orbital wall (S02.84-) medial orbital wall (S02.83-) orbital floor (S02.3-) orbital roof (S02.12-)

S02.9 Fracture of unspecified skull and facial bones

S02.91X- Unspecified fracture of skull

S02.92X- Unspecified fracture of facial bones

S03 DISLOCATION AND SPRAIN OF JOINTS AND LIGAMENTS OF HEAD

Includes: avulsion of joint (capsule) or ligament of head
laceration of cartilage, joint (capsule) or ligament of head
sprain of cartilage, joint (capsule) or ligament of head
traumatic hemarthrosis of joint or ligament of head
traumatic rupture of joint or ligament of head
traumatic subluxation of joint or ligament of head
traumatic tear of joint or ligament of head

Code also any associated open wound

Excludes2: Strain of muscle or tendon of head (S09.1)

S03.0 Dislocation of jaw,

Dislocation of jaw (cartilage) (meniscus) Dislocation of mandible or of temporomandibular (joint)

S03.00X- unspecified side

S03.01X- right side

S03.02X- left side

S03.03X- bilateral

S03.1XX- Dislocation of septal cartilage of nose

S03.2XX- Dislocation of tooth

S03.4 Sprain of jaw,

Sprain of temporomandibular (joint) (ligament)

S03.40X- unspecified side

S03.41X- right side

S03.42X- left side

S03.43X- bilateral

S04 INJURY OF CRANIAL NERVE

The selection of side should be based on the side of the body being affected

Code first any associated intracranial injury (S06.-)

Code also any associated: open wound of head (S01.-) skull fracture (S02.-)

S04.5 Injury of facial nerve,

Injury of 7th cranial nerve

S04.51X- right side

S04.52X- left side

S05 INJURY OF EYE AND ORBIT

Includes: open wound of eye and orbit
Excludes2: 2nd cranial [optic] nerve injury (S04.0-)
3rd cranial [oculomotor] nerve injury (S04.1-)
open wound of eyelid and periocular area (S01.1-)
orbital bone fracture (S02.1-, S02.3-, S02.8-)
superficial injury of eyelid (S00.1-S00.2)

S05.0 Injury of conjunctiva and corneal abrasion without FB,
Excludes1: FB in conjunctival sac (T15.1)
FB in cornea (T15.0)
S05.01X- right eye
S05.02X- left eye

S05.1 Contusion of eyeball and orbital tissues,
Traumatic hyphema
Excludes2: black eye NOS (S00.1)
contusion of eyelid and periocular area (S00.1)
S05.11X- right eye
S05.12X- left eye

S05.8 Other injuries of eye and orbit
Lacrimal duct injury
S05.8X Other injuries of eye and orbit
S05.8X1- Other injuries of right eye and orbit
S05.8X2- Other injuries of left eye and orbit

S05.9 Unspecified injury of eye and orbit
Injury of eye NOS
S05.91X- Unspecified injury of right eye and orbit
S05.92X- Unspecified injury of left eye and orbit

S06 INTRACRANIAL INJURY

Includes: traumatic brain injury
Code also any associated:
open wound of head (S01.-)
skull fracture (S02.-)
Excludes1: head injury NOS (S09.90)

S06.0 Concussion
Commotio cerebri
Excludes1: concussion with other intracranial injuries classified in subcategories S06.1- to S06.6-, S06.81- and S06.82- code to specified intracranial injury
S06.0X Concussion
S06.0X0- without loss of consciousness
S06.0X1- with LOC of 30 min or less
S06.0XA- with LOC status unknown
S06.0X9- with LOC unspecified duration
Concussion NOS

S06.1 Traumatic cerebral edema
Diffuse traumatic cerebral edema
Focal traumatic cerebral edema
S06.1X Traumatic cerebral edema
S06.1X0- without loss of consciousness
S06.1X1- with LOC of 30 min or less
Traumatic cerebral edema with brief LOC
S06.1X2- with LOC of 31 min to 59 min
S06.1X3- with LOC of 1 h to 5 h 59 min
S06.1X4- with LOC of 6 h to 24 h
S06.1X5- with LOC greater than 24 h with return to pre-existing conscious level

S06.1X6- with LOC greater than 24 h without return to pre-existing conscious level with patient surviving
S06.1X7A with LOC of any duration with death due to brain injury prior to regaining consciousness
S06.1X8A with LOC of any duration with death due to other cause prior to regaining consciousness
S06.1XA- with LOC status unknown
Traumatic cerebral edema NOS
S06.1X9- with LOC of unspecified duration

S06.2 Diffuse traumatic brain injury
Diffuse axonal brain injury
Use additional code, if applicable, for traumatic brain compression or herniation (S06.A-)
Excludes1: traumatic diffuse cerebral edema (S06.1X-)
S06.2X Diffuse traumatic brain injury
S06.2X0- without loss of consciousness
S06.2X1- with LOC of 30 m or less
Diffuse traumatic brain injury with brief LOC
S06.2X2- with LOC of 31 min to 59 min
S06.2X3- with LOC of 1 h to 5 h 59 min
S06.2X4- with LOC of 6 h to 24 h
S06.2X5- with LOC greater than 24 h with return to pre-existing conscious levels
S06.2X6- with LOC greater than 24 h without return to pre-existing conscious level with patient surviving
S06.2X7A with LOC of any duration with death due to brain injury prior to regaining consciousness
S06.2X8A with LOC of any duration with death due to other cause prior to regaining consciousness
S06.2XA- with LOC status unknown
Diffuse traumatic brain injury NOS
S06.2X9- with LOC of unspecified duration

S06.3 Focal traumatic brain injury
Use additional code, if applicable, for traumatic brain compression or herniation (S06.A-)
Excludes2: any condition classifiable to S06.4-S06.6
focal cerebral edema (S06.1)
S06.30 Unspecified focal traumatic brain injury
S06.300- without loss of consciousness
S06.301- with LOC of; 30 min or less
S06.302- 31 min to 59 min
S06.303- 1 hour to 5 h 59 min
S06.304- 6 h to 24 h
S06.305- greater than 24 h with return to pre-existing conscious level
S06.306- greater than 24 h without return to pre-existing conscious level with patient surviving
S06.307A any duration with death due to brain injury prior to regaining consciousness
S06.308A any duration with death due to other cause prior to regaining consciousness
S06.30A- status unknown
S06.309- unspecified duration
Unspecified focal traumatic brain injury NOS
S06.31 Contusion and laceration of right cerebrum
S06.310- without LOC

S06.311- with LOC of; 30 min or less
S06.312- 31 min to 59 min
S06.313- 1 hour to 5 h 59 min
S06.314- 6 h to 24 h

S06.315- greater than 24 h with return to pre-existing conscious level
S06.316- greater than 24 h without return to pre-existing conscious level with patient surviving
S06.317A any duration with death due to brain injury prior to regaining consciousness
S06.318A any duration with death due to other cause prior to regaining consciousness
S06.31A- with LOC status unknown

S06.319- unspecified duration
Contusion and laceration of right cerebrum NOS

S06.32 Contusion and laceration of left cerebrum

S06.320- without loss of consciousness

S06.321- with LOC of; 30 min or less

S06.322- 31 min to 59 min

S06.323- 1 hour to 5 h 59 min

S06.324- 6 h to 24 h

S06.325- greater than 24 h with return to pre-existing conscious level
S06.326- greater than 24 h without return to pre-existing conscious level with patient surviving
S06.327A any duration with death due to brain injury prior to regaining consciousness
S06.328A any duration with death due to other cause prior to regaining consciousness
S06.32A- with loss of consciousness status unknown
S06.329- unspecified duration
Contusion and laceration of left cerebrum NOS

S06.33 Contusion and laceration of cerebrum, unspecified

S06.330- without LOC

S06.331- with LOC of 30 min or less
Contusion and laceration of cerebrum, unspecified, with brief LOC
S06.332- with LOC of 31 min to 59 min

S06.333- with LOC of 1 h to 5 h 59 min

S06.334- with LOC of 6 h to 24 h

S06.335- with LOC greater than 24 h with return to pre-existing conscious level
S06.336- with LCO greater than 24 h without return to pre-existing conscious level with patient surviving
S06.337A with LOC of any duration with death due to brain injury prior to regaining consciousness
S06.338A with LOC of any duration with death due to other cause prior to regaining consciousness
S06.33A- with LOC status unknown
Contusion and laceration of cerebrum NOS

S06.34 Traumatic hemorrhage of right cerebrum
Traumatic intracerebral hemorrhage and hematoma of right cerebrum

S06.340- without loss of consciousness

S06.341- with brief LOC of; 30 min or less

S06.342- 31 min to 59 min

S06.343- 1 h to 5 h 59 min

S06.344- 6 h to 24 h

S06.345- greater than 24 h with return to pre-existing conscious level
S06.346- greater than 24 h without return to pre-existing conscious level with patient surviving
S06.347A any duration with death due to brain injury prior to regaining consciousness
S06.348A any duration with death due to other cause prior to regaining consciousness
S06.34A with LOC status unknown

S06.349- unspecified duration
Traumatic hemorrhage of right cerebrum NOS

S06.35 Traumatic hemorrhage of left cerebrum
Traumatic intracerebral hemorrhage and hematoma of left cerebrum

S06.350- Traumatic hemorrhage of left cerebrum without loss of consciousness
S06.351- with LOC of; 30 min or less

S06.352- 31 min to 59 min

S06.353- 1 h to 5 h 59 min

S06.354- 6 h to 24 h

S06.355- greater than 24 h with return to pre-existing conscious level
S06.356- greater than 24 h without return to pre-existing conscious level with patient surviving
S06.357A any duration with death due to brain injury prior to regaining consciousness
S06.358A any duration with death due to other cause prior to regaining consciousness
S06.35A- with LOC status unknown

S06.359- unspecified duration
Traumatic hemorrhage of left cerebrum NOS

S06.36 Traumatic hemorrhage of cerebrum, unspecified;
Traumatic intracerebral hemorrhage and hematoma, unspecified

S06.360- without loss of consciousness

S06.361- with LOC of 30 min or less
Traumatic hemorrhage of cerebrum, unspecified, with brief LOC
S06.362- with LOC of 31 min to 59 min

S06.363- with LOC of 1 h to 5 h 59 min

S06.364- with LOC of 6 h to 24 h

S06.365- with LOC greater than 24 h with return to pre-existing conscious level
S06.366- with LOC greater than 24 h without return to pre-existing conscious level with patient surviving

S06.339- with LOC of unspecified duration

S06.367A with LOC of any duration with death due to brain injury prior to regaining consciousness

S06.368A with LOC of any duration with death due to other cause prior to regaining consciousness

S06.36A- with LOC status unknown

Traumatic hemorrhage of cerebrum NOS

S06.369- with LOC of unspecified duration

S06.37 Contusion, laceration, and hemorrhage of cerebellum

S06.370- without loss of consciousness

S06.371- Contusion, laceration, and hemorrhage of cerebellum with LOC of; 30 min or less

S06.372- 31 min to 59 min

S06.373- 1 hour to 5 h 59 min

S06.374- 6 h to 24 h

S06.375- greater than 24 h with return to pre-existing conscious level

S06.376- greater than 24 h without return to pre-existing conscious level with patient surviving

S06.377A any duration with death due to brain injury prior to regaining consciousness

S06.378A any duration with death due to other cause prior to regaining consciousness

S06.37A- with LOC status unknown

S06.379- unspecified duration

Contusion, laceration, and hemorrhage of cerebellum NOS

S06.38 Contusion, laceration, and hemorrhage of brainstem

S06.380- without loss of consciousness

S06.381- with LOC of; 30 min or less

S06.382- 31 min to 59 min

S06.383- 1 hour to 5 h 59 min

S06.384- 6 h to 24 h

S06.385- greater than 24 h with return to pre-existing conscious level

S06.386- greater than 24 h without return to pre-existing conscious level with patient surviving

S06.387A any duration with death due to brain injury prior to regaining consciousness

S06.388A any duration with death due to other cause prior to regaining consciousness

S06.38A- with LOC status unknown

S06.389- unspecified duration

Contusion, laceration, and hemorrhage of brainstem NOS

S06.4 Epidural hemorrhage

Extradural hemorrhage NOS

Extradural hemorrhage (traumatic)

S06.4X Epidural hemorrhage

S06.4X0- without loss of consciousness

S06.4X1- with LOC of 30 min or less

S06.4X2- with LOC of 31 min to 59 min

S06.4X3- with LOC of 1 h to 5 h 59 min

S06.4X4- with LOC of 6 h to 24 h

S06.4X5- with LOC greater than 24 h with return to pre-existing conscious level

S06.4X6- with LOC greater than 24 h without return to pre-existing conscious level with patient surviving

S06.4X7A with loss of consciousness of any duration with death due to brain injury prior to regaining consciousness

S06.4X8A with LOC of any duration with death due to other causes prior to regaining consciousness

S06.4XA- with LOC status unknown

S06.4X9- with LOC of unspecified duration

Epidural hemorrhage NOS

S06.5 Traumatic subdural hemorrhage

Use additional code, if applicable, for traumatic brain compression or herniation (S06.A-)

S06.5X Traumatic subdural hemorrhage

S06.5X0- without loss of consciousness

S06.5X1- with LOC of; 30 min or less

S06.5X2- 31 min to 59 min

S06.5X3- 1 hour to 5 h 59 min

S06.5X4- 6 h to 24 h

S06.5X5- greater than 24 h with return to pre-existing conscious level

S06.5X6- greater than 24 h without return to pre-existing conscious level with patient surviving

S06.5X7A any duration with death due to brain injury before regaining consciousness

S06.5X8A any duration with death due to other cause before regaining consciousness

S06.5XA- with LOC status unknown

S06.5X9- unspecified duration

Traumatic subdural hemorrhage NOS

S06.6 Traumatic subarachnoid hemorrhage

Use additional code, if applicable, for traumatic brain compression or herniation (S06.A-)

S06.6X Traumatic subarachnoid hemorrhage

S06.6X0- without loss of consciousness

S06.6X1- with LOC of; 30 min or less

S06.6X2- 31 min to 59 min

S06.6X3- 1 hour to 5 h 59 min

S06.6X4- 6 h to 24 h

S06.6X5- greater than 24 h with return to pre-existing conscious level

S06.6X6- greater than 24 h without return to pre-existing conscious level with patient surviving

S06.6X7A any duration with death due to brain injury prior to regaining consciousness

S06.6X8A any duration with death due to other cause prior to regaining consciousness

S06.6XA- with LOC status unknown
S06.6X9- unspecified duration
7th Traumatic suba-rachnoid hemorrhage NOS

S06.8 Other specified intracranial injuries
5th **S06.81 Injury of right internal carotid artery, intracranial**
6th **portion, not elsewhere classified**
S06.810- without loss of consciousness
7th
S06.811- with LOC of 30 min or less
7th Injury of right internal carotid artery, intracranial portion, not elsewhere classified with brief LOC
S06.812- with LOC of 31 min to 59 min
7th
S06.813- with LOC of 1 h to 5 h 59 min
7th
S06.814- with LOC of 6 h to 24 h
7th
S06.815- with LOC greater than 24 h with return
7th to pre-existing conscious level
S06.816- with LOC greater than 24 h without
7th return to pre-existing conscious level with patient surviving
S06.817A with LOC of any duration with death
7th due to brain injury prior to regaining consciousness
S06.818A with LOC of any duration with death
7th due to other cause prior to regaining consciousness
S06.81A- with LOC status unknown
7th Injury of right internal carotid artery, intracranial portion, not elsewhere classified NOS
S06.819- with LOC of unspecified duration
7th

S06.82 Injury of left internal carotid artery, intracranial
6th **portion, not elsewhere classified**
S06.820- without LOC
7th
S06.821- with LOC of 30 min or less
7th Injury of left internal carotid artery, intracranial portion, not elsewhere classified with brief LOC
S06.822- with LOC of 31 min to 59 min
7th
S06.823- with LOC of 1 h to 5 h 59 min
7th
S06.824- with LOC of 6 h to 24 h
7th
S06.825- with LOC greater than 24 h with return
7th to pre-existing conscious level
S06.826- with LOC greater than 24 h without
7th return to pre-existing conscious level with patient surviving
S06.827A with LOC of any duration with death
7th due to brain injury prior to regaining consciousness
S06.828A with LOC of any duration with death
7th due to other cause prior to regaining consciousness
S06.82A- with LOC status unknown
7th Injury of left internal carotid artery, intracranial portion, not elsewhere classified NOS

S06.829- with LOC of unspecified duration
7th

S06.8A Primary blast injury of brain, not elsewhere
6th **classified**
Code also, if applicable, focal traumatic brain injury (S06.3-)
Excludes2: traumatic cerebral edema (S06.1)
S06.8A0- Primary blast injury of brain, NEC without
6th loss of consciousness
S06.8A1- Primary blast injury of brain, NEC with LOC
6th
S06.8A2- with LOC of 31 min to 59 min
7th
S06.8A3- with LOC of 1 h to 5 h 59 min
7th
S06.8A4- with LOC of 6 h to 24 h
7th
S06.8A5- with LOC greater than 24 h with return
7th to pre-existing conscious level
S06.8A6- with LOC greater than 24 h without
7th return to pre-existing conscious level with patient surviving
S06.8A7A with LOC of any duration with death
7th due to brain injury prior to regaining consciousness
S06.8A8A with LOC of any duration with death
7th due to other cause prior to regaining consciousness
S06.8AA- with LOC status unknown
7th
S06.8A9- with LOC of unspecified duration
7th

S06.89 Other specified intracranial injury
6th *Excludes1:* concussion (S06.0X-)
S06.890- without LOC
7th
S06.891- with LOC of 30 min or less
7th
S06.892- with LOC of; 31 min to 59 min
7th
S06.893- 1 hour to 5 h 59 min
7th
S06.894- 6 h to 24 h
7th
S06.895- greater than 24 h with return to pre-
7th existing conscious level
S06.896- greater than 24 h without return to pre-
7th existing conscious level with patient surviving
S06.897A any duration with death due to brain
7th injury prior to regaining consciousness
S06.898A any duration with death due to other
7th cause prior to regaining consciousness
S06.89A- with LOC status unknown
7th
S06.899- unspecified duration
7th

S06.9 Unspecified intracranial injury
5th Brain injury NOS
Head injury NOS with LOC
Traumatic brain injury NOS
Excludes1: conditions classifiable to S06.0- to S06.8- code to specified intracranial injury
head injury NOS (S09.90)
S06.9X Unspecified intracranial injury
6th S06.9X0- without loss of consciousness
7th
S06.9X1- with LOC of; 30 min or less
7th
S06.9X2- 31 min to 59 min
7th
S06.9X3- 1 hour to 5 h 59 min
7th

S06.9X4- 6 h to 24 h

S06.9X5- greater than 24 h with return to pre-existing conscious level

S06.9X6- greater than 24 h without return to pre-existing conscious level with patient surviving

S06.9X7A any duration with death due to brain injury prior to regaining consciousness

S06.9X8A any duration with death due to other cause prior to regaining consciousness

S06.9XA- with LOC status unknown

S06.9X9- unspecified duration

S06.A Traumatic brain compression

Traumatic cerebral compression

Code first the underlying traumatic brain injury, such as:
diffuse traumatic brain injury (S06.2-)
focal traumatic brain injury (S06.3-)
traumatic subdural hemorrhage (S06.5-)
traumatic subarachnoid hemorrhage (S06.6-)

S06.A0X- without herniation

Traumatic brain or cerebral compression NOS

S06.A1X- with herniation

Traumatic brain herniation
Traumatic brainstem or cerebellar or cerebral compression with herniation

S09 OTHER AND UNSPECIFIED INJURIES OF HEAD

S09.0XX- Injury of blood vessels of head, NEC

Excludes1: injury of cerebral blood vessels (S06.-)
injury of precerebral blood vessels (S15.-)

S09.1 Injury of muscle and tendon of head

Code also any associated open wound (S01.-)

Excludes2: sprain to joints and ligament of head (S03.9)

S09.10X- Unspecified injury of muscle and tendon of head

Injury of muscle and tendon of head NOS

S09.11X- Strain of muscle and tendon of head

S09.12X- Laceration of muscle and tendon of head

S09.19X- Other specified injury of muscle and tendon of head

S09.2 Traumatic rupture of ear drum

Excludes1: traumatic rupture of ear drum due to blast injury (S09.31-)

S09.21X- Traumatic rupture of right ear drum

S09.22X- Traumatic rupture of left ear drum

S09.8XX- Other specified injuries of head

S09.9 Unspecified injury of face and head

S09.90X- Unspecified injury of head

Head injury NOS

Excludes1: brain injury NOS (S06.9-)
head injury NOS with LOC (S06.9-)
intracranial injury NOS (S06.9-)

S09.91X- Unspecified injury of ear

Injury of ear NOS

S09.92X- Unspecified injury of nose

Injury of nose NOS

S09.93X- Unspecified injury of face

Injury of face NOS

Injuries to the neck (S10–S19)

Includes: injuries of nape
injuries of supraclavicular region
injuries of throat

Excludes2: burns and corrosions (T20–T32)
effects of FB in esophagus (T18.1)
effects of FB in larynx (T17.3)
effects of FB in pharynx (T17.2)
effects of FB in trachea (T17.4)
frostbite (T33–T34)
insect bite or sting, venomous (T63.4)

Includes: injuries of nape
injuries of supraclavicular region
injuries of throat

Excludes2: burns and corrosions (T20–T32)
effects of FB in esophagus (T18.1)
effects of FB in larynx (T17.3)
effects of FB in pharynx (T17.2)
effects of FB in trachea (T17.4)
frostbite (T33–T34)
insect bite or sting, venomous (T63.4)

S10 SUPERFICIAL INJURY OF NECK

S10.0XX- Contusion of throat

Contusion of cervical esophagus
Contusion of larynx
Contusion of pharynx
Contusion of trachea

S10.1 Other and unspecified superficial injuries of throat

S10.10X- Unspecified superficial injuries of throat

S10.11X- Abrasion of throat

S10.12X- Blister (nonthermal) of throat

S10.14X- External constriction of part of throat

S10.15X- Superficial FB of throat

Splinter in the throat

S10.16X- Insect bite (nonvenomous) of throat

S10.17X- Other superficial bite of throat

Excludes1: open bite of throat (S11.85)

S10.8 Superficial injury of other specified parts of neck

S10.80X- Unspecified superficial injury of other specified part of neck

S10.81X- Abrasion of other specified part of neck

S10.82X- Blister (nonthermal) of other specified part of neck

S10.83X- Contusion of other specified part of neck

S10.84X- External constriction of other specified part of neck

S10.85X- Superficial FB of other specified part of neck

Splinter in other specified part of neck

S10.86X- Insect bite of other specified part of neck

S10.87X- Other superficial bite of other specified part of neck

Excludes1: open bite of other specified parts of neck (S11.85)

S10.9 Superficial injury of unspecified part of neck

S10.90X- Unspecified superficial injury of unspecified part of neck

S10.91X- Abrasion of unspecified part of neck

S10.92X- Blister (nonthermal) of unspecified part of neck

S10.93X- Contusion of unspecified part of neck

S10.94X- External constriction of unspecified part of neck
7th

S10.95X- Superficial FB of unspecified part of neck
7th

S10.96X- Insect bite of unspecified part of neck
7th

S10.97X- Other superficial bite of unspecified part of neck
7th

S11 OPEN WOUND OF NECK
4th

S11 requires a 7th character
A—initial encounter
D—subsequent encounter
S—sequela

Code also any associated:
spinal cord injury (S14.0, S14.1-)
wound infection

Excludes2: open fracture of vertebra
(S12.- with 7th character B)

S11.8 Open wound of other specified parts of neck

5th **S11.80X-** Unspecified open wound of other specified part of neck
7th

S11.81X- Laceration without foreign body of other specified part of neck
7th

S11.82X- Laceration with foreign body of other specified part of neck
7th

S11.83X- Puncture wound without foreign body of other specified part of neck
7th

S11.84X- Puncture wound with foreign body of other specified part of neck
7th

S11.85X- Open bite of other specified part of neck
7th Bite of other specified part of neck NOS
Excludes1: superficial bite of other specified part of neck (S10.87)

S11.9 Open wound of unspecified part of neck

5th **S11.91X-** Laceration without FB of unspecified part of neck
7th

S11.92X- Laceration with FB of unspecified part of neck
7th

S11.93X- Puncture wound without FB of unspecified part of neck
7th neck

S11.94X- Puncture wound with FB of unspecified part of neck
7th

S11.95X- Open bite of unspecified part of neck
7th Bite of neck NOS
Excludes1: superficial bite of neck (S10.97)

S12 FRACTURE OF CERVICAL VERTEBRA AND OTHER PARTS OF NECK
4th

S12.0-S12.6 requires a 7th character
A—initial encounter for closed fracture
B—initial encounter for open fracture
D—subsequent encounter for fracture with routine healing
G—subsequent encounter for fracture with delayed healing
K—subsequent encounter for fracture with nonunion
S—sequela

Note: A fracture not indicated as displaced or nondisplaced should be coded to displaced

A fracture not indicated as open or closed should be coded to closed

Includes: fracture of cervical neural arch
fracture of cervical spine
fracture of cervical spinous process
fracture of cervical transverse process
fracture of cervical vertebral arch
fracture of neck

Code first any associated cervical spinal cord injury (S14.0, S14.1-)

S12.0 Fracture of first cervical vertebra
5th Atlas

S12.00 Unspecified fracture of first cervical vertebra
6th

S12.000- Unspecified displaced fracture of first cervical vertebra
7th

S12.001- Unspecified nondisplaced fracture of first cervical vertebra
7th

S12.03 Posterior arch fracture of first cervical vertebra
6th

S12.030- Displaced posterior arch fracture of first cervical vertebra
7th

S12.031- Nondisplaced posterior arch fracture of first cervical vertebra
7th

S12.1 Fracture of second cervical vertebra
5th Axis

S12.10 Unspecified fracture of second cervical vertebra
6th

S12.100- Unspecified displaced fracture of second cervical vertebra
7th

S12.101- Unspecified nondisplaced fracture of second cervical vertebra
7th

S12.2 Fracture of third cervical vertebra
5th

S12.20 Unspecified fracture of third cervical vertebra
6th

S12.200- Unspecified displaced fracture of third cervical vertebra
7th

S12.201- Unspecified nondisplaced fracture of third cervical vertebra
7th

S12.3 Fracture of fourth cervical vertebra
5th

S12.30 Unspecified fracture of fourth cervical vertebra
6th

S12.300- Unspecified displaced fracture of fourth cervical vertebra
7th

S12.301- Unspecified nondisplaced fracture of fourth cervical vertebra
7th

S12.4 Fracture of fifth cervical vertebra
5th

S12.40 Unspecified fracture of fifth cervical vertebra
6th

S12.400- Unspecified displaced fracture of fifth cervical vertebra
7th

S12.401- Unspecified nondisplaced fracture of fifth cervical vertebra
7th

S12.5 Fracture of sixth cervical vertebra
5th

S12.50 Unspecified fracture of sixth cervical vertebra
6th

S12.500- Unspecified displaced fracture of sixth cervical vertebra
7th

S12.501- Unspecified nondisplaced fracture of sixth cervical vertebra
7th

S12.6 Fracture of seventh cervical vertebra
5th

S12.60 Unspecified fracture of seventh cervical vertebra
6th

S12.600- Unspecified displaced fracture of seventh cervical vertebra
7th

S12.601- Unspecified nondisplaced fracture of seventh cervical vertebra
7th

S12.8XX- Fracture of other parts of neck
7th Hyoid bone
Larynx
Thyroid cartilage
Trachea

S12.8 and S12.9 require a 7th character
A—initial encounter
D—subsequent encounter
S—sequela

S12.9XX- Fracture of neck, unspecified
7th Fracture of neck NOS
Fracture of cervical spine NOS
Fracture of cervical vertebra NOS

S13 DISLOCATION AND SPRAIN OF JOINTS AND LIGAMENTS AT NECK LEVEL
4th

S13 requires a 7th character
A—initial encounter
D—subsequent encounter
S—sequela

Includes: avulsion of joint or ligament at neck level
laceration of cartilage, joint or ligament at neck level
sprain of cartilage, joint or ligament at neck level
traumatic hemarthrosis of joint or ligament at neck level
traumatic rupture of joint or ligament at neck level
traumatic subluxation of joint or ligament at neck level
traumatic tear of joint or ligament at neck level

Code also any associated open wound

Excludes2: strain of muscle or tendon at neck level (S16.1)

S13.4XX- Sprain of ligaments of cervical spine
7th Sprain of anterior longitudinal (ligament), cervical
Sprain of atlanto-axial (joints)
Sprain of atlanto-occipital (joints)
Whiplash injury of cervical spine

S13.8XX- Sprain of joints and ligaments of other parts of neck
7th

S13.9XX- Sprain of joints and ligaments of unspecified parts of neck
7th

S14 INJURY OF NERVES AND SPINAL CORD AT NECK LEVEL
4th

S14 requires a 7th character
A—initial encounter
D—subsequent encounter
S—sequela

Note: Code to highest level of cervical cord injury

Code also any associated:
fracture of cervical vertebra (S12.0–S12.6.-)
open wound of neck (S11.-)
transient paralysis (R29.5)

S14.0XX- Concussion and edema of cervical spinal cord
7th

S14.1 Other and unspecified injuries of cervical spinal cord

S14.10 Unspecified injury of cervical spinal cord

S14.101- Unspecified injury at; C1 level of cervical spinal cord

S14.102- C2 level of cervical spinal cord

S14.103- C3 level of cervical spinal cord

S14.104- C4 level of cervical spinal cord

S14 requires a 7th character
A—initial encounter
D—subsequent encounter
S—sequela

S14.105- C5 level of cervical spinal cord

S14.106- C6 level of cervical spinal cord

S14.107- C7 level of cervical spinal cord

S14.108- C8 level of cervical spinal cord

S14.109- unspecified level of cervical spinal cord
Injury of cervical spinal cord NOS

S14.2XX- Injury of nerve root of cervical spine

S14.3XX- Injury of brachial plexus

S14.4XX- Injury of peripheral nerves of neck

S14.5XX- Injury of cervical sympathetic nerves

S14.8XX- Injury of other specified nerves of neck

S14.9XX- Injury of unspecified nerves of neck

S15 INJURY OF BLOOD VESSELS AT NECK LEVEL

Code **also** any associated open wound (S11.-)

S15 requires a 7th character
A—initial encounter
D—subsequent encounter
S—sequela

S15.8XX- Injury of other specified blood vessels at neck level

S15.9XX- Injury of unspecified blood vessel at neck level

S16 INJURY OF MUSCLE, FASCIA AND TENDON AT NECK LEVEL

Code **also** any associated open wound (S11.-)

Excludes2: sprain of joint or ligament at neck level (S13.9)

S16 requires a 7th character
A—initial encounter
D—subsequent encounter
S—sequela

S16.1XX- Strain of muscle, fascia and tendon at neck level

S16.2XX- Laceration of muscle, fascia and tendon at neck level

S16.8XX- Other specified injury of muscle, fascia and tendon at neck level

S16.9XX- Unspecified injury of muscle, fascia and tendon at neck level

---

(S20–S29) INJURIES TO THE THORAX

Includes: injuries of breast
injuries of chest (wall)
injuries of interscapular area

Excludes2: burns and corrosions (T20–T32)
effects of FB in bronchus (T17.5)
effects of FB in esophagus (T18.1)
effects of FB in lung (T17.8)
effects of FB in trachea (T17.4)
frostbite (T33–T34)
injuries of axilla
injuries of clavicle
injuries of scapular region
injuries of shoulder
insect bite or sting, venomous (T63.4)

S20 SUPERFICIAL INJURY OF THORAX

S20 requires a 7th character
A—initial encounter
D—subsequent encounter
S—sequela

S20.0 Contusion of breast;

S20.00X- unspecified breast

S20.01X- right breast

S20.02X- left breast

S20.1 Other and unspecified superficial injuries of breast

S20.11 Abrasion of breast,

S20.111- right breast

S20.112- left breast

S20.119- unspecified breast

S20.12 Blister (nonthermal) of breast,

S20.121- right breast

S20.122- left breast

S20.129- unspecified breast

S20.14 External constriction of part of breast,

S20.141- right breast

S20.142- left breast

S20.15 Superficial FB of breast,
Splinter in the breast

S20.151- right breast

S20.152- left breast

S20.16 Insect bite (nonvenomous) of breast,

S20.161- right breast

S20.162- left breast

S20.17 Other superficial bite of breast,
Excludes1: open bite of breast (S21.05-)

S20.171- right breast

S20.172- left breast

S20.2 Contusion of thorax

S20.20X- Contusion of thorax, unspecified

S20.21 Contusion of front wall of thorax

S20.211- Contusion of right front wall of thorax

S20.212- Contusion of left front wall of thorax

S20.213- Contusion of bilateral front wall of thorax

S20.214- Contusion of middle front wall of thorax

S20.219- Contusion of unspecified front wall of thorax

S20.22 Contusion of back wall of thorax

S20.221- Contusion of right back wall of thorax

S20.222- Contusion of left back wall of thorax

S20.223- Contusion of bilateral back wall of thorax

S20.224- Contusion of middle back wall of thorax

S20.229- Contusion of unspecified back wall of thorax
Interscapular contusion

S20.3 Other and unspecified superficial injuries of front wall of thorax

S20.30 Unspecified superficial injuries of front wall of thorax

S20.301- Unspecified superficial injuries of right front wall of thorax

S20.302- Unspecified superficial injuries of left front wall of thorax

S20.303- Unspecified superficial injuries of bilateral front wall of thorax

S20.304- Unspecified superficial injuries of middle front wall of thorax

S20.309- Unspecified superficial injuries of unspecified front wall of thorax

S20.31 Abrasion of front wall of thorax

S20.311- Abrasion of right front wall of thorax

S20.312- Abrasion of left front wall of thorax

S20.313- Abrasion of bilateral front wall of thorax

S20.314- Abrasion of middle front wall of thorax

S20.319- Abrasion of unspecified front wall of thorax

S20.32 Blister (nonthermal) of front wall of thorax

S20.321- Blister (nonthermal) of right front wall of thorax

S20.322- Blister (nonthermal) of left front wall of thorax

S20.323- Blister (nonthermal) of bilateral front wall of thorax

S20.324- Blister (nonthermal) of middle front wall of thorax

S20.329- Blister (nonthermal) of unspecified front wall of thorax

S20.34 External constriction of front wall of thorax

S20.341- External constriction of right front wall of thorax

S20.342- External constriction of left front wall of thorax

S20.343- External constriction of bilateral front wall of thorax

S20.344- External constriction of middle front wall of thorax

S20.349- External constriction of unspecified front wall of thorax

S20.35 Superficial foreign body of front wall of thorax Splinter in front wall of thorax

S20.351- Superficial foreign body of right front wall of thorax

S20.352- Superficial foreign body of left front wall of thorax

S20.353- Superficial foreign body of bilateral front wall of thorax

S20.354- Superficial foreign body of middle front wall of thorax

S20.359- Superficial foreign body of unspecified front wall of thorax

S20.36 Insect bite (nonvenomous) of front wall of thorax

S20.361- Insect bite (nonvenomous) of right front wall of thorax

S20.362- Insect bite (nonvenomous) of left front wall of thorax

S20.363- Insect bite (nonvenomous) of bilateral front wall of thorax

S20.364- Insect bite (nonvenomous) of middle front wall of thorax

S20.369- Insect bite (nonvenomous) of unspecified front wall of thorax

S20.37 Other superficial bite of front wall of thorax *Excludes1:* open bite of front wall of thorax (S21.14)

S20.371- Other superficial bite of right front wall of thorax

S20.372- Other superficial bite of left front wall of thorax

S20.373- Other superficial bite of bilateral front wall of thorax

S20.374- Other superficial bite of middle front wall of thorax

S20.379- Other superficial bite of unspecified front wall of thorax

S20.4 Other and unspecified superficial injuries of back wall of thorax

S20.40 Unspecified superficial injuries of back wall of thorax

S20.401- Unspecified superficial injuries of right back wall of thorax

S20.402- Unspecified superficial injuries of left back wall of thorax

S20.409- Unspecified superficial injuries of unspecified back wall of thorax

S20.41 Abrasion of back wall of thorax

S20.411- Right back wall of thorax

S20.412- Left back wall of thorax

S20.419- Unspecified back wall of thorax

S20.42 Blister (nonthermal) of back wall of thorax

S20.421- Blister (nonthermal) of right back wall of thorax

S20.422- Blister (nonthermal) of left back wall of thorax

S20.429- Blister (nonthermal) of unspecified back wall of thorax

S20.44 External constriction of back wall of thorax

S20.441- External constriction of right back wall of thorax

S20.442- External constriction of left back wall of thorax

S20.449- External constriction of unspecified back wall of thorax

S20.46 Insect bite (nonvenomous) of back wall of thorax

S20.461- Insect bite (nonvenomous) of right back wall of thorax

S20.462- Insect bite (nonvenomous) of left back wall of thorax

S20.469- Insect bite (nonvenomous) of unspecified back wall of thorax

S20.47 Other superficial bite of back wall of thorax *Excludes1:* open bite of back wall of thorax (S21.24)

S20.471- Other superficial bite of right back wall of thorax

S20.472- Other superficial bite of left back wall of thorax

S20.479- Other superficial bite of unspecified back wall of thorax

S20.9 Superficial injury of unspecified parts of thorax *Excludes1:* contusion of thorax NOS (S20.20)

S20.90X- Unspecified superficial injury of unspecified parts of thorax Superficial injury of thoracic wall NOS

S20.91X- Abrasion of unspecified parts of thorax

S20.92X- Blister (nonthermal) of unspecified parts of thorax

S20.94X- External constriction of unspecified parts of thorax

S20.95X- Superficial FB of unspecified parts of thorax Splinter in thorax NOS

S20.96X- Insect bite (nonvenomous) of unspecified parts of thorax
 7th

S20.97X- Other superficial bite of unspecified parts of thorax
 7th *Excludes1:* open bite of thorax NOS (S21.95)

S21 OPEN WOUND OF THORAX
4th

Code also any associated injury, such as:
rib fracture (S22.3-, S22.4-)
wound infection

Excludes1: traumatic amputation (partial) of thorax (S28.1)

S21 requires a 7th character
A—initial encounter
D—subsequent encounter
S—sequela

S21.1 Open wound of front wall of thorax without penetration into thoracic cavity
 5th

S21.11 Laceration without FB of front wall of thorax without penetration into thoracic cavity
 6th

S21.111- right front wall of thorax without penetration into thoracic cavity
 7th

S21.112- left front wall of thorax without penetration into thoracic cavity
 7th

S21.119- unspecified front wall of thorax without penetration into thoracic cavity
 7th

S21.12 Laceration with FB of; front wall of thorax without penetration into thoracic cavity
 6th

S21.121- right front wall of thorax without penetration into thoracic cavity
 7th

S21.122- left front wall of thorax without penetration into thoracic cavity
 7th

S21.129- unspecified front wall of thorax without penetration into thoracic cavity
 7th

S21.13 Puncture wound without FB of; front wall of thorax without penetration into thoracic cavity
 6th

S21.131- right front wall of thorax without penetration into thoracic cavity
 7th

S21.132- left front wall of thorax without penetration into thoracic cavity
 7th

S21.139- unspecified front wall of thorax without penetration into thoracic cavity
 7th

S21.14 Puncture wound with FB of; front wall of thorax without penetration into thoracic cavity
 6th

S21.141- right front wall of thorax without penetration into thoracic cavity
 7th

S21.142- left front wall of thorax without penetration into thoracic cavity
 7th

S21.149- unspecified front wall of thorax without penetration into thoracic cavity
 7th

S21.2 Open wound of back wall of thorax without penetration into thoracic cavity
 5th

S21.21 Laceration without FB of; back wall of thorax without penetration into thoracic cavity
 6th

S21.211- right back wall of thorax without penetration into thoracic cavity
 7th

S21.212- left back wall of thorax without penetration into thoracic cavity
 7th

S21.219- unspecified back wall of thorax without penetration into thoracic cavity
 7th

S21.22 Laceration with FB of; back wall of thorax without penetration into thoracic cavity
 6th

S21.221- right back wall of thorax without penetration into thoracic cavity
 7th

S21.222- left back wall of thorax without penetration into thoracic cavity
 7th

S21.229- unspecified back wall of thorax without penetration into thoracic cavity
 7th

S21.23 Puncture wound without FB of; back wall of thorax without penetration into thoracic cavity
 6th

S21.231- right back wall of thorax without penetration into thoracic cavity
 7th

S21.232- left back wall of thorax without penetration into thoracic cavity
 7th

S21.239- unspecified back wall of thorax without penetration into thoracic cavity
 7th

S21.24 Puncture wound with FB of; back wall of thorax without penetration into thoracic cavity
 6th

S21.241- right back wall of thorax without penetration into thoracic cavity
 7th

S21.242- left back wall of thorax without penetration into thoracic cavity
 7th

S21.249- unspecified back wall of thorax without penetration into thoracic cavity
 7th

S21.9 Open wound of unspecified part of thorax
 5th Open wound of thoracic wall NOS

S21.91X- Laceration without FB of unspecified part of thorax
 7th

S21.92X- Laceration with FB of unspecified part of thorax
 7th

S21.93X- Puncture wound without FB of unspecified part of thorax
 7th

S21.94X- Puncture wound with FB of unspecified part of thorax
 7th

S21.95X- Open bite of unspecified part of thorax
 7th *Excludes1:* superficial bite of thorax (S20.97)

S22 FRACTURE OF RIB(S), STERNUM AND THORACIC SPINE
4th

Note: A fracture not indicated as displaced or nondisplaced should be coded to displaced

A fracture not indicated as open or closed should be coded to closed

Includes: fracture of thoracic neural arch
fracture of thoracic spinous process
fracture of thoracic transverse process
fracture of thoracic vertebra
fracture of thoracic vertebral arch

Code also, if applicable, any associated condition such as:
injury of intrathoracic organ (S27.-)
spinal cord injury (S24.0-, S24.1-)
traumatic hemopneumothorax (S27.2)
traumatic hemothorax (S27.1-)
traumatic pneumothorax (S27.0)

Excludes1: transection of thorax (S28.1)

Excludes2: fracture of clavicle (S42.0-)
fracture of scapula (S42.1-)

S22 requires a 7th character
A—initial encounter for closed fracture
B—initial encounter for open fracture
D—subsequent encounter for fracture with routine healing
G—subsequent encounter for fracture with delayed healing
K—subsequent encounter for fracture with nonunion
S—sequela

S22.2 Fracture of sternum
 5th

S22.20X- Unspecified fracture of sternum
 7th

S22.21X- Fracture of manubrium
 7th

S22.22X- Fracture of body of sternum
 7th

S22.23X- Sternal manubrial dissociation
 7th

S22.24X- Fracture of xiphoid process
 7th

S22.3 Fracture of one rib
 5th

S22.31X- Fracture of one rib, right side
 7th

S22.32X- Fracture of one rib, left side
 7th

S22.39X- Fracture of one rib, unspecified side
 7th

S22.4 Multiple fractures of ribs
 5th Fractures of two or more ribs
Excludes1: flail chest (S22.5-)

S22.41X- Multiple fractures of ribs, right side
 7th

S22.42X- Multiple fractures of ribs, left side
 7th

S22.43X- Multiple fractures of ribs, bilateral
 7th

S22.49X- Multiple fractures of ribs, unspecified side
 7th

S22.5XX- Flail chest
 7th

S22.9XX- Fracture of bony thorax, part unspecified
 7th

S24 INJURY OF NERVES AND SPINAL CORD AT THORAX LEVEL

Note: Code to highest level of thoracic spinal cord injury

Injuries to the spinal cord (S24.0 and S24.1) refer to the cord level and not bone level injury, and can affect nerve roots at and below the level given.

Code also any associated:
fracture of thoracic vertebra (S22.0-)
open wound of thorax (S21.-)
transient paralysis (R29.5)

Excludes2: injury of brachial plexus (S14.3)

S24.0XX- Concussion and edema of thoracic spinal cord

S24.1 Other and unspecified injuries of thoracic spinal cord

S24.10 Unspecified injury of thoracic spinal cord

S24.101- Unspecified injury at T1 level of thoracic spinal cord

S24.102- Unspecified injury at T2-T6 level of thoracic spinal cord

S24.103- Unspecified injury at T7-T10 level of thoracic spinal cord

S24.104- Unspecified injury at T11-T12 level of thoracic spinal cord

S24.109- Unspecified level of thoracic spinal cord Injury of thoracic spinal cord NOS

S27 INJURY OF OTHER AND UNSPECIFIED INTRATHORACIC ORGANS

Code also any associated open wound of thorax (S21.-)

Excludes2: injury of cervical esophagus (S10-S19)
injury of trachea (cervical) (S10-S19)

S27.0XX Traumatic pneumothorax

Excludes1: spontaneous pneumothorax (J93.-)

S27.3 Other and unspecified injuries of lung

S27.30 Unspecified injury of lung,

S27.301- unilateral

S27.302- bilateral

S27.32 Contusion of lung,

S27.321- unilateral

S27.322- bilateral

S27.329- unspecified

(S30-S39) INJURIES TO THE ABDOMEN, LOWER BACK, LUMBAR SPINE, PELVIS AND EXTERNAL GENITALS

Includes: injuries to the abdominal wall
injuries to the anus
injuries to the buttock
injuries to the external genitalia
injuries to the flank
injuries to the groin

Excludes2: burns and corrosions (T20-T32)
effects of FB in anus and rectum (T18.5)
effects of FB in genitourinary tract (T19.-)
effects of FB in stomach, small intestine and colon (T18.2-T18.4)
frostbite (T33-T34)
insect bite or sting, venomous (T63.4)

S30 SUPERFICIAL INJURY OF ABDOMEN, LOWER BACK, PELVIS AND EXTERNAL GENITALS

Excludes2: superficial injury of hip (S70.-)

S30.0XX- Contusion of lower back and pelvis
Contusion of buttock

S30.1XX- Contusion of abdominal wall
Contusion of flank
Contusion of groin

S30.2 Contusion of external genital organs

S30.20 Contusion of unspecified external genital organ

S30.201- Contusion of unspecified external genital organ, male

S30.202- Contusion of unspecified external genital organ, female

S30.21X- Contusion of penis

S30.22X- Contusion of scrotum and testes

S30.23X- Contusion of vagina and vulva

S30.3XX- Contusion of anus

S30.8 Other superficial injuries of abdomen, lower back, pelvis and external genitals

S30.81 Abrasion of abdomen, lower back, pelvis and external genitals

S30.810- Abrasion of lower back and pelvis

S30.811- Abrasion of abdominal wall

S30.812- Abrasion of penis

S30.813- Abrasion of scrotum and testes

S30.814- Abrasion of vagina and vulva

S30.815- Abrasion of unspecified external genital organs, male

S30.816- Abrasion of unspecified external genital organs, female

S30.817- Abrasion of anus

S30.82 Blister (nonthermal) of abdomen, lower back, pelvis and external genitals

S30.820- Blister (non-thermal) of lower back and pelvis

S30.821- Blister (nonthermal) of abdominal wall

S30.822- Blister (nonthermal) of penis

S30.823- Blister (nonthermal) of scrotum and testes

S30.824- Blister (nonthermal) of vagina and vulva

S30.825- Blister (nonthermal) of unspecified external genital organs, male

S30.826- Blister (nonthermal) of unspecified external genital organs, female

S30.827- Blister (nonthermal) of anus

S30.84 External constriction of abdomen, lower back, pelvis and external genitals

S30.840- External constriction of lower back and pelvis

S30.841- External constriction of abdominal wall

S30.842- External constriction of penis
Hair tourniquet syndrome of penis
Use additional cause code to identify the constricting item (W49.0-)

S30.843- External constriction of scrotum and testes

S30.844- External constriction of vagina and vulva

S30.845- External constriction of unspecified external genital organs, male

S30.846- External constriction of unspecified external genital organs, female

S24 requires a 7th character
A—initial encounter
D—subsequent encounter
S—sequela

S27 requires a 7th character
A—initial encounter
D—subsequent encounter
S—sequela

S30 requires a 7th character
A—initial encounter
D—subsequent encounter
S—sequela

S30.85 **Superficial FB of abdomen, lower back, pelvis and external genitals**

S30 requires a 7th character
A—initial encounter
D—subsequent encounter
S—sequela

Splinter in the abdomen, lower back, pelvis and external genitals

S30.850- Superficial FB of lower back and pelvis

S30.851- Superficial FB of abdominal wall

S30.852- Superficial FB of penis

S30.853- Superficial FB of scrotum and testes

S30.854- Superficial FB of vagina and vulva

S30.855- Superficial FB of unspecified external genital organs, male

S30.856- Superficial FB of unspecified external genital organs, female

S30.857- Superficial FB of anus

S30.86 **Insect bite (nonvenomous) of abdomen, lower back, pelvis and external genitals**

S30.860- Insect bite (nonvenomous) of lower back and pelvis

S30.861- Insect bite (nonvenomous) of abdominal wall

S30.862- Insect bite (nonvenomous) of penis

S30.863- Insect bite (nonvenomous) of scrotum and testes

S30.864- Insect bite (nonvenomous) of vagina and vulva

S30.865- Insect bite (nonvenomous) of unspecified external genital organs, male

S30.866- Insect bite (nonvenomous) of unspecified external genital organs, female

S30.867- Insect bite (nonvenomous) of anus

S30.87 **Other superficial bite of abdomen, lower back, pelvis and external genitals**

Excludes1: open bite of abdomen, lower back, pelvis and external genitals (S31.05, S31.15, S31.25, S31.35, S31.45, S31.55)

S30.870- Other superficial bite of lower back and pelvis

S30.871- Other superficial bite of abdominal wall

S30.872- Other superficial bite of penis

S30.873- Other superficial bite of scrotum and testes

S30.874- Other superficial bite of vagina and vulva

S30.875- Other superficial bite of unspecified external genital organs, male

S30.876- Other superficial bite of unspecified external genital organs, female

S30.877- Other superficial bite of anus

S30.9 **Unspecified superficial injury of abdomen, lower back, pelvis and external genitals**

S30.91X- Unspecified superficial injury of lower back and pelvis

S30.92X- Unspecified superficial injury of abdominal wall

S30.93X- Unspecified superficial injury of penis

S30.94X- Unspecified superficial injury of scrotum and testes

S30.95X- Unspecified superficial injury of vagina and vulva

S30.96X- Unspecified superficial injury of unspecified external genital organs, male

S30.97X- Unspecified superficial injury of unspecified external genital organs, female

S30.98X- Unspecified superficial injury of anus

S31 OPEN WOUND OF ABDOMEN, LOWER BACK, PELVIS AND EXTERNAL GENITALS

S31 requires a 7th character
A—initial encounter
D—subsequent encounter
S—sequela

Code also any associated:
spinal cord injury (S24.0, S24.1-, S34.0-, S34.1-)
wound infection

Excludes1: traumatic amputation of part of abdomen, lower back and pelvis (S38.2-, S38.3)

Excludes2: open wound of hip (S71.00–S71.02)
open fracture of pelvis (S32.1–S32.9 with 7th character B)

S31.0 **Open wound of lower back and pelvis**

S31.01 **Laceration without FB of lower back and pelvis;**

For subcategory S31.0, use 6th character of 1 for penetration into the retroperitoneum, along with the appropriate 7th character.

S31.010- without penetration into retroperitoneum
Laceration without FB of lower back and pelvis NOS

S31.011- with penetration into retroperitoneum

S31.02 **Laceration with FB of lower back and pelvis**

S31.020- without penetration into retroperitoneum
Laceration with FB of lower back and pelvis NOS

S31.021- with penetration into retroperitoneum

S31.03 **Puncture wound without FB of lower back and pelvis**

S31.030- without penetration into retroperitoneum
Puncture wound without FB of lower back and pelvis NOS

S31.031- with penetration into retroperitoneum

S31.04 **Puncture wound with FB of lower back and pelvis**

S31.040- without penetration into retroperitoneum
Puncture wound with FB of lower back and pelvis NOS

S31.041- with penetration into retroperitoneum

S31.05 **Open bite of lower back and pelvis**
Bite of lower back and pelvis NOS
Excludes1: superficial bite of lower back and pelvis (S30.860, S30.870)

S31.050- without penetration into retroperitoneum
Open bite of lower back and pelvis NOS

S31.051- with penetration into retroperitoneum

S31.1 **Open wound of abdominal wall without penetration into peritoneal cavity**
Open wound of abdominal wall NOS
Excludes2: open wound of abdominal wall with penetration into peritoneal cavity (S31.6-)

S31.11 **Laceration without FB of abdominal wall without penetration into peritoneal cavity**

S31.110- Laceration without foreign body of abdominal wall, right upper quadrant without penetration into peritoneal cavity

S31.111- Laceration without foreign body of abdominal wall, left upper quadrant without penetration into peritoneal cavity

S31.112- Laceration without foreign body of abdominal wall, epigastric region without penetration into peritoneal cavity

S31.113- Laceration without foreign body of abdominal wall, right lower quadrant without penetration into peritoneal cavity

S31.114- Laceration without foreign body of abdominal wall, left lower quadrant without penetration into peritoneal cavity

S31.115- Laceration without foreign body of abdominal wall, periumbilic region without penetration into peritoneal cavity

S31.119- Laceration without foreign body of abdominal wall, unspecified quadrant without penetration into peritoneal cavity

S31.12 Laceration with FB of abdominal wall without penetration into peritoneal cavity

S31.120- Laceration of abdominal wall with foreign body, right upper quadrant without penetration into peritoneal cavity

S31.121- Laceration of abdominal wall with foreign body, left upper quadrant without penetration into peritoneal cavity

S31.122- Laceration of abdominal wall with foreign body, epigastric region without penetration into peritoneal cavity

S31.123- Laceration of abdominal wall with foreign body, right lower quadrant without penetration into peritoneal cavity

S31.124- Laceration of abdominal wall with foreign body, left lower quadrant without penetration into peritoneal cavity

S31.125- Laceration of abdominal wall with foreign body, periumbilic region without penetration into peritoneal cavity

S31.129- Laceration of abdominal wall with foreign body, unspecified quadrant without penetration into peritoneal cavity

S31.13 Puncture wound of abdominal wall without FB without penetration into peritoneal cavity

S31.130- Puncture wound of abdominal wall without foreign body, right upper quadrant without penetration into peritoneal cavity

S31.131- Puncture wound of abdominal wall without foreign body, left upper quadrant without penetration into peritoneal cavity

S31.132- Puncture wound of abdominal wall without foreign body, epigastric region without penetration into peritoneal cavity

S31.133- Puncture wound of abdominal wall without foreign body, right lower quadrant without penetration into peritoneal cavity

S31.134- Puncture wound of abdominal wall without foreign body, left lower quadrant without penetration into peritoneal cavity

S31.135- Puncture wound of abdominal wall without foreign body, periumbilic region without penetration into peritoneal cavity

S31.139- Puncture wound of abdominal wall without foreign body, unspecified quadrant without penetration into peritoneal cavity

S31.14 Puncture wound of abdominal wall with FB without penetration into peritoneal cavity

S31.140- Puncture wound of abdominal wall with foreign body, right upper quadrant without penetration into peritoneal cavity

S31.141- Puncture wound of abdominal wall with foreign body, left upper quadrant without penetration into peritoneal cavity

S31.142- Puncture wound of abdominal wall with foreign body, epigastric region without penetration into peritoneal cavity

S31.143- Puncture wound of abdominal wall with foreign body, right lower quadrant without penetration into peritoneal cavity

S31.144- Puncture wound of abdominal wall with foreign body, left lower quadrant without penetration into peritoneal cavity

S31.145- Puncture wound of abdominal wall with foreign body, periumbilic region without penetration into peritoneal cavity

S31.149- Puncture wound of abdominal wall with foreign body, unspecified quadrant without penetration into peritoneal cavity

S31.15 Open bite of abdominal wall without penetration into peritoneal cavity

Bite of abdominal wall NOS

Excludes1: superficial bite of abdominal wall (S30.871)

S31.150- Open bite of abdominal wall, right upper quadrant without penetration into peritoneal cavity

S31.151- Open bite of abdominal wall, left upper quadrant without penetration into peritoneal cavity

S31.152- Open bite of abdominal wall, epigastric region without penetration into peritoneal cavity

S31.153- Open bite of abdominal wall, right lower quadrant without penetration into peritoneal cavity

S31.154- Open bite of abdominal wall, left lower quadrant without penetration into peritoneal cavity

S31.155- Open bite of abdominal wall, periumbilic region without penetration into peritoneal cavity

S31.159- Open bite of abdominal wall, unspecified quadrant without penetration into peritoneal cavity

S31.2 Open wound of penis

S31.21X- Laceration without FB of penis

S31.23X- Puncture wound without foreign body of penis

S31.24X- Puncture wound with foreign body of penis

S31.25X- Open bite of penis

Bite of penis NOS

Excludes1: superficial bite of penis (S30.862, S30.872)

S31.3 Open wound of scrotum and testes

S31.31X- Laceration without FB of scrotum and testes

S31.33X- Puncture wound without foreign body of scrotum and testes

S31.34X- Puncture wound with foreign body of scrotum and testes

S31.35X- Open bite of scrotum and testes

Bite of scrotum and testes NOS

Excludes1: superficial bite of scrotum and testes (S30.863, S30.873)

S31.4 Open wound of vagina and vulva

Excludes1: injury to vagina and vulva during delivery (O70.-, O71.4)

S31.41X- Laceration without FB of vagina and vulva

S31.42X- Laceration with FB of vagina and vulva

S31.43X- Puncture wound without FB of vagina and vulva

S31.44X- Puncture wound with FB of vagina and vulva

S31.45X- Open bite of vagina and vulva

Bite of vagina and vulva NOS

Excludes1: superficial bite of vagina and vulva (S30.864, S30.874)

S31.8 Open wound of other parts of abdomen, lower back and pelvis

S31.81 Open wound of right buttock

S31.811- Laceration without FB of right buttock

S31.812- Laceration with FB of right buttock

S31.813- Puncture wound without FB of right buttock

S31.814- Puncture wound with FB of right buttock

S31.815- Open bite of right buttock
Bite of right buttock NOS
Excludes1: superficial bite of buttock (S30.870)

S31.82 Open wound of left buttock

S31.821- Laceration without FB of left buttock

S31.822- Laceration with FB of left buttock

S31.823- Puncture wound without FB of left buttock

S31.824- Puncture wound with FB of left buttock

S31.825- Open bite of left buttock
Bite of left buttock NOS
Excludes1: superficial bite of buttock (S30.870)

S31.83 Open wound of anus

S31.831- Laceration without FB of anus

S31.832- Laceration with FB of anus

S31.833- Puncture wound without FB of anus

S31.834- Puncture wound with FB of anus

S31.835- Open bite of anus
Bite of anus NOS
Excludes1: superficial bite of anus (S30.877)

S32 FRACTURE OF LUMBAR SPINE AND PELVIS

Note: A fracture not indicated as displaced or nondisplaced should be coded to displaced

A fracture not indicated as opened or closed should be coded to closed

Includes: fracture of lumbosacral neural arch
fracture of lumbosacral spinous process
fracture of lumbosacral transverse process
fracture of lumbosacral vertebra or of lumbosacral vertebral arch

Code first any associated spinal cord and spinal nerve injury (S34.-)

Excludes1: transection of abdomen (S38.3)

Excludes2: fracture of hip NOS (S72.0-)

S32.1 Fracture of sacrum

For vertical fractures, code to most medial fracture extension

Use two codes if both a vertical and transverse fracture are present

Code also any associated fracture of pelvic ring (S32.8-)

S32.10X- Unspecified fracture of sacrum

S32.11 Zone I fracture of sacrum
Vertical sacral ala fracture of sacrum

S32.110- Nondisplaced Zone I fracture of sacrum

S32.111- Minimally displaced Zone I fracture of sacrum

S32.112- Severely displaced Zone I fracture of sacrum

S32.119- Unspecified Zone I fracture of sacrum

S32.12 Zone II fracture of sacrum
Vertical foraminal region fracture of sacrum

S32.120- Nondisplaced Zone II fracture of sacrum

S32.121- Minimally displaced Zone II fracture of sacrum

S32.122- Severely displaced Zone II fracture of sacrum

S32.129- Unspecified Zone II fracture of sacrum

S32.13 Zone III fracture of sacrum
Vertical fracture into spinal canal region of sacrum

S32.130- Nondisplaced Zone III fracture of sacrum

S32.131- Minimally displaced Zone III fracture of sacrum

S32.132- Severely displaced Zone III fracture of sacrum

S32.139- Unspecified Zone III fracture of sacrum

S32.14X- Type 1 fracture of sacrum
Transverse flexion fracture of sacrum without displacement

S32.15X- Type 2 fracture of sacrum
Transverse flexion fracture of sacrum with posterior displacement

S32.16X- Type 3 fracture of sacrum
Transverse extension fracture of sacrum with anterior displacement

S32.17X- Type 4 fracture of sacrum
Transverse segmental comminution of upper sacrum

S32.19X- Other fracture of sacrum

S32.2XX- Fracture of coccyx

S32.3 Fracture of ilium
Excludes1: fracture of ilium with associated disruption of pelvic ring (S32.8-)

S32.30 Unspecified fracture of ilium

S32.301- Unspecified fracture of right ilium

S32.302- Unspecified fracture of left ilium

S32.309- Unspecified fracture of unspecified ilium

S32.31 Avulsion fracture of ilium

S32.311- Displaced avulsion fracture of right ilium

S32.312- Displaced avulsion fracture of left ilium

S32.313- Displaced avulsion fracture of unspecified ilium

S32.314- Nondisplaced avulsion fracture of right ilium

S32.315- Nondisplaced avulsion fracture of left ilium

S32.316- Nondisplaced avulsion fracture of unspecified ilium

S32.39 Other fracture of ilium

S32.391- Other fracture of right ilium

S32.392- Other fracture of left ilium

S32.399- Other fracture of unspecified ilium

S32.4 Fracture of acetabulum

Code also any associated fracture of pelvic ring (S32.8-)

S32.40 Unspecified fracture of acetabulum

S32.401- Unspecified fracture of right acetabulum

S32.402- Unspecified fracture of left acetabulum

S32.41 Fracture of anterior wall of acetabulum

S32.411- Displaced fracture of anterior wall of right acetabulum

S32.412- Displaced fracture of anterior wall of left acetabulum

S32.414- Nondisplaced fracture of anterior wall of right acetabulum

S32.415- Nondisplaced fracture of anterior wall of left acetabulum

S32.42 Fracture of posterior wall of acetabulum

S32.421- Displaced fracture of posterior wall of right acetabulum

S32.422- Displaced fracture of posterior wall of left acetabulum

S32.424- Nondisplaced fracture of posterior wall of right acetabulum

S32.425- Nondisplaced fracture of posterior wall of left acetabulum

S32.43 Fracture of anterior column [iliopubic] of acetabulum

S32.431- Displaced fracture of anterior column [iliopubic] of right acetabulum

S32.432- Displaced fracture of anterior column [iliopubic] of left acetabulum

S32.434- Nondisplaced fracture of anterior column [iliopubic] of right aceta-bulum

S32.435- Nondisplaced fracture of anterior column [iliopubic] of left aceta-bulum

S32.44 Fracture of posterior column [ilioischial] of acetabulum

S32.441- Displaced fracture of posterior column [ilioischial] of right acetabulum

S32.442- Displaced fracture of posterior column [ilioischial] of left acetabulum

S32.444- Nondisplaced fracture of posterior column [ilioischial] of right acetabulum

S32.445- Nondisplaced fracture of posterior column [ilioischial] of left acetabulum

S32.45 Transverse fracture of acetabulum

S32.451- Displaced transverse fracture of right acetabulum

S32.452- Displaced transverse fracture of left acetabulum

S32.454- Nondisplaced transverse fracture of right acetabulum

S32.455- Nondisplaced transverse fracture of left acetabulum

S32.456- Nondisplaced transverse fracture of unspecified acetabulum

S32.46 Associated transverse-posterior fracture of acetabulum

S32.461- Displaced associated transverse-posterior fracture of right acetabulum

S32.462- Displaced associated transverse-posterior fracture of left acetabulum

S32.464- Nondisplaced associated transverse-posterior fracture of right acetabulum

S32.465- Nondisplaced associated transverse-posterior fracture of left acetabulum

S32.47 Fracture of medial wall of acetabulum

S32.471- Displaced fracture of medial wall of right acetabulum

S32.472- Displaced fracture of medial wall of left acetabulum

S32.474- Nondisplaced fracture of medial wall of right acetabulum

S32.475- Nondisplaced fracture of medial wall of left acetabulum

S32.48 Dome fracture of acetabulum

S32.481- Displaced dome fracture of right acetabulum

S32.482- Displaced dome fracture of left acetabulum

S32.484- Nondisplaced dome fracture of right acetabulum

S32.485- Nondisplaced dome fracture of left acetabulum

S32.49 Other specified fracture of acetabulum

S32.491- Other specified fracture of right acetabulum

S32.492- Other specified fracture of left acetabulum

S32.5 Fracture of pubis

Excludes1: fracture of pubis with associated disruption of pelvic ring (S32.8-)

S32.50 Unspecified fracture of pubis

S32.501- Unspecified fracture of right pubis

S32.502- Unspecified fracture of left pubis

S32.51 Fracture of superior rim of pubis

S32.511- Fracture of superior rim of right pubis

S32.512- Fracture of superior rim of left pubis

S32.59 Other specified fracture of pubis

S32.591- Other specified fracture of right pubis

S32.592- Other specified fracture of left pubis

S32.6 Fracture of ischium

Excludes1: fracture of ischium with associated disruption of pelvic ring (S32.8-)

S32.60 Unspecified fracture of ischium

S32.601- Unspecified fracture of right ischium

S32.602- Unspecified fracture of left ischium

S32.61 Avulsion fracture of ischium

S32.611- Displaced avulsion fracture of right ischium

S32.612- Displaced avulsion fracture of left ischium

S32.614- Nondisplaced avulsion fracture of right ischium

S32.615- Nondisplaced avulsion fracture of left ischium

S32.69 Other specified fracture of ischium

S32.691- Other specified fracture of right ischium

S32.692- Other specified fracture of left ischium

S32.8 Fracture of other parts of pelvis

Code also any associated: fracture of acetabulum (S32.4-) sacral fracture (S32.1-)

S32.81 Multiple fractures of pelvis with disruption of pelvic ring

Multiple pelvic fractures with disruption of pelvic circle

S32.810- Multiple fractures of pelvis with stable disruption of pelvic ring

S32.811- Multiple fractures of pelvis with unstable disruption of pelvic ring

S32.82X- Multiple fractures of pelvis without disruption of pelvic ring

Multiple pelvic fractures without disruption of pelvic circle

S32.89X- Fracture of other parts of pelvis

S32.9XX- Fracture of unspecified parts of lumbosacral spine and pelvis

7th

Fracture of lumbosacral spine NOS
Fracture of pelvis NOS

S33 DISLOCATION AND SPRAIN OF JOINTS AND LIGAMENTS OF LUMBAR SPINE AND PELVIS

Includes: avulsion of joint or ligament of lumbar spine and pelvis
laceration of cartilage, joint or ligament of lumbar spine and pelvis
sprain of cartilage, joint or ligament of lumbar spine and pelvis
traumatic hemarthrosis of joint or ligament of lumbar spine and pelvis
traumatic rupture of joint or ligament of lumbar spine and pelvis
traumatic subluxation of joint or ligament of lumbar spine and pelvis
traumatic tear of joint or ligament of lumbar spine and pelvis

Code also any associated open wound

Excludes1: nontraumatic rupture or displacement of lumbar intervertebral disc NOS (M51.-)
obstetric damage to pelvic joints and ligaments (O71.6)

Excludes2: dislocation and sprain of joints and ligaments of hip (S73.-)
strain of muscle of lower back and pelvis (S39.01-)

S33.2XX- Dislocation of sacroiliac and sacrococcygeal joint

7th

S33.5XX- Sprain of ligaments of lumbar spine

7th

S33.6XX- Sprain of sacroiliac joint

7th

S33.8XX- Sprain of other parts of lumbar spine and pelvis

7th

S33.9XX- Sprain of unspecified parts of lumbar spine and pelvis

7th

S34 INJURY OF LUMBAR AND SACRAL SPINAL CORD AND NERVES AT ABDOMEN, LOWER BACK AND PELVIS LEVEL

Note: Code to highest level of lumbar cord injury

Injuries to the spinal cord (S34.0 and S34.1) refer to the cord level and not bone level injury, and can affect nerve roots at and below the level given.

Code also any associated: fracture of vertebra (S22.0-, S32.0-)
open wound of abdomen, lower back and pelvis (S31.-)
transient paralysis (R29.5)

- **S34.0** Concussion and edema of lumbar and sacral spinal cord
  - 5th **S34.01X-** Concussion and edema of lumbar spinal cord
    - 7th
  - **S34.02X-** Concussion and edema of sacral spinal cord
    - 7th Concussion and edema of conus medullaris
- **S34.1** Other and unspecified injury of lumbar and sacral spinal cord
  - 5th **S34.10** Unspecified injury to lumbar spinal cord
    - 6th **S34.101-** Unspecified injury to L1 level of lumbar spinal cord
      - 7th
    - **S34.102-** Unspecified injury to L2 level of lumbar spinal cord
      - 7th
    - **S34.103-** Unspecified injury to L3 level of lumbar spinal cord
      - 7th
    - **S34.104-** Unspecified injury to L4 level of lumbar spinal cord
      - 7th
    - **S34.105-** Unspecified injury to L5 level of lumbar spinal cord
      - 7th
    - **S34.109-** Unspecified injury to unspecified level of lumbar spinal cord
      - 7th
  - **S34.12** Incomplete lesion of lumbar spinal cord
    - 6th **S34.121-** Incomplete lesion of L1 level of lumbar spinal cord
      - 7th
    - **S34.122-** Incomplete lesion of L2 level of lumbar spinal cord
      - 7th
    - **S34.123-** Incomplete lesion of L3 level of lumbar spinal cord
      - 7th
    - **S34.124-** Incomplete lesion of L4 level of lumbar spinal cord
      - 7th
    - **S34.125-** Incomplete lesion of L5 level of lumbar spinal cord
      - 7th

S34.129- Incomplete lesion of unspecified level of lumbar spinal cord

7th

- **S34.13** Other and unspecified injury to sacral spinal cord
  - 6th Other injury to conus medullaris
  - **S34.131-** Complete lesion of sacral spinal cord
    - 7th Complete lesion of conus medullaris
  - **S34.132-** Incomplete lesion of sacral spinal cord
    - 7th Incomplete lesion of conus medullaris
  - **S34.139-** Unspecified injury to sacral spinal cord
    - 7th Unspecified injury of conus medullaris
- **S34.2** Injury of nerve root of lumbar and sacral spine
  - 5th **S34.21X-** Injury of nerve root of lumbar spine
    - 7th
  - **S34.22X-** Injury of nerve root of sacral spine
    - 7th

S34.3XX- Injury of cauda equina

7th

S34.4XX- Injury of lumbosacral plexus

7th

- **S34.5XX-** Injury of lumbar, sacral and pelvic sympathetic nerves
  - 7th Injury of celiac ganglion or plexus
  - Injury of hypogastric plexus
  - Injury of mesenteric plexus (inferior) (superior)
  - Injury of splanchnic nerve

S34.6XX- Injury of peripheral nerve(s) at abdomen, lower back and pelvis level

7th

S34.8XX- Injury of other nerves at abdomen, lower back and pelvis level

7th

S34.9XX- Injury of unspecified nerves at abdomen, lower back and pelvis level

7th

S36 INJURY OF INTRA-ABDOMINAL ORGANS

Code also any associated open wound (S31.-)

- **S36.0** Injury of spleen
  - 5th **S36.02** Contusion of spleen
    - 6th **S36.020-** Minor contusion of spleen
      - 7th Contusion of spleen less than 2 cm
    - **S36.021-** Major contusion of spleen
      - 7th Contusion of spleen greater than 2 cm
  - **S36.03** Laceration of spleen
    - 6th **S36.030-** Superficial (capsular) laceration of spleen
      - 7th Laceration of spleen less than 1 cm
      - Minor laceration of spleen
    - **S36.032-** Major laceration of spleen
      - 7th Avulsion of spleen
      - Laceration of spleen greater than 3 cm
      - Massive laceration of spleen
      - Multiple moderate lacerations of spleen
      - Stellate laceration of spleen
- **S36.3** Injury of stomach
  - 5th **S36.30X-** Unspecified injury of stomach
    - 7th
  - **S36.32X-** Contusion of stomach
    - 7th
- **S36.6** Injury of rectum
  - 5th **S36.60X-** Unspecified injury of rectum
    - 7th
  - **S36.62X-** Contusion of rectum
    - 7th
  - **S36.63X-** Laceration of rectum
    - 7th
- **S36.9** Injury of unspecified intra-abdominal organ
  - 5th **S36.90X-** Unspecified injury of unspecified intra-abdominal organ
    - 7th
  - **S36.92X-** Contusion of unspecified intra-abdominal organ
    - 7th
  - **S36.93X-** Laceration of unspecified intra-abdominal organ
    - 7th
  - **S36.99X-** Other injury of unspecified intra-abdominal organ
    - 7th

S37 INJURY OF URINARY AND PELVIC ORGANS

S37 requires a 7th character
A—initial encounter
D—subsequent encounter
S—sequela

Code also any associated open wound (S31.-)

Excludes1: obstetric trauma to pelvic organs (O71.-)

Excludes2: injury of peritoneum (S36.81)
injury of retroperitoneum (S36.89-)

S37.0 Injury of kidney

Excludes2: acute kidney injury (nontraumatic) (N17.9)

S37.01 Minor contusion of kidney
Contusion of kidney less than 2 cm
Contusion of kidney NOS

S37.011- Minor contusion of right kidney

S37.012- Minor contusion of left kidney

S37.02 Major contusion of kidney
Contusion of kidney greater than 2 cm

S37.021- Major contusion of right kidney

S37.022- Major contusion of left kidney

S39 OTHER AND UNSPECIFIED INJURIES OF ABDOMEN, LOWER BACK, PELVIS AND EXTERNAL GENITALS

S39 requires a 7th character
A—initial encounter
D—subsequent encounter
S—sequela

Code also any associated open wound (S31.-)

Excludes2: sprain of joints and ligaments of lumbar spine and pelvis (S33.-)

S39.0 Injury of muscle, fascia and tendon of abdomen, lower back and pelvis

S39.01 Strain of muscle, fascia and tendon of abdomen, lower back and pelvis

S39.011- Strain of muscle, fascia and tendon of abdomen

S39.012- Strain of muscle, fascia and tendon of lower back

S39.8 Other specified injuries of abdomen, lower back, pelvis and external genitals

S39.83X- Other specified injuries of pelvis

S39.84 Other specified injuries of external genitals

S39.848- Other specified injuries of external genitals

S39.9 Unspecified injury of abdomen, lower back, pelvis and external genitals

S39.91X- Unspecified injury of abdomen

S39.92X- Unspecified injury of lower back

S39.93X- Unspecified injury of pelvis

S39.94X- Unspecified injury of external genitals

(S40–S49) INJURIES TO THE SHOULDER AND UPPER ARM

Includes: injuries of axilla
injuries of scapular region

Excludes2: burns and corrosions (T20-T32)
frostbite (T33-T34)
injuries of elbow (S50-S59)
insect bite or sting, venomous (T63.4)

S40 SUPERFICIAL INJURY OF SHOULDER AND UPPER ARM

S40 requires a 7th character
A—initial encounter
D—subsequent encounter
S—sequela

S40.0 Contusion of shoulder and upper arm

S40.01 Contusion of shoulder

S40.011- Contusion of right shoulder

S40.012- Contusion of left shoulder

S40.02 Contusion of upper arm

S40.021- Contusion of right upper arm

S40.022- Contusion of left upper arm

S40.2 Other superficial injuries of shoulder

S40.21 Abrasion of shoulder

S40.211- Abrasion of right shoulder

S40.212- Abrasion of left shoulder

S40.22 Blister (nonthermal) of shoulder

S40.221- Blister (nonthermal) of right shoulder

S40.222- Blister (nonthermal) of left shoulder

S40.24 External constriction of shoulder

S40.241- External constriction of right shoulder

S40.242- External constriction of left shoulder

S40.25 Superficial FB of shoulder
Splinter in the shoulder

S40.251- Superficial FB of right shoulder

S40.252- Superficial FB of left shoulder

S40.26 Insect bite (nonvenomous) of shoulder

S40.261- Insect bite (nonvenomous) of right shoulder

S40.262- Insect bite (nonvenomous) of left shoulder

S40.27 Other superficial bite of shoulder

Excludes1: open bite of shoulder (S41.05)

S40.271- Other superficial bite of right shoulder

S40.272- Other superficial bite of left shoulder

S40.8 Other superficial injuries of upper arm

S40.81 Abrasion of upper arm

S40.811- Abrasion of right upper arm

S40.812- Abrasion of left upper arm

S40.82 Blister (nonthermal) of upper arm

S40.821- Blister (nonthermal) of right upper arm

S40.822- Blister (nonthermal) of left upper arm

S40.84 External constriction of upper arm

S40.841- External constriction of right upper arm

S40.842- External constriction of left upper arm

S40.85 Superficial FB of upper arm
Splinter in the upper arm

S40.851- Superficial FB of right upper arm

S40.852- Superficial FB of left upper arm

S40.86 Insect bite (nonvenomous) of upper arm

S40.861- Insect bite (nonvenomous) of right upper arm

S40.862- Insect bite (nonvenomous) of left upper arm

S40.87 Other superficial bite of upper arm

Excludes1: open bite of upper arm (S41.14)

Excludes2: other superficial bite of shoulder (S40.27-)

S40.871- Other superficial bite of right upper arm

S40.872- Other superficial bite of left upper arm

S40.9 Unspecified superficial injury of shoulder and upper arm

S40.91 Unspecified superficial injury of shoulder

S40.911- Unspecified superficial injury of right shoulder

S40.912- Unspecified superficial injury of left shoulder

S40.92 Unspecified superficial injury of upper arm

S40.921- Unspecified superficial injury of right upper arm

S40.922- Unspecified superficial injury of left upper arm

S41 OPEN WOUND OF SHOULDER AND UPPER ARM

S41 requires a 7th character
A—initial encounter
D—subsequent encounter
S—sequela

Code also any associated wound infection

Excludes1: traumatic amputation of shoulder and upper arm (S48.-)

Excludes2: open fracture of shoulder and upper arm (S42.- with 7th character B or C)

S41.0 Open wound of shoulder

S41.01 Laceration without FB of shoulder

S41.011- Laceration without FB of right shoulder

S41.012- Laceration without FB of left shoulder

S41.02 Laceration with FB of shoulder

S41.021- Laceration with FB of right shoulder

S41.022- Laceration with FB of left shoulder

S41.03 Puncture wound without FB of shoulder

S41.031- Puncture wound without FB of right shoulder

S41.032- Puncture wound without FB of left shoulder

S41.04 Puncture wound with FB of shoulder

S41.041- Puncture wound with FB of right shoulder

S41.042- Puncture wound with FB of left shoulder

S41.05 Open bite of shoulder

Bite of shoulder NOS

Excludes1: superficial bite of shoulder (S40.27)

S41.051- Open bite of right shoulder

S41.052- Open bite of left shoulder

S41.1 Open wound of upper arm

S41.11 Laceration without FB of upper arm

S41.111- Laceration without FB of right upper arm

S41.112- Laceration without FB of left upper arm

S41.12 Laceration with FB of upper arm

S41.121- Laceration with FB of right upper arm

S41.122- Laceration with FB of left upper arm

S41.13 Puncture wound without FB of upper arm

S41.131- Puncture wound without FB of right upper arm

S41.132- Puncture wound without FB of left upper arm

S41.14 Puncture wound with FB of upper arm

S41.141- Puncture wound with FB of right upper arm

S41.142- Puncture wound with FB of left upper arm

S41.15 Open bite of upper arm

Bite of upper arm NOS

Excludes1: superficial bite of upper arm (S40.87)

S41.151- Open bite of right upper arm

S41.152- Open bite of left upper arm

S42 FRACTURE OF SHOULDER AND UPPER ARM

S42 requires a 7th character
A—initial encounter for closed fracture
B—initial encounter for open fracture
D—subsequent encounter for fracture with routine healing
G—subsequent encounter for fracture with delayed healing
K—subsequent encounter for fracture with nonunion
P—subsequent encounter for fracture with malunion
S—sequela

Note: A fracture not indicated as displaced or nondisplaced should be coded to displaced

A fracture not indicated as open or closed should be coded to closed

Excludes1: traumatic amputation of shoulder and upper arm (S48.-)

Excludes2: periprosthetic fracture around internal prosthetic shoulder joint (M97.3)

S42.0 Fracture of clavicle

S42.00 Fracture of unspecified part of clavicle

S42.001- Fracture of unspecified part of right clavicle

S42.002- Fracture of unspecified part of left clavicle

S42.01 Fracture of sternal end of clavicle

S42.011- Anterior displaced fracture of sternal end of right clavicle

S42.012- Anterior displaced fracture of sternal end of left clavicle

S42.014- Posterior displaced fracture of sternal end of right clavicle

S42.015- Posterior displaced fracture of sternal end of left clavicle

S42.017- Nondisplaced fracture of sternal end of right clavicle

S42.018- Nondisplaced fracture of sternal end of left clavicle

S42.02 Fracture of shaft of clavicle

S42.021- Displaced fracture of shaft of right clavicle

S42.022- Displaced fracture of shaft of left clavicle

S42.024- Nondisplaced fracture of shaft of right clavicle

S42.025- Nondisplaced fracture of shaft of left clavicle

S42.03 Fracture of lateral end of clavicle

Fracture of acromial end of clavicle

S42.031- Displaced fracture of lateral end of right clavicle

S42.032- Displaced fracture of lateral end of left clavicle

S42.034- Nondisplaced fracture of lateral end of right clavicle

S42.035- Nondisplaced fracture of lateral end of left clavicle

S42.2 Fracture of upper end of humerus

Fracture of proximal end of humerus

Excludes2: fracture of shaft of humerus (S42.3-)

physeal fracture of upper end of humerus (S49.0-)

S42.20 Unspecified fracture of upper end of humerus

S42.201- Unspecified fracture of upper end of; right humerus

S42.202- Unspecified fracture of upper end of; left humerus

S42.21 Unspecified fracture of surgical neck of humerus

Fracture of neck of humerus NOS

S42.211- Unspecified displaced fracture of surgical neck of right humerus

S42.212- Unspecified displaced fracture of surgical neck of left humerus

S42.214- Unspecified nondisplaced fracture of surgical neck of right humerus

S42.215- Unspecified nondisplaced fracture of surgical neck of left humerus

S42.22 2-part fracture of surgical neck of humerus

S42.221- 2-part displaced fracture of surgical neck of right humerus
S42.222- 2-part displaced fracture of surgical neck of left humerus
S42.224- 2-part nondisplaced fracture of surgical neck of right humerus
S42.225- 2-part nondisplaced fracture of surgical neck of left humerus
S42.23 3-part fracture of surgical neck of humerus
S42.231- 3-part fracture of surgical neck of right humerus
S42.232- 3-part fracture of surgical neck of left humerus
S42.24 4-part fracture of surgical neck of humerus
S42.241- 4-part fracture of surgical neck of right humerus
S42.242- 4-part fracture of surgical neck of left humerus
S42.25 Fracture of greater tuberosity of humerus
S42.251- Displaced fracture of greater tuberosity of right humerus
S42.252- Displaced fracture of greater tuberosity of left humerus
S42.254- Nondisplaced fracture of greater tuberosity of right humerus
S42.255- Nondisplaced fracture of greater tuberosity of left humerus
S42.26 Fracture of lesser tuberosity of humerus
S42.261- Displaced fracture of lesser tuberosity of right humerus
S42.262- Displaced fracture of lesser tuberosity of left humerus
S42.264- Nondisplaced fracture of lesser tuberosity of right humerus
S42.265- Nondisplaced fracture of lesser tuberosity of left humerus
S42.27 Torus fracture of upper end of humerus
S42.271- Torus fracture of upper end of right humerus
S42.272- Torus fracture of upper end of left humerus

S42 requires a 7th character
A—initial encounter for closed fracture
B—initial encounter for open fracture
D—subsequent encounter for fracture with routine healing
G—subsequent encounter for fracture with delayed healing
K—subsequent encounter for fracture with nonunion
P—subsequent encounter for fracture with malunion
S—sequela

S42.27 requires a 7th character
A—initial encounter for closed fracture
D—subsequent encounter for fracture with routine healing
G—subsequent encounter for fracture with delayed healing
K—subsequent encounter for fracture with nonunion
P—subsequent encounter for fracture with malunion
S—sequela

S42.29 Other fracture of upper end of humerus
Fracture of anatomical neck of humerus
Fracture of articular head of humerus
S42.291- Other displaced fracture of upper end of right humerus
S42.292- Other displaced fracture of upper end of left humerus
S42.293- Other displaced fracture of upper end of unspecified humerus
S42.294- Other nondisplaced fracture of upper end of right humerus
S42.295- Other nondisplaced fracture of upper end of left humerus

S42.3 Fracture of shaft of humerus
Fracture of humerus NOS
Fracture of upper arm NOS
Excludes2: physeal fractures of upper end of humerus (S49.0-)
physeal fractures of lower end of humerus (S49.1-)
S42.30 Unspecified fracture of shaft of humerus
S42.301- Unspecified fracture of shaft of humerus, right arm
S42.302- Unspecified fracture of shaft of humerus, left arm
S42.31 Greenstick fracture of shaft of humerus
S42.311- Greenstick fracture of shaft of humerus, right arm
S42.312- Greenstick fracture of shaft of humerus, left arm

S42.31 requires a 7th character
A—initial encounter for closed fracture
D—subsequent encounter for fracture with routine healing
G—subsequent encounter for fracture with delayed healing
K—subsequent encounter for fracture with nonunion
P—subsequent encounter for fracture with malunion
S—sequela

S42.32 Transverse fracture of shaft of humerus
S42.321- Displaced transverse fracture of shaft of humerus, right arm
S42.322- Displaced transverse fracture of shaft of humerus, left arm
S42.324- Nondisplaced transverse fracture of shaft of humerus, right arm
S42.325- Nondisplaced transverse fracture of shaft of humerus, left arm
S42.33 Oblique fracture of shaft of humerus
S42.331- Displaced oblique fracture of shaft of humerus, right arm
S42.332- Displaced oblique fracture of shaft of humerus, left arm
S42.334- Nondisplaced oblique fracture of shaft of humerus, right arm
S42.335- Nondisplaced oblique fracture of shaft of humerus, left arm
S42.34 Spiral fracture of shaft of humerus
S42.341- Displaced spiral fracture of shaft of humerus, right arm
S42.342- Displaced spiral fracture of shaft of humerus, left arm
S42.343- Displaced spiral fracture of shaft of humerus, unspecified arm
S42.344- Nondisplaced spiral fracture of shaft of humerus, right arm
S42.345- Nondisplaced spiral fracture of shaft of humerus, left arm
S42.35 Comminuted fracture of shaft of humerus
S42.351- Displaced comminuted fracture of shaft of humerus, right arm
S42.352- Displaced comminuted fracture of shaft of humerus, left arm
S42.354- Nondisplaced comminuted fracture of shaft of humerus, right arm
S42.355- Nondisplaced comminuted fracture of shaft of humerus, left arm
S42.36 Segmental fracture of shaft of humerus
S42.361- Displaced segmental fracture of shaft of humerus, right arm
S42.362- Displaced segmental fracture of shaft of humerus, left arm
S42.364- Nondisplaced segmental fracture of shaft of humerus, right arm
S42.365- Nondisplaced segmental fracture of shaft of humerus, left arm
S42.39 Other fracture of shaft of humerus
S42.391- Other fracture of shaft of right humerus
S42.392- Other fracture of shaft of left humerus

Additional Character Required ✓ 3-character code

Unspecified laterality codes were excluded here.

* =New Code
▲ =Revised Code
◻ =Social determinants of health

Excludes1—Not coded here, do not use together
Excludes2—Not included here

S42.4 Fracture of lower end of humerus

5th Fracture of distal end of humerus

Excludes2: fracture of shaft of humerus (S42.3-)
physeal fracture of lower end of humerus (S49.1-)

S42 requires a 7th character
A—initial encounter for closed fracture
B—initial encounter for open fracture
D—subsequent encounter for fracture with routine healing
G—subsequent encounter for fracture with delayed healing
K—subsequent encounter for fracture with nonunion
P—subsequent encounter for fracture with malunion
S—sequela

S42.40 Unspecified fracture of lower end of humerus

6th Fracture of elbow NOS

S42.401- Unspecified fracture of lower end of right humerus

7th

S42.402- Unspecified fracture of lower end of left humerus

7th

S42.41 Simple supracondylar fracture without intercondylar fracture of humerus

6th

S42.411- Displaced simple supracondylar fracture without intercondylar fracture of right humerus

7th

S42.412- Displaced simple supracondylar fracture without intercondylar fracture of left humerus

7th

S42.414- Nondisplaced simple supracondylar fracture without intercondylar fracture of right humerus

7th

S42.415- Nondisplaced simple supracondylar fracture without intercondylar fracture of left humerus

7th

S42.42 Comminuted supracondylar fracture without intercondylar fracture of humerus

6th

S42.421- Displaced comminuted supracon-dylar fracture without intercondylar fracture of right humerus

7th

S42.422- Displaced comminuted supracon-dylar fracture without intercondylar fracture of left humerus

7th

S42.424- Nondisplaced comminuted supracondylar fracture without intercondylar fracture of right humerus

7th

S42.425- Nondisplaced comminuted supracondylar fracture without intercondylar fracture of left humerus

7th

S42.43 Fracture (avulsion) of lateral epicondyle of humerus

6th

S42.431- Displaced fracture (avulsion) of lateral epicondyle of right humerus

7th

S42.432- Displaced fracture (avulsion) of lateral epicondyle of left humerus

7th

S42.434- Nondisplaced fracture (avulsion) of lateral epicondyle of right humerus

7th

S42.435- Nondisplaced fracture (avulsion) of lateral epicondyle of left humerus

7th

S42.44 Fracture (avulsion) of medial epicondyle of humerus

6th

S42.441- Displaced fracture (avulsion) of medial epicondyle of right humerus

7th

S42.442- Displaced fracture (avulsion) of medial epicondyle of left humerus

7th

S42.444- Nondisplaced fracture (avulsion) of medial epicondyle of right humerus

7th

S42.445- Nondisplaced fracture (avulsion) of medial epicondyle of left humerus

7th

S42.447- Incarcerated fracture (avulsion) of medial epicondyle of right humerus

7th

S42.448- Incarcerated fracture (avulsion) of medial epicondyle of left humerus

7th

S42.45 Fracture of lateral condyle of humerus

6th Fracture of capitellum of humerus

S42.451- Displaced fracture of lateral condyle of right humerus

7th

S42.452- Displaced fracture of lateral condyle of left humerus

7th

S42.454- Nondisplaced fracture of lateral condyle of right humerus

7th

S42.455- Nondisplaced fracture of lateral condyle of left humerus

7th

S42.46 Fracture of medial condyle of humerus

6th Trochlea fracture of humerus

S42.461- Displaced fracture of medial condyle of right humerus

7th

S42.462- Displaced fracture of medial condyle of left humerus

7th

S42.464- Nondisplaced fracture of medial condyle of right humerus

7th

S42.465- Nondisplaced fracture of medial condyle of left humerus

7th

S42.47 Transcondylar fracture of humerus

6th

S42.471- Displaced transcondylar fracture of right humerus

7th

S42.472- Displaced transcondylar fracture of left humerus

7th

S42.474- Nondisplaced transcondylar fracture of right humerus

7th

S42.475- Nondisplaced transcondylar fracture of left humerus

7th

S42.48 Torus fracture of lower end of humerus

6th

S42.48 requires a 7th character
A—initial encounter for closed fracture
D—subsequent encounter for fracture with routine healing
G—subsequent encounter for fracture with delayed healing
K—subsequent encounter for fracture with nonunion
P—subsequent encounter for fracture with malunion
S—sequela

S42.481- Torus fracture of lower end of right humerus

7th

S42.482- Torus fracture of lower end of left humerus

7th

S42.49 Other fracture of lower end of humerus

6th

S42.491- Other displaced fracture of lower end of right humerus

7th

S42.492- Other displaced fracture of lower end of left humerus

7th

S42.494- Other nondisplaced fracture of lower end of right humerus

7th

S42.495- Other nondisplaced fracture of lower end of left humerus

7th

S42.9 Fracture of shoulder girdle, part unspecified

5th Fracture of shoulder NOS

S42.91X- Fracture of right shoulder girdle, part unspecified

7th

S42.92X- Fracture of left shoulder girdle, part unspecified

7th

S43 DISLOCATION AND SPRAIN OF JOINTS AND LIGAMENTS OF SHOULDER GIRDLE

4th

S43 requires a 7th character
A—initial encounter
D—subsequent encounter
S—sequela

Includes: avulsion of joint or ligament of shoulder girdle
laceration of cartilage, joint or ligament of shoulder girdle
sprain of cartilage, joint or ligament of shoulder girdle
traumatic hemarthrosis of joint or ligament of shoulder girdle
traumatic rupture of joint or ligament of shoulder girdle
traumatic subluxation of joint or ligament of shoulder girdle
traumatic tear of joint or ligament of shoulder girdle

Code also any associated open wound

Excludes2: strain of muscle, fascia and tendon of shoulder and upper arm (S46.-)

S43.0 Subluxation and dislocation of shoulder joint

5th Dislocation of glenohumeral joint
Subluxation of glenohumeral joint

S43.00 Unspecified subluxation and dislocation of shoulder joint

6th

Dislocation of humerus NOS
Subluxation of humerus NOS

S43.001- Unspecified subluxation of right shoulder joint

7th

S43.002- Unspecified subluxation of left shoulder joint

7th

S43.004- Unspecified dislocation of right shoulder joint

S43.005- Unspecified dislocation of left shoulder joint

S43.01 Anterior subluxation and dislocation of humerus

S43.011- Anterior subluxation of right humerus

S43.012- Anterior subluxation of left humerus

S43.014- Anterior dislocation of right humerus

S43.015- Anterior dislocation of left humerus

S43.02 Posterior subluxation and dislocation of humerus

S43.021- Posterior subluxation of right humerus

S43.022- Posterior subluxation of left humerus

S43.024- Posterior dislocation of right humerus

S43.025- Posterior dislocation of left humerus

S43.03 Inferior subluxation and dislocation of humerus

S43.031- Inferior subluxation of right humerus

S43.032- Inferior subluxation of left humerus

S43.034- Inferior dislocation of right humerus

S43.035- Inferior dislocation of left humerus

S43.08 Other subluxation and dislocation of shoulder joint

S43.081- Other subluxation of right shoulder joint

S43.082- Other subluxation of left shoulder joint

S43.084- Other dislocation of right shoulder joint

S43.085- Other dislocation of left shoulder joint

S43.1 Subluxation and dislocation of acromioclavicular joint

S43.10 Unspecified dislocation of acromioclavicular joint

S43.101- Unspecified dislocation of right acromioclavicular joint

S43.102- Unspecified dislocation of left acromioclavicular joint

S43.11 Subluxation of acromioclavicular joint

S43.111- Subluxation of right acromioclavicular joint

S43.112- Subluxation of left acromioclavicular joint

S43.12 Dislocation of acromioclavicular joint, 100%–200% displacement

S43.121- Dislocation of right acromioclavicular joint, 100%–200% displacement

S43.122- Dislocation of left acromioclavicular joint, 100%–200% displacement

S43.13 Dislocation of acromioclavicular joint, greater than 200% displacement

S43.131- Dislocation of right acromioclavicular joint, greater than 200% displacement

S43.132- Dislocation of left acromioclavicular joint, greater than 200% displacement

S43.14 Inferior dislocation of acromioclavicular joint

S43.141- Inferior dislocation of right acromioclavicular joint

S43.142- Inferior dislocation of left acromioclavicular joint

S43.15 Posterior dislocation of acromioclavicular joint

S43.151- Posterior dislocation of right acromioclavicular joint

S43.152- Posterior dislocation of left acromioclavicular joint

S43.2 Subluxation and dislocation of sternoclavicular joint

S43.20 Unspecified subluxation and dislocation of sternoclavicular joint

S43.201- Unspecified subluxation of right sternoclavicular joint

S43.202- Unspecified subluxation of left sternoclavicular joint

S43.204- Unspecified dislocation of right sternoclavicular joint

S43.205- Unspecified dislocation of left sternoclavicular joint

S43.21 Anterior subluxation and dislocation of sternoclavicular joint

S43.211- Anterior subluxation of right sternoclavicular joint

S43.212- Anterior subluxation of left sternoclavicular joint

S43.214- Anterior dislocation of right sternoclavicular joint

S43.215- Anterior dislocation of left sternoclavicular joint

S43.22 Posterior subluxation and dislocation of sternoclavicular joint

S43.221- Posterior subluxation of right sternoclavicular joint

S43.222- Posterior subluxation of left sternoclavicular joint

S43.224- Posterior dislocation of right sternoclavicular joint

S43.225- Posterior dislocation of left sternoclavicular joint

S43.3 Subluxation and dislocation of other and unspecified parts of shoulder girdle

S43.30 Subluxation and dislocation of unspecified parts of shoulder girdle

Dislocation/subluxation of shoulder girdle NOS

S43.301- Subluxation of unspecified parts of right shoulder girdle

S43.302- Subluxation of unspecified parts of left shoulder girdle

S43.304- Dislocation of unspecified parts of right shoulder girdle

S43.305- Dislocation of unspecified parts of left shoulder girdle

S43.31 Subluxation and dislocation of scapula

S43.311- Subluxation of right scapula

S43.312- Subluxation of left scapula

S43.314- Dislocation of right scapula

S43.315- Dislocation of left scapula

S43.39 Subluxation and dislocation of other parts of shoulder girdle

S43.391- Subluxation of other parts of right shoulder girdle

S43.392- Subluxation of other parts of left shoulder girdle

S43.394- Dislocation of other parts of right shoulder girdle

S43.395- Dislocation of other parts of left shoulder girdle

S43.4 Sprain of shoulder joint

S43.40 Unspecified sprain of shoulder joint

S43.401- Unspecified sprain of right shoulder joint

S43.402- Unspecified sprain of left shoulder joint

S43.41 Sprain of coracohumeral (ligament)

S43.411- Sprain of right coracohumeral (ligament)

S43.412- Sprain of left coracohumeral (ligament)

S43.42 Sprain of rotator cuff capsule

Excludes1: rotator cuff syndrome (complete) (incomplete), not specified as traumatic (M75.1-)

Excludes2: injury of tendon of rotator cuff (S46.0-)

S43.421- Sprain of right rotator cuff capsule

S43.422- Sprain of left rotator cuff capsule

S43.43 Superior glenoid labrum lesion SLAP lesion

S43.431- Superior glenoid labrum lesion of right shoulder

S43.432- Superior glenoid labrum lesion of left shoulder

S43.49 Other sprain of shoulder joint

S43.491- Other sprain of right shoulder joint

S43.492- Other sprain of left shoulder joint

S43.5 Sprain of acromioclavicular joint Sprain of acromioclavicular ligament

S43.51X- Sprain of right acromioclavicular joint

S43.52X- Sprain of left acromioclavicular joint

S43.6 Sprain of sternoclavicular joint

S43.61X- Sprain of right sternoclavicular joint

S43.62X- Sprain of left sternoclavicular joint

S43.8 Sprain of other specified parts of shoulder girdle

S43.81X- Sprain of other specified parts of right shoulder girdle

S43.82X- Sprain of other specified parts of left shoulder girdle

S46 INJURY OF MUSCLE, FASCIA AND TENDON AT SHOULDER AND UPPER ARM LEVEL

Code also any associated open wound (S41.-)

Excludes2: injury of muscle, fascia and tendon at elbow (S56.-)
sprain of joints and ligaments of shoulder girdle (S43.9)

S46.0 Injury of muscle(s) and tendon(s) of the rotator cuff of shoulder

S46.00 Unspecified injury of muscle(s) and tendon(s) of the rotator cuff of shoulder

S46.001- Unspecified injury of muscle(s) and tendon(s) of the rotator cuff of right shoulder

S46.002- Unspecified injury of muscle(s) and tendon(s) of the rotator cuff of left shoulder

S46.01 Strain of muscle(s) and tendon(s) of the rotator cuff of shoulder

S46.011- Strain of muscle(s) and tendon(s) of the rotator cuff of right shoulder

S46.012- Strain of muscle(s) and tendon(s) of the rotator cuff of left shoulder

S46.02 Laceration of muscle(s) and tendon(s) of the rotator cuff of shoulder

S46.021- Laceration of muscle(s) and tendon(s) of the rotator cuff of right shoulder

S46.022- Laceration of muscle(s) and tendon(s) of the rotator cuff of left shoulder

S46.09 Other injury of muscle(s) and tendon(s) of the rotator cuff of shoulder

S46.091- Other injury of muscle(s) and tendon(s) of the rotator cuff of right shoulder

S46.092- Other injury of muscle(s) and tendon(s) of the rotator cuff of left shoulder

S46.91 Strain of unspecified muscle, fascia and tendon at shoulder and upper arm level

S46.911- Strain of unspecified muscle, fascia and tendon at shoulder and upper arm level, right arm

S46.912- Strain of unspecified muscle, fascia and tendon at shoulder and upper arm level, left arm

S46.92 Laceration of unspecified muscle, fascia and tendon at shoulder and upper arm level

S46.921- Laceration of unspecified muscle, fascia and tendon at shoulder and upper arm level, right arm

S46.922- Laceration of unspecified muscle, fascia and tendon at shoulder and upper arm level, left arm

S46.99 Other injury of unspecified muscle, fascia and tendon at shoulder and upper arm level

S46.991- Other injury of unspecified muscle, fascia and tendon at shoulder and upper arm level, right arm

S46.992- Other injury of unspecified muscle, fascia and tendon at shoulder and upper arm level, left arm

S49 OTHER AND UNSPECIFIED INJURIES OF SHOULDER AND UPPER ARM

S49.0 Physeal fracture of upper end of humerus

S49.00 Unspecified physeal fracture of upper end of humerus

S49.001- Unspecified physeal fracture of upper end of humerus, right arm

S49.002- Unspecified physeal fracture of upper end of humerus, left arm

S49.01 Salter-Harris Type I physeal fracture of upper end of humerus,

S49.011- right arm

S49.012- left arm

S49.02 Salter-Harris Type II physeal fracture of upper end of humerus,

S49.021- right arm

S49.022- left arm

S49.03 Salter-Harris Type III physeal fracture of upper end of humerus,

S49.031- right arm

S49.032- left arm

S49.04 Salter-Harris Type IV physeal fracture of upper end of humerus,

S49.041- right arm

S49.042- left arm

S49.09 Other physeal fracture of upper end of humerus,

S49.091- Other physeal fracture of upper end of humerus, right arm

S49.092- Other physeal fracture of upper end of humerus, left arm

S49.1 Physeal fracture of lower end of humerus

S49.10 Unspecified physeal fracture of lower end of humerus

S49.101- right arm

S49.102- left arm

S49.11 Salter-Harris Type I physeal fracture of lower end of humerus,
S49.111- right arm

S49.112- left arm

S49.12 Salter-Harris Type II physeal fracture of lower end of humerus,
S49.121- right arm

S49.122- left arm

S49.13 Salter-Harris Type III physeal fracture of lower end of humerus,
S49.131- right arm

S49.132- left arm

S49.14 Salter-Harris Type IV physeal fracture of lower end of humerus,
S49.141- right arm

S49.142- left arm

S49.19 Other physeal fracture of lower end of humerus,
S49.191- right arm

S49.192 left arm

S49 requires a 7th character
A—initial encounter for closed fracture
D—subsequent encounter for fracture with routine healing
G—subsequent encounter for fracture with delayed healing
K—subsequent encounter for fracture with nonunion
P—subsequent encounter for fracture with malunion
S—sequela

(S50–S59) INJURIES TO THE ELBOW AND FOREARM

Excludes2: burns and corrosions (T20–T32)
frostbite (T33–T34)
injuries of wrist and hand (S60–S69)
insect bite or sting, venomous (T63.4)

S50 SUPERFICIAL INJURY OF ELBOW AND FOREARM

Excludes2: superficial injury of wrist and hand (S60.-)

S50 requires a 7th character
A—initial encounter
D—subsequent encounter
S—sequela

S50.0 Contusion of elbow
S50.01X- Contusion of right elbow

S50.02X- Contusion of left elbow

S50.1 Contusion of forearm
S50.11X- Contusion of right forearm

S50.12X- Contusion of left forearm

S50.3 Other superficial injuries of elbow
S50.31 Abrasion of elbow
S50.311- Abrasion of right elbow

S50.312- Abrasion of left elbow

S50.32 Blister (nonthermal) of elbow
S50.321- Blister (nonthermal) of right elbow

S50.322- Blister (nonthermal) of left elbow

S50.34 External constriction of elbow
S50.341- External constriction of right elbow

S50.342- External constriction of left elbow

S50.35 Superficial FB of elbow
Splinter in the elbow
S50.351- Superficial FB of right elbow

S50.352- Superficial FB of left elbow

S50.36 Insect bite (nonvenomous) of elbow
S50.361- Insect bite (nonvenomous) of right elbow

S50.362- Insect bite (nonvenomous) of left elbow

S50.37 Other superficial bite of elbow
Excludes1: open bite of elbow (S51.04)
S50.371- Other superficial bite of right elbow

S50.372- Other superficial bite of left elbow

S50.8 Other superficial injuries of forearm
S50.81 Abrasion of forearm
S50.811- Abrasion of right forearm

S50.812- Abrasion of left forearm

S50.82 Blister (nonthermal) of forearm
S50.821- Blister (nonthermal) of right forearm

S50.822- Blister (nonthermal) of left forearm

S50.84 External constriction of forearm
S50.841- External constriction of right forearm

S50.842- External constriction of left forearm

S50.85 Superficial FB of forearm
Splinter in the forearm
S50.851- Superficial FB of right forearm

S50.852- Superficial FB of left forearm

S50.86 Insect bite (nonvenomous) of forearm
S50.861- Insect bite (nonvenomous) of right forearm

S50.862- Insect bite (nonvenomous) of left forearm

S50.87 Other superficial bite of forearm
Excludes1: open bite of forearm (S51.84)
S50.871- Other superficial bite of right forearm

S50.872- Other superficial bite of left forearm

S51 OPEN WOUND OF ELBOW AND FOREARM

Code also any associated wound infection
Excludes1: open fracture of elbow and forearm (S52.- with open fracture 7th character)
traumatic amputation of elbow and forearm (S58.-)
Excludes2: open wound of wrist and hand (S61.-)

S51 requires a 7th character
A—initial encounter
D—subsequent encounter
S—sequela

S51.0 Open wound of elbow
S51.01 Laceration without FB of elbow
S51.011- Laceration without FB of right elbow

S51.012- Laceration without FB of left elbow

S51.02 Laceration with FB of elbow
S51.021- Laceration with FB of right elbow

S51.022- Laceration with FB of left elbow

S51.03 Puncture wound without FB of elbow
S51.031- Puncture wound without FB of right elbow

S51.032- Puncture wound without FB of left elbow

S51.04 Puncture wound with FB of elbow
S51.041- Puncture wound with FB of right elbow

S51.042- Puncture wound with FB of left elbow

S51 requires a 7th character
A—initial encounter
D—subsequent encounter
S—sequela

S51.05 Open bite of elbow
Bite of elbow NOS
Excludes1: superficial bite of elbow (S50.36, S50.37)
S51.051- Open bite, right elbow

S51.052- Open bite, left elbow

S51.8 Open wound of forearm
Excludes2: open wound of elbow (S51.0-)

S51.81 Laceration without FB of forearm
S51.811- Laceration without FB of right forearm

S51.812- Laceration without FB of left forearm

S51.82 Laceration with FB of forearm
S51.821- Laceration with FB of right forearm

S51.822- Laceration with FB of left forearm

S51.83 Puncture wound without FB of forearm
S51.831- Puncture wound without FB of right forearm
S51.832- Puncture wound without FB of left forearm

S51.84 Puncture wound with FB of forearm
S51.841- Puncture wound with FB of right forearm

S51.842- Puncture wound with FB of left forearm

S51.85 Open bite of forearm
Bite of forearm NOS
Excludes1: superficial bite of forearm (S50.86, S50.87)
S51.851- Open bite of right forearm

S51.852- Open bite of left forearm

S52 FRACTURE OF FOREARM

Note: A fracture not indicated as displaced or nondisplaced should be coded to displaced

A fracture not indicated as open or closed should be coded to closed

The open fracture designations are based on the Gustilo open fracture classification

Excludes1: traumatic amputation of forearm (S58.-)
Excludes2: fracture at wrist and hand level (S62.-)
periprosthetic fracture around internal prosthetic elbow joint (M97.4)

S52.0 Fracture of upper end of ulna
Fracture of proximal end of ulna
Excludes2: fracture of elbow NOS (S42.40-)
fractures of shaft of ulna (S52.2-)

S52.00 Unspecified fracture of upper end of ulna
S52.001- Unspecified fracture of upper end of right ulna
S52.002- Unspecified fracture of upper end of left ulna

S52 requires a 7th character
A—initial encounter for closed fracture
B—initial encounter for open fracture type I or II initial encounter for open fracture NOS
C—initial encounter for open fracture type IIIA, IIIB, or IIIC
D—subsequent encounter for closed fracture with routine healing
E—subsequent encounter for open fracture type I or II with routine healing
F—subsequent encounter for open fracture type IIIA, IIIB, or IIIC with routine healing
G—subsequent encounter for closed fracture with delayed healing
H—subsequent encounter for open fracture type I or II with delayed healing
J—subsequent encounter for open fracture type IIIA, IIIB, or IIIC with delayed healing
K—subsequent encounter for closed fracture with nonunion
M—subsequent encounter for open fracture type I or II with nonunion
N—subsequent encounter for open fracture type IIIA, IIIB, or IIIC with nonunion
P—subsequent encounter for closed fracture with malunion
Q—subsequent encounter for open fracture type I or II with malunion
R—subsequent encounter for open fracture type IIIA, IIIB, or IIIC with malunion
S—sequela

S52.01 Torus fracture of upper end of ulna
S52.011- Torus fracture of upper end of right ulna
S52.012- Torus fracture of upper end of left ulna

S52.01 requires a 7th character
A—initial encounter for closed fracture
D—subsequent encounter for fracture with routine healing
G—subsequent encounter for fracture with delayed healing
K—subsequent encounter for fracture with nonunion
P—subsequent encounter for fracture with malunion
S—sequela

S52.02 Fracture of olecranon process without intraarticular extension of ulna
S52.021- Displaced fracture of olecranon process without intraarticular extension of right ulna
S52.022- Displaced fracture of olecranon process without intraarticular extension of left ulna
S52.024- Nondisplaced fracture of olecranon process without intraarticular extension of right ulna
S52.025- Nondisplaced fracture of olecranon process without intraarticular extension of left ulna

S52.03 Fracture of olecranon process with intraarticular extension of ulna
S52.031- Displaced fracture of olecranon process with intraarticular extension of right ulna
S52.032- Displaced fracture of olecranon process with intraarticular extension of left ulna
S52.034- Nondisplaced fracture of olecranon process with intraarticular extension of right ulna
S52.035- Nondisplaced fracture of olecranon process with intraarticular extension of left ulna

S52.04 Fracture of coronoid process of ulna
S52.041- Displaced fracture of coronoid process of right ulna
S52.042- Displaced fracture of coronoid process of left ulna
S52.044- Nondisplaced fracture of coronoid process of right ulna
S52.045- Nondisplaced fracture of coronoid process of left ulna

S52.09 Other fracture of upper end of ulna
S52.091- Other fracture of upper end of right ulna

S52.092- Other fracture of upper end of left ulna

S52.1 Fracture of upper end of radius
Fracture of proximal end of radius
Excludes2: physeal fractures of upper end of radius (S59.2-)
fracture of shaft of radius (S52.3-)

S52.10 Unspecified fracture of upper end of radius
S52.101- Unspecified fracture of upper end of right radius
S52.102- Unspecified fracture of upper end of left radius

S52.11 Torus fracture of upper end of radius
S52.111- Torus fracture of upper end of right radius
S52.112- Torus fracture of upper end of left radius

S52.11 requires a 7th character
A—initial encounter for closed fracture
D—subsequent encounter for fracture with routine healing
G—subsequent encounter for fracture with delayed healing
K—subsequent encounter for fracture with nonunion
P—subsequent encounter for fracture with malunion
S—sequela

S52.12 Fracture of head of radius
S52.121- Displaced fracture of head of right radius

CHAPTER 19. INJURY, POISONING AND CERTAIN OTHER CONSEQUENCES OF EXTERNAL CAUSES (S00–T88)

(S52.122–S52.331)

S52.122- Displaced fracture of head of left radius

S52.124- Nondisplaced fracture of head of right radius

S52.125- Nondisplaced fracture of head of left radius

S52.13 Fracture of neck of radius

S52.131- Displaced fracture of neck of right radius

S52.132- Displaced fracture of neck of left radius

S52.134- Nondisplaced fracture of neck of right radius

S52.135- Nondisplaced fracture of neck of left radius

S52.18 Other fracture of upper end of radius

S52.181- Other fracture of upper end of right radius

S52.182- Other fracture of upper end of left radius

S52 requires a 7th character
A—initial encounter for closed fracture
B—initial encounter for open fracture type I or II initial encounter for open fracture NOS
C—initial encounter for open fracture type IIIA, IIIB, or IIIC
D—subsequent encounter for closed fracture with routine healing
E—subsequent encounter for open fracture type I or II with routine healing
F—subsequent encounter for open fracture type IIIA, IIIB, or IIIC with routine healing
G—subsequent encounter for closed fracture with delayed healing
H— subsequent encounter for open fracture type I or II with delayed healing
J—subsequent encounter for open fracture type IIIA, IIIB, or IIIC with delayed healing
K—subsequent encounter for closed fracture with nonunion
M—subsequent encounter for open fracture type I or II with nonunion
N—subsequent encounter for open fracture type IIIA, IIIB, or IIIC with nonunion
P—subsequent encounter for closed fracture with malunion
Q—subsequent encounter for open fracture type I or II with malunion
R—subsequent encounter for open fracture type IIIA, IIIB, or IIIC with malunion
S—sequela

S52.2 Fracture of shaft of ulna

S52.20 Unspecified fracture of shaft of ulna
Fracture of ulna NOS

S52.201- Unspecified fracture of shaft of right ulna

S52.202- Unspecified fracture of shaft of left ulna

S52.21 Greenstick fracture of shaft of ulna

S52.211- Greenstick fracture of shaft of right ulna

S52.212- Greenstick fracture of shaft of left ulna

S52.21 requires a 7th character
A—initial encounter for closed fracture
D—subsequent encounter for fracture with routine healing
G—subsequent encounter for fracture with delayed healing
K—subsequent encounter for fracture with nonunion
P—subsequent encounter for fracture with malunion
S—sequela

S52.22 Transverse fracture of shaft of ulna

S52.221- Displaced transverse fracture of shaft of right ulna

S52.222- Displaced transverse fracture of shaft of left ulna

S52.224- Nondisplaced transverse fracture of shaft of right ulna

S52.225- Nondisplaced transverse fracture of shaft of left ulna

S52.23 Oblique fracture of shaft of ulna

S52.231- Displaced oblique fracture of shaft of right ulna

S52.232- Displaced oblique fracture of shaft of left ulna

S52.234- Nondisplaced oblique fracture of shaft of right ulna

S52.235- Nondisplaced oblique fracture of shaft of left ulna

S52.24 Spiral fracture of shaft of ulna

S52.241- Displaced spiral fracture of shaft of ulna, right arm

S52.242- Displaced spiral fracture of shaft of ulna, left arm

S52.244- Nondisplaced spiral fracture of shaft of ulna, right arm

S52.245- Nondisplaced spiral fracture of shaft of ulna, left arm

S52.25 Comminuted fracture of shaft of ulna

S52.251- Displaced comminuted fracture of shaft of ulna, right arm

S52.252- Displaced comminuted fracture of shaft of ulna, left arm

S52.254- Nondisplaced comminuted fracture of shaft of ulna, right arm

S52.255- Nondisplaced comminuted fracture of shaft of ulna, left arm

S52.26 Segmental fracture of shaft of ulna

S52.261- Displaced segmental fracture of shaft of ulna, right arm

S52.262- Displaced segmental fracture of shaft of ulna, left arm

S52.264- Nondisplaced segmental fracture of shaft of ulna, right arm

S52.265- Nondisplaced segmental fracture of shaft of ulna, left arm

S52.27 Monteggia's fracture of ulna
Fracture of upper shaft of ulna with dislocation of radial head

S52.271- Monteggia's fracture of right ulna

S52.272- Monteggia's fracture of left ulna

S52.28 Bent bone of ulna

S52.281- Bent bone of right ulna

S52.282- Bent bone of left ulna

S52.29 Other fracture of shaft of ulna

S52.291- Other fracture of shaft of right ulna

S52.292- Other fracture of shaft of left ulna

S52.3 Fracture of shaft of radius

S52.30 Unspecified fracture of shaft of radius

S52.301- Unspecified fracture of shaft of right radius

S52.302- Unspecified fracture of shaft of left radius

S52.31 Greenstick fracture of shaft of radius

S52.311- Greenstick fracture of shaft of radius, right arm

S52.312- Greenstick fracture of shaft of radius, left arm

S52.31 requires a 7th character
A—initial encounter for closed fracture
D—subsequent encounter for fracture with routine healing
G—subsequent encounter for fracture with delayed healing
K—subsequent encounter for fracture with nonunion
P—subsequent encounter for fracture with malunion
S—sequela

S52.32 Transverse fracture of shaft of radius

S52.321- Displaced transverse fracture of shaft of right radius

S52.322- Displaced transverse fracture of shaft of left radius

S52.324- Nondisplaced transverse fracture of shaft of right radius

S52.325- Nondisplaced transverse fracture of shaft of left radius

S52.33 Oblique fracture of shaft of radius

S52.331- Displaced oblique fracture of shaft of right radius

S52.332- Displaced oblique fracture of shaft of left radius

S52.334- Nondisplaced oblique fracture of shaft of right radius

S52.335- Nondisplaced oblique fracture of shaft of left radius

S52.34 Spiral fracture of shaft of radius

S52.341- Displaced spiral fracture of shaft of radius, right arm

S52.342- Displaced spiral fracture of shaft of radius, left arm

S52.344- Nondisplaced spiral fracture of shaft of radius, right arm

S52.345- Nondisplaced spiral fracture of shaft of radius, left arm

S52.35 Comminuted fracture of shaft of radius

S52.351- Displaced comminuted fracture of shaft of radius, right arm

S52.352- Displaced comminuted fracture of shaft of radius, left arm

S52.354- Nondisplaced comminuted fracture of shaft of radius, right arm

S52.355- Nondisplaced comminuted fracture of shaft of radius, left arm

S52.36 Segmental fracture of shaft of radius

S52.361- Displaced segmental fracture of shaft of radius, right arm

S52.362- Displaced segmental fracture of shaft of radius, left arm

S52.364- Nondisplaced segmental fracture of shaft of radius, right arm

S52.365- Nondisplaced segmental fracture of shaft of radius, left arm

S52.37 Galeazzi's fracture

Fracture of lower shaft of radius with radioulnar joint dislocation

S52.371- Galeazzi's fracture of right radius

S52.372- Galeazzi's fracture of left radius

S52.38 Bent bone of radius

S52.381- Bent bone of right radius

S52.382- Bent bone of left radius

S52.39 Other fracture of shaft of radius

S52.391- Other fracture of shaft of radius, right arm

S52.392- Other fracture of shaft of radius, left arm

S52 requires a 7th character
A—initial encounter for closed fracture
B—initial encounter for open fracture type I or II initial encounter for open fracture NOS
C—initial encounter for open fracture type IIIA, IIIB, or IIIC
D—subsequent encounter for closed fracture with routine healing
E—subsequent encounter for open fracture type I or II with routine healing
F—subsequent encounter for open fracture type IIIA, IIIB, or IIIC with routine healing
G—subsequent encounter for closed fracture with delayed healing
H— subsequent encounter for open fracture type I or II with delayed healing
J—subsequent encounter for open fracture type IIIA, IIIB, or IIIC with delayed healing
K—subsequent encounter for closed fracture with nonunion
M—subsequent encounter for open fracture type I or II with nonunion
N—subsequent encounter for open fracture type IIIA, IIIB, or IIIC with nonunion
P—subsequent encounter for closed fracture with malunion
Q—subsequent encounter for open fracture type I or II with malunion
R—subsequent encounter for open fracture type IIIA, IIIB, or IIIC with malunion
S—sequela

S52.5 Fracture of lower end of radius

Fracture of distal end of radius

Excludes: physeal fractures of lower end of radius (S59.2-)

S52.50 Unspecified fracture of the lower end of radius

S52.501- Unspecified fracture of the lower end of right radius

S52.502- Unspecified fracture of the lower end of left radius

S52.51 Fracture of radial styloid process

S52.511- Displaced fracture of right radial styloid process

S52.512- Displaced fracture of left radial styloid process

S52.514- Nondisplaced fracture of right radial styloid process

S52.515- Nondisplaced fracture of left radial styloid process

S52.52 Torus fracture of lower end of radius

S52.521- Torus fracture of lower end of right radius

S52.522- Torus fracture of lower end of left radius

S52.52 requires a 7th character
A—initial encounter for closed fracture
D—subsequent encounter for fracture with routine healing
G—subsequent encounter for fracture with delayed healing
K—subsequent encounter for fracture with nonunion
P—subsequent encounter for fracture with malunion
S—sequela

S52.53 Colles' fracture

S52.531- Colles' fracture of right radius

S52.532- Colles' fracture of left radius

S52.54 Smith's fracture

S52.541- Smith's fracture of right radius

S52.542- Smith's fracture of left radius

S52.55 Other extraarticular fracture of lower end of radius

S52.551- Other extra-articular fracture of lower end of right radius

S52.552- Other extra-articular fracture of lower end of left radius

S52.56 Barton's fracture

S52.561- Barton's fracture of right radius

S52.562- Barton's fracture of left radius

S52.57 Other intraarticular fracture of lower end of radius

S52.571- Other intraarticular fracture of lower end of right radius

S52.572- Other intraarticular fracture of lower end of left radius

S52.59 Other fractures of lower end of radius

S52.591- Other fractures of lower end of right radius

S52.592- Other fractures of lower end of left radius

S52.6 Fracture of lower end of ulna

S52.60 Unspecified fracture of lower end of ulna

S52.601- Unspecified fracture of lower end of right ulna

S52.602- Unspecified fracture of lower end of left ulna

S52.61 Fracture of ulna styloid process

S52.611- Displaced fracture of right ulna styloid process

S52.612- Displaced fracture of left ulna styloid process

S52.614- Nondisplaced fracture of right ulna styloid process

S52.615- Nondisplaced fracture of left ulna styloid process

S52.62 Torus fracture of lower end of ulna

S52.621- Torus fracture of lower end of right ulna

S52.622- Torus fracture of lower end of left ulna

S52.69 Other fracture of lower end of ulna

S52.691- Other fracture of lower end of right ulna

S52.692- Other fracture of lower end of left ulna

S52.9 Unspecified fracture of forearm

S52.91X- Unspecified fracture of right forearm

S52.92X- Unspecified fracture of left forearm

S53 DISLOCATION AND SPRAIN OF JOINTS AND LIGAMENTS OF ELBOW

Includes: avulsion of joint or ligament of elbow
laceration of cartilage, joint or ligament of elbow
sprain of cartilage, joint or ligament of elbow
traumatic hemarthrosis of joint or ligament of elbow
traumatic rupture of joint or ligament of elbow
traumatic subluxation of joint or ligament of elbow
traumatic tear of joint or ligament of elbow

Code also any associated open wound

Excludes2: strain of muscle, fascia and tendon at forearm level (S56.-)

S53.0 Subluxation and dislocation of radial head

Dislocation of radiohumeral joint
Subluxation of radiohumeral joint

Excludes1: Monteggia's fracture-dislocation (S52.27-)

S53.00 Unspecified subluxation and dislocation of radial head

S53.001- Unspecified subluxation of right radial head

S53.002- Unspecified subluxation of left radial head

S53.004- Unspecified dislocation of right radial head

S53.005- Unspecified dislocation of left radial head

S53.02 Posterior subluxation and dislocation of radial head
Posteriolateral subluxation and dislocation of radial head

S53.021- Posterior subluxation of right radial head

S53.022- Posterior subluxation of left radial head

S53.024- Posterior dislocation of right radial head

S53.025- Posterior dislocation of left radial head

S53.03 Nursemaid's elbow,

S53.031- right elbow

S53.032- left elbow

S53.09 Other subluxation and dislocation of radial head

S53.091- Other subluxation of right radial head

S53.092- Other subluxation of left radial head

S53.094- Other dislocation of right radial head

S53.095- Other dislocation of left radial head

S53.4 Sprain of elbow

Excludes2: traumatic rupture of radial collateral ligament (S53.2-)
traumatic rupture of ulnar collateral ligament (S53.3-)

S53.40 Unspecified sprain of elbow

S53.401- Unspecified sprain of right elbow

S53.402- Unspecified sprain of left elbow

S53.41 Radiohumeral (joint) sprain

S53.411- Radiohumeral (joint) sprain of right elbow

S53.412- Radiohumeral (joint) sprain of left elbow

S53.42 Ulnohumeral (joint) sprain

S53.421- Ulnohumeral (joint) sprain of right elbow

S53.422- Ulnohumeral (joint) sprain of left elbow

S53.43 Radial collateral ligament sprain

S53.431- Radial collateral ligament sprain of right elbow

S53.432- Radial collateral ligament sprain of left elbow

S53.44 Ulnar collateral ligament sprain

S53.441- Ulnar collateral ligament sprain of right elbow

S53.442- Ulnar collateral ligament sprain of left elbow

S53.49 Other sprain of elbow

S53.491- Other sprain of right elbow

S53.492- Other sprain of left elbow

S56 INJURY OF MUSCLE, FASCIA AND TENDON AT FOREARM LEVEL

Code also any associated open wound (S51.-)

Excludes2: injury of muscle, fascia and tendon at or below wrist (S66.-)
sprain of joints and ligaments of elbow (S53.4-)

S56.0 Injury of flexor muscle, fascia and tendon of thumb at forearm level

S56.01 Strain of flexor muscle, fascia and tendon of thumb at forearm level

S56.011- Strain of flexor muscle, fascia and tendon of right thumb at forearm level

S56.012- Strain of flexor muscle, fascia and tendon of left thumb at forearm level

S56.02 Laceration of flexor muscle, fascia and tendon of thumb at forearm level

S56.021- Laceration of flexor muscle, fascia and tendon of right thumb at forearm level

S56.022- Laceration of flexor muscle, fascia and tendon of left thumb at forearm level

S56.1 Injury of flexor muscle, fascia and tendon of other and unspecified finger at forearm level

S56.11 Strain of flexor muscle, fascia and tendon of other and unspecified finger at forearm level

S56.111- Strain of flexor muscle, fascia and tendon of right index finger at forearm level

S56.112- Strain of flexor muscle, fascia and tendon of left index finger at forearm level

S56.113- Strain of flexor muscle, fascia and tendon of right middle finger at forearm level

S56.114- Strain of flexor muscle, fascia and tendon of left middle finger at forearm level

S56.115- Strain of flexor muscle, fascia and tendon of right ring finger at forearm level

S56.116- Strain of flexor muscle, fascia and tendon of left ring finger at forearm level

S56.117- Strain of flexor muscle, fascia and tendon of right little finger at forearm level

S56.118- Strain of flexor muscle, fascia and tendon of left little finger at forearm level

S56.12 Laceration of flexor muscle, fascia and tendon of other and unspecified finger at forearm level

S56.121- Laceration of flexor muscle, fascia and tendon of right index finger at forearm level

S56.122- Laceration of flexor muscle, fascia and tendon of left index finger at forearm level

S56.123- Laceration of flexor muscle, fascia and tendon of right middle finger at forearm level

S56.124- Laceration of flexor muscle, fascia and tendon of left middle finger at forearm level

S56.125- Laceration of flexor muscle, fascia and tendon of right ring finger at forearm level

S56.126- Laceration of flexor muscle, fascia and tendon of left ring finger at forearm level

S56.127- Laceration of flexor muscle, fascia and tendon of right little finger at forearm level

S56.128- Laceration of flexor muscle, fascia and tendon of left little finger at forearm level

S56.2 Injury of other flexor muscle, fascia and tendon at forearm level

S56.21 Strain of other flexor muscle, fascia and tendon at forearm level

S56.211- Strain of other flexor muscle, fascia and tendon at forearm level, right arm

S56.212- Strain of other flexor muscle, fascia and tendon at forearm level, left arm

S56.22 Laceration of other flexor muscle, fascia and tendon at forearm level

S56.221- Laceration of other flexor muscle, fascia and tendon at forearm level, right arm

S56.222- Laceration of other flexor muscle, fascia and tendon at forearm level, left arm

S56.3 Injury of extensor or abductor muscles, fascia and tendons of thumb at forearm level

S56.31 Strain of extensor or abductor muscles, fascia and tendons of thumb at forearm level

S56.311- Strain of extensor or abductor muscles, fascia and tendons of right thumb at forearm level

S56.312- Strain of extensor or abductor muscles, fascia and tendons of left thumb at forearm level

S56.32 Laceration of extensor or abductor muscles, fascia and tendons of thumb at forearm level

S56.321- Laceration of extensor or abductor muscles, fascia and tendons of right thumb at forearm level

S56.322- Laceration of extensor or abductor muscles, fascia and tendons of left thumb at forearm level

S56.39 Other injury of extensor or abductor muscles, fascia and tendons of thumb at forearm level

S56.391- Other injury of extensor or abductor muscles, fascia and tendons of right thumb at forearm level

S56.392- Other injury of extensor or abductor muscles, fascia and tendons of left thumb at forearm level

S56.4 Injury of extensor muscle, fascia and tendon of other and unspecified finger at forearm level

S56.41 Strain of extensor muscle, fascia and tendon of other and unspecified finger at forearm level

S56.411- Strain of extensor muscle, fascia and tendon of right index finger at forearm level

S56.412- Strain of extensor muscle, fascia and tendon of left index finger at forearm level

S56.413- Strain of extensor muscle, fascia and tendon of right middle finger at forearm level

S56.414- Strain of extensor muscle, fascia and tendon of left middle finger at forearm level

S56.415- Strain of extensor muscle, fascia and tendon of right ring finger at forearm level

S56.416- Strain of extensor muscle, fascia and tendon of left ring finger at forearm level

S56.417- Strain of extensor muscle, fascia and tendon of right little finger at forearm level

S56.418- Strain of extensor muscle, fascia and tendon of left little finger at forearm level

S56.42 Laceration of extensor muscle, fascia and tendon of other and unspecified finger at forearm level

S56.421- Laceration of extensor muscle, fascia and tendon of right index finger at forearm level

S56.422- Laceration of extensor muscle, fascia and tendon of left index finger at forearm level

S56.423- Laceration of extensor muscle, fascia and tendon of right middle finger at forearm level

S56.424- Laceration of extensor muscle, fascia and tendon of left middle finger at forearm level

S56.425- Laceration of extensor muscle, fascia and tendon of right ring finger at forearm level

S56.426- Laceration of extensor muscle, fascia and tendon of left ring finger at forearm level

S56.427- Laceration of extensor muscle, fascia and tendon of right little finger at forearm level

S56.428- Laceration of extensor muscle, fascia and tendon of left little finger at forearm level

S56.5 Injury of other extensor muscle, fascia and tendon at forearm level

S56.51 Strain of other extensor muscle, fascia and tendon at forearm level

S56.511- Strain of other extensor muscle, fascia and tendon at forearm level, right arm

S56.512- Strain of other extensor muscle, fascia and tendon at forearm level, left arm

S56.52 Laceration of other extensor muscle, fascia and tendon at forearm level

S56.521- Laceration of other extensor muscle, fascia and tendon at forearm level, right arm

S56.522- Laceration of other extensor muscle, fascia and tendon at forearm level, left arm

S56.8 Injury of other muscles, fascia and tendons at forearm level

S56.81 Strain of other muscles, fascia and tendons at forearm level

S56.811- Strain of other muscles, fascia and tendons at forearm level, right arm

S56.812- Strain of other muscles, fascia and tendons at forearm level, left arm

S56.82 Laceration of other muscles, fascia and tendons at forearm level

S56.821- Laceration of other muscles, fascia and tendons at forearm level, right arm

S56.822- Laceration of other muscles, fascia and tendons at forearm level, left arm

S56.9 Injury of unspecified muscles, fascia and tendons at forearm level

S56.90 Unspecified injury of unspecified muscles, fascia and tendons at forearm level

S56.901- Unspecified injury of unspecified muscles, fascia and tendons at forearm level, right arm

S56.902- Unspecified injury of unspecified muscles, fascia and tendons at forearm level, left arm

S56.91 Strain of unspecified muscles, fascia and tendons at forearm level
S56.911- Strain of unspecified muscles, fascia and tendons at forearm level, right arm
S56.912- Strain of unspecified muscles, fascia and tendons at forearm level, left arm

S56.92 Laceration of unspecified muscles, fascia and tendons at forearm level
S56.921- Laceration of unspecified muscles, fascia and tendons at forearm level, right arm
S56.922- Laceration of unspecified muscles, fascia and tendons at forearm level, left arm

S59 OTHER AND UNSPECIFIED INJURIES OF ELBOW AND FOREARM

Excludes2: other and unspecified injuries of wrist and hand (S69.-)

S59.0 Physeal fracture of lower end of ulna

S59.00 Unspecified physeal fracture of lower end of ulna,
S59.001- right arm
S59.002- left arm

S59.01 Salter-Harris Type I physeal fracture of lower end of ulna,
S59.011- right arm
S59.012- left arm

S59.02 Salter-Harris Type II physeal fracture of lower end of ulna,
S59.021- right arm
S59.022- left arm

S59.03 Salter-Harris Type III physeal fracture of lower end of ulna,
S59.031- right arm
S59.032- left arm

S59.04 Salter-Harris Type IV physeal fracture of lower end of ulna,
S59.041- right arm
S59.042- left arm

S59.09 Other physeal fracture of lower end of ulna,
S59.091- right arm
S59.092- left arm

S59.1 Physeal fracture of upper end of radius

S59.10 Unspecified physeal fracture of upper end of radius,
S59.101- right arm
S59.102- left arm

S59.11 Salter-Harris Type I physeal fracture of upper end of radius,
S59.111- right arm
S59.112- left arm

S59.12 Salter-Harris Type II physeal fracture of upper end of radius,
S59.121- right arm
S59.122- left arm

S59.13 Salter-Harris Type III physeal fracture of upper end of radius,
S59.131- right arm
S59.132- left arm

S59.14 Salter-Harris Type IV physeal fracture of upper end of radius,
S59.141- right arm
S59.142- left arm

S59.19 Other physeal fracture of upper end of radius,
S59.191- right arm
S59.192- left arm

S59.2 Physeal fracture of lower end of radius

S59.20 Unspecified physeal fracture of lower end of radius,
S59.201- right arm
S59.202- left arm

S59.21 Salter-Harris Type I physeal fracture of lower end of radius,
S59.211- right arm
S59.212- left arm

S59.22 Salter-Harris Type II physeal fracture of lower end of radius,
S59.221- right arm
S59.222- left arm

S59.23 Salter-Harris Type III physeal fracture of lower end of radius,
S59.231- right arm
S59.232- left arm

S59.24 Salter-Harris Type IV physeal fracture of lower end of radius,
S59.241- right arm
S59.242- left arm

S59.29 Other physeal fracture of lower end of radius,
S59.291- right arm
S59.292- left arm

S59.8 Other specified injuries of elbow and forearm

S59.80 Other specified injuries of elbow
S59.801- Other specified injuries of right elbow
S59.802- Other specified injuries of left elbow

S59.81 Other specified injuries of forearm
S59.811- Other specified injuries right forearm
S59.812- Other specified injuries left forearm

(S60–S69) INJURIES TO THE WRIST, HAND AND FINGERS

Excludes2: burns and corrosions (T20–T32)
frostbite (T33–T34)
insect bite or sting, venomous (T63.4)

S60 SUPERFICIAL INJURY OF WRIST, HAND AND FINGERS

S60 requires a 7th character
A—initial encounter
D—subsequent encounter
S—sequela

S60.0 Contusion of finger without damage to nail

Excludes1: contusion involving nail (matrix) (S60.1)

S60.00X- Contusion of unspecified finger without damage to nail

Contusion of finger(s) NOS

S60.01 Contusion of thumb without damage to nail

S60.011- Contusion of right thumb without damage to nail

S61.012- Laceration without foreign body of left thumb without damage to nail

S60.02 Contusion of index finger without damage to nail

S60.021- Contusion of right index finger without damage to nail

S60.022- Contusion of left index finger without damage to nail

S60.03 Contusion of middle finger without damage to nail

S60.031- Contusion of right middle finger without damage to nail

S60.032- Contusion of left middle finger without damage to nail

S60.04 Contusion of ring finger without damage to nail

S60.041- Contusion of right ring finger without damage to nail

S60.042- Contusion of left ring finger without damage to nail

S60.05 Contusion of little finger without damage to nail

S60.051- Contusion of right little finger without damage to nail

S60.052- Contusion of left little finger without damage to nail

S60.1 Contusion of finger with damage to nail

S60.11 Contusion of thumb with damage to nail

S60.111- Contusion of right thumb with damage to nail

S60.112- Contusion of left thumb with damage to nail

S60.12 Contusion of index finger with damage to nail

S60.121- Contusion of right index finger with damage to nail

S60.122- Contusion of left index finger with damage to nail

S60.13 Contusion of middle finger with damage to nail

S60.131- Contusion of right middle finger with damage to nail

S60.132- Contusion of left middle finger with damage to nail

S60.14 Contusion of ring finger with damage to nail

S60.141- Contusion of right ring finger with damage to nail

S60.142- Contusion of left ring finger with damage to nail

S60.15 Contusion of little finger with damage to nail

S60.151- Contusion of right little finger with damage to nail

S60.152- Contusion of left little finger with damage to nail

S60.2 Contusion of wrist and hand

Excludes2: contusion of fingers (S60.0-, S60.1-)

S60.21 Contusion of wrist

S60.211- Contusion of right wrist

S60.212- Contusion of left wrist

S60.22 Contusion of hand

S60.221- Contusion of right hand

S60.222- Contusion of left hand

S60.3 Other superficial injuries of thumb

S60.31 Abrasion of thumb

S60.311- Abrasion of right thumb

S60.312- Abrasion of left thumb

S60.32 Blister (nonthermal) of thumb

S60.321- Blister (nonthermal) of right thumb

S60.322- Blister (nonthermal) of left thumb

S60.34 External constriction of thumb

Hair tourniquet syndrome of thumb

Use additional cause code to identify the constricting item (W49.0-)

S60.341- External constriction of right thumb

S60.342- External constriction of left thumb

S60.35 Superficial FB of thumb

Splinter in the thumb

S60.351- Superficial FB of right thumb

S60.352- Superficial FB of left thumb

S60.36 Insect bite (nonvenomous) of thumb

S60.361- Insect bite (nonvenomous) of right thumb

S60.362- Insect bite (nonveno-mous) of left thumb

S60.37 Other superficial bite of thumb

Excludes1: open bite of thumb (S61.05-, S61.15-)

S60.371- Other superficial bite of right thumb

S60.372- Other superficial bite of left thumb

S60.4 Other superficial injuries of other fingers

S60.41 Abrasion of fingers

S60.410- Abrasion of right index finger

S60.411- Abrasion of left index finger

S60.412- Abrasion of right middle finger

S60.413- Abrasion of left middle finger

S60.414- Abrasion of right ring finger

S60.415- Abrasion of left ring finger

S60.416- Abrasion of right little finger

S60.417- Abrasion of left little finger

S60.42 Blister (nonthermal) of fingers

S60.420- Blister (nonthermal) of right index finger

S60.421- Blister (nonthermal) of left index finger

S60.422- Blister (nonthermal) of right middle finger

S60.423- Blister (nonthermal) of left middle finger

S60.424- Blister (nonthermal) of right ring finger

S60.425- Blister (nonthermal) of left ring finger

S60.426- Blister (nonthermal) of right little finger

S60.427- Blister (nonthermal) of left little finger

S60.44 External constriction of fingers

Hair tourniquet syndrome of finger

Use additional cause code to identify the constricting item (W49.0-)

S60.440- External constriction of right index finger

S60.441- External constriction of left index finger

S60.442- External constriction of right middle finger

S60.443- External constriction of left middle finger

S60.444- External constriction of right ring finger

S60.445- External constriction of left ring finger

S60.446- External constriction of right little finger

S60.447- External constriction of left little finger

S60.45 Superficial FB of fingers

Splinter in the finger(s)

S60.450- Superficial FB of right index finger

S60.451- Superficial FB of left index finger

S60.452- Superficial FB of right middle finger

S60.453- Superficial FB of left middle finger

S60.454- Superficial FB of right ring finger

S60.455- Superficial FB of left ring finger

S60.456- Superficial FB of right little finger

S60.457- Superficial FB of left little finger

S60.46 Insect bite (nonvenomous) of fingers

S60.460- Insect bite (nonvenomous) of right index finger

S60.461- Insect bite (nonvenomous) of left index finger

S60.462- Insect bite (nonvenomous) of right middle finger

S60.463- Insect bite (nonvenomous) of left middle finger

S60.464- Insect bite (nonvenomous) of right ring finger

S60.465- Insect bite (nonveno-mous) of left ring finger

S60.466- Insect bite (nonvenomous) of right little finger

S60.467- Insect bite (nonvenomous) of left little finger

S60.47 Other superficial bite of fingers

Excludes1: open bite of fingers (S61.25-, S61.35-)

S60.470- Other superficial bite of right index finger

S60.471- Other superficial bite of left index finger

S60.472- Other superficial bite of right middle finger

S60.473- Other superficial bite of left middle finger

S60.474- Other superficial bite of right ring finger

S60.475- Other superficial bite of left ring finger

S60.476- Other superficial bite of right little finger

S60.477- Other superficial bite of left little finger

S60.5 Other superficial injuries of hand

Excludes2: superficial injuries of fingers (S60.3-, S60.4-)

S60.51 Abrasion of hand

S60.511- Abrasion of right hand

S60.512- Abrasion of left hand

S60.52 Blister (nonthermal) of hand

S60.521- Blister (nonthermal) of right hand

S60.522- Blister (nonthermal) of left hand

S60.54 External constriction of hand

S60.541- External constriction of right hand

S60.542- External constriction of left hand

S60.55 Superficial FB of hand

Splinter in the hand

S60.551- Superficial FB of right hand

S60.552- Superficial FB of left hand

S60.56 Insect bite (nonvenomous) of hand

S60.561- Insect bite (nonvenomous) of right hand

S60.562- Insect bite (nonvenomous) of left hand

S60.57 Other superficial bite of hand

Excludes1: open bite of hand (S61.45-)

S60.571- Other superficial bite of hand of right hand

S60.572- Other superficial bite of hand of left hand

S60.8 Other superficial injuries of wrist

S60.81 Abrasion of wrist

S60.811- Abrasion of right wrist

S60.812- Abrasion of left wrist

S60.82 Blister (nonthermal) of wrist

S60.821- Blister (nonthermal) of right wrist

S60.822- Blister (nonthermal) of left wrist

S60.84 External constriction of wrist

S60.841- External constriction of right wrist

S60.842- External constriction of left wrist

S60.85 Superficial FB of wrist

Splinter in the wrist

S60.851- Superficial FB of right wrist

S60.852- Superficial FB of left wrist

S60.86 Insect bite (nonvenomous) of wrist

S60.861- Insect bite (nonvenomous) of right wrist

S60.862- Insect bite (nonveno-mous) of left wrist

S60.87 Other superficial bite of wrist

Excludes1: open bite of wrist (S61.55)

S60.871- Other superficial bite of right wrist

S60.872- Other superficial bite of left wrist

S61 OPEN WOUND OF WRIST, HAND AND FINGERS

Code also any associated wound infection
Excludes1: open fracture of wrist, hand and finger (S62.- with 7th character B)
traumatic amputation of wrist and hand (S68.-)

S61.0 Open wound of thumb without damage to nail

5th *Excludes1:* open wound of thumb with damage to nail (S61.1-)

S61.01 Laceration without FB of thumb without damage to nail

6th

S61.011- Laceration without FB of right thumb
7th without damage to nail

S61.012- Laceration without FB of left thumb
7th without damage to nail

S61.02 Laceration with FB of
6th **thumb without damage to nail**

S61.021- Laceration with FB of right thumb without
7th damage to nail

S61.022- Laceration with FB of left thumb without
7th damage to nail

S61.03 Puncture wound without FB of thumb without
6th **damage to nail**

S61.031- Puncture wound without FB of right thumb
7th without damage to nail

S61.032- Puncture wound without FB of left thumb
7th without damage to nail

S61.04 Puncture wound with FB of thumb without damage
6th **to nail**

S61.041- Puncture wound with FB of right thumb
7th without damage to nail

S61.042- Puncture wound with FB of left thumb
7th without damage to nail

S61.05 Open bite of thumb without damage to nail
6th Bite of thumb NOS

Excludes1: superficial bite of thumb (S60.36-, S60.37-)

S61.051- Open bite of right thumb without damage
7th to nail

S61.052- Open bite of left thumb without damage to
7th nail

S61.1 Open wound of thumb with damage to nail

5th

S61.11 Laceration without FB of thumb with damage to nail
6th

S61.111- Laceration without FB of right thumb with
7th damage to nail

S61.112- Laceration without FB of left thumb with
7th damage to nail

S61.12 Laceration with FB of thumb with damage to nail
6th

S61.121- Laceration with FB of right thumb with
7th damage to nail

S61.122- Laceration with FB of left thumb with
7th damage to nail

S61.13 Puncture wound without FB of thumb with damage
6th **to nail**

S61.131- Puncture wound without FB of right thumb
7th with damage to nail

S61.132- Puncture wound without FB of left thumb
7th with damage to nail

S61.14 Puncture wound with FB of thumb with damage to
6th **nail**

S61.141- Puncture wound with FB of right thumb
7th with damage to nail

S61.142- Puncture wound with FB of left thumb
7th with damage to nail

S61.15 Open bite of thumb with damage to nail
6th Bite of thumb with damage to nail NOS

Excludes1: superficial bite of thumb (S60.36-, S60.37-)

S61.151- Open bite of right thumb with damage to
7th nail

S61.152- Open bite of left thumb with damage to
7th nail

S61.2 Open wound of other finger without damage to nail

5th *Excludes1:* open wound of finger involving nail (matrix) (S61.3-)
Excludes2: open wound of thumb without damage to nail (S61.0-)

S61.21 Laceration without FB of finger without damage
6th **to nail**

S61.210- Laceration without FB of right index finger
7th without damage to nail

S61.211- Laceration without FB of left index finger
7th without damage to nail

S61.212- Laceration without FB of right middle
7th finger without damage to nail

S61.213- Laceration without FB of left middle finger
7th without damage to nail

S61.214- Laceration without FB of right ring finger
7th without damage to nail

S61.215- Laceration without FB
7th of left ring finger without damage to nail

S61.216- Laceration without FB of right little finger
7th without damage to nail

S61.217- Laceration without FB of left little finger
7th without damage to nail

S61.22 Laceration with FB of finger without damage to nail
6th

S61.220- Laceration with FB of right index finger
7th without damage to nail

S61.221- Laceration with FB of left index finger
7th without damage to nail

S61.222- Laceration with FB of right middle finger
7th without damage to nail

S61.223- Laceration with FB of left middle finger
7th without damage to nail

S61.224- Laceration with FB of right ring finger
7th without damage to nail

S61.225- Laceration with FB of left ring finger
7th without damage to nail

S61.226- Laceration with FB of right little finger
7th without damage to nail

S61.227- Laceration with FB of left little finger
7th without damage to nail

S61.23 Puncture wound without FB of finger without
6th **damage to nail**

S61.230- Puncture wound without FB of right index
7th finger without damage to nail

S61.231- Puncture wound without FB of left index
7th finger without damage to nail

S61.232- Puncture wound without FB of right
7th middle finger without damage to nail

S61.233- Puncture wound without FB of left middle
7th finger without damage to nail

S61.234- Puncture wound without FB of right ring
7th finger without damage to nail

S61.235- Puncture wound without FB of left ring
7th finger without damage to nail

S61.236- Puncture wound without FB of right little
7th finger without damage to nail

S61.237- Puncture wound without FB of left little
7th finger without damage to nail

S61.24 Puncture wound with FB of finger without damage
6th **to nail**

S61.240- Puncture wound with FB of right index
7th finger with-out damage to nail

S61.241- Puncture wound with FB of left index
7th finger without damage to nail

S61.242- Puncture wound with FB of right middle
7th finger without damage to nail

S61.243- Puncture wound with FB of left middle
7th finger without damage to nail

S61.244- Puncture wound with FB of right ring
7th finger without damage to nail

S61.245- Puncture wound with FB of left ring finger
7th without damage to nail

S61.246- Puncture wound with FB of right little
7th finger without damage to nail

S61.247- Puncture wound with FB of left little finger
7th without damage to nail

S61.25 Open bite of finger without damage to nail
6th Bite of finger without damage to nail NOS

Excludes1: superficial bite of finger (S60.46-, S60.47-)

S61.250- Open bite of right index finger without
7th damage to nail

S61.251- Open bite of left index finger without damage to nail

S61.252- Open bite of right middle finger without damage to nail

S61.253- Open bite of left middle finger without damage to nail

S61.254- Open bite of right ring finger without damage to nail

S61.255- Open bite of left ring finger without damage to nail

S61.256- Open bite of right little finger without damage to nail

S61.257- Open bite of left little finger without damage to nail

S61.3 Open wound of other finger with damage to nail

S61.31 Laceration without FB of finger with damage to nail

S61.310- Laceration without FB of right index finger with damage to nail

S61.311- Laceration without FB of left index finger with damage to nail

S61.312- Laceration without FB of right middle finger with damage to nail

S61.313- Laceration without FB of left middle finger with damage to nail

S61.314- Laceration without FB of right ring finger with damage to nail

S61.315- Laceration without FB of left ring finger with damage to nail

S61.316- Laceration without FB of right little finger with damage to nail

S61.317- Laceration without FB of left little finger with damage to nail

S61.32 Laceration with FB of finger with damage to nail

S61.320- Laceration with FB of right index finger with damage to nail

S61.321- Laceration with FB of left index finger with damage to nail

S61.322- Laceration with FB of right middle finger with damage to nail

S61.323- Laceration with FB of left middle finger with damage to nail

S61.324- Laceration with FB of right ring finger with damage to nail

S61.325- Laceration with FB of left ring finger with damage to nail

S61.326- Laceration with FB of right little finger with damage to nail

S61.327- Laceration with FB of left little finger with damage to nail

S61.33 Puncture wound without FB of finger with damage to nail

S61.330- Puncture wound without FB of right index finger with damage to nail

S61.331- Puncture wound without FB of left index finger with damage to nail

S61.332- Puncture wound without FB of right middle finger with damage to nail

S61.333- Puncture wound without FB of left middle finger with damage to nail

S61.334- Puncture wound without FB of right ring finger with damage to nail

S61.335- Puncture wound without FB of left ring finger with damage to nail

S61.336- Puncture wound without FB of right little finger with damage to nail

S61.337- Puncture wound without FB of left little finger with damage to nail

S61.34 Puncture wound with FB of finger with damage to nail

S61.340- Puncture wound with FB of right index finger with damage to nail

S61.341- Puncture wound with FB of left index finger with damage to nail

S61.342- Puncture wound with FB of right middle finger with damage to nail

S61.343- Puncture wound with FB of left middle finger with damage to nail

S61.344- Puncture wound with FB of right ring finger with damage to nail

S61.345- Puncture wound with FB of left ring finger with damage to nail

S61.346- Puncture wound with FB of right little finger with damage to nail

S61.347- Puncture wound with FB of left little finger with damage to nail

S61.35 Open bite of finger with damage to nail

Bite of finger with damage to nail NOS

Excludes1: superficial bite of finger (S60.46-, S60.47-)

S61.350- Open bite of right index finger with damage to nail

S61.351- Open bite of left index finger with damage to nail

S61.352- Open bite of right middle finger with damage to nail

S61.353- Open bite of left middle finger with damage to nail

S61.354- Open bite of right ring finger with damage to nail

S61.355- Open bite of left ring finger with damage to nail

S61.356- Open bite of right little finger with damage to nail

S61.357- Open bite of left little finger with damage to nail

S61.4 Open wound of hand

S61.41 Laceration without FB of hand

S61.411- Laceration without FB of right hand

S61.412- Laceration without FB of left hand

S61.42 Laceration with FB of hand

S61.421- Laceration with FB of right hand

S61.422- Laceration with FB of left hand

S61.43 Puncture wound without FB of hand

S61.431- Puncture wound without FB of right hand

S61.432- Puncture wound without FB of left hand

S61.44 Puncture wound with FB of hand

S61.441- Puncture wound with FB of right hand

S61.442- Puncture wound with FB of left hand

S61.45 Open bite of hand

Bite of hand NOS

Excludes1: superficial bite of hand (S60.56-, S60.57-)

S61.451- Open bite of right hand

S61.452- Open bite of left hand

S61.5 Open wound of wrist

S61.51 Laceration without FB of wrist

S61.511- Laceration without FB of right wrist

S61.512- Laceration without FB of left wrist

S61.52 Laceration with FB of wrist

S61.521- Laceration with FB of right wrist

S61.522- Laceration with FB of left wrist

S61.53 Puncture wound without FB of wrist

S61.531- Puncture wound without FB of right wrist
S61.532- Puncture wound without FB of left wrist

S61.54 Puncture wound with FB of wrist
S61.541- Puncture wound with FB of right wrist
S61.542- Puncture wound with FB of left wrist

S61.55 Open bite of wrist
Bite of wrist NOS
Excludes1: superficial bite of wrist (S60.86-, S60.87-)
S61.551- Open bite of right wrist
S61.552- Open bite of left wrist

S62 FRACTURE AT WRIST AND HAND LEVEL

Note: A fracture not indicated as displaced or nondisplaced should be coded to displaced
A fracture not indicated as open or closed should be coded to closed
Excludes1: traumatic amputation of wrist and hand (S68.-)
Excludes2: fracture of distal parts of ulna and radius (S52.-)

S62.0 Fracture of navicular [scaphoid] bone of wrist

S62.00 Unspecified fracture of navicular [scaphoid] bone of wrist
S62.001- Unspecified fracture of navicular [scaphoid] bone of right wrist
S62.002- Unspecified fracture of navicular [scaphoid] bone of left wrist

S62.01 Fracture of distal pole of navicular [scaphoid] bone of wrist
Fracture of volar tuberosity of navicular [scaphoid] bone of wrist
S62.011- Displaced fracture of distal pole of navicular [scaphoid] bone of right wrist
S62.012- Displaced fracture of distal pole of navicular [scaphoid] bone of left wrist
S62.014- Nondisplaced fracture of distal pole of navicular [scaphoid] bone of right wrist
S62.015- Nondisplaced fracture of distal pole of navicular [scaphoid] bone of left wrist

S62.02 Fracture of middle third of navicular [scaphoid] bone of wrist
S62.021- Displaced fracture of middle third of navicular [scaphoid] bone of right wrist
S62.022- Displaced fracture of middle third of navicular [scaphoid] bone of left wrist
S62.024- Nondisplaced fracture of middle third of navicular [scaphoid] bone of right wrist
S62.025- Nondisplaced fracture of middle third of navicular [scaphoid] bone of left wrist

S62.03 Fracture of proximal third of navicular [scaphoid] bone of wrist
S62.031- Displaced fracture of proximal third of navicular [scaphoid] bone of right wrist
S62.032- Displaced fracture of proximal third of navicular [scaphoid] bone of left wrist
S62.034- Nondisplaced fracture of proximal third of navicular [scaphoid] bone of right wrist
S62.035- Nondisplaced fracture of proximal third of navicular [scaphoid] bone of left wrist

S62.1 Fracture of other and unspecified carpal bone(s)
Excludes2: fracture of scaphoid of wrist (S62.0-)

S62.10 Fracture of unspecified carpal bone
Fracture of wrist NOS
S62.101- Fracture of unspecified carpal bone, right wrist
S62.102- Fracture of unspecified carpal bone, left wrist

S62.11 Fracture of triquetrum [cuneiform] bone of wrist
S62.111- Displaced fracture of triquetrum [cuneiform] bone, right wrist
S62.112- Displaced fracture of triquetrum [cuneiform] bone, left wrist
S62.114- Nondisplaced fracture of triquetrum [cuneiform] bone, right wrist
S62.115- Nondisplaced fracture of triquetrum [cuneiform] bone, left wrist

S62.12 Fracture of lunate [semilunar]
S62.121- Displaced fracture of lunate [semilunar], right wrist
S62.122- Displaced fracture of lunate [semilunar], left wrist
S62.124- Nondisplaced fracture of lunate [semilunar], right wrist
S62.125- Nondisplaced fracture of lunate [semilunar], left wrist

S62.13 Fracture of capitate [os magnum] bone
S62.131- Displaced fracture of capitate [os magnum] bone, right wrist
S62.132- Displaced fracture of capitate [os magnum] bone, left wrist
S62.134- Nondisplaced fracture of capitate [os magnum] bone, right wrist
S62.135- Nondisplaced fracture of capitate [os magnum] bone, left wrist

S62.14 Fracture of body of hamate [unciform] bone
Fracture of hamate [unciform] bone NOS
S62.141- Displaced fracture of body of hamate [unciform] bone, right wrist
S62.142- Displaced fracture of body of hamate [unciform] bone, left wrist
S62.144- Nondisplaced fracture of body of hamate [unciform] bone, right wrist
S62.145- Nondisplaced fracture of body of hamate [unciform] bone, left wrist

S62.15 Fracture of hook process of hamate [unciform] bone
Fracture of unciform process of hamate [unciform] bone
S62.151- Displaced fracture of hook process of hamate [unciform] bone, right wrist
S62.152- Displaced fracture of hook process of hamate [unciform] bone, left wrist
S62.154- Nondisplaced fracture of hook process of hamate [unciform] bone, right wrist
S62.155- Nondisplaced fracture of hook process of hamate [unciform] bone, left wrist

S62.16 Fracture of pisiform
S62.161- Displaced fracture of pisiform, right wrist
S62.162- Displaced fracture of pisiform, left wrist
S62.164- Nondisplaced fracture of pisiform, right wrist
S62.165- Nondisplaced fracture of pisiform, left wrist

S62.17 Fracture of trapezium [larger multangular]
S62.171- Displaced fracture of trapezium [larger multangular], right wrist
S62.172- Displaced fracture of trapezium [larger multangular], left wrist
S62.174- Nondisplaced fracture of trapezium [larger multangular], right wrist
S62.175- Nondisplaced fracture of trapezium [larger multangular], left wrist

S62.18 Fracture of trapezoid [smaller multangular]
S62.181- Displaced fracture of trapezoid [smaller multangular], right wrist

S62.182- Displaced fracture of trapezoid [smaller multangular], left wrist

S62.184- Nondisplaced fracture of trapezoid [smaller multangular], right wrist

S62.185- Nondisplaced fracture of trapezoid [smaller multangular], left wrist

S62.2 Fracture of first metacarpal bone

S62.20 Unspecified fracture of first metacarpal bone

S62.201- Unspecified fracture of first metacarpal bone, right hand

S62.202- Unspecified fracture of first metacarpal bone, left hand

S62.21 Bennett's fracture,

S62.211- right hand

S62.212- left hand

S62.22 Rolando's fracture

S62.221- Displaced Rolando's fracture, right hand

S62.222- Displaced Rolando's fracture, left hand

S62.224- Nondisplaced Rolando's fracture, right hand

S62.225- Nondisplaced Rolando's fracture, left hand

S62.23 Other fracture of base of first metacarpal bone

S62.231- Other displaced fracture of base of first metacarpal bone, right hand

S62.232- Other displaced fracture of base of first metacarpal bone, left hand

S62.234- Other nondisplaced fracture of base of first metacarpal bone, right hand

S62.235- Other nondisplaced fracture of base of first metacarpal bone, left hand

S62.24 Fracture of shaft of first metacarpal bone

S62.241- Displaced fracture of shaft of first metacarpal bone, right hand

S62.242- Displaced fracture of shaft of first metacarpal bone, left hand

S62.244- Nondisplaced fracture of shaft of first metacarpal bone, right hand

S62.245- Nondisplaced fracture of shaft of first metacarpal bone, left hand

S62.25 Fracture of neck of first metacarpal bone

S62.251- Displaced fracture of neck of first metacarpal bone, right hand

S62.252- Displaced fracture of neck of first metacarpal bone, left hand

S62.254- Nondisplaced fracture of neck of first metacarpal bone, right hand

S62.255- Nondisplaced fracture of neck of first metacarpal bone, left hand

S62.29 Other fracture of first metacarpal bone

S62.291- Other fracture of first metacarpal bone, right hand

S62.292- Other fracture of first metacarpal bone, left hand

S62.3 Fracture of other and unspecified metacarpal bone

Excludes2: fracture of first metacarpal bone (S62.2-)

S62.30 Unspecified fracture of other metacarpal bone

S62.300- Unspecified fracture of second metacarpal bone, right hand

S62.301- Unspecified fracture of second metacarpal bone, left hand

S62.302- Unspecified fracture of third metacarpal bone, right hand

S62.303- Unspecified fracture of third metacarpal bone, left hand

S62.304- Unspecified fracture of fourth metacarpal bone, right hand

S62.305- Unspecified fracture of fourth metacarpal bone, left hand

S62.306- Unspecified fracture of fifth metacarpal bone, right hand

S62.307- Unspecified fracture of fifth metacarpal bone, left hand

S62.31 Displaced fracture of base of other metacarpal bone

S62.310- Displaced fracture of base of second metacarpal bone, right hand

S62.311- Displaced fracture of base of second metacarpal bone, left hand

S62.312- Displaced fracture of base of third metacarpal bone, right hand

S62.313- Displaced fracture of base of third metacarpal bone, left hand

S62.314- Displaced fracture of base of fourth metacarpal bone, right hand

S62.315- Displaced fracture of base of fourth metacarpal bone, left hand

S62.316- Displaced fracture of base of fifth metacarpal bone, right hand

S62.317- Displaced fracture of base of fifth metacarpal bone, left hand

S62.32 Displaced fracture of shaft of other metacarpal bone

S62.320- Displaced fracture of shaft of second metacarpal bone, right hand

S62.321- Displaced fracture of shaft of second metacarpal bone, left hand

S62.322- Displaced fracture of shaft of third metacarpal bone, right hand

S62.323- Displaced fracture of shaft of third metacarpal bone, left hand

S62.324- Displaced fracture of shaft of fourth metacarpal bone, right hand

S62.325- Displaced fracture of shaft of fourth metacarpal bone, left hand

S62.326- Displaced fracture of shaft of fifth metacarpal bone, right hand

S62.327- Displaced fracture of shaft of fifth metacarpal bone, left hand

S62.33 Displaced fracture of neck of other metacarpal bone

S62.330- Displaced fracture of neck of second metacarpal bone, right hand

S62.331- Displaced fracture of neck of second metacarpal bone, left hand

S62.332- Displaced fracture of neck of third metacarpal bone, right hand

S62.333- Displaced fracture of neck of third metacarpal bone, left hand

S62.334- Displaced fracture of neck of fourth metacarpal bone, right hand

S62.335- Displaced fracture of neck of fourth metacarpal bone, left hand

S62.336- Displaced fracture of neck of fifth metacarpal bone, right hand

S62.337- Displaced fracture of neck of fifth metacarpal bone, left hand

S62.34 Nondisplaced fracture of base of other metacarpal bone

S62.340- Nondisplaced fracture of base of second metacarpal bone, right hand

S62.341- Nondisplaced fracture of base of second metacarpal bone left hand

S62.342- Nondisplaced fracture of base of third metacarpal bone, right hand

S62.343- Nondisplaced fracture of base of third metacarpal bone, left hand

S62.344- Nondisplaced fracture of base of fourth metacarpal bone, right hand

S62.345- Nondisplaced fracture of base of fourth metacarpal bone, left hand

S62.346- Nondisplaced fracture of base of fifth metacarpal bone, right hand

S62.347- Nondisplaced fracture of base of fifth metacarpal bone, left hand

S62.35 Nondisplaced fracture of shaft of other metacarpal bone

S62.350- Nondisplaced fracture of shaft of second metacarpal bone, right hand

S62.351- Nondisplaced fracture of shaft of second metacarpal bone, left hand

S62.352- Nondisplaced fracture of shaft of third metacarpal bone, right hand

S62.353- Nondisplaced fracture of shaft of third metacarpal bone, left hand

S62.354- Nondisplaced fracture of shaft of fourth metacarpal bone, right hand

S62.355- Nondisplaced fracture of shaft of fourth metacarpal bone, left hand

S62.356- Nondisplaced fracture of shaft of fifth metacarpal bone, right hand

S62.357- Nondisplaced fracture of shaft of fifth metacarpal bone, left hand

S62.36 Nondisplaced fracture of neck of other metacarpal bone

S62.360- Nondisplaced fracture of neck of second metacarpal bone, right hand

S62.361- Nondisplaced fracture of neck of second metacarpal bone, left hand

S62.362- Nondisplaced fracture of neck of third metacarpal bone, right hand

S62.363- Nondisplaced fracture of neck of third metacarpal bone, left hand

S62.364- Nondisplaced fracture of neck of fourth metacarpal bone, right hand

S62.365- Nondisplaced fracture of neck of fourth metacarpal bone, left hand

S62.366- Nondisplaced fracture of neck of fifth metacarpal bone, right hand

S62.367- Nondisplaced fracture of neck of fifth metacarpal bone, left hand

S62.39 Other fracture of other metacarpal bone

S62.390- Other fracture of second metacarpal bone, right hand

S62.391- Other fracture of second metacarpal bone, left hand

S62.392- Other fracture of third metacarpal bone, right hand

S62.393- Other fracture of third metacarpal bone, left hand

S62.394- Other fracture of fourth metacarpal bone, right hand

S62.395- Other fracture of fourth metacarpal bone, left hand

S62.396- Other fracture of fifth metacarpal bone, right hand

S62.397- Other fracture of fifth metacarpal bone, left hand

S62.5 Fracture of thumb

S62.50 Fracture of unspecified phalanx of thumb

S62 requires a 7th character
A—initial encounter for closed fracture
B—initial encounter for open fracture
D—subsequent encounter for fracture with routine healing
G—subsequent encounter for fracture with delayed healing
K—subsequent encounter for fracture with nonunion
P—subsequent encounter for fracture with malunion
S—sequela

S62.501- Fracture of unspecified phalanx of right thumb

S62.502- Fracture of unspecified phalanx of left thumb

S62.51 Fracture of proximal phalanx of thumb

S62.511- Displaced fracture of proximal phalanx of right thumb

S62.512- Displaced fracture of proximal phalanx of left thumb

S62.514- Nondisplaced fracture of proximal phalanx of right thumb

S62.515- Nondisplaced fracture of proximal phalanx of left thumb

S62.52 Fracture of distal phalanx of thumb

S62.521- Displaced fracture of distal phalanx of right thumb

S62.522- Displaced fracture of distal phalanx of left thumb

S62.524- Nondisplaced fracture of distal phalanx of right thumb

S62.525- Nondisplaced fracture of distal phalanx of left thumb

S62.6 Fracture of other and unspecified finger(s)

Excludes2: fracture of thumb (S62.5-)

S62.61 Displaced fracture of proximal phalanx of finger

S62.610- Displaced fracture of proximal phalanx of right index finger

S62.611- Displaced fracture of proximal phalanx of left index finger

S62.612- Displaced fracture of proximal phalanx of right middle finger

S62.613- Displaced fracture of proximal phalanx of left middle finger

S62.614- Displaced fracture of proximal phalanx of right ring finger

S62.615- Displaced fracture of proximal phalanx of left ring finger

S62.616- Displaced fracture of proximal phalanx of right little finger

S62.617- Displaced fracture of proximal phalanx of left little finger

S62.62 Displaced fracture of middle phalanx of finger

S62.620- Displaced fracture of middle phalanx of right index finger

S62.621- Displaced fracture of middle phalanx of left index finger

S62.622- Displaced fracture of middle phalanx of right middle finger

S62.623- Displaced fracture of middle phalanx of left middle finger

S62.624- Displaced fracture of middle phalanx of right ring finger

S62.625- Displaced fracture of middle phalanx of left ring finger

S62.626- Displaced fracture of middle phalanx of right little finger

S62.627- Displaced fracture of middle phalanx of left little finger

S62.63 Displaced fracture of distal phalanx of finger

S62.630- Displaced fracture of distal phalanx of right index finger

S62.631- Displaced fracture of distal phalanx of left index finger

S62.632- Displaced fracture of distal phalanx of right middle finger

S62.633- Displaced fracture of distal phalanx of left middle finger

S62.634- Displaced fracture of distal phalanx of right ring finger

S62.635- Displaced fracture of distal phalanx of left ring finger

S62.636- Displaced fracture of distal phalanx of right little finger

S62.637- Displaced fracture of distal phalanx of left little finger

S62.64 Nondisplaced fracture of proximal phalanx of finger

S62.640- Nondisplaced fracture of proximal phalanx of right index finger

S62.641- Nondisplaced fracture of proximal phalanx of left index finger

S62.642- Nondisplaced fracture of proximal phalanx of right middle finger

S62.643- Nondisplaced fracture of proximal phalanx of left middle finger

S62.644- Nondisplaced fracture of proximal phalanx of right ring finger

S62.645- Nondisplaced fracture of proximal phalanx of left ring finger

S62.646- Nondisplaced fracture of proximal phalanx of right little finger

S62.647- Nondisplaced fracture of proximal phalanx of left little finger

S62.65 Nondisplaced fracture of medial phalanx of finger

S62.650- Nondisplaced fracture of middle phalanx of right index finger

S62.651- Nondisplaced fracture of middle phalanx of left index finger

S62.652- Nondisplaced fracture of middle phalanx of right middle finger

S62.653- Nondisplaced fracture of middle phalanx of left middle finger

S62.654- Nondisplaced fracture of middle phalanx of right ring finger

S62.655- Nondisplaced fracture of middle phalanx of left ring finger

S62.656- Nondisplaced fracture of middle phalanx of right little finger

S62.657- Nondisplaced fracture of middle phalanx of left little finger

S62.66 Nondisplaced fracture of distal phalanx of finger

S62.660- Nondisplaced fracture of distal phalanx of right index finger

S62.661- Nondisplaced fracture of distal phalanx of left index finger

S62.662- Nondisplaced fracture of distal phalanx of right middle finger

S62.663- Nondisplaced fracture of distal phalanx of left middle finger

S62.664- Nondisplaced fracture of distal phalanx of right ring finger

S62.665- Nondisplaced fracture of distal phalanx of left ring finger

S62.666- Nondisplaced fracture of distal phalanx of right little finger

S62.667- Nondisplaced fracture of distal phalanx of left little finger

S63 DISLOCATION AND SPRAIN OF JOINTS AND LIGAMENTS AT WRIST AND HAND LEVEL

Includes: avulsion of joint or ligament at wrist and hand level
laceration of cartilage, joint or ligament at wrist and hand level
sprain of cartilage, joint or ligament at wrist and hand level
traumatic hemarthrosis of joint or ligament at wrist and hand level
traumatic rupture of joint or ligament at wrist and hand level
traumatic subluxation of joint or ligament at wrist and hand level
traumatic tear of joint or ligament at wrist and hand level

Code also any associated open wound
Excludes2: strain of muscle, fascia and tendon of wrist and hand (S66.-)

S63.0 Subluxation and dislocation of wrist and hand joints

S63.06 Subluxation and dislocation of metacarpal (bone), proximal end

S63.061- Subluxation of metacarpal (bone), proximal end of right hand

S63.062- Subluxation of meta-carpal (bone), proximal end of left hand

S63.063- Subluxation of metacarpal (bone), proximal end of unspecified hand

S63.064- Dislocation of metacarpal (bone), proximal end of right hand

S63.065- Dislocation of metacarpal (bone), proximal end of left hand

S63.1 Subluxation and dislocation of thumb

S63.10 Unspecified subluxation and dislocation of thumb

S63.101- Unspecified subluxation of right thumb

S63.102- Unspecified subluxation of left thumb

S63.104- Unspecified dislocation of right thumb

S63.105- Unspecified dislocation of left thumb

S63.11 Subluxation and dislocation of metacarpophalangeal joint of thumb

S63.111- Subluxation of metacarpophalangeal joint of right thumb

S63.112- Subluxation of metacarpophalangeal joint of left thumb

S63.114- Dislocation of metacarpophalangeal joint of right thumb

S63.115- Dislocation of metacarpophalangeal joint of left thumb

S63.12 Subluxation and dislocation of interphalangeal joint of thumb

S63.121- Subluxation of interphalangeal joint of right thumb

S63.122- Subluxation of interphalangeal joint of left thumb

S63.124- Dislocation of interphalangeal joint of right thumb

S63.125- Dislocation of interphalangeal joint of left thumb

S63.2 Subluxation and dislocation of other finger(s)

Excludes2: subluxation and dislocation of thumb (S63.1-)

S63.20 Unspecified subluxation of other finger

S63.200- Unspecified subluxation of right index finger

S63.201- Unspecified subluxation of left index finger

S63.202- Unspecified subluxation of right middle finger

S63.203- Unspecified subluxation of left middle finger

S63.204- Unspecified subluxation of right ring finger

S63.205- Unspecified subluxation of left ring finger

S63.206- Unspecified subluxation of right little finger

S63.207- Unspecified subluxation of left little finger

S63.21 Subluxation of metacarpophalangeal joint of finger

S63.210- Subluxation of metacarpophalangeal joint of right index finger

S63.211- Subluxation of metacar-pophalan-geal joint of left index finger

S63.212- Subluxation of metacarpophalangeal joint of right middle finger

S63.213- Subluxation of metacarpophalangeal joint of left middle finger

S63.214- Subluxation of metacar-pophalangeal joint of right ring finger

S63.215- Subluxation of metacarpophalangeal joint of left ring finger

S63.216- Subluxation of metacarpophalangeal joint of right little finger

S63.217- Subluxation of metacarpophalangeal joint of left little finger

S63.23 Subluxation of proximal interphalangeal joint of finger

S63.230- Subluxation of proximal interphalangeal joint of right index finger

S63.231- Subluxation of proximal interphalangeal joint of left index finger

S63.232- Subluxation of proximal interphalan-geal joint of right middle finger

S63.233- Subluxation of proximal interphalangeal joint of left middle finger

S63.234- Subluxation of proximal interphalangeal joint of right ring finger

S63.235- Subluxation of proximal interphalangeal joint of left ring finger

S63.236- Subluxation of proximal interphalangeal joint of right little finger

S63.237- Subluxation of proximal interphalangeal joint of left little finger

S63.24 Subluxation of distal interphalangeal joint of finger

S63.240- Subluxation of distal interphalangeal joint of right index finger

S63.241- Subluxation of distal interphalangeal joint of left index finger

S63.242- Subluxation of distal interphalangeal joint of right middle finger

S63.243- Subluxation of distal interphalangeal joint of left middle finger

S63.244- Subluxation of distal interphalangeal joint of right ring finger

S63.245- Subluxation of distal interphalangeal joint of left ring finger

S63.246- Subluxation of distal interphalangeal joint of right little finger

S63.247- Subluxation of distal interphalangeal joint of left little finger

S63.26 Dislocation of metacarpophalangeal joint of finger

S63.260- Dislocation of metacarpophalangeal joint of right index finger

S63.261- Dislocation of metacarpophalangeal joint of left index finger

S63.262- Dislocation of metacarpophalangeal joint of right middle finger

S63.263- Dislocation of metacarpophalangeal joint of left middle finger

S63.264- Dislocation of metacarpophalangeal joint of right ring finger

S63.265- Dislocation of metacarpophalangeal joint of left ring finger

S63.266- Dislocation of metacarpophalangeal joint of right little finger

S63.267- Dislocation of metacarpophalangeal joint of left little finger

S63.28 Dislocation of proximal interphalangeal joint of finger

S63.280- Dislocation of proximal interphalangeal joint of right index finger

S63.281- Dislocation of proximal interphalangeal joint of left index finger

S63.282- Dislocation of proximal interphalangeal joint of right middle finger

S63.283- Dislocation of proximal interphalangeal joint of left middle finger

S63.284- Dislocation of proximal interphalangeal joint of right ring finger

S63.285- Dislocation of proximal interphalangeal joint of left ring finger

S63.286- Dislocation of proximal interphalangeal joint of right little finger

S63.287- Dislocation of proximal interphalangeal joint of left little finger

S63.29 Dislocation of distal interphalangeal joint of finger

S63.290- Dislocation of distal interphalangeal joint of right index finger

S63.291- Dislocation of distal interphalangeal joint of left index finger

S63.292- Dislocation of distal interphalangeal joint of right middle finger

S63.293- Dislocation of distal interphalangeal joint of left middle finger

S63.294- Dislocation of distal interphalangeal joint of right ring finger

S63.295- Dislocation of distal interphalangeal joint of left ring finger

S63.296- Dislocation of distal interphalangeal joint of right little finger

S63.297- Dislocation of distal inter-phalangeal joint of left little finger

S63.5 Other and unspecified sprain of wrist

S63.50 Unspecified sprain of wrist

S63.501- Unspecified sprain of right wrist

S63.502- Unspecified sprain of left wrist

S63.51 Sprain of carpal (joint)

S63.511- Sprain of carpal joint of right wrist

S63.512- Sprain of carpal joint of left wrist

S63.52 Sprain of radiocarpal joint

Excludes1: traumatic rupture of radiocarpal ligament (S63.32-)

S63.521- Sprain of radiocarpal joint of right wrist

S63.522- Sprain of radiocarpal joint of left wrist

S63.59 Other specified sprain of wrist

S63.591- Other specified sprain of right wrist

S63.592- Other specified sprain of left wrist

S63.6 Other and unspecified sprain of finger(s)

Excludes1: traumatic rupture of ligament of finger at metacarpophalangeal and interphalangeal joint(s) (S63.4-)

S63.60 Unspecified sprain of thumb

S63.601- Unspecified sprain of right thumb

S63.602- Unspecified sprain of left thumb

S63.61 Unspecified sprain of other and unspecified finger(s)

S63.610- Unspecified sprain of right index finger

S63.611- Unspecified sprain of left index finger

S63.612- Unspecified sprain of right middle finger

S63.613- Unspecified sprain of left middle finger

S63.614- Unspecified sprain of right ring finger

S63.615- Unspecified sprain of left ring finger

S63.616- Unspecified sprain of right little finger

S63.617- Unspecified sprain of left little finger

S63.62 Sprain of interphalangeal joint of thumb

S63.621- Sprain of interphalangeal joint of right thumb

S63.622- Sprain of interphalangeal joint of left thumb

S63.63 Sprain of interphalangeal joint of other and unspecified finger(s)

S63.630- Sprain of interphalangeal joint of right index finger

S63.631- Sprain of interphalangeal joint of left index finger

S63.632- Sprain of interphalangeal joint of right middle finger

S63.633- Sprain of interphalan-geal joint of left middle finger

S63.634- Sprain of interphalangeal joint of right ring finger

S63.635- Sprain of interphalangeal joint of left ring finger

S63.636- Sprain of interphalangeal joint of right little finger

S63.637- Sprain of interphalangeal joint of left little finger

S63.64 Sprain of metacarpophalangeal joint of thumb

S63.641- Sprain of metacarpophalangeal joint of right thumb

S63.642- Sprain of metacarpophalangeal joint of left thumb

S63.65 Sprain of metacarpophalangeal joint of other and unspecified finger(s)

S63.650- Sprain of metacarpophalangeal joint of right index finger

S63.651- Sprain of metacarpophalangeal joint of left index finger

S63.652- Sprain of metacarpophalangeal joint of right middle finger

S63.653- Sprain of metacarpophalangeal joint of left middle finger

S63.654- Sprain of metacarpophalangeal joint of right ring finger

S63.655- Sprain of metacarpophalangeal joint of left ring finger

S63.656- Sprain of metacarpophalangeal joint of right little finger

S63.657- Sprain of metacarpophalangeal joint of left little finger

S63.68 Other sprain of thumb

S63.681- Other sprain of right thumb

S63.682- Other sprain of left thumb

S63.69 Other sprain of other and unspecified finger(s)

S63.690- Other sprain of right index finger

S63.691- Other sprain of left index finger

S63.692- Other sprain of right middle finger

S63.693- Other sprain of left middle finger

S63.694- Other sprain of right ring finger

S63.695- Other sprain of left ring finger

S63.696- Other sprain of right little finger

S63.697- Other sprain of left little finger

S63.8 Sprain of other part of wrist and hand

S63.8X Sprain of other part of wrist and hand

S63.8X1- Sprain of other part of right wrist and hand

S63.8X2- Sprain of other part of left wrist and hand

S63.9 Sprain of unspecified part of wrist and hand

S63.91X- Sprain of unspecified part of right wrist and hand

S63.92X- Sprain of unspecified part of left wrist and hand

S65 INJURY OF BLOOD VESSELS AT WRIST AND HAND LEVEL

Code also any associated open wound (S61.-)

S65.2 Injury of superficial palmar arch

S65.21 Laceration of superficial palmar arch

S65.211- Laceration of superficial palmar arch of right hand

S65.212- Laceration of superficial palmar arch of left hand

S65.29 Other specified injury of superficial palmar arch

S65.291- Other specified injury of superficial palmar arch of right hand

S65.292- Other specified injury of superficial palmar arch of left hand

S65.3 Injury of deep palmar arch

S65.30 Unspecified injury of deep palmar arch

S65.301- Unspecified injury of deep palmar arch of right hand

S65.302- Unspecified injury of deep palmar arch of left hand

S65.31 Laceration of deep palmar arch

S65.311- Laceration of deep palmar arch of right hand

S65.312- Laceration of deep palmar arch of left hand

S65.39 Other specified injury of deep palmar arch

S65.391- Other specified injury of deep palmar arch of right hand

S65.392- Other specified injury of deep palmar arch of left hand

S65.9 Injury of unspecified blood vessel at wrist and hand level

S65.91 Laceration of unspecified blood vessel at wrist and hand level

S65.911- Laceration of unspecified blood vessel at wrist and hand level of right arm

S65.912- Laceration of unspecified blood vessel at wrist and hand level of left arm

S65.99 Other specified injury of unspecified blood vessel at wrist and hand level

S65.991- Other specified injury of unspecified blood vessel at wrist and hand of right arm

S65.992- Other specified injury of unspecified blood vessel at wrist and hand of left arm

S66 INJURY OF MUSCLE, FASCIA AND TENDON AT WRIST AND HAND LEVEL

Code also any associated open wound (S61.-)

Excludes2: sprain of joints and ligaments of wrist and hand (S63.-)

S66.0 Injury of long flexor muscle, fascia, and tendon of thumb at wrist and hand level

S66.01 Strain of long flexor muscle, fascia and tendon of thumb at wrist and hand level

S66.011- Strain of long flexor muscle, fascia and tendon of right thumb at wrist and hand level

S66.012- Strain of long flexor muscle, fascia and tendon of left thumb at wrist and hand level

S66.02 Laceration of long flexor muscle, fascia and tendon of thumb at wrist and hand level

S66.021- Laceration of long flexor muscle, fascia and tendon of right thumb at wrist and hand level

S66.022- Laceration of long flexor muscle, fascia and tendon of left thumb at wrist and hand level

S66.11 Strain of flexor muscle, fascia and tendon of other and unspecified finger at wrist and hand level

S66.110- Strain of flexor muscle, fascia and tendon of right index finger at wrist and hand level

S66.111- Strain of flexor muscle, fascia and tendon of left index finger at wrist and hand level

S66.112- Strain of flexor muscle, fascia and tendon of right middle finger at wrist and hand level

S66.113- Strain of flexor muscle, fascia and tendon of left middle finger at wrist and hand level

S66.114- Strain of flexor muscle, fascia and tendon of right ring finger at wrist and hand level

S66.115- Strain of flexor muscle, fascia and tendon of left ring finger at wrist and hand level

S66.116- Strain of flexor muscle, fascia and tendon of right little finger at wrist and hand level

S66.117- Strain of flexor muscle, fascia and tendon of left little finger at wrist and hand level

S66.21 Strain of extensor muscle, fascia and tendon of thumb at wrist and hand level

S66.211- Strain of extensor muscle, fascia and tendon of right thumb at wrist and hand level

S66.212- Strain of extensor muscle, fascia and tendon of left thumb at wrist and hand level

S66.31 Strain of extensor muscle, fascia and tendon of other and unspecified finger at wrist and hand level

S66.310- Strain of extensor muscle, fascia and tendon of right index finger at wrist and hand level

S66.311- Strain of extensor muscle, fascia and tendon of left index finger at wrist and hand level

S66.312- Strain of extensor muscle, fascia and tendon of right middle finger at wrist and hand level

S66.313- Strain of extensor muscle, fascia and tendon of left middle finger at wrist and hand level

S66.314- Strain of extensor muscle, fascia and tendon of right ring finger at wrist and hand level

S66.315- Strain of extensor muscle, fascia and tendon of left ring finger at wrist and hand level

S66.316- Strain of extensor muscle, fascia and tendon of right little finger at wrist and hand level

S66.317- Strain of extensor muscle, fascia and tendon of left little finger at wrist and hand level

S66.41 Strain of intrinsic muscle, fascia and tendon of thumb at wrist and hand level

S66.411- Strain of intrinsic muscle, fascia and tendon of right thumb at wrist and hand level

S66.412- Strain of intrinsic muscle, fascia and tendon of left thumb at wrist and hand level

S66.51 Strain of intrinsic muscle, fascia and tendon of other and unspecified finger at wrist and hand level

S66.510- Strain of intrinsic muscle, fascia and tendon of right index finger at wrist and hand level

S66.511- Strain of intrinsic muscle, fascia and tendon of left index finger at wrist and hand level

S66.512- Strain of intrinsic muscle, fascia and tendon of right middle finger at wrist and hand level

S66.513- Strain of intrinsic muscle, fascia and tendon of left middle finger at wrist and hand level

S66.514- Strain of intrinsic muscle, fascia and tendon of right ring finger at wrist and hand level

S66.515- Strain of intrinsic muscle, fascia and tendon of left ring finger at wrist and hand level

S66.516- Strain of intrinsic muscle, fascia and tendon of right little finger at wrist and hand level

S66.517- Strain of intrinsic muscle, fascia and tendon of left little finger at wrist and hand level

S66.91 Strain of unspecified muscle, fascia and tendon at wrist and hand level

S66.911- Strain of unspecified muscle, fascia and tendon at wrist and hand level, right hand

S66.912- Strain of unspecified muscle, fascia and tendon at wrist and hand level, left hand

S67 CRUSHING INJURY OF WRIST, HAND AND FINGERS

Use additional code for all associated injuries, such as: fracture of wrist and hand (S62.-) open wound of wrist and hand (S61.-)

S67.0 Crushing injury of thumb

S67.01X- Crushing injury of right thumb

S67.02X- Crushing injury of left thumb

S67.1 Crushing injury of other and unspecified finger(s)

Excludes2: crushing injury of thumb (S67.0-)

S67.19 Crushing injury of other finger(s)

S67.190- Crushing injury of right index finger

S67.191- Crushing injury of left index finger

S67.192- Crushing injury of right middle finger

S67.193- Crushing injury of left middle finger

S67.194- Crushing injury of right ring finger

S67.195- Crushing injury of left ring finger

S67.196- Crushing injury of right little finger

S67.197- Crushing injury of left little finger, initial encounter

S67.198- Crushing injury of other finger- Crushing injury of specified finger with unspecified laterality

S67.2 Crushing injury of hand

Excludes2: crushing injury of fingers (S67.1-) crushing injury of thumb (S67.0-)

S67.21X- Crushing injury of right hand

S67.22X- Crushing injury of left hand

S67.3 Crushing injury of wrist

S67 requires a 7th character
A—initial encounter
D—subsequent encounter
S—sequela

S67.31X- Crushing injury of right wrist

S67.32X- Crushing injury of left wrist

S67.4 Crushing injury of wrist and hand

Excludes1: crushing injury of hand alone (S67.2-)
crushing injury of wrist alone (S67.3-)

Excludes2: crushing injury of fingers (S67.1-)
crushing of thumb (S67.0-)

S67.41X- Crushing injury of right wrist and hand

S67.42X- Crushing injury of left wrist and hand

(S70–S79) INJURIES TO THE HIP AND THIGH

Excludes2: burns and corrosions (T20–T32)
frostbite (T33–T34)
snake bite (T63.0-)
venomous insect bite or sting (T63.4-)

S70 SUPERFICIAL INJURY OF HIP AND THIGH

S70 requires a 7th character
A—initial encounter
D—subsequent encounter
S—sequela

S70.0 Contusion of hip

S70.01X- Contusion of right hip

S70.02X- Contusion of left hip

S70.1 Contusion of thigh

S70.11X- Contusion of right thigh

S70.12X- Contusion of left thigh

S70.2 Other superficial injuries of hip

S70.21 Abrasion of hip

S70.211- Abrasion, right hip

S70.212- Abrasion, left hip

S70.22 Blister (nonthermal) of hip

S70.221- Blister (nonthermal), right hip

S70.222- Blister (nonthermal), left hip

S70.24 External constriction of hip

S70.241- External constriction, right hip

S70.242- External constriction, left hip

S70.25 Superficial FB of hip
Splinter in the hip

S70.251- Superficial FB, right hip

S70.252- Superficial FB, left hip

S70.26 Insect bite (nonvenomous) of hip

S70.261- Insect bite (nonvenomous), right hip

S70.262- Insect bite (nonvenomous), left hip

S70.27 Other superficial bite of hip
Excludes1: open bite of hip (S71.05-)

S70.271- Other superficial bite of hip, right hip

S70.272- Other superficial bite of hip, left hip

S70.3 Other superficial injuries of thigh

S70.31 Abrasion of thigh

S70.311- Abrasion, right thigh

S70.312- Abrasion, left thigh

S70.32 Blister (nonthermal) of thigh

S70.321- Blister (nonthermal), right thigh

S70.322- Blister (nonthermal), left thigh

S70.34 External constriction of thigh

S70.341- External constriction, right thigh

S70.342- External constriction, left thigh

S70.35 Superficial FB of thigh
Splinter in the thigh

S70.351- Superficial FB, right thigh

S70.352- Superficial FB, left thigh

S70.36 Insect bite (nonvenomous) of thigh

S70.361- Insect bite (nonvenomous), right thigh

S70.362- Insect bite (nonvenomous), left thigh

S70.37 Other superficial bite of thigh
Excludes1: open bite of thigh (S71.15)

S70.371- Other superficial bite of right thigh

S70.372- Other superficial bite of left thigh

S71 OPEN WOUND OF HIP AND THIGH

S71 requires a 7th character
A—initial encounter
D—subsequent encounter
S—sequela

Code also any associated wound infection

Excludes1: open fracture of hip and thigh (S72.-)
traumatic amputation of hip and thigh (S78.-)

Excludes2: bite of venomous animal (T63.-)
open wound of ankle, foot and toes (S91.-)
open wound of knee and lower leg (S81.-)

S71.0 Open wound of hip

S71.01 Laceration without FB of hip

S71.011- Laceration without FB, right hip

S71.012- Laceration without FB, left hip

S71.02 Laceration with FB of hip

S71.021- Laceration with FB, right hip

S71.022- Laceration with FB, left hip

S71.03 Puncture wound without FB of hip

S71.031- Puncture wound without FB, right hip

S71.032- Puncture wound without FB, left hip

S71.04 Puncture wound with FB of hip

S71.041- Puncture wound with FB, right hip

S71.042- Puncture wound with FB, left hip

S71.05 Open bite of hip
Bite of hip NOS
Excludes1: superficial bite of hip (S70.26, S70.27)

S71.051- Open bite, right hip

S71.052- Open bite, left hip

S71.1 Open wound of thigh

S71.11 Laceration without FB of thigh

S71.111- Laceration without FB, right thigh

S71.112- Laceration without FB, left thigh

S71.12 Laceration with FB of thigh

S71.121- Laceration with FB, right thigh

S71.122- Laceration with FB, left thigh

S71.13 Puncture wound without FB of thigh

S71.131- Puncture wound without FB, right thigh

S71.132- Puncture wound without FB, left thigh

S71.14 Puncture wound with FB of thigh

S71.141- Puncture wound with FB, right thigh

S71.142- Puncture wound with FB, left thigh

S71.15 Open bite of thigh

Bite of thigh NOS

Excludes1: superficial bite of thigh (S70.37-)

S71.151- Open bite, right thigh

S71.152- Open bite, left thigh

S72 FRACTURE OF FEMUR

Please see full *ICD-10-CM* manual for seventh characters applicable to open fracture types IIIA, IIIB, or IIIC.

Note: A fracture not indicated as displaced or nondisplaced should be coded to displaced

A fracture not indicated as open or closed should be coded to closed

The open fracture designations are based on the Gustilo open fracture classification

Excludes1: traumatic amputation of hip and thigh (S78.-)

Excludes2: fracture of lower leg and ankle (S82.-) fracture of foot (S92.-) periprosthetic fracture of prosthetic implant of hip (M97.0-)

S72.0 Fracture of head and neck of femur

Excludes2: physeal fracture of lower end of femur (S79.1-) physeal fracture of upper end of femur (S79.0-)

S72.00 Fracture of unspecified part of neck of femur

Fracture of hip NOS Fracture of neck of femur NOS

S72.001- Fracture of unspecified part of neck of right femur

S72.002- Fracture of unspecified part of neck of left femur

S72.01 Unspecified intracapsular fracture of femur

Subcapital fracture of femur

S72.011- Unspecified intracapsular fracture of right femur

S72.012- Unspecified intracapsular fracture of left femur

S72.02 Fracture of epiphysis (separation) (upper) of femur

Transepiphyseal fracture of femur

Excludes1: capital femoral epiphyseal fracture (pediatric) of femur (S79.01-) Salter-Harris Type I physeal fracture of upper end of femur (S79.01-)

S72.021- Displaced fracture of epiphysis (separation) (upper) of right femur

S72.022- Displaced fracture of epiphysis (separation) (upper) of left femur

S72.023- Displaced fracture of epiphysis (separation) (upper) of unspecified femur

S72.024- Nondisplaced fracture of epiphysis (separation) (upper) of right femur

S72.025- Nondisplaced fracture of epiphysis (separation) (upper) of left femur

S72.03 Midcervical fracture of femur

Transcervical fracture of femur NOS

S72.031- Displaced midcervical fracture of right femur

S72.032- Displaced midcervical fracture of left femur

S72.034- Nondisplaced midcervical fracture of right femur

S72.035- Nondisplaced midcervical fracture of left femur

S72.04 Fracture of base of neck of femur

Cervicotrochanteric fracture of femur

S72.041- Displaced fracture of base of neck of right femur

S72.042- Displaced fracture of base of neck of left femur

S72.044- Nondisplaced fracture of base of neck of right femur

S72.045- Nondisplaced fracture of base of neck of left femur

S72.3 Fracture of shaft of femur

S72.30 Unspecified fracture of shaft of femur

S72.301- Unspecified fracture of shaft of right femur

S72.302- Unspecified fracture of shaft of left femur

S72.32 Transverse fracture of shaft of femur

S72.321- Displaced transverse fracture of shaft of right femur

S72.322- Displaced transverse fracture of shaft of left femur

S72.324- Nondisplaced transverse fracture of shaft of right femur

S72.325- Nondisplaced transverse fracture of shaft of left femur

S72.33 Oblique fracture of shaft of femur

S72.331- Displaced oblique fracture of shaft of right femur

S72.332- Displaced oblique fracture of shaft of left femur

S72.334- Nondisplaced oblique fracture of shaft of right femur

S72.335- Nondisplaced oblique fracture of shaft of left femur

S72.34 Spiral fracture of shaft of femur

S72.341- Displaced spiral fracture of shaft of right femur

S72.342- Displaced spiral fracture of shaft of left femur

S72.344- Nondisplaced spiral fracture of shaft of right femur

S72.345- Nondisplaced spiral fracture of shaft of left femur

S72.35 Comminuted fracture of shaft of femur

S72.351- Displaced comminuted fracture of shaft of right femur

S72.352- Displaced comminuted fracture of shaft of left femur

S72.354- Nondisplaced comminuted fracture of shaft of right femur

S72.355- Nondisplaced comminuted fracture of shaft of left femur

S72.36 Segmental fracture of shaft of femur

S72.361- Displaced segmental fracture of shaft of right femur

S72.362- Displaced segmental fracture of shaft of left femur

S72.364- Nondisplaced segmental fracture of shaft of right femur

S72.365- Nondisplaced segmental fracture of shaft of left femur

S72.39 Other fracture of shaft of femur

S72.391- Other fracture of shaft of right femur

S72.392- Other fracture of shaft of left femur

S72.4 Fracture of lower end of femur

Fracture of distal end of femur

Excludes2: fracture of shaft of femur (S72.3-)

physeal fracture of lower end of femur (S79.1-)

S72.40 Unspecified fracture of lower end of femur

S72.401- Unspecified fracture of lower end of right femur

S72.402- Unspecified fracture of lower end of left femur

S72.41 Unspecified condyle fracture of lower end of femur

Condyle fracture of femur NOS

S72.411- Displaced unspecified condyle fracture of lower end of right femur

S72.412- Displaced unspecified condyle fracture of lower end of left femur

S72.414- Nondisplaced unspecified condyle fracture of lower end of right femur

S72.415- Nondisplaced unspecified condyle fracture of lower end of left femur

S72.42 Fracture of lateral condyle of femur

S72.421- Displaced fracture of lateral condyle of right femur

S72.422- Displaced fracture of lateral condyle of left femur

S72.424- Nondisplaced fracture of lateral condyle of right femur

S72.425- Nondisplaced fracture of lateral condyle of left femur

S72.43 Fracture of medial condyle of femur

S72.431- Displaced fracture of medial condyle of right femur

S72.432- Displaced fracture of medial condyle of left femur

S72.434- Nondisplaced fracture of medial condyle of right femur

S72.435- Nondisplaced fracture of medial condyle of left femur

S72.44 Fracture of lower epiphysis (separation) of femur

Excludes1: Salter-Harris Type I physeal fracture of lower end of femur (S79.11-)

S72.441- Displaced fracture of lower epiphysis (separation) of right femur

S72 requires a 7th character
A—initial encounter for closed fracture
B—initial encounter for open fracture type I or II initial encounter for open fracture NOS
C—initial encounter for open fracture type IIIA, IIIB, or IIIC
D—subsequent encounter for closed fracture with routine healing
E—subsequent encounter for open fracture type I or II with routine healing
F—subsequent encounter for open fracture type IIIA, IIIB, or IIIC with routine healing
G—subsequent encounter for closed fracture with delayed healing
H—subsequent encounter for open fracture type I or II with delayed healing
J—subsequent encounter for open fracture type IIIA, IIIB, or IIIC with delayed healing
K—subsequent encounter for closed fracture with nonunion
M—subsequent encounter for open fracture type I or II with nonunion
N—subsequent encounter for open fracture type IIIA, IIIB, or IIIC with nonunion
P—subsequent encounter for closed fracture with malunion
Q—subsequent encounter for open fracture type I or II with malunion
R—subsequent encounter for open fracture type IIIA, IIIB, or IIIC with malunion
S—sequela

S72.442- Displaced fracture of lower epiphysis (separation) of left femur

S72.444- Nondisplaced fracture of lower epiphysis (separation) of right femur

S72.445- Nondisplaced fracture of lower epiphysis (separation) of left femur

S72.45 Supracondylar fracture without intracondylar extension of lower end of femur

Supracondylar fracture of lower end of femur NOS

Excludes1: supracondylar fracture with intracondylar extension of lower end of femur (S72.46-)

S72.451- Displaced supracondylar fracture without intracondylar extension of lower end of right femur

S72.452- Displaced supracondylar fracture without intracondylar extension of lower end of left femur

S72.454- Nondisplaced supracondylar fracture without intracondylar extension of lower end of right femur

S72.455- Nondisplaced supracondylar fracture without intracondylar extension of lower end of left femur

S72.46 Supracondylar fracture with intracondylar extension of lower end of femur

Excludes1: supracondylar fracture without intracondylar extension of lower end of femur (S72.45-)

S72.461- Displaced supracondylar fracture with intracondylar extension of lower end of right femur

S72.462- Displaced supracondylar fracture with intracondylar extension of lower end of left femur

S72.464- Nondisplaced supracondylar fracture with intracondylar extension of lower end of right femur

S72.465- Nondisplaced supracondylar fracture with intracondylar extension of lower end of left femur

S72.47 Torus fracture of lower end of femur

S72.471- Torus fracture of lower end of right femur

S72.472- Torus fracture of lower end of left femur

S72.47 requires a 7th character
A—initial encounter for closed fracture
D—subsequent encounter for closed fracture with routine healing
G—subsequent encounter for closed fracture with delayed healing
K—subsequent encounter for closed fracture with nonunion
P—subsequent encounter for closed fracture with malunion
S—sequela

S72.49 Other fracture of lower end of femur

S72.491- Other fracture of lower end of right femur

S72.492- Other fracture of lower end of left femur

S72.8 Other fracture of femur

S72.8X Other fracture of femur

S72.8X1- Other fracture of right femur

S72.8X2- Other fracture of left femur

S72.9 Unspecified fracture of femur

Fracture of thigh NOS

Fracture of upper leg NOS

Excludes1: fracture of hip NOS (S72.00-, S72.01-)

S72.91X- Unspecified fracture of right femur

S72.92X- Unspecified fracture of left femur

S73 DISLOCATION AND SPRAIN OF JOINT AND LIGAMENTS OF HIP

S73 requires a 7th character)
A—initial encounter
D—subsequent encounter
S—sequela

Includes: avulsion of joint or ligament of hip
laceration of cartilage, joint or ligament of hip
sprain of cartilage, joint or ligament of hip
traumatic hemarthrosis of joint or ligament of hip
traumatic rupture of joint or ligament of hip
traumatic subluxation of joint or ligament of hip
traumatic tear of joint or ligament of hip

Code also any associated open wound

Excludes2: strain of muscle, fascia and tendon of hip and thigh (S76.-)

S73.0 Subluxation and dislocation of hip

S73.01 Posterior subluxation and dislocation of hip

S73.011- Posterior subluxation of right hip

S73.012- Posterior subluxation of left hip

S73.014- Posterior dislocation of right hip

S73.015- Posterior dislocation of left hip

S73.02 Obturator subluxation and dislocation of hip

S73.021- Obturator subluxation of right hip

S73.022- Obturator subluxation of left hip

S73.024- Obturator dislocation of right hip

S73.025- Obturator dislocation of left hip

S73.03 Other anterior subluxation and dislocation of hip

S73.031- Other anterior subluxation of right hip

S73.032- Other anterior subluxation of left hip

S73.034- Other anterior dislocation of right hip

S73.035- Other anterior dislocation of left hip

S73.04 Central subluxation and dislocation of hip

S73.041- Central subluxation of right hip

S73.042- Central subluxation of left hip

S73.044- Central dislocation of right hip

S73.045- Central dislocation of left hip

S73.1 Sprain of hip

S73.10 Unspecified sprain of hip

S73.101- Unspecified sprain of right hip

S73.102- Unspecified sprain of left hip

S73.11 Iliofemoral ligament sprain of hip

S73.111- Iliofemoral ligament sprain of right hip

S73.112- Iliofemoral ligament sprain of left hip

S73.12 Ischiocapsular (ligament) sprain of hip

S73.121- Ischiocapsular ligament sprain of right hip

S73.122- Ischiocapsular ligament sprain of left hip

S73.19 Other sprain of hip

S73.191- Other sprain of right hip

S73.192- Other sprain of left hip

S76 INJURY OF MUSCLE, FASCIA AND TENDON AT HIP AND THIGH LEVEL

S76 requires a 7th character
A—initial encounter
D—subsequent encounter
S—sequela

Code also any associated open wound (S71.-)

Excludes2: injury of muscle, fascia and tendon at lower leg level (S86)
sprain of joint and ligament of hip (S73.1)

S76.0 Injury of muscle, fascia and tendon of hip

S76.01 Strain of muscle, fascia and tendon of hip

S76.011- Strain of muscle, fascia and tendon of right hip

S76.012- Strain of muscle, fascia and tendon of left hip

S76.1 Injury of quadriceps muscle, fascia and tendon
Injury of patellar ligament (tendon)

S76.11 Strain of quadriceps muscle, fascia and tendon

S76.111- Strain of right quadriceps muscle, fascia and tendon

S76.112- Strain of left quadriceps muscle, fascia and tendon

S76.21 Strain of adductor muscle, fascia and tendon of thigh

S76.211- Strain of adductor muscle, fascia and tendon of right thigh

S76.212- Strain of adductor muscle, fascia and tendon of left thigh

S76.31 Strain of muscle, fascia and tendon of the posterior muscle group at thigh level

S76.311- Strain of muscle, fascia and tendon of the posterior muscle group at thigh level, right thigh

S76.312- Strain of muscle, fascia and tendon of the posterior muscle group at thigh level, left thigh

S76.91 Strain of unspecified muscles, fascia and tendons at thigh level

S76.911- Strain of unspecified muscles, fascia and tendons at thigh level, right thigh

S76.912- Strain of unspecified muscles, fascia and tendons at thigh level, left thigh

---

S79 OTHER AND UNSPECIFIED INJURIES OF HIP AND THIGH

S79.0 requires a 7th character
A—initial encounter for closed fracture
D—subsequent encounter for fracture with routine healing
G—subsequent encounter for fracture with delayed healing
K—subsequent encounter for fracture with nonunion
P—subsequent encounter for fracture with malunion
S—sequela

Note: A fracture not indicated as open or closed should be coded to closed

S79.0 Physeal fracture of upper end of femur

Excludes1: apophyseal fracture of upper end of femur (S72.13-)
nontraumatic slipped upper femoral epiphysis (M93.0-)

S79.00 Unspecified physeal fracture of upper end of femur

S79.001- Unspecified physeal fracture of upper end of right femur

S79.002- Unspecified physeal fracture of upper end of left femur

S79.01 Salter-Harris Type I physeal fracture of upper end of femur
Acute on chronic slipped capital femoral epiphysis (traumatic)
Acute slipped capital femoral epiphysis (traumatic)
Capital femoral epiphyseal fracture
Excludes1: chronic slipped upper femoral epiphysis (nontraumatic) (M93.02-)

S79.011- Salter-Harris Type I physeal fracture of upper end of right femur,

S79.012- Salter-Harris Type I physeal fracture of upper end of left femur

S79.09 Other physeal fracture of upper end of femur

S79.091- Other physeal fracture of upper end of right femur

S79.092- Other physeal fracture of upper end of left femur

S79.1 Physeal fracture of lower end of femur

S79.10 Unspecified physeal fracture of lower end of femur

S79.101- Unspecified physeal fracture of lower end of right femur

S79.102- Unspecified physeal fracture of lower end of left femur

S79.11 Salter-Harris Type I physeal fracture of lower end of femur

S79.111- Salter-Harris Type I physeal fracture of lower end of right femur

S79.112- Salter-Harris Type I physeal fracture of lower end of left femur

S79.12 Salter-Harris Type II physeal fracture of lower end of femur

S79.121- Salter-Harris Type II physeal fracture of lower end of right femur

S79.122- Salter-Harris Type II physeal fracture of lower end of left femur

S79.13 Salter-Harris Type III physeal fracture of lower end of femur

S79.131- Salter-Harris Type III physeal fracture of lower end of right femur

S79.132- Salter-Harris Type III physeal fracture of lower end of left femur

S79.14 Salter-Harris Type IV physeal fracture of lower end of femur

S79.141- Salter-Harris Type IV physeal fracture of lower end of right femur

S79.142- Salter-Harris Type IV physeal fracture of lower end of left femur

S79.19 Other physeal fracture of lower end of femur

S79.191- Other physeal fracture of lower end of right femur

S79.192- Other physeal fracture of lower end of left femur

S79.8 Other specified injuries of hip and thigh

S79.81 Other specified injuries of hip

S79.811- Other specified injuries of right hip

S79.812- Other specified injuries of left hip

S79.82 Other specified injuries of thigh

S79.821- Other specified injuries of right thigh

S79.822- Other specified injuries of left thigh

Excludes2: burns and corrosions (T20–T32)
frostbite (T33–T34)
injuries of ankle and foot, except fracture of ankle and malleolus (S90–S99)
insect bite or sting, venomous (T63.4)

S80 SUPERFICIAL INJURY OF KNEE AND LOWER LEG

Excludes2: superficial injury of ankle and foot (S90.-)

S80.0 Contusion of knee

S80.01X- Contusion of right knee

S80.02X- Contusion of left knee

S80.1 Contusion of lower leg

S80.11X- Contusion of right lower leg

S80.12X- Contusion of left lower leg

S80.2 Other superficial injuries of knee

S80.21 Abrasion of knee

S80.211- Abrasion, right knee

S80.212- Abrasion, left knee

S80.22 Blister (nonthermal) of knee

S80.221- Blister (nonthermal), right knee

S80.222- Blister (nonthermal), left knee

S80.24 External constriction of knee

S80.241- External constriction, right knee

S80.242- External constriction, left knee

S80.25 Superficial FB of knee
Splinter in the knee

S80.251- Superficial FB, right knee

S80.252- Superficial FB, left knee

S80.26 Insect bite (nonvenomous) of knee

S80.261- Insect bite (nonvenomous), right knee

S80.262- Insect bite (nonvenomous), left knee

S80.27 Other superficial bite of knee
Excludes1: open bite of knee (S81.05-)

S80.271- Other superficial bite of right knee

S80.272- Other superficial bite of left knee

S80.8 Other superficial injuries of lower leg

S80.81 Abrasion of lower leg

S80.811- Abrasion, right lower leg

S80.812- Abrasion, left lower leg

S80.82 Blister (nonthermal) of lower leg

S80.821- Blister (nonthermal), right lower leg

S80.822- Blister (nonthermal), left lower leg

S80.84 External constriction of lower leg

S80.841- External constriction, right lower leg

S80.842- External constriction, left lower leg

S80.85 Superficial FB of lower leg
Splinter in the lower leg

S80.851- Superficial FB, right lower leg

S80.852- Superficial FB, left lower leg

S80.86 Insect bite (nonvenomous) of lower leg

S80.861- Insect bite (nonvenomous), right lower leg

S80.862- Insect bite (nonvenomous), left lower leg

S80.87 Other superficial bite of lower leg
Excludes1: open bite of lower leg (S81.85-)

S80.871- Other superficial bite, right lower leg

S80.872- Other superficial bite, left lower leg

S81 OPEN WOUND OF KNEE AND LOWER LEG

S81 requires a 7th character
A—initial encounter
D—subsequent encounter
S—sequela

Code also any associated wound infection
Excludes1: open fracture of knee and lower leg (S82.-)
traumatic amputation of lower leg (S88.-)
Excludes2: open wound of ankle and foot (S91.-)

S81.0 Open wound of knee

S81.01 Laceration without FB of knee

S81.011- Laceration without FB, right knee

S81.012- Laceration without FB, left knee

S81.02 Laceration with FB of knee

S81.021- Laceration with FB, right knee

S81.022- Laceration with FB, left knee

S81.03 Puncture wound without FB of knee

S81.031- Puncture wound without FB, right knee

S81.032- Puncture wound without FB, left knee

S81.04 Puncture wound with FB of knee

S81.041- Puncture wound with FB, right knee

S81.042- Puncture wound with FB, left knee

S81.05 Open bite of knee
Bite of knee NOS
Excludes1: superficial bite of knee (S80.27-)

S81.051- Open bite, right knee

S81.052- Open bite, left knee

S81.8 Open wound of lower leg

S81.81 Laceration without FB of lower leg

S81.811- Laceration without FB, right lower leg

S81.812- Laceration without FB, left lower leg

S81.82 Laceration with FB of lower leg

S81.821- Laceration with FB, right lower leg

S81.822- Laceration with FB, left lower leg

S81.83 Puncture wound without FB of lower leg

S81.831- Puncture wound without FB, right lower leg

S81.832- Puncture wound without FB, left lower leg

S81.84 Puncture wound with FB of lower leg

S81.841- Puncture wound with FB, right lower leg

S81.842- Puncture wound with FB, left lower leg

S81.85 Open bite of lower leg
Bite of lower leg NOS
Excludes1: superficial bite of lower leg (S80.86-, S80.87-)

S81.851- Open bite, right lower leg

S81.852- Open bite, left lower leg

S82 FRACTURE OF LOWER LEG, INCLUDING ANKLE

S82 requires a 7th character
A—initial encounter for closed fracture
B— initial encounter for open fracture type I or II initial encounter for open fracture NOS
C— initial encounter for open fracture type IIIA, IIIB, or IIIC
D—subsequent encounter for closed fracture with routine healing
E—subsequent encounter for open fracture type I or II with routine healing
F—subsequent encounter for open fracture type IIIA, IIIB, or IIIC with routine healing
G—subsequent encounter for closed fracture with delayed healing
H—subsequent encounter for open fracture type I or II with delayed healing
J—subsequent encounter for open fracture type IIIA, IIIB, or IIIC with delayed healing
K—subsequent encounter for closed fracture with nonunion
M—subsequent encounter for open fracture type I or II with nonunion
N— subsequent encounter for open fracture type IIIA, IIIB, or IIIC with nonunion
P—subsequent encounter for closed fracture with malunion
Q—subsequent encounter for open fracture type I or II with malunion
R—subsequent encounter for open fracture type IIIA, IIIB, or IIIC with malunion
S—sequela

Please see full *ICD-10-CM* manual for seventh characters applicable to open fracture types IIIA, IIIB, or IIIC.

Note: A fracture not indicated as displaced or nondisplaced should be coded to displaced

A fracture not indicated as open or closed should be coded to closed

The open fracture designations are based on the Gustilo open fracture classification

Includes: fracture of malleolus
Excludes1: traumatic amputation of lower leg (S88.-)
Excludes2: fracture of foot, except ankle (S92.-)
periprosthetic fracture around internal prosthetic ankle joint (M97.2)
periprosthetic fracture around internal prosthetic implant of knee joint (M97.1-)

S82.0 Fracture of patella
Knee cap

S82.00 Unspecified fracture of patella

S82.001- Unspecified fracture of right patella

S82.002- Unspecified fracture of left patella

S82.1 Fracture of upper end of tibia
Fracture of proximal end of tibia
Excludes2: fracture of shaft of tibia (S82.2-)
physeal fracture of upper end of tibia (S89.0-)

S82.10 Unspecified fracture of upper end of tibia

S82.101- Unspecified fracture of upper end of right tibia

S82.102- Unspecified fracture of upper end of left tibia

S82.16 Torus fracture of upper end of tibia

S82.16 requires a 7th character
A—initial encounter for closed fracture
D—subsequent encounter for fracture with routine healing
G—subsequent encounter for fracture with delayed healing
K—subsequent encounter for fracture with nonunion
P—subsequent encounter for fracture with malunion
S—sequela

S82.161- Torus fracture of upper end of right tibia

S82.162- Torus fracture of upper end of left tibia

S82.19 Other fracture of upper end of tibia

S82.191- Other fracture of upper end of right tibia

S82.192- Other fracture of upper end of left tibia

S82.2 Fracture of shaft of tibia

S82.20 Unspecified fracture of shaft of tibia
Fracture of tibia NOS

S82.201- Unspecified fracture of shaft of right tibia

S82.202- Unspecified fracture of shaft of left tibia

S82.24 Spiral fracture of shaft of tibia
Toddler fracture

S82.241- Displaced spiral fracture of shaft of right tibia

S82.242- Displaced spiral fracture of shaft of left tibia

S82.244- Nondisplaced spiral fracture of shaft of right tibia

S82.245- Nondisplaced spiral fracture of shaft of left tibia

S82.3 Fracture of lower end of tibia

Excludes1: bimalleolar fracture of lower leg (S82.84-)
fracture of medial malleolus alone (S82.5-)
Maisonneuve's fracture (S82.86-)
pilon fracture of distal tibia (S82.87-)
trimalleolar fractures of lower leg (S82.85-)

S82.30 Unspecified fracture of lower end of tibia

S82.301- Unspecified fracture of lower end of right tibia

S82.302- Unspecified fracture of lower end of left tibia

S82.31 Torus fracture of lower end of tibia

S82.311- Torus fracture of lower end of right tibia

S82.312- Torus fracture of lower end of left tibia

S82.39 Other fracture of lower end of tibia

S82.391- Other fracture of lower end of right tibia

S82.392- Other fracture of lower end of left tibia

S82.4 Fracture of shaft of fibula

Excludes2: fracture of lateral malleolus alone (S82.6-)

S82.40 Unspecified fracture of shaft of fibula

S82.401- Unspecified fracture of shaft of right fibula

S82.402- Unspecified fracture of shaft of left fibula

S82.5 Fracture of medial malleolus

Excludes1: pilon fracture of distal tibia (S82.87-)
Salter-Harris type III of lower end of tibia (S89.13-)
Salter-Harris type IV of lower end of tibia (S89.14-)

S82.51X- Displaced fracture of medial malleolus of right tibia

S82.52X- Displaced fracture of medial malleolus of left tibia

S82.54X- Nondisplaced fracture of medial malleolus of right tibia

S82.55X- Nondisplaced fracture of medial malleolus of left tibia

S82.6 Fracture of lateral malleolus

Excludes1: pilon fracture of distal tibia (S82.87-)

S82.61X- Displaced fracture of lateral malleolus of right fibula

S82.62X- Displaced fracture of lateral malleolus of left fibula

S82.64X- Nondisplaced fracture of lateral malleolus of right fibula

S82.65X- Nondisplaced fracture of lateral malleolus of left fibula

S82.31 requires a 7th character
A—initial encounter for closed fracture
D—subsequent encounter for fracture with routine healing
G—subsequent encounter for fracture with delayed healing
K—subsequent encounter for fracture with nonunion
P—subsequent encounter for fracture with malunion
S—sequela

S82 requires a 7th character
A—initial encounter for closed fracture
B— initial encounter for open fracture type I or II initial encounter for open fracture NOS
C— initial encounter for open fracture type IIIA, IIIB, or IIIC
D—subsequent encounter for closed fracture with routine healing
E—subsequent encounter for open fracture type I or II with routine healing
F—subsequent encounter for open fracture type IIIA, IIIB, or IIIC with routine healing
G —subsequent encounter for closed fracture with delayed healing
H—subsequent encounter for open fracture type I or II with delayed healing
J—subsequent encounter for open fracture type IIIA, IIIB, or IIIC with delayed healing
K—subsequent encounter for closed fracture with nonunion
M—subsequent encounter for open fracture type I or II with nonunion
N— subsequent encounter for open fracture type IIIA, IIIB, or IIIC with nonunion
P—subsequent encounter for closed fracture with malunion
Q—subsequent encounter for open fracture type I or II with malunion
R—subsequent encounter for open fracture type IIIA, IIIB, or IIIC with malunion
S—sequela

S82.8 Other fractures of lower leg

S82.81 Torus fracture of upper end of fibula

S82.811- Torus fracture of upper end of right fibula

S82.812- Torus fracture of upper end of left fibula

S82.82 Torus fracture of lower end of fibula

S82.821- Torus fracture of lower end of right fibula

S82.822- Torus fracture of lower end of left fibula

S82.83 Other fracture of upper and lower end of fibula

S82.831- Other fracture of upper and lower end of right fibula

S82.832- Other fracture of upper and lower end of left fibula

S82.84 Bimalleolar fracture of lower leg

S82.841- Displaced bimalleolar fracture of right lower leg

S82.842- Displaced bimalleolar fracture of left lower leg

S82.844- Nondisplaced bimalleolar fracture of right lower leg

S82.845- Nondisplaced bimalleolar fracture of left lower leg

S82.85 Trimalleolar fracture of lower leg

S82.851- Displaced trimalleolar fracture of right lower leg

S82.852- Displaced trimalleolar fracture of left lower leg

S82.854- Nondisplaced trimalleolar fracture of right lower leg

S82.855- Nondisplaced trimalleolar fracture of left lower leg

S82.86 Maisonneuve's fracture

S82.861- Displaced Maisonneuve's fracture of right leg

S82.862- Displaced Maisonneuve's fracture of left leg

S82.864- Nondisplaced Maisonneuve's fracture of right leg

S82.865- Nondisplaced Maisonneuve's fracture of left leg

S82.87 Pilon fracture of tibia

S82.871- Displaced pilon fracture of right tibia

S82.872- Displaced pilon fracture of left tibia

S82.874- Nondisplaced pilon fracture of right tibia

S82.875- Nondisplaced pilon fracture of left tibia

S82.89 Other fractures of lower leg
Fracture of ankle NOS

S82.891- Other fracture of right lower leg

S82.892- Other fracture of left lower leg

S82.81 and S82.82 require a 7th character
A—initial encounter for closed fracture
D—subsequent encounter for fracture with routine healing
G—subsequent encounter for fracture with delayed healing
K—subsequent encounter for fracture with nonunion
P—subsequent encounter for fracture with malunion
S— sequela

S83 **DISLOCATION AND SPRAIN OF JOINTS AND LIGAMENTS OF KNEE**

Includes: avulsion of joint or ligament of knee
laceration of cartilage, joint or ligament of knee
sprain of cartilage, joint or ligament of knee
traumatic hemarthrosis of joint or ligament of knee
traumatic rupture of joint or ligament of knee

S83 requires a 7th character
A—initial encounter
D—subsequent encounter
S—sequela

traumatic subluxation of joint or ligament of knee
traumatic tear of joint or ligament of knee

Code also any associated open wound
Excludes1: derangement of patella (M22.0–M22.3)
injury of patellar ligament (tendon) (S76.1-)
internal derangement of knee (M23.-)
old dislocation of knee (M24.36)
pathological dislocation of knee (M24.36)
recurrent dislocation of knee (M22.0)
Excludes2: strain of muscle, fascia and tendon of lower leg (S86.-)

S83.0 Subluxation and dislocation of patella

S83.00 Unspecified subluxation and dislocation of patella

S83.001- Unspecified subluxation of right patella

S83.002- Unspecified subluxation of left patella

S83.004- Unspecified dislocation of right patella

S83.005- Unspecified dislocation of left patella

S83.01 Lateral subluxation and dislocation of patella

S83.011- Lateral subluxation of right patella

S83.012- Lateral subluxation of left patella

S83.014- Lateral dislocation of right patella

S83.015- Lateral dislocation of left patella

S83.09 Other subluxation and dislocation of patella

S83.091- Other subluxation of right patella

S83.092- Other subluxation of left patella

S83.094- Other dislocation of right patella

S83.095- Other dislocation of left patella

S83.1 Subluxation and dislocation of knee

Excludes2: instability of knee prosthesis (T84.022, T84.023)

S83.10 Unspecified subluxation and dislocation of knee

S83.101- Unspecified subluxation of right knee

S83.102- Unspecified subluxation of left knee

S83.104- Unspecified dislocation of right knee

S83.105- Unspecified dislocation of left knee

S83.11 Anterior subluxation and dislocation of proximal end of tibia

Posterior subluxation and dislocation of distal end of femur

S83.111- Anterior subluxation of proximal end of tibia, right knee

S83.112- Anterior subluxation of proximal end of tibia, left knee

S83.114- Anterior dislocation of proximal end of tibia, right knee

S83.115- Anterior dislocation of proximal end of tibia, left knee

S83.12 Posterior subluxation and dislocation of proximal end of tibia

Anterior dislocation of distal end of femur

S83.121- Posterior subluxation of proximal end of tibia, right knee

S83.122- Posterior subluxation of proximal end of tibia, left knee

S83.124- Posterior dislocation of proximal end of tibia, right knee

S83.125- Posterior dislocation of proximal end of tibia, left knee

S83.13 Medial subluxation and dislocation of proximal end of tibia

S83.131- Medial subluxation of proximal end of tibia, right knee

S83.132- Medial subluxation of proximal end of tibia, left knee

S83.134- Medial dislocation of proximal end of tibia, right knee

S83.135- Medial dislocation of proximal end of tibia, left knee

S83.14 Lateral subluxation and dislocation of proximal end of tibia

S83.141- Lateral subluxation of proximal end of tibia, right knee

S83.142- Lateral subluxation of proximal end of tibia, left knee

S83.144- Lateral dislocation of proximal end of tibia, right knee

S83.145- Lateral dislocation of proximal end of tibia, left knee

S83.19 Other subluxation and dislocation of knee

S83.191- Other subluxation of right knee

S83.192- Other subluxation of left knee

S83.194- Other dislocation of right knee

S83.195- Other dislocation of left knee

S83.4 Sprain of collateral ligament of knee

S83.40 Sprain of unspecified collateral ligament of knee

S83.401- Sprain of unspecified collateral ligament of right knee

S83.402- Sprain of unspecified collateral ligament of left knee

S83.41 Sprain of medial collateral ligament of knee

Sprain of tibial collateral ligament

S83.411- Sprain of medial collateral ligament of right knee

S83.412- Sprain of medial collateral ligament of left knee

S83.42 Sprain of lateral collateral ligament of knee

Sprain of fibular collateral ligament

S83.421- Sprain of lateral collateral ligament of right knee

S83.422- Sprain of lateral collateral ligament of left knee

S83.5 Sprain of cruciate ligament of knee

S83.50 Sprain of unspecified cruciate ligament of knee

S83.501- Sprain of unspecified cruciate ligament of right knee

S83.502- Sprain of unspecified cruciate ligament of left knee

S83.51 Sprain of anterior cruciate ligament of knee

S83.511- Sprain of anterior cruciate ligament of right knee

S83.512- Sprain of anterior cruciate ligament of left knee

S83.52 Sprain of posterior cruciate ligament of knee

S83.521- Sprain of posterior cruciate ligament of right knee

S83.522- Sprain of posterior cruciate ligament of left knee

S83.6 Sprain of the superior tibiofibular joint and ligament

S83.60X- Sprain of the superior tibiofibular joint and ligament, unspecified knee

S83.61X- Sprain of the superior tibiofibular joint and ligament, right knee

S83.62X- Sprain of the superior tibiofibular joint and ligament, left knee

S83.8 Sprain of other specified parts of knee

S83.8X Sprain of other specified parts of knee

S83.8X1- Sprain of other specified parts of right knee

S83.8X2- Sprain of other specified parts of left knee

S83 requires a 7th character
A—initial encounter
D—subsequent encounter
S—sequela

S83.9 Sprain of unspecified site of knee

5th S83.91X- Sprain of unspecified site of right knee

7th

S83.92X- Sprain of unspecified site of left knee

7th

S86 INJURY OF MUSCLE, FASCIA AND TENDON AT LOWER LEG LEVEL

4th

S86 requires a 7th character
A—initial encounter
D—subsequent encounter
S—sequela

Code also any associated open wound (S81.-)

Excludes2: injury of muscle, fascia and tendon at ankle (S96.-)
injury of patellar ligament (tendon) (S76.1-)
sprain of joints and ligaments of knee (S83.-)

S86.0 Injury of Achilles tendon

5th S86.00 Unspecified injury of Achilles tendon

6th S86.001- Unspecified injury of right Achilles tendon

7th

S86.002- Unspecified injury of left Achilles tendon

7th

S86.01 Strain of Achilles tendon

6th S86.011- Strain of right Achilles tendon

7th

S86.012- Strain of left Achilles tendon

7th

S86.02 Laceration of Achilles tendon

6th S86.021- Laceration of right Achilles tendon

7th

S86.022- Laceration of left Achilles tendon

7th

S86.09 Other specified injury of Achilles tendon

6th S86.091- Other specified injury of right Achilles tendon

7th

S86.092- Other specified injury of left Achilles tendon

7th

S86.1 Injury of other muscle(s) and tendon(s) of posterior muscle group at lower leg level

5th

S86.11 Strain of other muscle(s) and tendon(s) of posterior muscle group at lower leg level,

6th

S86.111- right leg

7th

S86.112- left leg

7th

S86.2 Injury of muscle(s) and tendon(s) of anterior muscle group at lower leg level

5th

S86.21 Strain of muscle(s) and tendon(s) of anterior muscle group at lower leg level,

6th

S86.211- right leg

7th

S86.212- left leg

7th

S86.3 Injury of muscle(s) and tendon(s) of peroneal muscle group at lower leg level

5th

S86.31 Strain of muscle(s) and tendon(s) of peroneal muscle group at lower leg level,

6th

S86.311- right leg

7th

S86.312- left leg

7th

S86.32 Laceration of muscle(s) and tendon(s) of peroneal muscle group at lower leg level,

6th

S86.321- right leg

7th

S86.322- left leg

7th

S86.39 Other injury of muscle(s) and tendon(s) of peroneal muscle group at lower leg level,

6th

S86.391- right leg

7th

S86.392- left leg

7th

S86.8 Injury of other muscles and tendons at lower leg level

5th S86.81 Strain of other muscles and tendons at lower leg level,

6th

S86.811- right leg

7th

S86.812- left leg

7th

S86.82 Laceration of other muscles and tendons at lower leg level,

6th

S86.821- right leg

7th

S86.822- left leg

7th

S86.89 Other injury of other muscles and tendons at lower leg level,

6th

S86.891- right leg

7th

S86.892- left leg

7th

S86.9 Injury of unspecified muscle and tendon at lower leg level

5th S86.91 Strain of unspecified muscle and tendon at lower leg level,

6th

S86.911- right leg

7th

S86.912- left leg

7th

S89 OTHER AND UNSPECIFIED INJURIES OF LOWER LEG

4th

Note: A fracture not indicated as open or closed should be coded to closed

Excludes2: other and unspecified injuries of ankle and foot (S99.-)

S89.0 Physeal fracture of upper end of tibia

5th

S89.0, S89.1, S89.2, and S89.3 require a 7th character
A—initial encounter for closed fracture
D—subsequent encounter for fracture with routine healing
G—subsequent encounter for fracture with delayed healing
K—subsequent encounter for fracture with nonunion
P—subsequent encounter for fracture with malunion
S—sequela

S89.00 Unspecified physeal fracture of upper end of tibia

6th

S89.001- Unspecified physeal fracture of upper end of right tibia

7th

S89.002- Unspecified physeal fracture of upper end of left tibia

7th

S89.01 Salter-Harris Type I physeal fracture of upper end of tibia

6th

S89.011- Salter-Harris Type I physeal fracture of upper end of right tibia

7th

S89.012- Salter-Harris Type I physeal fracture of upper end of left tibia

7th

S89.02 Salter-Harris Type II physeal fracture of upper end of tibia

6th

S89.021- Salter-Harris Type II physeal fracture of upper end of right tibia

7th

S89.022- Salter-Harris Type II physeal fracture of upper end of left tibia

7th

S89.03 Salter-Harris Type III physeal fracture of upper end of tibia

6th

S89.031- Salter-Harris Type III physeal fracture of upper end of right tibia

7th

S89.032- Salter-Harris Type III physeal fracture of upper end of left tibia

7th

S89.04 Salter-Harris Type IV physeal fracture of upper end of tibia

6th

S89.041- Salter-Harris Type IV physeal fracture of upper end of right tibia

7th

S89.042- Salter-Harris Type IV physeal fracture of upper end of left tibia

7th

S89.09 Other physeal fracture of upper end of tibia

6th

S89.091- Other physeal fracture of upper end of right tibia

7th

S89.092- Other physeal fracture of upper end of left tibia

S89.0, S89.1, S89.2, and S89.3 require a 7th character
A—initial encounter for closed fracture
D—subsequent encounter for fracture with routine healing
G—subsequent encounter for fracture with delayed healing
K—subsequent encounter for fracture with nonunion
P—subsequent encounter for fracture with malunion
S—sequela

S89.1 Physeal fracture of lower end of tibia

S89.10 Unspecified physeal fracture of lower end of tibia

S89.101- Unspecified physeal fracture of lower end of right tibia

S89.102- Unspecified physeal fracture of lower end of left tibia

S89.11 Salter-Harris Type I physeal fracture of lower end of tibia

S89.111- Salter-Harris Type I physeal fracture of lower end of right tibia

S89.112- Salter-Harris Type I physeal fracture of lower end of left tibia

S89.12 Salter-Harris Type II physeal fracture of lower end of tibia

S89.121- Salter-Harris Type II physeal fracture of lower end of right tibia

S89.122- Salter-Harris Type II physeal fracture of lower end of left tibia

S89.13 Salter-Harris Type III physeal fracture of lower end of tibia

Excludes1: fracture of medial malleolus (adult) (S82.5-)

S89.131- Salter-Harris Type III physeal fracture of lower end of right tibia

S89.132- Salter-Harris Type III physeal fracture of lower end of left tibia

S89.14 Salter-Harris Type IV physeal fracture of lower end of tibia

Excludes1: fracture of medial malleolus (adult) (S82.5-)

S89.141- Salter-Harris Type IV physeal fracture of lower end of right tibia

S89.142- Salter-Harris Type IV physeal fracture of lower end of left tibia

S89.19 Other physeal fracture of lower end of tibia

S89.191- Other physeal fracture of lower end of right tibia

S89.192- Other physeal fracture of lower end of left tibia

S89.2 Physeal fracture of upper end of fibula

S89.20 Unspecified physeal fracture of upper end of fibula

S89.201- Unspecified physeal fracture of upper end of right fibula

S89.202- Unspecified physeal fracture of upper end of left fibula

S89.21 Salter-Harris Type I physeal fracture of upper end of fibula

S89.211- Salter-Harris Type I physeal fracture of upper end of right fibula

S89.212- Salter-Harris Type I physeal fracture of upper end of left fibula

S89.22 Salter-Harris Type II physeal fracture of upper end of fibula

S89.221- Salter-Harris Type II physeal fracture of upper end of right fibula

S89.222- Salter-Harris Type II physeal fracture of upper end of left fibula

S89.29 Other physeal fracture of upper end of fibula

S89.291- Other physeal fracture of upper end of right fibula

S89.292- Other physeal fracture of upper end of left fibula

S89.3 Physeal fracture of lower end of fibula

S89.30 Unspecified physeal fracture of lower end of fibula

S89.301- Unspecified physeal fracture of lower end of right fibula

S89.302- Unspecified physeal fracture of lower end of left fibula

S89.31 Salter-Harris Type I physeal fracture of lower end of fibula

S89.311- Salter-Harris Type I physeal fracture of lower end of right fibula

S89.312- Salter-Harris Type I physeal fracture of lower end of left fibula

S89.32 Salter-Harris Type II physeal fracture of lower end of fibula

S89.321- Salter-Harris Type II physeal fracture of lower end of right fibula

S89.322- Salter-Harris Type II physeal fracture of lower end of left fibula

S89.39 Other physeal fracture of lower end of fibula

S89.391- Other physeal fracture of lower end of right fibula

S89.392- Other physeal fracture of lower end of left fibula

S89.8 Other specified injuries of lower leg

S89.8 requires a 7th character
A—initial encounter
D—subsequent encounter
S—sequela

S89.81X- Other specified injuries of right lower leg

S89.82X- Other specified injuries of left lower leg

(S90–S99) INJURIES TO THE ANKLE AND FOOT

Excludes2: burns and corrosions (T20–T32)
fracture of ankle and malleolus (S82.-)
frostbite (T33–T34)
insect bite or sting, venomous (T63.4)

S90 SUPERFICIAL INJURY OF ANKLE, FOOT AND TOES

S90 requires a 7th character
A—initial encounter
D—subsequent encounter
S—sequela

S90.0 Contusion of ankle

S90.01X- Contusion of right ankle

S90.02X- Contusion of left ankle

S90.1 Contusion of toe without damage to nail

S90.11 Contusion of great toe without damage to nail

S90.111- Contusion of right great toe without damage to nail

S90.112- Contusion of left great toe without damage to nail

S90.12 Contusion of lesser toe without damage to nail

S90.121- Contusion of right lesser toe(s) without damage to nail

S90.122- Contusion of left lesser toe(s) without damage to nail

S90.2 Contusion of toe with damage to nail

S90.21 Contusion of great toe with damage to nail

S90.211- Contusion of right great toe with damage to nail

S90.212- Contusion of left great toe with damage to nail

S90.22 Contusion of lesser toe with damage to nail

S90.221- Contusion of right lesser toe(s) with damage to nail

S90.222- Contusion of left lesser toe(s) with damage to nail

S90.3 Contusion of foot

Excludes2: contusion of toes (S90.1-, S90.2-)

S90.31X- Contusion of right foot

S90.32X- Contusion of left foot

S90.4 Other superficial injuries of toe

S90.41 Abrasion of toe

S90.411- Abrasion, right great toe

S90.412- Abrasion, left great toe

S90.414- Abrasion, right lesser toe(s)

S90.415- Abrasion, left lesser toe(s)

S90.42 Blister (nonthermal) of toe

S90.421- Blister (nonthermal), right great toe

S90.422- Blister (nonthermal), left great toe

S90.424- Blister (nonthermal), right lesser toe(s)

S90.425- Blister (nonthermal), left lesser toe(s)

S90.44 External constriction of toe

Hair tourniquet syndrome of toe

S90.441- External constriction, right great toe

S90.442- External constriction, left great toe

S90.444- External constriction, right lesser toe(s)

S90.445- External constriction, left lesser toe(s)

S90.45 Superficial FB of toe

Splinter in the toe

S90.451- Superficial FB, right great toe

S90.452- Superficial FB, left great toe

S90.454- Superficial FB, right lesser toe(s)

S90.455- Superficial FB, left lesser toe(s)

S90.46 Insect bite (nonvenomous) of toc

S90.461- Insect bite (nonvenomous), right great toe

S90.462- Insect bite (nonvenomous), left great toe

S90.464- Insect bite (nonvenomous), right lesser toe(s)

S90.465- Insect bite (nonvenomous), left lesser toe(s)

S90.47 Other superficial bite of toe

Excludes1: open bite of toe (S91.15-, S91.25-)

S90.471- Other superficial bite of right great toe

S90.472- Other superficial bite of left great toe

S90.474- Other superficial bite of right lesser toe(s)

S90.475- Other superficial bite of left lesser toe(s)

S90.5 Other superficial injuries of ankle

S90.51 Abrasion of ankle

S90.511- Abrasion, right ankle

S90.512- Abrasion, left ankle

S90.52 Blister (nonthermal) of ankle

S90.521- Blister (nonthermal), right ankle

S90.522- Blister (nonthermal), left ankle

S90.54 External constriction of ankle

S90.541- External constriction, right ankle

S90.542- External constriction, left ankle

S90.55 Superficial FB of ankle

Splinter in the ankle

S90.551- Superficial FB, right ankle

S90.552- Superficial FB, left ankle

S90.56 Insect bite (nonvenomous) of ankle

S90.561- Insect bite (nonvenomous), right ankle

S90.562- Insect bite (nonvenomous), left ankle

S90.57 Other superficial bite of ankle,

Excludes1: open bite of ankle (S91.05-)

S90.571- right ankle

S90.572- left ankle

S90.8 Other superficial injuries of foot

S90.81 Abrasion of foot

S90.811- Abrasion, right foot

S90.812- Abrasion, left foot

S90.82 Blister (nonthermal) of foot

S90.821- Blister (nonthermal), right foot

S90.822- Blister (nonthermal), left foot

S90.84 External constriction of foot

S90.841- External constriction, right foot

S90.842- External constriction, left foot

S90.85 Superficial FB of foot

Splinter in the foot

S90.851- Superficial FB, right foot

S90.852- Superficial FB, left foot

S90.86 Insect bite (nonvenomous) of foot

S90.861- Insect bite (nonvenomous), right foot

S90.862- Insect bite (nonvenomous), left foot

S90.87 Other superficial bite of foot

Excludes1: open bite of foot (S91.35-)

S90.871- Other superficial bite of right foot

S90.872- Other superficial bite of left foot

S91 OPEN WOUND OF ANKLE, FOOT AND TOES

Code also any associated wound infection

Excludes1: open fracture of ankle, foot and toes (S92.-with 7th character B)

traumatic amputation of ankle and foot (S98.-)

S91.0 Open wound of ankle

S91.01 Laceration without FB of ankle

S91.011- Laceration without FB, right ankle

S91.012- Laceration without FB, left ankle

S91.02 Laceration with FB of ankle

S91.021- Laceration with FB, right ankle

S91.022- Laceration with FB, left ankle

S91.03 Puncture wound without FB of ankle

S91.031- Puncture wound without FB, right ankle

S91.032- Puncture wound without FB, left ankle

S91.04 Puncture wound with FB of ankle

S91.041- Puncture wound with FB, right ankle

S91.042- Puncture wound with FB, left ankle

S91.05 Open bite of ankle

6th *Excludes1:* superficial bite of ankle (S90.56-, S90.57-)

S91.051- Open bite, right ankle

7th

S91.052- Open bite, left ankle

7th

S91.1 Open wound of toe without damage to nail

5th **S91.11** Laceration without FB of toe without damage to nail

6th **S91.111-** Laceration without FB of right great toe

7th without damage to nail

S91.112- Laceration without FB of left great toe

7th without damage to nail

S91.114- Laceration without FB of right lesser toe(s)

7th without damage to nail

S91.115- Laceration without FB of left lesser toe(s)

7th without damage to nail

S91.12 Laceration with FB of toe without damage to nail

6th **S91.121-** Laceration with FB of right great toe

7th without damage to nail

S91.122- Laceration with FB of left great toe

7th without damage to nail

S91.124- Laceration with FB of right lesser toe(s)

7th without damage to nail

S91.125- Laceration with FB of left lesser toe(s)

7th without damage to nail

S91.13 Puncture wound without FB of toe without damage

6th to nail

S91.131- Puncture wound without FB of right great

7th toe without damage to nail

S91.132- Puncture wound without FB of left great

7th toe without damage to nail

S91.134- Puncture wound without FB of right lesser

7th toe(s) without damage to nail

S91.135- Puncture wound without FB of left lesser

7th toe(s) without damage to nail

S91.14 Puncture wound with FB of toe without damage to

6th nail

S91.141- Puncture wound with FB of right great toe

7th without damage to nail

S91.142- Puncture wound with FB of left great toe

7th without damage to nail

S91.144- Puncture wound with FB of right lesser

7th toe(s) without damage to nail

S91.145- Puncture wound with FB of left lesser

7th toe(s) without damage to nail

S91.15 Open bite of toe without damage to nail

6th Bite of toe NOS

Excludes1: superficial bite of toe (S90.46-, S90.47-)

S91.151- Open bite of right great toe without

7th damage to nail

S91.152- Open bite of left great toe without damage

7th to nail

S91.154- Open bite of right lesser toe(s) without

7th damage to nail

S91.155- Open bite of left lesser toe(s) without

7th damage to nail

S91.2 Open wound of toe with damage to nail

5th **S91.21** Laceration without FB of toe with damage to nail

6th **S91.211-** Laceration without FB of right great toe

7th with damage to nail

S91.212- Laceration without FB of left great toe

7th with damage to nail

S91.214- Laceration without FB of right lesser toe(s)

7th with damage to nail

S91.215- Laceration without FB of left lesser toe(s)

7th with damage to nail

S91.22 Laceration with FB of toe with damage to nail

6th **S91.221-** Laceration with FB of right great toe with

7th damage to nail

S91.222- Laceration with FB of left great toe with

7th damage to nail

S91.224- Laceration with FB of right lesser toe(s)

7th with damage to nail

S91.225- Laceration with FB of left lesser toe(s)

7th with damage to nail

S91.23 Puncture wound without FB of toe with damage to

6th nail

S91.231- Puncture wound without FB of right great

7th toe with damage to nail

S91.232- Puncture wound without FB of left great

7th toe with damage to nail

S91.234- Puncture wound without FB of right lesser

7th toe(s) with damage to nail

S91.235- Puncture wound without FB of left lesser

7th toe(s) with damage to nail

S91.24 Puncture wound with FB of toe with damage to nail

6th **S91.241-** Puncture wound with FB of right great toe

7th with damage to nail

S91.242- Puncture wound with FB of left great toe

7th with damage to nail

S91.244- Puncture wound with FB of right lesser

7th toe(s) with damage to nail

S91.245- Puncture wound with FB of left lesser

7th toe(s) with damage to nail

S91.25 Open bite of toe with damage to nail

6th Bite of toe with damage to nail NOS

Excludes1: superficial bite of toe (S90.46-, S90.47-)

S91.251- Open bite of right great toe with damage

7th to nail

S91.252- Open bite of left great toe with damage to

7th nail

S91.254- Open bite of right lesser toe(s) with

7th damage to nail

S91.255- Open bite of left lesser toe(s) with damage

7th to nail

S91.3 Open wound of foot

5th **S91.31** Laceration without FB of foot

6th **S91.311-** Laceration without FB, right foot

7th

S91.312- Laceration without FB, left foot

7th

S91.32 Laceration with FB of foot

6th **S91.321-** Laceration with FB, right foot

7th

S91.322- Laceration with FB, left foot

7th

S91.33 Puncture wound without FB of foot

6th **S91.331-** Puncture wound without FB, right foot

7th

S91.332- Puncture wound without FB, left foot

7th

S91.34 Puncture wound with FB of foot

6th **S91.341-** Puncture wound with FB, right foot

7th

S91.342- Puncture wound with FB, left foot

7th

S91.35 Open bite of foot

6th *Excludes1:* superficial bite of foot (S90.86-, S90.87-)

S91.351- Open bite, right foot

7th

S91.352- Open bite, left foot

7th

S92 FRACTURE OF FOOT AND TOE, EXCEPT ANKLE

Note: A fracture not indicated as displaced or nondisplaced should be coded to displaced

A fracture not indicated as open or closed should be coded to closed

Excludes2: traumatic amputation of ankle and foot (S98.-)
fracture of ankle (S82.-)
fracture of malleolus (S82.-)

S92.0 Fracture of calcaneus

Heel bone
Os calcis

Excludes2: physeal fracture of calcaneus (S99.0-)

S92.00 Unspecified fracture of calcaneus

S92.001- Unspecified fracture of right calcaneus

S92.002- Unspecified fracture of left calcaneus

S92.01 Fracture of body of calcaneus

S92.011- Displaced fracture of body of right calcaneus

S92.012- Displaced fracture of body of left calcaneus

S92.014- Nondisplaced fracture of body of right calcaneus

S92.015- Nondisplaced fracture of body of left calcaneus

S92.02 Fracture of anterior process of calcaneus

S92.021- Displaced fracture of anterior process of right calcaneus

S92.022- Displaced fracture of anterior process of left calcaneus

S92.024- Nondis-placed fracture of anterior process of right calcaneus

S92.025- Nondisplaced fracture of anterior process of left calcaneus

S92.03 Avulsion fracture of tuberosity of calcaneus

S92.031- Displaced avulsion fracture of tuberosity of right calcaneus

S92.032- Displaced avulsion fracture of tuberosity of left calcaneus

S92.034- Nondisplaced avulsion fracture of tuberosity of right calcaneus

S92.035- Nondisplaced avulsion fracture of tuberosity of left calcaneus

S92.04 Other fracture of tuberosity of calcaneus

S92.041- Displaced other fracture of tuberosity of right calcaneus

S92.042- Displaced other fracture of tuberosity of left calcaneus

S92.044- Nondisplaced other fracture of tuberosity of right calcaneus

S92.045- Nondisplaced other fracture of tuberosity of left calcaneus

S92.05 Other extraarticular fracture of calcaneus

S92.051- Displaced other extraarticular fracture of right calcaneus

S92.052- Displaced other extraarticular fracture of left calcaneus

S92.054- Nondisplaced other extraarticular fracture of right calcaneus

S92.055- Nondisplaced other extraarticular fracture of left calcaneus

S92.06 Intraarticular fracture of calcaneus

S92.061- Displaced intraarticular fracture of right calcaneus

S92.062- Displaced intraarticular fracture of left calcaneus

S92.064- Nondisplaced intraarticular fracture of right calcaneus

S92.065- Nondisplaced intraarticular fracture of left calcaneus

S92.1 Fracture of talus

Astragalus

S92.10 Unspecified fracture of talus

S92.101- Unspecified fracture of right talus

S92.102- Unspecified fracture of left talus

S92.11 Fracture of neck of talus

S92.111- Displaced fracture of neck of right talus

S92.112- Displaced fracture of neck of left talus

S92.114- Nondisplaced fracture of neck of right talus

S92.115- Nondisplaced fracture of neck of left talus

S92.12 Fracture of body of talus

S92.121- Displaced fracture of body of right talus

S92.122- Displaced fracture of body of left talus

S92.124- Nondisplaced fracture of body of right talus

S92.125- Nondisplaced fracture of body of left talus

S92.13 Fracture of posterior process of talus

S92.131- Displaced fracture of posterior process of right talus

S92.132- Displaced fracture of posterior process of left talus

S92.134- Nondisplaced fracture of posterior process of right talus

S92.135- Nondisplaced fracture of posterior process of left talus

S92.14 Dome fracture of talus

Excludes1: osteochondritis dissecans (M93.2)

S92.141- Displaced dome fracture of right talus

S92.142- Displaced dome fracture of left talus

S92.144- Nondisplaced dome fracture of right talus

S92.145- Nondisplaced dome fracture of left talus

S92.15 Avulsion fracture (chip fracture) of talus

S92.151- Displaced avulsion fracture (chip fracture) of right talus

S92.152- Displaced avulsion fracture (chip fracture) of left talus

S92.154- Nondisplaced avulsion fracture (chip fracture) of right talus

S92.155- Nondisplaced avulsion fracture (chip fracture) of left talus

S92.19 Other fracture of talus

S92.191- Other fracture of right talus

S92.192- Other fracture of left talus

S92.2 Fracture of other and unspecified tarsal bone(s)

S92.20 Fracture of unspecified tarsal bone(s)

S92.201- Fracture of unspecified tarsal bone(s) of right foot

S92.202- Fracture of unspecified tarsal bone(s) of left foot

S92.21 Fracture of cuboid bone

S92.211- Displaced fracture of cuboid bone of right foot

S92.212- Displaced fracture of cuboid bone of left foot

S92.214- Nondisplaced fracture of cuboid bone of right foot

S92.215- Nondisplaced fracture of cuboid bone of left foot

S92.22 Fracture of lateral cuneiform

S92.221- Displaced fracture of lateral cuneiform of right foot

S92.222- Displaced fracture of lateral cuneiform of left foot

S92.224- Nondisplaced fracture of lateral cuneiform of right foot

S92.225- Nondisplaced fracture of lateral cuneiform of left foot

S92.23 Fracture of intermediate cuneiform

S92.231- Displaced fracture of intermediate cuneiform of right foot

S92.232- Displaced fracture of intermediate cuneiform of left foot

S92.234- Nondisplaced fracture of intermediate cuneiform of right foot

S92.235- Nondisplaced fracture of intermediate cuneiform of left foot

S92.24 Fracture of medial cuneiform

S92.241- Displaced fracture of medial cuneiform of right foot

S92.242- Displaced fracture of medial cuneiform of left foot

S92.244- Nondisplaced fracture of medial cuneiform of right foot

S92.245- Nondisplaced fracture of medial cuneiform of left foot

S92.25 Fracture of navicular [scaphoid] of foot

S92.251- Displaced fracture of navicular [scaphoid] of right foot

S92.252- Displaced fracture of navicular [scaphoid] of left foot

S92.254- Nondisplaced fracture of navicular [scaphoid] of right foot

S92.255- Nondisplaced fracture of navicular [scaphoid] of left foot

S92.3 Fracture of metatarsal bone(s)

Excludes2: physeal fracture of metatarsal (S99.1-)

S92.30 Fracture of unspecified metatarsal bone(s),

S92.301- right foot

S92.302- left foot

S92.31 Fracture of first metatarsal bone

S92.311- Displaced fracture of first metatarsal bone, right foot

S92.312- Displaced fracture of first metatarsal bone, left foot

S92.314- Nondisplaced fracture of first metatarsal bone, right foot

S92.315- Nondisplaced fracture of first metatarsal bone, left foot

S92.32 Fracture of second metatarsal bone

S92.321- Displaced fracture of second metatarsal bone, right foot

S92.322- Displaced fracture of second metatarsal bone, left foot

S92.324- Nondisplaced fracture of second metatarsal bone, right foot

S92.325- Nondisplaced fracture of second metatarsal bone, left foot

S92.33 Fracture of third metatarsal bone

S92.331- Displaced fracture of third metatarsal bone, right foot

S92.332- Displaced fracture of third metatarsal bone, left foot

S92.334- Nondisplaced fracture of third metatarsal bone, right foot

S92.335- Nondisplaced fracture of third metatarsal bone, left foot

S92.34 Fracture of fourth metatarsal bone

S92.341- Displaced fracture of fourth metatarsal bone, right foot

S92.342- Displaced fracture of fourth metatarsal bone, left foot

S92.344- Nondisplaced fracture of fourth metatarsal bone, right foot

S92.345- Nondisplaced fracture of fourth metatarsal bone, left foot

S92.35 Fracture of fifth metatarsal bone

S92.351- Displaced fracture of fifth metatarsal bone, right foot

S92.352- Displaced fracture of fifth metatarsal bone, left foot

S92.354- Nondisplaced fracture of fifth metatarsal bone, right foot

S92.355- Nondisplaced fracture of fifth metatarsal bone, left foot

S92.4 Fracture of great toe

Excludes2: physeal fracture of phalanx of toe (S99.2-)

S92.41 Fracture of proximal phalanx of great toe

S92.411- Displaced fracture of proximal phalanx of right great toe

S92.412- Displaced fracture of proximal phalanx of left great toe

S92.414- Nondisplaced fracture of proximal phalanx of right great toe

S92.415- Nondisplaced fracture of proximal phalanx of left great toe

S92.42 Fracture of distal phalanx of great toe

S92.421- Displaced fracture of distal phalanx of right great toe

S92.422- Displaced fracture of distal phalanx of left great toe

S92.424- Nondisplaced fracture of distal phalanx of right great toe

S92.425- Nondisplaced fracture of distal phalanx of left great toe

S92.49 Other fracture of great toe

S92.491- Other fracture of right great toe

S92.492- Other fracture of left great toe

S92.5 Fracture of lesser toe(s)

Excludes2: physeal fracture of toe (S99.2-)

S92.51 Fracture of proximal phalanx of lesser toe(s)

S92.511- Displaced fracture of proximal phalanx of right lesser toe(s)

S92.512- Displaced fracture of proximal phalanx of left lesser toe(s)

S92.514- Nondisplaced fracture of proximal phalanx of right lesser toe(s)

S92.515- Nondisplaced fracture of proximal phalanx of left lesser toe(s)

S92.52 Fracture of middle phalanx of lesser toe(s)

S92.521- Displaced fracture of middle phalanx of right lesser toe(s)

S92.522- Displaced fracture of middle phalanx of left lesser toe(s)

S92.524- Nondisplaced fracture of middle phalanx of right lesser toe(s)

S92.525- Nondisplaced fracture of middle phalanx of left lesser toe(s)

S92.53 Fracture of distal phalanx of lesser toe(s)

S92.531- Displaced fracture of distal phalanx of right lesser toe(s)

S92.532- Displaced fracture of distal phalanx of left lesser toe(s)

S92.534- Nondisplaced fracture of distal phalanx of right lesser toe(s)

S92.535- Nondisplaced fracture of distal phalanx of left lesser toe(s)

S92.59 Other fracture of lesser toe(s)

S92.591- Other fracture of right lesser toe(s)

S92.592- Other fracture of left lesser toe(s)

S92.8 Other fracture of foot

S92.81 Other fracture of foot

Sesamoid fracture of foot

S92.811- Other fracture of right foot

S92.812- Other fracture of left foot

S92.9 Unspecified fracture of foot and toe

S92.90 Unspecified fracture of foot

S92.901- Unspecified fracture of right foot

S92.902- Unspecified fracture of left foot

S92.91 Unspecified fracture of toe

S92.911- Unspecified fracture of right toe(s)

S92.912- Unspecified fracture of left toe(s)

S93 DISLOCATION AND SPRAIN OF JOINTS AND LIGAMENTS AT ANKLE, FOOT AND TOE LEVEL

Includes: avulsion of joint or ligament of ankle, foot and toe

laceration of cartilage, joint or ligament of ankle, foot and toe

sprain of cartilage, joint or ligament of foot and toe

traumatic hemarthrosis of joint or ligament of ankle, foot and toe

traumatic rupture of joint or ligament of ankle, foot and toe

traumatic subluxation of joint or ligament of ankle, foot and toe

traumatic tear of joint or ligament of ankle, foot and toe

Code also any associated open wound

Excludes2: strain of muscle and tendon of ankle and foot (S96.-)

S93.0 Subluxation and dislocation of ankle joint

Subluxation and dislocation of astragalus

Subluxation and dislocation of fibula, lower end

Subluxation and dislocation of talus or of tibia, lower end

S93.01X- Subluxation of right ankle joint

S93.02X- Subluxation of left ankle joint

S93.04X- Dislocation of right ankle joint

S93.05X- Dislocation of left ankle joint

S93.1 Subluxation and dislocation of toe

S93.10 Unspecified subluxation and dislocation of toe

Dislocation/subluxation of toe NOS

S93.101- Unspecified subluxation of right toe(s)

S93.102- Unspecified subluxation of left toe(s)

S93.104- Unspecified dislocation of right toe(s)

S93.105- Unspecified dislocation of left toe(s)

S93.11 Dislocation of interphalangeal joint

S93.111- Dislocation of interphalangeal joint of right great toe

S93.112- Dislocation of interphalangeal joint of left great toe

S93.114- Dislocation of inter-phalangeal joint of right lesser toe(s)

S93.115- Dislocation of interphalangeal joint of left lesser toe(s)

S93.12 Dislocation of metatarsophalangeal joint

S93.121- Dislocation of metatarsophalangeal joint of right great toe

S93.122- Dislocation of metatarsophalangeal joint of left great toe

S93.124- Dislocation of metatarsophalangeal joint of right lesser toe(s)

S93.125- Dislocation of metatarsophalangeal joint of left lesser toe(s)

S93.13 Subluxation of interphalangeal joint

S93.131- of right great toe

S93.132- of left great toe

S93.134- of right lesser toe(s)

S93.135- of left lesser toe(s)

S93.14 Subluxation of metatarsophalangeal joint

S93.141- of right great toe

S93.142- of left great toe

S93.144- of right lesser toe(s)

S93.145- of left lesser toe(s)

S93.3 Subluxation and dislocation of foot

Excludes2: dislocation of toe (S93.1-)

S93.30 Unspecified subluxation and dislocation of foot

Dislocation of foot NOS

Subluxation of foot NOS

S93.301- Unspecified subluxation of right foot

S93.302- Unspecified subluxation of left foot

S93.304- Unspecified dislocation of right foot

S93.305- Unspecified dislocation of left foot

S93.31 Subluxation and dislocation of tarsal joint

S93.311- Subluxation of tarsal joint of right foot

S93.312- Subluxation of tarsal joint of left foot

S93.314- Dislocation of tarsal joint of right foot

S93.315- Dislocation of tarsal joint of left foot

S93.32 Subluxation and dislocation of tarsometatarsal joint

S93.321- Subluxation of tarsometatarsal joint of right foot

S93.322- Subluxation of tarsometatarsal joint of left foot

S93.324- Dislocation of tarsometatarsal joint of right foot

S93.325- Dislocation of tarsometatarsal joint of left foot

S93.33 Other subluxation and dislocation of foot

S93.331- Other subluxation of right foot

S93.332- Other subluxation of left foot

S93.334- Other dislocation of right foot

S93.335- Other dislocation of left foot

S93.4 Sprain of ankle

Excludes2: injury of Achilles tendon (S86.0-)

S93.40 Sprain of unspecified ligament of ankle
Sprain of ankle NOS
Sprained ankle NOS

S93 requires a 7th character
A—initial encounter
D—subsequent encounter
S—sequela

S93.401- Sprain of unspecified ligament of right ankle
S93.402- Sprain of unspecified ligament of left ankle

S93.41 Sprain of calcaneofibular ligament
S93.411- of right ankle
S93.412- of left ankle

S93.42 Sprain of deltoid ligament
S93.421- of right ankle
S93.422- of left ankle

S93.43 Sprain of tibiofibular ligament
S93.431- of right ankle
S93.432- of left ankle

S93.49 Sprain of other ligament of ankle
Sprain of internal collateral ligament
Sprain of talofibular ligament
S93.491- Sprain of other ligament of right ankle
S93.492- Sprain of other ligament of left ankle

S93.5 Sprain of toe

S93.50 Unspecified sprain of toe
S93.501- Unspecified sprain of right great toe
S93.502- Unspecified sprain of left great toe
S93.504- Unspecified sprain of right lesser toe(s)
S93.505- Unspecified sprain of left lesser toe(s)

S93.51 Sprain of interphalangeal joint of toe
S93.511- Sprain of interphalangeal joint of right great toe
S93.512- Sprain of interphalangeal joint of left great toe
S93.514- Sprain of interphalangeal joint of right lesser toe(s)
S93.515- Sprain of interphalangeal joint of left lesser toe(s)

S93.52 Sprain of metatarsophalangeal joint of toe
S93.521- Sprain of metatarsophalangeal joint of right great toe
S93.522- Sprain of metatarsophalangeal joint of left great toe
S93.524- Sprain of metatarsophalangeal joint of right lesser toe(s)
S93.525- Sprain of metatarsophalangeal joint of left lesser toe(s)

S93.6 Sprain of foot
Excludes2: sprain of metatarsophalangeal joint of toe (S93.52-)
sprain of toe (S93.5-)

S93.60 Unspecified sprain of foot
S93.601- Unspecified sprain of right foot
S93.602- Unspecified sprain of left foot

S93.61 Sprain of tarsal ligament of foot
S93.611- Sprain of tarsal ligament of right foot
S93.612- Sprain of tarsal ligament of left foot

S93.62 Sprain of tarsometatarsal ligament of foot

S93.621- Sprain of tarsometatarsal ligament of right foot
S93.622- Sprain of tarsometatarsal ligament of left foot

S93.69 Other sprain of foot
S93.691- Other sprain of right foot
S93.692- Other sprain of left foot

S96 INJURY OF MUSCLE AND TENDON AT ANKLE AND FOOT LEVEL

S96 requires a 7th character
A—initial encounter
D—subsequent encounter
S—sequela

Code also any associated open wound (S91.-)

Excludes2: injury of Achilles tendon (S86.0-)
sprain of joints and ligaments of ankle and foot (S93.-)

S96.0 Injury of muscle and tendon of long flexor muscle of toe, ankle and foot level

S96.01 Strain of muscle and tendon of long flexor muscle of toe at ankle and foot level,
S96.011- right foot
S96.012- left foot

S96.02 Laceration of muscle and tendon of long flexor muscle of toe at ankle and foot level,
S96.021- right foot
S96.022- left foot

S96.11 Strain of muscle and tendon of long extensor muscle of toe at ankle and foot level,
S96.111- right foot
S96.112- left foot

S96.12 Laceration of muscle and tendon of long extensor muscle of toe at ankle and foot level,
S96.121- right foot
S96.122- left foot

S96.21 Strain of intrinsic muscle and tendon at ankle and foot level,
S96.211- right foot
S96.212- left foot

S96.22 Laceration of intrinsic muscle and tendon at ankle and foot level,
S96.221- right foot
S96.222- left foot

S96.81 Strain of other specified muscles and tendons at ankle and foot level,
S96.811- right foot
S96.812- left foot

S96.91 Strain of unspecified muscle and tendon at ankle and foot level,
S96.911- right foot
S96.912- left foot

S96.92 Laceration of unspecified muscle and tendon at ankle and foot level,
S96.921- right foot
S96.922- left foot

S97 CRUSHING INJURY OF ANKLE AND FOOT

Use additional code(s) for all associated injuries

S97.0 Crushing injury of ankle

S97.01X- Crushing injury of right ankle

S97.02X- Crushing injury of left ankle

S97.1 Crushing injury of toe

S97.10 Crushing injury of unspecified toe(s)

S97.101- Crushing injury of unspecified right toe(s)

S97.102- Crushing injury of unspecified left toe(s)

S97.11 Crushing injury of great toe

S97.111- Crushing injury of right great toe

S97.112- Crushing injury of left great toe

S97.12 Crushing injury of lesser toe(s)

S97.121- Crushing injury of right lesser toe(s)

S97.122- Crushing injury of lesser toe(s)

S97.8 Crushing injury of foot

S97.81X- Crushing injury of right foot

S97.82X- Crushing injury of left foot

S99 OTHER AND UNSPECIFIED INJURIES OF ANKLE AND FOOT

S99.0 Physeal fracture of calcaneus

S99.00 Unspecified physeal fracture

S99.001- of right calcaneus

S99.002- of left calcaneus

S99.01 Salter-Harris Type I physeal fracture

S99.011- of right calcaneus

S99.012- of left calcaneus

S99.02 Salter-Harris Type II physeal fracture

S99.021- of right calcaneus

S99.022- of left calcaneus

S99.03 Salter-Harris Type III physeal fracture

S99.031- of right calcaneus

S99.032- of left calcaneus

S99.04 Salter-Harris Type IV physeal fracture

S99.041- of right calcaneus

S99.042- of left calcaneus

S99.09 Other physeal fracture

S99.091- of right calcaneus

S99.092- of left calcaneus

S99.1 Physeal fracture of right metatarsal

S99.10 Unspecified physeal fracture

S99.101- Unspecified physeal fracture of right metatarsal

S99.102- Unspecified physeal fracture of left metatarsal

S99.11 Salter-Harris Type I physeal fracture of metatarsal

S99.111- Salter-Harris Type I physeal fracture of right metatarsal

S99.112- Salter-Harris Type I physeal fracture of left metatarsal

S99.12 Salter-Harris Type II physeal fracture of metatarsal

S99.121- Salter-Harris Type II physeal fracture of right metatarsal

S99.122- Salter-Harris Type II physeal fracture of left metatarsal

S99.13 Salter-Harris Type III physeal fracture of metatarsal

S99.131- Salter-Harris Type III physeal fracture of right metatarsal

S99.132- Salter-Harris Type III physeal fracture of left metatarsal

S99.14 Salter-Harris Type IV physeal fracture of metatarsal

S99.141- Salter-Harris Type IV physeal fracture of right metatarsal

S99.142- Salter-Harris Type IV physeal fracture of left metatarsal

S99.19 Other physeal fracture of metatarsal

S99.191- Other physeal fracture of right metatarsal

S99.192- Other physeal fracture of left metatarsal

S99.2 Physeal fracture of phalanx of toe

S99.20 Unspecified physeal fracture of phalanx of toe

S99.201- Unspecified physeal fracture of phalanx of right toe

S99.202- Unspecified physeal fracture of phalanx of left toe

S99.21 Salter-Harris Type I physeal fracture of phalanx of toe

S99.211- Salter-Harris Type I physeal fracture of phalanx of right toe

S99.212- Salter-Harris Type I physeal fracture of phalanx of left toe

S99.22 Salter-Harris Type II physeal fracture of phalanx of toe

S99.221- Salter-Harris Type II physeal fracture of phalanx of right toe

S99.222- Salter-Harris Type II physeal fracture of phalanx of left toe

S99.23 Salter-Harris Type III physeal fracture of phalanx of toe

S99.231- Salter-Harris Type III physeal fracture of phalanx of right toe

S99.232- Salter-Harris Type III physeal fracture of phalanx of left toe

S99.24 Salter-Harris Type IV physeal fracture of phalanx of toe

S99.241- Salter-Harris Type IV physeal fracture of phalanx of right toe

S99.242- Salter-Harris Type IV physeal fracture of phalanx of left toe

S99.29 Other physeal fracture of phalanx of toe

S99.291- Other physeal fracture of phalanx of right toe

S99.292- Other physeal fracture of phalanx of left toe

S99.8 Other specified injuries of ankle and foot

S99.81 Other specified injuries of ankle

S99.811- Other specified injuries of right ankle

S99.812- Other specified injuries of left ankle

S99.82 Other specified injuries of foot

S99.821- Other specified injuries of right foot

S99.822- Other specified injuries of left foot

S99.9 Unspecified injury of ankle and foot

S99.91 Unspecified injury of ankle

S99.911- Unspecified injury of right ankle

S99.912- Unspecified injury of left ankle

S99.92 Unspecified injury of foot

S99.921- Unspecified injury of right foot

S99.922- Unspecified injury of left foot

S99.8- and S99.9- require a 7th character
A—initial encounter
D—subsequent encounter
S—sequela

(T07–T88) INJURY, POISONING AND CERTAIN OTHER CONSEQUENCES OF EXTERNAL CAUSES

(T07) INJURIES INVOLVING MULTIPLE BODY REGIONS

Excludes1: burns and corrosions (T20–T32)
frostbite (T33–T34)
insect bite or sting, venomous (T63.4)
sunburn (L55.-)

T07.XXX- UNSPECIFIED MULTIPLE INJURIES

Excludes1: injury NOS (T14.90)

T07 requires a 7th character
A—initial encounter
D—subsequent encounter
S—sequela

(T14) INJURY OF UNSPECIFIED BODY REGION

T14 INJURY OF UNSPECIFIED BODY REGION

Excludes1: multiple unspecified injuries (T07)

T14.8XX- Other injury of unspecified body region

Abrasion NOS
Contusion NOS
Crush injury NOS
Fracture NOS
Skin injury NOS
Vascular injury NOS
Wound NOS

T14.9 Unspecified injury

T14.90X- Injury, unspecified

Injury NOS

T14.91X- Suicide attempt

Attempted suicide NOS

T14 requires a 7th character-
A—initial encounter
D—subsequent encounter
S—sequela

(T15–T19) EFFECTS OF FB ENTERING THROUGH NATURAL ORIFICE

Excludes2: FB accidentally left in operation wound (T81.5-)
FB in penetrating wound—See open wound by body region
residual FB in soft tissue (M79.5)
splinter, without open wound—See superficial injury by body region

T15 FB ON EXTERNAL EYE

Excludes2: FB in penetrating wound of orbit and eye ball (S05.4-, S05.5-)
open wound of eyelid and periocular area (S01.1-)
retained FB in eyelid (H02.8-)
retained (old) FB in penetrating wound of orbit and eye ball (H05.5-, H44.6-, H44.7-)
superficial FB of eyelid and periocular area (S00.25-)

T15 requires a 7th character
A—initial encounter
D—subsequent encounter
S—sequela

T15.0 FB in cornea,

T15.01X- right eye

T15.02X- left eye

T15.1 FB in conjunctival sac,

T15.11X- right eye

T15.12X- left eye

T16 FB IN EAR

Includes: FB in auditory canal

T16.1XX- FB in right ear

T16.2XX- FB in left ear

T16 requires a 7th character
A—initial encounter
D—subsequent encounter
S—sequela

T17 FB IN RESPIRATORY TRACT

T17.0XX- FB in nasal sinus

T17.1XX- FB in nostril

FB in nose NOS

T17.2 FB in pharynx

FB in nasopharynx
FB in throat NOS

T17.20 Unspecified FB in pharynx

T17.200- causing asphyxiation

T17.208- causing other injury

T17.21 Gastric contents in pharynx

Aspiration of gastric contents into pharynx
Vomitus in pharynx

T17.210- causing asphyxiation

T17.218- causing other injury

T17.22 Food in pharynx

Bones in pharynx
Seeds in pharynx

T17.220- causing asphyxiation

T17.228- causing other injury

T17.29 Other foreign object in pharynx

T17.290- causing asphyxiation

T17.298- causing other injury

T17.3 FB in larynx

T17.30 Unspecified FB in larynx

T17.300- causing asphyxiation

T17.308- causing other injury

T17.31 Gastric contents in larynx

Aspiration of gastric contents into larynx
Vomitus in larynx

T17.310- causing asphyxiation

T17.318- causing other injury

T17.32 Food in larynx

Bones in larynx
Seeds in larynx

T17.320- causing asphyxiation

T17.328- causing other injury

T17.39 Other foreign object in larynx

T17.390- causing asphyxiation

T17.398- causing other injury

T17.8 Foreign body in other parts of respiratory tract

Foreign body in bronchioles
Foreign body in lung

T17.80 Unspecified foreign body in other parts of respiratory tract

T17 requires a 7th character
A—initial encounter
D—subsequent encounter
S—sequela

T17.800 Unspecified foreign body in other parts of respiratory tract causing asphyxiation

T17.808 Unspecified foreign body in other parts of respiratory tract causing other injury

T17.9 FB in respiratory tract, part unspecified

T17.90 Unspecified FB in respiratory tract, part unspecified

T17.900- causing asphyxiation

T17.908- causing other injury

T17.91 Gastric contents in respiratory tract, part unspecified

Aspiration of gastric contents into respiratory tract, part unspecified

Vomitus in trachea respiratory tract, part unspecified

T17.910- causing asphyxiation

T17.918- causing other injury

T17.92 Food in respiratory tract, part unspecified

Bones in respiratory tract, part unspecified

Seeds in respiratory tract, part unspecified

T17.920- causing asphyxiation

T17.928- causing other injury

T17.99 Other foreign object in respiratory tract, part unspecified

T17.990- causing asphyxiation

T17.998- causing other injury

T17 requires a 7th character
A—initial encounter
D—subsequent encounter
S—sequela

T18 FB IN ALIMENTARY TRACT

Excludes2: FB in pharynx (T17.2-)

T18.0XX- Foreign body in mouth

T18 requires a 7th character
A—initial encounter
D—subsequent encounter
S—sequela

T18.1 FB in esophagus

Excludes2: FB in respiratory tract (T17.-)

T18.10 Unspecified FB in esophagus

T18.100- causing compression of trachea

Unspecified FB in esophagus causing obstruction of respiration

T18.108- causing other injury

T18.11 Gastric contents in esophagus

Vomitus in esophagus

T18.110- causing compression of trachea

Gastric contents in esophagus causing obstruction of respiration

T18.118- causing other injury

T18.12 Food in esophagus

Bones in esophagus

Seeds in esophagus

T18.120- causing compression of trachea

T18.128- causing other injury

T18.19 Other foreign object in esophagus

T18.190- causing compression of trachea

Other FB in esophagus causing obstruction of respiration

T18.198- causing other injury

T18.2XX- FB in stomach

T18.3XX- FB in small intestine

T18.4XX- FB in colon

T18.5XX- FB in anus and rectum

FB in rectosigmoid (junction)

T18.8XX- FB in other parts of alimentary tract

T18.9XX- FB of alimentary tract, part unspecified

FB in digestive system NOS

Swallowed FB NOS

T19 FB IN GENITOURINARY TRACT

Excludes2: complications due to implanted mesh (T83.7-) mechanical complications of contraceptive device (intrauterine) (vaginal) (T83.3-) presence of contraceptive device (intrauterine) (vaginal) (Z97.5)

T19 requires a 7th character
A—initial encounter
D—subsequent encounter
S—sequela

T19.0XX- FB in urethra

T19.2XX- FB in vulva and vagina

T19.4XX- FB in penis

T19.8XX- FB in other parts of genitourinary tract

T19.9XX- FB in genitourinary tract, part unspecified

(T20–T32) BURNS AND CORROSIONS

GUIDELINES

The *ICD-10-CM* makes a distinction between burns and corrosions. The burn codes are for thermal burns, except sunburns, that come from a heat source, such as a fire or hot appliance. The burn codes are also for burns resulting from electricity and radiation. Corrosions are burns due to chemicals. The guidelines are the same for burns and corrosions.

Current burns (T20–T25) are classified by depth, extent and by agent (X code). Burns are classified by depth as first degree (erythema), second degree (blistering), and third degree (full-thickness involvement). Burns of the eye and internal organs (T26–T28) are classified by site, but not by degree.

Sequencing of burn and related condition codes

Sequence first the code that reflects the highest degree of burn when more than one burn is present.

When the reason for the admission or encounter is for treatment of external multiple burns, sequence first the code that reflects the burn of the highest degree.

When a patient has both internal and external burns, the circumstances of admission govern the selection of the principal diagnosis or first-listed diagnosis.

When a patient is admitted for burn injuries and other related conditions such as smoke inhalation and/or respiratory failure, the circumstances of admission govern the selection of the principal or first-listed diagnosis.

Burns of the same anatomic site

Classify burns of the same anatomic site and on the same side but of different degrees to the subcategory identifying the highest degree recorded in the diagnosis (eg, for second and third degree burns of right thigh, assign only code T24.311-).

Non-healing burns

Non-healing burns are coded as acute burns.
Necrosis of burned skin should be coded as a non-healed burn.

Infected burn

For any documented infected burn site, use an additional code for the infection.

Assign separate codes for each burn site

When coding burns, assign separate codes for each burn site. Category T30, Burn and corrosion, body region unspecified is extremely vague and should rarely be used.

Codes for burns of "multiple sites" should only be assigned when the medical record documentation does not specify the individual sites.

Burns and corrosions classified according to extent of body surface involved

See category T31.

Encounters for treatment of sequela of burns

Encounters for the treatment of the late effects of burns or corrosions (ie, scars or joint contractures) should be coded with a burn or corrosion code with the 7th character S for sequela.

Sequela with a late effect code and current burn

When appropriate, both a code for a current burn or corrosion with 7th character A or D and a burn or corrosion code with 7th character S may be assigned on the same record (when both a current burn and sequela of an old burn exist). Burns and corrosions do not heal at the same rate and a current healing wound may still exist with sequela of a healed burn or corrosion.

See Section I.B.10. Sequela (Late Effects)

Use of an external cause code with burns and corrosions

An external cause code should be used with burns and corrosions to identify the source and intent of the burn, as well as the place where it occurred.

Includes: burns (thermal) from electrical heating appliances
burns (thermal) from electricity
burns (thermal) from flame
burns (thermal) from friction
burns (thermal) from hot air and hot gases
burns (thermal) from hot objects
burns (thermal) from lightning
burns (thermal) from radiation
chemical burn [corrosion] (external) (internal)
scalds

Excludes2: erythema [dermatitis] ab igne (L59.0)
radiation-related disorders of the skin and subcutaneous tissue (L55–L59)
sunburn (L55.-)

(T20–T25) BURNS AND CORROSIONS OF EXTERNAL BODY SURFACE, SPECIFIED BY SITE

Includes: burns and corrosions of first degree [erythema]
burns and corrosions of second degree [blisters] [epidermal loss]
burns and corrosions of third degree [deep necrosis of underlying tissue] [full- thickness skin loss]

Use additional code from category T31 or T32 to identify extent of body surface involved

T20 BURN AND CORROSION OF HEAD, FACE, AND NECK

T20 requires a 7th character
A—initial encounter
D—subsequent encounter
S—sequela

Excludes2: burn and corrosion of ear drum (T28.41, T28.91)
burn and corrosion of eye and adnexa (T26.-)
burn and corrosion of mouth and pharynx (T28.0)

T20.0 Burn of unspecified degree of head, face, and neck

Use additional external cause code to identify the source, place and intent of the burn (X00–X19, X75–X77, X96–X98, Y92)

- **T20.00X-** Burn of unspecified degree of head, face, and neck, unspecified site
- **T20.01** Burn of unspecified degree of ear [any part, except ear drum]
  - *Excludes2:* burn of ear drum (T28.41-)
  - **T20.011-** Burn of unspecified degree of right ear [any part, except ear drum]
  - **T20.012-** Burn of unspecified degree of left ear [any part, except ear drum]
- **T20.02X-** Burn of unspecified degree of lip(s)
- **T20.03X-** Burn of unspecified degree of chin
- **T20.04X-** Burn of unspecified degree of nose (septum)
- **T20.05X-** Burn of unspecified degree of scalp [any part]
- **T20.06X-** Burn of unspecified degree of forehead and cheek
- **T20.07X-** Burn of unspecified degree of neck, initial encounter
- **T20.09X-** Burn of unspecified degree of multiple sites of head, face, and neck

T20.1 Burn of first degree of head, face, and neck

Use additional external cause code to identify the source, place and intent of the burn (X00–X19, X75–X77, X96–X98, Y92)

- **T20.10X-** Burn of first degree of head, face, and neck, unspecified site
- **T20.11** Burn of first degree of ear [any part, except ear drum]
  - *Excludes2:* burn of ear drum (T28.41-)
  - **T20.111-** Burn of first degree of right ear [any part, except ear drum]
  - **T20.112-** Burn of first degree of left ear [any part, except ear drum]
- **T20.119-** Burn of first degree of unspecified ear [any part, except ear drum]
- **T20.12X-** Burn of first degree of lip(s)
- **T20.13X-** Burn of first degree of chin
- **T20.14X-** Burn of first degree of nose (septum)
- **T20.15X-** Burn of first degree of scalp [any part]
- **T20.16X-** Burn of first degree of forehead and cheek
- **T20.17X-** Burn of first degree of neck
- **T20.19X-** Burn of first degree of multiple sites of head, face, and neck

T20.2 Burn of second degree of head, face, and neck

Use additional external cause code to identify the source, place and intent of the burn (X00–X19, X75–X77, X96–X98, Y92)

- **T20.20X-** Burn of second degree of head, face, and neck, unspecified site
- **T20.21** Burn of second degree of ear [any part, except ear drum]
  - *Excludes2:* burn of ear drum (T28.41-)
  - **T20.211-** Burn of second degree of right ear [any part, except ear drum]
  - **T20.212-** Burn of second degree of left ear [any part, except ear drum]
  - **T20.219-** Burn of second degree of unspecified ear [any part, except ear drum]
- **T20.22X-** Burn of second degree of lip(s)
- **T20.23X-** Burn of second degree of chin
- **T20.24X-** Burn of second degree of nose (septum)
- **T20.25X-** Burn of second degree of scalp [any part]
- **T20.26X-** Burn of second degree of forehead and cheek
- **T20.27X-** Burn of second degree of neck
- **T20.29X-** Burn of second degree of multiple sites of head, face, and neck

T20.3 Burn of third degree of head, face, and neck

Use additional external cause code to identify the source, place and intent of the burn (X00–X19, X75–X77, X96–X98, Y92)

- **T20.30X-** Burn of third degree of head, face, and neck, unspecified site
- **T20.31** Burn of third degree of ear [any part, except ear drum]
  - *Excludes2:* burn of ear drum (T28.41-)
  - **T20.311-** Burn of third degree of right ear [any part, except ear drum]
  - **T20.312-** Burn of third degree of left ear [any part, except ear drum]

T20.319- Burn of third degree of unspecified ear [any part, except ear drum]

T20.32X- Burn of third degree of lip(s)

T20.33X- Burn of third degree of chin

T20.34X- Burn of third degree of nose (septum)

T20.35X- Burn of third degree of scalp [any part]

T20.36X- Burn of third degree of forehead and cheek

T20.37X- Burn of third degree of neck

T20.39X- Burn of third degree of multiple sites of head, face, and neck

T21 BURN AND CORROSION OF TRUNK

Includes: burns and corrosion of hip region

Excludes2: burns and corrosion of axilla (T22.- with fifth character 4)

burns and corrosion of scapular region (T22.- with fifth character 6)

burns and corrosion of shoulder (T22.- with fifth character 5)

T21.0 Burn of unspecified degree of trunk

Use additional external cause code to identify the source, place and intent of the burn (X00-X19, X75-X77, X96-X98, Y92)

T21.00X- Burn of unspecified degree of trunk, unspecified site

T21.01X- Burn of unspecified degree of chest wall

Burn of unspecified degree of breast

T21.02X- Burn of unspecified degree of abdominal wall

Burn of unspecified degree of flank or of groin

T21.03X- Burn of unspecified degree of upper back

Burn of unspecified degree of interscapular region

T21.04X- Burn of unspecified degree of lower back

T21.05X- Burn of unspecified degree of buttock

Burn of unspecified degree of anus

T21.06X- Burn of unspecified degree of male genital region

Burn of unspecified degree of penis or of scrotum or of testis

T21.07X- Burn of unspecified degree of female genital region

Burn of unspecified degree of labium (majus) (minus) or of perineum

Burn of unspecified degree of vulva

Excludes2: burn of vagina (T28.3)

T21.09X- Burn of unspecified degree of other site of trunk

T21.1 Burn of first degree of trunk

Use additional external cause code to identify the source, place and intent of the burn (X00-X19, X75-X77, X96-X98, Y92)

T21.10X- Burn of first degree of trunk, unspecified site

T21.11X- Burn of first degree of chest wall

Burn of first degree of breast

T21.12X- Burn of first degree of abdominal wall

Burn of first degree of flank or of groin

T21.13X- Burn of first degree of upper back

Burn of first degree of interscapular region

T21.14X- Burn of first degree of lower back

T21.15X- Burn of first degree of buttock

Burn of first degree of anus

T21.16X- Burn of first degree of male genital region

Burn of first degree of penis or of scrotum or of testis

T21.17X- Burn of first degree of female genital region

Burn of first degree of labium (majus) (minus) or of perineum

Burn of first degree of vulva

Excludes2: burn of vagina (T28.3)

T21.19X- Burn of first degree of other site of trunk

T21.2 Burn of second degree of trunk

Use additional external cause code to identify the source, place and intent of the burn (X00-X19, X75-X77, X96-X98, Y92)

T21.20X- Burn of second degree of trunk, unspecified site

T21.21X- Burn of second degree of chest wall

Burn of second degree of breast

T21.22X- Burn of second degree of abdominal wall

Burn of second degree of flank or of groin

T21.23X- Burn of second degree of upper back

Burn of second degree of interscapular region

T21.24X- Burn of second degree of lower back

T21.25X- Burn of second degree of buttock

Burn of second degree of anus

T21.26X- Burn of second degree of male genital region

Burn of second degree of penis or of scrotum or of testis

T21.27X- Burn of second degree of female genital region

Burn of second degree of labium (majus) (minus) or of perineum

Burn of second degree of vulva

Excludes2: burn of vagina (T28.3)

T21.29X- Burn of second degree of other site of trunk

T21.3 Burn of third degree of trunk

Use additional external cause code to identify the source, place and intent of the burn (X00-X19, X75-X77, X96-X98, Y92)

T21.30X- Burn of third degree of trunk, unspecified site

T21.31X- Burn of third degree of chest wall

Burn of third degree of breast

T21.32X- Burn of third degree of abdominal wall

Burn of third degree of flank OR GROIN

T21.33X- Burn of third degree of upper back

Burn of third degree of interscapular region

T21.34X- Burn of third degree of lower back

T21.35X- Burn of third degree of buttock

Burn of third degree of anus

T21.36X- Burn of third degree of male genital region

Burn of third degree of penis or of scrotum or of testis

T21.37X- Burn of third degree of female genital region

Burn of third degree of labium (majus) (minus)

Burn of third degree of perineum

Burn of third degree of vulva

Excludes2: burn of vagina (T28.3)

T21.39X- Burn of third degree of other site of trunk

T22 BURN AND CORROSION OF SHOULDER AND UPPER LIMB, EXCEPT WRIST AND HAND

Excludes2: burn and corrosion of interscapular region (T21.-)

burn and corrosion of wrist and hand (T23.-)

T22.0 Burn of unspecified degree of shoulder and upper limb, except wrist and hand

Use additional external cause code to identify the source, place and intent of the burn (X00-X19, X75-X77, X96-X98, Y92)

T22.00X- Burn of unspecified degree of shoulder and upper limb, except wrist and hand, unspecified site

T22.01 Burn of unspecified degree of forearm

T22.011- Burn of unspecified degree of right forearm

T22.012- Burn of unspecified degree of left forearm

T22.02 Burn of unspecified degree of elbow

T22.021- Burn of unspecified degree of right elbow

T22.022- Burn of unspecified degree of left elbow

T22.03 Burn of unspecified degree of upper arm

T22.031- Burn of unspecified degree of right upper arm

T22.032- Burn of unspecified degree of left upper arm

T22.04 Burn of unspecified degree of axilla

T22.041- Burn of unspecified degree of right axilla

T22.042- Burn of unspecified degree of left axilla

T22.05 Burn of unspecified degree of shoulder

T22.051- Burn of unspecified degree of right shoulder

T22.052- Burn of unspecified degree of left shoulder

T22.06 Burn of unspecified degree of scapular region

T22.061- Burn of unspecified degree of right scapular region

T22.062- Burn of unspecified degree of left scapular region

T22.09 Burn of unspecified degree of multiple sites of shoulder and upper limb, except wrist and hand

T22.091- Burn of unspecified degree of multiple sites of right shoulder and upper limb, except wrist and hand

T22.092- Burn of unspecified degree of multiple sites of left shoulder and upper limb, except wrist and hand

T22.1 Burn of first degree of shoulder and upper limb, except wrist and hand

Use additional external cause code to identify the source, place and intent of the burn (X00-X19, X75-X77, X96-X98, Y92)

T22.10X Burn of first degree of shoulder and upper limb, except wrist and hand, unspecified site

T22.11 Burn of first degree of forearm

T22.111- Burn of first degree of right forearm

T22.112- Burn of first degree of left forearm

T22.12 Burn of first degree of elbow

T22.121- Burn of first degree of right elbow

T22.122- Burn of first degree of left elbow

T22.13 Burn of first degree of upper arm

T22.131- Burn of first degree of right upper arm

T22.132- Burn of first degree of left upper arm

T22.14 Burn of first degree of axilla

T22.141- Burn of first degree of right axilla

T22.142- Burn of first degree of left axilla

T22.15 Burn of first degree of shoulder

T22.151- Burn of first degree of right shoulder

T22.152- Burn of first degree of left shoulder

T22.16 Burn of first degree of scapular region

T22.161- Burn of first degree of right scapular region

T22.162- Burn of first degree of left scapular region

T22.19 Burn of first degree of multiple sites of shoulder and upper limb, except wrist and hand

T22.191- Burn of first degree of multiple sites of right shoulder and upper limb, except wrist and hand

T22.192- Burn of first degree of multiple sites of left shoulder and upper limb, except wrist and hand

T22.199- Burn of first degree of multiple sites of unspecified shoulder and upper limb, except wrist and hand

T22.2 Burn of second degree of shoulder and upper limb, except wrist and hand

Use additional external cause code to identify the source, place and intent of the burn (X00-X19, X75-X77,X96-X98, Y92)

T22.20X- Burn of second degree of shoulder and upper limb, except wrist and hand, unspecified site

T22.21 Burn of second degree of forearm

T22.211- Burn of second degree of right forearm

T22.212- Burn of second degree of left forearm

T22.219- Burn of second degree of unspecified forearm

T22.22 Burn of second degree of elbow

T22.221- Burn of second degree of right elbow

T22.222- Burn of second degree of left elbow

T22.23 Burn of second degree of upper arm

T22.231- Burn of second degree of right upper arm

T22.232- Burn of second degree of left upper arm

T22.24 Burn of second degree of axilla

T22.241- Burn of second degree of right axilla

T22.242- Burn of second degree of left axilla

T22.25 Burn of second degree of shoulder

T22.251- Burn of second degree of right shoulder

T22.252- Burn of second degree of left shoulder

T22.26 Burn of second degree of scapular region

T22.261- Burn of second degree of right scapular region

T22.262- Burn of second degree of left scapular region

T22.29 Burn of second degree of multiple sites of shoulder and upper limb, except wrist and hand

T22.291- Burn of second degree of multiple sites of right shoulder and upper limb, except wrist and hand

T22.292- Burn of second degree of multiple sites of left shoulder and upper limb, except wrist and hand

T22.3 Burn of third degree of shoulder and upper limb, except wrist and hand

Use additional external cause code to identify the source, place and intent of the burn (X00-X19, X75-X77, X96-X98, Y92)

T22.31 Burn of third degree of forearm

T22.311- Burn of third degree of right forearm

T22.312- Burn of third degree of left forearm

T22.319- Burn of third degree of unspecified forearm

T22.32 Burn of third degree of elbow

T22.321- Burn of third degree of right elbow

T22.322- Burn of third degree of left elbow

T22.33 Burn of third degree of upper arm

T22.331- Burn of third degree of right upper arm

T22.332- Burn of third degree of left upper arm

T22.34 Burn of third degree of axilla

T22.341- Burn of third degree of right axilla

T22.342- Burn of third degree of left axilla

T22.35 Burn of third degree of shoulder

T22.351- Burn of third degree of right shoulder

T22.352- Burn of third degree of left shoulder

T22.36 Burn of third degree of scapular region

T22.361- Burn of third degree of right scapular region

T22.362- Burn of third degree of left scapular region

T22.39 Burn of third degree of multiple sites of shoulder and upper limb, except wrist and hand

T22.391- Burn of third degree of multiple sites of right shoulder and upper limb, except wrist and hand

T22.392- Burn of third degree of multiple sites of left shoulder and upper limb, except wrist and hand

T23 BURN AND CORROSION OF WRIST AND HAND

T23.0 Burn of unspecified degree of wrist and hand

Use additional external cause code to identify the source, place and intent of the burn (X00-X19, X75-X77, X96-X98, Y92)

T23.00 Burn of unspecified degree of hand, unspecified site

T23.001- Burn of unspecified degree of right hand, unspecified site

T23.002- Burn of unspecified degree of left hand, unspecified site

T23.009- Burn of unspecified degree of unspecified hand, unspecified site

T23.01 Burn of unspecified degree of thumb (nail)

T23.011- Burn of unspecified degree of right thumb (nail)

T23.012- Burn of unspecified degree of left thumb (nail)

T23.02 Burn of unspecified degree of single finger (nail) except thumb

T23.021- Burn of unspecified degree of single right finger (nail) except thumb

T23.022- Burn of unspecified degree of single left finger (nail) except thumb

T23.03 Burn of unspecified degree of multiple fingers (nail), not including thumb

T23.031- Burn of unspecified degree of multiple right fingers (nail), not including thumb

T23.032- Burn of unspecified degree of multiple left fingers (nail), not including thumb

T23.04 Burn of unspecified degree of multiple fingers (nail), including thumb

T23.041- Burn of unspecified degree of multiple right fingers (nail), including thumb

T23.042- Burn of unspecified degree of multiple left fingers (nail), including thumb

T23.05 Burn of unspecified degree of palm

T23.051- Burn of unspecified degree of right palm

T23.052- Burn of unspecified degree of left palm

T23.06 Burn of unspecified degree of back of hand

T23.061- Burn of unspecified degree of back of right hand

T23.062- Burn of unspecified degree of back of left hand

T23.07 Burn of unspecified degree of wrist

T23.071- Burn of unspecified degree of right wrist

T23.072- Burn of unspecified degree of left wrist

T23.09 Burn of unspecified degree of multiple sites of wrist and hand

T23.091- Burn of unspecified degree of multiple sites of right wrist and hand

T23.092- Burn of unspecified degree of multiple sites of left wrist and hand

T23.1 Burn of first degree of wrist and hand

Use additional external cause code to identify the source, place and intent of the burn (X00-X19, X75-X77, X96-X98, Y92)

T23.10 Burn of first degree of hand, unspecified site

T23.101- Burn of first degree of right hand, unspecified site

T23.102- Burn of first degree of left hand, unspecified site

T23.11 Burn of first degree of thumb (nail)

T23.111- Burn of first degree of right thumb (nail)

T23.112- Burn of first degree of left thumb (nail)

T23.12 Burn of first degree of single finger (nail) except thumb

T23.121- Burn of first degree of single right finger (nail) except thumb

T23.122- Burn of first degree of single left finger (nail) except thumb

T23.13 Burn of first degree of multiple fingers (nail), not including thumb

T23.131- Burn of first degree of multiple right fingers (nail), not including thumb

T23.132- Burn of first degree of multiple left fingers (nail), not including thumb

T23.14 Burn of first degree of multiple fingers (nail), including thumb

T23.141- Burn of first degree of multiple right fingers (nail), including thumb

T23.142- Burn of first degree of multiple left fingers (nail), including thumb

T23.15 Burn of first degree of palm

T23.151- Burn of first degree of right palm

T23.152- Burn of first degree of left palm

T23.16 Burn of first degree of back of hand

T23.161- Burn of first degree of back of right hand

T23.162- Burn of first degree of back of left hand

T23.17 Burn of first degree of wrist

T23.171- Burn of first degree of right wrist

T23.172- Burn of first degree of left wrist

T23.19 Burn of first degree of multiple sites of wrist and hand

T23.191- Burn of first degree of multiple sites of right wrist and hand

T23.192- Burn of first degree of multiple sites of left wrist and hand

T23.2 Burn of second degree of wrist and hand

Use additional external cause code to identify the source, place and intent of the burn (X00-X19, X75-X77, X96-X98, Y92)

T23.20 Burn of second degree of hand, unspecified site

T23.201- Burn of second degree of right hand, unspecified site

T23.202- Burn of second degree of left hand, unspecified site

T23.21 Burn of second degree of thumb (nail)

T23.211- Burn of second degree of right thumb (nail)

T23.212- Burn of second degree of left thumb (nail)

T23.22 Burn of second degree of single finger (nail) except thumb

T23.221- Burn of second degree of single right finger (nail) except thumb

T23.222- Burn of second degree of single left finger (nail) except thumb

T23.23 Burn of second degree of multiple fingers (nail), not including thumb

T23.231- Burn of second degree of multiple right fingers (nail), not including thumb

T23.232- Burn of second degree of multiple left fingers (nail), not including thumb

T23.24 Burn of second degree of multiple fingers (nail), including thumb

T23.241- Burn of second degree of multiple right fingers (nail), including thumb

T23.242- Burn of second degree of multiple left fingers (nail), including thumb

T23.25 Burn of second degree of palm

T23.251- Burn of second degree of right palm

T23.252- Burn of second degree of left palm

T23.26 Burn of second degree of back of hand

T23.261- Burn of second degree of back of right hand

T23.262- Burn of second degree of back of left hand

T23.27 Burn of second degree of wrist

T23.271- Burn of second degree of right wrist

T23.272- Burn of second degree of left wrist

T23.29 Burn of second degree of multiple sites of wrist and hand

T23.291- Burn of second degree of multiple sites of right wrist and hand

T23.292- Burn of second degree of multiple sites of left wrist and hand

T23.3 Burn of third degree of wrist and hand

Use additional external cause code to identify the source, place and intent of the burn (X00-X19, X75-X77, X96-X98, Y92)

T23.30 Burn of third degree of hand, unspecified site

T23.301- Burn of third degree of right hand, unspecified site

T23.302- Burn of third degree of left hand, unspecified site

T23.31 Burn of third degree of thumb (nail)

T23.311- Burn of third degree of right thumb (nail)

T23.312- Burn of third degree of left thumb (nail)

T23.32 Burn of third degree of single finger (nail) except thumb

T23.321- Burn of third degree of single right finger (nail) except thumb

T23.322- Burn of third degree of single left finger (nail) except thumb

T23.33 Burn of third degree of multiple fingers (nail), not including thumb

T23.331- Burn of third degree of multiple right fingers (nail), not including thumb

T23.332- Burn of third degree of multiple left fingers (nail), not including thumb

T23.34 Burn of third degree of multiple fingers (nail), including thumb

T23.341- Burn of third degree of multiple right fingers (nail), including thumb

T23.342- Burn of third degree of multiple left fingers (nail), including thumb

T23.35 Burn of third degree of palm

T23.351- Burn of third degree of right palm

T23.352- Burn of third degree of left palm

T23.36 Burn of third degree of back of hand

T23.361- Burn of third degree of back of right hand

T23.362- Burn of third degree of back of left hand

T23.37 Burn of third degree of wrist

T23.371- Burn of third degree of right wrist

T23.372- Burn of third degree of left wrist

T23.39 Burn of third degree of multiple sites of wrist and hand

T23.391- Burn of third degree of multiple sites of right wrist and hand

T23.392- Burn of third degree of multiple sites of left wrist and hand

T24 BURN AND CORROSION OF LOWER LIMB, EXCEPT ANKLE AND FOOT

Excludes2: burn and corrosion of ankle and foot (T25.-)

burn and corrosion of hip region (T21.-)

T24.0 Burn of unspecified degree of lower limb, except ankle and foot

Use additional external cause code to identify the source, place and intent of the burn (X00-X19, X75-X77, X96-X98, Y92)

T24.00 Burn of unspecified degree of unspecified site of lower limb, except ankle and foot

T24.001- Burn of unspecified degree of unspecified site of right lower limb, except ankle and foot

T24.002- Burn of unspecified degree of unspecified site of left lower limb, except ankle and foot

T24.01 Burn of unspecified degree of thigh

T24.011- Burn of unspecified degree of right thigh

T24.012- Burn of unspecified degree of left thigh

T24.02 Burn of unspecified degree of knee

T24.021- Burn of unspecified degree of right knee

T24.022- Burn of unspecified degree of left knee

T24.03 Burn of unspecified degree of lower leg

T24.031- Burn of unspecified degree of right lower leg

T24.032- Burn of unspecified degree of left lower leg

T24.09 Burn of unspecified degree of multiple sites of lower limb, except ankle and foot

T24.091- Burn of unspecified degree of multiple sites of right lower limb, except ankle and foot

T24.092- Burn of unspecified degree of multiple sites of left lower limb, except ankle and foot

T24.1 Burn of first degree of lower limb, except ankle and foot

Use additional external cause code to identify the source, place and intent of the burn (X00-X19, X75-X77, X96-X98, Y92)

T24.10 Burn of first degree of unspecified site of lower limb, except ankle and foot

T24.101- Burn of first degree of unspecified site of right lower limb, except ankle and foot

T24.102- Burn of first degree of unspecified site of left lower limb, except ankle and foot

T24.11 Burn of first degree of thigh

T24.111- Burn of first degree of right thigh

T24.112- Burn of first degree of left thigh

T24.12 Burn of first degree of knee

T24.121- Burn of first degree of right knee

T24.122- Burn of first degree of left knee

T24.13 Burn of first degree of lower leg

T24.131- Burn of first degree of right lower leg

T24.132- Burn of first degree of left lower leg

T24.19 Burn of first degree of multiple sites of lower limb, except ankle and foot

T24.191- Burn of first degree of multiple sites of right lower limb, except ankle and foot

T24.192- Burn of first degree of multiple sites of left lower limb, except ankle and foot

T24.2 Burn of second degree of lower limb, except ankle and foot

Use additional external cause code to identify the source, place and intent of the burn (X00-X19, X75-X77, X96-X98, Y92)

T24.20 Burn of second degree of unspecified site of lower limb, except ankle and foot

T24.201- Burn of second degree of unspecified site of right lower limb, except ankle and foot

T24.202- Burn of second degree of unspecified site of left lower limb, except ankle and foot

T24.21 Burn of second degree of thigh

T24.211- Burn of second degree of right thigh

T24.212- Burn of second degree of left thigh

T24.22 Burn of second degree of knee

T24.221- Burn of second degree of right knee

T24.222- Burn of second degree of left knee

T24.23 Burn of second degree of lower leg

T24.231- Burn of second degree of right lower leg

T24.232- Burn of second degree of left lower leg

T24.29 Burn of second degree of multiple sites of lower limb, except ankle and foot

T24.291- Burn of second degree of multiple sites of right lower limb, except ankle and foot

T24.292- Burn of second degree of multiple sites of left lower limb, except ankle and foot

T24.3 Burn of third degree of lower limb, except ankle and foot

Use additional external cause code to identify the source, place and intent of the burn (X00-X19, X75-X77, X96-X98, Y92)

T24.30 Burn of third degree of unspecified site of lower limb, except ankle and foot

T24.301- Burn of third degree of unspecified site of right lower limb, except ankle and foot

T24.302- Burn of third degree of unspecified site of left lower limb, except ankle and foot

T24.31 Burn of third degree of thigh

T24.311- Burn of third degree of right thigh

T24.312- Burn of third degree of left thigh

T24.32 Burn of third degree of knee

T24.321- Burn of third degree of right knee

T24.322- Burn of third degree of left knee

T24.33 Burn of third degree of lower leg

T24.331- Burn of third degree of right lower leg

T24.332- Burn of third degree of left lower leg

T24.39 Burn of third degree of multiple sites of lower limb, except ankle and foot

T24.391- Burn of third degree of multiple sites of right lower limb, except ankle and foot

T24.392- Burn of third degree of multiple sites of left lower limb, except ankle and foot

T25 BURN AND CORROSION OF ANKLE AND FOOT

T25.0 Burn of unspecified degree of ankle and foot

Use additional external cause code to identify the source, place and intent of the burn (X00-X19, X75-X77, X96-X98, Y92)

T25.01 Burn of unspecified degree of ankle

T25.011- Burn of unspecified degree of right ankle

T25.012- Burn of unspecified degree of left ankle

T25.02 Burn of unspecified degree of foot

Excludes2: burn of unspecified degree of toe(s) (nail) (T25.03-)

T25.021- Burn of unspecified degree of right foot

T25.022- Burn of unspecified degree of left foot

T25.03 Burn of unspecified degree of toe(s) (nail)

T25.031- Burn of unspecified degree of right toe(s) (nail)

T25.032- Burn of unspecified degree of left toe(s) (nail)

T25.09 Burn of unspecified degree of multiple sites of ankle and foot

T25.091- Burn of unspecified degree of multiple sites of right ankle and foot

T25.092- Burn of unspecified degree of multiple sites of left ankle and foot

T25.1 Burn of first degree of ankle and foot

Use additional external cause code to identify the source, place and intent of the burn (X00-X19, X75-X77, X96-X98, Y92)

T25.11 Burn of first degree of ankle

T25.111- Burn of first degree of right ankle

T25.112- Burn of first degree of left ankle

T25.12 Burn of first degree of foot

Excludes2: burn of first degree of toe(s) (nail) (T25.13-)

T25.121- Burn of first degree of right foot

T25.122- Burn of first degree of left foot

T25.13 Burn of first degree of toe(s) (nail)

T25.131- Burn of first degree of right toe(s) (nail)

T25.132- Burn of first degree of left toe(s) (nail)

T25.19 Burn of first degree of multiple sites of ankle and foot

T25.191- Burn of first degree of multiple sites of right ankle and foot

T25.192- Burn of first degree of multiple sites of left ankle and foot

T25.2 Burn of second degree of ankle and foot

Use additional external cause code to identify the source, place and intent of the burn (X00-X19, X75-X77, X96-X98, Y92)

T25.21 Burn of second degree of ankle

T25.211- Burn of second degree of right ankle

T25.212- Burn of second degree of left ankle

T25.22 Burn of second degree of foot

Excludes2: burn of second degree of toe(s) (nail) (T25.23-)

T25.221- Burn of second degree of right foot

T25.222- Burn of second degree of left foot

T25.23 Burn of second degree of toe(s) (nail)

T25.231- Burn of second degree of right toe(s) (nail)

T25.232- Burn of second degree of left toe(s) (nail)

T25.29 Burn of second degree of multiple sites of ankle and foot

T25 requires a 7th character
A—initial encounter
D—subsequent encounter
S—sequela

T25.291- Burn of second degree of multiple sites of right ankle and foot

T25.292- Burn of second degree of multiple sites of left ankle and foot

T25.3 Burn of third degree of ankle and foot

Use additional external cause code to identify the source, place and intent of the burn (X00-X19, X75-X77, X96-X98, Y92)

T25.31 Burn of third degree of ankle

T25.311- Burn of third degree of right ankle

T25.312- Burn of third degree of left ankle

T25.32 Burn of third degree of foot

Excludes2: burn of third degree of toe(s) (nail) (T25.33-)

T25.321- Burn of third degree of right foot

T25.322- Burn of third degree of left foot

T25.33 Burn of third degree of toe(s) (nail)

T25.331- Burn of third degree of right toe(s) (nail)

T25.332- Burn of third degree of left toe(s) (nail)

T25.39 Burn of third degree of multiple sites of ankle and foot

T25.391- Burn of third degree of multiple sites of right ankle and foot

T25.392- Burn of third degree of multiple sites of left ankle and foot

(T26-T28) BURNS AND CORROSIONS CONFINED TO EYE AND INTERNAL ORGANS

T26 BURN AND CORROSION CONFINED TO EYE AND ADNEXA

T26 requires a 7th character
A—initial encounter
D—subsequent encounter
S—sequela

T26.0 Burn of eyelid and periocular area

Use additional external cause code to identify the source, place and intent of the burn (X00-X19, X75-X77, X96-X98, Y92)

T26.01X- Burn of right eyelid and periocular area

T26.02X- Burn of left eyelid and periocular area

T28 BURN AND CORROSION OF OTHER INTERNAL ORGANS

T28 requires a 7th character
A—initial encounter
D—subsequent encounter
S—sequela

Use additional external cause code to identify the source and intent of the burn (X00-X19, X75-X77, X96-X98) and external cause code to identify place (Y92)

T28.0XX- Burn of mouth and pharynx

T28.1XX- Burn of esophagus

(T30-T32) BURNS AND CORROSIONS OF MULTIPLE AND UNSPECIFIED BODY REGIONS

T30 BURN AND CORROSION, BODY REGION UNSPECIFIED

T30.0 Burn of unspecified body region, unspecified degree

This code is not for inpatient use. Code to specified site and degree of burns
Burn NOS
Multiple burns NOS

Note: No 7th characters are required for categories T30, T31, and T32.

T30.4 Corrosion of unspecified body region, unspecified degree

This code is not for inpatient use. Code to specified site and degree of corrosion
Corrosion NOS
Multiple corrosion NOS

T31 BURNS CLASSIFIED ACCORDING TO EXTENT OF BODY SURFACE INVOLVED

GUIDELINES

Assign codes from category T31, Burns classified according to extent of body surface involved, or T32, Corrosions classified according to extent of body surface involved, for acute burns or corrosions when the site of the burn or corrosion is not specified or when there is a need for additional data. It is advisable to use category T31 as additional coding when needed to provide data for evaluating burn mortality, such as that needed by burn units. It is also advisable to use category T31 as an additional code for reporting purposes when there is mention of a third-degree burn involving 20 percent or more of the body surface. Codes from categories T31 and T32 should not be used for sequelae of burns or corrosions. Categories T31 and T32 are based on the classic "rule of nines" in estimating body surface involved: head and neck are assigned nine percent, each arm nine percent, each leg 18 percent, the anterior trunk 18 percent, posterior trunk 18 percent, and genitalia one percent. Providers may change these percentage assignments where necessary to accommodate infants and children who have proportionately larger heads than adults, and patients who have large buttocks, thighs, or abdomen that involve burns.

Note: This category is to be used as the primary code only when the site of the burn is unspecified. It should be used as a supplementary code with categories T20 – T25 when the site is specified.

Please see full *ICD-10-CM* manual if reporting burns classified according to extent of body surface beyond 10% of body surface.

T31.0 Burns involving less than 10% of body surface

T31.1 Burns involving 10-19% of body surface

T31.10 with 0% to 9% third degree burns

Burns involving 10-19% of body surface NOS

T31.11 with 10-19% third degree burns

T32 CORROSIONS CLASSIFIED ACCORDING TO EXTENT OF BODY SURFACE INVOLVED

Note: This category is to be used as the primary code only when the site of the corrosion is unspecified. It may be used as a supplementary code with categories T20-T25 when the site is specified.

T32.0 Corrosions involving less than 10% of body surface

T32.1 Corrosions involving 10-19% of body surface

T32.10 with 0% to 9% third degree corrosion

Corrosions involving 10-19% of body surface NOS

T32.11 with 10-19% third degree corrosion

(T36-T50) POISONING BY, ADVERSE EFFECTS OF AND UNDERDOSING OF DRUGS, MEDICAMENTS AND BIOLOGICAL SUBSTANCES

GUIDELINES

Codes in categories T36-T65 are combination codes that include the substance that was taken as well as the intent. No additional external cause code is required for poisonings, toxic effects, adverse effects and underdosing codes.

Do not code directly from the Table of Drugs

Do not code directly from the Table of Drugs and Chemicals. Always refer back to the Tabular List. *Refer to the ICD-10-CM manual for the Table of Drugs.*

Use as many codes as necessary to describe

Use as many codes as necessary to describe completely all drugs, medicinal or biological substances.

If the same code would describe the causative agent

If the same code would describe the causative agent for more than one adverse reaction, poisoning, toxic effect or underdosing, assign the code only once.

If two or more drugs, medicinal or biological substances

If two or more drugs, medicinal or biological substances are taken, code each individually unless a combination code is listed in the Table of Drugs and Chemicals. If multiple unspecified drugs, medicinal or biological substances were taken, assign the appropriate code from subcategory T50.91, Poisoning by, adverse effect of and underdosing of multiple unspecified drugs, medicaments and biological substances.

The occurrence of drug toxicity is classified in *ICD-10-CM* as follows:

ADVERSE EFFECT

When coding an adverse effect of a drug that has been correctly prescribed and properly administered, assign the appropriate code for the nature of the adverse effect followed by the appropriate code for the adverse effect of the drug (T36–T50). The code for the drug should have a 5th or 6th character "5" (for example T36.0X5-). Examples of the nature of an adverse effect are tachycardia, delirium, gastrointestinal hemorrhaging, vomiting, hypokalemia, hepatitis, renal failure, or respiratory failure.

POISONING

When coding a poisoning or reaction to the improper use of a medication (eg, overdose, wrong substance given or taken in error, wrong route of administration), first assign the appropriate code from categories T36–T50. The poisoning codes have an associated intent as their 5th or 6th character (accidental, intentional self-harm, assault and undetermined). If the intent of the poisoning is unknown or unspecified, code the intent as accidental intent. The undetermined intent is only for use if the documentation in the record specifies that the intent cannot be determined. Use additional code(s) for all manifestations of poisonings.

If there is also a diagnosis of abuse or dependence of the substance, the abuse or dependence is assigned as an additional code.

Examples of poisoning include:

Error was made in drug prescription
Errors made in drug prescription or in the administration of the drug by provider, nurse, patient, or other person.

Overdose of a drug intentionally taken
If an overdose of a drug was intentionally taken or administered and resulted in drug toxicity, it would be coded as a poisoning.

Nonprescribed drug taken with correctly prescribed and properly administered drug
If a nonprescribed drug or medicinal agent was taken in combination with a correctly prescribed and properly administered drug, any drug toxicity or other reaction resulting from the interaction of the two drugs would be classified as a poisoning.

Interaction of drug(s) and alcohol
When a reaction results from the interaction of a drug(s) and alcohol, this would be classified as poisoning.

See Chapter 4 if poisoning is the result of insulin pump malfunctions.

UNDERDOSING

Underdosing refers to taking less of a medication than is prescribed by a provider or a manufacturer's instruction. Discontinuing the use of a prescribed medication on the patient's own initiative (not directed by the patient's provider) is also classified as an underdosing. For underdosing, assign the code from categories

T36–T50 (fifth or sixth character "6"). Documentation of a change in the patient's condition is not required in order to assign an underdosing code. Documentation that the patient is taking less of a medication than is prescribed or discontinued the prescribed medication is sufficient for code assignment.

Codes for underdosing should never be assigned as principal or first-listed codes. If a patient has a relapse or exacerbation of the medical condition for which the drug is prescribed because of the reduction in dose, then the medical condition itself should be coded.

Noncompliance (Z91.12-, Z91.13-, Z91.14- and Z91.A4-) or complication of care (Y63.6–Y63.9) codes are to be used with an underdosing code to indicate intent, if known.

Toxic Effects

When a harmful substance is ingested or comes in contact with a person, this is classified as a toxic effect. The toxic effect codes are in categories T51–T65.

Toxic effect codes have an associated intent: accidental, intentional self-harm, assault and undetermined.

Includes: adverse effect of correct substance properly administered
poisoning by overdose of substance
poisoning by wrong substance given or taken in error
underdosing by (inadvertently) (deliberately) taking less substance than prescribed or instructed

Code first, for adverse effects, the nature of the adverse effect, such as:
adverse effect NOS (T88.7)
aspirin gastritis (K29.-)
blood disorders (D56–D76)
contact dermatitis (L23–L25)
dermatitis due to substances taken internally (L27.-)
nephropathy (N14.0–N14.2)

Note: The drug giving rise to the adverse effect should be identified by use of codes from categories T36–T50 with fifth or sixth character 5.

Use additional code(s) to specify: manifestations of poisoning underdosing or failure in dosage during medical and surgical care (Y63.6, Y63.8–Y63.9)
underdosing of medication regimen (Z91.12-, Z91.13-)

Excludes1: toxic reaction to local anesthesia in pregnancy (O29.3-)

Excludes2: abuse and dependence of psychoactive substances (F10–F19)
abuse of non-dependence-producing substances (F55.-)
drug reaction and poisoning affecting newborn (P00–P96)
immunodeficiency due to drugs (D84.821)
pathological drug intoxication (inebriation) (F10–F19)

		6th characters for categories T36–T50
T36	**POISONING BY, ADVERSE EFFECT OF AND UNDERDOSING OF SYSTEMIC ANTIBIOTICS**	1—accidental (unintentional), NOS
	Excludes1: antineoplastic antibiotics (T45.1-)	2—intentional (self-harm)
	locally applied antibiotic NEC (T49.0)	3—assault
	topically used antibiotic for ear, nose and throat (T49.6)	4—undetermined
	topically used antibiotic for eye (T49.5)	5—adverse effect
T36.0	Poisoning by, adverse effect of and underdosing of penicillins	6—underdosing
	T36.0X- Poisoning by,	7th characters for categories T36–T50
	adverse effect of and underdosing of penicillins	A—initial encounter
T36.1	Poisoning by, adverse effect of and underdosing of cephalosporins and other beta-lactam antibiotics	D—subsequent encounter
	T36.1X- Poisoning by, adverse effect of and underdosing of cephalosporins and other beta-lactam antibiotics	S—sequela
T36.3	Poisoning by, adverse effect of and underdosing of macrolides	
	T36.3X- Poisoning by, adverse effect of and underdosing of macrolides	
T36.6	Poisoning by, adverse effect of and underdosing of rifampicins	
	T36.6X- Poisoning by, adverse effect of and underdosing of rifampicins	
T36.8	Poisoning by, adverse effect of and underdosing of other systemic antibiotics	
	T36.8X- Poisoning by, adverse effect of and underdosing of other systemic antibiotics	

T37 POISONING BY, ADVERSE EFFECT OF AND UNDERDOSING OF OTHER SYSTEMIC ANTI-INFECTIVES AND ANTIPARASITICS

Excludes1: anti-infectives topically used for ear, nose and throat (T49.6-)
anti-infectives topically used for eye (T49.5-)
locally applied anti-infectives NEC (T49.0-)

T37.0 Poisoning by, adverse effect of and underdosing of sulfonamides
- **T37.0X-** Poisoning by, adverse effect of and underdosing of sulfonamides

T38 POISONING BY, ADVERSE EFFECT OF AND UNDERDOSING OF HORMONES AND THEIR SYNTHETIC SUBSTITUTES AND ANTAGONISTS, NEC

Excludes1: mineralocorticoids and their antagonists (T50.0-)
oxytocic hormones (T48.0-)
parathyroid hormones and derivatives (T50.9-)

T38.2 Poisoning by, adverse effect of and underdosing of antithyroid drugs
- **T38.2X-** Poisoning by, adverse effect of and underdosing of antithyroid drugs

T38.3 Poisoning by, adverse effect of and underdosing of insulin and oral hypoglycemic [antidiabetic] drugs
- **T38.3X-** Poisoning by, adverse effect of and underdosing of insulin and oral hypoglycemic [antidiabetic] drugs

T39 POISONING BY, ADVERSE EFFECT OF AND UNDERDOSING OF NONOPIOID ANALGESICS, ANTIPYRETICS AND ANTIRHEUMATICS

T39.0 Poisoning by, adverse effect of and underdosing of salicylates
- **T39.01-** Poisoning by, adverse effect of and underdosing of aspirin
  Poisoning by, adverse effect of and underdosing of acetylsalicylic acid
- **T39.09-** Poisoning by, adverse effect of and underdosing of other salicylates

T39.1 Poisoning by, adverse effect of and underdosing of 4-Aminophenol derivatives
- **T39.1X-** Poisoning by, adverse effect of and underdosing of 4-Aminophenol derivatives

T39.3 Poisoning by, adverse effect of and underdosing of other nonsteroidal anti-inflammatory drugs [NSAID]
- **T39.31-** Poisoning by, adverse effect of and underdosing of propionic acid derivatives
  Poisoning by, adverse effect of and underdosing of fenoprofen/flurbiprofen/ibuprofen/ketoprofen/naproxen/oxaprozin
- **T39.39-** Poisoning by, adverse effect of and under-dosing of other nonsteroidal anti-inflammatory drugs [NSAID]

T40 POISONING BY, ADVERSE EFFECT OF AND UNDERDOSING OF NARCOTICS AND PSYCHODYSLEPTICS [HALLUCINOGENS]

Excludes2: drug dependence and related mental and behavioral disorders due to psychoactive substance use (F10.–F19.-)

T40.2 Poisoning by, adverse effect of and underdosing of other opioids
- **T40.2X-** Poisoning by, adverse effect of and underdosing of other opioids

T40.4 Poisoning by, adverse effect of and underdosing of other synthetic narcotics
- **T40.41-** Poisoning by fentanyl or fentanyl analogs
- **T40.42-** Poisoning by, adverse effect of and underdosing of tramadol
- **T40.49-** Poisoning by, adverse effect of and underdosing of other synthetic narcotics

T40.5 Poisoning by, adverse effect of and underdosing of cocaine
- **T40.5X-** Poisoning by, adverse effect of and underdosing of cocaine

T40.7 Poisoning by, adverse effect of and underdosing of cannabis (derivatives)
- **T40.71-** Poisoning by, adverse effect of and underdosing of cannabis (derivatives)
- **T40.72-** Poisoning by, adverse effect of and underdosing of synthetic cannabinoids

T42 POISONING BY, ADVERSE EFFECT OF AND UNDERDOSING OF ANTI-EPILEPTIC, SEDATIVE-HYPNOTIC AND ANTI-PARKINSONISM DRUGS

Excludes2: drug dependence and related mental and behavioral disorders due to psychoactive substance use (F10. - – F19.-)

T42.0 Poisoning by, adverse effect of and underdosing of hydantoin derivatives
- **T42.0X-** Poisoning by, adverse effect of and underdosing of hydantoin derivatives

T42.3 Poisoning by, adverse effect of and underdosing of barbiturates
Excludes1: poisoning by, adverse effect of and underdosing of thiobarbiturates (T41.1-)
- **T42.3X-** Poisoning by, adverse effect of and underdosing of barbiturates

T42.4 Poisoning by, adverse effect of and underdosing of benzodiazepines
- **T42.4X-** Poisoning by, adverse effect of and underdosing of benzodiazepines

T42.6 Poisoning by, adverse effect of and underdosing of other antiepileptic and sedative-hypnotic drugs
Poisoning by, adverse effect of and underdosing of methaqualone
Poisoning by, adverse effect of and underdosing of valproic acid
Excludes1: poisoning by, adverse effect of and underdosing of carbamazepine (T42.1-)
- **T42.6X-** Poisoning by, adverse effect of and underdosing of other antiepileptic and sedative-hypnotic drugs

T43 POISONING BY, ADVERSE EFFECT OF AND UNDERDOSING OF PSYCHOTROPIC DRUGS, NEC

Excludes1: appetite depressants (T50.5-)
barbiturates (T42.3-)
benzodiazepines (T42.4-)
methaqualone (T42.6-)
psychodysleptics [hallucinogens] (T40.7–T40.9-)

Excludes2: drug dependence and related mental and behavioral disorders due to psychoactive substance use (F10.––F19.-)

T43.0 Poisoning by, adverse effect of and underdosing of tricyclic and tetracyclic antidepressants
- **T43.01-** Poisoning by, adverse effect of and underdosing of tricyclic antidepressants
- **T43.02-** Poisoning by, adverse effect of and underdosing of tetracyclic antidepressants

T43.3 Poisoning by, adverse effect of and underdosing of phenothiazine antipsychotics and neuroleptics
- **T43.3X-** Poisoning by, adverse effect of and underdosing of phenothiazine antipsychotics and neuroleptics

T43.6 Poisoning by, adverse effect of and underdosing of psychostimulants
Excludes1: poisoning by, adverse effect of and underdosing of cocaine (T40.5-)
- **T43.62-** Poisoning by, adverse effect of and underdosing of amphetamines
  Poisoning by, adverse effect of and underdosing of methamphetamines
- **T43.63-** Poisoning by, adverse effect of and underdosing of methylphenidate
- **T43.64-** Poisoning by ecstasy
  Poisoning by MDMA
  Poisoning by 3,4-methylenedioxymethamphetamine
- **T43.65-** Poisoning by, adverse effect of and underdosing of methamphetamines

T43.9 Poisoning by, adverse effect of and underdosing of unspecified psychotropic drug

CHAPTER 19. INJURY, POISONING AND CERTAIN OTHER CONSEQUENCES OF EXTERNAL CAUSES (S00–T88)

(T43.91–T52.0)

- T43.91- Poisoning by unspecified psychotropic drug, accidental (unintentional)
  - 7th
  - Poisoning by psychotropic drug NOS
- T43.92- Poisoning by unspecified psychotropic drug, intentional self-harm
  - 7th
- T43.95- Adverse effect of unspecified psychotropic drug
  - 7th
- T43.96- Underdosing of unspecified psychotropic drug
  - 7th

T44 POISONING BY, ADVERSE EFFECT OF AND UNDERDOSING OF DRUGS PRIMARILY AFFECTING THE AUTONOMIC NERVOUS SYSTEM

- **4th**
- T44.5 Poisoning by, adverse effect
  - **5th** of and underdosing of predominantly beta-adrenoreceptor agonists
  - *Excludes1:* poisoning by, adverse effect of and underdosing of beta-adrenoreceptor agonists used in asthma therapy (T48.6-)
- T44.5X- Poisoning by, adverse effect of and underdosing of
  - **7th** predominantly beta-adrenoreceptor agonists

T45 POISONING BY, ADVERSE EFFECT OF AND UNDERDOSING OF PRIMARILY SYSTEMIC AND HEMATOLOGICAL AGENTS, NEC

- **4th**
- T45.0 Poisoning by, adverse effect of
  - **5th** and underdosing of antiallergic and antiemetic drugs
  - *Excludes1:* poisoning by, adverse effect of and underdosing of phenothiazine-based neuroleptics (T43.3)
- T45.0X- Poisoning by,
  - **7th** adverse effect of and underdosing of antiallergic and antiemetic drugs
- T45.4 Poisoning by, adverse effect of and underdosing of iron and its
  - **5th** compounds
  - T45.4X- Poisoning by, adverse effect of and underdosing of
    - **7th** iron and its compounds

T46 POISONING BY, ADVERSE EFFECT OF AND UNDERDOSING OF AGENTS PRIMARILY AFFECTING THE CARDIOVASCULAR SYSTEM

- **4th**
- *Excludes1:* poisoning by, adverse effect of and underdosing of metaraminol (T44.4)
- T46.0 Poisoning by, adverse effect of and underdosing of cardiac-
  - **5th** stimulant glycosides and drugs of similar action
  - T46.0X- Poisoning by, adverse effect of and underdosing of
    - **7th** cardiac-stimulant glycosides and drugs of similar action

T47 POISONING BY, ADVERSE EFFECT OF AND UNDERDOSING OF AGENTS PRIMARILY AFFECTING THE GASTROINTESTINAL SYSTEM

- **4th**
- T47.8 Poisoning by, adverse effect of and underdosing of other
  - **5th** agents primarily affecting gastrointestinal system
  - T47.8X- Poisoning by, adverse effect of and underdosing of
    - **7th** other agents primarily affecting gastro-intestinal system

T48 POISONING BY, ADVERSE EFFECT OF AND UNDERDOSING OF AGENTS PRIMARILY ACTING ON SMOOTH AND SKELETAL MUSCLES AND THE RESPIRATORY SYSTEM

- **4th**
- T48.3 Poisoning by, adverse effect of and underdosing of
  - **5th** antitussives
  - T48.3X- Poisoning by, adverse effect of and underdosing of
    - **7th** antitussives
- T48.5 Poisoning by, adverse effect of and underdosing of other anti-
  - **5th** common-cold drugs
  - Poisoning by, adverse effect of and underdosing of decongestants
  - *Excludes2:* poisoning by, adverse effect of and underdosing of antipyretics, NEC (T39.9-)
    - poisoning by, adverse effect of and underdosing of non-steroidal antiinflammatory drugs (T39.3-)
    - poisoning by, adverse effect of and underdosing of salicylates (T39.0-)

- T48.5X- Poisoning by, adverse effect of and underdosing of
  - **7th** other anti-common-cold drugs
- T48.6 Poisoning by, adverse effect of and underdosing of
  - **5th** antiasthmatics, NEC
  - Poisoning by, adverse effect of and underdosing of beta-adrenoreceptor agonists used in asthma therapy
  - *Excludes1:* poisoning by, adverse effect of and underdosing of beta-adrenoreceptor agonists not used in asthma therapy (T44.5)
  - poisoning by, adverse effect of and underdosing of anterior pituitary [adenohypophyseal] hormones (T38.8)
- T48.6X- Poisoning by, adverse effect of and underdosing of
  - **7th** antiasthmatics

T50 POISONING BY, ADVERSE EFFECT OF AND UNDERDOSING OF DIURETICS AND OTHER AND UNSPECIFIED DRUGS, MEDICAMENTS AND BIOLOGICAL SUBSTANCES

- **4th**
- T50.0 Poisoning by, adverse effect of and underdosing of
  - **5th** mineralocorticoids and their antagonists
- T50.0X- Poisoning by, adverse effect of and underdosing of
  - **7th** mineralocorticoids and their antagonists
- T50.A Poisoning by, adverse effect of and underdosing of bacterial
  - **5th** vaccines
  - T50.A1- Poisoning by, adverse effect of and underdosing of
    - **7th** pertussis vaccine, including combinations with a pertussis component
  - T50.A2- Poisoning by, adverse effect of and underdosing
    - **7th** of mixed bacterial vaccines without a pertussis component
  - T50.A9- Poisoning by, adverse effect of and underdosing of
    - **7th** other bacterial vaccines
- T50.B Poisoning by, adverse effect of and underdosing of viral
  - **5th** vaccines
  - T50.B9- Poisoning by, adverse effect of and underdosing of
    - **7th** other viral vaccines
- T50.9 Poisoning by, adverse effect of and underdosing of other and
  - **5th** unspecified drugs, medicaments and biological substances
  - T50.90- Poisoning by, adverse effect of and underdosing
    - **7th** of unspecified drugs, medicaments and biological substances
  - T50.91- Poisoning by multiple unspecified drugs,
    - **7th** medicaments and biological substances
  - T50.99- Poisoning by, adverse effect of and underdosing of
    - **7th** other drugs, medicaments and biological substances

(T51–T65) TOXIC EFFECTS OF SUBSTANCES CHIEFLY NONMEDICINAL AS TO SOURCE

Note: When no intent is indicated code to accidental. Undetermined intent is only for use when there is specific documentation in the record that the intent of the toxic effect cannot be determined.

Note: Refer to the Table of Drugs first for a complete listing of chemicals and drugs. If the code is not listed in the tabular, please refer to the complete *ICD-10-CM Manual*.

Use additional code(s): for all associated manifestations of toxic effect, such as: respiratory conditions due to external agents (J60–J70) personal history of FB fully removed (Z87.821) to identify any retained FB, if applicable (Z18.-)

Excludes1: contact with and (suspected) exposure to toxic substances (Z77.-)

T52 TOXIC EFFECT OF ORGANIC SOLVENTS

- **4th**
- *Excludes1:* halogen derivatives of aliphatic and aromatic hydrocarbons (T53.-)
- T52.0 Toxic effects of petroleum
  - **5th** products
  - Toxic effects of gasoline [petrol]
  - Toxic effects of kerosene [paraffin oil]
  - Toxic effects of paraffin wax
  - Toxic effects of ether petroleum
  - Toxic effects of naphtha petroleum
  - Toxic effects of spirit petroleum

4th **5th** **6th** **7th** Additional Character Required ✓ 3-character code Unspecified laterality codes were excluded here.

* =New Code ▲ =Revised Code ◻ =Social determinants of health *Excludes1*—Not coded here, do not use together *Excludes2*—Not included here

T52.0X Toxic effects of petroleum products,

T52.0X1- accidental (unintentional)

Toxic effects of petroleum products NOS

T52.0X2- intentional self-harm

T52.8 Toxic effects of other organic solvents

T52.8X Toxic effects of other organic solvents,

T52.8X1- accidental (unintentional)

Toxic effects of other organic solvents NOS

T52.8X2- intentional self-harm

T54 TOXIC EFFECT OF CORROSIVE SUBSTANCES

T54 requires a 7th character
A—initial encounter
D—subsequent encounter
S—sequela

T54.3 Toxic effects of corrosive alkalis and alkali-like substances

Toxic effects of potassium hydroxide

Toxic effects of sodium hydroxide

T54.3X Toxic effects of corrosive alkalis and alkali-like substances,

T54 requires a 7th character
A—initial encounter
D—subsequent encounter
S—sequela

T54.3X1- accidental (unintentional)

Toxic effects of corrosive alkalis and alkali-like substances NOS

T54.3X2- intentional self-harm

T56 TOXIC EFFECT OF METALS

Includes: toxic effects of fumes and vapors of metals
toxic effects of metals from all sources, except medicinal substances

Use additional code to identify any retained metal FB, if applicable (Z18.0-, T18.1-)

Excludes1: arsenic and its compounds (T57.0) manganese and its compounds (T57.2)

T56 requires a 7th character
A—initial encounter
D—subsequent encounter
S—sequela

T56.0 Toxic effects of lead and its compounds,

T56.0X Toxic effects of lead and its compounds,

T56.0X1- accidental (unintentional)

Toxic effects of lead and its compounds NOS

T58 TOXIC EFFECT OF CARBON MONOXIDE

Includes: asphyxiation from carbon monoxide
toxic effect of carbon monoxide from all sources

T58 requires a 7th character
A—initial encounter
D—subsequent encounter
S—sequela

T58.0 Toxic effect of carbon monoxide from motor vehicle exhaust,

Toxic effect of exhaust gas from gas engine
Toxic effect of exhaust gas from motor pump

T58.01X- accidental (unintentional)

T58.02X- intentional self-harm

T58.03X- assault

T58.04X- undetermined

T58.1 Toxic effect of carbon monoxide from utility gas,

Toxic effect of acetylene
Toxic effect of gas NOS used for lighting, heating, cooking
Toxic effect of water gas

T58.11X- accidental (unintentional)

T58.12X- intentional self-harm

T58.13X- assault

T58.14X- undetermined

T58.9 Toxic effect of carbon monoxide from unspecified source,

---

T58.91X- accidental (unintentional)

T58.92X- intentional self-harm

T58.93X- assault

T58.94X- undetermined

T59 TOXIC EFFECT OF OTHER GASES, FUMES AND VAPORS

Includes: aerosol propellants

Excludes1: chlorofluorocarbons (T53.5)

T59 requires a 7th character
A—initial encounter
D—subsequent encounter
S—sequela

T59.8 Toxic effect of other specified gases, fumes and vapors

T59.89 Toxic effect of other specified gases, fumes and vapors,

T59.891- accidental (unintentional)

T59.892- intentional self-harm

T59.894- undetermined

T60 TOXIC EFFECT OF PESTICIDES

Includes: toxic effect of wood preservatives

T60 requires a 7th character
A—initial encounter
D—subsequent encounter
S—sequela

T60.0 Toxic effect of organophosphate and carbamate insecticides

T60.0X Toxic effect of organophosphate and carbamate insecticides,

T60.0X1- accidental (unintentional)

Toxic effect of organophosphate and carbamate insecticides NOS

T60.0X2- intentional self-harm

T60.0X3- assault

T60.0X4- undetermined

T62 TOXIC EFFECT OF OTHER NOXIOUS SUBSTANCES EATEN AS FOOD

Excludes1: allergic reaction to food, such as:
anaphylactic shock (reaction) due to adverse food reaction (T78.0-)
bacterial food borne intoxications (A05.-)
dermatitis (L23.6, L25.4, L27.2)
food protein-induced enterocolitis syndrome (K52.21)
food protein-induced enteropathy (K52.22)
gastroenteritis (noninfective) (K52.29)
toxic effect of aflatoxin and other mycotoxins (T64)
toxic effect of cyanides (T65.0-)
toxic effect of hydrogen cyanide (T57.3-)
toxic effect of mercury (T56.1-)

T62 requires a 7th character
A—initial encounter
D—subsequent encounter
S—sequela

T62.0 Toxic effect of ingested mushrooms

T62.0X Toxic effect of ingested mushrooms,

T62.0X1- accidental (unintentional)

Toxic effect of ingested mushrooms NOS

T62.0X2- intentional self-harm

T63 TOXIC EFFECT OF CONTACT WITH VENOMOUS ANIMALS AND PLANTS

Includes: bite or touch of venomous animal
pricked or stuck by thorn or leaf

Excludes2: ingestion of toxic animal or plant (T61.-, T62.-)

T63 requires a 7th character
A—initial encounter
D—subsequent encounter
S—sequela

T63.0 Toxic effect of snake venom

T63.00 Toxic effect of unspecified snake venom,

T63.001- accidental (unintentional)

Toxic effect of unspecified snake venom NOS

T63.3 Toxic effect of venom of spider

T63.30 Toxic effect of unspecified spider venom,

T63.301- accidental (unintentional)

T63.33 Toxic effect of venom of brown recluse spider,

T63.331- accidental (unintentional)

T63.332- intentional self-harm

T63.333- assault

T63.334- undetermined

T63.4 Toxic effect of venom of other arthropods

Use additional code, if applicable, for anaphylactic shock (T78.2)

T63.42 Toxic effect of venom of ants,

T63.421- accidental (unintentional)

T63.44 Toxic effect of venom of bees,

T63.441- accidental (unintentional)

T63.45 Toxic effect of venom of hornets,

T63.451- accidental (unintentional)

T63 requires a 7th character
A—initial encounter
D—subsequent encounter
S—sequela

T63.46 Toxic effect of venom of wasps

Toxic effect of yellow jacket

T63.461- accidental (unintentional)

T63.48 Toxic effect of venom of other arthropod,

T63.481- accidental (unintentional)

T63.6 Toxic effect of contact with other venomous marine animals

Excludes1: sea-snake venom (T63.09)

Excludes2: poisoning by ingestion of shellfish (T61.78-)

T63.62 Toxic effect of contact with other jellyfish,

T63.621- accidental (unintentional)

T63.9 Toxic effect of contact with unspecified venomous animal,

T63.91X- accidental (unintentional)

T65 TOXIC EFFECT OF OTHER AND UNSPECIFIED SUBSTANCES

T65 requires a 7th character
A—initial encounter
D—subsequent encounter
S—sequela

T65.8 Toxic effect of other specified substances

T65.82 Toxic effect of harmful algae and algae toxins,

Toxic effect of (harmful) algae bloom NOS
Toxic effect of blue-green algae bloom
Toxic effect of brown tide
Toxic effect of cyanobacteria bloom
Toxic effect of Florida red tide
Toxic effect of pfiesteria piscicida
Toxic effect of red tide

T65.821- accidental (unintentional)

Toxic effect of harmful algae and algae toxins NOS

T65.9 Toxic effect of unspecified substance,

T65.91X- accidental (unintentional)

Poisoning NOS

T65.92X- intentional self-harm

(T66–T78) OTHER AND UNSPECIFIED EFFECTS OF EXTERNAL CAUSES

T67 EFFECTS OF HEAT AND LIGHT

Excludes1: erythema [dermatitis] ab igne (L59.0)

malignant hyperpyrexia due to anesthesia (T88.3)

radiation-related disorders of the skin and subcutaneous tissue (L55–L59)

T67 requires a 7th character
A—initial encounter
D—subsequent encounter
S—sequela

Excludes2: burns (T20–T31)

sunburn (L55.-)

sweat disorder due to heat (L74–L75)

T67.0 Heatstroke and sunstroke

Use additional code(s) to identify any associated complications of heatstroke, such as:

coma and stupor (R40.-)

rhabdomyolysis (M62.82)

SIRS (R65.1-)

T67.01X- Heatstroke and sunstroke

Heat apoplexy
Heat pyrexia
Siriasis
Thermoplegia

T67.02X- Exertional heatstroke

T67.09X- Other heatstroke and sunstroke

T67.1XX- Heat syncope

Heat collapse

T67.2XX- Heat cramp

T67.3XX- Heat exhaustion, anhydrotic

Heat prostration due to water depletion

Excludes1: heat exhaustion due to salt depletion (T67.4)

T67.4XX- Heat exhaustion due to salt depletion

Heat prostration due to salt (and water) depletion

T67.5XX- Heat exhaustion, unspecified

Heat prostration NOS

T67.6XX- Heat fatigue, transient

T67.8XX- Other effects of heat and light

T67.9XX- Effect of heat and light, unspecified

T68.XXX- HYPOTHERMIA

Accidental hypothermia
Hypothermia NOS

Use additional code to identify source of exposure:

Exposure to excessive cold of man-made origin (W93)

Exposure to excessive cold of natural origin (X31)

Excludes1: hypothermia following anesthesia (T88.51)

hypothermia not associated with low environmental temperature (R68.0)

hypothermia of newborn (P80.-)

Excludes2: frostbite (T33–T34)

T68 requires a 7th character
A—initial encounter
D—subsequent encounter
S—sequela

T70 EFFECTS OF AIR PRESSURE AND WATER PRESSURE

T70 requires a 7th character
A—initial encounter
D—subsequent encounter
S—sequela

T70.0XX- Otitic barotrauma

Aero-otitis media

Effects of change in ambient atmospheric pressure or water pressure on ears

T70.1XX- Sinus barotrauma

Aerosinusitis

Effects of change in ambient atmospheric pressure on sinuses

T70.2 Other and unspecified effects of high altitude

Excludes2: polycythemia due to high altitude (D75.1)

T70.20X- Unspecified effects of high altitude

T70.29X- Other effects of high altitude

Alpine sickness
Anoxia due to high altitude
Barotrauma NOS
Hypobaropathy
Mountain sickness

T71 ASPHYXIATION

Mechanical suffocation
Traumatic suffocation

Excludes1: acute respiratory distress (syndrome) (J80)

anoxia due to high altitude (T70.2)

T71 requires a 7th character
A—initial encounter
D—subsequent encounter
S—sequela

asphyxia NOS (R09.01)
asphyxia from carbon monoxide (T58.-)
asphyxia from inhalation of food or FB (T17.-)
asphyxia from other gases, fumes and vapors (T59.-)
respiratory distress (syndrome) in newborn (P22.-)

T71.1 Asphyxiation due to mechanical threat to breathing

Suffocation due to mechanical threat to breathing

T71.11 Asphyxiation due to smothering under pillow,

T71.111- accidental

Asphyxiation due to smothering under pillow NOS

T71.112- intentional self-harm

T71.113- assault

T71.114- undetermined, initial encounter

T71.12 Asphyxiation due to plastic bag,

T71.121- accidental

Asphyxiation due to plastic bag NOS

T71.122- intentional self-harm

T71.123- assault

T71.124- undetermined

T71.13 Asphyxiation due to being trapped in bed linens,

T71.131- accidental

Asphyxiation due to being trapped in bed linens NOS

T71.132- intentional self-harm

T71.133- assault

T71.134- undetermined

T71.14 Asphyxiation due to smothering under another person's body (in bed),

T71.141- accidental

Asphyxiation due to smothering under another person's body (in bed) NOS

T71.143- assault

T71.144- undetermined

T71.15 Asphyxiation due to smothering in furniture,

T71.151- accidental

Asphyxiation due to smothering in furniture NOS

T71.152- intentional self-harm

T71.153- assault

T71.154- undetermined

T71.16 Asphyxiation due to hanging,

Hanging by window shade cord

Use additional code for any associated injuries, such as: crushing injury of neck (S17.-) fracture of cervical vertebrae (S12.0-S12.2-) open wound of neck (S11.-)

T71.161- accidental

Asphyxiation due to hanging NOS Hanging NOS

T71.162- intentional self-harm

T71.163- assault

T71.164- undetermined

T71.19 Asphyxiation due to mechanical threat to breathing due to other causes,

T71.191- accidental

Asphyxiation due to other causes NOS

T71.192- intentional self-harm

T71.193- assault

T71.194- undetermined

T71.2 Asphyxiation due to systemic oxygen deficiency due to low oxygen content in ambient air

Suffocation due to systemic oxygen deficiency due to low oxygen content in ambient air

T71.21X- Asphyxiation due to cave-in or falling earth

Use additional code for any associated cataclysm (X34-X38)

T71.22 Asphyxiation due to being trapped in a car trunk,

T71.221- accidental

T71.222- intentional self-harm

T71.223- assault

T71.224- undetermined

T71.23 Asphyxiation due to being trapped in a (discarded) refrigerator,

T71.231- accidental

T71.232- intentional self-harm

T71.233- assault

T71.234- undetermined

T71.29 Asphyxiation due to being trapped in other low oxygen environment

T71.9XX- Asphyxiation due to unspecified cause

Suffocation (by strangulation) due to unspecified cause Suffocation NOS Systemic oxygen deficiency due to low oxygen content in ambient air or due to due to mechanical threat to breathing due to unspecified cause Traumatic asphyxia NOS

T73 EFFECTS OF OTHER DEPRIVATION

T73.0XX- Starvation

Deprivation of food

T73.1XX- Deprivation of water

T73.2XX- Exhaustion due to exposure

T73.3XX- Exhaustion due to excessive exertion

Exhaustion due to overexertion

T73.8XX- Other effects of deprivation

T74 ADULT AND CHILD ABUSE, NEGLECT AND OTHER MALTREATMENT, CONFIRMED

GUIDELINES

Sequence first the appropriate code from categories T74, Adult and child abuse, neglect and other maltreatment, confirmed, or T76, Adult and child abuse, neglect and other maltreatment, suspected, for abuse, neglect and other maltreatment, followed by any accompanying mental health or injury code(s).

If the documentation in the medical record states abuse or neglect, it is coded as confirmed (T74.-). It is coded as suspected if it is documented as suspected (T76.-).

For cases of confirmed abuse or neglect an external cause code from the assault section (X92-Y09) should be added to identify the cause of any physical injuries. A perpetrator code (Y07) should be added when the perpetrator of the abuse is known. For suspected cases of abuse or neglect, do not report external cause or perpetrator code.

If a suspected case of abuse, neglect or mistreatment is ruled out during an encounter code Z04.71, Encounter for examination and observation following alleged physical adult abuse, ruled out, or code Z04.72, Encounter for examination and observation following alleged child physical abuse, ruled out, should be used, not a code from T76.

If a suspected case of alleged rape or sexual abuse is ruled out during an encounter for examination and observation following alleged physical adult abuse, ruled out, or code Z04.41, Encounter for examination and observation following alleged rape or sexual abuse, ruled out, should be used, not a code from T76.

If a suspected case of forced sexual exploitation or forced labor exploitation is ruled out during an encounter, code Z04.81, Encounter for examination and observation of victim following forced sexual exploitation, or code Z04.82, Encounter for examination and observation of victim following forced labor exploitation, should be used, not a code from T76.

See Chapter 15, "Abuse in a pregnant patient."

Use additional code, if applicable, to identify any associated current injury

Use additional external cause code to identify perpetrator, if known (Y07.-)

Excludes1: abuse and maltreatment in pregnancy (O9A.3-, O9A.4-, O9A.5-)

adult and child maltreatment, suspected (T76.-)

▪T74.0 **Neglect or abandonment, confirmed**

5th ▪T74.02X- **Child neglect or abandonment, confirmed**

7th

▪T74.1 **Physical abuse, confirmed**

5th ***Excludes2:*** sexual abuse (T74.2-)

▪T74.12X- **Child physical abuse, confirmed**

7th ***Excludes2:*** shaken infant syndrome (T74.4)

▪T74.2 **Sexual abuse, confirmed**

5th Rape, confirmed

Sexual assault, confirmed

▪T74.22X- **Child sexual abuse, confirmed**

7th

▪T74.3 **Psychological abuse, confirmed**

5th Bullying and intimidation, confirmed

Intimidation through social media, confirmed

Target of threatened harm, confirmed

Target of threatened physical violence, confirmed

Target of threatened sexual abuse, confirmed

▪T74.32X- **Child psychological abuse, confirmed**

7th

▪T74.4XX- **Shaken infant syndrome**

7th

▪T74.5 **Forced sexual exploitation, confirmed**

5th ▪T74.51X- **Adult forced sexual exploitation, confirmed**

7th

▪T74.52X- **Child sexual exploitation, confirmed**

7th

▪T74.6 **Forced labor exploitation, confirmed**

5th ▪T74.61X- **Adult forced labor exploitation, confirmed**

7th

▪T74.62X- **Child forced labor exploitation, confirmed**

7th

▪T74.9 **Unspecified maltreatment, confirmed**

5th ▪T74.92X- **Unspecified child maltreatment, confirmed**

7th

T74.A **Financial abuse, confirmed**

5th T74.A2X- **Child financial abuse, confirmed**

7th

T75 OTHER AND UNSPECIFIED EFFECTS OF OTHER EXTERNAL CAUSES

4th

Excludes1: adverse effects NEC (T78.-)

Excludes2: burns (electric) (T20–T31)

T75.0XX- Effects of lightning

Struck by lightning

Use additional code for other effects of lightning

T75.1XX- Unspecified effects of drowning and nonfatal submersion

7th Immersion

Excludes1: specified effects of drowning —*code to* effects

T75.3XX- Motion sickness

7th Airsickness

Seasickness

Travel sickness

Use additional external cause code to identify vehicle or type of motion (Y92.81-)

T75.4XX- Electrocution

7th Shock from electric current

Shock from electroshock gun (taser)

T75.8 Other specified effects of external causes

5th **T75.89X- Other specified effects of external causes**

7th

T76 ADULT AND CHILD ABUSE, NEGLECT AND OTHER MALTREATMENT, SUSPECTED

4th

GUIDELINES

See T74 for full guidelines.

Use additional code, if applicable, to identify any associated current injury

Excludes1: adult and child maltreatment, confirmed (T74.-)

suspected abuse and maltreatment in pregnancy (O9A.3-, O9A.4-, O9A.5-)

suspected adult physical abuse, ruled out (Z04.71)

suspected adult sexual abuse, ruled out (Z04.41)

suspected child physical abuse, ruled out (Z04.72)

suspected child sexual abuse, ruled out (Z04.42)

▪T76.0 **Neglect or abandonment, suspected**

5th ▪T76.02X- **Child neglect or abandonment, suspected**

7th

▪T76.1 **Physical abuse, suspected**

5th ▪T76.12X- **Child physical abuse, suspected**

7th

▪T76.2 **Sexual abuse, suspected**

5th Rape, suspected

Excludes1: alleged abuse, ruled out (Z04.7)

▪T76.22X- **Child sexual abuse, suspected**

7th

▪T76.3 **Psychological abuse, suspected**

5th Target of threatened harm, suspected

Target of threatened physical violence, suspected

Target of threatened sexual abuse, suspected

▪T76.32X- **Child psychological abuse, suspected**

7th Bullying and intimidation, suspected

Intimidation through social media, suspected

▪T76.5 **Forced sexual exploitation, suspected**

5th ▪T76.52X- **Child sexual exploitation, suspected**

7th

▪T76.6 **Forced labor exploitation, suspected**

5th ▪T76.62X- **Child forced labor exploitation, suspected**

7th

▪T76.9 **Unspecified maltreatment, suspected**

5th ▪T76.92X- **Unspecified child maltreatment, suspected**

7th

▪T76.A **Financial abuse, suspected**

5th ▪T76.A1X- **Adult financial abuse, suspected**

7th

▪T76.A2X- **Child financial abuse, suspected**

7th

T78 ADVERSE EFFECTS, NEC

4th

Excludes2: complications of surgical and medical care NEC (T80–T88)

T78.0 Anaphylactic reaction due to food

5th Anaphylactic reaction due to adverse food reaction

Anaphylactic shock or reaction due to nonpoisonous foods

Anaphylactoid reaction due to food

T78.00X- Anaphylactic reaction due to unspecified food
7th

T78.01X- Anaphylactic reaction due to peanuts
7th

T78.02X- Anaphylactic reaction due to shellfish (crustaceans)
7th

T78.03X- Anaphylactic reaction due to other fish
7th

T78.04X- Anaphylactic reaction due to fruits and vegetables
7th

T78.05X- Anaphylactic reaction due to tree nuts and seeds
7th *Excludes2:* anaphylactic reaction due to peanuts (T78.01)

T78.06X- Anaphylactic reaction due to food additives
7th

T78.07X- Anaphylactic reaction due to milk and dairy products
7th

T78.08X- Anaphylactic reaction due to eggs
7th

T78.09X- Anaphylactic reaction due to other food products
7th

T78.1XX- Other adverse food reactions, NEC
7th Use **additional code** to identify the type of reaction, if applicable
Excludes1: anaphylactic reaction or shock due to adverse food reaction (T78.0-)
anaphylactic reaction due to food (T78.0-)
bacterial food borne intoxications (A05.-)
Excludes2: allergic and dietetic gastroenteritis and colitis (K52.29)
allergic rhinitis due to food (J30.5)
dermatitis due to food in contact with skin (L23.6, L24.6, L25.4)
dermatitis due to ingested food (L27.2)
food protein-induced enterocolitis syndrome (K52.21)
food protein-induced enteropathy (K52.22)

T78.2XX- Anaphylactic shock, unspecified
7th Allergic shock
Anaphylactic reaction
Anaphylaxis
Excludes1: anaphylactic reaction or shock due to adverse effect of correct medicinal substance properly administered (T88.6)
anaphylactic reaction or shock due to adverse food reaction (T78.0-)
anaphylactic reaction or shock due to serum (T80.5-)

T78.3XX- Angioneurotic edema
7th Allergic angioedema
Giant urticaria
Quincke's edema
Excludes1: serum urticaria (T80.6-)
urticaria (L50.-)

T78.4 Other and unspecified allergy
5th *Excludes1:* specified types of allergic reaction such as:
allergic diarrhea (K52.29)
allergic gastroenteritis and colitis (K52.29)
food protein-induced enterocolitis syndrome (K52.21)
food protein-induced enteropathy (K52.22)
dermatitis (L23–L25, L27.-)
hay fever (J30.1)

T78.40X- Allergy, unspecified
7th Allergic reaction NOS
Hypersensitivity NOS

T78.49X- Other allergy
7th

T78.8XX- Other adverse effects, NEC
7th

(T79) CERTAIN EARLY COMPLICATIONS OF TRAUMA

T79 CERTAIN EARLY COMPLICATIONS OF TRAUMA, NEC
4th

Excludes2: acute respiratory distress syndrome (J80)
complications occurring during or following medical procedures (T80–T88)
complications of surgical and medical care NEC (T80–T88)
newborn respiratory distress syndrome (P22.0)

T79.4XX- Traumatic shock
7th Shock (immediate) (delayed) following injury
Excludes1: anaphylactic shock due to adverse food reaction (T78.0-)
anaphylactic shock due to correct medicinal substance properly administered (T88.6)
anaphylactic shock due to serum (T80.5-)
anaphylactic shock NOS (T78.2)
electric shock (T75.4)
nontraumatic shock NEC (R57.-)
obstetric shock (O75.1)
postprocedural shock (T81.1-)
septic shock (R65.21)
shock complicating abortion or ectopic or molar pregnancy (O00–O07, O08.3)
shock due to anesthetic (T88.2)
shock due to lightning (T75.01)
shock NOS (R57.9)

T79.7XX- Traumatic subcutaneous emphysema
7th *Excludes2:* emphysema NOS (J43)
emphysema (subcutaneous) resulting from a procedure (T81.82)

(T80–T88) COMPLICATIONS OF SURGICAL AND MEDICAL CARE, NEC

Use additional code for adverse effect, if applicable, to identify drug (T36–T50 with fifth or sixth character 5)

Use additional code(s) to identify the specified condition resulting from the complication

Use additional code to identify devices involved and details of circumstances (Y62–Y82)

Excludes2: any encounters with medical care for postprocedural conditions in which no complications are present, such as:
artificial opening status (Z93.-)
closure of external stoma (Z43.-)
fitting and adjustment of external prosthetic device (Z44.-)
burns and corrosions from local applications and irradiation (T20–T32)
complications of surgical procedures during pregnancy, childbirth and the puerperium (O00–O9A)
mechanical complication of respirator [ventilator] (J95.850)
poisoning and toxic effects of drugs and chemicals (T36–T65 with fifth or sixth character 1–4 or 6)
postprocedural fever (R50.82)
specified complications classified elsewhere, such as:
cerebrospinal fluid leak from spinal puncture (G97.0)
colostomy malfunction (K94.0-)
disorders of fluid and electrolyte imbalance (E86–E87)
functional disturbances following cardiac surgery (I97.0–I97.1)
intraoperative and postprocedural complications of specified body systems (D78.-, E36.-, E89.-, G97.3-, G97.4, H59.3-, H59.-, H95.2-, H95.3, I97.4-, I97.5, J95.6-, J95.7, K91.6-, L76.-, M96.-, N99.-)
ostomy complications (J95.0-, K94.-, N99.5-)
postgastric surgery syndromes (K91.1)
postlaminectomy syndrome NEC (M96.1)
postmastectomy lymphedema syndrome (I97.2)
postsurgical blind-loop syndrome (K91.2)
ventilator associated pneumonia (J95.851)

T80 COMPLICATIONS FOLLOWING INFUSION, TRANSFUSION AND THERAPEUTIC INJECTION

T80 requires a 7th character
A—initial encounter
D—subsequent encounter
S—sequela

Includes: complications following perfusion

Excludes2: bone marrow transplant rejection (T86.01)
febrile nonhemolytic transfusion reaction (R50.84)
fluid overload due to transfusion (E87.71)
posttransfusion purpura (D69.51)
transfusion associated circulatory overload (TACO) (E87.71)
transfusion (red blood cell) associated hemochromatosis (E83.111)
transfusion related acute lung injury (TRALI) (J95.84)

T80.0XX- Air embolism following infusion, transfusion and
7th **therapeutic injection**

T80.2 Infections following infusion, transfusion and therapeutic
5th **injection**

Use additional code to identify the specific infection, such as: sepsis (A41.9)

Use additional code (R65.2-) to identify severe sepsis, if applicable

Excludes2: infections specified as due to prosthetic devices, implants and grafts (T82.6–T82.7, T83.5–T83.6, T84.5–T84.7, T85.7)
postprocedural infections (T81.4-)

T80.21 Infection due to central
6th **venous catheter**

T80 requires a 7th character
A—initial encounter
D—subsequent encounter
S—sequela

Infection due to pulmonary artery catheter (Swan-Ganz catheter)

T80.211- Bloodstream infection due to central
7th **venous catheter**
Catheter-related bloodstream infection (CRBSI) NOS
Central line-associated blood-stream infection (CLABSI)
Bloodstream infection due to Hickman catheter/peripherally inserted central catheter (PICC)/portacath (port-a-cath)/ pulmonary artery catheter/triple lumen catheter/umbilical venous catheter

T80.212- Local infection due to central venous
7th **catheter**
Exit or insertion site infection
Local infection due to Hickman catheter/ peripherally inserted central catheter (PICC)/portacath (port-a-cath)/pulmonary artery catheter/triple lumen catheter/ umbilical venous catheter
Port or reservoir infection
Tunnel infection

T80.218- Other infection due to central venous
7th **catheter**
Other central line–associated infection/ Hickman catheter/peripherally inserted central catheter (PICC)/portacath (port-a-cath)/pulmonary artery catheter/triple lumen catheter/umbilical venous catheter

T80.219- Unspecified infection due to central
7th **venous catheter**
Central line-associated infection NOS
Unspecified infection due to Hickman catheter/peripherally inserted central catheter (PICC)/portacath (port-a-cath)/ pulmonary artery catheter/triple lumen catheter/umbilical venous catheter

T80.22X- Acute infection following transfusion, infusion, or
7th **injection of blood and blood products**

T80.29X- Infection following other infusion, transfusion and
7th **therapeutic injection**

T80.3 ABO incompatibility reaction due to transfusion of blood or
5th **blood products**

Excludes1: minor blood group antigens reactions (Duffy) (E) (K(ell)) (Kidd) (Lewis) (M) (N) (P) (S) (T80.A-)

T80.30X- ABO incompatibility
7th **reaction due to transfusion of blood or blood products, unspecified**
ABO incompatibility blood transfusion NOS
Reaction to ABO incompatibility from transfusion NOS

T80.5 Anaphylactic reaction due to serum
5th Allergic shock due to serum
Anaphylactic shock due to serum
Anaphylactoid reaction due to serum
Anaphylaxis due to serum

Excludes1: ABO incompatibility reaction due to transfusion of blood or blood products (T80.3-)
allergic reaction or shock NOS (T78.2)
anaphylactic reaction or shock NOS (T78.2)
anaphylactic reaction or shock due to adverse effect of correct medicinal substance properly administered (T88.6)
other serum reaction (T80.6-)

T80.51X- Anaphylactic reaction due to administration of blood
7th **and blood products**

T80.52X- Anaphylactic reaction due to vaccination
7th

T80.59X- Anaphylactic reaction due to other serum
7th

T80.6 Other serum reactions
5th Intoxication by serum
Protein sickness
Serum rash
Serum sickness
Serum urticaria

Excludes2: serum hepatitis (B16–B19)

T80.61X- Other serum reaction due to administration of blood
7th **and blood products**

T80.62X- Other serum reaction due to vaccination
7th

T80.69X- Other serum reaction due to other serum
7th **Code also**, if applicable, arthropathy in hypersensitivity reactions classified elsewhere (M36.4)

T80.8 Other complications following infusion, transfusion and
5th **therapeutic injection**

T80.81 Extravasation of vesicant agent
6th **Infiltration of vesicant agent**

T80.810- Extravasation of vesicant antineoplastic
7th **chemotherapy**
Infiltration of vesicant antineoplastic chemotherapy

T80.818- Extravasation of other vesicant agent
7th Infiltration of other vesicant agent
Use additional code to identify the specific infection, such as:
sepsis (A41.9)
Use additional code (R65.2-) to identify severe sepsis, if applicable
Excludes2: infections specified as due to prosthetic devices, implants and grafts (T82.6-T82.7, T83.5-T83.6, T84.5-T84.7, T85.7)
postprocedural infections (T81.4-)

T80.82X- Complication of immune effector cellular therapy
7th Complication of chimeric antigen receptor (CAR-T) cell therapy
Complication of IEC therapy

Excludes2: adverse effect of immune checkpoint inhibitors and immunostimulant drugs (T45.AX5)
complication of bone marrow transplant (T86.0)
complication of stem cell transplant (T86.5)

Use additional code to identify the specific complication, such as:
Cytokine release syndrome (D89.83-)
Immune effector cell-associated neurotoxicity syndrome (G92.0-)

T80.89X- Other complications following infusion, transfusion and therapeutic injection

Delayed serologic transfusion reaction (DSTR), unspecified incompatibility

Use additional code to identify graft-versus-host reaction, if applicable, (D89.81-)

T80.9 Unspecified complication following infusion, transfusion and therapeutic injection

T80.90X- Unspecified complication following infusion and therapeutic injection

T80.91 Hemolytic transfusion reaction, unspecified incompatibility

Excludes1: ABO incompatibility with hemolytic transfusion reaction (T80.31-)

Non-ABO incompatibility with hemolytic transfusion reaction (T80.A1-)

Rh incompatibility with hemolytic transfusion reaction (T80.41-)

T80.910- Acute hemolytic transfusion reaction, unspecified incompatibility

T80.911- Delayed hemolytic transfusion reaction, unspecified incompatibility

T80.919- Hemolytic transfusion reaction, unspecified incompatibility, unspecified as acute or delayed

Hemolytic transfusion reaction NOS

T80.92X- Unspecified transfusion reaction

Transfusion reaction NOS

T81 COMPLICATIONS OF PROCEDURES, NEC

Use additional code for adverse effect, if applicable, to identify drug (T36–T50 with fifth or sixth character 5)

Excludes2: complications following immunization (T88.0–T88.1) complications following infusion, transfusion and therapeutic injection (T80.-)

complications of transplanted organs and tissue (T86.-)

specified complications classified elsewhere, such as:

complication of prosthetic devices, implants and grafts (T82–T85)

dermatitis due to drugs and medicaments (L23.3, L24.4, L25.1, L27.0–L27.1)

endosseous dental implant failure (M27.6-)

floppy iris syndrome (IFIS) (intraoperative) H21.81

intraoperative and postprocedural complications of specific body system (D78.-, E36.-, E89.-, G97.3-, G97.4, H59.3-, H59.-, H95.2-, H95.3, I97.4-, I97.5, J95, K91.-, L76.-, M96.-, N99.-)

ostomy complications (J95.0-, K94.-, N99.5-)

plateau iris syndrome (post-iridectomy) (postprocedural) H21.82

poisoning and toxic effects of drugs and chemicals (T36–T65 with fifth or sixth character 1–4)

T81.1 Postprocedural shock

Shock during or resulting from a procedure, NEC

Excludes1: anaphylactic shock NOS (T78.2)

anaphylactic shock due to correct substance properly administered (T88.6)

anaphylactic shock due to serum (T80.5-)

electric shock (T75.4)

obstetric shock (O75.1)

shock due to anesthetic (T88.2)

shock following abortion or ectopic or molar pregnancy (O00–O07, O08.3)

traumatic shock (T79.4)

T81.10X- Postprocedural shock unspecified

Collapse NOS during or resulting from a procedure, NEC

Postprocedural failure of peripheral circulation

Postprocedural shock NOS

T81.11X- Postprocedural cardiogenic shock

T81.12X- Postprocedural septic shock

Postprocedural endotoxic shock resulting from a procedure, NEC

Postprocedural gram-negative shock resulting from a procedure, NEC

Code first underlying infection

Use additional code, to identify any associated acute organ dysfunction, if applicable

T81.19X- Other postprocedural shock

Postprocedural hypovolemic shock

T81.3 Disruption of wound, NEC

Disruption of any suture materials or other closure methods

Excludes1: breakdown (mechanical) of permanent sutures (T85.612)

displacement of permanent sutures (T85.622)

disruption of cesarean delivery wound (O90.0)

disruption of perineal obstetric wound (O90.1)

mechanical complication of permanent sutures NEC (T85.692)

T81.30X- Disruption of wound, unspecified

Disruption of wound NOS

T81.31X- Disruption of external operation (surgical) wound, NEC

Dehiscence of operation wound NOS

Disruption of operation wound NOS

Disruption or dehis-cence of closure of cornea

Disruption or dehiscence of closure of mucosa

Disruption or dehiscence of closure of skin and subcutaneous tissue

Full-thickness skin disruption or dehiscence

Superficial disruption or dehiscence of operation wound

Excludes1: dehiscence of amputation stump (T87.81)

T81.33X- Disruption of traumatic injury wound repair

Disruption or dehiscence of closure of traumatic laceration (external) (internal)

T81.4 Infection following a procedure

Wound abscess following a procedure

Code also, if applicable, disruption of internal operation (surgical) wound (T81.32-)

Use additional code to identify infection

Use additional code (R65.2-) to identify severe sepsis, if applicable

Excludes2: bleb associated endophthalmitis (H59.4-)

infection due to infusion, transfusion and therapeutic injection (T80.2-)

infection due to prosthetic devices, implants and grafts (T82.6-T82.7, T83.5-T83.6, T84.5-T84.7,T85.7)

obstetric surgical wound infection (O86.0-)

postprocedural fever NOS (R50.82)

postprocedural retroperitoneal abscess (K68.11)

T81.40X- Infection following a procedure, unspecified

T81.41X- Infection following a procedure, superficial incisional surgical site

Subcutaneous abscess following a procedure

Stitch abscess following a procedure

T81.42X- Infection following a procedure, deep incisional surgical site

Intra-muscular abscess following a procedure

T81.43X- Infection following a procedure, organ and space surgical site

Intra-abdominal abscess following a procedure

Subphrenic abscess following a procedure

T81.44X- Sepsis following a procedure

Use additional code to identify the sepsis

T81.49X- Infection following a procedure, other surgical site

T81.8 Other complications of procedures, NEC

Excludes2: hypothermia following anesthesia (T88.51)

malignant hyperpyrexia due to anesthesia (T88.3)

T81.89X- Other complications of procedures, NEC

Use additional code to specify complication, such as: postprocedural delirium (F05)

T81.9XX- Unspecified complication of procedure

T82 COMPLICATIONS OF CARDIAC AND VASCULAR PROSTHETIC DEVICES, IMPLANTS AND GRAFTS

T82 requires a 7th character
A—initial encounter
D—subsequent encounter
S—sequela

Excludes2: failure and rejection of transplanted organs and tissue (T86.-)

T82.7XX- Infection and inflammatory reaction due to other cardiac and vascular devices, implants and grafts
Use additional code to identify infection

T82.8 Other specified complications of cardiac and vascular prosthetic devices, implants and grafts

T82.84 Pain due to cardiac and vascular prosthetic devices, implants and grafts

T82.847- Pain due to cardiac prosthetic devices, implants and grafts

T82.848- Pain due to vascular prosthetic devices, implants and grafts

T82.89 Other specified complication of cardiac and vascular prosthetic devices, implants and grafts

T82.897- Other specified complication of cardiac prosthetic devices, implants and grafts

T82.898- Other specified complication of vascular prosthetic devices, implants and grafts

T82.9XX- Unspecified complication of cardiac and vascular prosthetic device, implant and graft

---

T83 COMPLICATIONS OF GENITOURINARY PROSTHETIC DEVICES, IMPLANTS AND GRAFTS

T83 requires a 7th character
A—initial encounter
D—subsequent encounter
S—sequela

Excludes2: failure and rejection of transplanted organs and tissue (T86.-)

T83.0 Mechanical complication of urinary catheter

T83.09 Other mechanical complication of urinary catheter

S43 requires a 7th character
A—initial encounter
D—subsequent encounter
S—sequela

Obstruction (mechanical) of urinary catheter
Perforation of urinary catheter
Protrusion of urinary catheter

T83.090- Other mechanical complication of cystostomy catheter

T83.091- Other mechanical complication of indwelling urethral catheter

T83.098- Other mechanical complication of other urinary catheter

Other mechanical complication of Hopkins catheter
Other mechanical complication of ileostomy catheter
Other mechanical complication of urostomy catheter

T83.5 Infection and inflammatory reaction due to prosthetic device, implant and graft in urinary system

Use additional code to identify infection

T83.51 Infection and inflammatory reaction due to urinary catheter

Excludes2: complications of stoma of urinary tract (N99.5-)

T83.510- Infection and inflammatory reaction due to cystostomy catheter

T83.511- Infection and inflammatory reaction due to indwelling urethral catheter

T83.512- Infection and inflammatory reaction due to nephrostomy catheter

T83.518- Infection and inflammatory reaction due to other urinary catheter

Infection and inflammatory reaction due to Hopkins catheter or ileostomy catheter or urostomy catheter

T83.59 Infection and inflammatory reaction due to prosthetic device, implant and graft in urinary system

T83.591- Infection and inflammatory reaction due to implanted urinary sphincter

T83.593- Infection and inflammatory reaction due to other urinary stents

Infection and inflammatory reaction due to ileal conduit stents
Infection and inflammatory reaction due to nephroureteral stent

T83.598- Infection and inflammatory reaction due to other prosthetic device, implant and graft in urinary system

T83.9XX- Unspecified complication of genitourinary prosthetic device, implant and graft

---

T85 COMPLICATIONS OF OTHER INTERNAL PROSTHETIC DEVICES, IMPLANTS AND GRAFTS

T85 requires a 7th character
A—initial encounter
D—subsequent encounter
S—sequela

Excludes2: failure and rejection of transplanted organs and tissue (T86.-)

T85.0 Mechanical complication of ventricular intracranial (communicating) shunt

T85.01X- Breakdown (mechanical) of ventricular intracranial (communicating) shunt

T85.02X- Displacement of ventricular intracranial (communicating) shunt

Malposition of ventricular intracranial (communicating) shunt

T85.03X- Leakage of ventricular intracranial (communicating) shunt

T85.09X- Other mechanical complication of ventricular intracranial (communicating) shunt

Obstruction (mechanical) of ventricular intracranial (communicating) shunt
Perforation of ventricular intracranial (communicating) shunt
Protrusion of ventricular intracranial (communicating) shunt

T85.6 Mechanical complication of other specified internal and external prosthetic devices, implants and grafts

T85.62 Displacement of other specified internal prosthetic devices, implants and grafts

Malposition of other specified internal prosthetic devices, implants and grafts

T85.624- Displacement of insulin pump

T85.628- Displacement of other specified internal prosthetic devices, implants and grafts

T85.69 Other mechanical complication of other specified internal prosthetic devices, implants and grafts

Obstruction, mechanical of other specified internal prosthetic devices, implants and grafts
Perforation of other specified internal prosthetic devices, implants and grafts
Protrusion of other specified internal prosthetic devices, implants and grafts

T85.694- Other mechanical complication of insulin pump

T85.695- Other mechanical complication of other nervous system device, implant or graft

Other mechanical complication of intrathecal infusion pump

T85.698- Other mechanical complication of other specified internal prosthetic devices, implant and grafts

Mechanical complication of nonabsorbable surgical material NOS

T85.7 Infection and inflammatory reaction due to other internal prosthetic devices, implants and grafts

Use additional code to identify infection

T85.79X- Infection and inflammatory reaction due to other internal prosthetic devices, implants and grafts

T86 COMPLICATIONS OF TRANSPLANTED ORGANS AND TISSUE

GUIDELINES

Codes under category T86, Complications of transplanted organs and tissues, are for use for both complications and rejection of transplanted organs. A transplant complication code is only assigned if the complication affects the function of the transplanted organ. Two codes are required to fully describe a transplant complication: the appropriate code from category T86 and a secondary code that identifies the complication.

Pre-existing conditions or conditions that develop after the transplant are not coded as complications unless they affect the function of the transplanted organs.

See Chapter 21 for transplant organ removal status.
See Chapter 2 for malignant neoplasm associated with transplanted organ.

See Chapter 1 for sequencing of sepsis due to infection in transplanted organ

Use additional code to identify other transplant complications, such as:
graft-versus-host disease (D89.81-)
malignancy associated with organ transplant (C80.2)
post-transplant lymphoproliferative disorders (PTLD) (D47.Z1)

T86.0 Complications of bone marrow transplant

- **T86.01 Bone marrow transplant rejection**
- **T86.02 Bone marrow transplant failure**

T86.1 Complications of kidney transplant

GUIDELINES

Patients who have undergone kidney transplant may still have some form of chronic kidney disease (CKD) because the kidney transplant may not fully restore kidney function. Code T86.1- should be assigned for documented complications of a kidney transplant, such as transplant failure or rejection or other transplant complication. Code T86.1- should not be assigned for post kidney transplant patients who have CKD unless a transplant complication such as transplant failure or rejection is documented. If the documentation is unclear as to whether the patient has a complication of the transplant, query the provider.

Conditions that affect the function of the transplanted kidney, other than CKD, should be assigned a code from subcategory T86.1, Complications of transplanted organ, Kidney, and a secondary code that identifies the complication.

For patients with CKD following a kidney transplant, but who do not have a complication such as failure or rejection, see Chapter 14.

See Chapter 1 for sequencing of sepsis due to infection in transplanted organ

- **T86.10 Unspecified complication of kidney transplant**
- **T86.11 Kidney transplant rejection**
- **T86.12 Kidney transplant failure**
- **T86.13 Kidney transplant infection**
  - **Use additional code** to specify infection
- **T86.19 Other complication of kidney transplant**

T86.2 Complications of heart transplant

Excludes1: complication of:
artificial heart device (T82.5-)
heart-lung transplant (T86.3-)

- **T86.21 Heart transplant rejection**
- **T86.22 Heart transplant failure**
- **T86.29 Other complications of heart transplant**
  - **T86.290 Cardiac allograft vasculopathy**
    - *Excludes1:* atherosclerosis of coronary arteries (I25.75-, I25.76-, I25.81-)
  - **T86.298 Other complications of heart transplant**

T86.3 Complications of heart-lung transplant

- **T86.30 Unspecified complication of heart-lung transplant**
- **T86.31 Heart-lung transplant rejection**
- **T86.32 Heart-lung transplant failure**
- **T86.3X Heart-lung transplant infection**
  - **Use additional code** to specify infection
- **T86.39 Other complications of heart-lung transplant**

T86.4 Complications of liver transplant

- **T86.41 Liver transplant rejection**
- **T86.42 Liver transplant failure**

T86.5 Complications of stem cell transplant

Complications from stem cells from peripheral blood
Complications from stem cells from umbilical cord

T86.8 Complications of other transplanted organs and tissues

- **T86.81 Complications of lung transplant**
  - *Excludes1:* complication of heart-lung transplant (T86.3-)
  - **T86.810 Lung transplant rejection**
  - **T86.811 Lung transplant failure**

T86.9 Complication of unspecified transplanted organ and tissue

- **T86.90 Unspecified complication of unspecified transplanted organ and tissue**

T88 OTHER COMPLICATIONS OF SURGICAL AND MEDICAL CARE, NEC

T88 requires a 7th character
A—initial encounter
D—subsequent encounter
S—sequela

Excludes2: complication following infusion, transfusion and therapeutic injection (T80.-)

complication following procedure NEC (T81.-)
complications of anesthesia in labor and delivery (O74.-)
complications of anesthesia in pregnancy (O29.-)
complications of anesthesia in puerperium (O89.-)
complications of devices, implants and grafts (T82–T85)
complications of obstetric surgery and procedure (O75.4)
dermatitis due to drugs and medicaments (L23.3, L24.4, L25.1, L27.0–L27.1)
poisoning and toxic effects of drugs and chemicals (T36–T65 with fifth or sixth character 1–4)
specified complications classified elsewhere

T88.0XX- Infection following immunization

Sepsis following immunization

T88.1XX- Other complications following immunization, NEC

Generalized vaccinia
Rash following immunization

Excludes1: vaccinia not from vaccine (B08.011)

Excludes2: anaphylactic shock due to serum (T80.5-)
other serum reactions (T80.6-)
postimmunization arthropathy (M02.2)
postimmunization encephalitis (G04.02)
postimmunization fever (R50.83)

Use additional code to identify the complication

T88.6XX- Anaphylactic reaction due to adverse effect of correct drug or medicament properly administered

Anaphylactic shock due to adverse effect of correct drug or medicament properly administered
Anaphylactoid reaction NOS

Use additional code for adverse effect, if applicable, to identify drug (T36–T50 with fifth or sixth character 5)

Excludes1: anaphylactic reaction due to serum (T80.5-)
anaphylactic shock or reaction due to adverse food reaction (T78.0-)

T88.7XX- Unspecified adverse effect of drug or medicament

Drug hypersensitivity NOS
Drug reaction NOS

Use additional code for adverse effect, if applicable, to identify drug (T36–T50 with fifth or sixth character 5)

Excludes1: specified adverse effects of drugs and medicaments (A00–R94 and T80–T88.6, T88.8)

T88.8XX- Other specified complications of surgical and medical care, NEC

T88.9XX- Complication of surgical and medical care, unspecified

Chapter 20. External causes of morbidity (V00–Y99)

GUIDELINES

The external causes of morbidity codes should never be sequenced as the first-listed or principal diagnosis.

External cause codes are intended to provide data for injury research and evaluation of injury prevention strategies. These codes capture how the injury or health condition happened (cause), the intent (unintentional or accidental; or intentional, such as suicide or assault), the place where the event occurred, the activity of the patient at the time of the event, and the person's status (eg, civilian, military).

There is no national requirement for mandatory *ICD-10-CM* external cause code reporting. Unless a provider is subject to a state-based external cause code reporting mandate or these codes are required by a particular payer, reporting of *ICD-10-CM* codes in Chapter 20, External Causes of Morbidity, is not required. In the absence of a mandatory reporting requirement, providers are encouraged to voluntarily report external cause codes, as they provide valuable data for injury research and evaluation of injury prevention strategies.

General External Cause Coding Guidelines

USED WITH ANY CODE IN THE RANGE OF A00.0–T88.9, Z00–Z99

An external cause code may be used with any code in the range of A00.0–T88.9, Z00–Z99, classification that represents a health condition due to an external cause. Though they are most applicable to injuries, they are also valid for use with such things as infections or diseases due to an external source, and other health conditions, such as a heart attack that occurs during strenuous physical activity.

EXTERNAL CAUSE CODE USED FOR LENGTH OF TREATMENT

Assign the external cause code, with the appropriate 7th character (initial encounter, subsequent encounter or sequela) for each encounter for which the injury or condition is being treated.

Most categories in Chapter 20 have a 7th character requirement for each applicable code. Most categories in this chapter have three 7th character values: A, initial encounter, D, subsequent encounter and S, sequela. While the patient may be seen by a new or different provider over the course of treatment for an injury or condition, assignment of the 7th character of the code assigned for external cause should match the 7th character of the code assigned for the associated injury or condition for the encounter.

USE THE FULL RANGE OF EXTERNAL CAUSE CODES

Use the full range of external cause codes to completely describe the cause, the intent, the place of occurrence, and if applicable, the activity of the patient at the time of the event, and the patient's status, for all injuries, and other health conditions due to an external cause.

ASSIGN AS MANY EXTERNAL CAUSE CODES AS NECESSARY

Assign as many external cause codes as necessary to fully explain each cause. If only one external code can be recorded, assign the code most related to the principal diagnosis.

THE SELECTION OF THE APPROPRIATE EXTERNAL CAUSE CODE

The selection of the appropriate external cause code is guided by the Alphabetic Index of External Causes and by Inclusion and Exclusion notes in the Tabular List.

EXTERNAL CAUSE CODE CAN NEVER BE A PRINCIPAL DIAGNOSIS

An external cause code can never be a principal (first-listed) diagnosis.

COMBINATION EXTERNAL CAUSE CODES

Certain of the external cause codes are combination codes that identify sequential events that result in an injury, such as a fall which results in striking against an object. The injury may be due to either event or both. The combination external cause code used should correspond to the sequence of events regardless of which caused the most serious injury.

NO EXTERNAL CAUSE CODE NEEDED IN CERTAIN CIRCUMSTANCES

No external cause code from Chapter 20 is needed if the external cause and intent are included in a code from another chapter (eg, T36.0X1- Poisoning by penicillins, accidental [unintentional]).

Place of Occurrence Guideline

See category Y92.

Activity Code

See category Y93.

Place of Occurrence, Activity, and Status Codes Used with other External Cause Code

When applicable, place of occurrence, activity, and external cause status codes are sequenced after the main external cause code(s). Regardless of the number of external cause codes assigned, generally there should be only one place of occurrence code, one activity code, and one external cause status code assigned to an encounter. However, in the rare instance that a new injury occurs during hospitalization, an additional place of occurrence code may be assigned.

If the Reporting Format Limits the Number of External Cause Codes

If the reporting format limits the number of external cause codes that can be used in reporting clinical data, report the code for the cause/intent most related to the principal diagnosis. If the format permits capture of additional external cause codes, the cause/intent, including medical misadventures, of the additional events should be reported rather than the codes for place, activity, or external status.

Multiple External Cause Coding Guidelines

More than one external cause code is required to fully describe the external cause of an illness or injury. The assignment of external cause codes should be sequenced in the following priority:

If two or more events cause separate injuries, an external cause code should be assigned for each cause. The first-listed external cause code will be selected in the following order:

External codes for child and adult abuse take priority over all other external cause codes.

See Chapter 19, Child and Adult abuse guidelines.

External cause codes for terrorism events take priority over all other external cause codes except child and adult abuse.

External cause codes for cataclysmic events take priority over all other external cause codes except child and adult abuse and terrorism.

External cause codes for transport accidents take priority over all other external cause codes except cataclysmic events, child and adult abuse and terrorism.

Activity and external cause status codes are assigned following all causal (intent) external cause codes.

The first-listed external cause code should correspond to the cause of the most serious diagnosis due to an assault, accident, or self-harm, following the order of hierarchy listed above.

Child and Adult Abuse Guideline

See category Y07.

Unknown or Undetermined Intent Guideline

If the intent (accident, self-harm, assault) of the cause of an injury or other condition is unknown or unspecified, code the intent as accidental intent. All transport accident categories assume accidental intent.

USE OF UNDETERMINED INTENT

External cause codes for events of undetermined intent are only for use if the documentation in the record specifies that the intent cannot be determined.

Sequelae (Late Effects) of External Cause Guidelines

SEQUELAE EXTERNAL CAUSE CODES

Sequela are reported using the external cause code with the 7th character "S" for sequela. These codes should be used with any report of a late effect or sequela resulting from a previous injury.

See *ICD-10-CM* Official Guidelines for Coding and Reporting FY 2024 in front matter, "Sequela (Late Effects)."

SEQUELA EXTERNAL CAUSE CODE WITH A RELATED CURRENT INJURY

A sequela external cause code should never be used with a related current nature of injury code.

USE OF SEQUELA EXTERNAL CAUSE CODES FOR SUBSEQUENT VISITS

Use a late effect external cause code for subsequent visits when a late effect of the initial injury is being treated. Do not use a late effect external cause code for subsequent visits for follow-up care (eg, to assess healing, to receive rehabilitative therapy) of the injury when no late effect of the injury has been documented.

Terrorism Guidelines

CAUSE OF INJURY IDENTIFIED BY THE FEDERAL GOVERNMENT (FBI) AS TERRORISM

When the cause of an injury is identified by the FBI as terrorism, the first-listed external cause code should be a code from category Y38, Terrorism. The definition of terrorism employed by the FBI is found at the inclusion note at the beginning of category Y38. Use additional code for place of occurrence (Y92.-). More than one Y38 code may be assigned if the injury is the result of more than one mechanism of terrorism. See *ICD-10-CM* manual for full guidelines.

External cause status

See category Y99.

Note: This chapter permits the classification of environmental events and circumstances as the cause of injury, and other adverse effects. Where a code from this section is applicable, it is intended that it shall be used secondary to a code from another chapter of the Classification indicating the nature of the condition. Most often, the condition will be classifiable to Chapter 19, Injury, poisoning and certain other consequences of external causes (S00–T88). Other conditions that may be stated to be due to external causes are classified in Chapters 1 to 18. For these conditions, codes from Chapter 20 should be used to provide additional information as to the cause of the condition.

ACCIDENTS (V00–X58)

(V00–V99) TRANSPORT ACCIDENTS

Note: This section is structured in 12 groups. Those relating to land transport accidents (V01–V89) reflect the victim's mode of transport and are subdivided to identify the victim's 'counterpart' or the type of event. The vehicle of which the injured person is an occupant is identified in the first two characters since it is seen as the most important factor to identify for prevention purposes. A transport accident is one in which the vehicle involved must be moving or running or in use for transport purposes at the time of the accident.

Use additional code to identify:
Airbag injury (W22.1)
Type of street or road (Y92.4-)
Use of cellular telephone and other electronic equipment at the time of the transport accident (Y93.C-)

Excludes1: agricultural vehicles in stationary use or maintenance (W31.-)
assault by crashing of motor vehicle (Y03.-)
automobile or motor cycle in stationary use or maintenance- code to type of accident
crashing of motor vehicle, undetermined intent (Y32)
intentional self-harm by crashing of motor vehicle (X82)

Excludes2: transport accidents due to cataclysm (X34–X38)
A traffic accident is any vehicle accident occurring on the public highway [ie, originating on, terminating on, or involving a vehicle partially on the highway]. A vehicle accident is assumed to have occurred on the public highway unless another place is specified, except in the case of accidents involving only off-road motor vehicles, which are classified as nontraffic unless the contrary is stated.

A nontraffic accident is any vehicle accident that occurs entirely in any place other than a public highway. Please see full *ICD-10-CM* manual for definitions of transport vehicles.

(V00–V09) PEDESTRIAN INJURED IN TRANSPORT ACCIDENT

Includes: person changing tire on transport vehicle
person examining engine of vehicle broken down in (on side of) road
Excludes1: fall due to non-transport collision with other person (W03)
pedestrian on foot falling (slipping) on ice and snow (W00.-)
struck or bumped by another person (W51)
See External Cause of Injuries Table.

V00 PEDESTRIAN CONVEYANCE ACCIDENT

Use additional place of occurrence and activity external cause codes, if known (Y92.-, Y93.-)

Excludes1: collision with another person without fall (W51)
fall due to person on foot colliding with another person on foot (W03)
fall from non-moving wheelchair, nonmotorized scooter and motorized mobility scooter without collision (W05.-)
pedestrian (conveyance) collision with other land transport vehicle (V01–V09)
pedestrian on foot falling (slipping) on ice and snow (W00.-)

V00.0 Pedestrian on foot injured in collision with pedestrian conveyance

V00.01X- Pedestrian on foot injured in collision with roller-skater

V00.02X- Pedestrian on foot injured in collision with skateboarder

V00.031- Pedestrian on foot injured in collision with rider of standing electric scooter

V00.038- Pedestrian on foot injured in collision with rider of other standing micro-mobility pedestrian conveyance

V00.09X- Pedestrian on foot injured in collision with other pedestrian conveyance

V00.1 Rolling-type pedestrian conveyance accident

Excludes1: accident with baby stroller (V00.82-)
accident with wheelchair (powered) (V00.81-)
accident with motorized mobility scooter (V00.83-)

V00.11 In-line roller-skate accident

V00.111- Fall from in-line roller-skates

V00.112- In-line roller-skater colliding with stationary object

V00.118- Other in-line roller-skate accident
Excludes1: roller-skater collision with other land transport vehicle (V01–V09 with 5th character 1)

V00.12 Non-in-line roller-skate accident

V00.121- Fall from non-in-line roller-skates

V00.122- Non-in-line roller-skater colliding with stationary object

V00.128- Other non-in-line roller-skating accident
Excludes1: roller-skater collision with other land transport vehicle (V01–V09 with 5th character 1)

V00.13 Skateboard accident

V00.131- Fall from skateboard

V00.132- Skateboarder colliding with stationary object

V00.138- Other skateboard accident
Excludes1: skateboarder collision with other land transport vehicle (V01–V09 with 5th character 2)

V00.14 Scooter (nonmotorized) accident
Excludes1: motorscooter accident (V20–V29)

V00.141- Fall from scooter (nonmotorized)

V00.142- Scooter (nonmotorized) colliding with stationary object

V00.148- Other scooter (nonmotorized) accident
Excludes1: scooter (nonmotorized) collision with other land transport vehicle (V01–V09 with fifth character 9)

V00.15 Heelies accident
Rolling shoe
Wheeled shoe
Wheelies accident

V00.151- Fall from heelies

V00.152- Heelies colliding with stationary object

V00.158- Other heelies accident

V00.18 Accident on other rolling-type pedestrian conveyance

V00.181- Fall from other rolling-type pedestrian conveyance

V00.182- Pedestrian on other rolling-type pedestrian conveyance colliding with stationary object

V00.188- Other accident on other rolling-type pedestrian conveyance

V00.2 Gliding-type pedestrian conveyance accident

V00.21 Ice-skates accident

V00.211- Fall from ice-skates

V00.212- Ice-skater colliding with stationary object

V00.218- Other ice-skates accident

Excludes1: ice-skater collision with other land transport vehicle (V01–V09 with 5th character 9)

V00.22 Sled accident

V00.221- Fall from sled

V00.222- Sledder colliding with stationary object

V00.228- Other sled accident

Excludes1: sled collision with other land transport vehicle (V01–V09 with 5th character 9)

V00.3 Flat-bottomed pedestrian conveyance accident

V00.31 Snowboard accident

V00.311- Fall from snowboard

V00.312- Snowboarder colliding with stationary object

V00.318- Other snowboard accident

Excludes1: snowboarder collision with other land transport vehicle (V01–V09 with 5th character 9)

V00.32 Snow-ski accident

V00.321- Fall from snow-skis

V00.322- Snow-skier colliding with stationary object

V00.328- Other snow-ski accident

Excludes1: snow-skier collision with other land transport vehicle (V01–V09 with 5th character 9)

V00.38 Other flat-bottomed pedestrian conveyance accident

V00.381- Fall from other flat-bottomed pedestrian conveyance

V00.382- Pedestrian on other flat-bottomed pedestrian conveyance colliding with stationary object

V00.388- Other accident on other flat-bottomed pedestrian conveyance

V00.8 Accident on other pedestrian conveyance

V00.81 Accident with wheelchair (powered)

V00.811- Fall from moving wheelchair (powered)

Excludes1: fall from non-moving wheelchair (W05.0)

V00.812- Wheelchair (powered) colliding with stationary object

V00.818- Other accident with wheelchair (powered)

V00.82 Accident with baby stroller

V00.821- Fall from baby stroller

V00.822- Baby stroller colliding with stationary object

V00.828- Other accident with baby stroller

V00.84 Accident with standing micro-mobility pedestrian conveyance

V00.841- Fall from standing electric scooter

V00.842- Pedestrian on standing electric scooter colliding with stationary object

V00.848- Other accident with standing micro-mobility pedestrian conveyance

Accident with hoverboard

Accident with segway

V00.89 Accident on other pedestrian conveyance

V00.891- Fall from other pedestrian conveyance

V00.892- Pedestrian on other pedestrian conveyance colliding with stationary object

V00.898- Other accident on other pedestrian conveyance

Excludes1: other pedestrian (conveyance) collision with other land transport vehicle (V01–V09 with 5th character 9)

V01 PEDESTRIAN INJURED IN COLLISION WITH PEDAL CYCLE

See External Cause of Injuries Table.

V01.0 Pedestrian injured in collision with pedal cycle in nontraffic accident

V01.00X- Pedestrian on foot injured in collision with pedal cycle in nontraffic accident

Pedestrian NOS injured in collision with pedal cycle in nontraffic accident

V01.01X- Pedestrian on roller-skates injured in collision with pedal cycle in nontraffic accident

V01.02X- Pedestrian on skateboard injured in collision with pedal cycle in nontraffic accident

V01.03 Pedestrian on standing micro-mobility pedestrian conveyance injured in collision with pedal cycle in nontraffic accident

V01.031- Pedestrian on standing electric scooter injured in collision with pedal cycle in nontraffic accident

V01.038- Pedestrian on other standing micro-mobility pedestrian conveyance injured in collision with pedal cycle in nontraffic accident

Pedestrian on hoverboard injured in collision with pedal cycle in nontraffic accident

Pedestrian on segway injured in collision with pedal cycle in nontraffic accident

V01.09X- Pedestrian with other conveyance injured in collision with pedal cycle in nontraffic accident

Pedestrian with baby stroller injured in collision with pedal cycle in nontraffic accident

Pedestrian on ice-skates or nonmotorized scooter or motorized mobility scooter or sled or snowboard or snow-skis or wheelchair (powered) injured in collision with pedal cycle in nontraffic accident

V01.1 Pedestrian injured in collision with pedal cycle in traffic accident

V01.10X- Pedestrian on foot injured in collision with pedal cycle in traffic accident

Pedestrian NOS injured in collision with pedal cycle in traffic accident

V01.11X- Pedestrian on roller-skates injured in collision with pedal cycle in traffic accident

V01.12X- Pedestrian on skateboard injured in collision with pedal cycle in traffic accident

V01.13 Pedestrian on standing micro-mobility pedestrian conveyance injured in collision with pedal cycle in traffic accident

V01.131- Pedestrian collision with pedal cycle in traffic accident

V01.138- Pedestrian on other standing micro-mobility pedestrian conveyance injured in collision with pedal cycle in traffic accident

V01.19X- Pedestrian with other conveyance injured in collision with pedal cycle in traffic accident

Pedestrian with baby stroller injured in collision with pedal cycle in traffic accident

Pedestrian on ice-skates or nonmotorized scooter or motorized mobility scooter or sled or snowboard or snow-ski or wheelchair (powered) injured in collision with pedal cycle in traffic accident

V01.9 Pedestrian injured in collision with pedal cycle, unspecified whether traffic or nontraffic accident

V01.90X- Pedestrian on foot injured in collision with pedal cycle, unspecified whether traffic or nontraffic accident

Pedestrian NOS injured in collision with pedal cycle, unspecified whether traffic or nontraffic accident

V01.91X- Pedestrian on roller-skates injured in collision with pedal cycle, unspecified whether traffic or nontraffic accident

V01.92X- Pedestrian on skateboard injured in collision with pedal cycle, unspecified whether traffic or nontraffic accident

V01.93 Pedestrian on standing micro-mobility pedestrian conveyance injured in collision with pedal cycle, unspecified whether traffic or nontraffic accident

V01.931- Pedestrian on standing electric scooter injured in collision with pedal cycle, unspecified whether traffic or nontraffic accident

V01.938- Pedestrian on other standing micro-mobility pedestrian conveyance injured in collision with pedal cycle, unspecified whether traffic or nontraffic accident

Pedestrian on hoverboard or segway injured in collision with pedal cycle, unspecified whether traffic or nontraffic accident

V01.99X- Pedestrian with other conveyance injured in collision with pedal cycle, unspecified whether traffic or nontraffic accident

Includes: Pedestrian with baby stroller, on ice-skates or nonmotorized scooter or motorized mobility scooter or sled or snowboard or snow-skis or wheelchair (powered) injured in collision with pedal cycle unspecified, whether traffic or nontraffic accident

V02 PEDESTRIAN INJURED IN COLLISION WITH TWO- OR THREE-WHEELED MOTOR VEHICLE

See *External Cause of Injuries Table.*

V03 PEDESTRIAN INJURED IN COLLISION WITH CAR, PICK-UP TRUCK OR VAN

See *External Cause of Injuries Table.*

V03.0 Pedestrian injured in collision with car, pick-up truck or van in nontraffic accident

V03.00X- Pedestrian on foot injured in collision with car, pick-up truck or van in nontraffic accident

Pedestrian NOS injured in collision with car, pick-up truck or van in nontraffic accident

V03.01X- Pedestrian on roller-skates injured in collision with car, pick-up truck or van in nontraffic accident

V03.02X- Pedestrian on skateboard injured in collision with car, pick-up truck or van in nontraffic accident

V03.03 Pedestrian on standing micro-mobility pedestrian conveyance injured in collision with car, pick-up or van in nontraffic accident

V03.031- Pedestrian on standing electric scooter injured in collision with car, pick-up or van in nontraffic accident

V03.038- Pedestrian on other standing micro-mobility pedestrian conveyance injured in collision with car, pick-up or van in nontraffic accident

V03.09X- Pedestrian with other conveyance injured in collision with car, pick-up truck or van in nontraffic accident

Includes: Pedestrian with baby stroller or on ice-skates or nonmotorized scooter or motorized mobility scooter or sled or snowboard or snow-skis or wheelchair (powered) injured

V03.1 Pedestrian injured in collision with car, pick-up truck or van in traffic accident

V03.10X- Pedestrian on foot injured in collision with car, pick-up truck or van in traffic accident

Pedestrian NOS injured in collision with car, pick-up truck or van in traffic accident

V03.11X- Pedestrian on roller-skates injured in collision with car, pick-up truck or van in traffic accident

V03.12X- Pedestrian on skateboard injured in collision with car, pick-up truck or van in traffic accident

V03.13 Pedestrian on standing micro-mobility pedestrian conveyance injured in collision with car, pick-up or van in traffic accident

V03.131- Pedestrian on standing electric scooter injured in collision with car, pick-up or van in traffic accident

V03.138- Pedestrian on other standing micro-mobility pedestrian conveyance injured in collision with car, pick-up or van in traffic accident

Includes: Pedestrian on hoverboard or segway injured

V03.19X- Pedestrian with other conveyance injured in collision with car, pick-up truck or van in traffic accident

Pedestrian with baby stroller or on ice-skates or nonmotorized scooter or motorized mobility scooter or sled or snowboard or snow-skis or wheelchair (powered) injured in collision with car, pick-up truck or van in traffic accident

V03.9 Pedestrian injured in collision with car, pick-up truck or van, unspecified whether traffic or nontraffic accident

V03.90X- Pedestrian on foot injured in collision with car, pick-up truck or van, unspecified whether traffic or nontraffic accident

Pedestrian NOS injured in collision with car, pick-up truck or van, unspecified whether traffic or nontraffic accident

V03.91X- Pedestrian on roller-skates injured in collision with car, pick-up truck or van, unspecified whether traffic or nontraffic accident

V03.92X- Pedestrian on skateboard injured in collision with car, pick-up truck or van, unspecified whether traffic or nontraffic accident

V03.93 Pedestrian on standing micro-mobility pedestrian conveyance injured in collision with car, pick-up or van, unspecified whether traffic or nontraffic accident

V03.931- Pedestrian on standing electric scooter injured in collision with car, pick-up or van, unspecified whether traffic or nontraffic accident

V03.938- Pedestrian on other standing micro-mobility pedestrian conveyance injured in collision with car, pick-up or van, unspecified whether traffic or nontraffic accident

Includes: Pedestrian on hoverboard or segway injured

V03.99- Pedestrian with other conveyance injured in collision with car, pick-up truck or van, unspecified whether traffic or nontraffic accident

V04 PEDESTRIAN INJURED IN COLLISION WITH HEAVY TRANSPORT VEHICLE OR BUS

Excludes1: pedestrian injured in collision with military vehicle (V09.01, V09.21). *See External Cause of Injuries Table.*

V04–V09 require a 7th character
A—initial encounter
D—subsequent encounter
S—sequela

V04.0 Pedestrian injured in collision with heavy transport vehicle or bus in nontraffic accident

V04.00X- Pedestrian on foot injured in collision with heavy transport vehicle or bus in nontraffic accident Pedestrian NOS injured in collision with heavy transport vehicle or bus in nontraffic accident

V04.01X- Pedestrian on roller-skates injured in collision with heavy transport vehicle or bus in nontraffic accident

V04.02X- Pedestrian on skateboard injured in collision with heavy transport vehicle or bus in nontraffic accident

V04.03 Pedestrian on standing micro-mobility pedestrian conveyance injured in collision with heavy transport vehicle or bus in nontraffic accident

V04.031- Pedestrian on standing electric scooter injured in collision with heavy transport vehicle or bus in nontraffic accident

V04.038- Pedestrian on other standing micro-mobility pedestrian conveyance injured in collision with heavy transport vehicle or bus in nontraffic accident Pedestrian on hoverboard or segway injured in collision with heavy transport vehicle or bus in nontraffic accident

V04.09X- Pedestrian with other conveyance injured in collision with heavy transport vehicle or bus in nontraffic accident *Includes:* Pedestrian with baby stroller or on ice-skates or nonmotorized scooter or motorized mobility scooter or sled or snowboard or snow-skis or wheelchair (powered) injured

V04.1 Pedestrian injured in collision with heavy transport vehicle or bus in traffic accident

V04.10X- Pedestrian on foot injured in collision with heavy transport vehicle or bus in traffic accident Pedestrian NOS injured in collision with heavy transport vehicle or bus in traffic accident

V04.11X- Pedestrian on roller-skates injured in collision with heavy transport vehicle or bus in traffic accident

V04.12X- Pedestrian on skateboard injured in collision with heavy transport vehicle or bus in traffic accident

V04.13 Pedestrian on standing micro-mobility pedestrian conveyance injured in collision with heavy transport vehicle or bus in traffic accident

V04.131- Pedestrian on standing electric scooter injured in collision with heavy transport vehicle or bus in traffic accident

V04.138- Pedestrian on other standing micro-mobility pedestrian conveyance injured in collision with heavy transport vehicle or bus in traffic accident Pedestrian on hoverboard or segway injured in collision with heavy transport vehicle or bus intraffic accident

V04.19X- Pedestrian with other conveyance injured in collision with heavy transport vehicle or bus in traffic accident *Includes:* Pedestrian with baby stroller or on ice-skates or nonmotorized scooter or motorized mobility scooter or sled or snowboard or snow-skis or wheelchair (powered) injured

V04.9- Pedestrian injured in collision with heavy transport vehicle or bus, unspecified whether traffic or nontraffic accident *See External Cause of Injuries Table.*

V05 PEDESTRIAN INJURED IN COLLISION WITH RAILWAY TRAIN OR RAILWAY VEHICLE

See External Cause of Injuries Table.

V06 PEDESTRIAN INJURED IN COLLISION WITH OTHER NONMOTOR VEHICLE

Includes: collision with animal-drawn vehicle, animal being ridden, nonpowered streetcar

Excludes1: pedestrian injured in collision with pedestrian conveyance (V00.0-)

See External Cause of Injuries Table.

V09 PEDESTRIAN INJURED IN OTHER AND UNSPECIFIED TRANSPORT ACCIDENTS

See External Cause of Injuries Table.

(V10–V19) PEDAL CYCLE RIDER INJURED IN TRANSPORT ACCIDENT

Includes: any non-motorized vehicle, excluding an animal-drawn vehicle, or a sidecar or trailer attached to the pedal cycle

Excludes2: rupture of pedal cycle tire (W37.0)

V10–V18 require a 7th character
A—initial encounter
D—subsequent encounter
S—sequela

V10 PEDAL CYCLE RIDER INJURED IN COLLISION WITH PEDESTRIAN OR ANIMAL

Excludes1: pedal cycle rider collision with animal-drawn vehicle or animal being ridden (V16.-) *See External Cause of Injuries Table.*

V11 PEDAL CYCLE RIDER INJURED IN COLLISION WITH OTHER PEDAL CYCLE

See External Cause of Injuries Table.

V12 PEDAL CYCLE RIDER INJURED IN COLLISION WITH TWO- OR THREE-WHEELED MOTOR VEHICLE

See External Cause of Injuries Table.

V13 PEDAL CYCLE RIDER INJURED IN COLLISION WITH CAR, PICK-UP TRUCK OR VAN

See External Cause of Injuries Table.

V14 PEDAL CYCLE RIDER INJURED IN COLLISION WITH HEAVY TRANSPORT VEHICLE OR BUS

Excludes1: pedal cycle rider injured in collision with military vehicle (V19.81)

See External Cause of Injuries Table

V15 PEDAL CYCLE RIDER INJURED IN COLLISION WITH RAILWAY TRAIN OR RAILWAY VEHICLE

See External Cause of Injuries Table.

V16 PEDAL CYCLE RIDER INJURED IN COLLISION WITH OTHER NONMOTOR VEHICLE

Includes: collision with animal-drawn vehicle, animal being ridden, streetcar

See External Cause of Injuries Table.

V17 PEDAL CYCLE RIDER INJURED IN COLLISION WITH FIXED OR STATIONARY OBJECT

See External Cause of Injuries Table.

V18 PEDAL CYCLE RIDER INJURED IN NONCOLLISION TRANSPORT ACCIDENT

Includes: fall or thrown from pedal cycle (without antecedent collision) overturning pedal cycle NOS overturning pedal cycle without collision

V18.0XX- Pedal cycle driver injured in noncollision transport accident in nontraffic accident

V18.1XX- Pedal cycle passenger injured in noncollision transport accident in nontraffic accident

V18.2XX- Unspecified pedal cyclist injured in noncollision transport accident in nontraffic accident

V18.3XX- Person boarding or alighting a pedal cycle injured in noncollision transport accident

V18.4XX- Pedal cycle driver injured in noncollision transport accident in traffic accident

V18.5XX- Pedal cycle passenger injured in noncollision transport accident in traffic accident

V18.9XX- Unspecified pedal cyclist injured in noncollision transport accident in traffic accident

●=New Code
▲=Revised Code

Excludes1—Not coded here, do not use together
Excludes2—Not included here

TABULAR LIST — CHAPTER 20. EXTERNAL CAUSES OF MORBIDITY (V00–Y99)

V19 PEDAL CYCLE RIDER INJURED IN OTHER AND UNSPECIFIED TRANSPORT ACCIDENTS

V19 requires a 7th character
A—initial encounter
D—subsequent encounter
S—sequela

See External Cause of Injuries Table.

(V20–V29) MOTORCYCLE RIDER INJURED IN TRANSPORT ACCIDENT

Includes: moped
motorcycle with sidecar
motorized bicycle
motor scooter

V20–V29 require a 7th character
A—initial encounter
D—subsequent encounter
S—sequela

Excludes1: three-wheeled motor vehicle (V30–V39)

V20 MOTORCYCLE RIDER INJURED IN COLLISION WITH PEDESTRIAN OR ANIMAL

Excludes1: motorcycle rider collision with animal-drawn vehicle or animal being ridden (V26.-)
See External Cause of Injuries Table.

V21 MOTORCYCLE RIDER INJURED IN COLLISION WITH PEDAL CYCLE

Excludes1: motorcycle rider collision with animal-drawn vehicle or animal being ridden (V26.-)
See External Cause of Injuries Table.

V22 MOTORCYCLE RIDER INJURED IN COLLISION WITH TWO- OR THREE-WHEELED MOTOR VEHICLE

See External Cause of Injuries Table.

V23 MOTORCYCLE RIDER INJURED IN COLLISION WITH CAR, PICK-UP TRUCK OR VAN

See External Cause of Injuries Table.

V24 MOTORCYCLE RIDER INJURED IN COLLISION WITH HEAVY TRANSPORT VEHICLE OR BUS

Excludes1: motorcycle rider injured in collision with military vehicle (V29.81)
See External Cause of Injuries Table.

V25 MOTORCYCLE RIDER INJURED IN COLLISION WITH RAILWAY TRAIN OR RAILWAY VEHICLE

See External Cause of Injuries Table.

V26 MOTORCYCLE RIDER INJURED IN COLLISION WITH OTHER NONMOTOR VEHICLE

Includes: collision with animal-drawn vehicle, animal being ridden, streetcar
See External Cause of Injuries Table.

V27 MOTORCYCLE RIDER INJURED IN COLLISION WITH FIXED OR STATIONARY OBJECT

See External Cause of Injuries Table.

V28 MOTORCYCLE RIDER INJURED IN NONCOLLISION TRANSPORT ACCIDENT

Includes: fall or thrown from motorcycle (without antecedent collision)
overturning motorcycle NOS
overturning motorcycle without collision

- V28.0 Motorcycle driver injured in noncollision transport accident in nontraffic accident
  - V28.01X- Electric (assisted) bicycle driver injured in noncollision transport accident in nontraffic accident
  - V28.09X- Other motorcycle driver injured in noncollision transport accident in nontraffic accident
- V28.1 Motorcycle passenger injured in noncollision transport accident in nontraffic accident
  - V28.11X- Electric (assisted) bicycle passenger injured in noncollision transport accident in nontraffic accident
  - V28.19X- Other motorcycle passenger injured in noncollision transport accident in nontraffic accident
- V28.2 Unspecified motorcycle rider injured in noncollision transport accident in nontraffic accident
  - V28.21X- Unspecified electric (assisted) bicycle rider injured in noncollision transport accident in nontraffic accident
  - V28.29X- Unspecified rider of other motorcycle injured in

noncollision transport accident in nontraffic accident

- V28.3 Person boarding or alighting a motorcycle injured in noncollision transport accident
  - V28.31X- Person boarding or alighting an electric (assisted) bicycle injured in noncollision transport accident
  - V28.39X- Person boarding or alighting other motorcycle injured in noncollision transport accident
- V28.4 Motorcycle driver injured in noncollision transport accident in traffic accident
  - V28.41X- Electric (assisted) bicycle driver injured in noncollision transport accident in traffic accident
  - V28.49X- Other motorcycle driver injured in noncollision transport accident in traffic accident
- V28.5 Motorcycle passenger injured in noncollision transport accident in traffic accident
  - V28.51X- Electric (assisted) bicycle passenger injured in noncollision transport accident in traffic accident
  - V28.59X- Other motorcycle passenger injured in noncollision transport accident in traffic accident
- V28.9 Unspecified motorcycle rider injured in noncollision transport accident in traffic accident
  - V28.91X- Unspecified electric (assisted) bicycle rider injured in noncollision transport accident in traffic accident
  - V28.99X- Unspecified rider of other motorcycle injured in noncollision transport accident in traffic accident

V29 MOTORCYCLE RIDER INJURED IN OTHER AND UNSPECIFIED TRANSPORT ACCIDENTS

- V29.0 Motorcycle driver injured in collision with other and unspecified motor vehicles in nontraffic accident
  - V29.00 Motorcycle driver injured in collision with unspecified motor vehicles in nontraffic accident
    - V29.001- Electric (assisted) bicycle driver injured in collision with unspecified motor vehicles in nontraffic accident
    - V29.008- Other motorcycle driver injured in collision with unspecified motor vehicles in nontraffic accident
  - V29.09 Motorcycle driver injured in collision with other motor vehicles in nontraffic accident
    - V29.091- Electric (assisted) bicycle driver injured in collision with other motor vehicles in nontraffic accident
    - V29.098- Other motorcycle driver injured in collision with other motor vehicles in nontraffic accident
- V29.1 Motorcycle passenger injured in collision with other and unspecified motor vehicles in nontraffic accident
  - V29.10 Motorcycle passenger injured in collision with unspecified motor vehicles in nontraffic accident
    - V29.101- Electric (assisted) bicycle passenger injured in collision with unspecified motor vehicles in nontraffic accident
    - V29.108- Other motorcycle passenger injured in collision with unspecified motor vehicles in nontraffic accident
  - V29.19 Motorcycle passenger injured in collision with other motor vehicles in nontraffic accident
    - V29.191- Electric (assisted) bicycle passenger injured in collision with other motor vehicles in nontraffic accident
    - V29.198- Other motorcycle passenger injured in collision with other motor vehicles in nontraffic accident
- V29.2 Unspecified motorcycle rider injured in collision with other and unspecified motor vehicles in nontraffic accident
  - V29.20 Unspecified motorcycle rider injured in collision with unspecified motor vehicles in nontraffic accident
    Motorcycle collision NOS, nontraffic
    - V29.201- Unspecified electric (assisted) bicycle rider injured in collision with unspecified motor vehicles in nontraffic accident

●=New Code ▲=Revised Code

Excludes1—Not coded here, do not use together
Excludes2—Not included here

PEDIATRIC ICD-10-CM 2024: A MANUAL FOR PROVIDER-BASED CODING

V29.208- Unspecified rider of other motorcycle injured in collision with unspecified motor vehicles in nontraffic accident

V29 requires a 7th character
A—initial encounter
D—subsequent encounter
S—sequela

V29.29 Unspecified motorcycle rider injured in collision with other motor vehicles in nontraffic accident

V29.291- Unspecified electric (assisted) bicycle rider injured in collision with other motor vehicles in nontraffic accident

V29.298- Unspecified rider of other motorcycle injured in collision with other motor vehicles in nontraffic accident

V29.3 Motorcycle rider (driver) (passenger) injured in unspecified nontraffic accident

Motorcycle accident NOS, nontraffic
Motorcycle rider injured in nontraffic accident NOS

V29.31X- Electric (assisted) bicycle (driver) (passenger) injured in unspecified nontraffic accident

V29.39X- Other motorcycle (driver) (passenger) injured in unspecified nontraffic accident

V29.4 Motorcycle driver injured in collision with other and unspecified motor vehicles in traffic accident

V29.40 Motorcycle driver injured in collision with unspecified motor vehicles in traffic accident

V29.401- Electric (assisted) bicycle driver injured in collision with unspecified motor vehicles in traffic accident

V29.408- Other motorcycle driver injured in collision with unspecified motor vehicles in traffic accident

V29.49 Motorcycle driver injured in collision with other motor vehicles in traffic accident

V29.491- Electric (assisted) bicycle driver injured in collision with other motor vehicles in traffic accident

V29.498- Other motorcycle driver injured in collision with other motor vehicles in traffic accident

V29.5 Motorcycle passenger injured in collision with other and unspecified motor vehicles in traffic accident

V29.50 Motorcycle passenger injured in collision with unspecified motor vehicles in traffic accident

V29.501- Electric (assisted) bicycle passenger injured in collision with unspecified motor vehicles in traffic accident

V29.508- Other motorcycle passenger injured in collision with unspecified motor vehicles in traffic accident

V29.59 Motorcycle passenger injured in collision with other motor vehicles in traffic accident

V29.591- Electric (assisted) bicycle passenger injured in collision with other motor vehicles in traffic accident

V29.598- Other motorcycle passenger injured in collision with other motor vehicles in traffic accident

V29.6 Unspecified motorcycle rider injured in collision with other and unspecified motor vehicles in traffic accident

V29.60 Unspecified motorcycle rider injured in collision with unspecified motor vehicles in traffic accident
Motorcycle collision NOS (traffic)

V29.601- Unspecified electric (assisted) bicycle rider injured in collision with unspecified motor vehicles in traffic accident

V29.608- Unspecified rider of other motorcycle injured in collision with unspecified motor vehicles in traffic accident

V29.69 Unspecified motorcycle rider injured in collision with other motor vehicles in traffic accident

V29.691- Unspecified electric (assisted) bicycle rider injured in collision with other motor vehicles in traffic accident

V29.698- Unspecified rider of other motorcycle injured in collision with other motor vehicles in traffic accident

V29.8 Motorcycle rider (driver) (passenger) injured in other specified transport accidents

V29.81 Motorcycle rider (driver) (passenger) injured in transport accident with military vehicle

V29.811- Electric (assisted) bicycle rider (driver) (passenger) injured in transport accident with military vehicle

V29.818- Rider (driver) (passenger) of other motorcycle injured in transport accident with military vehicle

V29.88 Motorcycle rider (driver) (passenger) injured in other specified transport accidents

V29.881- Electric (assisted) bicycle rider (driver) (passenger) injured in other specified transport accidents

V29.888- Rider (driver) (passenger) of other motorcycle injured in other specified transport accidents

V29.9 Motorcycle rider (driver) (passenger) injured in unspecified traffic accident
Motorcycle accident NOS

V29.91X- Electric (assisted) bicycle rider (driver) (passenger) injured in unspecified traffic accident

V29.99X- Rider (driver) (passenger) of other motorcycle injured in unspecified traffic accident
Motorcycle accident NOS

(V30–V39) OCCUPANT OF THREE-WHEELED MOTOR VEHICLE INJURED IN TRANSPORT ACCIDENT

Includes: motorized tricycle
motorized rickshaw
three-wheeled motor car

V30–V35 require a 7th character
A—initial encounter
D—subsequent encounter
S—sequela

Excludes1: all-terrain vehicles (V86.-)
motorcycle with sidecar (V20–V29)
vehicle designed primarily for off-road use (V86.-)

V30 **OCCUPANT OF THREE-WHEELED MOTOR VEHICLE INJURED IN COLLISION WITH PEDESTRIAN OR ANIMAL**
Excludes1: three-wheeled motor vehicle collision with animal-drawn vehicle or animal being ridden (V36.-)
See External Cause of Injuries Table.

V31 **OCCUPANT OF THREE-WHEELED MOTOR VEHICLE INJURED IN COLLISION WITH PEDAL CYCLE**
See External Cause of Injuries Table.

V32 **OCCUPANT OF THREE-WHEELED MOTOR VEHICLE INJURED IN COLLISION WITH TWO- OR THREE-WHEELED MOTOR VEHICLE**
See External Cause of Injuries Table.

V33 **OCCUPANT OF THREE-WHEELED MOTOR VEHICLE INJURED IN COLLISION WITH CAR, PICK-UP TRUCK OR VAN**
See External Cause of Injuries Table.

V34 **OCCUPANT OF THREE-WHEELED MOTOR VEHICLE INJURED IN COLLISION WITH HEAVY TRANSPORT VEHICLE OR BUS**
Excludes1: occupant of three-wheeled motor vehicle injured in collision with military vehicle (V39.81)
See External Cause of Injuries Table.

V35 **OCCUPANT OF THREE-WHEELED MOTOR VEHICLE INJURED IN COLLISION WITH RAILWAY TRAIN OR RAILWAY VEHICLE**
See External Cause of Injuries Table.

V36 OCCUPANT OF THREE-WHEELED MOTOR VEHICLE INJURED IN COLLISION WITH OTHER NONMOTOR VEHICLE

7th

V36–V39 require a 7th character
A—initial encounter
D—subsequent encounter
S—sequela

Includes: collision with animal-drawn vehicle, animal being ridden, streetcar
See External Cause of Injuries Table.

V37 OCCUPANT OF THREE-WHEELED MOTOR VEHICLE INJURED IN COLLISION WITH FIXED OR STATIONARY OBJECT

7th

See External Cause of Injuries Table.

V38 OCCUPANT OF THREE-WHEELED MOTOR VEHICLE INJURED IN NONCOLLISION TRANSPORT ACCIDENT

4th

Includes: fall or thrown from three-wheeled motor vehicle overturning of three-wheeled motor vehicle NOS overturning of three-wheeled motor vehicle without collision

V38.0XX- Driver of three-wheeled motor vehicle injured in 7th noncollision transport accident in nontraffic accident

V38.1XX- Passenger in three-wheeled 7th motor vehicle injured in noncollision transport accident in nontraffic accident

V38.2XX- Person on outside of three-wheeled motor vehicle injured in 7th noncollision transport accident in nontraffic accident

V38.3XX- Unspecified occupant of three-wheeled motor vehicle 7th injured in noncollision transport accident in nontraffic accident

V38.4XX- Person boarding or alighting a three-wheeled motor vehicle 7th injured in noncollision transport accident

V38.5XX- Driver of three-wheeled motor vehicle injured in 7th noncollision transport accident in traffic accident

V38.6XX- Passenger in three-wheeled motor vehicle injured in 7th noncollision transport accident in traffic accident

V38.7XX- Person on outside of three-wheeled motor vehicle injured in 7th noncollision transport accident in traffic accident

V38.9XX- Unspecified occupant of three-wheeled motor vehicle 7th injured in noncollision transport accident in traffic accident

V39 OCCUPANT OF THREE-WHEELED MOTOR VEHICLE INJURED IN OTHER AND UNSPECIFIED TRANSPORT ACCIDENTS

4th

V39.0 Driver of three-wheeled motor vehicle injured in collision with 5th other and unspecified motor vehicles in nontraffic accident

V39.00X- Driver of three-wheeled motor vehicle injured 7th in collision with unspecified motor vehicles in nontraffic accident

V39.09X- Driver of three-wheeled motor vehicle injured in 7th collision with other motor vehicles in nontraffic accident

V39.1 Passenger in three-wheeled motor vehicle injured in collision 5th with other and unspecified motor vehicles in nontraffic accident

V39.10X- Passenger in three-wheeled motor vehicle injured 7th in collision with unspecified motor vehicles in nontraffic accident

V39.19X- Passenger in three-wheeled motor vehicle injured 7th in collision with other motor vehicles in nontraffic accident

V39.2 Unspecified occupant of three-wheeled motor vehicle injured 5th in accident

V39.20X- Unspecified occupant of three-wheeled motor 7th vehicle injured in collision with unspecified motor vehicles in nontraffic accident Collision NOS involving three-wheeled motor vehicle, nontraffic

V39.29X- Unspecified occupant of three-wheeled 7th

V39.3XX- Occupant (driver) (passenger) of three-wheeled motor 7th vehicle injured in unspecified nontraffic accident Accident NOS involving three-wheeled motor vehicle, nontraffic Occupant of three-wheeled motor vehicle injured in nontraffic accident NOS

V39.4 Driver of three-wheeled motor vehicle injured in collision with 5th other and unspecified motor vehicles in traffic accident

V39.40X- Driver of three-wheeled motor vehicle injured in 7th collision with unspecified motor vehicles in traffic accident

V39.49X- Driver of three-wheeled motor vehicle injured in 7th collision with other motor vehicles in traffic accident

V39.5 Passenger in three-wheeled motor vehicle injured in collision 5th with other and unspecified motor vehicles in traffic accident

V39.50X- Passenger in three-wheeled motor vehicle injured in 7th collision with unspecified motor vehicles in traffic accident

V39.59X- Passenger in three-wheeled motor vehicle injured in 7th collision with other motor vehicles in traffic accident

V39.6 Unspecified occupant of three-wheeled motor vehicle injured 5th in collision with other and unspecified motor vehicles in traffic accident

V39.60X- Unspecified occupant of three-wheeled motor 7th vehicle injured in collision with unspecified motor vehicles in traffic accident Collision NOS involving three-wheeled motor vehicle (traffic)

V39.69X- Unspecified occupant of three-wheeled motor 7th vehicle injured in collision with other motor vehicles in traffic accident

V39.8 Occupant (driver) (passenger) of three-wheeled motor vehicle 5th injured in other specified transport accidents

V39.81X- Occupant (driver) (passenger) of three-wheeled 7th motor vehicle injured in transport accident with military vehicle

V39.89X- Occupant (driver) 7th (passenger) of three-wheeled motor vehicle injured in other specified transport accidents

V39.9XX- Occupant (driver) (passenger) of three-wheeled motor 7th vehicle injured in unspecified traffic accident Accident NOS involving three-wheeled motor vehicle

(V40–V49) CAR OCCUPANT INJURED IN TRANSPORT ACCIDENT

Includes: a four-wheeled motor vehicle designed primarily for carrying passengers automobile (pulling a trailer or camper)

Excludes1: bus (V50–V59) minibus (V50–V59) minivan (V50–V59) motorcoach (V70–V79) pick-up truck (V50–V59) sport utility vehicle (SUV) (V50–V59)

V40–V43 require a 7th character
A—initial encounter
D—subsequent encounter
S—sequela

V40 CAR OCCUPANT INJURED IN COLLISION WITH PEDESTRIAN OR ANIMAL

7th

Excludes1: car collision with animal-drawn vehicle or animal being ridden (V46.-)
See External Cause of Injuries Table.

V41 CAR OCCUPANT INJURED IN COLLISION WITH PEDAL CYCLE

7th

See External Cause of Injuries Table.

V42 CAR OCCUPANT INJURED IN COLLISION WITH TWO- OR THREE-WHEELED MOTOR VEHICLE

7th

See External Cause of Injuries Table.

V43 CAR OCCUPANT INJURED IN COLLISION WITH CAR, PICK-UP TRUCK OR VAN

4th

V43.0 Car driver injured in collision with car, pick-up truck or van in 5th nontraffic accident

V43.01X- Car driver injured in collision with sport utility 7th vehicle in nontraffic accident

V43.02X- Car driver injured in collision with other type car in 7th nontraffic accident

V43.03X- Car driver injured in collision with pick-up truck in 7th nontraffic accident

V43.04X- Car driver injured in collision with van in nontraffic 7th accident

4th 5th 6th 7th Additional Character Required ✓ 3-character code

●=New Code ▲=Revised Code *Excludes1*—Not coded here, do not use together *Excludes2*—Not included here

V43.1 Car passenger injured in collision with car, pick-up truck or van in nontraffic accident

V43.11X- Car passenger injured in collision with sport utility vehicle in nontraffic accident

V43.12X- Car passenger injured in collision with other type car in nontraffic accident

V43.13X- Car passenger injured in collision with pick-up in nontraffic accident

V43.14X- Car passenger injured in collision with van in nontraffic accident

V43.2 Person on outside of car injured in collision with car, pick-up truck or van in nontraffic accident

V43.21X- Person on outside of car injured in collision with sport utility vehicle in nontraffic accident

V43.22X- Person on outside of car injured in collision with other type car in nontraffic accident

V43.23X- Person on outside of car injured in collision with pick-up truck in nontraffic accident

V43.24X- Person on outside of car injured in collision with van in nontraffic accident

V43.3 Unspecified car occupant injured in collision with car, pick-up truck or van in nontraffic accident

V43.31X- Unspecified car occupant injured in collision with sport utility vehicle in nontraffic accident

V43.32X- Unspecified car occupant injured in collision with other type car in nontraffic accident

V43.33X- Unspecified car occupant injured in collision with pick-up truck in nontraffic accident

V43.34X- Unspecified car occupant injured in collision with van in nontraffic accident

V43.4 Person boarding or alighting a car injured in collision with car, pick-up truck or van

V43.41X- Person boarding or alighting a car injured in collision with sport utility vehicle, initial encounter

V43.42X- Person boarding or alighting a car injured in collision with other type car

V43.43X- Person boarding or alighting a car injured in collision with pick-up truck

V43.44X- Person boarding or alighting a car injured in collision with van

V43.5 Car driver injured in collision with car, pick-up truck or van in traffic accident

V43.51X- Car driver injured in collision with sport utility vehicle in traffic accident

V43.52X- Car driver injured in collision with other type car in traffic accident

V43.53X- Car driver injured in collision with pick-up truck in traffic accident

V43.54X- Car driver injured in collision with van in traffic accident

V43.6 Car passenger injured in collision with car, pick-up truck or van in traffic accident

V43.61X- Car passenger injured in collision with sport utility vehicle in traffic accident

V43.62X- Car passenger injured in collision with other type car in traffic accident

V43.63X- Car passenger injured in collision with pick-up truck in traffic accident

V43.64X- Car passenger injured in collision with van in traffic accident

V43.7 Person on outside of car injured in collision with car, pick-up truck or van in traffic accident

V43.71X- Person on outside of car injured in collision with sport utility vehicle in traffic accident

V43.72X- Person on outside of car injured in collision with other type car in traffic accident

V43.73X- Person on outside of car injured in collision with pick-up truck in traffic accident

V43.74X- Person on outside of car injured in collision with van in traffic accident

V43.9 Unspecified car occupant injured in collision with car, pick-up truck or van in traffic accident

V43.91X- Unspecified car occupant injured in collision with sport utility vehicle in traffic accident

V43.92X- Unspecified car occupant injured in collision with other type car in traffic accident

V43.93X- Unspecified car occupant injured in collision with pick-up truck in traffic accident

V43.94X- Unspecified car occupant injured in collision with van in traffic accident

V44 CAR OCCUPANT INJURED IN COLLISION WITH HEAVY TRANSPORT VEHICLE OR BUS

Excludes1: car occupant injured in collision with military vehicle (V49.81) *See External Cause of Injuries Table.*

V45 CAR OCCUPANT INJURED IN COLLISION WITH RAILWAY TRAIN OR RAILWAY VEHICLE

See External Cause of Injuries Table.

V46 CAR OCCUPANT INJURED IN COLLISION WITH OTHER NONMOTOR VEHICLE

Includes: collision with animal-drawn vehicle, animal being ridden, streetcar *See External Cause of Injuries Table.*

V47 CAR OCCUPANT INJURED IN COLLISION WITH FIXED OR STATIONARY OBJECT

See External Cause of Injuries Table.

V48 CAR OCCUPANT INJURED IN NONCOLLISION TRANSPORT ACCIDENT

Includes: overturning car NOS overturning car without collision

V48.0XX- Car driver injured in noncollision transport accident in nontraffic accident

V48.1XX- Car passenger injured in noncollision transport accident in nontraffic accident

V48.2XX- Person on outside of car injured in noncollision transport accident in nontraffic accident

V48.3XX- Unspecified car occupant injured in noncollision transport accident in nontraffic accident

V48.4XX- Person boarding or alighting a car injured in noncollision transport accident

V48.5XX- Car driver injured in noncollision transport accident in traffic accident

V48.6XX- Car passenger injured in noncollision transport accident in traffic accident

V48.7XX- Person on outside of car injured in noncollision transport accident in traffic accident

V48.9XX- Unspecified car occupant injured in noncollision transport accident in traffic accident

V49 CAR OCCUPANT INJURED IN OTHER AND UNSPECIFIED TRANSPORT ACCIDENTS

V49.0 Driver injured in collision with other and unspecified motor vehicles in nontraffic accident

V49.00X- Driver injured in collision with unspecified motor vehicles in nontraffic accident

V49.09X- Driver injured in collision with other motor vehicles in nontraffic accident

V49.1 Passenger injured in collision with other and unspecified motor vehicles in nontraffic accident

V49.10X- Passenger injured in collision with unspecified motor vehicles in nontraffic accident

V49.19X- Passenger injured in collision with other motor vehicles in nontraffic accident

V49.2 Unspecified car occupant injured in collision with other and unspecified motor vehicles in nontraffic accident

V49.20X- Unspecified car occupant injured in collision with unspecified motor vehicles in nontraffic accident Car collision NOS, nontraffic

V49.29X- Unspecified car occupant injured in collision with other motor vehicles in nontraffic accident

V49.3XX- Car occupant (driver) (passenger) injured in unspecified nontraffic accident

V49 requires a 7th character
A—initial encounter
D—subsequent encounter
S—sequela

Car accident NOS, nontraffic
Car occupant injured in nontraffic accident NOS

V49.4 Driver injured in collision with other and unspecified motor vehicles in traffic accident

V49.40X- Driver injured in collision with unspecified motor vehicles in traffic accident

V49.49X- Driver injured in collision with other motor vehicles in traffic accident

V49.5 Passenger injured in collision with other and unspecified motor vehicles in traffic accident

V49.50X- Passenger injured in collision with unspecified motor vehicles in traffic accident

V49.59X- Passenger injured in collision with other motor vehicles in traffic accident

V49.6 Unspecified car occupant injured in collision with other and unspecified motor vehicles in traffic accident

V49.60X- Unspecified car occupant injured in collision with other and unspecified motor vehicles in traffic accident

Car collision NOS (traffic)

V49.69X- Unspecified car occupant injured in collision with other motor vehicles in traffic accident

V49.8 Car occupant (driver) (passenger) injured in other specified transport accidents

V49.81X- Car occupant (driver) (passenger) injured in transport accident with military vehicle

V49.88X- Car occupant (driver) (passenger) injured in other specified transport accidents

V49.9XX- Car occupant (driver) (passenger) injured in unspecified traffic accident

Car accident NOS

(V50–V59) OCCUPANT OF PICK-UP TRUCK OR VAN OR SUV INJURED IN TRANSPORT ACCIDENT

Includes: a four or six wheel motor vehicle designed primarily for carrying passengers and property but weighing less than the local limit for classification as a heavy goods vehicle
Minibus, minivan, sport utility vehicle (SUV), truck, van

V50–V59 require a 7th character
A—initial encounter
D—subsequent encounter
S—sequela

Excludes1: heavy transport vehicle (V60–V69)

V50 OCCUPANT OF PICK-UP TRUCK OR VAN OR SUV INJURED IN COLLISION WITH PEDESTRIAN OR ANIMAL

Excludes1: pick-up truck or van collision with animal-drawn vehicle or animal being ridden (V56.-)
See External Cause of Injuries Table.

V51 OCCUPANT OF PICK-UP TRUCK OR VAN INJURED IN COLLISION WITH PEDAL CYCLE

See External Cause of Injuries Table.

V52 OCCUPANT OF PICK-UP TRUCK OR VAN OR SUV INJURED IN COLLISION WITH TWO- OR THREE-WHEELED MOTOR VEHICLE

See External Cause of Injuries Table.

V53 OCCUPANT OF PICK-UP TRUCK OR VAN OR SUV INJURED IN COLLISION WITH CAR, PICK-UP TRUCK OR VAN

See External Cause of Injuries Table.

V54 OCCUPANT OF PICK-UP TRUCK OR VAN OR SUV INJURED IN COLLISION WITH HEAVY TRANSPORT VEHICLE OR BUS

Excludes1: occupant of pick-up truck or van injured in collision with military vehicle (V59.81)
See External Cause of Injuries Table.

V55 OCCUPANT OF PICK-UP TRUCK OR VAN OR SUV INJURED IN COLLISION WITH RAILWAY TRAIN OR RAILWAY VEHICLE

See External Cause of Injuries Table.

V56 OCCUPANT OF PICK-UP TRUCK OR VAN INJURED IN COLLISION WITH OTHER NONMOTOR VEHICLE

Includes: collision with animal-drawn vehicle, animal being ridden, streetcar
See External Cause of Injuries Table.

V57 OCCUPANT OF PICK-UP TRUCK OR VAN OR SUV INJURED IN COLLISION WITH FIXED OR STATIONARY OBJECT

See External Cause of Injuries Table.

V58 OCCUPANT OF PICK-UP TRUCK OR VAN OR SUV INJURED IN NONCOLLISION TRANSPORT ACCIDENT

Includes: overturning pick-up truck or van NOS overturning pick-up truck or van without collision

V58.0XX- Driver of pick-up truck or van injured in noncollision transport accident in nontraffic accident

V58.1XX- Passenger in pick-up truck or van injured in noncollision transport accident in nontraffic accident

V58.2XX- Person on outside of pick-up truck or van injured in noncollision transport accident in nontraffic accident

V58.3XX- Unspecified occupant of pick-up truck or van injured in noncollision transport accident in nontraffic accident

V58.4XX- Person boarding or alighting a pick-up truck or van injured in a noncollision transport accident

V58.5XX- Driver of pick-up truck or van injured in noncollision transport accident in traffic accident

V58.6XX- Passenger in pick-up truck or van injured in noncollision transport accident in traffic accident

V58.7XX- Person on outside of pick-up truck or van injured in noncollision transport accident in traffic accident

V58.9XX- Unspecified occupant of pick-up truck or van injured in noncollision transport accident in traffic accident

V59 OCCUPANT OF PICK-UP TRUCK OR VAN OR SUV INJURED IN OTHER AND UNSPECIFIED TRANSPORT ACCIDENTS

V59.0 Driver of pick-up truck or van injured in collision with other and unspecified motor vehicles in nontraffic accident

V59.00X- Driver of pick-up truck or van injured in collision with unspecified motor vehicles in nontraffic accident

V59.09X- Driver of pick-up truck or van injured in collision with other motor vehicles in nontraffic accident

V59.1 Passenger in pick-up truck or van injured in collision with other and unspecified motor vehicles in nontraffic accident

V59.10X- Passenger in pick-up truck or van injured in collision with unspecified motor vehicles in nontraffic accident

V59.19X- Passenger in pick-up truck or van injured in collision with other motor vehicles in nontraffic accident

V59.2 Unspecified occupant of pick-up truck or van injured in collision with other and unspecified motor vehicles in nontraffic accident

V59.20X- Unspecified occupant of pick-up truck or van injured in collision with unspecified motor vehicles in nontraffic accident

Collision NOS involving pick-up truck or van, nontraffic

V59.29X- Unspecified occupant of pick-up truck or van injured in collision with other motor vehicles in nontraffic accident

V59.3XX- Occupant (driver) (passenger) of pick-up truck or van injured in unspecified nontraffic accident

Accident NOS involving pick-up truck or van, nontraffic
Occupant of pick-up truck or van injured in nontraffic accident NOS

V59.4 Driver of pick-up truck or van injured in collision with other and unspecified motor vehicles in traffic accident

V59.40X- Driver of pick-up truck or van injured in collision with unspecified motor vehicles in traffic accident

V59.49X- Driver of pick-up truck or van injured in collision with other motor vehicles in traffic accident

V59 requires a 7th character
A—initial encounter
D—subsequent encounter
S—sequela

V59.5 Passenger in pick-up truck or van injured in collision with other and unspecified motor vehicles in traffic accident

V59.50X- Passenger in pick-up truck or van injured in collision with unspecified motor vehicles in traffic accident

V59.59X- Passenger in pick-up truck or van injured in collision with other motor vehicles in traffic accident

V59.6 Unspecified occupant of pick-up truck or van injured in collision with other and unspecified motor vehicles in traffic accident

V59.60X- Unspecified occupant of pick-up truck or van injured in collision with unspecified motor vehicles in traffic accident
Collision NOS involving pick-up truck or van (traffic)

V59.69X- Unspecified occupant of pick-up truck or van injured in collision with other motor vehicles in traffic accident

V59.8 Occupant (driver) (passenger) of pick-up truck or van injured in other specified transport accidents

V59.81X- Occupant (driver) (passenger) of pick-up truck or van injured in transport accident with military vehicle

V59.88X- Occupant (driver) (passenger) of pick-up truck or van injured in other specified transport accidents

V59.9XX- Occupant (driver) (passenger) of pick-up truck or van injured in unspecified traffic accident
Accident NOS involving pick-up truck or van

(V60-V69) OCCUPANT OF HEAVY TRANSPORT VEHICLE INJURED IN TRANSPORT ACCIDENT

V60 **OCCUPANT OF HEAVY TRANSPORT VEHICLE INJURED IN COLLISION WITH PEDESTRIAN OR ANIMAL**

Excludes1: heavy transport vehicle collision with animal-drawn vehicle or animal being ridden (V66.-)

See complete *ICD-10-CM* manual for codes in category V60.

V60-V69 require a 7th character
A—initial encounter
D—subsequent encounter
S—sequela

V61 **OCCUPANT OF HEAVY TRANSPORT VEHICLE INJURED IN COLLISION WITH PEDAL CYCLE**

See complete *ICD-10-CM* manual for codes in category V61.

V62 **OCCUPANT OF HEAVY TRANSPORT VEHICLE INJURED IN COLLISION WITH TWO- OR THREE-WHEELED MOTOR VEHICLE**

See complete *ICD-10-CM* manual for codes in category V62.

V63 **OCCUPANT OF HEAVY TRANSPORT VEHICLE INJURED IN COLLISION WITH CAR, PICK-UP TRUCK OR VAN**

See complete *ICD-10-CM* manual for codes in category V63.

V64 **OCCUPANT OF HEAVY TRANSPORT VEHICLE INJURED IN COLLISION WITH HEAVY TRANSPORT VEHICLE OR BUS**

Excludes1: occupant of heavy transport vehicle injured in collision with military vehicle (V69.81)

See complete *ICD-10-CM* manual for codes in category V64.

V65 **OCCUPANT OF HEAVY TRANSPORT VEHICLE INJURED IN COLLISION WITH RAILWAY TRAIN OR RAILWAY VEHICLE**

See complete *ICD-10-CM* manual for codes in category V65.

V66 **OCCUPANT OF HEAVY TRANSPORT VEHICLE INJURED IN COLLISION WITH OTHER NONMOTOR VEHICLE**

Includes: collision with animal-drawn vehicle, animal being ridden, streetcar

See complete *ICD-10-CM* manual for codes in category V66.

V67 **OCCUPANT OF HEAVY TRANSPORT VEHICLE INJURED IN COLLISION WITH FIXED OR STATIONARY OBJECT**

See complete *ICD-10-CM* manual for codes in category V67.

V68 **OCCUPANT OF HEAVY TRANSPORT VEHICLE INJURED IN NONCOLLISION TRANSPORT ACCIDENT**

Includes: overturning heavy transport vehicle NOS overturning heavy transport vehicle without collision

See complete *ICD-10-CM* manual for codes in category V68

V69 **OCCUPANT OF HEAVY TRANSPORT VEHICLE INJURED IN OTHER AND UNSPECIFIED TRANSPORT ACCIDENTS**

See complete *ICD-10-CM* manual for codes in category V69

(V70-V79) BUS OCCUPANT INJURED IN TRANSPORT ACCIDENT

Includes: motorcoach
Excludes1: minibus (V50-V59)

V70-V78 require a 7th character
A—initial encounter
D—subsequent encounter
S—sequela

V70 **BUS OCCUPANT INJURED IN COLLISION WITH PEDESTRIAN OR ANIMAL**

Excludes1: bus collision with animal-drawn vehicle or animal being ridden (V76.-)

See External Cause of Injuries Table.

V71 **BUS OCCUPANT INJURED IN COLLISION WITH PEDAL CYCLE**

See External Cause of Injuries Table.

V72 **BUS OCCUPANT INJURED IN COLLISION WITH TWO- OR THREE-WHEELED MOTOR VEHICLE**

See External Cause of Injuries Table.

V73 **BUS OCCUPANT INJURED IN COLLISION WITH CAR, PICK-UP TRUCK OR VAN**

See External Cause of Injuries Table.

V74 **BUS OCCUPANT INJURED IN COLLISION WITH HEAVY TRANSPORT VEHICLE OR BUS**

Excludes1: bus occupant injured in collision with military vehicle (V79.81)

See External Cause of Injuries Table.

V75 **BUS OCCUPANT INJURED IN COLLISION WITH RAILWAY TRAIN OR RAILWAY VEHICLE**

See External Cause of Injuries Table.

V76 **BUS OCCUPANT INJURED IN COLLISION WITH OTHER NONMOTOR VEHICLE**

See External Cause of Injuries Table.

V77 **BUS OCCUPANT INJURED IN COLLISION WITH FIXED OR STATIONARY OBJECT**

See External Cause of Injuries Table.

V78 **BUS OCCUPANT INJURED IN NONCOLLISION TRANSPORT ACCIDENT**

Includes: overturning bus NOS overturning bus without collision

V78.0XX- Driver of bus injured in noncollision transport accident in nontraffic accident

V78.1XX- Passenger on bus injured in noncollision transport accident in nontraffic accident

V78.2XX- Person on outside of bus injured in noncollision transport accident in nontraffic accident

V78.3XX- Unspecified occupant of bus injured in noncollision transport accident in nontraffic accident

V78.4XX- Person boarding or alighting from bus injured in noncollision transport accident

V78.5XX- Driver of bus injured in noncollision transport accident in traffic accident

V78.6XX- Passenger on bus injured in noncollision transport accident in traffic accident

V78.7XX- Person on outside of bus injured in noncollision transport accident in traffic accident

V78.9XX- Unspecified occupant of bus injured in noncollision transport accident in traffic accident

V79 BUS OCCUPANT INJURED IN OTHER AND UNSPECIFIED TRANSPORT ACCIDENTS

V79 requires a 7th character
A—initial encounter
D—subsequent encounter
S—sequela

V79.0 Driver of bus injured in collision with other and unspecified motor vehicles in nontraffic accident

V79.00X- Driver of bus injured in collision with unspecified motor vehicles in nontraffic accident

V79.09X- Driver of bus injured in collision with other motor vehicles in nontraffic accident

V79.1 Passenger on bus injured in collision with other and unspecified motor vehicles in nontraffic accident

V79.10X- Passenger on bus injured in collision with unspecified motor vehicles in nontraffic accident

V79.19X- Passenger on bus injured in collision with other motor vehicles in nontraffic accident

V79.2 Unspecified bus occupant injured in collision with other and unspecified motor vehicles in nontraffic accident

V79.20X- Unspecified bus occupant injured in collision with unspecified motor vehicles in nontraffic accident

V79.29X- Unspecified bus occupant injured in collision with other motor vehicles in nontraffic accident

V79.3XX- Bus occupant (driver) (passenger) injured in unspecified nontraffic accident
Bus accident NOS, nontraffic
Bus occupant injured in nontraffic accident NOS

V79.4 Driver of bus injured in collision with other and unspecified motor vehicles in traffic accident

V79.40X- Driver of bus injured in collision with unspecified motor vehicles in traffic accident

V79.49X- Driver of bus injured in collision with other motor vehicles in traffic accident

V79.5 Passenger on bus injured in collision with other and unspecified motor vehicles in traffic accident

V79.50X- Passenger on bus injured in collision with unspecified motor vehicles in traffic accident

V79.59X- Passenger on bus injured in collision with other motor vehicles in traffic accident

V79.6 Unspecified bus occupant injured in collision with other and unspecified motor vehicles in traffic accident

V79.60X- Unspecified bus occupant injured in collision with unspecified motor vehicles in traffic accident
Bus collision NOS (traffic)

V79.69X- Unspecified bus occupant injured in collision with other motor vehicles in traffic accident

V79.8 Bus occupant (driver) (passenger) injured in other specified transport accidents

V79.81X- Bus occupant (driver) (passenger) injured in transport accidents with military vehicle

V79.88X- Bus occupant (driver) (passenger) injured in other specified transport accidents

V79.9XX- Bus occupant (driver) (passenger) injured in unspecified traffic accident
Bus accident NOS

(V80–V89) OTHER LAND TRANSPORT ACCIDENTS

V80 ANIMAL-RIDER OR OCCUPANT OF ANIMAL-DRAWN VEHICLE INJURED IN TRANSPORT ACCIDENT

V80 requires a 7th character
A—initial encounter
D—subsequent encounter
S—sequela

V80.0 Animal-rider or occupant of animal-drawn vehicle injured by fall from or being thrown from animal or animal-drawn vehicle in noncollision accident

V80.01 Animal-rider injured by fall from or being thrown from animal in noncollision accident

V80.010- Animal-rider injured by fall from or being thrown from horse in noncollision accident

V80.018- Animal-rider injured by fall from or being thrown from other animal in noncollision accident

V80.02X- Occupant of animal-drawn vehicle injured by fall from or being thrown from animal-drawn vehicle in noncollision accident
Overturning animal-drawn vehicle NOS
Overturning animal-drawn vehicle without collision

V80.1 Animal-rider or occupant of animal-drawn vehicle injured in collision with pedestrian or animal

Excludes1: animal-rider or animal-drawn vehicle collision with animal-drawn vehicle or animal being ridden (V80.7)

V80.11X- Animal-rider injured in collision with pedestrian or animal

V80.12X- Occupant of animal-drawn vehicle injured in collision with pedestrian or animal

V80.4 Animal-rider or occupant of animal-drawn vehicle injured in collision with car, pick-up truck, van, heavy transport vehicle or bus

Excludes1: animal-rider injured in collision with military vehicle (V80.910)
occupant of animal-drawn vehicle injured in collision with military vehicle (V80.920)

V80.41X- Animal-rider injured in collision with car, pick-up truck, van, heavy transport vehicle or bus

V80.42X- Occupant of animal-drawn vehicle injured in collision with car, pick-up truck, van, heavy transport vehicle or bus

V80.7 Animal-rider or occupant of animal-drawn vehicle injured in collision with other nonmotor vehicles

V80.71 Animal-rider or occupant of animal-drawn vehicle injured in collision with animal being ridden

V80.710- Animal-rider injured in collision with other animal being ridden

V80.711- Occupant of animal-drawn vehicle injured in collision with animal being ridden

V80.72 Animal-rider or occupant of animal-drawn vehicle injured in collision with other animal-drawnvehicle

V80.720- Animal-rider injured in collision with animal-drawn vehicle

V80.721- Occupant of animal-drawn vehicle injured in collision with other animal-drawn vehicle

V80.73 Animal-rider or occupant of animal-drawn vehicle injured in collision with streetcar

V80.730- Animal-rider injured in collision with streetcar

V80.731- Occupant of animal-drawn vehicle injured in collision with streetcar

V80.79 Animal-rider or occupant of animal-drawn vehicle injured in collision with other nonmotorvehicles

V80.790- Animal-rider injured in collision with other nonmotor vehicles

V80.791- Occupant of animal-drawn vehicle injured in collision with other nonmotor vehicles

V80.8 Animal-rider or occupant of animal-drawn vehicle injured in collision with fixed or stationary object

V80.81X- Animal-rider injured in collision with fixed or stationary object

V80.82X- Occupant of animal-drawn vehicle injured in collision with fixed or stationary object

V80.9 Animal-rider or occupant of animal-drawn vehicle injured in other and unspecified transport accidents

V80.91 Animal-rider injured in other and unspecified transport accidents

V80.918- Animal-rider injured in other transport accident

V80.919- Animal-rider injured in unspecified transport accident
Animal rider accident NOS

V80.92 Occupant of animal-drawn vehicle injured in other and unspecified transport accidents

V80.928- Occupant of animal-drawn vehicle injured in other transport accident

V80.929- Occupant of animal-drawn vehicle injured in unspecified transport accident
Animal-drawn vehicle accident NOS

V81 OCCUPANT OF RAILWAY TRAIN OR RAILWAY VEHICLE INJURED IN TRANSPORT ACCIDENT

Includes: derailment of railway train or railway vehicle
person on outside of train

Excludes1: streetcar (V82.-)

See complete *ICD-10-CM* manual for codes in category V81.

V82 OCCUPANT OF POWERED STREETCAR INJURED IN TRANSPORT ACCIDENT

Includes: interurban electric car
person on outside of streetcar
tram (car)
trolley (car)

Excludes1: bus (V70–V79)
motorcoach (V70–V79)
nonpowered streetcar (V76.-)
train (V81.-)

See complete *ICD-10-CM* manual for codes in category V82.

V83 OCCUPANT OF SPECIAL VEHICLE MAINLY USED ON INDUSTRIAL PREMISES INJURED IN TRANSPORT ACCIDENT

Includes: battery-powered airport passenger vehicle
battery-powered truck (baggage) (mail)
coal-car in mine
forklift (truck)
logging car
self-propelled industrial truck
station baggage truck (powered)
tram, truck, or tub (powered) in mine or quarry

Excludes1: special construction vehicles (V85.-)
special industrial vehicle in stationary use or maintenance (W31.-)

See complete *ICD-10-CM* manual for codes in category V83.

V84 OCCUPANT OF SPECIAL VEHICLE MAINLY USED IN AGRICULTURE INJURED IN TRANSPORT ACCIDENT

Includes: self-propelled farm machinery
tractor (and trailer)

Excludes1: animal-powered farm machinery accident (W30.8-)
contact with combine harvester (W30.0)
special agricultural vehicle in stationary use or maintenance (W30.-)

See External Cause of Injuries Table.

V86 OCCUPANT OF SPECIAL ALL-TERRAIN OR OTHER OFF-ROAD MOTOR VEHICLE, INJURED IN TRANSPORT ACCIDENT

Excludes1: special all-terrain vehicle in stationary use or maintenance (W31.-)
sport-utility vehicle (V50–V59)
three-wheeled motor vehicle designed for on-road use (V30–V39)

V86.0 Driver of special all-terrain or other off-road motor vehicle injured in traffic accident

V86.02X- Driver of snowmobile injured in traffic accident

V86.03X- Driver of dune buggy injured in traffic accident

V86.05X- Driver of 3- or 4- wheeled all-terrain vehicle (ATV) injured in traffic accident

V86.06X- Driver of dirt bike or motor/cross bike injured in traffic accident

V86.09X- Driver of other special all-terrain or other off-road motor vehicle injured in traffic accident
Driver of go cart injured in traffic accident
Driver of golf cart injured in traffic accident

V86.1 Passenger of special all-terrain or other off-road motor vehicle injured in traffic accident

V86.12X- Passenger of snowmobile injured in traffic accident

V86.13X- Passenger of dune buggy injured in traffic accident

V86.15X- Passenger of 3- or 4- wheeled ATV injured in traffic accident

V86.16X- Passenger of dirt bike or motor/cross bike injured in traffic accident

V86.19X- Passenger of other special all-terrain or other off-road motor vehicle injured in traffic accident
Passenger of go cart injured in traffic accident
Passenger of golf cart injured in traffic accident

V86.3 Unspecified occupant of special all-terrain or other off-road motor vehicle injured in traffic accident

V86.32X- Unspecific occupant of snowmobile injured in traffic accident

V86.33X- Unspecified occupant of dune buggy injured in traffic accident

V86.35X- Unspecified occupant of 3- or 4- wheeled ATV injured in traffic accident

V86.36X- Unspecified occupant of dirt bike or motor/cross bike injured in traffic accident

V86.39X- Unspecified occupant of other special all-terrain or other off-road motor vehicle injured in traffic accident
Person in go cart or golf cart injured in traffic accident

V86.5 Driver of special all-terrain or other off-road motor vehicle injured in nontraffic accident

V86.52X- Driver of snowmobile injured in nontraffic accident

V86.53X- Driver of dune buggy injured in nontraffic accident

V86.55X- Driver of 3- or 4- wheeled ATV injured in nontraffic accident

V86.56X- Driver of dirt bike or motor/cross bike injured in nontraffic accident

V86.59X- Driver of other special all-terrain or other off-road motor vehicle injured in nontraffic accident
Driver of go cart or golf cart injured in nontraffic accident

V86.6 Passenger of special all-terrain or other off-road motor vehicle injured in nontraffic accident

V86.62X- Passenger of snowmobile injured in nontraffic accident

V86.63X- Passenger of dune buggy injured in nontraffic accident

V86.65X- Passenger of 3- or 4- wheeled ATV injured in nontraffic accident

V86.66X- Passenger of dirt bike or motor/cross bike injured in nontraffic accident

V86.69X- Passenger of other special all-terrain or other off-road motor vehicle injured in nontraffic accident
Passenger of go cart or golf cart injured in nontraffic accident

V86.9 Unspecified occupant of special all-terrain or other off-road motor vehicle injured in nontraffic accident

V86.92X- Unspecific occupant of snowmobile injured in nontraffic accident

V86.93X- Unspecified occupant of dune buggy injured in nontraffic accident

V86.95X- Unspecified occupant of 3- or 4- wheeled ATV injured in nontraffic accident

V86.96X- Unspecified occupant of dirt bike or motor/cross bike injured in nontraffic accident

V86.99X- Unspecified occupant of other special all-terrain or other off-road motor vehicle injured in nontraffic accident
Off-road motor-vehicle accident NOS
Other motor-vehicle accident NOS
Unspecified occupant of go cart or golf cart injured in nontraffic accident

V87 TRAFFIC ACCIDENT OF SPECIFIED TYPE BUT VICTIM'S MODE OF TRANSPORT UNKNOWN

Excludes1: collision involving:
pedal cycle (V10–V19)
pedestrian (V01–V09)

See complete *ICD-10-CM* manual for codes in category V87.

V88 NONTRAFFIC ACCIDENT OF SPECIFIED TYPE BUT VICTIM'S MODE OF TRANSPORT UNKNOWN

V88 and V89 require a 7th character
A—initial encounter
D—subsequent encounter
S—sequela

Excludes1: collision involving:
pedal cycle (V10–V19)
pedestrian (V01–V09)
See complete *ICD-10-CM* manual for codes in category V88.

V89 MOTOR- OR NONMOTOR-VEHICLE ACCIDENT, TYPE OF VEHICLE UNSPECIFIED

V89.0XX- Person injured in unspecified motor-vehicle accident, nontraffic
Motor-vehicle accident NOS, nontraffic

V89.1XX- Person injured in unspecified nonmotor-vehicle accident, nontraffic
Nonmotor-vehicle accident NOS (nontraffic)

V89.2XX- Person injured in unspecified motor-vehicle accident, traffic
Motor-vehicle accident [MVA] NOS
Road (traffic) accident NOS

V89.3XX- Person injured in unspecified nonmotor-vehicle accident, traffic
Nonmotor-vehicle traffic accident NOS

V89.9XX- Person injured in unspecified vehicle accident
Collision NOS

(V90–V94) WATER TRANSPORT ACCIDENTS

V90 DROWNING AND SUBMERSION DUE TO ACCIDENT TO WATERCRAFT

V90–V94 require a 7th character
A—initial encounter
D—subsequent encounter
S—sequela

Excludes1: fall into water not from watercraft (W16.-)
water-transport-related drowning
or submersion without accident to watercraft (V92.-)
See complete *ICD-10-CM* manual for subcategory codes V90.1-, V90.2-, V90.3-, and V90.8-.

V90.0 Drowning and submersion due to watercraft overturning

V90.01X- Drowning and submersion due to; passenger ship overturning
Drowning and submersion due to Ferry-boat overturning
Drowning and submersion due to Liner overturning

V90.02X- fishing boat overturning

V90.03X- other powered watercraft overturning
Drowning and submersion due to Hovercraft (on open water)/Jet ski overturning

V90.04X- sailboat overturning

V90.05X- canoe or kayak overturning

V90.06X- (nonpowered) inflatable craft overturning

V90.08X- other unpowered watercraft overturning
Drowning and submersion due to windsurfer overturning

V90.09X- unspecified watercraft overturning
Drowning and submersion due to boat/ship/watercraft NOS overturning

V91 OTHER INJURY DUE TO ACCIDENT TO WATERCRAFT

Includes: any injury except drowning and submersion as a result of an accident to watercraft
Excludes1: civilian water transport accident involving military watercraft (V94.81-)
military watercraft accident in military or war operations (Y36, Y37.-)
Excludes2: drowning and submersion due to accident to watercraft (V90.-)
See complete *ICD-10-CM* manual for codes in category V91.

V92 DROWNING AND SUBMERSION DUE TO ACCIDENT ON BOARD WATERCRAFT, WITHOUT ACCIDENT TO WATERCRAFT

Excludes1: civilian water transport accident involving military watercraft (V94.81-)
drowning or submersion due to accident to watercraft (V90-V91)
drowning or submersion of diver who voluntarily jumps from boat not involved in an accident (W16.711, W16.721)

fall into water without watercraft (W16.-)
military watercraft accident in military or war operations (Y36, Y37)
See complete *ICD-10-CM* manual for codes in category V92.

V93 OTHER INJURY WHILE ON WATERCRAFT, WITHOUT ACCIDENT TO WATERCRAFT

See complete *ICD-10-CM* manual for subcategory codes V93.0-, V93.1-, V93.2-, V93.4-, V93.5-, V93.6- and V93.8-. codes in category V82.

V93.3 Fall on board watercraft
Excludes1: fall due to collision of watercraft (V91.2-)

V93.32X- Fall on board fishing boat

V93.33X- Fall on board other powered watercraft
Fall on board Hovercraft/Jet ski (on open water)

V93.34X- Fall on board sailboat

V93.35X- Fall on board canoe or kayak

V93.36X- Fall on board (nonpowered) inflatable craft

V93.38X- Fall on board other unpowered watercraft

V93.39X- Fall on board unspecified watercraft
Fall on board boat/ship/watercraft NOS

V93.8 Other injury due to other accident on board watercraft
Accidental poisoning by gases or fumes on watercraft

V93.82X- Other injury due to other accident on board fishing boat

V93.83X- Other injury due to other accident on board other powered watercraft
Other injury due to other accident on board Hovercraft
Other injury due to other accident on board Jet ski

V93.84X- Other injury due to other accident on board sailboat

V93.85X- Other injury due to other accident on board canoe or kayak

V93.86X- Other injury due to other accident on board (nonpowered) inflatable craft

V93.87X- Other injury due to other accident on board water-skis
Hit or struck by object while waterskiing

V93.88X- Other injury due to other accident on board other unpowered watercraft
Hit or struck by object while surfing
Hit or struck by object while on board windsurfer

V93.89X- Other injury due to other accident on board unspecified watercraft
Other injury due to other accident on board boat/ship/watercraft NOS

V94 OTHER AND UNSPECIFIED WATER TRANSPORT ACCIDENTS

Excludes1: military watercraft accidents in military or war operations (Y36, Y37)

V94.0XX- Hitting object or bottom of body of water due to fall from watercraft
Excludes2: drowning and submersion due to fall from watercraft (V92.0-)

V94.1 Bather struck by watercraft
Swimmer hit by watercraft

V94.11X- Bather struck by powered watercraft

V94.12X- Bather struck by nonpowered watercraft

V94.2 Rider of nonpowered watercraft struck by other watercraft

V94.21X- Rider of nonpowered watercraft struck by other nonpowered watercraft
Canoer hit by other nonpowered watercraft
Surfer hit by other nonpowered watercraft
Windsurfer hit by other nonpowered watercraft

V94.22X- Rider of nonpowered watercraft struck by powered watercraft
Canoer hit by motorboat
Surfer hit by motorboat
Windsurfer hit by motorboat

V94.3 Injury to rider of (inflatable) watercraft being pulled behind other watercraft

V94 requires a 7th character
A—initial encounter
D—subsequent encounter
S—sequela

V94.31X- Injury to rider of (inflatable) recreational watercraft being pulled behind other watercraft

Injury to rider of inner-tube pulled behind motor boat

V94.32X- Injury to rider of non-recreational watercraft being pulled behind other watercraft

Injury to occupant of dingy being pulled behind boat or ship

Injury to occupant of life-raft being pulled behind boat or ship

V94.4XX- Injury to barefoot water-skier

Injury to person being pulled behind boat or ship

V94.89X- Other water transport accident

V94.9XX- Unspecified water transport accident

Water transport accident NOS

initial encounter accident

for definitions of transport

(V95–V97) AIR AND SPACE TRANSPORT ACCIDENTS

Excludes1: military aircraft accidents in military or war operations (Y36, Y37)

V95 ACCIDENT TO POWERED AIRCRAFT CAUSING INJURY TO OCCUPANT

V95–V97 require a 7th character
A—initial encounter
D—subsequent encounter
S—sequela

See complete *ICD-10-CM* manual for codes in categories V95.

V96 ACCIDENT TO NONPOWERED AIRCRAFT CAUSING INJURY TO OCCUPANT

See complete *ICD-10-CM* manual for codes in categories V96.

V97 OTHER SPECIFIED AIR TRANSPORT ACCIDENTS

See complete *ICD-10-CM* manual for codes in categories V97.

(V98–V99) OTHER AND UNSPECIFIED TRANSPORT ACCIDENTS

Excludes1: vehicle accident, type of vehicle unspecified (V89.-)

V98 OTHER SPECIFIED TRANSPORT ACCIDENTS

V98–V99 require a 7th character
A—initial encounter
D—subsequent encounter
S—sequela

See complete *ICD-10-CM* manual for codes in categories V98.

V99 UNSPECIFIED TRANSPORT ACCIDENT

(W00–X58) OTHER EXTERNAL CAUSES OF ACCIDENTAL INJURY

(W00–W19) SLIPPING, TRIPPING, STUMBLING AND FALLS

Excludes1: assault involving a fall (Y01–Y02)
fall from animal (V80.-)
fall (in) (from) machinery (in operation) (W28–W31)
fall (in) (from) transport vehicle (V01–V99)
intentional self-harm involving a fall (X80–X81)

W00–W05 require a 7th character
A—initial encounter
D—subsequent encounter
S—sequela

Excludes2: at risk for fall (history of fall) Z91.81 fall (in) (from) burning building (X00.-)
fall into fire (X00–X04, X08)

W00 FALL DUE TO ICE AND SNOW

Includes: pedestrian on foot falling (slipping) on ice and snow

Excludes1: fall on (from) ice and snow involving pedestrian conveyance (V00.-)
fall from stairs and steps not due to ice and snow (W10.-)

W00.0XX- Fall on same level due to ice and snow

W00.1XX- Fall from stairs and steps due to ice and snow

W00.2XX- Other fall from one level to another due to ice and snow

W00.9XX- Unspecified fall due to ice and snow

W01 FALL ON SAME LEVEL FROM SLIPPING, TRIPPING AND STUMBLING

Includes: fall on moving sidewalk

Excludes1: fall due to bumping (striking) against object (W18.0-)
fall in shower or bathtub (W18.2-)
fall on same level NOS (W18.30)
fall on same level from slipping, tripping and stumbling due to ice or snow (W00.0)
fall off or from toilet (W18.1-)
slipping, tripping and stumbling NOS (W18.40)
slipping, tripping and stumbling without falling (W18.4-)

W01.0XX- Fall on same level from slipping, tripping and stumbling without subsequent striking against object

Falling over animal

W01.1 Fall on same level from slipping, tripping and stumbling with subsequent striking against object

W01.10X- Fall on same level from slipping, tripping and stumbling with subsequent striking against unspecified object

W01.11 Fall on same level from slipping, tripping and stumbling with subsequent striking against sharp object

W01.110- Fall on same level from slipping, tripping and stumbling with subsequent striking against sharp glass

W01.111- Fall on same level from slipping, tripping and stumbling with subsequent striking against power tool or machine

W01.118- Fall on same level from slipping, tripping and stumbling with subsequent striking against other sharp object

W01.119- Fall on same level from slipping, tripping and stumbling with subsequent striking against unspecified sharp object

W01.19 Fall on same level from slipping, tripping and stumbling with subsequent striking against other object

W01.190- Fall on same level from slipping, tripping and stumbling with subsequent striking against furniture

W01.198- Fall on same level from slipping, tripping and stumbling with subsequent striking against other object

W03.XXX- OTHER FALL ON SAME LEVEL DUE TO COLLISION WITH ANOTHER PERSON

Fall due to non-transport collision with other person

Excludes1: collision with another person without fall (W51)
crushed or pushed by a crowd or human stampede (W52)
fall involving pedestrian conveyance (V00-V09)
fall due to ice or snow (W00)
fall on same level NOS (W18.30)

W04.XXX- FALL WHILE BEING CARRIED OR SUPPORTED BY OTHER PERSONS

Accidentally dropped while being carried

W05 FALL FROM NON-MOVING WHEELCHAIR, NONMOTORIZED SCOOTER AND MOTORIZED MOBILITY SCOOTER

Excludes1: fall from moving wheelchair (powered) (V00.811)
fall from moving motorized mobility scooter (V00.831)
fall from nonmotorized scooter (V00.141)

W05.0XX- Fall from non-moving wheelchair

W05.1XX- Fall from non-moving nonmotorized scooter

W05.2XX- Fall from non-moving motorized mobility scooter

W06.XXX- FALL FROM BED

7th

W07.XXX- FALL FROM CHAIR

7th

W08.XXX- FALL FROM OTHER FURNITURE

7th Fall from stool

W09 FALL ON AND FROM PLAYGROUND EQUIPMENT

4th *Excludes1:* fall involving recreational machinery (W31)

W09.0XX- Fall on or from playground slide

7th

W09.1XX- Fall from playground swing

7th

W09.2XX- Fall on or from jungle gym

7th

W09.8XX- Fall on or from other playground equipment

7th

W10 FALL ON AND FROM STAIRS AND STEPS

4th *Excludes1:* Fall from stairs and steps due to ice and snow (W00.1)

W10.0XX- Fall (on) (from) escalator

7th

W10.1XX- Fall (on) (from) sidewalk curb

7th

W10.2XX- Fall (on) (from) incline

7th Fall (on) (from) ramp

W10.8XX- Fall (on) (from) other stairs and steps

7th

W10.9XX- Fall (on) (from) unspecified stairs and steps

7th

W11.XXX- FALL ON AND FROM LADDER

7th

W12.XXX- FALL ON AND FROM SCAFFOLDING

7th

W13 FALL FROM, OUT OF OR THROUGH BUILDING OR STRUCTURE

4th

W13.0XX- Fall from, out of or through balcony

7th Fall from, out of or through railing

W13.1XX- Fall from, out of or through bridge

7th

W13.2XX- Fall from, out of or through roof

7th

W13.3XX- Fall through floor

7th

W13.4XX- Fall from, out of or through window

7th *Excludes2:* fall with subsequent striking against sharp glass (W01.110-)

W13.8XX- Fall from, out of or through other building or structure

7th Fall from, out of or through viaduct
Fall from, out of or through wall
Fall from, out of or through flag-pole

W13.9XX- Fall from, out of or through building, not otherwise specified

7th *Excludes1:* collapse of a building or structure (W20.-)
fall or jump from burning building or structure (X00.-)

W14.XXX- FALL FROM TREE

7th

W15.XXX- FALL FROM CLIFF

7th

W16 FALL, JUMP OR DIVING INTO WATER

4th *Excludes1:* accidental non-watercraft drowning and submersion not involving fall (W65–W74)
effects of air pressure from diving (W94.-)
fall into water from watercraft (V90–V94)
hitting an object or against bottom when falling from watercraft (V94.0)

Excludes2: striking or hitting diving board (W21.4)

W16.0 Fall into swimming pool

5th *Excludes1:* fall into empty swimming pool (W17.3)

W16.01 Fall into swimming pool striking water surface

6th **W16.011-** Fall into swimming pool striking water

7th surface causing drowning and submersion

Excludes1: drowning and submersion while in swimming pool without fall (W67)

W16.012- Fall into swimming pool striking water

7th surface causing other injury

W16.02 Fall into swimming pool striking bottom

6th **W16.021-** Fall into swimming pool striking bottom

7th causing drowning and submersion

Excludes1: drowning and submersion while in swimming pool without fall (W67)

W16.022- Fall into swimming pool striking bottom

7th causing other injury

W16.03 Fall into swimming pool striking wall

6th **W16.031-** Fall into swimming pool striking wall

7th causing drowning and submersion

Excludes1: drowning and submersion while in swimming pool without fall (W67)

W16.032- Fall into swimming pool striking wall

7th causing other injury

W16.1 Fall into natural body of water

5th *Includes:* Fall into lake or open sea or river or stream

W16.11 Fall into natural body of water striking water surface

6th **W16.111-** Fall into natural body of water striking

7th water surface causing drowning and submersion

Excludes1: drowning and submersion while in natural body of water without fall (W69)

W16.112- Fall into natural body of water striking

7th water surface causing other injury

W16.12 Fall into natural body of water striking bottom

6th **W16.121-** Fall into natural body of water striking

7th bottom causing drowning and submersion

Excludes1: drowning and submersion while in natural body of water without fall (W69)

W16.122- Fall into natural body of water striking

7th bottom causing other injury

W16.13 Fall into natural body of water striking side

6th **W16.131-** Fall into natural body of water striking

7th side causing drowning and submersion

Excludes1: drowning and submersion while in natural body of water without fall (W69)

W16.132- Fall into natural body of water striking

7th side causing other injury

W16.2 Fall in (into) filled bathtub or bucket of water

5th **W16.21** Fall in (into) filled bathtub

6th *Excludes1:* fall into empty bathtub (W18.2)

W16.211- Fall in (into) filled bathtub causing

7th drowning and submersion

Excludes1: drowning and submersion while in filled bathtub without fall (W65)

W16.212- Fall in (into) filled bathtub causing other

7th injury

W16.22 Fall in (into) bucket of water

6th **W16.221-** Fall in (into) bucket of water causing

7th drowning and submersion

W16.222- Fall in (into) bucket of water causing other

7th injury

W16.3 Fall into other water

7th Fall into fountain
Fall into reservoir
See complete *ICD-10-CM* manual for codes in subcategory W16.3

W16.4 Fall into unspecified water

6th **W16.41X-** Fall into unspecified water causing drowning and

7th submersion

W16.42X- Fall into unspecified water causing other injury

7th

W16.5 Jumping or diving into swimming pool

5th **W16.51** Jumping or diving into swimming pool striking water

6th surface

W16.511- Jumping or diving into swimming pool

7th striking water surface causing drowning and submersion

Excludes1: drowning and submersion while in swimming pool without jumping or diving (W67)

W06–W16 require a 7th character
A—initial encounter
D—subsequent encounter
S—sequela

4th	5th	6th	7th	Additional Character Required	✓	3-character code

●=New Code
▲=Revised Code

Excludes1—Not coded here, do not use together
Excludes2—Not included here

W16.512- Jumping or diving into swimming pool striking water surface causing other injury

W16.52 Jumping or diving into swimming pool striking bottom

W16.521- Jumping or diving into swimming pool striking bottom causing drowning and submersion

Excludes1: drowning and submersion while in swimming pool without jumping or diving (W67)

W16.522- Jumping or diving into swimming pool striking bottom causing other injury

W16.53 Jumping or diving into swimming pool striking wall

W16.531- Jumping or diving into swimming pool striking wall causing drowning and submersion

Excludes1: drowning and submersion while in swimming pool without jumping or diving (W67)

W16.532- Jumping or diving into swimming pool striking wall causing other injury

W16.6 Jumping or diving into natural body of water

Includes: Jumping or diving into lake or open sea or river or stream

W16.61 Jumping or diving into natural body of water striking water surface

W16.611- Jumping or diving into natural body of water striking water surface causing drowning and submersion

Excludes1: drowning and submersion while in natural body of water without jumping or diving (W69)

W16.612- Jumping or diving into natural body of water striking water surface causing other injury

W16.62 Jumping or diving into natural body of water striking bottom

W16.621- Jumping or diving into natural body of water striking bottom causing drowning and submersion

Excludes1: drowning and submersion while in natural body of water without jumping or diving (W69)

W16.622- Jumping or diving into natural body of water striking bottom causing other injury

W16.7 Jumping or diving from boat

Excludes1: Fall from boat into water -see watercraft accident (V90 –V94)

See complete *ICD-10-CM* manual for codes in subcategory W16.7

W16.8 Jumping or diving into other water

Jumping or diving into fountain

Jumping or diving into reservoir

See complete *ICD-10-CM* manual for codes in subcategory W16.8

W16.9 Jumping or diving into unspecified water

See complete *ICD-10-CM* manual for codes in subcategory W16.9

W17 OTHER FALL FROM ONE LEVEL TO ANOTHER

W17.0XX- Fall into well

W17.1XX- Fall into storm drain or manhole

W17.2XX- Fall into hole

Fall into pit

W17.3XX- Fall into empty swimming pool

Excludes1: fall into filled swimming pool (W16.0-)

W17.4XX- Fall from dock

W17.8 Other fall from one level to another

W17.81X- Fall down embankment (hill)

W17.82X- Fall from (out of) grocery cart

Fall due to grocery cart tipping over

W17.89X- Other fall from one level to another

Fall from cherry picker/lifting device/sky lift

W18 OTHER SLIPPING, TRIPPING AND STUMBLING AND FALLS

W18.0 Fall due to bumping against object

Striking against object with subsequent fall

Excludes1: fall on same level due to slipping, tripping, or stumbling with subsequent striking against object (W01.1-)

W18.00X- Striking against unspecified object with subsequent fall

W18.01X- Striking against sports equipment with subsequent fall

W18.02X- Striking against glass with subsequent fall

W18.09X- Striking against other object with subsequent fall

W18.1 Fall from or off toilet

W18.11X- Fall from or off toilet without subsequent striking against object

Fall from (off) toilet NOS

W18.12X- Fall from or off toilet with subsequent striking against object

W18.2XX- Fall in (into) shower or empty bathtub

Excludes1: fall in full bathtub causing drowning or submersion (W16.21-)

W18.3 Other and unspecified fall on same level

W18.30X- Fall on same level, unspecified

W18.31X- Fall on same level due to stepping on an object

Fall on same level due to stepping on an animal

Excludes1: slipping, tripping and stumbling without fall due to stepping on animal (W18.41)

W18.39X- Other fall on same level

W18.4 Slipping, tripping and stumbling without falling

Excludes1: collision with another person without fall (W51)

W18.40X- Slipping, tripping and stumbling without falling, unspecified

W18.41X- Slipping, tripping and stumbling without falling due to stepping on object

Slipping, tripping and stumbling without falling due to stepping on animal

Excludes1: slipping, tripping and stumbling with fall due to stepping on animal (W18.31)

W18.42X- Slipping, tripping and stumbling without falling due to stepping into hole or opening

W18.43X- Slipping, tripping and stumbling without falling due to stepping from one level to another

W18.49X- Other slipping, tripping and stumbling without falling

W19.XXX- UNSPECIFIED FALL

Accidental fall NOS

(W20–W49) EXPOSURE TO INANIMATE MECHANICAL FORCES

Excludes1: assault (X92–Y08)
contact or collision with animals or persons (W50–W64)
exposure to inanimate mechanical forces involving military or war operations (Y36.-, Y37.-)
intentional self-harm (X71–X83)

W20 STRUCK BY THROWN, PROJECTED OR FALLING OBJECT

7th

Code first any associated:
cataclysm (X34-X39)
lightning strike (T75.00)

Excludes1: falling object in machinery accident (W24, W28-W31)
falling object in transport accident (V01-V99)
object set in motion by explosion (W35-W40)
object set in motion by firearm (W32-W34)
struck by thrown sports equipment (W21.-)
See complete *ICD-10-CM* manual for codes in category W20.

W21 STRIKING AGAINST OR STRUCK BY SPORTS EQUIPMENT

4th

Excludes1: assault with sports equipment (Y08.0-)
striking against or struck by sports equipment with subsequent fall (W18.01)

W21.0 Struck by hit or thrown ball

5th **W21.00X-Struck by hit or thrown ball, unspecified type**

7th

W21.01X-Struck by football

7th

W21.02X-Struck by soccer ball

7th

W21.03X-Struck by baseball

7th

W21.04X-Struck by golf ball

7th

W21.05X-Struck by basketball

7th

W21.06X-Struck by volleyball

7th

W21.07X-Struck by softball

7th

W21.09X-Struck by other hit or thrown ball

7th

W21.1 Struck by bat, racquet or club

6th **W21.11X-Struck by baseball bat**

7th

W21.12X-Struck by tennis racquet

7th

W21.13X-Struck by golf club

7th

W21.19X-Struck by other bat, racquet or club

7th

W21.2 Struck by hockey stick or puck

5th **W21.21 Struck by hockey stick**

6th **W21.210- Struck by ice hockey stick**

7th

W21.211- Struck by field hockey stick

7th

W21.22 Struck by hockey puck

6th **W21.220- Struck by ice hockey puck**

7th

W21.221- Struck by field hockey puck

7th

W21.3 Struck by sports foot wear

5th **W21.31X-Struck by shoe cleats**

7th Stepped on by shoe cleats

W21.32X-Struck by skate blades

7th Skated over by skate blades

W21.39X-Struck by other sports

7th foot wear

W21.4XX-Striking against diving board

7th Use additional code for subsequent falling into water, if applicable (W16.-)

W21.8 Striking against or struck by other sports equipment

5th **W21.81X-Striking against or struck by football helmet**

7th

W21.89X-Striking against or struck by other sports equipment

7th

W21.9XX-Striking against or struck by unspecified sports equipment

7th

W22 STRIKING AGAINST OR STRUCK BY OTHER OBJECTS

4th

Excludes1: striking against or struck by object with subsequent fall (W18.09)

W22.0 Striking against stationary object

5th *Excludes1:* striking against stationary sports equipment (W21.8)

W22.01X-Walked into wall

7th

W22.02X-Walked into lamppost

7th

W22.03X-Walked into furniture

7th

W22.04 Striking against wall of swimming pool

6th **W22.041- Striking against wall of swimming pool**

7th causing drowning and submersion

Excludes1: drowning and submersion while swimming without striking against wall (W67)

W22.042- Striking against wall of swimming pool

7th causing other injury

W22.09X-Striking against other stationary object

7th

W22.1 Striking against or struck by automobile airbag

5th **W22.10X-Striking against or struck by unspecified automobile**

7th airbag

W22.11X-Striking against or struck by driver side automobile

7th airbag

W22.12X-Striking against or struck by front passenger side

7th automobile airbag

W22.19X-Striking against or struck by other automobile airbag

7th

W22.8XX-Striking against or struck by other objects

7th Striking against or struck by object NOS

Excludes1: struck by thrown, projected or falling object (W20.-)

W23 CAUGHT, CRUSHED, JAMMED OR PINCHED IN OR BETWEEN OBJECTS

6th

Excludes1: injury caused by cutting or piercing instruments (W25-W27)
injury caused by firearms malfunction (W32.1, W33.1-, W34.1-)
injury caused by lifting and transmission devices (W24.-)
injury caused by machinery (W28-W31)
injury caused by nonpowered hand tools (W27.-)
injury caused by transport vehicle being used as a means of transportation (V01-V99)
injury caused by struck by thrown, projected or falling object (W20.-)

W23.0XX-Caught, crushed, jammed, or pinched between moving

7th objects

W23.1XX-Caught, crushed, jammed, or pinched between stationary

7th objects

W23.2XX-Caught, crushed, jammed or pinched between a moving and

7th stationary object

W24 CONTACT WITH LIFTING AND TRANSMISSION DEVICES, NOT ELSEWHERE CLASSIFIED

4th

Excludes1: transport accidents (V01-V99)

W24.0XX-Contact with lifting devices, not elsewhere classified

7th Contact with chain hoist
Contact with drive belt
Contact with pulley (block)

W24.1XX-Contact with transmission devices, not elsewhere classified

7th Contact with transmission belt or cable

W25.XXX- CONTACT WITH SHARP GLASS

7th **Code first** any associated:
injury due to flying glass from explosion or firearm discharge (W32-W40)
transport accident (V00-V99)

Excludes1: fall on same level due to slipping, tripping and stumbling with subsequent striking against sharp glass (W01.110-)
striking against sharp glass with subsequent fall (W18.02-)

Excludes 2: glass embedded in skin (W45)

| 4th | 5th | 6th | 7th | Additional Character Required | ✓ | 3-character code | ●=New Code △=Revised Code | *Excludes1*—Not coded here, do not use together *Excludes2*—Not included here |

W26 CONTACT WITH OTHER SHARP OBJECTS

Excludes 2: glass embedded in skin (W45.-)

W26.0XX-Contact with knife

W26.1XX-Contact with sword or dagger
Excludes1: contact with electric knife (W29.1)

W26.2XX-Contact with edge of stiff paper
Paper cut

W26.8XX-Contact with other sharp objects NEC
Contact with tin can lid

W26.9XX-Contact with unspecified sharp objects

W27 CONTACT WITH NONPOWERED HAND TOOL

W27.0XX-Contact with workbench tool
Includes: Contact with auger or axe or chisel or handsaw or screwdriver

W27.1XX-Contact with garden tool
Includes: Contact with hoe or nonpowered lawn mower or pitchfork or rake

W27.2XX-Contact with scissors

W27.3XX-Contact with needle (sewing)
Excludes1: contact with hypodermic needle (W46.-)

W27.4XX-Contact with kitchen utensil
Includes: Contact with fork or ice-pick or can-opener NOS

W27.5XX-Contact with paper-cutter

W27.8XX-Contact with other nonpowered hand tool
Contact with nonpowered sewing machine or shovel

W28.XXX- CONTACT WITH POWERED LAWN MOWER

Powered lawn mower (commercial) (residential)
Excludes1: contact with nonpowered lawn mower (W27.1)
Excludes2: exposure to electric current (W86.-)

W29 CONTACT WITH OTHER POWERED HAND TOOLS AND HOUSEHOLD MACHINERY

Excludes1: contact with commercial machinery (W31.82)
contact with hot household appliance (X15)
contact with nonpowered hand tool (W27.-)
exposure to electric current (W86)
See complete *ICD-10-CM* manual for codes in category W29.

W30 CONTACT WITH AGRICULTURAL MACHINERY

Includes: animal-powered farm machine
Excludes1: agricultural transport vehicle accident (V01-V99)
explosion of grain store (W40.8)
exposure to electric current (W86.-)
See complete *ICD-10-CM* manual for codes in category W30.

W31 CONTACT WITH OTHER AND UNSPECIFIED MACHINERY

Excludes1: contact with agricultural machinery (W30.-)
contact with machinery in transport under own power or being towed by a vehicle (V01-V99)
exposure to electric current (W86)
See complete *ICD-10-CM* manual for codes in category W31.

W32 ACCIDENTAL HANDGUN DISCHARGE AND MALFUNCTION

Includes: accidental discharge and malfunction of gun for single hand use
accidental discharge and malfunction of pistol
accidental discharge and malfunction of revolver
Handgun discharge and malfunction NOS
Excludes1: accidental airgun discharge and malfunction (W34.010, W34.110)
accidental BB gun discharge and malfunction (W34.010, W34.110)
accidental pellet gun discharge and malfunction (W34.010, W34.110)
accidental shotgun discharge and malfunction (W33.01, W33.11)
assault by handgun discharge (X93)
handgun discharge involving legal intervention (Y35.0-)
handgun discharge involving military or war operations (Y36.4-)
intentional self-harm by handgun discharge (X72)
Very pistol discharge and malfunction (W34.09, W34.19)
See complete *ICD-10-CM* manual for codes in category W32.

W33 ACCIDENTAL RIFLE, SHOTGUN AND LARGER FIREARM DISCHARGE AND MALFUNCTION

Includes: rifle, shotgun and larger firearm discharge and malfunction NOS
Excludes1: accidental airgun discharge and malfunction (W34.010, W34.110)
accidental BB gun discharge and malfunction (W34.010, W34.110)
accidental handgun discharge and malfunction (W32.-)
accidental pellet gun discharge and malfunction (W34.010, W34.110)
assault by rifle, shotgun and larger firearm discharge (X94)
firearm discharge involving legal intervention (Y35.0-)
firearm discharge involving military or war operations (Y36.4-)
intentional self-harm by rifle, shotgun and larger firearm discharge (X73)
See complete *ICD-10-CM* manual for codes in category W33.

W34 ACCIDENTAL DISCHARGE AND MALFUNCTION FROM OTHER AND UNSPECIFIED FIREARMS AND GUNS

See complete *ICD-10-CM* manual for codes in category W34.

W35 EXPLOSION AND RUPTURE OF BOILER

Excludes1: explosion and rupture of boiler on watercraft (V93.4)
See complete *ICD-10-CM* manual for codes in category W35.

W36 EXPLOSION AND RUPTURE OF GAS CYLINDER

See complete *ICD-10-CM* manual for codes in category W36.

W37 EXPLOSION AND RUPTURE OF PRESSURIZED TIRE, PIPE OR HOSE

See complete *ICD-10-CM* manual for codes in category W37.

W38 EXPLOSION AND RUPTURE OF OTHER SPECIFIED PRESSURIZED DEVICES

See complete *ICD-10-CM* manual for codes in category W38.

W39.XXX- DISCHARGE OF FIREWORK

W40 EXPLOSION OF OTHER MATERIALS

Excludes1: assault by explosive material (X96)
explosion involving legal intervention (Y35.1-)
explosion involving military or war operations (Y36.0-, Y36.2-)
intentional self-harm by explosive material (X75)
See complete *ICD-10-CM* manual for codes in category W40.

W42 EXPOSURE TO NOISE

See complete *ICD-10-CM* manual for codes in category W42.

W44 FOREIGN BODY ENTERING INTO OR THROUGH A NATURAL ORIFICE

Excludes2: contact with other sharp objects (W26)
contact with sharp glass (W25)
foreign body or object entering through skin (W45)
See complete *ICD-10-CM* manual for codes in category W44.

W45 FB OR OBJECT ENTERING THROUGH SKIN

Includes: foreign body or object embedded in skin
nail embedded in skin
Excludes2: contact with hand tools (nonpowered) (powered) (W27–W29)
contact with other sharp object(s) (W26.-)
contact with sharp glass (W25.-)
paper cut (W26.2-)
struck by objects (W20–W22)

W45.0XX-Nail entering through skin

W45.8XX-Other FB or object entering through skin
Splinter in skin NOS

W46 CONTACT WITH HYPODERMIC NEEDLE

W46.0XX-Contact with hypodermic needle
Hypodermic needle stick NOS

W46.1XX-Contact with contaminated hypodermic needle

W49 EXPOSURE TO OTHER INANIMATE MECHANICAL FORCES

Includes: exposure to abnormal gravitational [G] forces
exposure to inanimate mechanical forces NEC
Excludes1: exposure to inanimate mechanical forces involving military or war operations (Y36.-, Y37.-)

●=New Code *Excludes1*—Not coded here, do not use together
▲=Revised Code *Excludes2*—Not included here

W49.0 Item causing external constriction

W49 requires a 7th character
A—initial encounter
D—subsequent encounter
S—sequela

5th **W49.01X-Hair causing external constriction**

7th constriction

W49.02X-String or thread

7th causing external constriction

W49.03X-Rubber band causing external constriction

7th

W49.04X-Ring or other jewelry causing external constriction

7th

W49.09X-Other specified item causing external constriction

7th

W49.9XX- Exposure to other inanimate mechanical forces

7th

(W50–W64) EXPOSURE TO ANIMATE MECHANICAL FORCES

Excludes1: Toxic effect of contact with venomous animals and plants (T63.-)

W50–W55 require a 7th character
A—initial encounter
D—subsequent encounter
S—sequela

W50 ACCIDENTAL HIT, STRIKE, KICK, TWIST, OR SCRATCH BY ANOTHER PERSON

4th

Includes: hit, strike, kick, twist, bite, or scratch by another person NOS

Excludes1: assault by bodily force (Y04) struck by objects (W20–W22)

W50.0XX-Accidental hit or strike by another person

7th Hit or strike by another person NOS

W50.1XX-Accidental kick by another person

7th Kick by another person NOS

W50.2XX-Accidental twist by another person

7th Twist by another person NOS

W50.3XX-Accidental bite by another person

7th Human bite

Bite by another person NOS

W50.4XX-Accidental scratch by another person

7th Scratch by another person NOS

W51.XXX- ACCIDENTAL STRIKING AGAINST OR BUMPED INTO BY ANOTHER PERSON

7th

Excludes1: assault by striking against or bumping into by another person (Y04.2)

fall due to collision with another person (W03)

W52.XXX- CRUSHED, PUSHED OR STEPPED ON BY CROWD OR HUMAN STAMPEDE

7th

Crushed, pushed or stepped on by crowd or human stampede with or without fall

W53 CONTACT WITH RODENT

4th

Includes: contact with saliva, feces or urine of rodent

W53.0 Contact with mouse

5th **W53.01X-Bitten by mouse**

7th

W53.09X-Other contact with mouse

7th

W53.1 Contact with rat

5th **W53.11X-Bitten by rat**

7th

W53.19X-Other contact with rat

7th

W53.2 Contact with squirrel

5th **W53.21X-Bitten by squirrel**

7th

W53.29X-Other contact with squirrel

7th

W53.8 Contact with other rodent

5th **W53.81X-Bitten by other rodent**

7th

W53.89X-Other contact with other rodent

7th

W54 CONTACT WITH DOG

4th

Includes: contact with saliva, feces or urine of dog

Report the injury code as primary

W54.0XX-Bitten by dog

7th

W54.1XX-Struck by dog

7th Knocked over by dog

W54.8XX-Other contact with dog

7th

W55 CONTACT WITH OTHER MAMMALS

4th

Includes: contact with saliva, feces or urine of mammal

Excludes1: animal being ridden—see transport accidents bitten or struck by dog (W54) bitten or struck by rodent (W53.-) contact with marine mammals (W56.-)

See complete *ICD-10-CM* manual for code subcategories W55.1-, W55.2-, W55.3- W55.4-, W55.5-, and W55.8-.

W55.0 Contact with cat

5th **W55.01X-Bitten by cat**

7th

W55.03X-Scratched by cat

7th

W55.09X-Other contact with cat

7th

W56 CONTACT WITH NONVENOMOUS MARINE ANIMAL

7th

Excludes1: contact with venomous marine animal (T63.-)

See complete *ICD-10-CM* manual for codes in category W56.

W57.XXX- ACCIDENTAL BITTEN OR STUNG BY NONVENOMOUS INSECT AND OTHER NONVENOMOUS ARTHROPODS

7th

W57 requires a 7th character
A—initial encounter
D—subsequent encounter
S—sequela

Excludes1: contact with venomous insects and arthropods (T63.2-, T63.3-, T63.4-)

W58 CONTACT WITH CROCODILE OR ALLIGATOR

7th See complete *ICD-10-CM* manual for codes in category W58.

W59 CONTACT WITH OTHER NONVENOMOUS REPTILES

4th

W59 requires a 7th character
A—initial encounter
D—subsequent encounter
S—sequela

Excludes1: contact with venomous reptile (T63.0-, T63.1-)

W59.0 Contact with nonvenomous lizards

5th

W59.01X-Bitten by nonvenomous lizards

7th

W59.02X-Struck by nonvenomous lizards

7th

W59.09X-Other contact with nonvenomous lizards

7th Exposure to nonvenomous lizards

W59.1 Contact with nonvenomous snakes

5th **W59.11X-Bitten by nonvenomous snake**

7th

W59.12X-Struck by nonvenomous snake

7th

W59.13X-Crushed by nonvenomous snake

7th

W59.19X-Other contact with nonvenomous snake

7th

W59.2 Contact with turtles

5th Excludes1: contact with tortoises (W59.8-)

W59.21X-Bitten by turtle

7th

W59.22X-Struck by turtle

7th

W59.29X-Other contact with turtle

7th Exposure to turtles

W59.8 Contact with other nonvenomous reptiles

5th **W59.81X-Bitten by other nonvenomous reptiles**

7th

W59.82X-Struck by other nonvenomous reptiles

7th

W59.83X-Crushed by other nonvenomous reptiles

7th

W59.89X-Other contact with other nonvenomous reptiles

7th

4th **5th** **6th** **7th** Additional Character Required ✓ 3-character code

●=New Code *Excludes1*—Not coded here, do not use together
▲=Revised Code *Excludes2*—Not included here

W60.XXX- CONTACT WITH NON-VENOMOUS PLANT THORNS AND SPINES AND SHARP LEAVES

W60-W62 require a 7th character
A—initial encounter
D—subsequent encounter
S—sequela

Excludes1: Contact with venomous plants (T63.7-)

W61 CONTACT WITH BIRDS (DOMESTIC) (WILD)

Includes: contact with excreta of birds

W61.0 Contact with parrot

W61.01X-Bitten by parrot

W61.02X-Struck by parrot

W61.09X-Other contact with parrot

Exposure to parrots

W61.1 Contact with macaw

W61.11X-Bitten by macaw

W61.12X-Struck by macaw

W61.19X-Other contact with macaw

Exposure to macaws

W61.3 Contact with chicken

W61.32X-Struck by chicken

W61.33X-Pecked by chicken

W61.39X-Other contact with chicken

Exposure to chickens

W61.4 Contact with turkey

W61.42X-Struck by turkey

W61.43X-Pecked by turkey

W61.49X-Other contact with turkey

W61.5 Contact with goose

W61.51X-Bitten by goose

W61.52X-Struck by goose

W61.59X-Other contact with goose

W61.6 Contact with duck

W61.61X-Bitten by duck

W61.62X-Struck by duck

W61.69X-Other contact with duck

W61.9 Contact with other birds

W61.91X-Bitten by other birds

W61.92X-Struck by other birds

W61.99X-Other contact with other birds

Contact with bird NOS

W62 CONTACT WITH NONVENOMOUS AMPHIBIANS

Excludes1: contact with venomous amphibians (T63.81-T63.83)

W62.0XX-Contact with nonvenomous frogs

W62.1XX-Contact with nonvenomous toads

W62.9XX-Contact with other nonvenomous amphibians

(W65-W74) ACCIDENTAL NON-TRANSPORT DROWNING AND SUBMERSION

W65-W74 require a 7th character
A—initial encounter
D—subsequent encounter
S—sequela

Excludes1: accidental drowning and submersion due to fall into water (W16.-)
accidental drowning and submersion due to water transport accident (V90.-, V92.-)

Excludes2: accidental drowning and submersion due to cataclysm (X34-X39)

W65.XXX- ACCIDENTAL DROWNING AND SUBMERSION WHILE IN BATHTUB

Excludes1: accidental drowning and submersion due to fall in (into) bathtub (W16.211)

W67.XXX- ACCIDENTAL DROWNING AND SUBMERSION WHILE IN SWIMMING-POOL

Excludes1: accidental drowning and submersion due to fall into swimming pool (W16.011, W16.021, W16.031)
accidental drowning and submersion due to striking into wall of swimming pool (W22.041)

W69.XXX- ACCIDENTAL DROWNING AND SUBMERSION WHILE IN NATURAL WATER

Accidental drowning and submersion while in lake/open sea/river/stream

Excludes1: accidental drowning and submersion due to fall into natural body of water (W16.111, W16.121, W16.131)

W74.XXX- UNSPECIFIED CAUSE OF ACCIDENTAL DROWNING AND SUBMERSION

Drowning NOS

(W85-W99) EXPOSURE TO ELECTRIC CURRENT, RADIATION AND EXTREME AMBIENT AIR TEMPERATURE AND PRESSURE

W86-W93 require a 7th character
A—initial encounter
D—subsequent encounter
S—sequela

Excludes1: exposure to: failure in dosage of radiation or temperature during surgical and medical care (Y63.2-Y63.5)
lightning (T75.0-)
natural cold (X31)
natural heat (X30)
natural radiation NOS (X39)
radiological procedure and radiotherapy (Y84.2)
sunlight (X32)

W86 EXPOSURE TO OTHER SPECIFIED ELECTRIC CURRENT

W86.0XX-Exposure to domestic wiring and appliances

W86.1XX-Exposure to industrial wiring, appliances and electrical machinery

Includes: Exposure to conductors or control apparatus or electrical equipment and machinery or transformers

W86.8XX-Exposure to other electric current

Includes: Exposure to wiring and appliances in or on farm (not farmhouse) or public building or residential institutions or schools
Exposure to wiring and appliances outdoors

W89 EXPOSURE TO MAN-MADE VISIBLE AND ULTRAVIOLET LIGHT

Includes: exposure to welding light (arc)

Excludes2: exposure to sunlight (X32)

W89.1XX-Exposure to tanning bed

W93 EXPOSURE TO EXCESSIVE COLD OF MAN-MADE ORIGIN

W93.0 Contact with or inhalation of dry ice

W93.01X-Contact with dry ice

W93.02X-Inhalation of dry ice

W93.1 Contact with or inhalation of liquid air

W93.11X-Contact with liquid air

Contact with liquid hydrogen
Contact with liquid nitrogen

W93.12X- Inhalation of liquid air

7th Inhalation of liquid hydrogen or nitrogen

W93.2XX- Prolonged exposure in deep freeze unit or refrigerator

7th

W93.8XX- Exposure to other excessive cold of man-made origin

7th

W93 and W94 require a 7th character
A—initial encounter
D—subsequent encounter
S—sequela

W94 EXPOSURE TO HIGH AND LOW AIR PRESSURE AND CHANGES IN AIR PRESSURE

4th

W94.0XX- Exposure to prolonged high air pressure

7th

W94.1 Exposure to prolonged low air pressure

5th **W94.11X-** Exposure to residence or prolonged visit at high altitude

7th

W94.12X- Exposure to other prolonged low air pressure

7th

W94.2 Exposure to rapid changes in air pressure during ascent

5th **W94.21X-** Exposure to reduction in atmospheric pressure while surfacing from deep-water diving

7th

W94.22X- Exposure to reduction in atmospheric pressure while surfacing from underground

7th

W94.23X- Exposure to sudden change in air pressure in aircraft during ascent

7th

W94.29X- Exposure to other rapid changes in air pressure during ascent

7th

W94.3 Exposure to rapid changes in air pressure during descent

5th **W94.31X-** Exposure to sudden change in air pressure in aircraft during descent

7th

W94.32X- Exposure to high air pressure from rapid descent in water

7th

W94.39X- Exposure to other rapid changes in air pressure during descent

7th

(X00–X08) EXPOSURE TO SMOKE, FIRE AND FLAMES

Excludes1: arson (X97)

Excludes2: explosions (W35–W40)
lightning (T75.0-)
transport accident (V01–V99)

X00 EXPOSURE TO UNCONTROLLED FIRE IN BUILDING OR STRUCTURE

4th

X00 requires a 7th character
A—initial encounter
D—subsequent encounter
S—sequela

X00.0XX- Exposure to flames in uncontrolled fire in building or structure

7th

X00.1XX- Exposure to smoke in uncontrolled fire in building or structure

7th

X01 EXPOSURE TO UNCONTROLLED FIRE, NOT IN BUILDING OR STRUCTURE

7th

Includes: exposure to forest fire
See complete *ICD-10-CM* manual for codes in category X01.

X02 EXPOSURE TO CONTROLLED FIRE IN BUILDING OR STRUCTURE

7th

Includes: exposure to fire in fireplace
exposure to fire in stove
See complete *ICD-10-CM* manual for codes in category X02.

X03 EXPOSURE TO CONTROLLED FIRE, NOT IN BUILDING OR STRUCTURE

7th

X03–X06 require a 7th character
A—initial encounter
D—subsequent encounter
S—sequela

Includes: exposure to bonfire or camp-fire or trash fire

Includes: conflagration in building or structure

Code first any associated cataclysm

Excludes2: Exposure to ignition or melting of nightwear (X05)
Exposure to ignition or melting of other clothing and apparel (X06.-)
Exposure to other specified smoke, fire and flames (X08.-)

X03.0XX- Exposure to flames in controlled fire, not in building or structure

7th

X03.1XX- Exposure to smoke in controlled fire, not in building or structure

7th

X04.XXX- EXPOSURE TO IGNITION OF HIGHLY FLAMMABLE MATERIAL

7th

Includes: Exposure to ignition of gasoline or kerosene or petrol

Excludes2: exposure to ignition or melting of nightwear (X05)
exposure to ignition or melting of other clothing and apparel (X06)

X05.XXX- EXPOSURE TO IGNITION OR MELTING OF NIGHTWEAR

7th

Excludes2: exposure to uncontrolled fire in building or structure (X00.-)
exposure to uncontrolled fire, not in building or structure (X01.-)
exposure to controlled fire in building or structure (X02.-)
exposure to controlled fire, not in building or structure (X03.-)
exposure to ignition of highly flammable materials (X04.-)

X06 EXPOSURE TO IGNITION OR MELTING OF OTHER CLOTHING AND APPAREL

4th

X06.0XX- Exposure to ignition of plastic jewelry

7th

X06.1XX- Exposure to melting of plastic jewelry

7th

X06.2XX- Exposure to ignition of other clothing and apparel

7th

X06.3XX- Exposure to melting of other clothing and apparel

7th

X08 EXPOSURE TO OTHER SPECIFIED SMOKE, FIRE AND FLAMES

7th

See complete *ICD-10-CM* manual for codes in category X08.

(X10–X19) CONTACT WITH HEAT AND HOT SUBSTANCES

Excludes1: exposure to excessive natural heat (X30)
exposure to fire and flames (X00–X08)

X10–X15 require a 7th character
A—initial encounter
D—subsequent encounter
S—sequela

X10 CONTACT WITH HOT DRINKS, FOOD, FATS AND COOKING OILS

4th

X10.0XX- Contact with hot drinks

7th

X10.1XX- Contact with hot food

7th

X10.2XX- Contact with fats and cooking oils

7th

X11 CONTACT WITH HOT TAP-WATER

4th

Includes: contact with boiling tap-water or boiling water NOS

Excludes1: contact with water heated on stove (X12)

X11.0XX- Contact with hot water in bath or tub

7th *Excludes1:* contact with running hot water in bath or tub (X11.1)

X11.1XX- Contact with running hot water

7th Contact with hot water running out of hose or tap

X11.8XX- Contact with other hot tap-water

7th Contact with hot water in bucket
Contact with hot tap-water NOS

X12.XXX- CONTACT WITH OTHER HOT FLUIDS

7th Contact with water heated on stove

Excludes1: hot (liquid) metals (X18)

X13 CONTACT WITH STEAM AND OTHER HOT VAPORS

4th

X13.0XX- Inhalation of steam and other hot vapors

7th

X13.1XX- Other contact with steam and other hot vapors

7th

X15 CONTACT WITH HOT HOUSEHOLD APPLIANCES

4th

Excludes1: contact with heating appliances (X16)
contact with powered household appliances (W29.-)
exposure to controlled fire in building or structure due to household appliance (X02.8)
exposure to household appliances electrical current (W86.0)

X15.0XX- Contact with hot stove (kitchen)

7th

X15.1XX- Contact with hot toaster

7th

4th 5th 6th 7th Additional Character Required ✓ 3-character code

*=New Code
▲=Revised Code

Excludes1—Not coded here, do not use together
Excludes2—Not included here

PEDIATRIC ICD-10-CM 2024: A MANUAL FOR PROVIDER-BASED CODING

X15.2XX- Contact with hotplate

7th

X15-X19 require a 7th character
A—initial encounter
D—subsequent encounter
S—sequela

X15.3XX- Contact with hot saucepan or skillet

7th

X15.8XX- Contact with other hot household appliances

7th

Contact with cooker/kettle/light bulbs

X16.XXX- **CONTACT WITH HOT HEATING APPLIANCES, RADIATORS AND PIPES**

7th

Excludes1: contact with powered appliances (W29.-)
exposure to controlled fire in building or structure due to appliance (X02.8)
exposure to industrial appliances electrical current (W86.1)

X17.XXX- **CONTACT WITH HOT ENGINES, MACHINERY AND TOOLS**

7th

Excludes1: contact with hot heating appliances, radiators and pipes (X16)
contact with hot household appliances (X15)

X18.XXX- **CONTACT WITH OTHER HOT METALS**

7th

Contact with liquid metal

X19.XXX- **CONTACT WITH OTHER HEAT AND HOT SUBSTANCES**

7th

Excludes1: objects that are not normally hot, e.g., an object made hot by a house fire (X00–X08)

(X30–X39) EXPOSURE TO FORCES OF NATURE

X30.XXX- **EXPOSURE TO EXCESSIVE NATURAL HEAT**

7th

X30–X39 require a 7th character
A—initial encounter
D—subsequent encounter
S—sequela

Exposure to excessive heat as the cause of sunstroke
Exposure to heat NOS
Excludes1: excessive heat of man-made origin (W92)
exposure to man-made radiation (W89)
exposure to sunlight (X32)
exposure to tanning bed (W89)

X31.XXX- **EXPOSURE TO EXCESSIVE NATURAL COLD**

7th

Excessive cold as the cause of chilblains NOS
Excessive cold as the cause of immersion foot or hand
Exposure to cold NOS
Exposure to weather conditions
Excludes1: cold of man-made origin (W93.-)
contact with or inhalation of dry ice (W93.-)
contact with or inhalation of liquefied gas (W93.-)

X32.XXX- **EXPOSURE TO SUNLIGHT**

7th

Excludes1: man-made radiation (tanning bed) (W89)
Excludes2: radiation-related disorders of the skin and subcutaneous tissue (L55–L59)

X34.XXX- **EARTHQUAKE**

7th

Excludes2: tidal wave (tsunami) due to earthquake (X37.41)

X35.XXX- **VOLCANIC ERUPTION**

7th

Excludes2: tidal wave (tsunami) due to volcanic eruption (X37.41)

X36 **AVALANCHE, LANDSLIDE AND OTHER EARTH MOVEMENTS**

4th

Includes: victim of mudslide of cataclysmic nature
Excludes1: earthquake (X34)
Excludes2: transport accident involving collision with avalanche or landslide not in motion (V01–V99)

X36.0XX- Collapse of dam or man-made structure causing earth movement

7th

X36.1XX- Avalanche, landslide, or mudslide

7th

X37 **CATACLYSMIC STORM**

4th

X37.0XX- Hurricane

7th

Storm surge

X37.1XX- Tornado

7th

Cyclone
Twister

X37.2XX- Blizzard (snow) (ice)

7th

X37.3XX- Dust storm

7th

X37.4 Tidal wave

5th

X37.41X- Tidal wave due to earthquake or volcanic eruption

7th

Tidal wave NOS
Tsunami

X37.42X- Tidal wave due to storm

7th

X37.43X- Tidal wave due to landslide

7th

X37.8XX- Other cataclysmic storms

7th

Cloudburst
Torrential rain
Excludes2: flood (X38)

X37.9XX- Unspecified cataclysmic storm

7th

Storm NOS
Excludes1: collapse of dam or man-made structure causing earth movement (X36.0)

X38.XXX- **FLOOD**

7th

Flood arising from remote storm or of nature arising from melting snow
Flood resulting directly from storm
Excludes1: collapse of dam or man-made structure causing earth movement (X36.0)
tidal wave NOS (X37.41)
tidal wave caused by storm (X37.42)

X39 **EXPOSURE TO OTHER FORCES OF NATURE**

4th

X39.0 Exposure to natural radiation

5th

Excludes1: contact with and (suspected) exposure to radon and other naturally occurring radiation (Z77.123)
exposure to man-made radiation (W88–W90)
exposure to sunlight (X32)

X39.01X- Exposure to radon

7th

X39.08X- Exposure to other natural radiation

7th

X39.8XX- Other exposure to forces of nature

7th

(X50–X58) ACCIDENTAL EXPOSURE TO OTHER SPECIFIED FACTORS

X50 **OVEREXERTION FROM MOVEMENT**

4th

X50–X58 require a 7th character
A—initial encounter
D—subsequent encounter
S—sequela

X50.0XX- Overexertion from strenuous movement or load

7th

Lifting heavy objects
Lifting weights

X50.1XX- Overexertion from prolonged static or awkward postures

7th

Includes: Prolonged or static bending or kneeling or reaching or sitting or standing or twisting

X50.3XX- Overexertion from repetitive movements

7th

Use of hand as hammer

X50.9XX- Other and unspecified overexertion or strenuous movements or postures

7th

Contact pressure or contact stress

X58.XXX- **EXPOSURE TO OTHER SPECIFIED FACTORS**

7th

Accident NOS
Exposure NOS

(X71–X83) INTENTIONAL SELF-HARM

Purposely self-inflicted injury
Suicide (attempted)

X71 **INTENTIONAL SELF-HARM BY DROWNING AND SUBMERSION**

7th

See complete *ICD-10-CM* manual for codes in category X71.

4th 5th 6th 7th Additional Character Required ✓ 3-character code

● =New Code *Excludes1*—Not coded here, do not use together
▲=Revised Code *Excludes2*—Not included here

X72.XXX- INTENTIONAL SELF-HARM BY HANDGUN DISCHARGE

7th Intentional self-harm by gun/pistol/ revolver for single hand use
Excludes1: Very pistol (X74.8)

X72 requires a 7th character
A—initial encounter
D—subsequent encounter
S—sequela

X73 INTENTIONAL SELF-HARM BY RIFLE, SHOTGUN AND LARGER FIREARM DISCHARGE

7th *Excludes1:* airgun (X74.01)
See complete *ICD-10-CM* manual for codes in category X73.

X74 INTENTIONAL SELF-HARM BY OTHER AND UNSPECIFIED FIREARM AND GUN DISCHARGE

7th See complete *ICD-10-CM* manual for codes in category X74.

X75.XXX- INTENTIONAL SELF-HARM BY EXPLOSIVE MATERIAL

7th

X75 and X76 require a 7th character
A—initial encounter
D—subsequent encounter
S—sequela

X76.XXX- INTENTIONAL SELF-HARM BY SMOKE, FIRE AND FLAMES

7th

X77 INTENTIONAL SELF-HARM BY STEAM, HOT VAPORS AND HOT OBJECTS

7th See complete *ICD-10-CM* manual for codes in category X77.

X78 INTENTIONAL SELF-HARM BY SHARP OBJECT

4th

X78–X80 require a 7th character
A—initial encounter
D—subsequent encounter
S—sequela

X78.0XX- Intentional self-harm by sharp glass

7th

X78.1XX- Intentional self-harm by knife

7th

X78.2XX- Intentional self-harm by sword or dagger

7th

X78.8XX- Intentional self-harm by other sharp object

7th

X78.9XX- Intentional self-harm by unspecified sharp object

7th

X79.XXX- INTENTIONAL SELF-HARM BY BLUNT OBJECT

7th

X80.XXX- INTENTIONAL SELF-HARM BY JUMPING FROM A HIGH PLACE

7th Intentional fall from one level to another
See complete *ICD-10-CM* manual for codes in category X80.

X81 INTENTIONAL SELF-HARM BY JUMPING OR LYING IN FRONT OF MOVING OBJECT

7th See complete *ICD-10-CM* manual for codes in category X81.

X82 INTENTIONAL SELF-HARM BY CRASHING OF MOTOR VEHICLE

7th See complete *ICD-10-CM* manual for codes in category X82.

X83 INTENTIONAL SELF-HARM BY OTHER SPECIFIED MEANS

7th *Excludes1:* intentional self-harm by poisoning or contact with toxic substance — See Table of Drugs and Chemicals
See complete *ICD-10-CM* manual for codes in category X83.

(X92–Y09) ASSAULT

Adult and child abuse, neglect and maltreatment are classified as assault. Any of the assault codes may be used to indicate the external cause of any injury resulting from the confirmed abuse.

For confirmed cases of abuse, neglect and maltreatment, when the perpetrator is known, a code from Y07, Perpetrator of maltreatment and neglect, should accompany any other assault codes.

Includes: homicide
injuries inflicted by another person with intent to injure or kill, by any means
Excludes1: injuries due to legal intervention (Y35.-)
injuries due to operations of war (Y36.-)
injuries due to terrorism (Y38.-)

X92 ASSAULT BY DROWNING AND SUBMERSION

4th

X92–X95 requires a 7th character
A—initial encounter
D—subsequent encounter
S—sequela

X92.0XX- Assault by drowning and submersion while in bathtub

7th

X92.1XX- Assault by drowning and submersion while in swimming pool

7th

X92.2XX- Assault by drowning and submersion after push into swimming pool

7th

X92.3XX- Assault by drowning and submersion in natural water

7th

X92.8XX- Other assault by drowning and submersion

7th

X92.9XX- Assault by drowning and submersion, unspecified

7th

X93.XXX- ASSAULT BY HANDGUN DISCHARGE

7th *Excludes1:* Very pistol (X95.8)

X94 ASSAULT BY RIFLE, SHOTGUN AND LARGER FIREARM DISCHARGE

4th *Excludes1:* airgun (X95.01)

X94.0XX- Assault by shotgun

7th

X94.1XX- Assault by hunting rifle

7th

X94.2XX- Assault by machine gun

7th

X94.8XX- Assault by other larger firearm discharge

7th

X94.9XX- Assault by unspecified larger firearm discharge

7th

X95 ASSAULT BY OTHER AND UNSPECIFIED FIREARM AND GUN DISCHARGE

4th

X95.0 Assault by gas, air or spring-operated guns

5th **X95.01X- Assault by airgun discharge**

7th Assault by BB or pellet gun discharge

X95.02X- Assault by paintball gun discharge

7th

X95.09X- Assault by other gas, air or spring-operated gun

7th

X95.8XX- Assault by other firearm discharge

7th Assault by very pistol [flare] discharge

X95.9XX- Assault by unspecified firearm discharge

7th

X96 ASSAULT BY EXPLOSIVE MATERIAL

7th *Excludes1:* incendiary device (X97)
terrorism involving explosive material (Y38.2-)
See complete *ICD-10-CM* manual for codes in category X96.

X97.XXX- ASSAULT BY SMOKE, FIRE AND FLAMES

7th Assault by arson
Assault by cigarettes
Assault by incendiary device

X97–X99 require a 7th character
A—initial encounter
D—subsequent encounter
S—sequela

X98 ASSAULT BY STEAM, HOT VAPORS AND HOT OBJECTS

4th

X98.0XX- Assault by steam or hot vapors

7th

X98.1XX- Assault by hot tap water

7th

X98.2XX- Assault by hot fluids

7th

X98.3XX- Assault by hot household appliances

7th

X98.8XX- Assault by other hot objects

7th

X98.9XX- Assault by unspecified hot objects

7th

X99 ASSAULT BY SHARP OBJECT

4th *Excludes1:* assault by strike by sports equipment (Y08.0-)

X99.0XX- Assault by sharp glass

7th

X99.1XX- Assault by knife

7th

X99.2XX- Assault by sword or dagger

7th

X99.8XX- Assault by other sharp object

7th

X99.9XX- Assault by unspecified sharp object

7th Assault by stabbing NOS

Y00.XXX- ASSAULT BY BLUNT OBJECT
7th

Excludes1: assault by strike by sports equipment (Y08.0-)

Y01.XXX- ASSAULT BY PUSHING FROM HIGH PLACE
7th

Y02 ASSAULT BY PUSHING OR PLACING VICTIM IN FRONT OF MOVING OBJECT
6th

Y02.0XX- Assault by pushing or placing victim in front of motor vehicle **7th**

Y02.1XX- Assault by pushing or placing victim in front of (subway) train **7th**

Y02.8XX- Assault by pushing or placing victim in front of other moving object **7th**

Y03 ASSAULT BY CRASHING OF MOTOR VEHICLE
6th

Y03.0XX- Assault by being hit or run over by motor vehicle **7th**

Y03.8XX- Other assault by crashing of motor vehicle **7th**

Y04 ASSAULT BY BODILY FORCE
4th

Excludes1: assault by:
submersion (X92.-)
use of weapon (X93–X95, X99, Y00)

Y04.0XX- Assault by unarmed brawl or fight **7th**

Y04.1XX- Assault by human bite **7th**

Y04.2XX- Assault by strike against or bumped into by another person **7th**

Y04.8XX- Assault by other bodily force **7th** Assault by bodily force NOS

Y07 PERPETRATOR OF ASSAULT, MALTREATMENT AND NEGLECT
4th

GUIDELINES

Adult and child abuse, neglect and maltreatment are classified as assault. Any of the assault codes may be used to indicate the external cause of any injury resulting from the confirmed abuse.

For confirmed cases of abuse, neglect and maltreatment, when the perpetrator is known, a code from Y07, Perpetrator of maltreatment and neglect, should accompany any other assault codes.

See Chapter 19, "Adult and Child Abuse, Neglect and Other Maltreatment"

Note: Codes from this category are for use only in cases of confirmed abuse (T74.-)

Selection of the correct perpetrator code is based on the relationship between the perpetrator and the victim

Includes: perpetrator of abandonment, emotional neglect, mental cruelty, physical abuse, physical neglect, sexual abuse, torture, verbal abuse

Y07.0 Spouse or partner, perpetrator of maltreatment and neglect
5th Spouse or partner, perpetrator of maltreatment and neglect against spouse or partner

Y07.01 Husband, perpetrator of maltreatment and neglect
6th

Y07.010 Husband, current, perpetrator of maltreatment and neglect

Y07.011 Husband, former, perpetrator of maltreatment and neglect

Y07.02 Wife, perpetrator of maltreatment and neglect
6th

Y07.020 Wife, current, perpetrator of maltreatment and neglect

Y07.021 Wife, former, perpetrator of maltreatment and neglect

Y07.03 Male partner, perpetrator of maltreatment and neglect
6th Male intimate or dating partner, perpetrator of maltreatment and neglect

Y07.030 Male partner, current, perpetrator of maltreatment and neglect

Y07.031 Male partner, former, perpetrator of maltreatment and neglect

Y07.04 Female partner, perpetrator of maltreatment and neglect
6th Female intimate or dating partner, perpetrator of maltreatment and neglect

Y07.040 Female partner, current, perpetrator of maltreatment and neglect

Y07.041 Female partner, former, perpetrator of maltreatment and neglect

Y07.05 Non-binary partner, perpetrator of maltreatment and neglect
6th Gender non-conforming partner, perpetrator of maltreatment and neglect

Y07.050 Non-binary partner, current, perpetrator of maltreatment and neglect

Y07.051 Non-binary partner, former, perpetrator of maltreatment and neglect

Y07.1 Parent (adoptive) (biological), perpetrator of maltreatment and neglect
5th

Y07.11 Biological father, perpetrator of maltreatment and neglect

Y07.12 Biological mother, perpetrator of maltreatment and neglect

Y07.13 Adoptive father, perpetrator of maltreatment and neglect

Y07.14 Adoptive mother, perpetrator of maltreatment and neglect

Y07.4 Other family member, perpetrator of maltreatment and neglect
5th

Y07.41 Sibling, perpetrator of maltreatment and neglect
6th *Excludes1:* stepsibling, perpetrator of maltreatment and neglect (Y07.435, Y07.436)

Y07.410 Brother, perpetrator of maltreatment and neglect

Y07.411 Sister, perpetrator of maltreatment and neglect

Y07.42 Foster parent, perpetrator of maltreatment and neglect
6th

Y07.420 Foster father, perpetrator of maltreatment and neglect

Y07.421 Foster mother, perpetrator of maltreatment and neglect

Y07.43 Stepparent or stepsibling, perpetrator of maltreatment and neglect
6th

Y07.430 Stepfather, perpetrator of maltreatment and neglect

Y07.432 Male friend of parent (co-residing in household), perpetrator of maltreatment and neglect

Y07.433 Stepmother, perpetrator of maltreatment and neglect

Y07.434 Female friend of parent (co-residing in household), perpetrator of maltreatment and neglect

Y07.435 Stepbrother, perpetrator or maltreatment and neglect

Y07.436 Stepsister, perpetrator of maltreatment and neglect

Y07.44 Child, perpetrator of maltreatment and neglect
Adopted child, biological child, daughter, foster child, in-law child, non-binary child, son, stepchild

Y07.45 Grandchild, perpetrator of maltreatment and neglect
Adopted grandchild, biological grandchild, foster grandchild, granddaughter, grandson, in-law grandchild, non-binary grandchild, step grandchild

Y07.46 Grandparent, perpetrator of maltreatment and neglect
Grandfather, grandmother, non-binary grandparent.

Y07.47 Parental sibling, perpetrator of maltreatment and neglect
Aunt, uncle, or non-binary parental sibling

Y07.49 Other family member, perpetrator of maltreatment and neglect
6th

Y07.490 Male cousin, perpetrator of maltreatment and neglect

Y07.491 Female cousin, perpetrator of maltreatment and neglect

Y07.499 Other family member, perpetrator of maltreatment and neglect

Y07.5 Non-family member, perpetrator of maltreatment and neglect

Y07.50 Unspecified non-family member, perpetrator of maltreatment and neglect

Y07.51 Daycare provider, perpetrator of maltreatment and neglect

Y07.510 At-home childcare provider, perpetrator of maltreatment and neglect

Y07.511 Daycare center childcare provider, perpetrator of maltreatment and neglect

Y07.519 Unspecified daycare provider, perpetrator of maltreatment and neglect

Y07.53 Teacher or instructor, perpetrator of maltreatment and neglect

Coach, perpetrator of maltreatment and neglect

Y07.54 Acquaintance or friend, perpetrator of maltreatment and neglect

Y07.59 Other non-family member, perpetrator of maltreatment and neglect

Y07.6 Multiple perpetrators of maltreatment and neglect

Y07.9 Unspecified perpetrator of maltreatment and neglect

Y08 ASSAULT BY OTHER SPECIFIED MEANS

Y08 and Y09 require a 7th character
A—initial encounter
D—subsequent encounter
S—sequela

Y08.0 Assault by strike by sport equipment

Y08.01X- Assault by strike by hockey stick

Y08.02X- Assault by strike by baseball bat

Y08.09X- Assault by strike by other specified type of sport equipment

Y08.8 Assault by other specified means

Y08.81X- Assault by crashing of aircraft

Y08.89X- Assault by other specified means

Y09.XXX- ASSAULT BY UNSPECIFIED MEANS

Includes: Assassination (attempted) or homicide (attempted), manslaughter (attempted) or murder (attempted) NOS

(Y21–Y33) EVENT OF UNDETERMINED INTENT

Undetermined intent is only for use when there is specific documentation in the record that the intent of the injury cannot be determined. If no such documentation is present, code to accidental (unintentional).

Y21–Y33 require a 7th character
A—initial encounter
D—subsequent encounter
S—sequela

Y21 DROWNING AND SUBMERSION, UNDETERMINED INTENT

See complete *ICD-10-CM* manual for codes in category Y21.

Y22 HANDGUN DISCHARGE, UNDETERMINED INTENT

Discharge of gun for single hand use, undetermined intent
Discharge of pistol, undetermined intent
Discharge of revolver, undetermined intent
Excludes2: very pistol (Y24.8)
See complete *ICD-10-CM* manual for codes in category Y22.

Y23 RIFLE, SHOTGUN AND LARGER FIREARM DISCHARGE, UNDETERMINED INTENT

Excludes2: airgun (Y24.0)
See complete *ICD-10-CM* manual for codes in category Y23.

Y24 OTHER AND UNSPECIFIED FIREARM DISCHARGE, UNDETERMINED INTENT

See complete *ICD-10-CM* manual for codes in category Y24.

Y25 CONTACT WITH EXPLOSIVE MATERIAL, UNDETERMINED INTENT

See complete *ICD-10-CM* manual for codes in category Y25.

Y26 EXPOSURE TO SMOKE, FIRE AND FLAMES, UNDETERMINED INTENT

See complete *ICD-10-CM* manual for codes in category Y26.

Y27 CONTACT WITH STEAM, HOT VAPORS AND HOT OBJECTS, UNDETERMINED INTENT

See complete *ICD-10-CM* manual for codes in category Y27.

Y28 CONTACT WITH SHARP OBJECT, UNDETERMINED INTENT

See complete *ICD-10-CM* manual for codes in category Y28.

Y29 CONTACT WITH BLUNT OBJECT, UNDETERMINED INTENT

See complete *ICD-10-CM* manual for codes in category Y29.

Y30 FALLING, JUMPING OR PUSHED FROM A HIGH PLACE, UNDETERMINED INTENT

See complete *ICD-10-CM* manual for codes in category Y30.

Y31 FALLING, LYING OR RUNNING BEFORE OR INTO MOVING OBJECT, UNDETERMINED INTENT

See complete *ICD-10-CM* manual for codes in category Y31.

Y32 CRASHING OF MOTOR VEHICLE, UNDETERMINED INTENT

See complete *ICD-10-CM* manual for codes in category Y32.

Y33 OTHER SPECIFIED EVENTS, UNDETERMINED INTENT

See complete *ICD-10-CM* manual for codes in category Y33.

(Y35–Y38) LEGAL INTERVENTION, OPERATIONS OF WAR, MILITARY OPERATIONS, AND TERRORISM

Y35 LEGAL INTERVENTION

Y35–Y38 require a 7th character
A—initial encounter
D—subsequent encounter
S—sequela

Includes: any injury sustained as a result of an encounter with any law enforcement official, serving in any capacity at the time of the encounter, whether on-duty or off-duty.

Includes: injury to law enforcement official, suspect and bystander
See complete *ICD-10-CM* manual for codes in category Y35.

Y36 OPERATIONS OF WAR

Includes: injuries to military personnel and civilians caused by war, civil insurrection, and peacekeeping missions

Excludes1: injury to military personnel occurring during peacetime military operations (Y37.-)
military vehicles involved in transport accidents with non-military vehicle during peacetime (V09.01, V09.21, V19.81, V29.818, V39.81, V49.81, V59.81, V69.81, V79.81)

See complete *ICD-10-CM* manual for codes in category Y36.

Y37 MILITARY OPERATIONS

Includes: injuries to military personnel and civilians occurring during peacetime on military property and during routine military exercises and operations

Excludes1: military aircraft involved in aircraft accident with civilian aircraft (V97.81-)
military vehicles involved in transport accident with civilian vehicle (V09.01, V09.21, V19.81, V29.818,V39.81, V49.81, V59.81, V69.81, V79.81)
military watercraft involved in water transport accident with civilian watercraft (V94.81-)
war operations (Y36.-)

See complete *ICD-10-CM* manual for codes in category Y37.

Y38 TERRORISM

These codes are for use to identify injuries resulting from the unlawful use of force or violence against persons or property to intimidate or coerce a Government, the civilian population, or any segment thereof, in furtherance of political or social objective

Use additional code for place of occurrence (Y92.-)
See complete *ICD-10-CM* manual for codes in category Y38.

(Y62–Y69) MISADVENTURES TO PATIENTS DURING SURGICAL AND MEDICAL CARE

Excludes2: breakdown or malfunctioning of medical device (during procedure) (after implantation) (ongoing use) (Y70–Y82)

Excludes 1: surgical and medical procedures as the cause of abnormal reaction of the patient, without mention of misadventure at the time of the procedure (Y83–Y84)

Y62 FAILURE OF STERILE PRECAUTIONS DURING SURGICAL AND MEDICAL CARE
See complete *ICD-10-CM* manual for codes in category Y62.

Y63 FAILURE IN DOSAGE DURING SURGICAL AND MEDICAL CARE
Excludes2: accidental overdose of drug or wrong drug given in error (T36–T50)
See complete *ICD-10-CM* manual for codes in category Y63.

Y64 CONTAMINATED MEDICAL OR BIOLOGICAL SUBSTANCES
See complete *ICD-10-CM* manual for codes in category Y64.

Y65 OTHER MISADVENTURES DURING SURGICAL AND MEDICAL CARE
See complete *ICD-10-CM* manual for codes in category Y64.

Y66 NONADMINISTRATION OF SURGICAL AND MEDICAL CARE
Premature cessation of surgical and medical care
Excludes1: DNR status (Z66)
palliative care (Z51.5)
See complete *ICD-10-CM* manual for codes in category Y66.

Y69 UNSPECIFIED MISADVENTURE DURING SURGICAL AND MEDICAL CARE
Medical devices associated with adverse incidents in diagnostic and therapeutic use (Y70–Y82)
Includes: breakdown or malfunction of medical devices (during use) (after implantation) (ongoing use)
Excludes2: later complications following use of medical devices without breakdown or malfunctioning of device (Y83-Y84)
misadventure to patients during surgical and medical care, classifiable to (Y62–Y69)
surgical and other medical procedures as the cause of abnormal reaction of the patient, or of later complication, without mention of misadventure at the time of the procedure (Y83–Y84)
See complete *ICD-10-CM* manual for codes in category Y69.

(Y70–Y82) MEDICAL DEVICES ASSOCIATED WITH ADVERSE INCIDENTS IN DIAGNOSTIC AND THERAPEUTIC USE

Includes: breakdown or malfunction of medical devices (during use) (after implantation) (ongoing use)

Excludes2: misadventure to patients during surgical and medical care, classifiable to (Y62–Y69)
later complications following use of medical devices without breakdown or malfunctioning of device (Y83–Y84)
surgical and other medical procedures as the cause of abnormal reaction of the patient, or of later complication, without mention of misadventure at the time of the procedure (Y83–Y84)

Y70 ANESTHESIOLOGY DEVICES ASSOCIATED WITH ADVERSE INCIDENTS
See complete *ICD-10-CM* manual for codes in category Y70.

Y71 CARDIOVASCULAR DEVICES ASSOCIATED WITH ADVERSE INCIDENTS
See complete *ICD-10-CM* manual for codes in category Y71.

Y72 OTORHINOLARYNGOLOGICAL DEVICES ASSOCIATED WITH ADVERSE INCIDENTS
See complete *ICD-10-CM* manual for codes in category Y72.

Y73 GASTROENTEROLOGY AND UROLOGY DEVICES ASSOCIATED WITH ADVERSE INCIDENTS
See complete *ICD-10-CM* manual for codes in category Y73.

Y74 GENERAL HOSPITAL AND PERSONAL-USE DEVICES ASSOCIATED WITH ADVERSE INCIDENTS
See complete *ICD-10-CM* manual for codes in category Y74.

Y75 NEUROLOGICAL DEVICES ASSOCIATED WITH ADVERSE INCIDENTS
See complete *ICD-10-CM* manual for codes in category Y75.

Y76 OBSTETRIC AND GYNECOLOGICAL DEVICES ASSOCIATED WITH ADVERSE INCIDENTS
See complete *ICD-10-CM* manual for codes in category Y76.

Y77 OPHTHALMIC DEVICES ASSOCIATED WITH ADVERSE INCIDENTS
See complete *ICD-10-CM* manual for codes in category Y77.

Y78 RADIOLOGICAL DEVICES ASSOCIATED WITH ADVERSE INCIDENTS
See complete *ICD-10-CM* manual for codes in category Y78.

Y79 ORTHOPEDIC DEVICES ASSOCIATED WITH ADVERSE INCIDENTS
See complete *ICD-10-CM* manual for codes in category Y79.

Y80 PHYSICAL MEDICINE DEVICES ASSOCIATED WITH ADVERSE INCIDENTS
See complete *ICD-10-CM* manual for codes in category Y80.

Y81 GENERAL- AND PLASTIC-SURGERY DEVICES ASSOCIATED WITH ADVERSE INCIDENTS
See complete *ICD-10-CM* manual for codes in category Y81.

Y82 OTHER AND UNSPECIFIED MEDICAL DEVICES ASSOCIATED WITH ADVERSE INCIDENTS
See complete *ICD-10-CM* manual for codes in category Y82.

(Y83–Y84) SURGICAL AND OTHER MEDICAL PROCEDURES AS THE CAUSE OF ABNORMAL REACTION OF THE PATIENT, OR OF LATER COMPLICATION, WITHOUT MENTION OF MISADVENTURE AT THE TIME OF THE PROCEDURE

Excludes1: misadventures to patients during surgical and medical care, classifiable to (Y62–Y69)

Excludes2: breakdown or malfunctioning of medical device (after implantation) (during procedure) (ongoing use) (Y70–Y82)

Y83 SURGICAL OPERATION AND OTHER SURGICAL PROCEDURES AS THE CAUSE OF ABNORMAL REACTION OF THE PATIENT, OR OF LATER COMPLICATION, WITHOUT MENTION OF MISADVENTURE AT THE TIME OF THE PROCEDURE
See complete *ICD-10-CM* manual for codes in category Y83.

Y84 OTHER MEDICAL PROCEDURES AS THE CAUSE OF ABNORMAL REACTION OF THE PATIENT, OR OF LATER COMPLICATION, WITHOUT MENTION OF MISADVENTURE AT THE TIME OF THE PROCEDURE
See complete *ICD-10-CM* manual for codes in category Y84.

(Y90–Y99) SUPPLEMENTARY FACTORS RELATED TO CAUSES OF MORBIDITY CLASSIFIED ELSEWHERE

Note: These categories may be used to provide supplementary information concerning causes of morbidity. They are not to be used for single-condition coding.

Y90 EVIDENCE OF ALCOHOL INVOLVEMENT DETERMINED BY BLOOD ALCOHOL LEVEL
Code first any associated alcohol related disorders (F10)
- **Y90.0** Blood alcohol level of less than 20 mg/100 ml
- **Y90.1** Blood alcohol level of 20–39 mg/100 ml
- **Y90.2** Blood alcohol level of 40–59 mg/100 ml
- **Y90.3** Blood alcohol level of 60–79 mg/100 ml
- **Y90.4** Blood alcohol level of 80–99 mg/100 ml
- **Y90.5** Blood alcohol level of 100–119 mg/100 ml
- **Y90.6** Blood alcohol level of 120–199 mg/100 ml
- **Y90.7** Blood alcohol level of 200–239 mg/100 ml
- **Y90.8** Blood alcohol level of 240 mg/100 ml or more
- **Y90.9** Presence of alcohol in blood, level not specified

Y92 PLACE OF OCCURRENCE OF THE EXTERNAL CAUSE

GUIDELINE

Codes from category Y92, Place of occurrence of the external cause, are secondary codes for use after other external cause codes to identify the location of the patient at the time of injury or other condition.

Generally, a place of occurrence code is assigned only once, at the initial encounter for treatment. However, in the rare instance that a new injury occurs during hospitalization, an additional place of occurrence code may be assigned. No 7th characters are used for Y92.

Do not use place of occurrence code Y92.9 if the place is not stated or is not applicable.

The following category is for use, when relevant, to identify the place of occurrence of the external cause. Use in conjunction with an activity code. Place of occurrence should be recorded only at the **initial encounter** for treatment.

- **Y92.0** Non-institutional (private) residence as the place of occurrence of the external cause

Excludes1: abandoned or derelict house (Y92.89) home under construction but not yet occupied (Y92.6-) institutional place of residence (Y92.1-)

- **Y92.00** Unspecified non-institutional (private) residence
  - **Y92.000** Kitchen of unspecified non-institutional (private) residence
  - **Y92.001** Dining room of unspecified non-institutional (private) residence
  - **Y92.002** Bathroom of unspecified non-institutional (private) residence
  - **Y92.003** Bedroom of unspecified non-institutional (private) residence
  - **Y92.007** Garden or yard of unspecified non-institutional (private) residence
  - **Y92.008** Other place in unspecified non-institutional (private) residence
  - **Y92.009** Unspecified place in unspecified non-institutional (private) residence Home (NOS)
- **Y92.01** Single-family non-institutional (private) house Farmhouse
  Excludes1: barn (Y92.71) chicken coop or hen house (Y92.72) farm field (Y92.73) orchard (Y92.74) single family mobile home or trailer (Y92.02-) slaughter house (Y92.86)
  - **Y92.010** Kitchen of single-family (private) house
  - **Y92.011** Dining room of single-family (private) house
  - **Y92.012** Bathroom of single-family (private) house
  - **Y92.013** Bedroom of single-family (private) house
  - **Y92.014** Private driveway to single-family (private) house
  - **Y92.015** Private garage of single-family (private) house
  - **Y92.016** Swimming-pool in single-family (private) house or garden
  - **Y92.017** Garden or yard in single-family (private) house
  - **Y92.018** Other place in single-family (private) house
  - **Y92.019** Unspecified place in single-family (private) house
- **Y92.02** Mobile home
  - **Y92.020** Kitchen in mobile home
  - **Y92.021** Dining room in mobile home
  - **Y92.022** Bathroom in mobile home
  - **Y92.023** Bedroom in mobile home
  - **Y92.024** Driveway of mobile home
  - **Y92.025** Garage of mobile home
  - **Y92.026** Swimming-pool of mobile home
  - **Y92.027** Garden or yard of mobile home
  - **Y92.028** Other place in mobile home
  - **Y92.029** Unspecified place in mobile home
- **Y92.03** Apartment Condominium Co-op apartment
  - **Y92.030** Kitchen in apartment
  - **Y92.031** Bathroom in apartment
  - **Y92.032** Bedroom in apartment
  - **Y92.038** Other place in apartment
  - **Y92.039** Unspecified place in apartment
- **Y92.04** Boarding-house
  - **Y92.040** Kitchen in boarding-house
  - **Y92.041** Bathroom in boarding-house
  - **Y92.042** Bedroom in boarding-house
  - **Y92.043** Driveway of boarding-house
  - **Y92.044** Garage of boarding-house
  - **Y92.045** Swimming-pool of boarding-house
  - **Y92.046** Garden or yard of boarding-house
  - **Y92.048** Other place in boarding-house
  - **Y92.049** Unspecified place in boarding-house
- **Y92.09** Other non-institutional residence
  - **Y92.090** Kitchen in other non-institutional residence
  - **Y92.091** Bathroom in other non-institutional residence
  - **Y92.092** Bedroom in other non-institutional residence
  - **Y92.093** Driveway of other non-institutional residence
  - **Y92.094** Garage of other non-institutional residence
  - **Y92.095** Swimming-pool of other non-institutional residence
  - **Y92.096** Garden or yard of other non-institutional residence
  - **Y92.098** Other place in other non-institutional residence
  - **Y92.099** Unspecified place in other non-institutional residence
- **Y92.1** Institutional (nonprivate) residence
  - **Y92.10** Unspecified residential institution
  - **Y92.11** Children's home and orphanage
    - **Y92.110** Kitchen in children's home and orphanage
    - **Y92.111** Bathroom in children's home and orphanage
    - **Y92.112** Bedroom in children's home and orphanage
    - **Y92.113** Driveway of children's home and orphanage
    - **Y92.114** Garage of children's home and orphanage
    - **Y92.115** Swimming-pool of children's home and orphanage
    - **Y92.116** Garden or yard of children's home and orphanage
    - **Y92.118** Other place in children's home and orphanage
    - **Y92.119** Unspecified place in children's home and orphanage
  - **Y92.12** Nursing home Home for the sick Hospice Refer to the complete *ICD-10-CM* manual for subcategory Y92.12-
  - **Y92.15** Reform school
    - **Y92.150** Kitchen in reform school
    - **Y92.151** Dining room in reform school
    - **Y92.152** Bathroom in reform school
    - **Y92.153** Bedroom in reform school
    - **Y92.154** Driveway of reform school
    - **Y92.155** Garage of reform school
    - **Y92.156** Swimming-pool of reform school
    - **Y92.157** Garden or yard of reform school
    - **Y92.158** Other place in reform school
    - **Y92.159** Unspecified place in reform school

Y92.16 School dormitory

6th *Excludes1:* reform school (Y92.15-)
school buildings and grounds (Y92.2-)
school sports and athletic areas (Y92.3-)

Y92.160 Kitchen in school dormitory

Y92.161 Dining room in school dormitory

Y92.162 Bathroom in school dormitory

Y92.163 Bedroom in school dormitory

Y92.168 Other place in school dormitory

Y92.169 Unspecified place in school dormitory

Y92.19 Other specified residential institution

Refer to the complete *ICD-10-CM* manual for subcategory Y92.19-

Y92.2 School, other institution and public administrative area

5th Building and adjacent grounds used by the general public or by a particular group of the public

Excludes1: building under construction (Y92.6)
residential institution (Y92.1)
school dormitory (Y92.16-)
sports and athletics area of schools (Y92.3-)

Y92.21 School (private) (public) (state)

6th **Y92.210 Daycare center**

Y92.211 Elementary school

Kindergarten

Y92.212 Middle school

Y92.213 High school

Y92.214 College

University

Y92.215 Trade school

Y92.218 Other school

Y92.219 Unspecified school

Y92.22 Religious institution

Church
Mosque
Synagogue

Y92.23 Hospital

6th *Excludes1:* ambulatory (outpatient) health services establishments (Y92.53-)
home for the sick (Y92.12-)
hospice (Y92.12-)
nursing home (Y92.12-)

Y92.230 Patient room in hospital

Y92.231 Patient bathroom in hospital

Y92.232 Corridor of hospital

Y92.233 Cafeteria of hospital

Y92.234 Operating room of hospital

Y92.238 Other place in hospital

Y92.239 Unspecified place in hospital

Y92.24 Public administrative building

6th **Y92.240 Courthouse**

Y92.241 Library

Y92.242 Post office

Y92.25 Cultural building

6th **Y92.250 Art Gallery**

Y92.251 Museum

Y92.252 Music hall

Y92.253 Opera house

Y92.254 Theater (live)

Y92.258 Other cultural public building

Y92.26 Movie house or cinema

Y92.29 Other specified public building

Assembly hall
Clubhouse

Y92.3 Sports and athletics area

5th **Y92.31 Athletic court**

6th *Excludes1:* tennis court in private home or garden (Y92.09)

Y92.310 Basketball court

Y92.311 Squash court

Y92.312 Tennis court

Y92.318 Other athletic court

Y92.32 Athletic field

6th **Y92.320 Baseball field**

Y92.321 Football field

Y92.322 Soccer field

Y92.328 Other athletic field

Cricket field
Hockey field

Y92.33 Skating rink

6th **Y92.330 Ice skating rink (indoor) (outdoor)**

Y92.331 Roller skating rink

Y92.34 Swimming pool (public)

Excludes1: swimming pool in private home or garden (Y92.016)

Y92.39 Other specified sports and athletic area

Golf-course/gymnasium

Y92.4 Street, highway and other paved roadways

5th *Excludes1:* private driveway of residence (Y92.014, Y92.024, Y92.043, Y92.093, Y92.113, Y92.123, Y92.154, Y92.194)

Y92.41 Street and highway

6th **Y92.410 Unspecified street and highway**

Road NOS

Y92.411 Interstate highway

Freeway/Motorway

Y92.412 Parkway

Y92.413 State road

Y92.414 Local residential or business street

Y92.415 Exit ramp or entrance ramp of street or highway

Y92.48 Other paved roadways

6th **Y92.480 Sidewalk**

Y92.481 Parking lot

Y92.482 Bike path

Y92.488 Other paved roadways

Y92.5 Trade and service area

5th *Excludes1:* garage in private home (Y92.015)
schools and other public administration buildings (Y92.2-)

Y92.51 Private commercial establishments

6th **Y92.510 Bank**

Y92.511 Restaurant or café

Y92.512 Supermarket, store or market

Y92.513 Shop (commercial)

Y92.52 Service areas

6th **Y92.520 Airport**

Y92.521 Bus station

Y92.522 Railway station

Y92.523 Highway rest stop

Y92.524 Gas station

Petroleum station
Service station

Y92.53 Ambulatory health services establishments

6th **Y92.530 Ambulatory surgery center**

Outpatient surgery center, including that connected with a hospital
Same day surgery center, including that connected with a hospital

Y92.531 Health care provider office

Physician office

Y92.532 Urgent care center

Y92.538 Other ambulatory health services establishments

Y92.59 Other trade areas

Office building
Casino
Garage (commercial)
Hotel
Radio or television station
Shopping mall
Warehouse

Y92.6 Industrial and construction area

5th Refer to complete *ICD-10-CM* manual for subcategory Y92.6

Y92.7 Farm

5th Ranch

Excludes1: farmhouse and home premises of farm (Y92.01-)

Y92.71 **Barn**

Y92.72 **Chicken coop**

Hen house

Y92.73 **Farm field**

Y92.74 **Orchard**

Y92.79 **Other farm location**

Y92.8 Other places

Y92.81 **Transport vehicle**

Excludes1: transport accidents (V00-V99)

Y92.810 **Car**

Y92.811 **Bus**

Y92.812 **Truck**

Y92.813 **Airplane**

Y92.814 **Boat**

Y92.815 **Train**

Y92.816 **Subway car**

Y92.818 **Other transport vehicle**

Y92.82 **Wilderness area**

Y92.820 **Desert**

Y92.821 **Forest**

Y92.828 **Other wilderness area**

Swamp

Mountain

Marsh

Prairie

Y92.83 **Recreation area**

Y92.830 **Public park**

Y92.831 **Amusement park**

Y92.832 **Beach/Seashore**

Y92.833 **Campsite**

Y92.834 **Zoological garden (Zoo)**

Y92.838 **Other recreation area**

Y92.85 **Railroad track**

Y92.89 **Other specified places**

Derelict house

Y92.9 Unspecified place or not applicable

Y93 ACTIVITY CODES

GUIDELINE

Assign a code from category Y93, Activity code, to describe the activity of the patient at the time the injury or other health condition occurred.

An activity code is used only once, at the initial encounter for treatment. Only one code from Y93 should be recorded on a medical record.

The activity codes are not applicable to poisonings, adverse effects, misadventures or sequela.

Do not assign Y93.9, Unspecified activity, if the activity is not stated.

A code from category Y93 is appropriate for use with external cause and intent codes if identifying the activity provides additional information about the event.

Note: Category Y93 is provided for use to indicate the activity of the person seeking healthcare for an injury or health condition, such as a heart attack while shoveling snow, which resulted from, or was contributed to, by the activity. These codes are appropriate for use for both acute injuries, such as those from Chapter 19, and conditions that are due to the long-term, cumulative effects of an activity, such as those from Chapter 13. They are also appropriate for use with external cause codes for cause and intent if identifying the activity provides additional information on the event. These codes should be used in conjunction with codes for external cause status (Y99) and place of occurrence (Y92).

Y93.0 Activities involving walking and running

Excludes1: activity, walking an animal (Y93.K1)

activity, walking or running on a treadmill (Y93.A1)

Y93.01 Activity, walking, marching and hiking

Activity, walking, marching and hiking on level or elevated terrain

Excludes1: activity, mountain climbing (Y93.31)

Y93.02 Activity, running

Y93.1 Activities involving water and water craft

Excludes1: activities involving ice (Y93.2-)

Y93.11 Activity, swimming

Y93.12 Activity, springboard and platform diving

Y93.13 Activity, water polo

Y93.14 Activity, water aerobics and water exercise

Y93.15 Activity, underwater diving and snorkeling

Activity, SCUBA diving

Y93.16 Activity, rowing, canoeing, kayaking, rafting and tubing

Y93.17 Activity, water skiing and wake boarding

Y93.18 Activity, surfing, windsurfing and boogie boarding

Activity, water sliding

Y93.19 Activity, other involving water and watercraft

Activity involving water NOS

Activity, parasailing

Activity, water survival training and testing

Y93.2 Activities involving ice and snow

Excludes1: activity, shoveling ice and snow (Y93.H1)

Y93.21 Activity, ice skating

Activity, figure skating (singles) (pairs)

Activity, ice dancing

Excludes1: activity, ice hockey (Y93.22)

Y93.22 Activity, ice hockey

Y93.23 Activity, snow (alpine) (downhill) skiing, snowboarding, sledding, tobogganing and snow tubing

Excludes1: activity, cross country skiing (Y93.24)

Y93.24 Activity, cross country skiing

Activity, nordic skiing

Y93.29 Activity, other involving ice and snow

Activity involving ice and snow NOS

Y93.3 Activities involving climbing, rappelling and jumping off

Excludes1: activity, hiking on level or elevated terrain (Y93.01)

activity, jumping rope (Y93.56)

activity, trampoline jumping (Y93.44)

Y93.31 Activity, mountain climbing, rock climbing and wall climbing

Y93.32 Activity, rappelling

Y93.33 Activity, BASE jumping

Activity, Building, Antenna, Span, Earth jumping

Y93.34 Activity, bungee jumping

Y93.35 Activity, hang gliding

Y93.39 Activity, other involving climbing, rappelling and jumping off

Y93.4 Activities involving dancing and other rhythmic movement

Excludes1: activity, martial arts (Y93.75)

Y93.41 Activity, dancing

Y93.42 Activity, yoga

Y93.43 Activity, gymnastics

Activity, rhythmic gymnastics

Excludes1: activity, trampolining (Y93.44)

Y93.44 Activity, trampolining

Y93.45 Activity, cheerleading

Y93.49 Activity, other involving dancing and other rhythmic movements

Y93.5 Activities involving other sports and athletics played individually

Excludes1: activity, dancing (Y93.41)

activity, gymnastic (Y93.43)

activity, trampolining (Y93.44)

activity, yoga (Y93.42)

Y93.51 Activity, roller skating (inline) and skateboarding

Y93.52 Activity, horseback riding

Y93.53 Activity, golf

Y93.54 Activity, bowling

Y93.55 Activity, bike riding

Y93.56 Activity, jumping rope

Y93.57 Activity, non-running track and field events

Excludes1: activity, running (any form) (Y93.02)

Y93.59 Activity, other involving other sports and athletics played individually

Excludes1: activities involving climbing, rappelling, and jumping (Y93.3-)

activities involving ice and snow (Y93.2-)

activities involving walking and running (Y93.0-)

activities involving water and watercraft (Y93.1-)

Y93.6 Activities involving other sports and athletics played as a team or group

Excludes1: activity, ice hockey (Y93.22)

activity, water polo (Y93.13)

Y93.61 **Activity, American tackle football**
Activity, football NOS

Y93.62 **Activity, American flag or touch football**

Y93.63 Activity, rugby

Y93.64 **Activity, baseball**
Activity, softball

Y93.65 Activity, lacrosse and field hockey

Y93.66 Activity, soccer

Y93.67 Activity, basketball

Y93.68 Activity, volleyball (beach) (court)

Y93.6A **Activity, physical games generally associated with school recess, summer camp and children**
Including capture the flag/dodge ball/four square/kickball

Y93.69 **Activity, other involving other sports and athletics played as a team or group**
Activity, cricket

Y93.7 Activities involving other specified sports and athletics

Y93.71 Activity, boxing

Y93.72 Activity, wrestling

Y93.73 Activity, racquet and hand sports
Activity, handball/racquetball/squash/tennis

Y93.74 Activity, Frisbee

Y93.75 **Activity, martial arts**
Activity, combatives

Y93.79 **Activity, other specified sports and athletics**
Excludes1: sports and athletics activities specified in categories Y93.0–Y93.6

Y93.B Activities involving other muscle strengthening exercises

Y93.B1 **Activity, exercise machines primarily for muscle strengthening**

Y93.B2 **Activity, push-ups, pull-ups, sit-ups**

Y93.B3 **Activity, free weights**
Activity, barbells/dumbbells

Y93.B4 Activity, pilates

Y93.B9 **Activity, other involving muscle strengthening exercises**
Excludes1: activities involving muscle strengthening specified in categories Y93.0–Y93.A

Y93.C Activities involving computer technology and electronic devices

Excludes1: activity, electronic musical keyboard or instruments (Y93.J-)

Y93.C1 **Activity, computer keyboarding**
Activity, electronic game playing using keyboard or other stationary device

Y93.C2 **Activity, hand held interactive electronic device**
Activity, cellular telephone and communication device
Activity, electronic game playing using interactive device
Excludes1: activity, electronic game playing using keyboard or other stationary device (Y93.C1)

Y93.C9 **Activity, other involving computer technology and electronic devices**

Y93.D Activities involving arts and handcrafts

Excludes1: activities involving playing musical instrument (Y93.J-)

Y93.D1 **Activity, knitting and crocheting**

Y93.D2 **Activity, sewing**

Y93.D3 **Activity, furniture building and finishing**
Activity, furniture repair

Y93.D9 **Activity, other involving arts and handcrafts**

Y93.E Activities involving personal hygiene and interior property and clothing maintenance

Excludes1: activities involving cooking and grilling (Y93.G-)
activities involving exterior property and land maintenance, building and construction (Y93.H-)
activities involving caregiving (Y93.F-)
activity, dishwashing (Y93.G1)
activity, food preparation (Y93.G1)
activity, gardening (Y93.H2)

Y93.E1 **Activity, personal bathing and showering**

Y93.E2 **Activity, laundry**

Y93.E3 **Activity, vacuuming**

Y93.E4 **Activity, ironing**

Y93.E5 **Activity, floor mopping and cleaning**

Y93.E6 **Activity, residential relocation**

Activity, packing up and unpacking involved in moving to a new residence

Y93.E8 **Activity, other personal hygiene**

Y93.E9 **Activity, other interior property and clothing maintenance**

Y93.G Activities involving food preparation, cooking and grilling

Y93.G1 **Activity, food preparation and clean up**
Activity, dishwashing

Y93.G2 **Activity, grilling and smoking food**

Y93.G3 **Activity, cooking and baking**
Activity, use of stove, oven and microwave oven

Y93.G9 **Activity, other involving cooking and grilling**

Y93.I Activities involving roller coasters and other types of external motion

Y93.I1 **Activity, roller coaster riding**

Y93.I9 **Activity, other involving external motion**

Y93.J Activities involving playing musical instrument

Activity involving playing electric musical instrument

Y93.J1 **Activity, piano playing**
Activity, musical keyboard (electronic) playing

Y93.J2 **Activity, drum and other percussion instrument playing**

Y93.J3 **Activity, string instrument playing**

Y93.J4 **Activity, winds and brass instrument playing**

Y93.K Activities involving animal care

Excludes1: activity, horseback riding (Y93.52)

Y93.K1 **Activity, walking an animal**

Y93.K2 **Activity, milking an animal**

Y93.K3 **Activity, grooming and shearing an animal**

Y93.K9 **Activity, other involving animal care**

Y93.8 Activities, other specified

Y93.81 **Activity, refereeing a sports activity**

Y93.82 **Activity, spectator at an event**

Y93.83 **Activity, rough housing and horseplay**

Y93.84 **Activity, sleeping**

Y93.85 **Activity, choking game**
Activity, blackout or fainting or pass out game

Y93.89 **Activity, other specified**

Y95 NOSOCOMIAL CONDITION ✓

Y99 EXTERNAL CAUSE STATUS

GUIDELINE

A code from category Y99, External cause status, should be assigned whenever any other external cause code is assigned for an encounter, including an Activity code, except for the events noted below. Assign a code from category Y99, External cause status, to indicate the work status of the person at the time the event occurred. The status code indicates whether the event occurred during military activity, whether a non-military person was at work, whether an individual including a student or volunteer was involved in a non-work activity at the time of the causal event.

A code from Y99, External cause status, should be assigned, when applicable, with other external cause codes, such as transport accidents and falls. The external cause status codes are not applicable to poisonings, adverse effects, misadventures or late effects.

Do not assign a code from category Y99 if no other external cause codes (cause, activity) are applicable for the encounter.

An external cause status code is used only once, at the initial encounter for treatment. Only one code from Y99 should be recorded on a medical record.

Do not assign code Y99.9, Unspecified external cause status, if the status is not stated.

Note: A single code from category Y99 should be used in conjunction with the external cause code(s) assigned to a record to indicate the status of the person at the time the event occurred.

Y99.0 Civilian activity done for income or pay
Civilian activity done for financial or other compensation
Excludes1: military activity (Y99.1)
volunteer activity (Y99.2)

Y99.2 Volunteer activity
Excludes1: activity of child or other family member assisting in compensated work of other family member (Y99.8)

Y99.8 Other external cause status

Activity NEC
Activity of child or other family member assisting in compensated work of other family member
Hobby not done for income
Leisure activity
Off-duty activity of military personnel
Recreation or sport not for income or while a student
Student activity
Excludes1: civilian activity done for income or compensation (Y99.0)
military activity (Y99.1)

Y99.9 Unspecified external cause status

Chapter 21. Factors influencing health status and contact with health services (Z00–Z99)

GUIDELINES

Note: The chapter specific guidelines provide additional information about the use of Z codes for specified encounters.

Use of Z Codes in Any Healthcare Setting

Z codes are for use in any healthcare setting. Z codes may be used as either a first-listed (principal diagnosis code in the inpatient setting) or secondary code, depending on the circumstances of the encounter. Certain Z codes may only be used as first-listed or principal diagnosis.

Z Codes Indicate a Reason for an Encounter *or Provide Additional Information about a Patient Encounter*

Z codes are not procedure codes. A corresponding procedure code must accompany a Z code to describe any procedure performed.

Categories of Z codes

CONTACT/EXPOSURE

See categories Z20 and Z77.

INOCULATIONS AND VACCINATIONS

See category Z23.

STATUS

Status codes indicate that a patient is either a carrier of a disease or has the sequelae or residual of a past disease or condition. This includes such things as the presence of prosthetic or mechanical devices resulting from past treatment. A status code is informative, because the status may affect the course of treatment and its outcome. A status code is distinct from a history code. The history code indicates that the patient no longer has the condition.

A status code should not be used with a diagnosis code from one of the body system chapters, if the diagnosis code includes the information provided by the status code. For example, code Z94.1, Heart transplant status, should not be used with a code from subcategory T86.2, Complications of heart transplant. The status code does not provide additional information. The complication code indicates that the patient is a heart transplant patient.

For encounters for weaning from a mechanical ventilator, assign a code from subcategory J96.1, Chronic respiratory failure, followed by code Z99.11, Dependence on respirator [ventilator] status.

The status Z codes/categories are: Z14, Z15, Z16, Z17, Z18, Z19, Z21, Z22, Z28.3, Z33.1, Z66, Z67, Z68, Z74.01, Z76.82, Z78, Z79, Z88 (Except: Z88.9), Z89, Z90, Z91.0-, Z92.82, Z93, Z94, Z95, Z96, Z97, Z98, Z99

HISTORY (OF)

There are two types of history Z codes, personal and family. Personal and history codes explain a patient's past medical condition that no longer exists and is not receiving any treatment, but that has the potential for recurrence, and therefore may require continued monitoring.

Family history codes are for use when a patient has a family member(s) who has had a particular disease that causes the patient to be at higher risk of also contracting the disease.

Personal history codes may be used in conjunction with follow-up codes and family history codes may be used in conjunction with screening codes to explain the need for a test or procedure. History codes are also acceptable on any medical record regardless of the reason for visit. A history of an illness, even if no longer present, is important information that may alter the type of treatment ordered.

The reason for the encounter (for example, screening or counseling) should be sequenced first and the appropriate personal and/or family history code(s) should be assigned as additional diagnos(es). The history Z code categories are: *Z80, Z81, Z82, Z83, Z84, Z85, Z86, Z87, Z91.4-, Z91.5-, Z91.81, Z91.82, **Z91.85,** Z92 (Except: Z92.0 and Z92.82)*

SCREENING

Screening is the testing for disease or disease precursors in seemingly well individuals so that early detection and treatment can be provided for those who test positive for the disease (e.g., screening mammogram).

The testing of a person to rule out or confirm a suspected diagnosis because the patient has some sign or symptom is a diagnostic examination, not a screening. In these cases, the sign or symptom is used to explain the reason for the test.

A screening code may be a first-listed code if the reason for the visit is specifically the screening exam. It may also be used as an additional code if the screening is done during an office visit for other health problems. A screening code is not necessary if the screening is inherent to a routine examination, such as a pap smear done during a routine pelvic examination.

Should a condition be discovered during the screening then the code for the condition may be assigned as an additional diagnosis.

The Z code indicates that a screening exam is planned. A procedure code is required to confirm that the screening was performed.

The screening Z code categories: Z11, Z12 and Z13 (except: Z13.9).

OBSERVATION

There are three observation Z code categories. They are for use in very limited circumstances when a person is being observed for a suspected condition that is ruled out. The observation codes are not for use if an injury or illness or any signs or symptoms related to the suspected condition are present. In such cases the diagnosis/symptom code is used with the corresponding external cause code.

The observation codes are primarily to be used as a principal/first-listed diagnosis. An observation code may be assigned as a secondary diagnosis code when the patient is being observed for a condition that is ruled out and is unrelated to the principal/first-listed diagnosis. Also, when the principal diagnosis is required to be a code from category Z38, Liveborn infants according to place of birth and type of delivery, then a code from category Z05, Encounter for observation and evaluation of newborn for suspected diseases and conditions ruled out, is sequenced after the Z38 code. Additional codes may be used in addition to the observation code, but only if they are unrelated to the suspected condition being observed.

For encounters for suspected fetal condition that are inconclusive following testing and evaluation, assign the appropriate code from category O35, O36, O40 or O41.

The observation Z code categories: Z03, Z04, and Z05.

AFTERCARE

Aftercare visit codes cover situations when the initial treatment of a disease has been performed and the patient requires continued care during the healing or recovery phase, or for the long-term consequences of the disease. The aftercare Z code should not be used if treatment is directed at a current, acute disease. The diagnosis code is to be used in these cases. Exceptions to this rule are codes Z51.0, Encounter for antineoplastic radiation therapy, and codes from subcategory Z51.1, Encounter for antineoplastic chemotherapy and immunotherapy. These codes are to be first-listed, followed by the diagnosis code when a patient's encounter is solely to receive radiation therapy, chemotherapy, or immunotherapy for the treatment of a neoplasm. If the reason for the encounter is more than one type of antineoplastic therapy, code Z51.0 and a code from subcategory Z51.1 may be assigned together, in which case one of these codes would be reported as a secondary diagnosis.

The aftercare Z codes should also not be used for aftercare for injuries. For aftercare of an injury, assign the acute injury code with the appropriate 7th character (for subsequent encounter).

The aftercare codes are generally first-listed to explain the specific reason for the encounter. An aftercare code may be used as an additional code when some type of aftercare is provided in addition to the reason for admission and no diagnosis code is applicable. An example of this would be the closure of a colostomy during an encounter for treatment of another condition.

Aftercare codes should be used in conjunction with other aftercare codes or diagnosis codes to provide better detail on the specifics of an aftercare encounter visit, unless otherwise directed by the classification. The sequencing of multiple aftercare codes depends on the circumstances of the encounter.

Certain aftercare Z code categories need a secondary diagnosis code to describe the resolving condition or sequelae. For others, the condition is included in the code title.

Additional Z code aftercare category terms include fitting and adjustment, and attention to artificial openings.

Status Z codes may be used with aftercare Z codes to indicate the nature of the aftercare. For example, code Z95.1, Presence of aortocoronary bypass graft, may be used with code Z48.812, Encounter for surgical aftercare following surgery on the circulatory system, to indicate the surgery for which the aftercare is being performed. A status code should not be used when the aftercare code indicates the type of status, such as using Z43.0, Encounter for attention to tracheostomy, with Z93.0, Tracheostomy status.

The aftercare Z category/codes: Z42, Z43, Z44, Z45, Z46, Z47, Z48, Z49 and Z51

FOLLOW-UP

The follow-up codes are used to explain continuing surveillance following completed treatment of a disease, condition, or injury. They imply that the condition has been fully treated and no longer exists. They should not be confused with aftercare codes, or injury codes with a 7th character for subsequent encounter, that explain ongoing care of a healing condition or its sequelae. Follow-up codes may be used in conjunction with history codes to provide the full picture of the healed condition and its treatment. The follow-up code is sequenced first, followed by the history code.

A follow-up code may be used to explain multiple visits. Should a condition be found to have recurred on the follow-up visit, then the diagnosis code for the condition should be assigned in place of the follow-up code. *See categories Z08 and Z09.*

Codes Z08, Encounter for follow-up examination after completed treatment for malignant neoplasm, and Z09, Encounter for follow up examination after completed treatment for conditions other than malignant neoplasm, may be assigned following any type of completed treatment modality (including both medical and surgical treatments).

DONOR

Refer to the *ICD-10-CM* manual.

COUNSELING

Counseling Z codes are used when a patient or family member receives assistance in the aftermath of an illness or injury, or when support is required in coping with family or social problems.

The counseling Z codes/categories: Z30.0-, Z31.5, Z31.6-, Z32.2, Z32.3, Z69, Z70, Z71 and Z76.81

NEWBORNS AND INFANTS

See Chapter 16 for further instruction on the use of these codes. Newborn Z codes/ categories: Z76.1, Z00.1- and Z38

ROUTINE AND ADMINISTRATIVE EXAMINATIONS

The Z codes allow for the description of encounters for routine examinations, such as a general check-up or examinations for administrative purposes, such as a pre-employment physical. The codes are not to be used if the examination is for diagnosis of a suspected condition or for treatment purposes. In such cases the diagnosis code is used. During a routine exam, should a diagnosis or condition be discovered, it should be coded as an additional code. Pre-existing and chronic conditions and history codes may also be included as additional codes as long as the examination is for administrative purposes and not focused on any particular condition.

Some of the codes for routine health examinations distinguish between "with" and "without" abnormal findings. Code assignment depends on the information that is known at the time the encounter is being coded. For example, if no abnormal findings were found during the examination, but the encounter is being coded before test results are back, it is acceptable to assign the code for "without abnormal findings." When assigning a code for "with abnormal findings," additional code(s) should be assigned to identify the specific abnormal finding(s).

Pre-operative examination and pre-procedural laboratory examination Z codes are for use only in those situations when a patient is being cleared for a procedure or surgery and no treatment is given.

The Z codes/categories for routine and administrative examinations: Z00, Z01, Z02 (except: Z02.9) and Z32.0-

MISCELLANEOUS Z CODES

The miscellaneous Z codes capture a number of other health care encounters that do not fall into one of the other categories. Certain of these codes identify the reason for the encounter; others are for use as additional codes that provide useful information on circumstances that may affect a patient's care and treatment.

Prophylactic organ removal

For encounters specifically for prophylactic removal of an organ refer to the full *ICD-10-CM* manual guidelines.

Miscellaneous Z codes/categories: Z28 (except: Z28.3), Z29, Z40, Z41 (except: Z41.9), Z53, Z72, Z73, Z74 (except: Z74.01), Z75, Z76.0, Z76.3, Z76.4, Z76.5, Z91.1-, **Z91.A-** Z91.83, Z91.84-, and Z91.89

NONSPECIFIC Z CODES

Certain Z codes are so non-specific, or potentially redundant with other codes in the classification, that there can be little justification for their use in the inpatient setting. Their use in the outpatient setting should be limited to those instances when there is no further documentation to permit more precise coding. Otherwise,

any sign or symptom or any other reason for visit that is captured in another code should be used.

Nonspecific Z codes/categories: Z02.9, Z04.9, Z13.9, Z41.9, Z52.9, Z86.59, Z88.9 and Z92.0

Z CODES THAT MAY ONLY BE PRINCIPAL/FIRST-LISTED DIAGNOSIS

The following Z codes/categories may only be reported as the principal/first-listed diagnosis, except when there are multiple encounters on the same day and the medical records for the encounters are combined: Z00 (except: Z00.6), Z01, Z02, Z04, Z33.2, Z31.81, Z31.83, Z31.84, Z34, Z39, Z38, Z40, Z42, Z51.0, Z51.1-, Z52 (except: Z52.9), Z76.1, Z76.2, and Z99.12.

Note: Z codes represent reasons for encounters. A corresponding procedure code must accompany a Z code if a procedure is performed. Categories Z00–Z99 are provided for occasions when circumstances other than a disease, injury or external cause classifiable to categories A00–Y89 are recorded as 'diagnoses' or 'problems.' This can arise in two main ways:

- a) When a person who may or may not be sick encounters the health services for some specific purpose, such as to receive limited care or service for a current condition, to donate an organ or tissue, to receive prophylactic vaccination (immunization), or to discuss a problem which is in itself not a disease or injury.
- b) When some circumstance or problem is present which influences the person's health status but is not in itself a current illness or injury.

SOCIAL DETERMINANTS OF HEALTH

See categories Z55–Z65.

(Z00–Z13) PERSONS ENCOUNTERING HEALTH SERVICES FOR EXAMINATIONS

Note: Nonspecific abnormal findings disclosed at the time of these examinations are classified to categories R70–R94.

Excludes1: examinations related to pregnancy and reproduction (Z30–Z36, Z39.-)

Codes in categories Z00–Z04 "may only be reported as the principal/first-listed diagnosis, except when there are multiple encounters on the same day and the medical records for the encounters are combined."

- **Z00 ENCOUNTER FOR GENERAL EXAMINATION WITHOUT COMPLAINT, SUSPECTED OR REPORTED DIAGNOSIS**
  - ***Excludes1:*** encounter for examination for administrative purposes (Z02.-)
  - ***Excludes2:*** encounter for pre-procedural examinations (Z01.81-) special screening examinations (Z11–Z13)
  - **Z00.0 Encounter for general adult medical examination**
    - Encounter for adult periodic examination (annual) (physical) and any associated laboratory and radiologic examinations
    - ***Excludes1:*** encounter for examination of sign or symptom— code to sign or symptom
    - general health check-up of infant or child (Z00.12.-)
    - **Z00.00 Encounter for general adult medical examination without abnormal findings**
      - Encounter for adult health check-up NOS
    - **Z00.01 Encounter for general adult medical examination with abnormal findings**
      - **Use additional code to identify abnormal findings**
  - **Z00.1 Encounter for newborn, infant and child health examinations**
    - **Z00.11 Newborn health examination**
      - *See Chapter 16 for guidelines.*
      - Health check for child under 29 days old
      - **Use additional code to identify any abnormal findings**
      - ***Excludes1:*** health check for child over 28 days old (Z00.12-)
      - **Z00.110 Health examination for newborn; under 8 days old**
        - Health check for newborn under 8 days old
      - **Z00.111 8 to 28 days old**
        - Health check for newborn 8 to 28 days old
        - Newborn weight check
    - **Z00.12 Encounter for routine child health examination;**

Health check (routine) for child over 28 days old
Immunizations appropriate for age

Routine developmental screening of infant or child
Routine vision and hearing testing
Excludes1: health check for child under 29 days old (Z00.11-)
health supervision of foundling or other healthy infant or child (Z76.1-Z76.2)
newborn health examination (Z00.11-)

Z00.121 **with abnormal findings**
Use additional code to identify abnormal findings

Z00.129 **without abnormal findings**
Encounter for routine child health examination NOS

Z00.2 Encounter for examination for period of rapid growth in childhood

Z00.3 Encounter for examination for adolescent development state
Encounter for puberty development state

Z00.7 Encounter for examination for period of delayed growth in childhood

Z00.70 Encounter for examination for period of delayed growth in childhood without abnormal findings

Z00.71 Encounter for examination for period of delayed growth in childhood with abnormal findings
Use additional code to identify abnormal findings

Z01 ENCOUNTER FOR OTHER SPECIAL EXAMINATION WITHOUT COMPLAINT, SUSPECTED OR REPORTED DIAGNOSIS

Includes: routine examination of specific system
Note: Codes from category Z01 represent the reason for the encounter. A separate procedure code is required to identify any examinations or procedures performed
Excludes1: encounter for examination for administrative purposes (Z02.-)
encounter for examination for suspected conditions, proven not to exist (Z03.-)
encounter for laboratory and radiologic examinations as a component of general medical examinations (Z00.0-)
encounter for laboratory, radiologic and imaging examinations for sign(s) and symptom(s)—**code to the sign(s) or symptom(s)**
Excludes2: screening examinations (Z11-Z13)

Z01.0 Encounter for examination of eyes and vision;
Excludes1: examination for driving license (Z02.4)

Z01.00 **without abnormal findings**
Encounter for examination of eyes and vision NOS

Z01.01 **with abnormal findings**
Use additional code to identify abnormal findings

Z01.02 Encounter for examination of eyes and vision following failed vision screening;
Excludes1: encounter for examination of eyes and vision with abnormal findings (Z01.01)
encounter for examination of eyes and vision without abnormal findings (Z01.00)

Z01.020 **without abnormal findings**
Z01.021 **with abnormal findings**

Z01.1 Encounter for examination of ears and hearing;

Z01.10 Encounter for examination of ears and hearing without abnormal findings
Encounter for examination of ears and hearing NOS

Z01.11 Encounter for examination of ears and hearing with abnormal findings

Z01.110 Encounter for hearing examination following failed hearing screening

Z01.118 Encounter for examination of ears and hearing with other abnormal findings
Use additional code to identify abnormal findings

Z01.12 Encounter for hearing conservation and treatment

Z01.3 Encounter for examination of blood pressure

Z01.30 Encounter for examination of blood pressure without abnormal findings
Encounter for examination of blood pressure NOS

Z01.31 Encounter for examination of blood pressure with abnormal findings
Use additional code to identify abnormal findings

Z01.4 Encounter for gynecological examination
Excludes2: pregnancy examination or test (Z32.0-)
routine examination for contraceptive maintenance (Z30.4-)

Z01.41 Encounter for routine gynecological examination
Encounter for general gynecological examination with or without cervical smear
Encounter for gynecological examination (general) (routine) NOS
Encounter for pelvic examination (annual) (periodic)
Use additional code: for screening for human papillomavirus, if applicable, (Z11.51)
for screening vaginal pap smear, if applicable (Z12.72)
to identify acquired absence of uterus, if applicable (Z90.71-)
Excludes1: gynecologic examination status (Z08)
screening cervical pap smear not a part of a routine
gynecological examination (Z12.4)

Z01.411 Encounter for gynecological examination (general) (routine); with abnormal findings
Use additional code to identify abnormal findings

Z01.419 **without abnormal findings**

Z01.42 Encounter for cervical smear to confirm findings of recent normal smear following initial abnormal smear

Z01.8 Encounter for other specified special examinations

Z01.81 Encounter for preprocedural examinations
Pre-operative examination and pre-procedural laboratory examination Z codes are for use only in those situations when a patient is being cleared for a procedure or surgery and no treatment is given.
Encounter for preoperative examinations
Encounter for radiological and imaging examinations as part of preprocedural examination

Z01.810 Encounter for preprocedural; cardiovascular examination

Z01.811 **respiratory examination**

Z01.812 **laboratory examination**
Blood and urine tests prior to treatment or procedure

Z01.818 Encounter for other preprocedural examination
Encounter for preprocedural examination NOS
Encounter for examinations prior to antineoplastic chemotherapy

Z01.82 Encounter for allergy testing
Excludes1: encounter for antibody response examination (Z01.84)

Z01.84 Encounter for antibody response examination
Encounter for immunity status testing
Excludes1: encounter for allergy testing (Z01.82)

Z01.89 Encounter for other specified special examinations

Z02 ENCOUNTER FOR ADMINISTRATIVE EXAMINATION

Z02.0 Encounter for examination for admission to educational institution
Encounter for examination for admission to preschool (education)
Encounter for examination for re-admission to school following illness or medical treatment

Z02.1 Encounter for pre-employment examination

Z02.2 Encounter for examination for admission to residential institution
Excludes1: examination for admission to prison (Z02.89)

Z02.3 Encounter for examination for recruitment to armed forces

Z02.4 Encounter for examination for driving license

Z02.5 Encounter for examination for participation in sport
Excludes1: blood-alcohol and blood-drug test (Z02.83)

Z02.6 Encounter for examination for insurance purposes

Z02.7 Encounter for issue of medical certificate
Excludes1: encounter for general medical examination (Z00-Z01, Z02.0-Z02.6, Z02.8-Z02.9)

Z02.71 **Encounter for disability determination**
Encounter for issue of medical certificate of incapacity or invalidity

Z02.79 **Encounter for issue of other medical certificate**

Z02.8 **Encounter for other administrative examinations**

Z02.82 **Encounter for adoption services**

Z02.83 **Encounter for blood-alcohol and blood-drug test**
Use additional code for findings of alcohol or drugs in blood (R78.-)

Z02.84 **Encounter for child welfare exam**
Encounter for child welfare exam
Encounter for child welfare screening exam
Excludes2: encounter for examination and observation for alleged child physical abuse (Z04.72)
encounter for examination and observation for alleged child rape (Z04.42)

Z02.89 **Encounter for other administrative examinations**
Encounter for examination for admission to prison
Encounter for examination for admission to summer camp
Encounter for immigration or naturalization examination
Encounter for premarital examination
Excludes1: health supervision of foundling or other healthy infant or child (Z76.1–Z76.2)

Z02.9 **Encounter for administrative examinations, unspecified**

Z03 ENCOUNTER FOR MEDICAL OBSERVATION FOR SUSPECTED DISEASES AND CONDITIONS RULED OUT

Excludes1: contact with and (suspected) exposures hazardous to health (Z77.-)
encounter for observation and evaluation of newborn for suspected diseases and conditions ruled out (Z05.-)
person with feared complaint in whom no diagnosis is made (Z71.1)
signs or symptoms under study—code to signs or symptoms

Z03.6 **Encounter for observation for suspected toxic effect from ingested substance ruled out**
Encounter for observation for suspected adverse effect from drug
Encounter for observation for suspected poisoning

Z03.7 **Encounter for suspected maternal and fetal conditions ruled out**

GUIDELINES

Codes from subcategory Z03.7 may either be used as a first-listed or as an additional code assignment depending on the case. They are for use in very limited circumstances on a maternal record when an encounter is for a suspected maternal or fetal condition that is ruled out during that encounter (for example, a maternal or fetal condition may be suspected due to an abnormal test result).

These codes should not be used when the condition is confirmed. In those cases, the confirmed condition should be coded. In addition, these codes are not for use if an illness or any signs or symptoms related to the suspected condition or problem are present. In such cases the diagnosis/symptom code is used.

Additional codes may be used in addition to the code from subcategory Z03.7, but only if they are unrelated to the suspected condition being evaluated. Codes from subcategory Z03.7 may not be used for encounters for antenatal screening of mother.

Encounter for suspected maternal and fetal conditions not found
Excludes1: known or suspected fetal anomalies affecting management of mother, not ruled out (O26.-, O35.-, O36.-, O40.-, O41.-)

Z03.73 **Encounter for suspected; fetal anomaly ruled out**

Z03.74 **problem with fetal growth ruled out**

Z03.79 **maternal and fetal conditions ruled out**

Z03.8 **Encounter for observation for other suspected diseases and conditions ruled out**

Z03.81 **Encounter for observation for suspected exposure to; biological agents ruled out**

Z03.810 **anthrax ruled out**

Z03.818 **other biological agents ruled out**

Z03.82 **Encounter for observation for suspected foreign body ruled out**
Excludes1: retained foreign body (Z18.-)

retained foreign body in eyelid (H02.81)
residual foreign body in soft tissue (M79.5)
Excludes2: confirmed foreign body ingestion or aspiration including:
foreign body in alimentary tract (T18)
foreign body in ear (T16)
foreign body on external eye (T15)
foreign body in respiratory tract (T17)

Z03.821 **Encounter for observation for suspected ingested foreign body ruled out**

Z03.822 **Encounter for observation for suspected aspirated (inhaled) foreign body ruled out**

Z03.823 **Encounter for observation for suspected inserted (injected) foreign body ruled out**
Encounter for observation for suspected inserted (injected) foreign body in eye, orifice or skin ruled out

Z03.83 **Encounter for observation for suspected conditions related to home physiologic monitoring device ruled out**

Z03.89 **Encounter for observation for other suspected diseases and conditions ruled out**
Encounter for observation for suspected inserted (injected) foreign body in eye, orifice or skin ruled out

Z04 ENCOUNTER FOR EXAMINATION AND OBSERVATION FOR OTHER REASONS

Includes: encounter for examination for medicolegal reasons
This category is to be used when a person without a diagnosis is suspected of having an abnormal condition, without signs or symptoms, which requires study, but after examination and observation, is ruled out.
This category is also for use for administrative and legal observation status.

Z04.1 **Encounter for examination and observation following; transport accident**
Excludes1: encounter for examination and observation following work accident (Z04.2)
Do not report an external cause code with a Z04- code

Z04.2 **work accident**

Z04.3 **other accident**

Z04.4 **Encounter for examination and observation following alleged rape**
Encounter for examination and observation of victim following alleged rape
Encounter for examination and observation of victim following alleged sexual abuse

Z04.42 **Encounter for examination and observation following alleged child rape**
Suspected child rape, ruled out
Suspected child sexual abuse, ruled out

Z04.7 **Encounter for examination and observation following alleged; physical abuse**

Z04.72 **child physical abuse**
Suspected child physical abuse, ruled out
Excludes1: confirmed case of child physical abuse (T74.-)
encounter for examination and observation following alleged child sexual abuse (Z04.42)
suspected case of child physical abuse, not ruled out (T76.-)

Z04.8 **Encounter for examination and observation for other specified reasons**
Encounter for examination and observation for request for expert evidence

Z04.81 **Encounter for examination and observation of victim following forced sexual exploitation**

Z04.82 **Encounter for examination and observation of victim following forced labor exploitation**

Z04.89 **Encounter for examination and observation for other specified reasons**

Z04.9 **Encounter for examination and observation for unspecified reason**
Code is a nonspecific Z code, refer to Chapter 21 for guidelines.

Z05 ENCOUNTER FOR OBSERVATION AND EVALUATION OF NEWBORN FOR SUSPECTED DISEASES AND CONDITIONS RULED OUT

GUIDELINES

Use of Z05 codes

Assign a code from category Z05, Observation and evaluation of newborns and infants for suspected conditions ruled out, to identify those instances when a healthy newborn is evaluated for a suspected condition that is determined after study not to be present. Do not use a code from category Z05 when the patient has identified signs or symptoms of a suspected problem; in such cases code the sign or symptom.

Z05 on Other than the Birth Record

A code from category Z05 may also be assigned as a principal or first-listed code for readmissions or encounters when the code from category Z38 code no longer applies. Codes from category Z05 are for use only for healthy newborns and infants for which no condition after study is found to be present.

Z05 on a birth record

A code from category Z05 is to be used as a secondary code after the code from category Z38, Liveborn infants according to place of birth and type of delivery is listed first.

This category is to be used for newborns, within the neonatal period (the first 28 days of life), who are suspected of having an abnormal condition but without signs or symptoms, and which, after examination and observation, is ruled out.

An observation code may be assigned as a secondary diagnosis code when the patient is being observed for a condition that is ruled out and is unrelated to the principal/first-listed diagnosis (e.g., patient presents for treatment following injuries sustained in a motor vehicle accident and is also observed for suspected COVID-19 infection that is subsequently ruled out).

- **Z05.0 Observation and evaluation of newborn for suspected; cardiac condition ruled out**
- **Z05.1 infectious condition ruled out**
- **Z05.2 neurological condition ruled out**
- **Z05.3 respiratory condition ruled out**
- **Z05.4 genetic, metabolic or immunologic condition ruled out**
  - **Z05.41 genetic condition ruled out**
  - **Z05.42 metabolic condition ruled out**
  - **Z05.43 immunologic condition ruled out**
- **Z05.5 gastrointestinal condition ruled out**
- **Z05.6 genitourinary condition ruled out**
- **Z05.7 skin and subcutaneous tissue or musculoskeletal condition ruled out**
  - **Z05.71 skin and subcutaneous tissue condition ruled out**
  - **Z05.72 musculoskeletal condition ruled out**
  - **Z05.73 connective tissue condition ruled out**
- **Z05.8 Observation and evaluation of newborn for other specified suspected condition ruled out**
  - **Z05.81 Observation and evaluation of newborn for suspected condition related to home physiologic monitoring device ruled out**
    - Encounter for observation of newborn for apnea alarm without findings
    - Encounter for observation of newborn for bradycardia alarm without findings
    - Encounter for observation of newborn for malfunction of home cardiorespiratory monitor
    - Encounter for observation of newborn for non-specific findings home physiologic monitoring device
    - Encounter for observation of newborn for pulse oximeter alarm without findings
    - *Excludes1:* encounter for observation for suspected conditions related to home physiologic monitoring device ruled out (Z03.83)
    - neonatal bradycardia (P29.12)
    - other newborn apnea (P28.4-)
    - primary sleep apnea of newborn (P28.3-)
  - **Z05.89 Observation and evaluation of newborn for other specified suspected condition ruled out**
- **Z05.9 Observation and evaluation of newborn for unspecified suspected condition ruled out**

Z08 ENCOUNTER FOR FOLLOW-UP EXAMINATION AFTER COMPLETED TREATMENT FOR MALIGNANT NEOPLASM

Medical surveillance following completed treatment

Use additional code to identify any acquired absence of organs (Z90.-)

Use additional code to identify the personal history of malignant neoplasm (Z85.-)

Excludes1: aftercare following medical care (Z43–Z49, Z51)

Z09 ENCOUNTER FOR FOLLOW-UP EXAMINATION AFTER COMPLETED TREATMENT FOR CONDITIONS OTHER THAN MALIGNANT NEOPLASM

Medical surveillance following completed treatment

Use additional code to identify any applicable history of disease code (Z86.-, Z87.-)

Excludes1: aftercare following medical care (Z43–Z49, Z51)

surveillance of contraception (Z30.4-)

surveillance of prosthetic and other medical devices (Z44–Z46)

Z11 ENCOUNTER FOR SCREENING FOR INFECTIOUS AND PARASITIC DISEASES

Excludes1: encounter for diagnostic examination-code to sign or symptom

- **Z11.0 Encounter for screening for; intestinal infectious diseases**
- **Z11.1 respiratory tuberculosis**
  - Encounter for screening for active tuberculosis disease
- **Z11.2 other bacterial diseases**
- **Z11.3 infections with a predominantly sexual mode of transmission**
  - *Excludes2:* encounter for screening for HIV (Z11.4)
  - encounter for screening for human papillomavirus (Z11.51)
- **Z11.4 HIV**
- **Z11.5 Encounter for screening for; other viral diseases**
  - *Excludes2:* encounter for screening for viral intestinal disease (Z11.0)
  - **Z11.51 human papillomavirus (HPV)**
  - **Z11.52 COVID-19**
  - **Z11.59 other viral diseases**
- **Z11.6 Encounter for screening for other protozoal diseases and helminthiases**
  - *Excludes2:* encounter for screening for protozoal intestinal disease (Z11.0)
- **Z11.7 Encounter for testing for latent tuberculosis infection**
- **Z11.8 Encounter for screening for other infectious and parasitic diseases**
  - Encounter for screening for chlamydia or rickettsial or spirochetal or mycoses
- **Z11.9 Encounter for screening for infectious and parasitic diseases, unspecified**

Z12 ENCOUNTER FOR SCREENING FOR MALIGNANT NEOPLASMS

Use additional code to identify any family history of malignant neoplasm (Z80.-)

Excludes1: encounter for diagnostic examination-code to sign or symptom

- **Z12.3 Encounter for screening for malignant neoplasm of breast**
  - **Z12.31 Encounter for screening mammogram for malignant neoplasm of breast**
    - *Excludes1:* inconclusive mammogram (R92.2)
  - **Z12.39 Encounter for other screening for malignant neoplasm of breast**
- **Z12.4 Encounter for screening for malignant neoplasm of cervix**
  - Encounter for screening pap smear for malignant neoplasm of cervix
  - *Excludes1:* when screening is part of general gynecological examination (Z01.4-)
  - *Excludes2:* encounter for screening for human papillomavirus (Z11.51)
- **Z12.8 Encounter for screening for malignant neoplasm of; other sites**
  - **Z12.82 nervous system**
  - **Z12.89 other sites**
- **Z12.9 Encounter for screening for malignant neoplasm, site unspecified**

Z13 ENCOUNTER FOR SCREENING FOR OTHER DISEASES AND DISORDERS

Excludes Z13.9.

Excludes1: encounter for diagnostic examination-code to sign or symptom

Z13.0 Encounter for screening for; diseases of the blood and blood-forming organs and certain disorders involving the immune mechanism

Z13.1 DM

Z13.2 nutritional, metabolic and other endocrine disorders

5th **Z13.21** nutritional disorder

Z13.22 metabolic disorder

6th **Z13.220** lipid disorders

Encounter for screening for cholesterol level or hypercholesterolemia or hyperlipidemia

Z13.228 other metabolic disorders

Z13.29 other suspected endocrine disorder

Excludes2: encounter for screening for DM (Z13.1)

Z13.3 Encounter for screening for mental health and behavioral

5th disorders

Z13.30 Encounter for screening examination for mental health and behavioral disorders, unspecified

Z13.31 Encounter for screening for depression

Encounter for screening for depression, adult

Encounter for screening for depression for child or adolescent

Z13.32 Encounter for screening for maternal depression

Encounter for screening for perinatal depression

Z13.39 Encounter for screening examination for other mental health and behavioral disorders

Encounter for screening for alcoholism

Encounter for screening for intellectual disabilities

Z13.4 Encounter for screening for certain developmental disorders

5th in childhood

Encounter for screening for developmental handicaps in early childhood

Excludes2: encounter for routine child health examination (Z00.12-)

Z13.40 Encounter for screening for unspecified developmental delays

Z13.41 Encounter for autism screening

Z13.42 Encounter for screening for global developmental delays (milestones)

Encounter for screening for developmental handicaps in early childhood

Z13.49 Encounter for screening for other developmental delays

Z13.5 eye and ear disorders

Excludes2: encounter for general hearing examination (Z01.1-)

encounter for general vision examination (Z01.0-)

Z13.6 cardiovascular disorders

Z13.7 genetic and chromosomal anomalies

5th *Excludes1:* genetic testing for procreative management (Z31.4-)

Z13.71 Encounter for nonprocreative screening for genetic disease carrier status

Z13.79 Encounter for other screening for genetic and chromosomal anomalies

Z13.8 Encounter for screening for; other specified diseases

5th and disorders

Excludes2: screening for malignant neoplasms (Z12.-)

Z13.81 digestive system disorders

6th **Z13.810** upper gastrointestinal disorder

Z13.811 lower gastrointestinal disorder

Excludes1: encounter for screening for intestinal infectious disease (Z11.0)

Z13.818 other digestive system disorders

Z13.82 Encounter for screening for musculoskeletal disorder

6th **Z13.828** other musculoskeletal disorder

Z13.83 respiratory disorder NEC

Excludes1: encounter for screening for respiratory tuberculosis (Z11.1)

Z13.84 dental disorders

Z13.85 Encounter for screening for nervous system

6th disorders

Z13.850 traumatic brain injury

Z13.858 other nervous system disorders

Z13.88 disorder due to exposure to contaminants

Excludes1: those exposed to contaminants without suspected disorders (Z57.-, Z77.-)

Z13.89 other disorder

Encounter for screening for genitourinary disorders

Z13.9 Encounter for screening, unspecified

Code is a nonspecific Z code, refer to Chapter 21 for guidelines.

(Z14–Z15) GENETIC CARRIER AND GENETIC SUSCEPTIBILITY TO DISEASE

Z14 GENETIC CARRIER

4th Genetic carrier status indicates that a person carries a gene, associated with a particular disease, which may be passed to offspring who may develop that disease. The person does not have the disease and is not at risk of developing the disease. Refer to Chapter 21 for status guidelines.

Z14.0 Hemophilia A carrier

5th **Z14.01** Asymptomatic hemophilia A carrier

Z14.02 Symptomatic hemophilia A carrier

Z14.1 Cystic fibrosis carrier

Z14.8 Genetic carrier of other disease

Z15 GENETIC SUSCEPTIBILITY TO DISEASE

Includes: confirmed abnormal gene

Use additional code, if applicable, for any associated family history of the disease (Z80–Z84)

Excludes1: chromosomal anomalies (Q90–Q99)

Z15.0 Genetic susceptibility to malignant neoplasm

Code first, if applicable, any current malignant neoplasm (C00–C75, C81–C96)

Use additional code, if applicable, for any personal history of malignant neoplasm (Z85.-)

Z15.01 Genetic susceptibility to malignant neoplasm of breast

Z15.02 Genetic susceptibility to malignant neoplasm of ovary

Z15.03 Genetic susceptibility to malignant neoplasm of prostate

Z15.04 Genetic susceptibility to malignant neoplasm of endometrium

Z15.09 Genetic susceptibility to other malignant neoplasm

●**Z15.1** Genetic susceptibility to epilepsy and neurodevelopmental disorders

Code also, if applicable, related disorders such as:

developmental and epileptic encephalopathy (G93.45)

developmental disorder of speech and language (F80.-)

developmental disorders of scholastic skills (F81.-)

epilepsy, by specific type (G40.-)

intellectual disabilities (F70–F79)

other neurodevelopmental disorder (F88)

pervasive developmental disorders (F84.-)

●**Z15.2** Genetic susceptibility to obesity

Code also, if applicable, any associated manifestations, such as:

other obesity (E66.8-)

polyphagia (R63.2)

Use additional code to identify body mass index (BMI), if known (Z68.-)

Z15.8 Genetic susceptibility to other disease

Z15.81 Genetic susceptibility to multiple endocrine neoplasia [MEN]

Excludes1: multiple endocrine neoplasia [MEN] syndromes (E31.2-)

Z15.89 Genetic susceptibility to other disease

(Z16) RESISTANCE TO ANTIMICROBIAL DRUGS

Z16 RESISTANCE TO ANTIMICROBIAL DRUGS

4th This code indicates that a patient has a condition that is resistant to antimicrobial drug treatment. Sequence the infection code first.

Note: The codes in this category are provided for use as additional codes to identify the resistance and non-responsiveness of a condition to antimicrobial drugs.

Code first the infection

Excludes1: MRSA infection (A49.02)
MRSA infection in diseases classified elsewhere (B95.62)
MRSA pneumonia (J15.212)
Sepsis due to MRSA (A41.02)

Z16.1 Resistance to beta lactam antibiotics

5th Z16.10 Resistance to unspecified beta lactam antibiotics

Z16.11 Resistance to penicillins
Resistance to amoxicillin or ampicillin

Z16.12 Extended spectrum beta lactamase (ESBL) resistance
Excludes 2: MRSA infection in diseases classified elsewhere (B95.62)

Z16.13 Resistance to carbapenem

Z16.19 other specified beta lactam antibiotics
Resistance to cephalosporins

Z16.2 Resistance to; other antibiotics

5th Z16.20 unspecified antibiotic
Resistance to antibiotics NOS

Z16.21 vancomycin

Z16.22 vancomycin related antibiotics

Z16.23 quinolones and fluoroquinolones

Z16.24 multiple antibiotics

Z16.29 other single specified antibiotic
Resistance to aminoglycosides or macrolides or sulfonamides or tetracyclines

Z16.3 Resistance to; other antimicrobial drugs

5th *Excludes1:* resistance to antibiotics (Z16.1-, Z16.2-)

Z16.30 unspecified antimicrobial drugs
Drug resistance NOS

Z16.32 antifungal drug(s)

Z16.33 antiviral drug(s)

6th Z16.341 single antimycobacterial drug
Resistance to antimycobacterial drug NOS

Z16.342 multiple antimycobacterial drugs

Z16.34 Resistance to antimycobacterial drug(s)
Resistance to tuberculostatics

Z16.35 Resistance to multiple antimicrobial drugs
Excludes1: Resistance to multiple antibiotics only (Z16.24)

Z16.39 other specified antimicrobial drug

(Z18) RETAINED FB FRAGMENTS

Z18 RETAINED FB FRAGMENTS

4th *Includes:* embedded fragment (status)
embedded splinter (status)
retained FB status
Excludes1: artificial joint prosthesis status (Z96.6-)
FB accidentally left during a procedure (T81.5-)
FB entering through orifice (T15–T19)
in situ cardiac device (Z95.-)
organ or tissue replaced by means other than transplant (Z96.-, Z97.-)
organ or tissue replaced by transplant (Z94.-)
personal history of retained FB fully removed Z87.821
superficial FB (non-embedded splinter)—code to superficial FB, by site

Z18.1 Retained metal fragments;

5th *Excludes1:* retained radioactive metal fragments (Z18.01–Z18.09)

Z18.10 Retained metal fragments, unspecified
Retained metal fragment NOS

Z18.11 Retained magnetic metal fragments

Z18.12 Retained nonmagnetic metal fragments

Z18.2 Retained plastic fragments
Acrylics fragments
Diethylhexyl phthalates fragments
Isocyanate fragments

Z18.3 Retained organic fragments

5th Z18.31 Retained animal quills or spines

Z18.32 Retained tooth

Z18.33 Retained wood fragments

Z18.39 Other retained organic fragments

Z18.8 Other specified retained FB

5th Z18.81 Retained glass fragments

Z18.83 Retained stone or crystalline fragments
Retained concrete or cement fragments

Z18.89 Other specified retained FB fragments

Z18.9 Retained FB fragments, unspecified material

(Z20–Z29) PERSONS WITH POTENTIAL HEALTH HAZARDS RELATED TO COMMUNICABLE DISEASES

GUIDELINES

Category Z20 indicates contact with, and suspected exposure to, communicable diseases. These codes are for patients who are suspected to have been exposed to a disease by close personal contact with an infected individual or are in an area where a disease is epidemic.

Contact/exposure codes may be used as a first-listed code to explain an encounter for testing, or, more commonly, as a secondary code to identify a potential risk.

Z20 CONTACT WITH AND (SUSPECTED) EXPOSURE TO COMMUNICABLE DISEASES

4th *Excludes1:* carrier of infectious disease (Z22.-)
diagnosed current infectious or parasitic disease—see Alphabetic Index
Excludes2: personal history of infectious and parasitic diseases (Z86.1-)

Z20.0 Contact with and (suspected) exposure to intestinal infectious diseases;

5th Z20.01 due to E. coli

Z20.09 other intestinal infectious diseases

Z20.1 Contact with and (suspected) exposure to; tuberculosis

Z20.2 infections with a predominantly sexual mode of transmission

Z20.3 rabies

Z20.4 rubella

Z20.5 viral hepatitis

Z20.6 HIV
Excludes1: asymptomatic HIV
HIV infection status (Z21)

Z20.7 pediculosis, acariasis and other infestations

Z20.8 Contact with and (suspected) exposure to; other communicable diseases

5th Z20.81 other bacterial communicable diseases

6th Z20.810 anthrax

Z20.811 meningococcus

Z20.818 other bacterial communicable diseases
Use Z20.818 for exposure to strep throat

Z20.82 Contact with and (suspected) exposure to; other viral communicable diseases

6th Z20.820 varicella

Z20.821 Zika virus

GUIDELINE

See Code U07.1 for more information.

Z20.822 COVID-19

Z20.828 other viral communicable diseases

Z20.89 other communicable diseases

Z20.9 unspecified communicable disease

Z21 ASYMPTOMATIC HIV INFECTION STATUS

✓ This code indicates that a patient has tested positive for HIV but has manifested no signs or symptoms of the disease.
HIV positive NOS
Code first HIV disease complicating pregnancy, childbirth and the puerperium, if applicable (O98.7-)
Excludes1: acquired immunodeficiency syndrome (B20)
contact with HIV (Z20.6)
exposure to HIV (Z20.6)
HIV disease (B20)
inconclusive laboratory evidence of HIV (R75)

Z22 CARRIER OF INFECTIOUS DISEASE

4th Carrier status indicates that a person harbors the specific organisms of a disease without manifest symptoms and is capable of transmitting the infection.
Includes: colonization status
suspected carrier
Excludes2: carrier of viral hepatitis (B18.-)

Z22.1 Carrier of other intestinal infectious diseases

Z22.2 Carrier of diphtheria

Z22.3 Carrier of other specified bacterial diseases

5th **Z22.31** Carrier of bacterial disease due to; meningococci

Z22.32 Carrier of bacterial disease due to staphylococci

6th **Z22.321** Carrier or suspected carrier of MSSA
MSSA colonization

Z22.322 Carrier or suspected carrier of MRSA
MRSA colonization

Z22.33 Carrier of bacterial disease due to streptococci

6th **Z22.330** Carrier of Group B streptococcus
Excludes1: carrier of streptococcus group B (GBS) complicating pregnancy, childbirth and the puerperium (O99.82-)

Z22.338 Carrier of other streptococcus

Z22.34 Carrier of Acinetobacter baumannii

6th **Z22.340** Carrier of carbapenem-resistant Acinetobacter baumannii

Z22.341 Carrier of carbapenem-sensitive Acinetobacter baumannii

Z22.349 Carrier of Acinetobacter baumannii, unspecified

Z22.35 Carrier of Enterobacterales

6th Carrier of E. coli
Carrier of K. pneumoniae

Z22.350 Carrier of carbapenem-resistant Enterobacterales

Z22.358 Carrier of other Enterobacterales
Carrier of carbapenem-sensitive Enterobacterales
Carrier of ESBL-producing Enterobacterales
Carrier of extended-spectrum beta-lactamase producing Enterobacterales

Z22.359 Carrier of Enterobacterales, unspecified

Z22.39 Carrier of other specified bacterial diseases

Z22.4 Carrier of infections with a predominantly sexual mode of transmission

Z22.5 Carrier of viral hepatitis

Z22.6 Carrier of human T-lymphotropic virus type-1 [HTLV-1] infection

Z22.7 Latent tuberculosis
Latent tuberculosis infection (LTBI)
Excludes1: nonspecific reaction to cell mediated immunity measurement of gamma interferonantigen response without active tuberculosis (R76.12)
nonspecific reaction to tuberculin skin test without active tuberculosis (R76.11)

Z22.8 Carrier of other infectious diseases

Z22.9 Carrier of infectious disease, unspecified

Z23 ENCOUNTER FOR IMMUNIZATION

✔

GUIDELINES

Code Z23 is for encounters for inoculations and vaccinations. It indicates that a patient is being seen to receive a prophylactic inoculation against a disease. Procedure codes are required to identify the actual administration of the injection and the type(s) of immunizations given. Code Z23 may be used as a secondary code if the inoculation is given as a routine part of preventive health care, such as a well-baby visit.

Code first any routine childhood examination

Code also, if applicable, encounter for immunization safety counseling (Z71.85)

Note: procedure codes are required to identify the types of immunizations given

Z28 IMMUNIZATION NOT CARRIED OUT AND UNDERIMMUNIZATION STATUS

4th

Includes: vaccination not carried out

Code also, if applicable, encounter for immunization safety counseling (Z71.85)

Z28.0 Immunization not carried out due to; contraindication

5th **Z28.01** acute illness of patient

Z28.02 chronic illness or condition of patient

Z28.03 immune compromised state of patient

Z28.04 patient allergy to vaccine or component

Z28.09 other contraindication

Z28.1 Immunization not carried out due to patient decision for reasons of belief or group pressure
Immunization not carried out because of religious belief

Z28.2 Immunization not carried out due to; patient decision for other and unspecified reason

5th **Z28.20** patient decision for unspecified reason

Z28.21 patient refusal

Z28.29 patient decision for other reason

GUIDELINES

Code Z28.310, Unvaccinated for COVID-19, may be assigned when the patient has not received a COVID-19 vaccine of any type. Code Z28.311, Partially vaccinated for COVID-19, may be assigned when the patient has been partially vaccinated for COVID-19 as per the recommendations of the Centers for Disease Control and Prevention (CDC) in place at the time of the encounter. For information, visit the CDC's website https://www.cdc.gov/coronavirus/2019-ncov/vaccines/.

See *ICD-10-CM Official Guidelines for Coding and Reporting* FY 2024 in front matter, "Documentation by Clinicians Other than the Patient's Provider."

Z28.3 Underimmunization status

5th **Use Additional** code, if applicable, to identify:
immunization not carried out because of contraindication (Z28.0-)
immunization not carried out because of patient decision for other and unspecified reason (Z28.2-)
immunization not carried out because of patient decision for reasons of belief or group pressure (Z28.1)
immunization not carried out for other reason (Z28.8-)

Z28.31 Underimmunization for COVID-19 status

6th Note: These codes should not be used for individuals who are not eligible for the COVID-19 vaccines, as determined by the healthcare provider.

Z28.310 Unvaccinated for COVID-19

Z28.311 Partially vaccinated for COVID-19

Z28.39 Other underimmunization status
Delinquent immunization status
Lapsed immunization schedule status

Z28.8 Immunization not carried out; for other reason

5th **Z28.81** due to patient having had the disease

Z28.82 because of caregiver refusal
Immunization not carried out because of parental or guardian refusal
Excludes1: immunization not carried out because of caregiver refusal because of religious belief (Z28.1)

Z28.83 **due to unavailability of vaccine**
Delay in delivery of vaccine
Lack of availability of vaccine
Manufacturer delay of vaccine

Z28.89 for other reason

Z28.9 Immunization not carried out for unspecified reason

Z29 ENCOUNTER FOR PROPHYLACTIC MEASURES

4th *Excludes 1:* desensitization to allergens (Z51.6)
prophylactic surgery (Z40.-)

Z29.1 Encounter for prophylactic therapy

5th Encounter for administration of immunoglobulin

Z29.11 Encounter for prophylactic immunotherapy for RSV

Z29.12 Encounter for prophylactic antivenin

Z29.13 Encounter for prophylactic Rho(D) immune globulin

Z29.14 Encounter for prophylactic rabies immune globin

Z29.3 Encounter for prophylactic fluoride administration

Z29.8 Encounter for other specified prophylactic measures

5th **Z29.81** Encounter for HIV pre-exposure prophylaxis
Code also, if applicable, risk factors for HIV, such as:
contact with and (suspected) exposure to human immunodeficiency virus [HIV] (Z20.6)
high risk sexual behavior (Z72.5-)

Z29.89 Encounter for other specified prophylactic measures

Z29.9 Encounter for prophylactic measures, unspecified

(Z30–Z39) PERSONS ENCOUNTERING HEALTH SERVICES IN CIRCUMSTANCES RELATED TO REPRODUCTION

Z30 ENCOUNTER FOR CONTRACEPTIVE MANAGEMENT

Z30.0 Encounter for general counseling and advice on contraception

Refer to Chapter 21 for guidelines on counseling.

Z30.01 Encounter for initial prescription of; contraceptives

Excludes1: encounter for surveillance of contraceptives (Z30.4-)

Z30.011 contraceptive pills

Z30.012 emergency contraception

Encounter for postcoital contraception

Z30.013 injectable contraceptive

Z30.014 intrauterine contraceptive device

Excludes1: encounter for insertion of intrauterine contraceptive device (Z30.430, Z30.432)

Z30.015 vaginal ring hormonal contraceptive

Z30.016 transdermal patch hormonal contraceptive device

Z30.017 implantable subdermal contraceptive

Z30.018 other contraceptives

Encounter for initial prescription of barrier contraception or diaphragm

Z30.019 contraceptives, unspecified

Z30.02 Counseling and instruction in natural family planning to avoid pregnancy

Z30.09 Encounter for other general counseling and advice on contraception

Encounter for family planning advice NOS

Z30.4 Encounter for surveillance of contraceptives

Z30.40 Encounter for surveillance of unspecified

Z30.41 Encounter for surveillance of contraceptive pills

Encounter for repeat prescription for contraceptive pill

Z30.42 Encounter for surveillance of injectable contraceptive

Z30.43 Encounter for surveillance of intrauterine contraceptive device

Z30.430 Encounter for insertion of intrauterine contraceptive device

Z30.431 Encounter for routine checking of intrauterine contraceptive device

Z30.432 Encounter for removal of intrauterine contraceptive device

Z30.433 Encounter for removal and reinsertion of intrauterine contraceptive device replacement of intrauterine contraceptive device

Z30.44 Encounter for surveillance of vaginal ring hormonal contraceptive device

Z30.45 Encounter for surveillance of transdermal patch hormonal contraceptive device

Z30.46 Encounter for surveillance of implantable subdermal contraceptive

Encounter for checking, reinsertion or removal of implantable subdermal contraceptive

Z30.49 Encounter for surveillance of other contraceptives

Encounter for surveillance of barrier contraception

Encounter for surveillance of diaphragm

Z30.8 Encounter for other contraceptive management

Encounter for postvasectomy sperm count

Encounter for routine examination for contraceptive maintenance

Excludes1: sperm count following sterilization reversal (Z31.42) sperm count for fertility testing (Z31.41)

Z30.9 Encounter for contraceptive management, unspecified

Z31 ENCOUNTER FOR PROCREATIVE MANAGEMENT

Excludes2: complications associated with artificial fertilization (N98.-)

female infertility (N97.-)

male infertility (N46.-)

Z31.5 Encounter for procreative genetic counseling

See Chapter 21 for guidelines on counseling.

Z31.6 Encounter for general counseling and advice on procreation

See Chapter 21 for guidelines on counseling.

Z31.69 Encounter for other general counseling and advice on procreation

Z32 ENCOUNTER FOR PREGNANCY TEST AND CHILDBIRTH AND CHILDCARE INSTRUCTION

Z32.0 Encounter for pregnancy test

Z32.00 Encounter for pregnancy test, result unknown

Encounter for pregnancy test NOS

Z32.01 Encounter for pregnancy test, result positive

Z32.02 Encounter for pregnancy test, result negative

Z32.3 Encounter for childcare instruction

Encounter for prenatal or postpartum childcare instruction

Z33 PREGNANT STATE

Z33.1 Pregnant state, incidental

Pregnancy NOS

Pregnant state NOS

Excludes1: complications of pregnancy (O00–O9A)

Z38 LIVEBORN INFANTS ACCORDING TO PLACE OF BIRTH AND TYPE OF DELIVERY

GUIDELINES

When coding the birth episode in a newborn record, assign a code from category Z38 as the principal diagnosis. A code from category Z38 is assigned only once, to a newborn at the time of birth. If a newborn is transferred to another institution, a code from category Z38 should not be used at the receiving hospital.

A code from category Z38 is used only on the newborn record, not on the mother's record.

Z38.0 Single liveborn infant, born in hospital

Single liveborn infant, born in birthing center or other health care facility

Z38.00 Single liveborn infant, delivered vaginally

Z38.01 Single liveborn infant, delivered by cesarean

Z38.1 Single liveborn infant, born outside hospital

Z38.2 Single liveborn infant, unspecified as to place of birth

Single liveborn infant NOS

Z38.3 Twin liveborn infant, born in hospital

Z38.30 Twin liveborn infant, delivered vaginally

Z38.31 Twin liveborn infant, delivered by cesarean

Z38.4 Twin liveborn infant, born outside hospital

Z38.5 Twin liveborn infant, unspecified as to place of birth

Z38.6 Other multiple liveborn infant, born in hospital

Z38.61 Triplet liveborn infant, delivered vaginally

Z38.62 Triplet liveborn infant, delivered by cesarean

Z38.63 Quadruplet liveborn infant, delivered vaginally

Z38.64 Quadruplet liveborn infant, delivered by cesarean

Z38.65 Quintuplet liveborn infant, delivered vaginally

Z38.66 Quintuplet liveborn infant, delivered by cesarean

Z38.68 Other multiple liveborn infant, delivered vaginally

Z38.69 Other multiple liveborn infant, delivered by cesarean

Z38.7 Other multiple liveborn infant, born outside hospital

Z38.8 Other multiple liveborn infant, unspecified as to place of birth

Z39 ENCOUNTER FOR MATERNAL POSTPARTUM CARE

Use only when billing under the mother

Z39.1 Encounter for care and examination of lactating mother

Encounter for supervision of lactation

Excludes1: disorders of lactation (O92.-)

(Z40–Z53) ENCOUNTERS FOR OTHER SPECIFIC HEALTH CARE

Categories Z40–Z53 are intended for use to indicate a reason for care. They may be used for patients who have already been treated for a disease or injury, but who are receiving aftercare or prophylactic care, or care to consolidate the treatment, or to deal with a residual state.

Z41 ENCOUNTER FOR PROCEDURES FOR PURPOSES OTHER THAN REMEDYING HEALTH STATE

Z41.2 Encounter for routine and ritual male circumcision

Z41.3 Encounter for ear piercing

Z41.8 Encounter for other procedures for purposes other than remedying health state

Z41.9 Encounter for procedure for purposes other than remedying health state, unspecified

Z43 ENCOUNTER FOR ATTENTION TO ARTIFICIAL OPENINGS

Includes: closure of artificial openings
passage of sounds or bougies through artificial openings
reforming artificial openings
removal of catheter from artificial openings
toilet or cleansing of artificial openings

Excludes1: complications of external stoma (J95.0-, K94.-, N99.5-)

Excludes2: fitting and adjustment of prosthetic and other devices (Z44–Z46)

- Z43.0 Encounter for attention to tracheostomy
- Z43.1 Encounter for attention to gastrostomy
  - *Excludes 2:* artificial opening status only, without need for care (Z93.-)
- Z43.2 Encounter for attention to ileostomy
- Z43.3 Encounter for attention to colostomy
- Z43.4 Encounter for attention to other artificial openings of digestive tract
- Z43.5 Encounter for attention to cystostomy
- Z43.6 Encounter for attention to other artificial openings of urinary tract
  - Encounter for attention to nephrostomy or ureterostomy or urethrostomy
- Z43.7 Encounter for attention to artificial vagina
- Z43.8 Encounter for attention to other artificial openings
- Z43.9 Encounter for attention to unspecified artificial opening

Z45 ENCOUNTER FOR ADJUSTMENT AND MANAGEMENT OF IMPLANTED DEVICE

Includes: removal or replacement of implanted device

Excludes1: malfunction or other complications of device—see Alphabetical Index

Excludes2: encounter for fitting and adjustment of non-implanted device (Z46.-)

- Z45.0 Encounter for adjustment and management of cardiac device
  - Z45.01 Encounter for adjustment and management of cardiac pacemaker
    - Encounter for adjustment and management of cardiac resynchronization therapy pacemaker (CRT-P)
    - *Excludes1:* encounter for adjustment and management of automatic implantable cardiac defibrillator with synchronous cardiac pacemaker (Z45.02)
    - Z45.010 Encounter for checking and testing of cardiac pacemaker pulse generator [battery]
      - Encounter for replacing cardiac pacemaker pulse generator [battery]
    - Z45.018 Encounter for adjustment and management of other part of cardiac pacemaker
      - *Excludes1:* presence of other part of cardiac pacemaker (Z95.0)
      - *Excludes2:* presence of prosthetic and other devices (Z95.1–Z95.5, Z95.811–Z97)
  - Z45.02 Encounter for adjustment and management of automatic implantable cardiac defibrillator
    - Encounter for adjustment and management of automatic implantable cardiac defibrillator with synchronous cardiac pacemaker
    - Encounter for adjustment and management of cardiac resynchronization therapy defibrillator (CRT-D)
  - Z45.09 Encounter for adjustment and management of other cardiac device

Z46 ENCOUNTER FOR FITTING AND ADJUSTMENT OF OTHER DEVICES

Includes: removal or replacement of other device

Excludes1: malfunction or other complications of device — see Alphabetical Index

Excludes2: encounter for fitting and management of implanted devices (Z45.-)
issue of repeat prescription only (Z76.0)
presence of prosthetic and other devices (Z95–Z97)

- Z46.2 Encounter for fitting and adjustment of other devices related to nervous system and special senses
  - *Excludes2:* encounter for adjustment and management of implanted nervous system device (Z45.4-)
  - encounter for adjustment and management of implanted visual substitution device (Z45.31)
- Z46.6 Encounter for fitting and adjustment of urinary device
  - *Excludes2:* attention to artificial openings of urinary tract (Z43.5, Z43.6)
- Z46.8 Encounter for fitting and adjustment of other specified devices
  - Z46.81 Encounter for fitting and adjustment of insulin pump
    - Encounter for insulin pump instruction and training
    - Encounter for insulin pump titration
  - Z46.82 Encounter for fitting and adjustment of non-vascular catheter
  - Z46.89 Encounter for fitting and adjustment of other specified devices
    - Encounter for fitting and adjustment of wheelchair
- Z46.9 Encounter for fitting and adjustment of unspecified device

Z48 ENCOUNTER FOR OTHER POSTPROCEDURAL AFTERCARE

Excludes1: encounter for follow-up examination after completed treatment (Z08–Z09)
encounter for aftercare following injury - code to Injury, by site, with appropriate 7th character for subsequent encounter

Excludes2: encounter for attention to artificial openings (Z43.-)
encounter for fitting and adjustment of prosthetic and other devices (Z44–Z46)

- Z48.0 Encounter for; attention to dressings, sutures and drains
  - *Excludes1:* encounter for planned postprocedural wound closure (Z48.1)
  - Do not report a Z48 code for an injury. Use the appropriate injury code.
  - Z48.00 change or removal of nonsurgical wound dressing
    - change or removal of wound dressing NOS
  - Z48.01 change or removal of surgical wound dressing
  - Z48.02 removal of sutures
    - removal of staples
  - Z48.03 change or removal of drains
- Z48.1 Encounter for planned postprocedural wound closure
  - *Excludes1:* encounter for attention to dressings and sutures (Z48.0-)
- Z48.2 Encounter for aftercare following; organ transplant
  - Z48.21 heart transplant
  - Z48.22 kidney transplant
  - Z48.23 liver transplant
  - Z48.24 lung transplant
  - Z48.28 multiple organ transplant
    - Z48.280 heart-lung transplant
    - Z48.288 multiple organ transplant
  - Z48.29 other organ transplant
    - Z48.290 bone marrow transplant
    - Z48.298 other organ transplant
- Z48.3 Aftercare following surgery for neoplasm
  - Use additional code to identify the neoplasm
- Z48.8 Encounter for other specified postprocedural aftercare
  - Z48.81 Encounter for surgical aftercare following surgery on specified body systems
    - These codes identify the body system requiring aftercare. They are for use in conjunction with other aftercare codes to fully explain the aftercare encounter. The condition treated should also be coded if still present.
    - *Excludes1:* aftercare for injury — code the injury with 7th character D
    - aftercare following surgery for neoplasm (Z48.3)
    - *Excludes2:* aftercare following organ transplant (Z48.2-)
    - orthopedic aftercare (Z47.-)
    - Z48.810 Encounter for surgical aftercare following surgery on the sense organs

Z48.811 surgery on the nervous system

Excludes2: encounter for surgical aftercare following surgery on the sense organs (Z48.810)

Z48.812 surgery on the circulatory system

Z48.813 surgery on the respiratory system

Z48.814 surgery on the teeth or oral cavity

Z48.815 surgery on the digestive system

Z48.816 surgery on the genitourinary system

Excludes1: encounter for aftercare following sterilization reversal (Z31.42)

Z48.817 surgery on the skin and subcutaneous tissue

Z48.89 Encounter for other specified surgical aftercare

Z51 ENCOUNTER FOR OTHER AFTERCARE AND MEDICAL CARE

4th

Code **also** condition requiring care

Excludes1: follow-up examination after treatment (Z08–Z09)

Excludes2: follow-up examination for medical surveillance after treatment (Z08–Z09)

- Z51.0 Encounter for antineoplastic; radiation therapy

May only be reported as the principal/first-listed diagnosis, except when there are multiple encounters on the same day and the medical records for the encounters are combined.

- Z51.1 chemotherapy and immunotherapy

5th Codes Z51.1- may only be reported as the principal/first-listed diagnosis, except when there are multiple encounters on the same day and the medical records for the encounters are combined.

Excludes2: encounter for chemotherapy and immunotherapy for non-neoplastic condition—code to condition

Z51.11 chemotherapy

Z51.12 immunotherapy

- Z51.5 Encounter for palliative care
- Z51.6 Encounter for desensitization to allergens
- Z51.8 Encounter for other specified aftercare

5th **Excludes1:** holiday relief care (Z75.5)

Z51.81 Encounter for therapeutic drug level monitoring Code **also** any long-term (current) drug therapy (Z79.-)

Excludes1: encounter for blood-drug test for administrative or medicolegal reasons (Z02.83)

Z51.89 Encounter for other specified aftercare

●Z51.A Encounter for sepsis aftercare

Z53 PERSONS ENCOUNTERING HEALTH SERVICES FOR SPECIFIC PROCEDURES AND TREATMENT, NOT CARRIED OUT

4th

- Z53.0 Procedure and treatment not carried out because of contraindication

5th

Z53.01 Procedure and treatment not carried out due to patient smoking

Z53.09 Procedure and treatment not carried out because of other contraindication

- Z53.1 Procedure and treatment not carried out because of patient's decision for reasons of belief and group pressure
- Z53.2 Procedure and treatment not carried out because of patient's decision for other and unspecified reasons

5th

Z53.20 Procedure and treatment not carried out because of patient's decision for unspecified reasons

Z53.21 Procedure and treatment not carried out due to patient leaving prior to being seen by healthcare provider

Z53.29 Procedure and treatment not carried out because of patient's decision for other reasons

- Z53.3 Procedure converted to open procedure

5th

Z53.31 Laparoscopic surgical procedure converted to open procedure

Z53.32 Thoracoscopic surgical procedure converted to open procedure

Z53.33 Arthroscopic surgical procedure converted to open procedure

Z53.39 Other specified procedure converted to open procedure

- Z53.8 Procedure and treatment not carried out for other reasons
- Z53.9 Procedure and treatment not carried out, unspecified reason

(Z55–Z65) PERSONS WITH POTENTIAL HEALTH HAZARDS RELATED TO SOCIOECONOMIC AND PSYCHOSOCIAL CIRCUMSTANCES

GUIDELINES

Social determinants of health (SDOH) codes describing social problems, conditions, or risk factors that influence a patient's health should be assigned when this information is documented in the patient's medical record. Assign as many SDOH codes as are necessary to describe all of the social problems, conditions, or risk factors documented during the current episode of care. For example, a patient who lives alone may suffer an acute injury temporarily impacting their ability to perform routine activities of daily living.

When documented as such, this would support assignment of code Z60.2, Problems related to living alone. However, merely living alone, without documentation of a risk or unmet need for assistance at home, would not support assignment of code Z60.2. Documentation by a clinician (or patient-reported information that is signed off by a clinician) that the patient expressed concerns with access and availability of food would support assignment of code Z59.41, Food insecurity. Similarly, medical record documentation indicating the patient is homeless would support assignment of a code from subcategory Z59.0-, Homelessness.

For social determinants of health **classified to chapter 21**, such as information found in categories Z55-Z65, Persons with potential health hazards related to socioeconomic and psychosocial circumstances, code assignment may be based on medical record documentation from clinicians involved in the care of the patient who are not the patient's provider since this information represents social information, rather than medical diagnoses. For example, coding professionals may utilize documentation of social information from social workers, community health workers, case managers, or nurses, if their documentation is included in the official medical record.

Patient self-reported documentation may be used to assign codes for social determinants of health, as long as the patient self-reported information is signed-off by and incorporated into the medical record by either a clinician or provider.

Z55 PROBLEMS RELATED TO EDUCATION AND LITERACY

4th **Excludes1:** disorders of psychological development (F80–F89)

▫Z55.0 Illiteracy and low-level literacy

▫Z55.1 Schooling unavailable and unattainable

▫Z55.2 Failed school examinations

▫Z55.3 Underachievement in school

▫Z55.4 Educational maladjustment and discord with teachers and classmates

▲**Z55.5** Less than a high school diploma

No general equivalence degree (GED)

▫Z55.6 Problems related to health literacy

Difficulty understanding health related information

Difficulty understanding medication instructions

Problem completing medical forms

▫Z55.8 Other problems related to education and literacy

Problems related to inadequate teaching

▫Z55.9 Problems related to education and literacy, unspecified

Academic problems NOS

Z58 PROBLEMS RELATED TO PHYSICAL ENVIRONMENT

4th **Excludes2:** occupational exposure (Z57.-)

▫Z58.6 Inadequate drinking-water supply

Lack of safe drinking water

Excludes2: deprivation of water (T73.1)

▫**Z58.8** Other problems related to physical environment

5th ▫**Z58.81** Basic services unavailable in physical environment

Unable to obtain internet service, due to unavailability in geographic area

Unable to obtain telephone service, due to unavailability in geographic area

Unable to obtain utilities, due to inadequate physical environment

▫**Z58.89** Other problems related to physical environment

Z59 PROBLEMS RELATED TO HOUSING AND ECONOMIC CIRCUMSTANCES

Excludes2: problems related to upbringing (Z62.-)

- **□Z59.0 Homelessness**
  - **□Z59.00 Homelessness unspecified**
  - **□Z59.01 Sheltered homelessness**
    - Doubled up
    - Living in a shelter such as: motel, scattered site housing, temporary or transitional living situation
  - **□Z59.02 Unsheltered homelessness**
    - Residing in place not meant for human habitation such as: abandoned buildings, cars, parks, sidewalk
    - Residing on the street
- **□Z59.1 Inadequate housing**
  - *Excludes2:* problems related to the natural and physical environment (Z77.1-)
  - **□Z59.10 Inadequate housing, unspecified**
    - Inadequate housing NOS
  - **□Z59.11 Inadequate housing environmental temperature**
    - Lack of air conditioning or heating
  - **□Z59.12 Inadequate housing utilities**
    - Lack of electricity, gas, oil, or water services
    - *Excludes2:* basic services unavailable in physical environment (Z58.81)
    - lack of adequate food (Z59.4-)
    - other problems related to housing and economic circumstances (Z59.8-)
  - **□Z59.19 Other inadequate housing**
    - Pest infestation
    - Restriction of space
    - Technical defects in home preventing adequate care
    - Unsatisfactory surroundings
- **□Z59.4 Lack of adequate food**
  - *Excludes2:* deprivation of food/effects of hunger (T73.0)
  - inappropriate diet or eating habits (Z72.4)
  - malnutrition (E40-E46)
  - **□Z59.41 Food insecurity**
  - **□Z59.48 Other specified lack of adequate food**
    - Inadequate food
    - Lack of food
- **□Z59.5 Extreme poverty**
- **□Z59.6 Low income**
- **□Z59.7 Insufficient social insurance and welfare support**
  - Insufficient social and welfare insurance
  - **▪□Z59.71 Insufficient health insurance coverage**
    - Inadequate social insurance
    - Insufficient social insurance
    - No health insurance coverage
  - **▪□Z59.72 Insufficient welfare support**
    - Inadequate welfare support
- **□Z59.8 Other problems related to housing and economic circumstances**
  - **□Z59.81 Housing instability, housed**
    - Foreclosure on home loan
    - Past due on rent or mortgage
    - Unwanted multiple moves in the last 12 months
    - **□Z59.811 Housing instability, housed, with risk of homelessness**
      - Imminent risk of homelessness
    - **□Z59.812 Housing instability, housed, homelessness in past 12 months**
    - **□Z59.819 Housing instability, housed unspecified**
      - *Excludes2:* extreme poverty (Z59.5)
      - financial insecurity (Z59.86)
      - low income (Z59.6)
      - material hardship due to limited financial resources, not elsewhere classified (Z59.87)
  - **□Z59.82 Transportation insecurity**
    - *Excludes2:* unavailability and inaccessibility of healthcare facilities (Z75.3)
  - **□Z59.86 Financial insecurity**
- **□Z59.87 Material hardship due to limited financial resources, not elsewhere classified**
  - Material deprivation due to limited financial resources
  - Unable to obtain adequate childcare due to limited financial resources
  - Unable to obtain adequate clothing due to limited financial resources
  - Unable to obtain adequate utilities due to limited financial resources
  - Unable to obtain basic needs due to limited financial resources
  - *Excludes2:* extreme poverty (Z59.5)
  - financial insecurity, not elsewhere classified (Z59.86)
  - low income (Z59.6)
- **□Z59.89 Other problems related to housing and economic circumstances**
  - Foreclosure on loan
  - Isolated dwelling
  - Problems with creditors
- **□Z59.9 Problem related to housing and economic circumstances, unspecified**
  - Inadequate social support
  - Lack of emotional support

Z60 PROBLEMS RELATED TO SOCIAL ENVIRONMENT

- **□Z60.2 Problems related to living alone**
- **□Z60.3 Acculturation difficulty**
  - Problem with migration
  - Problem with social transplantation
- **□Z60.4 Social exclusion and rejection**
  - Exclusion and rejection on the basis of personal characteristics, such as unusual physical appearance, illness or behavior
  - Social isolation
  - *Excludes1:* target of adverse discrimination such as for racial or religious reasons (Z60.5)
- **□Z60.5 Target of (perceived) adverse discrimination and persecution**
  - *Excludes1:* social exclusion and rejection (Z60.4)
- **□Z60.8 Other problems related to social environment**
- **□Z60.9 Problem related to social environment, unspecified**
  - Inadequate social support
  - Lack of emotional support

Z62 PROBLEMS RELATED TO UPBRINGING

Includes: current and past negative life events in childhood current and past problems of a child related to upbringing

Excludes2: maltreatment syndrome (T74.-)

problems related to housing and economic circumstances (Z59.-)

- **□Z62.0 Inadequate parental supervision and control**
- **□Z62.1 Parental overprotection**
- **Z62.2 Upbringing away from parents**
  - *Excludes1:* problems with boarding school (Z59.3)
  - **□Z62.21 Child in welfare custody**
    - Child in foster care
    - Child in welfare guardianship
  - **□Z62.22 Institutional upbringing**
    - Child living in orphanage or group home
  - **□Z62.23 Child in custody of non-parental relative**
    - Child in care of non-parental family member
    - Child in custody of grandparent
    - Child in kinship care
    - Guardianship by non-parental relative
    - **Code also**, if applicable, child in welfare custody (Z62.21)
  - **□Z62.24 Child in custody of non-relative guardian**
    - **Code also**, if applicable, child in welfare custody (Z62.21)
  - **□Z62.29 Other upbringing away from parents**
- **Z62.8 Other specified problems related to upbringing**
  - **Code also**, if applicable:
  - absence of family member (Z63.3-)
  - disappearance and death of family member (Z63.4)
  - disruption of family by separation and divorce (Z63.5)
  - other specified problems related to primary support group (Z63.8)
  - other stressful life events affecting family and household (Z63.7-)

⊡Z62.81 **Personal history of abuse in childhood**

Personal history of abuse in adolescence

⊡Z62.810 **Personal history of; physical and sexual abuse in childhood**

Excludes1: current child physical abuse (T74.12, T76.12)

current child sexual abuse (T74.22, T76.22)

⊡Z62.811 **psychological abuse in childhood**

Excludes1: current child psychological abuse (T74.32, T76.32)

⊡Z62.812 **neglect in childhood**

Excludes1: current child neglect (T74.02, T76.02)

⊡Z62.813 **forced labor or sexual exploitation in childhood**

Excludes1: current exploitation or forced labor (T74.52-, T74.62-, T76.52-, T76.62-)

⊡Z62.814 **Personal history of child financial abuse**

Excludes1: current child financial abuse (T74.A2)

⊡Z62.815 **Personal history of intimate partner abuse in childhood**

Excludes2: adult and child abuse, neglect and other maltreatment, confirmed (T74.-)

⊡Z62.819 **unspecified abuse in childhood**

Excludes1: current child abuse NOS (T74.92, T76.92)

Z62.82 Parent-child conflict

⊡Z62.820 **Parent-biological child conflict**

Parent-child problem NOS

⊡Z62.821 **Parent-adopted child conflict**

⊡Z62.822 **Parent-foster child conflict**

⊡Z62.823 **Parent-step child conflict**

⊡Z62.83 **Non-parental relative or guardian-child conflict**

Z62.831 **Non-parental relative-child conflict**

Grandparent-child conflict

Kinship-care child conflict

Non-parental relative legal guardian-child conflict

Other relative-child conflict

Excludes1: group home staff-child conflict (Z62.833)

⊡Z62.832 **Non-relative guardian-child conflict**

Excludes1: group home staff-child conflict (Z62.833)

Z62.833 **Group home staff-child conflict**

Z62.89 Other specified problems related to upbringing

⊡Z62.890 **Parent-child estrangement NEC**

⊡Z62.891 **Sibling rivalry**

⊡Z62.892 **Runaway [from current living environment]**

Child leaving living situation without permission

⊡Z62.898 **Other specified problems related to upbringing**

⊡Z62.9 **Problem related to upbringing, unspecified**

Z63 OTHER PROBLEMS RELATED TO PRIMARY SUPPORT GROUP, INCLUDING FAMILY CIRCUMSTANCES

Excludes2: maltreatment syndrome (T74.-, T76)

parent-child problems (Z62.-)

problems related to negative life events in childhood (Z62.-)

problems related to upbringing (Z62.-)

Z63.0 Problems in relationship with spouse or partner

Relationship distress with spouse or intimate partner

Excludes1: counseling for spousal or partner abuse problems (Z69.1)

counseling related to sexual attitude, behavior, and orientation (Z70.-)

Z63.3 Absence of family member

Excludes1: absence of family member due to disappearance and death (Z63.4)

absence of family member due to separation and divorce (Z63.5)

⊡Z63.31 **Absence of family member due to military deployment**

Individual or family affected by other family member being on military deployment

Excludes1: family disruption due to return of family member from military deployment (Z63.71)

⊡Z63.32 **Other absence of family member**

⊡Z63.4 **Disappearance and death of family member**

Assumed death of family member

Bereavement

⊡Z63.5 **Disruption of family by separation and divorce**

Z63.6 **Dependent relative needing care at home**

Z63.7 Other stressful life events affecting family and household

⊡Z63.71 **Stress on family due to return of family member from military deployment**

Individual or family affected by family member having returned from military deployment (current or past conflict)

⊡Z63.72 **Alcoholism and drug addiction in family**

⊡Z63.79 **Other stressful life events affecting family and household**

Anxiety (normal) about sick person in family

Health problems within family

Ill or disturbed family member

Isolated family

⊡Z63.8 **Other specified problems related to primary support group**

Family discord NOS

Family estrangement NOS

High expressed emotional level within family

Inadequate family support NOS

Inadequate or distorted communication within family

⊡Z63.9 **Problem related to primary support group, unspecified**

Relationship disorder NOS

Z64 PROBLEMS RELATED TO CERTAIN PSYCHOSOCIAL CIRCUMSTANCES

⊡Z64.0 **Problems related to unwanted pregnancy**

⊡Z64.4 **Discord with counselors**

Discord with probation officer

Discord with social worker

Z65 PROBLEMS RELATED TO OTHER PSYCHOSOCIAL CIRCUMSTANCES

⊡Z65.3 **Problems related to other legal circumstances**

Arrest

Child custody or support proceedings

Litigation

Prosecution

⊡Z65.4 **Victim of crime and terrorism**

Victim of torture

⊡Z65.8 **Other specified problems related to psychosocial circumstances**

At risk for feeling loneliness

Religious or spiritual problem

⊡Z65.9 **Problem related to unspecified psychosocial circumstances**

(Z66) DO NOT RESUSCITATE STATUS

Z66 DO NOT RESUSCITATE

This code may be used when it is documented by the provider that a patient is on do not resuscitate status at any time during the stay.

DNR status

(Z67) BLOOD TYPE

Z67 BLOOD TYPE

Z67.1 Type A blood

Z67.10 Type A blood, Rh positive

Z67.11 Type A blood, Rh negative

Z67.2 Type B blood

Z67.20 Type B blood, Rh positive

Z67.21 Type B blood, Rh negative

Z67.3 Type AB blood

Z67.30 Type AB blood, Rh positive

Z67.31 Type AB blood, Rh negative

Z67.4 Type O blood

Z67.40 Type O blood, Rh positive

Z67.41 Type O blood, Rh negative

●Z67.A Duffy phenotype

●Z67.A1 Duffy null Duffy phenotype Fy(a-b-)

●Z67.A2 Duffy a positive Duffy phenotype Fy(a+b-)

●Z67.A3 Duffy b positive Duffy phenotype Fy(a-b+)

●Z67.A4 Duffy a and b positive Duffy phenotype Fy(a+b+)

(Z68) BODY MASS INDEX [BMI]

Z68 BODY MASS INDEX [BMI]

GUIDELINES

BMI codes should only be assigned when there is an associated, reportable diagnosis (such as obesity).

Do not assign BMI codes during pregnancy. See *ICD-10-CM Official Guidelines for Coding and Reporting FY 2024* in front matter, "Documentation by Clinicians Other than the Patient's Provider."

Kilograms per meters squared

Note: BMI adult codes are for use for persons 20 years of age or older. BMI pediatric codes are for use for persons 2–19 years of age. These percentiles are based on the growth charts published by the Centers for Disease Control and Prevention (CDC)

Z68.1 BMI 19.9 or less, adult

Z68.2 BMI 20-29, adult

Z68.20 BMI 20.0-20.9, adult

Z68.21 BMI 21.0-21.9, adult

Z68.22 BMI 22.0-22.9, adult

Z68.23 BMI 23.0-23.9, adult

Z68.24 BMI 24.0-24.9, adult

Z68.25 BMI 25.0-25.9, adult

Z68.26 BMI 26.0-26.9, adult

Z68.27 BMI 27.0-27.9, adult

Z68.28 BMI 28.0-28.9, adult

Z68.29 BMI 29.0-29.9, adult

Z68.3 BMI 30-39, adult

Z68.30 BMI 30.0-30.9, adult

Z68.31 BMI 31.0-31.9, adult

Z68.32 BMI 32.0-32.9, adult

Z68.33 BMI 33.0-33.9, adult

Z68.34 BMI 34.0-34.9, adult

Z68.35 BMI 35.0-35.9, adult

Z68.36 BMI 36.0-36.9, adult

Z68.37 BMI 37.0-37.9, adult

Z68.38 BMI 38.0-38.9, adult

Z68.39 BMI 39.0-39.9, adult

Z68.4 BMI 40 or greater, adult

Z68.41 BMI 40.0-44.9, adult

Z68.42 BMI 45.0-49.9, adult

Z68.43 BMI 50.0-59.9, adult

Z68.44 BMI 60.0-69.9, adult

Z68.45 BMI 70 or greater, adult

Z68.5 BMI pediatric

Z68.51 BMI pediatric, less than 5th percentile for age

Z68.52 BMI pediatric, 5th percentile to less than 85th percentile for age

Z68.53 BMI pediatric, 85th percentile to less than 95th percentile for age

▲Z68.54 BMI pediatric, 95th percentile for age to less than 120% of the 95th percentile for age

●Z68.55 BMI pediatric, 120% of the 95th percentile for age to less than 140% of the 95th percentile for age

●Z68.56 BMI pediatric, greater than or equal to 140% of the 95th percentile for age

(Z69–Z76) PERSONS ENCOUNTERING HEALTH SERVICES IN OTHER CIRCUMSTANCES

Z69 ENCOUNTER FOR MENTAL HEALTH SERVICES FOR VICTIM AND PERPETRATOR OF ABUSE

Includes: counseling for victims and perpetrators of abuse

Z69.0 Encounter for mental health services for child abuse problems

Z69.01 Encounter for mental health services for; parental child abuse

◻Z69.010 victim of parental child abuse Encounter for mental health services for victim of child abuse or neglect by parent Encounter for mental health services for victim of child psychological or sexual abuse by parent

◻Z69.011 perpetrator of parental child abuse Encounter for mental health services for perpetrator of parental child neglect Encounter for mental health services for perpetrator of parental child psychological or sexual abuse

Excludes1: encounter for mental health services for non-parental child abuse (Z69.02-)

Z69.02 Encounter for mental health services for; non-parental child abuse

◻Z69.020 victim of non-parental child abuse Encounter for mental health services for victim of non-parental child neglect Encounter for mental health services for victim of non-parental child psychological or sexual abuse

◻Z69.021 perpetrator of non-parental child abuse Encounter for mental health services for perpetrator of non-parental child neglect Encounter for mental health services for perpetrator of non-parental child psychological or sexual abuse

Z69.1 Encounter for mental health services for; spousal or partner abuse problems

Z69.11 victim of spousal or partner abuse Encounter for mental health services for victim of spouse or partner neglect Encounter for mental health services for victim of spouse or partner psychological abuse Encounter for mental health services for victim of spouse or partner violence, physical

Z69.12 perpetrator of spousal or partner abuse Encounter for mental health services for perpetrator of spouse or partner neglect Encounter for mental health services for perpetrator of spouse or partner psychological abuse Encounter for mental health services for perpetrator of spouse or partner violence, physical Encounter for mental health services for perpetrator of spouse or partner violence, sexual

Z69.8 Encounter for mental health services for victim or perpetrator of other abuse

◻Z69.81 Encounter for mental health services for victim of other abuse Encounter for mental health services for victim of non-spousal adult abuse Encounter for mental health services for victim of spouse or partner violence, sexual Encounter for rape victim counseling

Z69.82 Encounter for mental health services for perpetrator of other abuse Encounter for mental health services for perpetrator of non-spousal adult abuse

Z70 COUNSELING RELATED TO SEXUAL ATTITUDE, BEHAVIOR AND ORIENTATION

Includes: encounter for mental health services for sexual attitude, behavior and orientation

Excludes2: contraceptive or procreative counseling (Z30-Z31)

- **Z70.0** Counseling related to sexual attitude
- **Z70.1** Counseling related to patient's sexual behavior and orientation
  - Patient concerned regarding impotence
  - Patient concerned regarding non-responsiveness
  - Patient concerned regarding promiscuity
  - Patient concerned regarding sexual orientation
- **Z70.2** Counseling related to sexual behavior and orientation of third party
  - Advice sought regarding sexual behavior and orientation of child
  - Advice sought regarding sexual behavior and orientation of partner
  - Advice sought regarding sexual behavior and orientation of spouse
- **Z70.3** Counseling related to combined concerns regarding sexual attitude, behavior and orientation
- **Z70.8** Other sex counseling
  - Encounter for sex education
- **Z70.9** Sex counseling, unspecified

Z71 PERSONS ENCOUNTERING HEALTH SERVICES FOR OTHER COUNSELING AND MEDICAL ADVICE, NEC

See category Z69 for guideline.

Excludes2: contraceptive or procreative counseling (Z30-Z31) sex counseling (Z70.-)

- **Z71.0** Person encountering health services to consult on behalf of another person
  - Person encountering health services to seek advice or treatment for non-attending third party
  - **Excludes2:** anxiety (normal) about sick person in family (Z63.7) expectant (adoptive) parent(s) pre-birth pediatrician visit (Z76.81)
- **Z71.2** Person consulting for explanation of examination or test findings
- **Z71.3** Dietary counseling and surveillance
  - **Use additional code** for any associated underlying medical condition
  - **Use additional code** to identify body mass index (BMI), if known (Z68.-)
- **Z71.4** Alcohol abuse counseling and surveillance
  - **Use additional code** for alcohol abuse or dependence (F10.-)
  - **Z71.41** Alcohol abuse counseling and surveillance of alcoholic
  - ◻**Z71.42** Counseling for family member of alcoholic
    - Counseling for significant other, partner, or friend of alcoholic
- **Z71.5** Drug abuse counseling and surveillance
  - **Use additional code** for drug abuse or dependence (F11-F16, F18-F19)
  - **Z71.51** Drug abuse counseling and surveillance of drug abuser
  - ◻**Z71.52** Counseling for family member of drug abuser
    - Counseling for significant other, partner, or friend of drug abuser
- **Z71.6** Tobacco abuse counseling
  - **Use additional code** for nicotine dependence (F17.-)
- **Z71.7** HIV counseling
- **Z71.8** Other specified counseling
  - **Excludes2:** counseling for contraception (Z30.0-)
  - **Z71.81** Spiritual or religious counseling
  - **Z71.82** Exercise counseling
  - **Z71.83** Encounter for nonprocreative genetic counseling
    - **Excludes1:** counseling for genetics (Z31.5) counseling for procreative management (Z31.6)
  - **Z71.84** Encounter for health counseling related to travel
    - Encounter for health risk and safety counseling for (international) travel
    - **Code also**, if applicable, encounter for immunization (Z23)

Excludes2: encounter for administrative examination (Z02.-)
encounter for other special examination without complaint, suspected or reported diagnosis (Z01.-)

GUIDELINE

Code Z71.85, Encounter for immunization safety counseling, is to be used for counseling of the patient or caregiver regarding the safety of a vaccine. This code should not be used for the provision of general information regarding risks and potential side effects during routine encounters for the administration of vaccines.

- **Z71.85** Encounter for immunization safety counseling
  - Encounter for vaccine product safety counseling
  - **Code also**, if applicable, encounter for vaccine Z23
  - **Code also**, if applicable, immunization not carried out (Z28.-)
  - **Excludes1:** encounter for health counseling related to travel (Z71.84)

GUIDELINES

Code Z71.87, Encounter for pediatric-to-adult transition counseling, should be assigned when pediatric-to-adult transition counseling is the sole reason for the encounter or when this counseling is provided in addition to other services, such as treatment of a chronic condition. If both transition counseling and treatment of a medical condition are provided during the same encounter, the code(s) for the medical condition(s) treated and code Z71.87 should be assigned, with sequencing depending on the circumstances of the encounter.

- **Z71.87** Encounter for pediatric-to-adult transition counseling
- **Z71.88** Encounter for counseling for socioeconomic factors
- **Z71.89** Other specified counseling
  - Encounter for mental health services for victim of child abuse or neglect by parent
  - Encounter for mental health services for victim of child psychological or sexual abuse by parent
- **Z71.9** Counseling, unspecified
  - Encounter for medical advice NOS

Z72 PROBLEMS RELATED TO LIFESTYLE

Excludes2: problems related to life-management difficulty (Z73.-) problems related to socioeconomic and psychosocial circumstances (Z55-Z65)

- **Z72.0** Tobacco use
  - Tobacco use NOS
  - **Excludes1:** history of tobacco dependence (Z87.891) nicotine dependence (F17.2-) tobacco dependence (F17.2-) tobacco use during pregnancy (O99.33-)
- **Z72.3** Lack of physical exercise
- **Z72.4** Inappropriate diet and eating habits
  - **Excludes1:** behavioral eating disorders of infancy or childhood (F98.2.-F98.3) eating disorders (F50.-) lack of adequate food (Z59.48) malnutrition and other nutritional deficiencies (E40-E64)
- **Z72.5** High risk sexual behavior
  - Promiscuity
  - **Excludes1:** paraphilias (F65)
  - **Z72.51** High risk heterosexual behavior
  - **Z72.52** High risk homosexual behavior
  - **Z72.53** High risk bisexual behavior
- **Z72.6** Gambling and betting
  - **Excludes1:** compulsive or pathological gambling (F63.0)
- **Z72.8** Other problems related to lifestyle
  - **Z72.81** Antisocial behavior
    - **Excludes1:** conduct disorders (F91.-)
    - **Z72.810** Child and adolescent antisocial behavior
      - Antisocial behavior (child) (adolescent) without manifest psychiatric disorder
      - Delinquency NOS
      - Group delinquency
      - Offenses in the context of gang membership

Stealing in company with others
Truancy from school

Z72.82 Problems related to sleep

Z72.820 **Sleep deprivation**
Lack of adequate sleep
Excludes1: insomnia (G47.0-)

Z72.821 **Inadequate sleep hygiene**
Bad sleep habits
Irregular sleep habits
Unhealthy sleep wake schedule
Excludes1: insomnia (F51.0-, G47.0-)

Z72.823 **Risk of suffocation (smothering) under another while sleeping**

Z72.89 Other problems related to lifestyle
Self-damaging behavior

Z72.9 Problem related to lifestyle, unspecified

Z73 PROBLEMS RELATED TO LIFE MANAGEMENT DIFFICULTY

Excludes2: problems related to socioeconomic and psychosocial circumstances (Z55-Z65)

Z73.4 Inadequate social skills, NEC

Z73.6 Limitation of activities due to disability
Excludes1: care-provider dependency (Z74.-)

Z73.8 Other problems related to life management difficulty

Z73.81 **Behavioral insomnia of childhood**

Z73.810 **Behavioral insomnia of childhood, sleep-onset association type**

Z73.811 **Behavioral insomnia of childhood, limit setting type**

Z73.812 **Behavioral insomnia of childhood, combined type**

Z73.819 **Behavioral insomnia of childhood, unspecified type**

Z73.82 **Dual sensory impairment**

Z73.89 **Other problems related to life management difficulty**

Z73.9 Problem related to life management difficulty, unspecified

Z74 PROBLEMS RELATED TO CARE PROVIDER DEPENDENCY

Excludes2: dependence on enabling machines or devices NEC (Z99.-)

Z74.0 Reduced mobility

Z74.09 **Other reduced mobility**
Chair ridden
Reduced mobility NOS
Excludes2: wheelchair dependence (Z99.3)

Z74.1 Need for assistance with personal care

Z74.2 Need for assistance at home and no other household member able to render care

Z74.3 Need for continuous supervision

Z74.8 Other problems related to care provider dependency

Z74.9 Problem related to care provider dependency, unspecified

Z75 PROBLEMS RELATED TO MEDICAL FACILITIES AND OTHER HEALTH CARE

Z75.0 Medical services not available in home
Excludes1: no other household member able to render care (Z74.2)

Z75.3 Unavailability and inaccessibility of health-care facilities
Excludes1: bed unavailable (Z75.1)

Z76 PERSONS ENCOUNTERING HEALTH SERVICES IN OTHER CIRCUMSTANCES

Z76.0 Encounter for issue of repeat prescription
Encounter for issue of repeat prescription for appliance or medicaments or spectacles
Excludes2: issue of medical certificate (Z02.7)
repeat prescription for contraceptive (Z30.4-)
Codes Z76.1 and Z76.2 may only be reported as the principal/first-listed diagnosis, except when there are multiple encounters on the same day and the medical records for the encounters are combined.

Z76.1 Encounter for health supervision and care of foundling
See Chapter 16 for guidelines.

Z76.2 Encounter for health supervision and care of other healthy infant and child
Encounter for medical or nursing care or supervision of healthy infant under circumstances such as adverse socioeconomic conditions at home or such as awaiting foster or adoptive placement or such as maternal illness or such as number of children at home preventing or interfering with normal care

Z76.4 Other boarder to healthcare facility
Excludes1: homelessness (Z59.0-)

Z76.5 Malingerer [conscious simulation]
Person feigning illness (with obvious motivation)
Excludes1: factitious disorder (F68.1-, F68.A)
peregrinating patient (F68.1-)

Z76.8 Persons encountering health services in other specified circumstances

Z76.81 **Expectant parent(s) prebirth pediatrician visit**
See Chapter 21 for guidelines on counseling.
Pre-adoption pediatrician visit for adoptive parent(s)

Z76.82 **Awaiting organ transplant status**
Patient waiting for organ availability

Z76.89 Persons encountering health services in other specified circumstances
Persons encountering health services NOS

(Z77-Z99) PERSONS WITH POTENTIAL HEALTH HAZARDS RELATED TO FAMILY AND PERSONAL HISTORY AND CERTAIN CONDITIONS INFLUENCING HEALTH STATUS

GUIDELINES

Category Z77, Other contact with and (suspected) exposures hazardous to health, indicates contact with and suspected exposures hazardous to health. Contact/exposure codes may be used as a first-listed code to explain an encounter for testing, or, more commonly, as a secondary code to identify a potential risk. Code also any follow-up examination (Z08-Z09)

Z77 OTHER CONTACT WITH AND (SUSPECTED) EXPOSURES HAZARDOUS TO HEALTH

Includes: contact with and (suspected) exposures to potential hazards to health

Excludes2: contact with and (suspected) exposure to communicable diseases (Z20.-)
exposure to (parental) (environmental) tobacco smoke in the perinatal period (P96.81)
newborn affected by noxious substances transmitted via placenta or breast milk (P04.-)
occupational exposure to risk factors (Z57.-)
retained FB (Z18.-)
retained FB fully removed (Z87.821)
toxic effects of substances chiefly nonmedicinal as to source (T51-T65)

Z77.0 Contact with and (suspected) exposure to hazardous, chiefly nonmedicinal, chemicals

Z77.01 **Contact with and (suspected) exposure to; hazardous metals**

Z77.010 arsenic

Z77.011 lead

Z77.012 uranium
Excludes1: retained depleted uranium fragments (Z18.01)

Z77.018 other hazardous metals
Contact with and (suspected) exposure to chromium compounds or nickel dust

Z77.02 **Contact with and (suspected) exposure to; hazardous aromatic compounds**

Z77.020 amines

Z77.021 benzene

Z77.028 other hazardous aromatic compounds
Aromatic dyes NOS
Polycyclic aromatic hydrocarbons

Z77.09 **Contact with and (suspected) exposure to; other hazardous, chiefly nonmedicinal, chemicals**

Z77.090 asbestos

Z77.098 other hazardous, chiefly nonmedicinal, chemicals
Dyes NOS

Z77.1 Contact with and (suspected) exposure to; environmental pollution and hazards in the physical environment

Z77.12 hazards in the physical environment

Z77.120 mold (toxic)

Z77.128 other hazards in the physical environment

Z77.2 other hazardous substances

Z77.21 potentially hazardous body fluids

Z77.22 environmental tobacco smoke (acute) (chronic)

Exposure to second hand tobacco smoke (acute) (chronic)

Passive smoking (acute) (chronic)

Excludes1: nicotine dependence (F17.-)

tobacco use (Z72.0)

Excludes2: occupational exposure to environmental tobacco smoke (Z57.31)

Z77.29 other hazardous substances

Z77.9 Other contact with and (suspected) exposures hazardous to health

Z78 OTHER SPECIFIED HEALTH STATUS

Excludes2: asymptomatic HIV infection status (Z21) postprocedural status (Z93–Z99) sex reassignment status (Z87.890)

Z78.1 Physical restraint status

May be used when it is documented by the provider that a patient has been put in restraints during the current encounter. Please note that this code should not be reported when it is documented by the provider that a patient is temporarily restrained during a procedure.

Z78.9 Other specified health status

Z79 LONG TERM (CURRENT) DRUG THERAPY

GUIDELINES

Codes from this category indicate a patient's continuous use of a prescribed drug (including such things as aspirin therapy) for the long-term treatment of a condition or for prophylactic use. It is not for use for patients who have addictions to drugs. This subcategory is not for use of medications for detoxification or maintenance programs to prevent withdrawal symptoms (eg, methadone maintenance for opiate dependence). Assign the appropriate code for the drug dependence instead.

Assign a code from Z79 if the patient is receiving a medication for an extended period as a prophylactic measure (such as for the prevention of deep vein thrombosis) or as treatment of a chronic condition (such as arthritis) or a disease requiring a lengthy course of treatment (such as cancer). Do not assign a code from category Z79 for medication being administered for a brief period of time to treat an acute illness or injury (such as a course of antibiotics to treat acute bronchitis).

Includes: long term (current) drug use for prophylactic purposes

Code also any therapeutic drug level monitoring (Z51.81)

Excludes2: drug abuse and dependence (F11–F19) drug use complicating pregnancy, childbirth, and the puerperium (O99.32-)

Z79.1 Long term (current) use of; non-steroidal anti-inflammatories (NSAID)

Excludes2: long term (current) use of aspirin (Z79.82)

Z79.2 antibiotics

Z79.4 insulin

Excludes2: long term (current) use of oral antidiabetic drugs (Z79.84)

long term (current) use of oral hypoglycemic drugs (Z79.84)

Z79.5 steroids

Z79.51 inhaled steroids

Z79.52 systemic steroids

Z79.6 Long term (current) use of immunomodulators and immunosuppressants

Excludes2: long term (current) use of steroids (Z79.5-) long term (current) use of agents affecting estrogen receptors and estrogen levels (Z79.81-)

Z79.60 Long term (current) use of unspecified immunomodulators and immunosuppressants

Z79.61 Long term (current) use of immunomodulator

Z79.62 Long term (current) use of immunosuppressant

Z79.620 Long term (current) use of immunosuppressive biologic

Z79.621 Long term (current) use of calcineurin inhibitor

Z79.622 Long term (current) use of Janus kinase inhibitor

Z79.623 Long term (current) use of mammalian target of rapamycin (mTOR) inhibitor

Z79.624 Long term (current) use of inhibitors of nucleotide synthesis

Long term (current) use of azathioprine

Long term (current) use of mycophenolate

Long term (current) use of purine synthesis (IMDH) inhibitors

Z79.63 Long term (current) use of chemotherapeutic agent

Z79.630 Long term (current) use of alkylating agent

Z79.631 Long term (current) use of antimetabolite agent

Z79.632 Long term (current) use of antitumor antibiotic

Z79.633 Long term (current) use of mitotic inhibitor

Z79.634 Long term (current) use of topoisomerase inhibitor

Z79.64 Long term (current) use of myelosuppressive agent

Z79.69 Long term (current) use of other immunomodulators and immunosuppressants

Z79.8 Other long term (current) drug therapy

Z79.82 Long term (current) use of aspirin

Z79.84 Long term (current) use of oral hypoglycemic drugs

Long term use of oral antidiabetic drugs

Excludes2: long term (current) use of insulin (Z79.4)

Z79.85 Long-term (current) use of injectable non-insulin antidiabetic drugs

Z79.89 Other long term (current) drug therapy

Z79.899 Other long term (current) drug therapy

Z80 FAMILY HISTORY OF PRIMARY MALIGNANT NEOPLASM

Z80.0 Family history of malignant neoplasm of digestive organs

Conditions classifiable to C15-C26

Z80.1 Family history of malignant neoplasm of trachea, bronchus and lung

Conditions classifiable to C33-C34

Z80.2 Family history of malignant neoplasm of other respiratory and intrathoracic organs

Conditions classifiable to C30-C32, C37-C39

Z80.3 Family history of malignant neoplasm of breast

Conditions classifiable to C50.-

Z80.4 Family history of malignant neoplasm of genital organs

Conditions classifiable to C51-C63

Z80.41 Family history of malignant neoplasm of ovary

Z80.42 Family history of malignant neoplasm of prostate

Z80.43 Family history of malignant neoplasm of testis

Z80.49 Family history of malignant neoplasm of other genital organs

Z80.5 Family history of malignant neoplasm of urinary tract

Conditions classifiable to C64–C68

Z80.51 Family history of malignant neoplasm of kidney

Z80.52 Family history of malignant neoplasm of bladder

Z80.59 Family history of malignant neoplasm of other urinary tract organ

Z80.6 Family history of leukemia

Conditions classifiable to C91–C95

Z80.7 Family history of other malignant neoplasms of lymphoid, hematopoietic and related tissues

Conditions classifiable to C81–C90, C96.-

Z80.8 Family history of malignant neoplasm of other organs or systems

Conditions classifiable to C00-C14, C40-C49, C69-C79

Z80.9 Family history of malignant neoplasm, unspecified

Conditions classifiable to C80.1

Z81 FAMILY HISTORY OF MENTAL AND BEHAVIORAL DISORDERS

- **Z81.0** Family history of intellectual disabilities
  - Conditions classifiable to F70–F79
- °**Z81.1** Family history of alcohol abuse and dependence
  - Conditions classifiable to F10.
- **Z81.2** Family history of tobacco abuse and dependence
  - Conditions classifiable to F17.-
- **Z81.3** Family history of other psychoactive substance abuse and dependence
  - Conditions classifiable to F11-F16, F18-F19
- °**Z81.4** Family history of other substance abuse and dependence
  - Conditions classifiable to F55
- **Z81.8** Family history of other mental and behavioral disorders
  - Conditions classifiable elsewhere in F01–F99

Z82 FAMILY HISTORY OF CERTAIN DISABILITIES AND CHRONIC DISEASES (LEADING TO DISABLEMENT)

- **Z82.0** Family history of; epilepsy and other diseases of the nervous system
  - Conditions classifiable to G00–G99
- **Z82.1** blindness and visual loss
  - Conditions classifiable to H54.-
- **Z82.2** deafness and hearing loss
  - Conditions classifiable to H90–H91
- **Z82.3** Family history of stroke
  - Conditions classifiable to I60–I64
- **Z82.4** Family history of; ischemic heart disease and other diseases of the circulatory system
  - Conditions classifiable to I00–I5A, I65–I99
  - **Z82.41** sudden cardiac death
  - **Z82.49** ischemic heart disease and other diseases of the circulatory system
- **Z82.5** Family history of asthma and other chronic lower respiratory diseases
  - Conditions classifiable to J40–J47
  - *Excludes2:* family history of other diseases of the respiratory system (Z83.6)
- **Z82.6** Family history of; arthritis and other diseases of the musculoskeletal system and connective tissue
  - Conditions classifiable to M00–M99
  - **Z82.61** arthritis
  - **Z82.62** osteoporosis
  - **Z82.69** other diseases of the musculoskeletal system and connective tissue
- **Z82.7** Family history of; congenital malformations, deformations and chromosomal abnormalities
  - Conditions classifiable to Q00–Q99
  - **Z82.71** polycystic kidney
  - **Z82.79** other congenital malformations, deformations and chromosomal abnormalities
- **Z82.8** Family history of other disabilities and chronic diseases leading to disablement, NEC

Z83 FAMILY HISTORY OF OTHER SPECIFIC DISORDERS

Excludes2: contact with and (suspected) exposure to communicable disease in the family (Z20.-)

- **Z83.0** Family history of human immunodeficiency virus [HIV] disease
  - Conditions classifiable to B20
- **Z83.1** Family history of other infectious and parasitic diseases
  - Conditions classifiable to A00–B19, B25–B94, B99
- **Z83.2** Family history of; diseases of the blood and blood-forming organs and certain disorders involving the immune mechanism
  - Conditions classifiable to D50–D89
- **Z83.3** DM
  - Conditions classifiable to E08–E13
- **Z83.4** other endocrine, nutritional and metabolic diseases
  - Conditions classifiable to E00–E07, E15–E88
  - **Z83.41** multiple endocrine neoplasia syndrome
  - **Z83.42** familial hypercholesterolemia
  - **Z83.43** disorders of lipoprotein metabolism and other lipidemia
    - **Z83.430** elevated lipoprotein(a)
      - Family history of elevated Lp(a)

- **Z83.438** other disorder of lipoprotein metabolism and other lipidemia
  - Family history of familial combined hyperlipidemia
- **Z83.49** other endocrine, nutritional and metabolic diseases
- **Z83.5** Family history of eye and ear disorders
  - **Z83.51** Family history of eye disorders
    - Conditions classifiable to H00–H53, H55–H59
    - *Excludes2:* family history of blindness and visual loss (Z82.1)
    - **Z83.511** Family history of glaucoma
    - **Z83.518** Family history of other specified eye disorder
  - **Z83.52** Family history of ear disorders
    - Conditions classifiable to H60–H83, H92–H95
    - *Excludes2:* family history of deafness and hearing loss (Z82.2)
- **Z83.6** Family history of other diseases of the respiratory system
  - Conditions classifiable to J00–J39, J60–J99
  - *Excludes2:* family history of asthma and other chronic lower respiratory diseases (Z82.5)
- **Z83.7** Family history of diseases of the digestive system
  - Conditions classifiable to D12, K00–K93
  - **Z83.71** colonic polyps
    - *Excludes2:* family history of malignant neoplasm of digestive organs (Z80.0)
    - **Z83.710** Family history of adenomatous and serrated polyps
      - Conditions classifiable to D12.-
      - Family history of tubular adenoma polyps
      - Family history of tubulovillous adenoma polyps
      - Family history of villous adenoma polyps
    - **Z83.711** Family history of hyperplastic colon polyps
    - **Z83.718** Other family history of colon polyps
      - Family history of inflammatory colon polyps
    - **Z83.719** Family history of colon polyps, unspecified
      - Family history of colon polyps NOS
  - ***Z83.72** familial adenomatous polyposis
  - **Z83.79** other diseases of the digestive system

Z84 FAMILY HISTORY OF OTHER CONDITIONS

- **Z84.0** Family history of diseases of the skin and subcutaneous tissue
  - Conditions classifiable to L00–L99
- **Z84.1** Family history of disorders of kidney and ureter
  - Conditions classifiable to N00–N29
- **Z84.2** Family history of other diseases of the genitourinary system
  - Conditions classifiable to N30–N99
- **Z84.3** Family history of consanguinity
- **Z84.8** Family history of other specified conditions
  - **Z84.81** Family history of carrier of genetic disease
  - **Z84.82** Family history of sudden infant death syndrome
  - **Z84.89** Family history of other specified conditions

Z85 PERSONAL HISTORY OF MALIGNANT NEOPLASM

Code first any follow-up examination after treatment of malignant neoplasm (Z08)

Use additional code to identify: alcohol use and dependence (F10.-)
exposure to environmental tobacco smoke (Z77.22)
history of tobacco dependence (Z87.891)
occupational exposure to environmental tobacco smoke (Z57.31)
tobacco dependence (F17.-)
tobacco use (Z72.0)

Excludes2: personal history of benign neoplasm (Z86.01-)
personal history of carcinoma-in-situ (Z86.00-)

- **Z85.5** Personal history of malignant neoplasm of urinary tract
  - Conditions classifiable to C64–C68
  - **Z85.50** Personal history of malignant neoplasm of; unspecified urinary tract organ
  - **Z85.51** bladder
  - **Z85.52** kidney
    - *Excludes1:* personal history of malignant neoplasm of renal pelvis (Z85.53)

Z85.520 **Personal history of; malignant carcinoid tumor of kidney**
Conditions classifiable to C7A.093

Z85.528 **other malignant neoplasm of kidney**
Conditions classifiable to C64

Z85.6 Leukemia
Conditions classifiable to C91–C95
Excludes1: leukemia in remission C91.0–C95.9 with 5th character 1

Z85.7 Personal history of other malignant neoplasms of lymphoid, hematopoietic and related tissues

Z85.71 **Personal history of; Hodgkin lymphoma**
Conditions classifiable to C81

Z85.72 **non-Hodgkin lymphomas**
Conditions classifiable to C82–C85

Z85.79 **other malignant neoplasms of lymphoid, hematopoietic and related tissues**
Conditions classifiable to C88–C90, C96
Excludes1: multiple myeloma in remission (C90.01)
plasma cell leukemia in remission (C90.11)
plasmacytoma in remission (C90.21)

Z85.8 Malignant neoplasms of other organs and systems
Conditions classifiable to C00–C14, C40–C49, C69–C79, C7A.098

Z85.82 **Personal history of malignant neoplasm of skin**

Z85.820 **Personal history of malignant melanoma of skin**
Conditions classifiable to C43

Z85.83 **Personal history of malignant neoplasm of; bone and soft tissue**
Conditions classifiable to C40–C41; C45–C49

Z85.830 **bone**

Z85.831 **soft tissue**
Excludes2: personal history of malignant neoplasm of skin (Z85.82-)

Z85.84 **Personal history of; malignant neoplasm of eye and nervous tissue**
Conditions classifiable to C69–C72

Z85.840 **eye**

Z85.841 **brain**

Z85.848 **other parts of nervous tissue**

Z85.85 **Personal history of; malignant neoplasm of endocrine glands**
Conditions classifiable to C73–C75

Z85.850 **thyroid**

Z85.858 **other endocrine glands**

Z85.89 **other organs and systems**
Conditions classifiable to C7A.098, C76, C77–C79

Z85.9 Personal history of malignant neoplasm, unspecified
Conditions classifiable to C7A.00, C80.1

Z86 PERSONAL HISTORY OF CERTAIN OTHER DISEASES

Code first any follow-up examination after treatment (Z09)

Z86.0 Personal history of in-situ and benign neoplasms and neoplasms of uncertain behavior
Excludes2: personal history of malignant neoplasms (Z85.-)

Z86.00 **Personal history of in-situ neoplasm**
Conditions classifiable to D00–D09

Z86.000 **Personal history of in-situ neoplasm of breast**
Conditions classifiable to D05

Z86.001 **Personal history of in-situ neoplasm of cervix uteri**
Conditions classifiable to D06
Personal history of cervical intraepithelial neoplasia III [CIN III]

Z86.002 **Personal history of in-situ neoplasm of other and unspecified genital organs**
Conditions classifiable to D07
Personal history of high-grade prostatic intraepithelial neoplasia III [HGPIN III]
Personal history of vaginal intraepithelial neoplasia III [VAIN III]
Personal history of vulvar intraepithelial neoplasia III [VIN III]

Z86.003 **Personal history of in-situ neoplasm of oral cavity, esophagus and stomach**
Conditions classifiable to D00

Z86.004 **Personal history of in-situ neoplasm of other and unspecified digestive organs**
Conditions classifiable to D01
Personal history of anal intraepithelial neoplasia (AIN III)

Z86.005 **Personal history of in-situ neoplasm of middle ear and respiratory system**
Conditions classifiable to D02

Z86.006 **Personal history of melanoma in-situ**
Conditions classifiable to D03
Excludes2: sites other than skin—code to personal history of in-situ neoplasm of the site

Z86.007 **Personal history of in-situ neoplasm of skin**
Conditions classifiable to D04
Personal history of carcinoma in situ of skin

Z86.008 **Personal history of in-situ neoplasm of other site**
Conditions classifiable to D09

Z86.03 **Personal history of neoplasm of uncertain behavior**

Z86.1 Personal history of infectious and parasitic diseases
Conditions classifiable to A00–B89, B99
Excludes1: personal history of infectious diseases specific to a body system
sequelae of infectious and parasitic diseases (B90–B94)

Z86.11 **Personal history of; tuberculosis**

Z86.13 **malaria**

Z86.14 **MRSA infection**
Personal history of MRSA infection

Z86.15 **latent tuberculosis infection**

GUIDELINE

See code U07.1 for more information.

Z86.16 **COVID-19**
Excludes1: post COVID-19 condition (U09.9)

Z86.19 **other infectious and parasitic diseases**

Z86.2 Personal history of diseases of the blood and blood-forming organs and certain disorders involving the immune mechanism
Conditions classifiable to D50–D89

Z86.3 Personal history of endocrine, nutritional and metabolic diseases
Conditions classifiable to E00–E88

Z86.39 **other endocrine, nutritional and metabolic disease**

Z86.5 Personal history of; mental and behavioral disorders
Conditions classifiable to F40–F59

Z86.59 **other mental and behavioral disorders**
Code is a nonspecific Z code, refer to Chapter 21 for guidelines.

Z86.6 Personal history of; diseases of the nervous system and sense organs
Conditions classifiable to G00–G99, H00–H95

Z86.61 **infections of the central nervous system**
Personal history of encephalitis
Personal history of meningitis

Z86.69 **other diseases of the nervous system and sense organs**

Z86.7 Personal history of; diseases of the circulatory system
Conditions classifiable to I00–I99

Z86.73 **TIA and cerebral infarction without residual deficits**
Personal history of prolonged reversible ischemic neurological deficit (PRIND)
Personal history of stroke NOS without residual deficits
Excludes1: personal history of traumatic brain injury (Z87.820)
sequelae of cerebrovascular disease (I69.-)

Z86.74 sudden cardiac arrest
Personal history of sudden cardiac death successfully resuscitated

Z86.79 other diseases of the circulatory system

Z87 PERSONAL HISTORY OF OTHER DISEASES AND CONDITIONS

Code first any follow-up examination after treatment (Z09)

Z87.0 Personal history of; diseases of the respiratory system

Conditions classifiable to J00–J99

Z87.01 pneumonia (recurrent)

Z87.09 other diseases of the respiratory system

Z87.3 Personal history of diseases of the musculoskeletal system and connective tissue

Conditions classifiable to M00–M99

Excludes2: personal history of (healed) traumatic fracture (Z87.81)

Z87.39 other diseases of the musculoskeletal system and connective tissue

Z87.4 Personal history of; diseases of genitourinary system

Conditions classifiable to N00–N99

Z87.44 diseases of urinary system

Excludes1: personal history of malignant neoplasm of cervix uteri (Z85.41)

Z87.440 urinary (tract) infections

Z87.441 nephrotic syndrome

Z87.442 urinary calculi
Personal history of kidney stones

Z87.448 other diseases of urinary system

Z87. 6 Personal history of certain conditions arising in the perinatal period

Z87.61 Personal history of (corrected) necrotizing enterocolitis of newborn

Z87.68 Personal history of other (corrected) conditions arising in the perinatal period

Z87.7 Personal history of (corrected) congenital malformations

Conditions classifiable to Q00–Q89 that have been repaired or corrected

Excludes2: congenital malformations that have been partially corrected or repaired but which still require medical treatment—code to condition
other postprocedural states (Z98.-)
personal history of medical treatment (Z92.-)
presence of cardiac and vascular implants and grafts (Z95.-)
presence of other devices (Z97.-)
presence of other functional implants (Z96.-)
transplanted organ and tissue status (Z94.-)

Z87.71 Personal history of (corrected); congenital malformations of genitourinary system

Z87.710 hypospadias

Z87.718 other specified congenital malformations of genitourinary system

Z87.72 Personal history of (corrected) congenital malformations; of nervous system and sense organs

Z87.720 of eye

Z87.721 of ear

Z87.728 other specified of nervous system and sense organs

Z87.73 Personal history of (corrected); congenital malformations of digestive system

Z87.730 cleft lip and palate

Z87.731 tracheoesophageal fistula or atresia

Z87.732 persistent cloaca or cloacal malformations

Z87.738 other specified congenital malformations of digestive system

Z87.74 Personal history of; (corrected) congenital malformations of heart and circulatory system

Z87.75 (corrected) congenital malformations of respiratory system

Z87.76 (corrected) congenital malformations of integument, limbs and musculoskeletal system

Z87.760 (corrected) congenital diaphragmatic hernia or other congenital diaphragm malformations

Z87.761 (corrected) gastroschisis

Z87.762 (corrected) prune belly malformation

Z87.763 other (corrected) congenital abdominal wall malformations

Z87.768 other specified (corrected) congenital malformations of integument, limbs and musculoskeletal system

Z87.79 other (corrected) congenital malformations

Z87.790 (corrected) congenital malformations of face and neck

Z87.798 other (corrected) congenital malformations

Z87.8 Personal history of; other specified conditions

Excludes2: personal history of self harm (Z91.5-)

Z87.82 other (healed) physical injury and trauma

Conditions classifiable to S00–T88, except traumatic fractures

Z87.820 traumatic brain injury

Excludes1: personal history of TIA, and cerebral infarction without residual deficits (Z86.73)

Z87.821 retained FB fully removed

Z87.828 other (healed) physical injury and trauma

Z87.89 Personal history of; other specified conditions

Z87.891 nicotine dependence

Excludes1: current nicotine dependence (F17.2-)

Z87.892 anaphylaxis

Code also allergy status such as:
allergy status to drugs, medicaments and biological substances (Z88.-)
allergy status, other than to drugs and biological substances (Z91.0-)

Z87.898 other specified conditions

Z88 ALLERGY STATUS TO DRUGS, MEDICAMENTS AND BIOLOGICAL SUBSTANCES

Excludes2: Allergy status, other than to drugs and biological substances (Z91.0-)

Z88.0 Allergy status to; penicillin

Z88.1 other antibiotic agents

Z88.2 sulfonamides status

Z88.3 other anti-infective agents

Z88.4 anesthetic agent

Z88.5 narcotic agent

Z88.6 analgesic agent

Z88.7 serum and vaccine

Z88.8 other drugs, medicaments and biological substances

Z88.9 unspecified drugs, medicaments and biological substances

Code is a nonspecific Z code, refer to Chapter 21 for guidelines.

Z90 ACQUIRED ABSENCE OF ORGANS, NEC

Includes: postprocedural or post-traumatic loss of body part NEC

Excludes1: congenital absence—see Alphabetical Index

Excludes2: postprocedural absence of endocrine glands (E89.-)

Note: Use only if there are no complications or malfunctions of the organ or tissue replaced, the amputation site, or the equipment on which the patient is dependent.

Z90.4 Acquired absence of; other specified parts of digestive tract

Z90.49 other specified parts of digestive tract

Z90.5 Acquired absence of; kidney

Z90.7 genital organ(s)

Excludes1: personal history of sex reassignment (Z87.890)

Excludes2: female genital mutilation status (N90.81-)

Z90.79 other genital organ(s)

Z90.8 Acquired absence of; other organs

Z90.81 spleen

Z90.89 other organs

Z91 PERSONAL RISK FACTORS, NEC

Excludes2: contact with and (suspected) exposures hazardous to health (Z77.-)

exposure to pollution and other problems related to physical environment (Z77.1-)

personal history of physical injury and trauma (Z87.81, Z87.82-)

occupational exposure to risk factors (Z57.-)

Z91.0 Allergy status, other than to drugs and biological substances

Excludes2: Allergy status to drugs, medicaments, and biological substances (Z88.-)

Z91.01 Food allergy status

Excludes2: food additives allergy status (Z91.02)

Z91.010 Allergy to; peanuts

Z91.011 milk products

Excludes1: lactose intolerance (E73.-)

Z91.012 eggs

Z91.013 seafood

Allergy to shellfish or octopus or squid ink

Z91.014 mammalian meats

Allergy to beef, lamb, pork, red meats

Z91.018 other foods

nuts other than peanuts

Z91.02 Food additives allergy status

Z91.03 Insect allergy status

Z91.030 Bee allergy status

Z91.038 Other insect allergy status

Z91.04 Nonmedicinal substance allergy status

Z91.040 Latex allergy status

Latex sensitivity status

Z91.041 Radiographic dye allergy status

Allergy status to contrast media used for diagnostic X-ray procedure

Z91.048 Other nonmedicinal substance allergy status

Z91.1 Patient's noncompliance with medical treatment and regimen

Code also, if applicable, food insecurity (Z59.4-)

Code also, if applicable, to identify underdosing of specific drug (T36–T50 with final character 6)

Excludes2: caregiver noncompliance with patient's medical treatment and regimen (Z91.A-)

Z91.11 Patient's noncompliance with dietary regimen

⊡Z91.110 Patient's noncompliance with dietary regimen due to financial hardship

⊡Z91.118 Patient's noncompliance with dietary regimen for other reason

⊡Z91.119 Patient's noncompliance with dietary regimen due to unspecified reason

Z91.12 Patient's intentional underdosing of medication regimen

Code first underdosing of medication (T36–T50) with fifth or sixth character 6

⊡Z91.120 Patient's intentional underdosing of medication regimen due to financial hardship

Z91.128 Patient's intentional underdosing of medication regimen for other reason

Z91.13 Patient's unintentional underdosing of medication regimen

Code first underdosing of medication (T36–T50) with fifth or sixth character 6

Excludes1: adverse effect of prescribed drug taken as directed—code to adverse effect

poisoning (overdose)—code to poisoning

Z91.138 Patient's unintentional underdosing of medication regimen for other reason

Z91.14 Patient's other noncompliance with medication regimen

Patient's underdosing of medication NOS

⊡Z91.141 Patient's other noncompliance with medication regimen due to financial hardship

⊡Z91.148 Patient's other noncompliance with medication regimen for other reason

Z91.15 Patient's noncompliance with renal dialysis

⊡Z91.151 Patient's noncompliance with renal dialysis due to financial hardship

⊡Z91.158 Patient's noncompliance with renal dialysis for other reason

Z91.19 Patient's noncompliance with other medical treatment and regimen

Nonadherence to medical treatment

⊡Z91.190 Patient's noncompliance with other medical treatment and regimen due to financial hardship

Z91.198 Patient's noncompliance with other medical treatment and regimen for other reason

Z91.199 Patient's noncompliance with other medical treatment and regimen due to unspecified reason

Z91.A Caregiver's noncompliance with patient's medical treatment and regimen

Z91.A1 Caregiver's noncompliance with patient's dietary regimen

Caregiver's inability to comply with patient's dietary regimen

Code also, if applicable, food insecurity (Z59.4-)

⊡Z91.A10 Caregiver's noncompliance with patient's dietary regimen due to financial hardship

Z91.A18 Caregiver's noncompliance with patient's dietary regimen for other reason

Z91.A2 Caregiver's intentional underdosing of patient's medication regimen

Code first underdosing of medication (T36-T50) with fifth or sixth character 6

⊡Z91.A20 Caregiver's intentional underdosing of patient's medication regimen due to financial hardship

Z91.A28 Caregiver's intentional underdosing of medication regimen for other reason

Z91.A3 Caregiver's unintentional underdosing of patient's medication regimen

Z91.A4 Caregiver's other noncompliance with patient's medication regimen

Z91.A41 Caregiver's other noncompliance with patient's medication regimen due to financial hardship

Z91.A48 Caregiver's other noncompliance with patient's medication regimen for other reason

Z91.A5 Caregiver's noncompliance with patient's renal dialysis

Z91.A51 Caregiver's noncompliance with patient's renal dialysis due to financial hardship

Z91.A58 Caregiver's noncompliance with patient's renal dialysis for other reason

Z91.A9 Caregiver's noncompliance with patient's other medical treatment and regimen

Z91.A91 Caregiver's noncompliance with patient's other medical treatment and regimen due to financial hardship

Z91.A98 Caregiver's noncompliance with patient's other medical treatment and regimen for other reason

Z91.4 Personal history of psychological trauma, NEC

Z91.49 Other personal history of psychological trauma, NEC

⊡Z91.5 Personal history of self-harm

Code also mental health disorder, if known

Z91.51 Personal history of suicidal behavior

Personal history of parasuicide

Personal history of self-poisoning

Personal history of suicide attempt

Z91.52 Personal history of nonsuicidal self-harm

Personal history of nonsuicidal self-injury

Personal history of self-inflicted injury without suicidal intent

Personal history of self-mutilation

Z91.8 Other specified personal risk factors, NEC

Z91.81 History of falling
At risk for falling

Z91.83 Wandering in diseases classified elsewhere
Code first underlying disorder such as:
Alzheimer's disease (G30.-)
autism or pervasive developmental disorder (F84.-)
intellectual disabilities (F70–F79)
unspecified dementia with behavioral disturbance (F03.9-)

Z91.84 Oral health risk factors

Z91.841 Risk for dental caries, low
Z91.842 Risk for dental caries, moderate
Z91.843 Risk for dental caries, high
Z91.849 Unspecified risk for dental caries

Z91.89 Other specified personal risk factors, NEC

Z92 PERSONAL HISTORY OF MEDICAL TREATMENT

Excludes2: postprocedural states (Z98.-)

Z92.2 Personal history of; drug therapy

Excludes2: long term (current) drug therapy (Z79.-)

Z92.21 antineoplastic chemotherapy

Z92.22 monoclonal drug therapy

Excludes2: personal history of immune checkpoint inhibitor therapy (Z92.26)

Z92.24 steroid therapy

Z92.240 inhaled steroid therapy
Z92.241 systemic steroid therapy
steroid therapy NOS

Z92.25 immunosuppression therapy

Excludes2: personal history of steroid therapy (Z92.24)

●Z92.26 immune checkpoint inhibitor therapy
ICI drug therapy

Z92.29 other drug therapy

Z92.8 Personal history of; other medical treatment

Z92.81 extracorporeal membrane oxygenation (ECMO)
Z92.85 cellular therapy

Z92.850 Chimeric Antigen Receptor T-cell therapy
Personal history of CAR T-cell therapy
Z92.858 other cellular therapy
Z92.859 cellular therapy, unspecified

Z92.86 gene therapy

Z93 ARTIFICIAL OPENING STATUS

Note: Use only if there are no complications or malfunctions of the organ or tissue replaced, the amputation site, or the equipment on which the patient is dependent.

Excludes1: artificial openings requiring attention or management (Z43.-)
complications of external stoma (J95.0-, K94.-, N99.5-)

Z93.0 Tracheostomy status

Z93.1 Gastrostomy status

Z93.2 Ileostomy status

Z93.3 Colostomy status

Z93.4 Other artificial openings of gastrointestinal tract status

Z93.5 Cystostomy status

Z93.50 Unspecified cystostomy status
Z93.51 Cutaneous-vesicostomy status
Z93.52 Appendico-vesicostomy status
Z93.59 Other cystostomy status

Z93.8 Other artificial opening status

Z93.9 Artificial opening status, unspecified

Z94 TRANSPLANTED ORGAN AND TISSUE STATUS

Note: Use only if there are no complications or malfunctions of the organ or tissue replaced, the amputation site, or the equipment on which the patient is dependent.

Includes: organ or tissue replaced by heterogenous or homogenous transplant

Excludes1: complications of transplanted organ or tissue—see Alphabetical Index

Excludes2: presence of vascular grafts (Z95.-)

Z94.0 Kidney transplant status

Z94.1 Heart transplant status

Excludes1: artificial heart status (Z95.812)
heart-valve replacement status (Z95.2–Z95.4)

Z94.2 Lung transplant status

Z94.3 Heart and lungs transplant status

Z94.4 Liver transplant status

Z94.5 Skin transplant status
Autogenous skin transplant status

Z94.6 Bone transplant status

Z94.7 Corneal transplant status

Z94.8 Other transplanted organ and tissue status

Z94.81 Bone marrow transplant status
Z94.82 Intestine transplant status
Z94.83 Pancreas transplant status
Z94.84 Stem cells transplant status
Z94.89 Other transplanted organ and tissue status

Z94.9 Transplanted organ and tissue status, unspecified

Z95 PRESENCE OF CARDIAC AND VASCULAR IMPLANTS

Excludes2: complications of cardiac and vascular devices, implants and grafts (T82.-)

Z95.0 Presence of cardiac pacemaker
Presence of cardiac resynchronization therapy (CRT-P) pacemaker

Excludes1: adjustment or management of cardiac pacemaker (Z45.0-)
presence of automatic (implantable) cardiac defibrillator with synchronous cardiac pacemaker (Z95.810)

Z95.2 Presence of prosthetic heart valve
Presence of heart valve NOS

Z95.3 Presence of xenogenic heart valve

Z95.4 Presence of other heart-valve replacement

Z95.8 Presence of other cardiac and vascular implants and grafts

Z95.81 Presence of other cardiac implants and grafts

Z95.810 Presence of automatic (implantable) cardiac defibrillator
Presence of automatic (implantable) cardiac defibrillator with synchronous cardiac pacemaker
Presence of cardiac resynchronization therapy defibrillator (CRT-D)
Presence of cardioverter-defibrillator (ICD)

Z95.811 Presence of heart assist device
Z95.812 Presence of fully implantable artificial heart
Z95.818 Presence of other cardiac implants and grafts

Z96 PRESENCE OF OTHER FUNCTIONAL IMPLANTS

Excludes2: complications of internal prosthetic devices, implants and grafts (T82-T85)
fitting and adjustment of prosthetic and other devices (Z44-Z46)

Z96.0 Presence of urogenital implants

Z96.1 Presence of intraocular lens
Presence of pseudophakia

Z96.2 Presence of otological and audiological implants

Z96.21 Cochlear implant status
Z96.22 Myringotomy tube(s) status
Z96.29 Presence of other otological and audiological implants
Presence of bone-conduction hearing device
Presence of eustachian tube stent
Stapes replacement

Z96.3 Presence of artificial larynx

Z96.4 Presence of endocrine implants

Z96.41 Presence of insulin pump (external) (internal)
Z96.49 Presence of other endocrine implants

Z96.8 Presence of other specified functional implants

Z96.81 Presence of artificial skin
Z96.82 Presence of neurostimulator
Presence of brain neurostimulator
Presence of gastric neurostimulator
Presence of peripheral nerve neurostimulator
Presence of sacral nerve neurostimulator
Presence of spinal cord neurostimulator
Presence of vagus nerve neurostimulator

Z96.89 Presence of other specified functional implants

Z96.9 Presence of functional implant, unspecified

Z97 PRESENCE OF OTHER DEVICES

Excludes1: complications of internal prosthetic devices, implants and grafts (T82–T85)

Excludes 2: fitting and adjustment of prosthetic and other devices (Z44–Z46)

- **Z97.3** Presence of spectacles and contact lenses
- **Z97.4** Presence of external hearing-aid
- **Z97.5** Presence of (intrauterine) contraceptive device
  - checking, reinsertion or removal of contraceptive device (Z30.43)
  - **Excludes1:** checking, reinsertion or removal of implantable subdermal contraceptive (Z30.46)
  - checking, reinsertion or removal of intrauterine contraceptive device (Z30.43-)
- **Z97.8** Presence of other specified devices

Z98 OTHER POSTPROCEDURAL STATES

Excludes2: aftercare (Z43–Z49, Z51)

follow-up medical care (Z08–Z09)

postprocedural complication—see Alphabetical Index

- **Z98.2** Presence of cerebrospinal fluid drainage device
  - Presence of CSF shunt
- **Z98.8** Other specified postprocedural states
  - **Z98.85** **Transplanted organ removal status**
    - Assign code Z98.85, Transplanted organ removal status, to indicate that a transplanted organ has been previously removed. This code should not be assigned for the encounter in which the transplanted organ is removed. The complication necessitating removal of the transplant organ should be assigned for that encounter.
    - See Chapter 19 for information on the coding of organ transplant complications.
    - Transplanted organ previously removed due to complication, failure, rejection or infection
    - **Excludes1:** encounter for removal of transplanted organ—code to complication of transplanted organ (T86.-)
  - **Z98.87** **Personal history of in utero procedure**
    - **Z98.871** **Personal history of in utero procedure**

while a fetus

- **Z98.89** **Other specified postprocedural states**
  - **Z98.890** **Other specified postprocedural states**
    - Personal history of surgery, NEC

Z99 DEPENDENCE ON ENABLING MACHINES AND DEVICES, NEC

- **Z99.1** Dependence on respirator
  - Dependence on ventilator
  - **Z99.11** **Dependence on respirator [ventilator] status**
    - For encounters for weaning from a mechanical ventilator, assign a code from subcategory J96.1, Chronic respiratory failure, followed by code Z99.11, Dependence on respirator [ventilator] status.
- **Z99.2** Dependence on renal dialysis
  - Hemodialysis status
  - Peritoneal dialysis status
  - Presence of arteriovenous shunt for dialysis
  - Renal dialysis status NOS
  - **Excludes1:** encounter for fitting and adjustment of dialysis catheter (Z49.0-)
  - **Excludes2:** noncompliance with renal dialysis (Z91.15-)
- **Z99.3** Dependence on wheelchair
  - Wheelchair confinement status
  - **Code first** cause of dependence, such as:
    - muscular dystrophy (G71.0-)
    - obesity (E66.-)
- **Z99.8** Dependence on other enabling machines and devices
  - **Z99.81** **Dependence on supplemental oxygen**
    - Dependence on long-term oxygen
  - **Z99.89** **Dependence on other enabling machines and devices**
    - Dependence on machine or device NOS

Chapter 22. Codes for special purposes (U00–U85)

(U00–U49) PROVISIONAL ASSIGNMENT OF NEW DISEASES OF UNCERTAIN ETIOLOGY OR EMERGENCY USE

U07 EMERGENCY USE OF U07

4th

GUIDELINES

For patients presenting with condition(s) related to vaping, assign code U07.0, Vaping-related disorder, as the principal diagnosis. For lung injury due to vaping, assign only code U07.0. Assign additional codes for other manifestations, such as acute respiratory failure (subcategory J96.0-) or pneumonitis (code J68.0). Associated respiratory signs and symptoms due to vaping, such as cough, shortness of breath, etc., are not coded separately, when a definitive diagnosis has been established. However, it would be appropriate to code separately any gastrointestinal symptoms, such as diarrhea and abdominal pain.

U07.0 Vaping-related disorder

Dabbing related lung damage
Dabbing related lung injury
E-cigarette, or vaping, product use associated lung injury [EVALI]
Electronic cigarette related lung damage
Electronic cigarette related lung injury
Use additional code to identify manifestations, such as:
abdominal pain (R10.84)
acute respiratory distress syndrome (J80)
diarrhea (R19.7)
drug-induced interstitial lung disorder (J70.4)
lipoid pneumonia (J69.1)
weight loss (R63.4)

GUIDELINES

COVID-19 INFECTION (INFECTION DUE TO SARS-COV-2)

Code only confirmed cases

Code only a confirmed diagnosis of the 2019 novel coronavirus disease (COVID-19) as documented by the provider or documentation of a positive COVID-19 test result. For a confirmed diagnosis, assign code U07.1, COVID-19. This is an exception to the hospital inpatient guideline Section II, H. In this context, "confirmation" does not require documentation of a positive test result for COVID-19; the provider's documentation that the individual has COVID-19 is sufficient.

If the provider documents "suspected," "possible," "probable," or "inconclusive" COVID-19, do not assign code U07.1. Instead, code the signs and symptoms reported.

Sequencing of codes

When COVID-19 meets the definition of principal diagnosis, code U07.1, COVID-19, should be sequenced first, followed by the appropriate codes for associated manifestations, except when another guideline requires that certain codes be sequenced first, such as obstetrics, sepsis, or transplant complications.

For a COVID-19 infection that progresses to sepsis, see Section I.C.1.d. Sepsis, Severe Sepsis, and Septic Shock

See Section I.C.15.s. for COVID-19 infection in pregnancy, childbirth, and the puerperium

See Section I.C.16.h. for COVID-19 infection in newborn

For a COVID-19 infection in a lung transplant patient, see Section I.C.19.g.3.a. Transplant complications other than kidney.

Acute respiratory manifestations of COVID-19

When the reason for the encounter/admission is a respiratory manifestation of COVID-19, assign code U07.1, COVID-19, as the principal/first-listed diagnosis and assign code(s) for the respiratory manifestation(s) as additional diagnoses.

The following conditions are examples of common respiratory manifestations of COVID-19.

PNEUMONIA

For a patient with pneumonia confirmed as due to COVID-19, assign codes U07.1, COVID-19, and J12.82, Pneumonia due to coronavirus disease 2019.

ACUTE BRONCHITIS

For a patient with acute bronchitis confirmed as due to COVID-19, assign codes U07.1 and J20.8, Acute bronchitis due to other specified organisms. Bronchitis not otherwise specified (NOS) due to COVID-19 should be coded using code U07.1 and J40, Bronchitis, not specified as acute or chronic.

LOWER RESPIRATORY INFECTION

If the COVID-19 is documented as being associated with a lower respiratory infection, not otherwise specified (NOS), or an acute respiratory infection, NOS, codes U07.1 and J22, Unspecified acute lower respiratory infection, should be assigned. If the COVID-19 is documented as being associated with a respiratory infection, NOS, codes U07.1 and J98.8, Other specified respiratory disorders, should be assigned.

ACUTE RESPIRATORY DISTRESS SYNDROME

For acute respiratory distress syndrome (ARDS) due to COVID-19, assign codes U07.1, and J80, Acute respiratory distress syndrome.

ACUTE RESPIRATORY FAILURE

For acute respiratory failure due to COVID-19, assign code U07.1, and code J96.0-, Acute respiratory failure.

NON-RESPIRATORY MANIFESTATIONS OF COVID-19

When the reason for the encounter/admission is a non-respiratory manifestation (e.g., viral enteritis) of COVID-19, assign code U07.1, COVID-19, as the principal/first-listed diagnosis and assign code(s) for the manifestation(s) as additional diagnoses.

Exposure to COVID-19

For asymptomatic individuals with actual or suspected exposure to COVID-19, assign code Z20.822, Contact with and (suspected) exposure to COVID-19.

For symptomatic individuals with actual or suspected exposure to COVID-19 and the infection has been ruled out, or test results are inconclusive or unknown, assign code Z20.822, Contact with and (suspected) exposure to COVID-19. See Contact/Exposure guideline for additional guidance regarding the use of category Z20 codes. If COVID-19 is confirmed see the COVID infection guideline.

Screening for COVID-19

For screening for COVID-19, including preoperative testing, assign code Z11.52, Encounter for screening for COVID-19.

Signs and symptoms without definitive diagnosis of COVID-19

For patients presenting with any signs/symptoms associated with COVID-19 (such as fever, etc.) but a definitive diagnosis has not been established, assign the appropriate code(s) for each of the presenting signs and symptoms such as:

- R05.1 Acute Cough or R05.9, Cough, unspecified
- R06.02 Shortness of breath
- R50.9 Fever, unspecified

If a patient with signs/symptoms associated with COVID-19 also has an actual or suspected contact with or exposure to COVID-19, assign Z20.822, Contact with and (suspected) exposure to COVID-19, as an additional code.

Asymptomatic individuals who test positive for COVID-19

For asymptomatic individuals who test positive for COVID-19, see code only confirmed cases guideline. Although the individual is asymptomatic, the individual has tested positive and is considered to have the COVID-19 infection.

Personal history of COVID-19

For patients with a history of COVID-19, assign code Z86.16, Personal history of COVID-19.

Follow-up visits after COVID-19 infection has resolved

For individuals who previously had COVID-19, without residual symptom(s) or condition(s), and are being seen for follow-up evaluation, and COVID-19 test results are negative, assign codes Z09, Encounter for follow-up examination after completed treatment for conditions other than malignant neoplasm, and Z86.16, Personal history of COVID-19.

For follow-up visits for individuals with symptom(s) or condition(s) related to a previous COVID-19 infection, see U09.

Encounter for antibody testing

For an encounter for antibody testing that is not being performed to confirm a current COVID-19 infection, nor is a follow-up test after resolution of COVID-19, assign Z01.84, Encounter for antibody response examination.

Follow the applicable guidelines above if the individual is being tested to confirm a current COVID-19 infection. For follow-up testing after a COVID-19 infection, see follow-up visits after COVID-19 infection has resolved guideline.

Multisystem Inflammatory Syndrome

For individuals with multisystem inflammatory syndrome (MIS) and COVID-19, assign code U07.1, COVID-19, as the principal/ first-listed diagnosis and assign code M35.81, Multisystem inflammatory syndrome, as an additional diagnosis.

If an individual with a history of COVID-19 develops MIS, assign codes M35.81, Multisystem inflammatory syndrome, and U09.9, Post COVID-19 condition, unspecified.

If an individual with a known or suspected exposure to COVID-19, and no current COVID-19 infection or history of COVID-19, develops MIS, assign codes M35.81, Multisystem inflammatory syndrome, and Z20.822, Contact with and (suspected) exposure to COVID-19.

Additional codes should be assigned for any associated complications of MIS.

U07.1 COVID-19

Use additional code to identify pneumonia or other manifestations, such as:

pneumonia due to COVID-19 (J12.82)

Use additional code, if applicable, for associated conditions such as:

COVID-19 associated coagulopathy (D68.8)

disseminated intravascular coagulation (D65)

hypercoagulable states (D68.69)

thrombophilia (D68.69)

Excludes2: coronavirus as the cause of diseases classified elsewhere (B97.2-)

pneumonia due to SARS-associated coronavirus (J12.81)

U09 POST COVID-19 CONDITION

GUIDELINES

For sequela of COVID-19, or associated symptoms or conditions that develop following a previous COVID-19 infection, assign a code(s) for the specific symptom(s) or condition(s) related to the previous COVID-19 infection, if known, and code U09.9, Post COVID-19 condition, unspecified.

Code U09.9 should not be assigned for manifestations of an active (current) COVID-19 infection.

If a patient has a condition(s) associated with a previous COVID-19 infection and develops a new active (current) COVID-19 infection, code U09.9 may be assigned in conjunction with code U07.1, COVID-19, to identify that the patient also has a condition(s) associated with a previous COVID-19 infection. Code(s) for the specific condition(s) associated with the previous COVID-19 infection and code(s) for manifestation(s) of the new active (current) COVID-19 infection should also be assigned.

U09.9 Post COVID-19 condition, unspecified

Post-acute sequela of COVID-19

Code first the specific condition related to COVID-19 if known, such as:

chronic respiratory failure (J96.1-)

loss of smell (R43.8)

loss of taste (R43.8)

multisystem inflammatory syndrome (M35.81)

pulmonary embolism (I26.-)

pulmonary fibrosis (J84.10)

Note: This code enables establishment of a link with COVID-19. This code is not to be used in cases that are still presenting with active COVID-19. However, an exception is made in cases of re-infection with COVID-19, occurring with a condition related to prior COVID-19.

ICD-10-CM EXTERNAL CAUSE OF INJURIES DUE TO COLLISIONS TABLE

These tables are inserted for ease to locate an external cause code from a transport accident. If not listed here, refer to the index.

Note: All codes require additional characters.
4th, 5th, 6th characters are "X" if not listed and all 7th characters (A, D, S) refer to encounter.

ICD-10-CM EXTERNAL CAUSE OF INJURIES DUE TO COLLISIONS TABLE

	Pedestrian Conveyance	Car/Pick-up Truck/Van	Bike	Bus/HTV	Fixed Object	E-Scooter	Micro-Mobility	Train/Train Car	2 or 3 Motor Wheeler	Non-Motor Vehicle	Other (NOS)	Unspecified
Pedestrian on foot	V00.01- R V00.02- S V00.09- O	V03.00- N V03.10- T V03.90- U	V01.00- N V01.10- T V01.90- U	V04.00- N V04.10- T V04.90- U	Refer to W22	V00.031-	V00.038-	V05.00- N V05.10- T V05.90- U	V02.00- N V02.10- T V02.90- U	V06.00- N V06.10- T V06.90- U	V09.09- N V09.29- T	V09.00- N V09.1- N V09.20- T V09.3- N V09.9- T

Collides with	**Pedestrian or Animal**	**Car/Pick-up Truck/Van**	**Bike**	**Bus/HTV**	**Fixed Object**			**Train/Train Car**	**2 or 3 Motor Wheeler**	**Non-Motor Vehicle**	**Other (NOS)**	**Unspecified**
Activity of the Person Injured												
In-line skater (I)/Roller skater (R)	V00.118- I V00.128- R V00.138-	V03.01- N V03.11- T V03.91- U	V01.01- N V01.11- T V01.91- U	V04.01- N V04.11- T V04.91- U	V00.112- I V00.122- R V00.132-			V05.01- N V05.11- T V05.91- U	V02.01- N V02.11- T V02.91- U	V06.01- N V06.11- T V06.91- U	V00.118- I V00.128- R V00.138-	
Skateboarder		V03.02- N V03.12- T V03.92- U	V01.02- N V01.12- T V01.92- U	V04.02- N V04.12- T V04.92- U				V05.02- N V05.12- T V05.92- U	V02.02- N V02.12- T V02.92- U	V06.02- N V06.12- T V06.92- U		
E-Scooter		V03.031- N V03.131- T V03.931- U	V01.031- N V01.131- T V01.931- U	V04.031- N V04.131- T V04.931- U	V00.842-			V05.031- N V05.131- T V05.931- U	V02.031- N V02.131- T V02.931- U	V06.031- N V06.131- T V06.931- U		
Micro-mobility		V03.038- N V03.138- T V03.938- U	V01.038- N V01.138- T V01.938- U	V04.038- N V04.138- T V04.938- U				V05.038- N V05.138- T V05.938- U	V02.038- N V02.138- T V02.938- U	V06.038- N V06.138- T V06.938- U		
Other (NOS)		V03.09- N V03.19- T V03.99- U	V01.09- N V01.19- T V01.99- U	V04.09- N V04.19- T V04.99- U				V05.09- N V05.19- T V05.99- U	V02.09- N V02.19- T V02.99- U	V06.09- N V06.19- T V06.99- U	V00.848-	
Scooter (Non-motorized)		V03.09- N V03.19- T V03.99- U	V01.09- N V01.19- T V01.99- U	V04.09- N V04.19- T V04.99- U	V00.142-			V05.09- N V05.19- T V05.99- U	V02.09- N V02.19- T V02.99- U	V06.09- N V06.19- T V06.99- U		
Heelies		V03.09- N V03.19- T V03.99- U	V01.09- N V01.19- T V01.99- U	V04.09- N V04.19- T V04.99- U	V00.152-			V05.09- N V05.19- T V05.99- U	V02.09- N V02.19- T V02.99- U	V06.09- N V06.19- T V06.99- U		
Ice-skater		V03.09- N V03.19- T V03.99- U	V01.09- N V01.19- T V01.99- U	V04.09- N V04.19- T V04.99- U	V00.212-			V05.09- N V05.19- T V05.99- U	V02.09- N V02.19- T V02.99- U	V06.09- N V06.19- T V06.99- U		
Sledder		V03.09- N V03.19- T V03.99- U	V01.09- N V01.19- T V01.99- U	V04.09- N V04.19- T V04.99- U	V00.222-			V05.09- N V05.19- T V05.99- U	V02.09- N V02.19- T V02.99- U	V06.09- N V06.19- T V06.99- U		
Snowboarder		V03.09- N V03.19- T V03.99- U	V01.09- N V01.19- T V01.99- U	V04.09- N V04.19- T V04.99- U	V00.312-			V05.09- N V05.19- T V05.99- U	V02.09- N V02.19- T V02.99- U	V06.09- N V06.19- T V06.99- U		
Snowskier		V03.09- N V03.19- T V03.99- U	V01.09- N V01.19- T V01.99- U	V04.09- N V04.19- T V04.99- U	V00.322-			V05.09- N V05.19- T V05.99- U	V02.09- N V02.19- T V02.99- U	V06.09- N V06.19- T V06.99- U		

I = In-line skates; R = roller skates; N = nontraffic accident; T = traffic accident; U = unspecified whether traffic or not

ICD-10-CM EXTERNAL CAUSE OF INJURIES DUE TO COLLISIONS TABLE

Activity of the Person Injured	Car/Pick-up Truck/Van	Bike	Bus/HTV	Fixed Object	Pedestrian or Animal	Collides with Train/Train Car	2 or 3 Motor Wheeler	Non-Motor Vehicle	Other (NOS)	Unspecified
Wheelchair	V03.09- N V03.19- T V03.99- U	V01.09- N V01.19- T V01.99- U	V04.09- N V04.19- T V04.99- U	V00.812-		V05.09- N V05.19- T V05.99- U	V02.09- N V02.19- T V02.99- U	V06.09- N V06.19- T V06.99- U	V19.09- N V19.3- U V19.49- T V19.8- T V19.9- U	V19.00- N V19.40- T
Bike										
Driver	V13.0- N V13.4- T	V11.0- N V11.4- T	V14.0- N V14.4- T	V17.0- N V17.4- T	V10.0- N V10.4- T	V15.0- N V15.4- T	V12.0- N V12.4- T	V16.0- N V16.4- T		
Passenger	V13.1- N V13.5- T	V11.1- N V11.5- T	V14.1- N V14.5- T	V17.1- N V17.5- T	V10.1- N V10.5- T	V15.1- N V15.5- T	V12.1- N V12.5- T	V16.1- N V16.5- T	V19.19- N V19.59- T	V19.10- N V19.50- T
Boarding	V13.3-	V11.3-	V14.3-	V17.3-	V10.3-	V15.3-	V12.3-	V16.3-		
Unspecified	V13.2- N V13.9- T	V11.2- N V11.9- T	V14.2- N V14.9- T	V17.2- N V17.9- T	V10.2- N V10.9- T	V15.2- N V15.9- T	V12.2- N V12.9- T	V16.2- N V16.9- T	V19.29- N V19.69- T	V19.20- N V19.60- T
Other Motorcycle										
Driver	V23.09- N V23.49- T	V21.09- N V21.49- T	V24.09- N V24.49- T	V27.09- N V27.49- T	V20.09- N V20.49- T	V25.09- N V25.49- T	V22.09- N V22.49- T	V26.09- N V26.49- T	V29.098- N V29.498- T	V29.008- N V29.408- T
Passenger	V23.19- N V23.59- T	V21.19- N V21.59- T	V24.19- N V24.59- T	V27.19- N V27.59- T	V20.19- N V20.59- T	V25.19- N V25.59- T	V22.19- N V22.59- T	V26.19- N V26.59- T	V29.198- N V29.598- T	V29.108- N V29.508- T
Driver/Passenger										
Rider		V21.99- T							V29.888- T	V29.39- N V29.99- T
Unspecified rider	V23.29- N V23.99- T	V21.29- N V21.99- T	V24.29- N V24.99- T	V27.29- N V27.99- T	V20.29- N V20.99- T	V25.29- N V25.99- T	V22.29- N V22.99- T	V26.29- N V26.99- T	V29.298- N V29.698- T	V29.208- N V29.298- T
Person Boarding	V23.39-	V21.39-	V24.39-	V27.39-	V20.39-	V25.39-	V22.39-	V26.39-	V28.39-	V29.608- T
Motorcycle/Motor Scooter/ Moped										
Driver	V23.0 N V23.4 T	V21.0 N V21.4 T	V24.0 N V24.4 T	V27.0 N V27.4 T	V20.0 N V20.4 T	V25.0 N V25.4 T	V22.0 N V22.4 T	V26.0 N V26.4 T	V29.09 N V29.49 T	V29.00 N V29.40 N
Passenger	V23.1 N V23.5 T	V21.1 N V21.5 T	V24.1 N V24.5 T	V27.1 N V27.5 T	V20.1 N V20.5 T	V25.1 N V25.5 T	V22.1 N V22.5 T	V26.1 N V26.5 T	V29.19 T V29.59 T	V29.10 N V29.50 T
Boarding	V23.3	V21.3	V24.3	V27.3	V20.3	V25.3	V22.3	V26.3		
Unspecified	V23.2 N V23.9 T	V21.2 N V21.9 T	V24.2 N V24.9 T	V27.2 N V27.9 T	V20.2 N V20.9 T	V25.2 N V25.9 T	V22.2 N V22.9 T	V26.2 N V26.9 T	V29.29 N V29.69 T	V29.20 N V29.60 T
Electric (assisted) Bicycle										
Driver	V23.01- N V23.41- T	V21.01- N V21.41- T	V24.01- N V24.41- T	V27.01- N V27.41X- T	V20.01- N V20.41- T	V25.01- N V25.41- T	V22.01- N V22.41- T	V26.01- N V26.41- T	V29.091- N V29.491- T	V29.001- N V29.401- T
Rider		V21.21- N V21.29- N			V20.21- N V20.91- T				V29.291- T V29.691- T	V26.21- N V29.201- N V29.601- T V29.811- V29.818-

I = In-line skates; R = roller skates; N = nontraffic accident; T = traffic accident; U = unspecified whether traffic or not

ICD-10-CM EXTERNAL CAUSE OF INJURIES DUE TO COLLISIONS TABLE

Activity of the Person Injured	Car/Pick-up Truck/Van	Bike	Bus/HTV	Fixed Object	Pedestrian or Animal	Train/Train Car	2 or 3 Motor Wheeler	Non-Motor Vehicle	Other (NOS)	Unspecified
Electric (assisted) Bicycle										
Passenger	V23.11- N V23.51- T	V21.00- N V21.11- N V21.51- T	V24.11- N V24.51- T	V27.11- N V27.51- T	V20.11- N V20.51- T	V25.11- N V25.51- T	V22.11- N V22.51- T	V26.11- N V26.51- T	V29.191- N V29.591- T	V29.101- N V29.501- T
Driver/passenger	V23.31-	V21.31-	V24.31-	V27.31-	V20.31-	V25.31-	V22.31-		V29.881- T	V29.31- N V29.91- T
Person Boarding								V26.31-		
Unspecified Electric (assisted)										
Driver										
Rider	V23.21- N V23.91- T	V21.21- N V21.91- T	V24.21- N V24.91- T	V27.21- N V27.91- T	V20.21- N V20.91- T	V25.21- N V25.91- T	V22.21- N V22.91- T	V26.21- N V26.91- T	V29.291- N V29.691- T	V29.201- N V29.601- T
3-wheel vehicle										
Driver	V33.0- N V33.5- T	V31.0- N V31.5- T	V34.0- N V34.5- T	V37.0- N V37.5- T	V30.0- N V30.5- T	V35.0- N V35.5- T	V32.0- N V32.5- T	V36.0- N V36.5- T	V39.09- N V39.49- T	V39.00- N V39.40- T
Passenger	V33.1- N V33.6- T	V31.1- N V31.6- T	V34.1- N V34.6- T	V37.1- N V37.6- T	V30.1- N V30.6- T	V35.1- N V35.6- T	V32.1- N V32.6- T	V36.1- N V36.6- T	V39.19- N V39.59- T	V39.10- N V39.50- T
Rider on outside	V33.2- N V33.7- T	V31.2- N V31.7- T	V34.2- N V34.7- T	V37.2- N V37.7- T	V30.2- N V30.7- T	V35.2- N V35.7- T	V32.2- N V32.7- T	V36.2- N V36.7- T		
Boarding	V33.4-	V31.4-	V34.4-	V37.4-	V30.4-	V35.4-	V32.4-	V36.4-		
Unspecified	V33.3- N V33.9- T	V31.3- N V31.9- T	V34.3- N V34.9- T	V37.3- N V37.9- T	V30.3- N V30.9- T	V35.3- N V35.9- T	V32.3- N V32.9- T	V36.3- N V36.9- T	V39.29- N V39.69- T	V39.20- N V39.60- T
Car										
Driver	V43.0- N V43.5- T	V41.0- N V41.5- T	V44.0- N V44.5- T	V47.0- N V47.5- T	V40.0- N V40.5- T	V45.0- N V45.5- T	V42.0- N V42.5- T	V46.0- N V46.5- T	V49.09- N V49.49- T	V49.00- N V49.40- T
Passenger	V43.1- N V43.6- T	V41.1- N V41.6- T	V44.1- N V44.6- T	V47.1- N V47.6- T	V40.1- N V40.6- T	V45.1- N V45.6- T	V42.1- N V42.6- T	V46.1- N V46.6- T	V49.19- N V49.59- T	V49.10- N V49.50- T
Rider on outside	V43.2- N V43.7- T	V41.2- N V41.7- T	V44.2- N V44.7- T	V47.2- N V47.7- T	V40.2- N V40.7- T	V45.2- N V45.7- T	V42.2- N V42.7- T	V46.2- N V46.7- T		V59.3- N V59.9- T
Boarding	V43.4-	V41.4-	V44.4-	V47.4-	V40.4-	V45.4-	V42.4-	V46.4-		
Unspecified	V43.3- N V43.9- T	V41.3- N V41.9- T	V44.3- N V44.9- T	V47.3- N V47.9- T	V40.3- N V40.9- T	V45.3- N V45.9- T	V42.3- N V42.9- T	V46.3- N V46.9- T	V49.29- N V49.69- T	V49.20- N V49.60- T
Pick-up Truck/Van/SUV										
Driver	V53.0- N V53.5- T	V51.0- N V51.5- T	V54.0- N V54.5- T	V57.0- N V57.5- T	V50.0- N V50.5- T	V55.0- N V55.5- T	V52.0- N V52.5- T	V56.0- N V56.5- T	V59.09- N V59.49- T	V59.00- N V59.40- T
Passenger	V53.1- N V53.6- T	V51.1- N V51.6- T	V54.1- N V54.6- T	V57.1- N V57.6- T	V50.1- N V50.6- T	V55.1- N V55.6- T	V52.1- N V52.6- T	V56.1- N V56.6- T	V59.19- N V59.59- T	V59.10- N V59.50- T
Rider on outside	V53.2- N V53.7- T	V51.2- N V51.7- T	V54.2- N V54.7- T	V57.2- N V57.7- T	V50.2- N V50.7- T	V55.2- N V55.7- T	V52.2- N V52.7- T	V56.2- N V56.7- T		

[a] Collision with other animal being ridden
[b] Collision with animal-drawn vehicle
I = In-line skates; R = roller skates; N = nontraffic accident; T = traffic accident; U = unspecified whether traffic or not

ICD-10-CM EXTERNAL CAUSE OF INJURIES DUE TO COLLISIONS TABLE

Collides with

Activity of the Person Injured	Car/Pick-up Truck/Van	Bike	Bus/ATV	Fixed Object	Pedestrian or Animal	Train/Train Car	2 or 3 Motor Wheeler	Non-Motor Vehicle	Other (NOS)	Unspecified
Pick-up Truck/Van/SUV										
Boarding	V53.4-	V51.4-	V54.4-	V57.4-	V50.4-	V55.4-	V52.4-	V56.4-		V59.20- N
Unspecified	V53.3- N	V51.3- N	V54.3- N	V57.3- N	V50.3- N	V55.3- N	V52.3- N	V56.3- N	V59.29- N	V59.60- T
	V53.9- T	V51.9- T	V54.9- T	V57.9- T	V50.9- T	V55.9- T	V52.9- T	V56.9- T	V59.69- T	
Bus										
Driver	V73.0- N	V71.0- N	V74.0- N	V77.0- N	V70.0- N	V75.0- N	V72.0- N	V76.0- N	V79.09- N	V79.00- N
	V73.5- T	V71.5- T	V74.5- T	V77.5- T	V70.5- T	V75.5- T	V72.5- T	V76.5- T	V79.49- T	V79.40- T
Passenger	V73.1- N	V71.1- N	V74.1- N	V77.1- T	V70.1- N	V75.1- N	V72.1- N	V76.1- N	V79.19- N	V79.10- N
	V73.6- T	V71.6- T	V74.6- T	V77.6- T	V70.6- T	V75.6- T	V72.6- T	V76.6- T	V79.59- T	V79.50- T
Rider on outside	V73.2- N	V71.2- N	V74.2- N	V77.2- N	V70.2- N	V75.2- N	V72.2- N	V76.2- N		V79.3- N
	V73.7- T	V71.7- T	V74.7- T	V77.7- T	V70.7- T	V75.7- T	V72.7- T	V76.7- T		V79.9- T
Boarding	V73.4-	V71.4-	V74.4-	V77.4-	V70.4-	V75.4-	V72.4-	V76.4-		
Unspecified	V73.3- N	V71.3- N	V74.3- N	V77.3- N	V70.3- N	V75.3- N	V72.3- N	V76.3- N	V79.29- N	V79.20- N
	V73.9- T	V71.9- T	V74.9- T	V77.9- T	V70.9- T	V75.9- T	V72.9- T	V76.9- T	V79.69- T	V79.60- T
Animal Rider	V80.41-	V80.21-	V80.41-	V80.81-	V80.710-ᵃ	V80.61-	V80.3-1	V80.790-	V80.51-	V80.919-
					V80.720-ᵇ					
Animal-Drawn Vehicle	V80.42-	V80.22-	V80.42-	V80.82-	V80.711-ᵃ	V80.62-	V80.32-	V80.791-	V80.52-	V80.929-
					V80.721-ᵇ					

ᵃCollision with other animal being ridden
ᵇCollision with animal-drawn vehicle

I = In-line skates; R = roller skates; N = nontraffic accident; T = traffic accident; U = unspecified whether traffic or not

Vehicle	**Special Agriculture Vehicle**	**Snowmobile**	**Dune Buggy**	**3 or 4 Wheel ATV**	**Dirt Bike**	**Other ATV (eg, go-cart, golf cart)**
Injured Person						
Driver	V84.0- T	V86.02- T	V86.03- T	V86.05- T	V86.06- T	V86.09- T
	V84.5- N	V86.52- T	V86.53- N	V86.55- N	V86.56- N	V86.59- N
Passenger	V84.1- T	V86.12- T	V86.13- T	V86.15- T	V86.16- T	V86.19- T
	V84.6- N	V86.62- N	V86.63- N	V86.65- N	V86.66- N	V86.69- N
Outside rider	V84.2- T	V86.22- T	V86.23- T			V86.25- T
	V84.7- N	V86.72- N	V86.73- N			V86.75- N
Unspecified	V84.3- T	V86.32 T	V86.33- T	V86.35- T	V86.36- T	V86.39- T
	V84.9- N	V86.92- N	V86.93- N	V86.95- N	V86.96- N	V86.99- N
Boarding	V84.4-	V86.42-	V86.43-	V86.45-	V86.46-	V86.49-

I = In-line skates; R = roller skates; N = nontraffic accident; T = traffic accident; U = unspecified whether traffic or not

ICD-10-CM EXTERNAL CAUSE OF INJURIES INDEX

ICD-10-CM EXTERNAL CAUSE OF INJURIES INDEX

A

Refer to the External Cause of Injury Table first for those injuries resulting from a number of collisions (eg, cars, trucks, bikes, e-scooters).

Abandonment (causing exposure to weather conditions) (with intent to injure or kill) NEC X58.-

Abuse (adult) (child) (mental) (physical) (sexual) X58.-

Accident (to) X58.-

- aircraft (in transit) (powered)—*see also* Accident, transport, aircraft
  - due to, caused by cataclysm—*see* Forces of nature, by type
- animal-drawn vehicle—*see* Accident, transport, animal-drawn vehicle occupant
- animal-rider—*see* Accident, transport, animal-rider
- automobile—*see* Accident, transport, car occupant
- bare foot water skier V94.4-
- boat, boating—*see also* Accident, watercraft
  - striking swimmer
    - ■ powered V94.11-
    - ■ unpowered V94.12-
- bus—*see* Accident, transport, bus occupant
- cable car, not on rails V98.0-
  - on rails—*see* Accident, transport, streetcar occupant
- car—*see* Accident, transport, car occupant
- caused by, due to
  - chain hoist W24.0-
  - cold (excessive)—*see* Exposure, cold
  - corrosive liquid, substance—*see* Table of Drugs and Chemicals
  - cutting or piercing instrument—*see* Contact, with, by type of instrument
  - drive belt W24.0-
  - electric
    - ■ current—*see* Exposure, electric current
    - ■ motor (*see also* Contact, with, by type of machine) W31.3-
      - ~ current (of) W86.8-
  - environmental factor NEC X58.-
  - explosive material—*see* Explosion
  - fire, flames—*see* Exposure, fire
  - firearm missile—*see* Discharge, firearm by type
  - heat (excessive)—*see* Heat
  - hot—*see* Contact, with, hot
  - ignition—*see* Ignition
  - lifting device W24.0-
  - lightning—*see* subcategory T75.0-
    - ■ causing fire—*see* Exposure, fire
  - machine, machinery—*see* Contact, with, by type of machine
  - natural factor NEC X58.-
  - pulley (block) W24.0-
  - radiation—*see* Radiation
  - steam X13.1-
    - ■ inhalation X13.0-
    - ■ pipe X16.-
  - thunderbolt—*see* subcategory T75.0-
    - ■ causing fire—*see* Exposure, fire
  - transmission device W24.1-
- diving—*see also* Fall, into, water
  - with
    - ■ drowning or submersion—*see* Drowning
- ice yacht V98.2-
- in
  - medical, surgical procedure
    - ■ as, or due to misadventure—*see* Misadventure
    - ■ causing an abnormal reaction or later complication without mention of misadventure (*see also* Complication of or following, by type of procedure) Y84.9-
- land yacht V98.1-
- late effect of—*see* W00-X58 with 7th character S
- logging car—*see* Accident, transport, industrial vehicle occupant
- machine, machinery—*see also* Contact, with, by type of machine
  - on board watercraft V93.69-
    - ■ explosion—*see* Explosion, in, watercraft
    - ■ fire—*see* Burn, on board watercraft
    - ■ powered craft V93.63-
      - ~ ferry boat V93.61-
      - ~ fishing boat V93.62-

Accident (to), *continued*

- - ~ jet skis V93.63-
    - ~ liner V93.61-
    - ~ merchant ship V93.60-
    - ~ passenger ship V93.61-
    - ~ sailboat V93.64-
- mobility scooter (motorized)—*see* Accident, transport, pedestrian, conveyance, specified type NEC
- motor scooter—*see* Accident, transport, motorcyclist
- motor vehicle NOS (traffic) (*see also* Accident, transport) V89.2-
  - nontraffic V89.0-
  - three-wheeled NOS—*see* Accident, transport, three-wheeled motor vehicle occupant
- motorcycle NOS—*see* Accident, transport, motorcyclist
- nonmotor vehicle NOS (nontraffic) (*see also* Accident, transport) V89.1-
  - traffic NOS V89.3-
- nontraffic (victim's mode of transport NOS) V88.9-
  - collision (between) V88.7-
    - ■ bus and truck V88.5-
    - ■ car and:
      - ~ bus V88.3-
      - ~ pickup V88.2-
      - ~ three-wheeled motor vehicle V88.0-
      - ~ train V88.6-
      - ~ truck V88.4-
      - ~ two-wheeled motor vehicle V88.0-
      - ~ van V88.2-
    - ■ specified vehicle NEC and:
      - ~ three-wheeled motor vehicle V88.1-
      - ~ two-wheeled motor vehicle V88.1-
  - known mode of transport—*see* Accident, transport, by type of vehicle
  - noncollision V88.8-
- on board watercraft V93.8-
  - inflatable V93.86-
    - ■ in tow
      - ~ recreational V94.31-
      - ~ specified NEC V94.32-
- parachutist V97.29-
  - entangled in object V97.21-
  - injured on landing V97.22-
- pedal cycle—*see* Accident, transport, pedal cyclist
- pedestrian (on foot)
  - with
    - ■ another pedestrian W51.-
      - ~ with fall W03.-
        - ◊ due to ice or snow W00.0-
    - ■ rider of
      - ~ electric scooter V00.031-
      - ~ hoverboard V00.038-
      - ~ micro-mobility pedestrian conveyance NEC V00.038-
      - ~ Segway V00.038-
- transport vehicle—*see* Accident, transport
  - on pedestrian conveyance—*see* Accident, transport, pedestrian, conveyance
- quarry truck—*see* Accident, transport, industrial vehicle occupant
- railway vehicle (any) (in motion)—*see* Accident, transport, railway vehicle occupant
  - due to cataclysm—*see* Forces of nature, by type
- scooter (non-motorized)—*see* Accident, transport, pedestrian, conveyance, scooter
- skateboard—*see* Accident, transport, pedestrian, conveyance, skateboard
- ski(ing)—*see* Accident, transport, pedestrian, conveyance
  - lift V98.3-
- specified cause NEC X58.-
- streetcar—*see* Accident, transport, streetcar occupant
- traffic (victim's mode of transport NOS) V87.9-
  - collision (between) V87.7-
    - ■ bus and truck V87.5-
    - ■ car and:
      - ~ bus V87.3-
      - ~ pickup V87.2-
      - ~ three-wheeled motor vehicle V87.0-
      - ~ train V87.6-
      - ~ truck V87.4-
      - ~ two-wheeled motor vehicle V87.0-
      - ~ van V87.2-

Accident (to), *continued*

- - ■ specified vehicle NEC V86.39-
    - ~ three-wheeled motor vehicle V87.1-
    - ~ two-wheeled motor vehicle V87.1-
  - known mode of transport—*see* Accident, transport, by type of vehicle
  - noncollision V87.8-
- transport (involving injury to) V99.-
  - agricultural vehicle occupant (nontraffic) V84.-
  - aircraft V97.8-
    - ■ occupant injured (in)
      - ~ nonpowered craft accident V96.9-
        - ◊ balloon V96.0-.
        - ◊ glider V96.2-
        - ◊ hang glider V96.1-
        - ◊ specified craft NEC V96.8-
      - ~ powered craft accident V95.9-
        - ◊ fixed wing NEC
          - » commercial V95.3-
          - » private V95.2-
        - ◊ glider (powered) V95.1-
        - ◊ helicopter V95.0-
        - ◊ specified craft NEC V95.8-
        - ◊ ultralight V95.1-
      - ~ specified accident NEC V97.0-
      - ~ while boarding or alighting V97.1-
    - ■ person (injured by)
      - ~ falling from, in or on aircraft V97.0-
      - ~ machinery on aircraft V97.89-
      - ~ on ground with aircraft involvement V97.39-
      - ~ while boarding or alighting aircraft V97.1-
  - airport (battery-powered) passenger vehicle—*see* Accident, transport, industrial vehicle occupant
  - all-terrain vehicle occupant (nontraffic) V86.99-
    - ■ driver V86.59-
    - ■ dune buggy—*see* Accident, transport, dune buggy occupant
    - ■ passenger V86.69-
  - animal-drawn vehicle occupant (in) V80.929-
    - collision (with)
      - ~ animal V80.12-
        - ◊ being ridden V80.711-
      - ~ animal-drawn vehicle V80.721-
      - ~ fixed or stationary object V80.82-
      - ~ nonmotor vehicle V80.791-
      - ~ pedestrian V80.12-
      - ~ streetcar V80.731-
    - ■ noncollision V80.02-
    - ■ specified circumstance NEC V80.928-
  - animal-rider V80.919-
    - collision (with)
      - ~ animal V80.11-
        - ◊ being ridden V80.710-
      - ~ animal-drawn vehicle V80.720-
      - ~ fixed or stationary object V80.81-
      - ~ nonmotor vehicle V80.790-
      - ~ pedestrian V80.11-
      - ~ streetcar V80.730-
    - ■ noncollision V80.018-
      - ~ specified as horse rider V80.010-
    - ■ specified circumstance NEC V80.918-
  - bus occupant V79.9-
    - ■ collision (with)
      - ~ driver
        - ~ collision (with)
          - ~ noncollision accident (traffic) V78.5-
            - ◊ nontraffic V78.0-
          - ■ noncollision accident (traffic) V78.9-
            - ◊ nontraffic V78.3-
          - ~ while boarding or alighting V78.4-
        - ■ passenger
          - ~ collision (with)
            - ~ noncollision accident (traffic) V78.6-
              - ◊ nontraffic V78.1-
          - ■ specified type NEC V79.88-
            - ~ military vehicle V79.81-
        - cable car, not on rails V98.0-
          - ■ on rails—*see* Accident, transport, streetcar occupant

ICD-10-CM EXTERNAL CAUSE OF INJURIES INDEX

Accident (to), *continued*
- car occupant V49.9-
  - ■ ambulance occupant—*see* Accident, transport, ambulance occupant
  - ■ collision (with)
    - ~ animal being ridden (traffic) V46.9-
      - ◊ nontraffic V46.3-
      - ◊ while boarding or alighting V46.4-
    - ~ animal-drawn vehicle (traffic) V46.9-
      - ◊ nontraffic V46.3-
      - ◊ while boarding or alighting V46.4-
    - ~ car (traffic) V43.92-
      - ◊ nontraffic V43.32-
      - ◊ while boarding or alighting V43.42-
    - ~ motor vehicle NOS (traffic) V49.60-
      - ◊ nontraffic V49.20-
      - ◊ specified type NEC (traffic) V49.69-
        - » nontraffic V49.29-
    - ~ pickup truck (traffic) V43.93-
      - ◊ nontraffic V43.33-
      - ◊ while boarding or alighting V43.43-
    - ~ specified vehicle NEC (traffic) V46.9-
      - ◊ nontraffic V46.3-
      - ◊ while boarding or alighting V46.4-
    - ~ sport utility vehicle (traffic) V43.91-
      - ◊ nontraffic V43.31-
      - ◊ while boarding or alighting V43.41-
    - ~ stationary object (traffic) V47.92-
      - ◊ while boarding or alighting V47.4-
    - ~ streetcar (traffic) V46.9-
      - ◊ nontraffic V46.3-
      - ◊ while boarding or alighting V46.4-
    - ~ van (traffic) V43.94-
      - ◊ nontraffic V43.34-
      - ◊ while boarding or alighting V43.44-
  - ■ driver
    - ~ collision (with)
      - ◊ animal being ridden (traffic) V46.5-
        - » nontraffic V46.0-
      - ◊ animal-drawn vehicle (traffic) V46.5-
        - » nontraffic V46.0-
      - ◊ car (traffic) V43.52-
        - » nontraffic V43.02-
      - ◊ motor vehicle NOS (traffic) V49.40-
        - » nontraffic V49.00-
        - » specified type NEC (traffic) V49.49-
          - ❖ nontraffic V49.09-
      - ◊ pickup truck (traffic) V43.53-
        - » nontraffic V43.03-
      - ◊ specified vehicle NEC (traffic) V46.5-
        - » nontraffic V46.0-
      - ◊ sport utility vehicle (traffic) V43.51-
        - » nontraffic V43.01-
      - ◊ streetcar (traffic) V46.5-
        - » nontraffic V46.0-
      - ◊ van (traffic) V43.54-
        - » nontraffic V43.04-
    - ~ noncollision accident (traffic) V48.5-
      - ◊ nontraffic V48.0-
  - ■ hanger-on
    - ~ collision (with)
      - ◊ animal being ridden (traffic) V46.7-
        - » nontraffic V46.2-
      - ◊ animal-drawn vehicle (traffic) V46.7-
        - » nontraffic V46.2-
      - ◊ car (traffic) V43.72-
        - » nontraffic V43.22-
      - ◊ pickup truck (traffic) V43.73-
        - » nontraffic V43.23-
      - ◊ specified vehicle NEC (traffic) V46.7-
        - » nontraffic V46.2-
      - ◊ sport utility vehicle (traffic) V43.71-
        - » nontraffic V43.21-
      - ◊ stationary object (traffic) V47.7-
        - » nontraffic V47.2-
      - ◊ streetcar (traffic) V46.7-
        - » nontraffic V46.2-
      - ◊ van (traffic) V43.74-
        - » nontraffic V43.24-
    - ~ noncollision accident (traffic) V48.7-
      - ◊ nontraffic V48.2-

Accident (to), *continued*
- ■ noncollision accident (traffic) V48.9-
  - ~ nontraffic V48.3-
  - ~ while boarding or alighting V48.4-
  - ■ nontraffic V49.3-
- ■ passenger
  - ~ collision (with)
    - ◊ animal being ridden (traffic) V46.6-
      - » nontraffic V46.1-
    - ◊ animal-drawn vehicle (traffic) V46.6-
      - » nontraffic V46.1-
    - ◊ car (traffic) V43.62-
      - » nontraffic V43.12-
    - ◊ motor vehicle NOS (traffic) V49.50-
      - » nontraffic V49.10-
      - » specified type NEC (traffic) V49.59-
        - ❖ nontraffic V49.19-
    - ◊ pickup truck (traffic) V43.63-
      - » nontraffic V43.13-
    - ◊ specified vehicle NEC (traffic) V46.6-
      - » nontraffic V46.1-
    - ◊ sport utility vehicle (traffic) V43.61-
      - » nontraffic V43.11-
    - ◊ streetcar (traffic) V46.6-
      - » nontraffic V46.1-
    - ◊ van (traffic) V43.64-
      - » nontraffic V43.14-
  - ~ noncollision accident (traffic) V48.6-
    - ◊ nontraffic V48.1-
    - ◊ specified type NEC V49.88-
- due to cataclysm—*see* Forces of nature, by type
- hoverboard V00.848-
- ice yacht V98.2-
- industrial vehicle occupant (nontraffic) V83.-
- land yacht V98.1-
- logging car—*see* Accident, transport, industrial vehicle occupant
- motorcoach—*see* Accident, transport, bus occupant
- motorcyclist V29.9-
  - ■ collision (with)
    - ~ animal being ridden (traffic) V26.9-
      - ◊ nontraffic V26.2-
      - ◊ while boarding or alighting V26.3-
    - ~ animal-drawn vehicle (traffic) V26.9-
      - ◊ nontraffic V26.2-
      - ◊ while boarding or alighting V26.3-
    - ~ motor vehicle NOS (traffic) V29.60-
      - ◊ nontraffic V29.20-
      - ◊ specified type NEC (traffic) V29.69-
        - » nontraffic V29.29-
    - ~ specified vehicle NEC (traffic) V26.9-
      - ◊ nontraffic V26.2-
      - ◊ while boarding or alighting V26.3-
    - ~ streetcar (traffic) V26.9-
      - ◊ nontraffic V26.2-
      - ◊ while boarding or alighting V26.3-
  - ■ driver
    - ~ collision (with)
      - ◊ animal being ridden (traffic) V26.4-
        - » nontraffic V26.0-
      - ◊ animal-drawn vehicle (traffic) V26.4-
        - » nontraffic V26.0-
      - ◊ specified vehicle NEC (traffic) V26.4-
        - » nontraffic V26.0-
      - ◊ streetcar (traffic) V26.4-
        - » nontraffic V26.0-
    - ~ noncollision accident (traffic) V28.4-
      - ◊ nontraffic V28.0-
  - ■ noncollision accident (traffic) V28.9-
    - ~ nontraffic V28.2-
    - ~ while boarding or alighting V28.3-
  - ■ nontraffic V29.3-
  - ■ passenger
    - ~ collision (with)
      - ◊ animal being ridden (traffic) V26.5-
        - » nontraffic V26.1-
      - ◊ animal-drawn vehicle (traffic) V26.5-
        - » nontraffic V26.1-
      - ◊ specified vehicle NEC (traffic) V26.5-
      - ◊ streetcar (traffic) V26.5-
        - » nontraffic V26.1-
    - ~ noncollision accident (traffic) V28.5-
      - ◊ nontraffic V28.1-

Accident (to), *continued*
- ◊ specified type NEC V29.88-
  - ~ military vehicle V29.81-
- motor vehicle NEC occupant (traffic) V86.39-
- occupant (of)
  - ■ aircraft (powered) V95.9-
    - ~ nonpowered V96.9-
    - ~ specified NEC V95.8-
  - ■ airport battery-powered vehicle—*see* Accident, transport, industrial vehicle occupant
  - ■ all-terrain vehicle (ATV)—*see* Accident, transport, all-terrain vehicle occupant
  - ■ animal-drawn vehicle—*see* Accident, transport, animal-drawn vehicle occupant
  - ■ automobile—*see* Accident, transport, car occupant
  - ■ balloon V96.00-
  - ■ battery-powered vehicle—*see* Accident, transport, industrial vehicle occupant
  - ■ bicycle—*see* Accident, transport, pedal cyclist
    - ~ motorized—*see* Accident, transport, motorcycle rider
  - ■ boat NEC—*see* Accident, watercraft
  - ■ bus—*see* Accident, transport, bus occupant
  - ■ cable car (on rails)—*see also* Accident, transport, streetcar occupant
    - ~ not on rails V98.0-
  - ■ car—*see also* Accident, transport, car occupant
  - ■ cable (on rails)—*see also* Accident, transport, streetcar occupant
    - ◊ not on rails V98.0-
  - ■ coach—*see* Accident, transport, bus occupant
  - ■ farm machinery (self-propelled)—*see* Accident, transport, agricultural vehicle occupant
  - ■ forklift—*see* Accident, transport, industrial vehicle occupant
  - ■ glider (unpowered) V96.20-
    - ~ hang V96.10-
    - ~ powered (microlight) (ultralight)—*see* Accident, transport, aircraft, occupant, powered, glider
  - ■ glider (unpowered) NEC V96.20-
  - ■ hang-glider V96.10-
  - ■ heavy (transport) vehicle—*see* Accident, transport, truck occupant
  - ■ ice-yacht V98.2-
  - ■ kite (carrying person) V96.8-
  - ■ land-yacht V98.1-
  - ■ microlight—*see* Accident, transport, aircraft, occupant, powered, glider
  - ■ motor scooter—*see* Accident, transport, motorcycle
  - ■ motorcycle (with sidecar)—*see* Accident, transport, motorcycle
  - ■ pedal cycle—*see also* Accident, transport, pedal cyclist
  - ■ pick-up (truck)—*see* Accident, transport, pickup truck occupant
  - ■ railway (train) (vehicle) (subterranean) (elevated)—*see* Accident, transport, railway vehicle occupant
    - ~ motorized—*see* Accident, transport, three-wheeled motor vehicle
    - ~ pedal driven—*see* Accident, transport, pedal cyclist
  - ■ ship NOS V94.9-
  - ■ ski-lift (chair) (gondola) V98.3-
  - ■ sport utility vehicle—*see* Accident, transport, car occupant
  - ■ streetcar (interurban) (operating on public street or highway)—*see* Accident, transport, streetcar occupant
  - ■ three-wheeled vehicle (motorized)—*see also* Accident, transport, three-wheeled motor vehicle occupant
    - ~ nonmotorized—*see* Accident, transport, pedal cycle
  - ■ tractor (farm) (and trailer)—*see* Accident, transport, agricultural vehicle occupant
  - ■ train—*see* Accident, transport, railway vehicle occupant
  - ■ tram—*see* Accident, transport, streetcar occupant

ICD-10-CM EXTERNAL CAUSE OF INJURIES INDEX

Accident (to), *continued*

- ■ tricycle—*see* Accident, transport, pedal cycle
  - ~ motorized—*see* Accident, transport, three-wheeled motor vehicle
- ■ trolley—*see* Accident, transport, streetcar occupant
- ■ ultralight—*see* Accident, transport, aircraft, occupant, powered, glider
- ■ van—*see* Accident, transport, van occupant
- ■ vehicle NEC V89.9-
  - ~ heavy transport—*see* Accident, transport, truck occupant
  - ~ motor (traffic) NEC V89.2-
    - ◊ nontraffic NEC V89.0-
  - ~ watercraft NOS V94.9-
    - ~ causing drowning—*see* Drowning, resulting from accident to boat
- ~ parachutist V97.29-
  - ■ after accident to aircraft—*see* Accident, transport, aircraft
  - ■ entangled in object V97.21-
  - ■ injured on landing V97.22-
- ~ pedal cyclist V19.9-
  - ■ noncollision accident (traffic) V18.4-
    - ~ nontraffic V18.0-
  - ■ noncollision accident (traffic) V18.9-
    - ~ nontraffic V18.2-
    - ~ while boarding or alighting V18.3-
  - ■ nontraffic V19.3-
  - ■ passenger
    - ~ noncollision accident (traffic) V18.5-
      - ◊ nontraffic V18.1-
- ~ pedestrian
  - ■ conveyance (occupant) V09.9-
    - ~ baby stroller V00.828-
      - ◊ collision (with) V09.9-
        - » stationary object V00.822-
        - » vehicle V09.9-
          - ◆ nontraffic V09.00-
          - ◆ traffic V09.20-
      - ◊ fall V00.821-
      - ◊ nontraffic V09.1-
        - » involving motor vehicle NEC V09.00-
      - ◊ traffic V09.3-
        - » involving motor vehicle NEC V09.20-
    - ~ electric scooter (standing) (*see* External Cause of Injuries Table)
    - ~ flat-bottomed NEC V00.388-
      - ◊ collision (with) V09.9-
        - » stationary object V00.382-
        - » vehicle V09.9-
          - ◆ nontraffic V09.00-
          - ◆ traffic V09.20-
      - ◊ fall V00.381-
      - ◊ nontraffic V09.1-
        - » involving motor vehicle NEC V09.00-
      - ◊ snow
        - » board—*see* Accident, transport, pedestrian, conveyance, snow board
        - » ski—*see* Accident, transport, pedestrian, conveyance, skis (snow)
      - ◊ traffic V09.3-
        - » involving motor vehicle NEC V09.20-
    - ~ gliding type NEC
      - ◊ collision (with) V09.9-
        - » vehicle V09.9-
          - ◆ nontraffic V09.00-
          - ◆ traffic V09.20-
      - ◊ heelies—*see* Accident, transport, pedestrian, conveyance, heelies
      - ◊ ice skate—*see* Accident, transport, pedestrian, conveyance, ice skate
      - ◊ nontraffic V09.1-
        - » involving motor vehicle NEC V09.00-
      - ◊ sled—*see* Accident, transport, pedestrian, conveyance, sled
      - ◊ traffic V09.3-
        - » involving motor vehicle NEC V09.20-
        - » wheelies—*see* Accident, transport, pedestrian, conveyance, heelies
    - ~ heelies V00.158-
      - ◊ fall V00.151-

Accident (to), *continued*

- ~ hoverboard—*see* External Cause of Injuries Table
- ~ ice skates V00.218-
  - ◊ collision (with) V09.9-
    - » vehicle V09.9-
      - ◆ nontraffic V09.00-
      - ◆ traffic V09.20-
  - ◊ fall V00.211-
  - ◊ nontraffic V09.1-
    - » involving motor vehicle NEC V09.00-
  - ◊ traffic V09.3-
    - » involving motor vehicle NEC V09.20-
- ~ micro-mobility pedestrian conveyance—*see* External Cause of Injuries Table
- ~ nontraffic V09.1-
  - ◊ involving motor vehicle V09.00-
    - » military V09.01-
    - » specified type NEC V09.09-
- ~ roller skates (non in-line) V00.128-
  - ◊ collision (with) V09.9-
    - » stationary object V00.122-
    - » vehicle V09.9-
      - ◆ nontraffic V09.00-
      - ◆ traffic V09.20-
  - ◊ fall V00.121-
  - ◊ in-line V00.118-
    - » collision—see also Accident, transport, pedestrian, conveyance occupant, roller skates, collision
      - ◆ with stationary object V00.112-
    - » fall V00.111-
  - ◊ nontraffic V09.1-
    - » involving motor vehicle NEC V09.00-
  - ◊ traffic V09.3-
    - » involving motor vehicle NEC V09.20-
- ~ rolling shoes V00.158-
  - ◊ fall V00.151-
- ~ rolling type NEC V00.188-
  - ◊ collision (with) V09.9-
    - » stationary object V00.182-
    - » vehicle V09.9-
      - ◆ nontraffic V09.00
      - ◆ traffic V09.20-
  - ◊ fall V00.181-
  - ◊ in-line roller skate—*see* Accident, transport, pedestrian, conveyance, roller skate, in-line
  - ◊ nontraffic V09.1-
    - » involving motor vehicle NEC V09.00-
  - ◊ roller skate—*see* Accident, transport, conveyance, roller skate
  - ◊ scooter (non-motorized)—*see* Accident, transport, pedestrian, conveyance, scooter
  - ◊ skateboard—*see* Accident, transport, pedestrian, conveyance, skateboard
  - ◊ traffic V09.3-
    - » involving motor vehicle NEC V09.20-
- ~ scooter (non-motorized) V00.148-
  - ◊ collision (with) V09.9-
    - » vehicle V09.9-
      - ◆ nontraffic V09.00-
      - ◆ traffic V09.20-
  - ◊ fall V00.141-
  - ◊ nontraffic V09.1-
    - » involving motor vehicle NEC V09.00-
  - ◊ traffic V09.3-
    - » involving motor vehicle NEC V09.20-
- ~ Segway—*see* External Cause of Injuries Table
- ~ skate board V00.138-
  - ◊ collision (with) V09.9-
    - » stationary object V00.132-
    - » vehicle V09.9-
      - ◆ nontraffic V09.00-
      - ◆ traffic V09.20-
  - ◊ fall V00.131-
  - ◊ nontraffic V09.1-
    - » involving motor vehicle NEC V09.00-
  - ◊ traffic V09.3-
    - » involving motor vehicle NEC V09.20-
- ~ sled V00.228-
  - ◊ collision (with) V09.9-

Accident (to), *continued*

- » vehicle V09.9-
  - ◆ nontraffic V09.00-
  - ◆ traffic V09.20-
- ◊ fall V00.221-
- ◊ nontraffic V09.1-
  - » involving motor vehicle NEC V09.00-
- ◊ traffic V09.3-
  - » involving motor vehicle NEC V09.20-
- ~ skis (snow) V00.328-
  - ◊ collision (with) V09.9-
    - » vehicle V09.9-
      - ◆ nontraffic V09.00-
      - ◆ traffic V09.20-
  - ◊ fall V00.321-
  - ◊ nontraffic V09.1-
    - » involving motor vehicle NEC V09.00-
  - ◊ traffic V09.3-
    - » involving motor vehicle NEC V09.20-
- ~ snow board V00.318-
  - ◊ collision (with) V09.9-
    - » vehicle V09.9-
      - ◆ nontraffic V09.00-
      - ◆ traffic V09.20-
  - ◊ fall V00.311-
  - ◊ nontraffic V09.1-
    - » involving motor vehicle NEC V09.00-
  - ◊ traffic V09.3-
    - » involving motor vehicle NEC V09.20-
  - ~ specified type NEC V00.898-
    - ◊ collision (with) V09.9-
      - » stationary object V00.892-
      - » vehicle V09.9-
        - ◆ nontraffic V09.00-
        - ◆ traffic V09.20-
    - ◊ fall V00.891-
    - ◊ nontraffic V09.1-
      - » involving motor vehicle NEC V09.00-
    - ◊ traffic V09.3-
      - » involving motor vehicle NEC V09.20-
  - ~ traffic V09.3-
    - ◊ involving motor vehicle V09.20-
      - » specified type NEC V09.29-
  - ~ wheelchair (powered) V00.818-
    - ◊ collision (with) V09.9-
      - » stationary object V00.812-
      - » vehicle V09.9-
        - ◆ nontraffic V09.00-
        - ◆ traffic V09.20-
    - ◊ fall V00.811-
    - ◊ nontraffic V09.1-
      - » involving motor vehicle NEC V09.00-
    - ◊ traffic V09.3-
      - » involving motor vehicle NEC V09.20-
    - ~ wheeled shoe V00.158-
      - ◊ fall V00.151-
  - ■ on foot—*see also* Accident, pedestrian
    - ~ collision (with)
      - ◊ vehicle V09.9-
        - » nontraffic V09.00-
        - » traffic V09.20-
    - ~ nontraffic V09.1-
      - ◊ involving motor vehicle V09.00-
        - » military V09.01-
        - » specified type NEC V09.09-
    - ~ traffic V09.3-
      - ◊ involving motor vehicle V09.20-
        - » specified type NEC V09.29-
  - ~ person NEC (unknown way or transportation) V99.-
    - ■ collision (between)
      - ~ bus (with)
        - ◊ heavy transport vehicle (traffic) V87.5-
          - » nontraffic V88.5-
      - ~ car (with)
        - ◊ bus (traffic) V87.3-
          - » nontraffic V88.3-
        - ◊ heavy transport vehicle (traffic) V87.4
          - » nontraffic V88.4-
        - ◊ nontraffic V88.5-
        - ◊ pick-up truck or van (traffic) V87.2
          - » nontraffic V88.2-

ICD-10-CM EXTERNAL CAUSE OF INJURIES INDEX

Accident (to), *continued*
- ◊ train or railway vehicle (traffic) V87.6-
  - » nontraffic V88.6-
- ◊ two-or three-wheeled motor vehicle (traffic) V87.0-
  - » nontraffic V88.0-
- – motor vehicle (traffic) NEC V87.7-
  - ◊ nontraffic V88.7-
- – two-or three-wheeled vehicle (with) (traffic)
  - ◊ motor vehicle NEC V87.1-
    - » nontraffic V88.1-
- ■ nonmotor vehicle (collision) (noncollision) (traffic) V87.9-
  - – nontraffic V88.9-
- – pickup truck occupant V59.9-
  - ■ collision (with)
    - – animal (traffic) V50.9-
    - ◊ animal being ridden (traffic) V56.9-
      - » nontraffic V56.3-
      - » while boarding or alighting V56.4-
    - – animal-drawn vehicle (traffic) V56.9-
      - ◊ nontraffic V56.3-
      - ◊ while boarding or alighting V56.4-
    - – motor vehicle NOS (traffic) V59.60-
      - ◊ nontraffic V59.20-
      - ◊ specified type NEC (traffic) V59.69-
        - » nontraffic V59.29-
    - – specified vehicle NEC (traffic) V56.9-
      - ◊ nontraffic V56.3-
      - ◊ while boarding or alighting V56.4-
    - – streetcar (traffic) V56.9-
      - ◊ nontraffic V56.3-
      - ◊ while boarding or alighting V56.4-
  - ■ driver
    - – collision (with)
    - ◊ animal being ridden (traffic) V56.5-
      - » nontraffic V56.0-
    - ◊ animal-drawn vehicle (traffic) V56.5-
      - » nontraffic V56.0-
    - ◊ motor vehicle NOS (traffic) V59.40-
      - » nontraffic V59.00-
      - » specified type NEC (traffic) V59.49-
        - ◆ nontraffic V59.09-
    - ◊ specified vehicle NEC (traffic) V56.5-
      - » nontraffic V56.0-
    - ◊ streetcar (traffic) V56.5-
      - » nontraffic V56.0-
    - – noncollision accident (traffic) V58.5-
      - ◊ nontraffic V58.0-
  - ■ hanger-on
    - – collision (with)
    - ◊ animal being ridden (traffic) V56.7-
      - » nontraffic V56.2-
    - ◊ animal-drawn vehicle (traffic) V56.7-
      - » nontraffic V56.2-
    - ◊ specified vehicle NEC (traffic) V56.7-
      - » nontraffic V56.2-
    - ◊ streetcar (traffic) V56.7-
      - » nontraffic V56.2-
    - – noncollision accident (traffic) V58.7-
      - ◊ nontraffic V58.2-
  - ■ noncollision accident (traffic) V58.9-
    - – nontraffic V58.3-
    - – while boarding or alighting V58.4-
  - ■ nontraffic V59.3-
  - ■ passenger
    - – collision (with)
    - ◊ animal being ridden (traffic) V56.6-
      - » nontraffic V56.1-
    - ◊ animal-drawn vehicle (traffic) V56.6-
      - » nontraffic V56.1-
    - ◊ motor vehicle NOS (traffic) V59.50-
      - » nontraffic V59.10-
      - » specified type NEC (traffic) V59.59-
        - ◆ nontraffic V59.19-
    - ◊ specified vehicle NEC (traffic) V56.6-
      - » nontraffic V56.1-
    - ◊ streetcar (traffic) V56.6-
      - » nontraffic V56.1-
    - – noncollision accident (traffic) V58.6-
      - ◊ nontraffic V58.1-
  - ■ specified type NEC V59.88-
    - – military vehicle V59.81-

Accident (to), *continued*
- – railway vehicle occupant V81.9-
  - ■ collision (with) V81.3-
    - – motor vehicle (non-military) (traffic) V81.1-
      - ◊ military V81.83-
      - ◊ nontraffic V81.0-
    - – rolling stock V81.2-
    - – specified object NEC V81.3-
  - ■ during derailment V81.7-
  - ■ explosion V81.81-
  - ■ fall (in railway vehicle) V81.5-
    - – during derailment V81.7-
    - – from railway vehicle V81.6-
      - ◊ during derailment V81.7-
    - – while boarding or alighting V81.4-
  - ■ fire V81.81-
  - ■ object falling onto train V81.82-
  - ■ specified type NEC V81.89-
  - ■ while boarding or alighting V81.4-
- – ski lift V98.3-
  - ■ specified NEC V98.8-
- – sport utility vehicle occupant
  - ■ collision (with)
  - – streetcar occupant V82.9-
  - ■ collision (with) V82.3-
    - – motor vehicle (traffic) V82.1-
      - ◊ nontraffic V82.0-
    - – rolling stock V82.2-
  - ■ during derailment V82.7-
  - ■ fall (in streetcar) V82.5-
    - – during derailment V82.7-
    - – from streetcar V82.6-
      - ◊ during derailment V82.7-
    - – while boarding or alighting V82.4-
  - ■ specified type NEC V82.8-
  - ■ while boarding or alighting V82.4-
- – three-wheeled motor vehicle occupant V39.9-
  - ■ collision (with)
    - – motor vehicle NOS (traffic) V39.60-
      - ◊ nontraffic V39.20-
      - ◊ specified type NEC (traffic) V39.69-
        - » nontraffic V39.29-
  - ■ driver
    - – collision (with)
      - ◊ motor vehicle NOS (traffic) V39.40-
        - » nontraffic V39.00-
        - » specified type NEC (traffic) V39.49-
          - ◆ nontraffic V39.09-
    - – noncollision accident (traffic) V38.5-
      - ◊ nontraffic V38.0-
  - ■ hanger-on
    - – noncollision accident (traffic) V38.7-
      - ◊ nontraffic V38.2-
  - ■ noncollision accident (traffic) V38.9-
    - – nontraffic V38.3-
    - – while boarding or alighting V38.4-
  - ■ nontraffic V39.3-
  - ■ passenger
    - – collision (with)
      - ◊ motor vehicle NOS (traffic) V39.50-
        - » nontraffic V39.10-
        - » specified type NEC (traffic) V39.59-
          - ◆ nontraffic V39.19-
    - – noncollision accident (traffic) V38.6-
      - ◊ nontraffic V38.1-
  - ■ specified type NEC V39.89-
    - – military vehicle V39.81-
- – tractor (farm) (and trailer)—*see* Accident, transport, agricultural vehicle occupant
- – tram—*see* Accident, transport, streetcar
- – trolley—*see* Accident, transport, streetcar
- – truck (heavy) occupant V69.9
  - ■ collision (with)
    - – animal (traffic) V60.9-
      - ◊ being ridden (traffic) V66.9-
        - » nontraffic V66.3-
        - » while boarding or alighting V66.4-
      - ◊ nontraffic V60.3-
      - ◊ while boarding or alighting V60.4-
    - – animal-drawn vehicle (traffic) V66.9-
      - ◊ nontraffic V66.3-
      - ◊ while boarding or alighting V66.4-

Accident (to), *continued*
- – bus (traffic) V64.9-
  - ◊ nontraffic V64.3-
  - ◊ while boarding or alighting V64.4-
- – car (traffic) V63.9-
  - ◊ nontraffic V63.3-
  - ◊ while boarding or alighting V63.4-
- – motor vehicle NOS (traffic) V69.60
  - ◊ nontraffic V69.20
  - ◊ specified type NEC (traffic) V69.69
    - » nontraffic V69.29
- – pedal cycle (traffic) V61.9-
  - ◊ nontraffic V61.3-
  - ◊ while boarding or alighting V61.4-
- – pickup truck (traffic) V63.9-
  - ◊ nontraffic V63.3-
  - ◊ while boarding or alighting V63.4-
- – railway vehicle (traffic) V65.9-
  - ◊ nontraffic V65.3-
  - ◊ while boarding or alighting V65.4-
- – specified vehicle NEC (traffic) V66.9-
  - ◊ nontraffic V66.3-
  - ◊ while boarding or alighting V66.4-
- – stationary object (traffic) V67.9-
  - ◊ nontraffic V67.3-
  - ◊ while boarding or alighting V67.4-
- – streetcar (traffic) V66.9-
  - ◊ nontraffic V66.3-
  - ◊ while boarding or alighting V66.4-
- – three wheeled motor vehicle (traffic) V62.9-
  - ◊ nontraffic V62.3-
  - ◊ while boarding or alighting V62.4-
- – truck (traffic) V64.9-
  - ◊ nontraffic V64.3-
  - ◊ while boarding or alighting V64.4-
- – two wheeled motor vehicle (traffic) V62.9-
  - ◊ nontraffic V62.3-
  - ◊ while boarding or alighting V62.4-
- – van (traffic) V63.9-
  - ◊ nontraffic V63.3-
  - ◊ while boarding or alighting V63.4-
- ■ driver
  - – collision (with)
    - ◊ animal (traffic) V60.5-
      - » being ridden (traffic) V66.5-
        - ◆ nontraffic V66.0-
      - » nontraffic V60.0-
    - ◊ animal-drawn vehicle (traffic) V66.5-
      - » nontraffic V66.0-
    - ◊ bus (traffic) V64.5-
      - » nontraffic V64.0-
    - ◊ car (traffic) V63.5-
      - » nontraffic V63.0-
    - ◊ motor vehicle NOS (traffic) V69.40
      - » nontraffic V69.00
      - » specified type NEC (traffic) V69.49
        - ◆ nontraffic V69.09
    - ◊ pedal cycle (traffic) V61.5-
      - » nontraffic V61.0-
    - ◊ pickup truck (traffic) V63.5-
      - » nontraffic V63.0-
    - ◊ railway vehicle (traffic) V65.5-
      - » nontraffic V65.0-
    - ◊ specified vehicle NEC (traffic) V66.5-
      - » nontraffic V66.0-
    - ◊ stationary object (traffic) V67.5-
      - » nontraffic V67.0-
    - ◊ streetcar (traffic) V66.5-
      - » nontraffic V66.0-
    - ◊ three wheeled motor vehicle (traffic) V62.5-
      - » nontraffic V62.0-
    - ◊ truck (traffic) V64.5-
      - » nontraffic V64.0-
    - ◊ two wheeled motor vehicle (traffic) V62.5-
      - » nontraffic V62.0-
    - ◊ van (traffic) V63.5-
      - » nontraffic V63.0-
  - – noncollision accident (traffic) V68.5-
    - ◊ nontraffic V68.0-
- ■ hanger-on
  - – collision (with)

ICD-10-CM EXTERNAL CAUSE OF INJURIES INDEX

Accident (to), *continued*

◊ animal (traffic) V60.7-
» being ridden (traffic) V66.7-
◇ nontraffic V66.2-
» nontraffic V60.2-
◊ animal-drawn vehicle (traffic) V66.7-
» nontraffic V66.2-
◊ bus (traffic) V64.7-
» nontraffic V64.2-
◊ car (traffic) V63.7-
» nontraffic V63.2-
◊ pedal cycle (traffic) V61.7-
» nontraffic V61.2-
◊ pickup truck (traffic) V63.7-
» nontraffic V63.2-
◊ railway vehicle (traffic) V65.7-
» nontraffic V65.2-
◊ specified vehicle NEC (traffic) V66.7-
» nontraffic V66.2-
◊ stationary object (traffic) V67.7-
» nontraffic V67.2-
◊ streetcar (traffic) V66.7-
» nontraffic V66.2-
◊ three wheeled motor vehicle (traffic) V62.7-
» nontraffic V62.2-
◊ truck (traffic) V64.7-
» nontraffic V64.2-
◊ two wheeled motor vehicle (traffic) V62.7-
» nontraffic V62.2-
◊ van (traffic) V63.7-
» nontraffic V63.2-
~ noncollision accident (traffic) V68.7-
◊ nontraffic V68.2-
■ noncollision accident (traffic) V68.9-
~ nontraffic V68.3-
~ while boarding or alighting V68.4-
■ nontraffic V69.3
■ passenger
~ collision (with)
◊ animal (traffic) V60.6-
» being ridden (traffic) V66.6-
◇ nontraffic V66.1-
» nontraffic V60.1-
◊ animal-drawn vehicle (traffic) V66.6-
» nontraffic V66.1-
◊ bus (traffic) V64.6-
» nontraffic V64.1-
◊ car (traffic) V63.6-
» nontraffic V63.1-
◊ motor vehicle NOS (traffic) V69.50
» nontraffic V69.10
» specified type NEC (traffic) V69.59
◇ nontraffic V69.19
◊ pedal cycle (traffic) V61.6-
» nontraffic V61.1-
◊ pickup truck (traffic) V63.6-
» nontraffic V63.1-
◊ railway vehicle (traffic) V65.6-
» nontraffic V65.1-
◊ specified vehicle NEC (traffic) V66.6-
» nontraffic V66.1-
◊ stationary object (traffic) V67.6-
» nontraffic V67.1-
◊ streetcar (traffic) V66.6-
» nontraffic V66.1-
◊ three wheeled motor vehicle (traffic) V62.6-
» nontraffic V62.1-
◊ truck (traffic) V64.6-
» nontraffic V64.1-
◊ two wheeled motor vehicle (traffic) V62.6-
» nontraffic V62.1-
◊ van (traffic) V63.6-
» nontraffic V63.1-
~ noncollision accident (traffic) V68.6-
◊ nontraffic V68.1-
■ pickup—*see* Accident, transport, pickup truck occupant
■ specified type NEC V69.88
~ military vehicle V69.81
– van occupant V59.9-
■ collision (with)
~ animal (traffic) V50.9-
◊ being ridden (traffic) V56.9-

Accident (to), *continued*

» nontraffic V56.3-
» while boarding or alighting V56.4-
~ animal-drawn vehicle (traffic) V56.9-
◊ nontraffic V56.3-
◊ while boarding or alighting V56.4-
~ motor vehicle NOS (traffic) V59.60-
◊ nontraffic V59.20-
◊ specified type NEC (traffic) V59.69-
» nontraffic V59.29-
~ specified vehicle NEC (traffic) V56.9-
◊ nontraffic V56.3-
◊ while boarding or alighting V56.4-
~ streetcar (traffic) V56.9-
◊ nontraffic V56.3-
◊ while boarding or alighting V56.4-
■ driver
~ collision (with)
◊ animal being ridden (traffic) V56.5-
» nontraffic V56.0-
◊ animal-drawn vehicle (traffic) V56.5-
» nontraffic V56.0-
◊ motor vehicle NOS (traffic) V59.40-
» nontraffic V59.00-
» specified type NEC (traffic) V59.49-
◇ nontraffic V59.09-
◊ specified vehicle NEC (traffic) V56.5-
◊ streetcar (traffic) V56.5-
» nontraffic V56.0-
~ noncollision accident (traffic) V58.5-
◊ nontraffic V58.0-
■ hanger-on
~ collision (with)
◊ animal being ridden (traffic) V56.7-
» nontraffic V56.2-
◊ animal-drawn vehicle (traffic) V56.7-
» nontraffic V56.2-
◊ specified vehicle NEC (traffic) V56.7-
» nontraffic V56.2-
◊ streetcar (traffic) V56.7-
» nontraffic V56.2-
~ noncollision accident (traffic) V58.7-
◊ nontraffic V58.2-
■ noncollision accident (traffic) V58.9-
~ nontraffic V58.3-
~ while boarding or alighting V58.4-
» nontraffic V59.3-
■ passenger
~ collision (with)
◊ animal being ridden (traffic) V56.6-
» nontraffic V56.1-
◊ animal-drawn vehicle (traffic) V56.6-
◊ motor vehicle NOS (traffic) V59.50-
» nontraffic V59.10-
» specified type NEC (traffic) V59.59-
◇ nontraffic V59.19-
◊ specified vehicle NEC (traffic) V56.6-
» nontraffic V56.1-
◊ streetcar (traffic) V56.6-
» nontraffic V56.1-
~ noncollision accident (traffic) V58.6-
◊ nontraffic V58.1-
■ specified type NEC V59.88-
~ military vehicle V59.81-
– watercraft occupant—*see* Accident, watercraft
- vehicle NEC V89.9-
– animal-drawn NEC—*see* Accident, transport, animal-drawn vehicle occupant
– special
■ agricultural—*see* Accident, transport, agricultural vehicle occupant
– three-wheeled NEC (motorized)—*see* Accident, transport, three-wheeled motor vehicle occupant
- watercraft V94.9-
~ causing
■ drowning—*see* Drowning, due to, accident to, watercraft
■ injury NEC V91.89-
~ crushed between craft and object V91.19-
◊ powered craft V91.1-
◊ unpowered craft V91.1-
~ fall on board V91.29-
◊ powered craft V91.2-

Accident (to), *continued*

◊ unpowered craft V91.2-
~ fire on board causing burn V91.09-
◊ powered craft V91.0-
◊ unpowered craft V91.0-
~ hit by falling object V91.39-
◊ powered craft V91.3-
◊ unpowered craft V91.3-
~ specified type NEC V91.89-
◊ powered craft V91.8-
◊ unpowered craft V91.8-
– nonpowered, struck by
■ nonpowered vessel V94.22-
■ powered vessel V94.21-
– specified type NEC V94.89-
– striking swimmer
■ powered V94.11-
■ unpowered V94.12-

Acid throwing (assault) Y08.89-

Activity (involving) (of victim at time of event) Y93.9

- alpine skiing Y93.23
- animal care NEC Y93.K9
- arts and handcrafts NEC Y93.D9
- athletics NEC Y93.79
- athletics played as a team or group NEC Y93.69
- athletics played individually NEC Y93.59
- baking Y93.G3
- ballet Y93.41
- barbells Y93.B3
- BASE (Building, Antenna, Span, Earth) jumping Y93.33
- baseball Y93.64
- basketball Y93.67
- bathing (personal) Y93.E1
- beach volleyball Y93.68
- bike riding Y93.55
- blackout game Y93.85
- boogie boarding Y93.18
- bowling Y93.54
- boxing Y93.71
- brass instrument playing Y93.J4
- bungee jumping Y93.34
- canoeing (in calm and turbulent water) Y93.16
- capture the flag Y93.6A
- cellular
  – communication device Y93.C2
  – telephone Y93.C2
- cheerleading Y93.45
- choking game Y93.85
- cleaning
  – floor Y93.E5
- climbing NEC Y93.39
  – mountain Y93.31
  – rock Y93.31
  – wall Y93.31
- clothing care and maintenance NEC Y93.E9
- combatives Y93.75
- computer
  – keyboarding Y93.C1
  – technology NEC Y93.C9
- cooking and baking Y93.G3
- cricket Y93.69
- crocheting Y93.D1
- cross country skiing Y93.24
- dancing (all types) Y93.41
- dishwashing Y93.G1
- diving (platform) (springboard) Y93.12
  – underwater Y93.15
- dodge ball Y93.6A
- downhill skiing Y93.23
- drum playing Y93.J2
- dumbbells Y93.B3
- electronic
  – devices NEC Y93.C9
    ■ hand held interactive Y93.C2
  – game playing (using) (with)
    ■ interactive device Y93.C2
    ■ keyboard or other stationary device Y93.C1
- exercise(s)
  – machines (primarily) for)
    ■ muscle strengthening Y93.B1
  – muscle strengthening (non-machine) NEC Y93.B9

ICD-10-CM EXTERNAL CAUSE OF INJURIES INDEX

Activity (involving) (of victim at time of event), *continued*

- external motion NEC Y93.I9
  - rollercoaster Y93.I1
- fainting game Y93.85
- field hockey Y93.65
- figure skating (pairs) (singles) Y93.21
- flag football Y93.62
- floor mopping and cleaning Y93.E5
- food preparation and clean up Y93.G1
- football (American) NOS Y93.61
  - flag Y93.62
  - tackle Y93.61
  - touch Y93.62
- four square Y93.6A
- free weights Y93.B3
- frisbee (ultimate) Y93.74
- furniture
  - building Y93.D3
  - finishing Y93.D3
  - repair Y93.D3
- game playing (electronic)
  - using interactive device Y93.C2
  - using keyboard or other stationary device Y93.C1
- golf Y93.53
- grilling and smoking food Y93.G2
- grooming and shearing an animal Y93.K3
- gymnastics (rhythmic) Y93.43
- handball Y93.73
- handcrafts NEC Y93.D9
- hand held interactive electronic device Y93.C2
- hang gliding Y93.35
- hiking (on level or elevated terrain) Y93.01
- hockey (ice) Y93.22
  - field Y93.65
- horseback riding Y93.52
- household (interior) maintenance NEC Y93.E9
- ice NEC Y93.29
  - dancing or skating Y93.21
  - hockey Y93.22
- in-line roller skating Y93.51
- ironing Y93.E4
- judo Y93.75
- jumping (off) NEC Y93.39
  - BASE (Building, Antenna, Span, Earth) Y93.33
  - bungee Y93.34
  - rope Y93.56
- jumping rope Y93.56
- karate Y93.75
- kayaking (in calm and turbulent water) Y93.16
- keyboarding (computer) Y93.C1
- kickball Y93.6A
- knitting Y93.D1
- lacrosse Y93.65
- laundry Y93.E2
- machines (exercise)
  - primarily for muscle strengthening Y93.B1
- maintenance
  - household (interior) NEC Y93.E9
- marching (on level or elevated terrain) Y93.01
- martial arts Y93.75
- microwave oven Y93.G3
- milking an animal Y93.K2
- mopping (floor) Y93.E5
- mountain climbing Y93.31
- muscle strengthening
  - exercises (non-machine) NEC Y93.B9
  - machines Y93.B1
- musical keyboard (electronic) playing Y93.J1
- nordic skiing Y93.24
- oven (microwave) Y93.G3
- packing and unpacking in moving to a new residence Y93.E6
- parasailing Y93.19
- percussion instrument playing NEC Y93.J2
- personal
  - bathing and showering Y93.E1
  - hygiene NEC Y93.E8
  - showering Y93.E1
- physical games generally associated with school recess, summer camp and children Y93.6A
- piano playing Y93.J1
- pilates Y93.B4
- platform diving Y93.12

Activity (involving) (of victim at time of event), *continued*

- playing musical instrument
  - brass instrument Y93.J4
  - drum Y93.J2
  - musical keyboard (electronic) Y93.J1
  - percussion instrument NEC Y93.J2
  - piano Y93.J1
  - string instrument Y93.J3
  - winds instrument Y93.J4
- property maintenance
  - interior NEC Y93.E9
- pull-ups Y93.B2
- push-ups Y93.B2
- racquetball Y93.73
- rafting (in calm and turbulent water) Y93.16
- rappelling Y93.32
- refereeing a sports activity Y93.81
- residential relocation Y93.E6
- rhythmic gymnastics Y93.43
- rhythmic movement NEC Y93.49
- riding
  - horseback Y93.52
  - rollercoaster Y93.I1
- rock climbing Y93.31
- rollercoaster riding Y93.I1
- roller skating (in-line) Y93.51
- rough housing and horseplay Y93.83
- rowing (in calm and turbulent water) Y93.16
- rugby Y93.63
- running Y93.02
- SCUBA diving Y93.15
- sewing Y93.D2
- showering (personal) Y93.E1
- sit-ups Y93.B2
- skateboarding Y93.51
- skating (ice) Y93.21
  - roller Y93.51
- skiing (alpine) (downhill) Y93.23
  - cross country Y93.24
  - nordic Y93.24
  - water Y93.17
- sledding (snow) Y93.23
- sleeping (sleep) Y93.84
- smoking and grilling food Y93.G2
- snorkeling Y93.15
- snow NEC Y93.29
  - boarding Y93.23
  - sledding Y93.23
  - tubing Y93.23
- soccer Y93.66
- softball Y93.64
- specified NEC Y93.89
- spectator at an event Y93.82
- sports NEC Y93.79
  - sports played as a team or group NEC Y93.69
  - sports played individually NEC Y93.59
- springboard diving Y93.12
- squash Y93.73
- stove Y93.G3
- string instrument playing Y93.J3
- surfing Y93.18
  - wind Y93.18
- swimming Y93.11
- tap dancing Y93.41
- tennis Y93.73
- tobogganing Y93.23
- touch football Y93.62
- track and field events (non-running) Y93.57
  - running Y93.02
- trampoline Y93.44
- tubing (in calm and turbulent water) Y93.16
  - snow Y93.23
- ultimate frisbee Y93.74
- underwater diving Y93.15
- unpacking in moving to a new residence Y93.E6
- use of stove, oven and microwave oven Y93.G3
- vacuuming Y93.E3
- volleyball (beach) (court) Y93.68
- wake boarding Y93.17
- walking an animal Y93.K1
- walking (on level or elevated terrain) Y93.01
  - an animal Y93.K1
- wall climbing Y93.31

Activity (involving) (of victim at time of event), *continued*

- water NEC Y93.19
  - aerobics Y93.14
  - craft NEC Y93.19
  - exercise Y93.14
  - polo Y93.13
  - skiing Y93.17
  - sliding Y93.18
  - survival training and testing Y93.19
- wind instrument playing Y93.J4
- windsurfing Y93.18
- wrestling Y93.72
- yoga Y93.42

Adverse effect of drugs—*see* Table of Drugs and Chemicals

Air

- pressure
  - change, rapid
    - during
      - ascent W94.29-
      - ◊ while (in) (surfacing from)
        - » aircraft W94.23-
        - » deep water diving W94.21-
        - » underground W94.22-
      - descent W94.39-
    - ◊ in
      - » aircraft W94.31-
      - » water W94.32-
  - high, prolonged W94.0-
  - low, prolonged W94.12-
    - due to residence or long visit at high altitude W94.11-

Alpine sickness W94.11-

Altitude sickness W94.11-

Anaphylactic shock, anaphylaxis—*see* Table of Drugs and Chemicals

Andes disease W94.11-

Arachnidism, arachnoidism X58.-

Arson (with intent to injure or kill) X97.-

Asphyxia, asphyxiation

- by
  - food (bone) (seed) (*see* categories T17 and) T18
  - gas—*see also* Table of Drugs and Chemicals
- from
  - fire—*see also* Exposure, fire
  - ignition—*see* Ignition
  - vomitus T17.81-

Aspiration

- food (any type) (into respiratory tract) (with asphyxia, obstruction respiratory tract, suffocation) (*see* categories T17 and) T18
- foreign body—*see* Foreign body, aspiration
- vomitus (with asphyxia, obstruction respiratory tract, suffocation) T17.81-

Assassination (attempt)—*see* Assault

Assault (homicidal) (by) (in) Y09.-

- bite (of human being) Y04.1-
- bodily force Y04.8-
  - bite Y04.1-
  - bumping into Y04.2-
  - rape (confirmed) T74.2-
    - suspected T76.2-
  - sexual (by bodily force) T74.2-
    - suspected T76.2-
  - sexual (confirmed) T76.2
    - suspected T76.2-
  - unarmed fight Y04.0-
- brawl (hand) (fists) (foot) (unarmed) Y04.0-
- burning, burns (by fire) NEC X97.-
  - acid Y08.89-
  - caustic, corrosive substance Y08.89-
  - chemical from swallowing caustic, corrosive substance—*see* Table of Drugs and Chemicals
  - cigarette(s) X97.-
  - hot object X98.9-
    - fluid NEC X98.2-
    - household appliance X98.3-
    - specified NEC X98.8-
    - steam X98.0-
    - tap water X98.1-
    - vapors X98.0-

ICD-10-CM EXTERNAL CAUSE OF INJURIES INDEX

Assault (homicidal) (by) (in), *continued*

- scalding X97.-
- steam X98.0-
- vitriol Y08.89-
- caustic, corrosive substance (gas) Y08.89-
- crashing of
  - aircraft Y08.81-
  - motor vehicle Y03.8-
    - pushed in front of Y02.0-
    - run over Y03.0-
    - specified NEC Y03.8-
- cutting or piercing instrument X99.9-
  - dagger X99.2-
  - glass X99.0-
  - knife X99.1-
  - specified NEC X99.8-
  - sword X99.2-
- dagger X99.2-
- drowning (in) X92.9-
  - bathtub X92.0-
  - natural water X92.3-
  - specified NEC X92.8-
  - swimming pool X92.1-
    - following fall X92.2-
- dynamite X96.8-
- explosive(s) (material) X96.9-
- fight (hand) (fists) (foot) (unarmed) Y04.0-
  - with weapon—*see* Assault, by type of weapon
- fire X97.-
- firearm X95.9-
  - airgun X95.01-
  - handgun X93.-
  - hunting rifle X94.1-
  - specified NEC X95.8-
- gunshot (wound) NEC—*see* Assault, firearm, by type
- incendiary device X97.-
- injury Y09.-
  - to child due to criminal abortion attempt NEC Y08.89-
- knife X99.1-
- late effect of—*see* X92–Y08 with 7th character S
- placing before moving object NEC Y02.8-
  - motor vehicle Y02.0-
- poisoning—*see* categories T36-T65 with 7th character S
- puncture, any part of body—*see* Assault, cutting or piercing instrument
- pushing
  - before moving object NEC Y02.8-
    - motor vehicle Y02.0-
    - subway train Y02.1-
    - train Y02.1-
  - from high place Y01.-
- rape T74.2-
- scalding —X97.-
- sexual (by bodily force) T74.2-
- shooting—*see* Assault, firearm
- specified means NEC Y08.89-
- stab, any part of body—*see* Assault, cutting or piercing instrument
- steam X98.0-
- striking against
  - other person Y04.2-
  - sports equipment Y08.09-
    - baseball bat Y08.02-
    - hockey stick Y08.01-
- struck by
  - sports equipment Y08.09-
    - baseball bat Y08.02-
    - hockey stick Y08.01-
- submersion—*see* Assault, drowning
- violence Y09.-
- weapon Y09.-
  - blunt Y00.-
  - cutting or piercing—*see* Assault, cutting or piercing instrument
  - firearm—*see* Assault, firearm
- wound Y09.-
  - cutting—*see* Assault, cutting or piercing instrument
  - gunshot—*see* Assault, firearm
  - knife X99.1-
  - piercing—*see* Assault, cutting or piercing instrument

Assault (homicidal) (by) (in), *continued*

- puncture—*see* Assault, cutting or piercing instrument
- stab—*see* Assault, cutting or piercing instrument

Attack by mammals NEC W55.89-

Avalanche—*see* Landslide

B

Barotitis, barodontalgia, barosinusitis, barotrauma (otitic) (sinus)—*see* Air, pressure

Battered (baby) (child) (person) (syndrome) X58.-

Bean in nose (*see* categories T17 and) T18

Bed set on fire NEC—*see* Exposure, fire, uncontrolled, building, bed

Bending, injury in—*see* category Y93

Bends—*see* Air, pressure, change

Bite, bitten by

- alligator W58.01-
- arthropod (nonvenomous) NEC W57.-
- bull W55.21-
- cat W55.01-
- cow W55.21-
- crocodile W58.11-
- dog W54.0-
- goat W55.31-
- hoof stock NEC W55.31-
- horse W55.11-
- human being (accidentally) W50.3-
  - as, or caused by, a crowd or human stampede (with fall) W52.-
  - assault Y04.1-
  - in
    - fight Y04.1-
    - with intent to injure or kill Y04.1-
- insect (nonvenomous) W57.-
- lizard (nonvenomous) W59.01-
- mammal NEC W55.81-
  - marine W56.31-
- marine animal (nonvenomous) W56.81-
- millipede W57.-
- moray eel W56.51-
- mouse W53.01-
- person(s) (accidentally) W50.3-
  - as, or caused by, a crowd or human stampede (with fall) W52.-
  - assault Y04.1
  - in
    - fight Y04.1-
    - with intent to injure or kill Y04.1-
- pig W55.41-
- raccoon W55.51-
- rat W53.11-
- reptile W59.81-
  - lizard W59.01-
  - snake W59.11-
  - turtle W59.21-
    - terrestrial W59.81-
- rodent W53.81-
  - mouse W53.01-
  - rat W53.11-
  - specified NEC W53.81-
  - squirrel W53.21-
- shark W56.41-
- sheep W55.31-
- snake (nonvenomous) W59.11-
- spider (nonvenomous) W57.-
- squirrel W53.21-

Blizzard X37.2-

Blood alcohol level Y90.-

Blow X58.-

Blowing up—*see* Explosion

Brawl (hand) (fists) (foot) Y04.0-

Breakage (accidental) (part of)

- ladder (causing fall) W11.-
- scaffolding (causing fall) W12.-

Broken

- glass, contact with—*see* Contact, with, glass

Bumping against, into (accidentally)

- object NEC W22.8-
  - with fall—*see* Fall, due to, bumping against, object
  - caused by crowd or human stampede (with fall) W52.-
  - sports equipment W21.9-
- person(s) W51.-
  - with fall W03.-
    - due to ice or snow W00.0-
  - assault Y04.2-
  - caused by, a crowd or human stampede (with fall) W52.-
- sports equipment W21.9-

Burn, burned, burning (accidental) (by) (from) (on)

- acid NEC—*see* Table of Drugs and Chemicals
- bed linen—*see* Exposure, fire, uncontrolled, in building, bed
- blowtorch X08.8-
  - with ignition of clothing NEC X06.2-
    - nightwear X05.-
- bonfire, campfire (controlled)—*see also* Exposure, fire, controlled, not in building
  - uncontrolled—*see* Exposure, fire, uncontrolled, not in building
- candle X08.8-
  - with ignition of clothing NEC X06.2-
    - nightwear X05.-
- caustic liquid, substance (external) (internal) NEC—*see* Table of Drugs and Chemicals
- chemical (external) (internal)—*see also* Table of Drugs and Chemicals
- cigar(s) or cigarette(s) X08.8-
  - with ignition of clothing NEC X06.2-
    - nightwear X05.-
- clothes, clothing NEC (from controlled fire) X06.2-
  - with conflagration—*see* Exposure, fire, uncontrolled, building
    - not in building or structure—*see* Exposure, fire, uncontrolled, not in building
- cooker (hot) X15.8-
  - stated as undetermined whether accidental or intentional Y27.3-
- electric blanket X16.-
- engine (hot) X17.-
- fire, flames—*see* Exposure, fire
- flare, Very pistol—*see* Discharge, firearm NEC
- heat
  - from appliance (electrical) (household) (cooking object) X15.-
    - stated as undetermined whether accidental or intentional Y27.3-
  - in local application or packing during medical or surgical procedure Y63.5-
- heating
  - appliance, radiator or pipe X16.-
- hot
  - cooker X15.8-
  - drink X10.0-
  - engine X17.-
  - fat X10.2-
  - fluid NEC X12.-
  - food X10.1-
  - heating appliance X16.-
  - household appliance NEC X15.8-
  - kettle X15.8-
  - liquid NEC X12.-
  - machinery X17.-
  - metal (molten) (liquid) NEC X18.-
  - object (not producing fire or flames) NEC X19.-
  - oil (cooking) X10.2-
  - pipe(s) X16.-
  - radiator X16.-
  - saucepan (glass) (metal) X15.3-
  - stove (kitchen) X15.0-
  - substance NEC X19.-
    - caustic or corrosive NEC—*see* Table of Drugs and Chemicals
  - toaster X15.1-
  - tool X17.-
  - vapor X13.1-
  - water (tap)—*see* Contact, with, hot, tap water
- hotplate X15.2-
- ignition—*see* Ignition

Burn, burned, burning (accidental) (by) (from) (on), *continued*

- inflicted by other person X97.-
  - by hot objects, hot vapor, and steam—*see* Assault, burning, hot object
- internal, from swallowed caustic, corrosive liquid, substance—*see* Table of Drugs and Chemicals
- iron (hot) X15.8-
  - stated as undetermined whether accidental or intentional Y27.3-
- kettle (hot) X15.8-
  - stated as undetermined whether accidental or intentional Y27.3-
- lamp (flame) X08.8-
  - with ignition of clothing NEC X06.2-
    - nightwear X05.-
- lighter (cigar) (cigarette) X08.8-
  - with ignition of clothing NEC X06.2-
    - nightwear X05.-
- lightning—*see* subcategory T75.0-
  - causing fire—*see* Exposure, fire
- liquid (boiling) (hot) NEC X12.-
  - stated as undetermined whether accidental or intentional Y27.2-
- machinery (hot) X17.-
- matches X08.8-
  - with ignition of clothing NEC X06.2-
    - nightwear X05.-
- mattress—*see* Exposure, fire, uncontrolled, building, bed
- medicament, externally applied Y63.5-
- metal (hot) (liquid) (molten) NEC X18.-
- nightwear (nightclothes, nightdress, gown, pajamas, robe) X05.-
- object (hot) NEC X19.-
- on board watercraft
  - due to
    - accident to watercraft V91.09-
    - powered craft V91.0-
    - unpowered craft V91.0-
    - fire on board V93.0-
    - specified heat source NEC on board V93.19-
    - ferry boat V93.11-
    - fishing boat V93.12-
    - jet skis V93.13-
    - liner V93.11-
    - merchant ship V93.10-
    - passenger ship V93.11-
    - powered craft NEC V93.13-
    - sailboat V93.14-
- pipe (hot) X16.-
  - smoking X08.8-
    - with ignition of clothing NEC X06.2-
      - nightwear X05.-
- powder—*see* Powder burn
- radiator (hot) X16.-
- saucepan (hot) (glass) (metal) X15.3-
  - stated as undetermined whether accidental or intentional Y27.3-
- self-inflicted X76.-
  - stated as undetermined whether accidental or intentional Y26.-
- steam X13.1-
  - pipe X16.-
    - stated as undetermined whether accidental or intentional Y27.8-
    - stated as undetermined whether accidental or intentional Y27.0-
- stove (hot) (kitchen) X15.0-
  - stated as undetermined whether accidental or intentional Y27.3-
- substance (hot) NEC X19.-
  - boiling X12.-
    - stated as undetermined whether accidental or intentional Y27.2-
  - molten (metal) X18.-
  - hot
    - household appliance X77.3-
    - object X77.9-
- stated as undetermined whether accidental or intentional Y27.0-

Burn, burned, burning (accidental) (by) (from) (on), *continued*

- therapeutic misadventure
  - heat in local application or packing during medical or surgical procedure Y63.5-
  - overdose of radiation Y63.2-
- toaster (hot) X15.1-
  - stated as undetermined whether accidental or intentional Y27.3-
- tool (hot) X17.-
- torch, welding X08.8-
  - with ignition of clothing NEC X06.2-
    - nightwear X05.-
- trash fire (controlled)—*see* Exposure, fire, controlled, not in building
  - uncontrolled—*see* Exposure, fire, uncontrolled, not in building
- vapor (hot) X13.1-
  - stated as undetermined whether accidental or intentional Y27.0-
- Very pistol—*see* Discharge, firearm NEC

Butted by animal W55-

C

Caisson disease—*see* Air, pressure, change

Campfire (exposure to) (controlled)—*see also* Exposure, fire, controlled, not in building

- uncontrolled—*see* Exposure, fire, uncontrolled, not in building Car sickness T75.3-

Cat

- bite W55.01-
- scratch W55.03-

Cataclysm, cataclysmic (any injury) NEC—*see* Forces of nature

Catching fire—*see* Exposure, fire

Caught

- between
  - folding object W23.0-
  - objects (moving) (stationary and moving) W23.0-
  - and machinery—*see* Contact, with, by type of machine
    - stationary W23.1-
    - sliding door and door frame W23.0-
- by, in
  - machinery (moving parts of)—*see* Contact, with, by type of machine
  - washing-machine wringer W23.0-
  - under packing crate (due to losing grip) W23.1-

Cave-in caused by cataclysmic earth surface movement or eruption—*see* Landslide

Change(s) in air pressure—*see* Air, pressure, change

Choked, choking (on) (any object except food or vomitus)

- food (bone) (seed) (see categories T17 and) T18
- vomitus T17.81-

Cloudburst (any injury) X37.8-

Cold, exposure to (accidental) (excessive) (extreme) (natural) (place) NEC—*see* Exposure, cold

Collapse

- building W20.1-
  - burning (uncontrolled fire) X00.2-
- dam or man-made structure (causing earth movement) X36.0-
- machinery—*see* Contact, with, by type of machine
- structure W20.1-
  - burning (uncontrolled fire) X00.2-

Collision—*see also* **Accident, transport**

- car, pick-up truck, van
  - nontraffic accident
    - electric (assisted) bicycle driver V23.01-
    - electric (assisted) bicycle passenger V23.11-
    - other motorcycle driver V23.09-
    - other motorcycle passenger V23.19-
    - unspecified electric (assisted) bicycle rider V23.21-
    - unspecified rider of other motorcycle V23.29-
  - person boarding, alighting an electric (assisted) bicycle V23.31-
  - person boarding, alighting other motorcycle V23.39-

Collision, *continued*

- traffic accident
  - electric (assisted) bicycle driver V23.41-
  - electric (assisted) bicycle passenger V23.51-
  - other motorcycle driver V23.49-
  - other motorcycle passenger V23.59-
  - unspecified electric (assisted) bicycle rider V23.91-
  - unspecified rider of other motorcycle V23.99-
- fixed, stationary object
  - nontraffic accident
    - electric (assisted) bicycle passenger V27.11-
    - other motorcycle driver V27.19-
    - unspecified electric (assisted) bicycle rider V27.21-
    - unspecified rider of other motorcycle V27.29-
  - person boarding, alighting an electric (assisted) bicycle V27.31-
  - person boarding, alighting other motorcycle V27.39-
  - traffic accident
    - electric (assisted) bicycle driver V27.41-
    - electric (assisted) bicycle passenger V27.51-
    - other motorcycle driver V27.49-
    - other motorcycle passenger V27.59-
    - unspecified electric (assisted) bicycle rider V27.91-
    - unspecified rider of other motorcycle V27.99-
- heavy transport vehicle, bus
  - nontraffic accident
    - electric (assisted) bicycle driver V24.01-
    - electric (assisted) bicycle passenger V24.11-
    - other motorcycle driver V24.09-
    - other motorcycle passenger V24.19-
    - unspecified electric (assisted) bicycle rider V24.21-
    - unspecified rider of other motorcycle V24.29-
  - person boarding, alighting an electric (assisted) bicycle V24.31-
  - person boarding, alighting other motorcycle V24.39-
  - traffic accident
    - electric (assisted) bicycle driver V24.41-
    - electric (assisted) bicycle passenger V24.51-
    - other motorcycle driver V24.49-
    - other motorcycle passenger V24.59-
    - unspecified electric (assisted) bicycle rider V24.91-
    - unspecified rider of other motorcycle V24.99-
- military vehicle
  - electric (assisted) bicycle rider (driver) (passenger) V29.811-
  - rider (driver) (passenger) of other motorcycle V29.818-
- NEC V89.9-
- other motor vehicles
  - electric (assisted) bicycle rider (driver) (passenger) V29.881-
  - nontraffic accident
    - electric (assisted) bicycle driver V29.091-
    - electric (assisted) bicycle passenger V29.191-
    - other motorcycle driver V29.098-
    - other motorcycle passenger V29.198-
    - unspecified electric (assisted) bicycle rider V29.291-
    - unspecified rider of other motorcycle V29.298-
  - rider (driver) (passenger) of other motorcycle V29.888-
  - traffic accident
    - electric (assisted) bicycle driver V29.491-
    - electric (assisted) bicycle passenger V29.591-
    - other motorcycle driver V29.498-
    - other motorcycle passenger V29.598-
    - unspecified electric (assisted) bicycle rider V29.691-
    - unspecified rider of other motorcycle V29.698-
- other nonmotor vehicle
  - nontraffic accident
    - electric (assisted) bicycle driver V26.01-
    - electric (assisted) bicycle passenger V26.11-
    - other motorcycle driver V26.09-
    - other motorcycle passenger V26.19-
    - unspecified electric (assisted) bicycle rider V26.21-
    - unspecified rider of other motorcycle V26.29-
  - person boarding, alighting an electric (assisted) bicycle V26.31-
  - person boarding, alighting other motorcycle V26.39-
  - traffic accident
    - electric (assisted) bicycle driver V27.01-

ICD-10-CM EXTERNAL CAUSE OF INJURIES INDEX

Collision, *continued*

- ■ electric (assisted) bicycle driver V26.41-
- ■ electric (assisted) bicycle passenger V26.51-
- ■ other motorcycle driver V27.09-
- ■ other motorcycle driver V26.49-
- ■ other motorcycle passenger V26.59-
- ■ unspecified electric (assisted) bicycle rider V26.91-
- ■ unspecified rider of other motorcycle V26.99-
- pedal cycle
  - nontraffic accident
    - ■ electric (assisted) bicycle driver V21.01-
    - ■ electric (assisted) bicycle passenger V21.11-
    - ■ other motorcycle driver V21.09-
    - ■ other motorcycle passenger V21.19-
    - ■ unspecified electric (assisted) bicycle rider V21.21-
    - ■ unspecified rider of other motorcycle V21.29-
  - person boarding, alighting an electric (assisted) bicycle V21.31-
  - person boarding, alighting other motorcycle V21.39-
  - traffic accident
    - ■ electric (assisted) bicycle driver V21.41-
    - ■ electric (assisted) bicycle passenger V21.51-
    - ■ other motorcycle driver V21.49-
    - ■ other motorcycle passenger V21.59-
    - ■ unspecified electric (assisted) bicycle rider V21.91-
    - ■ unspecified rider of other motorcycle V21.99-
- pedestrian, animal
  - nontraffic accident
    - ■ electric (assisted) bicycle driver V20.01-
    - ■ electric (assisted) bicycle passenger V20.11-
    - ■ other motorcycle driver V20.09-
    - ■ other motorcycle passenger V20.19-
    - ■ unspecified electric (assisted) bicycle rider V20.21-
    - ■ unspecified rider other motorcycle V20.29-
  - person boarding, alighting electric (assisted) bicycle V20.31-
  - person boarding, alighting other motorcycle V20.39-
  - traffic accident
    - ■ electric (assisted) bicycle driver V20.41-
    - ■ electric (assisted) bicycle passenger V20.51-
    - ■ other motorcycle driver V20.49-
    - ■ other motorcycle passenger V20.59-
    - ■ unspecified electric (assisted) bicycle rider V20.91-
    - ■ unspecified rider of other motorcycle V20.29-
    - ■ unspecified rider of other motorcycle V20.99-
- pedestrian W51.-
  - with fall W03.-
    - ■ due to ice or snow W00.0-
    - ■ involving pedestrian conveyance—*see* Accident, transport, pedestrian, conveyance
  - and
    - ■ crowd or human stampede (with fall) W52.-
    - ■ object W22.8-
      - with fall — *see* Fall, due to, bumping against, object
- person(s)— *see* Collision, pedestrian
- railway train, railway vehicle
  - nontraffic accident
    - ■ electric (assisted) bicycle driver V25.01-
    - ■ electric (assisted) bicycle passenger V25.11-
    - ■ other motorcycle driver V25.09-
    - ■ other motorcycle passenger V25.19-
    - ■ unspecified electric (assisted) bicycle rider V25.21-
    - ■ unspecified rider of other motorcycle V25.29-
  - person boarding, alighting an electric (assisted) bicycle V25.31-
  - person boarding, alighting other motorcycle V25.39-
  - traffic accident
    - ■ electric (assisted) bicycle driver V25.41-
    - ■ electric (assisted) bicycle passenger V25.51-
    - ■ other motorcycle driver V25.49-
    - ■ other motorcycle passenger V25.59-
    - ■ unspecified electric (assisted) bicycle rider V25.91-
    - ■ unspecified rider of other motorcycle V25.99-
- transport vehicle NEC V89.9-
  - and
    - ■ avalanche, fallen or not moving—*see* Accident, transport
      - falling or moving—*see* Landslide
    - ■ landslide, fallen or not moving—*see* Accident, transport
      - falling or moving—*see* Landslide

Collision, *continued*

- due to cataclysm—*see* Forces of nature, by type
- two, three wheeled motor vehicles
  - nontraffic accident
    - ■ electric (assisted) bicycle driver V22.01-
    - ■ electric (assisted) bicycle passenger V22.11-
    - ■ other motorcycle driver V22.09-
    - ■ other motorcycle passenger V22.19-
    - ■ unspecified electric (assisted) bicycle rider V22.21-
    - ■ unspecified rider of other motorcycle V22.29-
  - person boarding, alighting an electric (assisted) bicycle V22.31-
  - person boarding, alighting other motorcycle V22.39-
  - traffic accident
    - ■ electric (assisted) bicycle driver V22.41-
    - ■ electric (assisted) bicycle passenger V22.51-
    - ■ other motorcycle driver V22.49-
    - ■ other motorcycle passenger V22.59-
    - ■ unspecified electric (assisted) bicycle rider V22.91-
    - ■ unspecified rider of other motorcycle V22.99-
- unspecified motor vehicles
  - nontraffic accident
    - ■ electric (assisted) bicycle (driver) (passenger) V29.31-
    - ■ electric (assisted) bicycle driver V29.001-
    - ■ electric (assisted) bicycle passenger V29.101-
    - ■ other motorcycle (driver) (passenger) V29.39-
    - ■ other motorcycle driver V29.008-
    - ■ other motorcycle passenger V29.108-
    - ■ unspecified electric (assisted) bicycle rider V29.201-
    - ■ unspecified rider of other motorcycle V29.208-
  - traffic accident
    - ■ electric (assisted) bicycle driver V29.401-
    - ■ electric (assisted) bicycle passenger V29.501-
    - ■ other motorcycle driver V29.408-
    - ■ other motorcycle passenger V29.508-
    - ■ unspecified electric (assisted) bicycle rider V29.601-
    - ■ unspecified rider of other motorcycle V29.608-
- unspecified traffic accident
  - electric (assisted) bicycle rider (driver) (passenger) V29.91-
  - rider (driver) (passenger) of other motorcycle V29.99-

Combustion, spontaneous—*see* Ignition

Complication (delayed) of or following (medical or surgical procedure) Y84.9-

- with misadventure—*see* Misadventure
- amputation of limb(s) Y83.5-
- anastomosis (arteriovenous) (blood vessel) (gastrojejunal) (tendon) (natural or artificial material) Y83.2-
- aspiration (of fluid) Y84.4-
  - tissue Y84.8-
- biopsy Y84.8-
- blood
  - sampling Y84.7-
  - transfusion
    - ■ procedure Y84.8-
- bypass Y83.2-
- catheterization (urinary) Y84.6-
  - cardiac Y84.0
- colostomy Y83.3-
- cystostomy Y83.3-
- dialysis (kidney) Y84.1
- drug—*see* Table of Drugs and Chemicals
  - due to misadventure—*see* Misadventure
- duodenostomy Y83.3-
- electroshock therapy Y84.3
- external stoma, creation of Y83.3-
- formation of external stoma Y83.3-
- gastrostomy Y83.3-
- graft Y83.2-
- hypothermia (medically-induced) Y84.8
- implant, implantation (of)
  - artificial
    - ■ internal device (cardiac pacemaker) (electrodes in brain) (heart valve prosthesis) (orthopedic) Y83.1-
    - ■ material or tissue (for anastomosis or bypass) Y83.2-
      - with creation of external stoma Y83.3-

Complication (delayed) of or following (medical or surgical procedure), *continued*

- natural tissues (for anastomosis or bypass) Y83.2-
  - ■ with creation of external stoma Y83.3-
- infusion
  - procedure Y84.8
- injection—*see* Table of Drugs and Chemicals
  - procedure Y84.8
- insertion of gastric or duodenal sound Y84.5
- insulin-shock therapy Y84.3
- paracentesis (abdominal) (thoracic) (aspirative) Y84.4
- procedures other than surgical operation—*see* Complication of or following, by type of procedure
- radiological procedure or therapy Y84.2
- removal of organ (partial) (total) NEC Y83.6-
- sampling
  - blood Y84.7
  - fluid NEC Y84.4
  - tissue Y84.8
- shock therapy Y84.3
- surgical operation NEC (*see also* Complication of or following, by type of operation) Y83.9-
  - reconstructive NEC Y83.4-
    - ■ with
      - anastomosis, bypass or graft Y83.2-
      - formation of external stoma Y83.3-
      - specified NEC Y83.8-
- transfusion—*see also* Table of Drugs and Chemicals
  - procedure Y84.8
- transplant, transplantation (heart) (kidney) (liver) (whole organ, any) Y83.0-
  - partial organ Y83.4-
- ureterostomy Y83.3-
- vaccination—*see also* Table of Drugs and Chemicals
  - procedure Y84.8

Compression

- divers' squeeze—*see* Air, pressure, change
- trachea by
  - food (lodged in esophagus) (*see* categories T17 and) T18
  - vomitus (lodged in esophagus) T17.81-
- Conflagration—*see* Exposure, fire, uncontrolled

Constriction (external)

- hair W49.01-
- jewelry W49.04-
- ring W49.04-
- rubber band W49.03-
- specified item NEC W49.09-
- string W49.02-
- thread W49.02-

Contact (accidental)

- with
  - abrasive wheel (metalworking) W31.1-
  - alligator W58.0-
  - amphibian W62.9-
    - ■ frog W62.0-
    - ■ toad W62.1-
  - animal (nonvenomous) (refer to specific animal by name in alphabetical order under "contact")
    - ■ marine W56.8-
  - arrow W21.89-
    - ■ not thrown, projected or falling W45.8-
  - arthropods (nonvenomous) W57.-
  - axe W27.0-
  - band-saw (industrial) W31.2-
  - bayonet—*see* Bayonet wound
  - bee(s) X58.-
  - bench-saw (industrial) W31.2-
  - bird W61.9-
  - blender W29.0.-
  - boiling water X12.-
    - ■ stated as undetermined whether accidental or intentional Y27.2-
  - bore, earth-drilling or mining (land) (seabed) W31.0-
  - buffalo W55.39-
  - bull W55.2-
  - bumper cars W31.81-
  - camel W55.39-
  - can
    - ■ lid W26.8-
    - ■ opener W27.4-
    - powered W29.0-

COLLISION-CONTACT (ACCIDENTAL)

ICD-10-CM EXTERNAL CAUSE OF INJURIES INDEX

Contact (accidental), *continued*

- cat W55.09-
  - ■ bite W55.01-
  - ■ scratch W55.03-
- caterpillar (venomous) X58.-
- centipede (venomous) X58.-
- chain
  - ■ hoist W24.0-
    - ~ agricultural operations W30.89-
  - ■ saw W29.3-
- chicken W61.3-
- chisel W27.0-
- circular saw W31.2-
- cobra X58.-
- combine (harvester) W30.0-
- conveyer belt W24.1-
- cooker (hot) X15.8-
  - ■ stated as undetermined whether accidental or intentional Y27.3-
- coral X58.-
- cotton gin W31.82-
- cow W55.2-
- crocodile W58.1-
- dagger W26.1-
  - ■ stated as undetermined whether accidental or intentional Y28.2-
- dairy equipment W31.82-
- dart W21.89-
  - ■ not thrown, projected or falling W26.8-
- deer W55.39-
- derrick W24.0-
  - ■ agricultural operations W30.89-
    - ~ hay W30.2-
- dog W54.-
- dolphin W56.0-
- donkey W55.39-
- drill (powered) W29.8-
  - ■ earth (land) (seabed) W31.0-
  - ■ nonpowered W27.8-
- drive belt W24.0-
  - ■ agricultural operations W30.89-
- dry ice—*see* Exposure, cold, man-made
- dryer (clothes) (powered) (spin) W29.2-
- duck W61.69-
- earth(-)
  - ■ drilling machine (industrial) W31.0-
  - ■ scraping machine in stationary use W31.83-
- edge of stiff paper W26.2-
- electric
  - ■ beater W29.0-
  - ■ blanket X16.-
  - ■ fan W29.2-
    - ~ commercial W31.82-
  - ■ knife W29.1-
  - ■ mixer W29.0-
- elevator (building) W24.0-
  - ■ agricultural operations W30.89-
    - ~ grain W30.3-
- engine(s), hot NEC X17.-
- excavating machine W31.0-
- farm machine W30.9-
- feces—*see* Contact, with, by type of animal
- fer de lance X58.-
- fish W56.5-
- flying horses W31.81-
- forging (metalworking) machine W31.1-
- fork W27.4-
- forklift (truck) W24.0-
  - ■ agricultural operations W30.89-
- frog W62.0-
- garden
  - ■ cultivator (powered) W29.3-
    - ~ riding W30.89-
  - ■ fork W27.1-
- gas turbine W31.3-
- Gila monster X58.-
- giraffe W55.39-
- glass (sharp) (broken) W25.-
  - ■ with subsequent fall W18.02-
  - ■ assault X99.0-
  - ■ due to fall—*see* Fall, by type
  - ■ stated as undetermined whether accidental or intentional Y28.0-

Contact (accidental), *continued*

- goat W55.3-
- goose W61.5-
- hand
  - ■ saw W27.0-
  - ■ tool (not powered) NEC W27.8-
    - ~ powered W29.8-
- harvester W30.0-
- hay-derrick W30.2-
- heat NEC X19.-
  - ■ from appliance (electrical) (household)—*see* Contact, with, hot, household appliance
    - ~ heating appliance X16.-
- heating
  - ■ appliance (hot) X16.-
  - ■ pad (electric) X16.-
- hedge-trimmer (powered) W29.3-
- hoe W27.1-
- hoist (chain) (shaft) NEC W24.0-
  - ■ agricultural W30.89-
- hoof stock NEC W55.3-
- hornet(s) X58.-
- horse W55.1-
- hot
  - ■ cooker X15.8-
  - ■ drinks X10.0-
  - ■ engine X17.-
  - ■ fats X10.2-
  - ■ fluids NEC X12.-
    - ~ assault X98.2-
    - ~ undetermined whether accidental or intentional Y27.2-
  - ■ food X10.1-
  - ■ heating appliance X16.-
  - ■ household appliance X15.-
    - ~ assault X98.3-
    - ~ object NEC X19.-
    - ◊ assault X98.8-
    - ◊ stated as undetermined whether accidental or intentional Y27.9-
    - ~ stated as undetermined whether accidental or intentional Y27.3-
  - ■ kettle X15.8-
  - ■ light bulb X15.8-
  - ■ liquid NEC (*see also* Burn) X12.-
    - ~ drinks X10.0-
    - ~ stated as undetermined whether accidental or intentional Y27.2-
    - ~ tap water X11.8-
    - ◊ stated as undetermined whether accidental or intentional Y27.1-
  - ■ machinery X17.-
  - ■ metal (molten) (liquid) NEC X18.-
  - ■ object (not producing fire or flames) NEC X19.-
  - ■ oil (cooking) X10.2-
  - ■ pipe X16.-
  - ■ plate X15.2-
  - ■ radiator X16.-
  - ■ saucepan (glass) (metal) X15.3-
  - ■ skillet X15.3-
  - ■ stove (kitchen) X15.0-
  - ■ substance NEC X19.-
  - ■ tap-water X11.8-
    - ~ assault X98.1-
    - ~ heated on stove X12.-
    - ◊ stated as undetermined whether accidental or intentional Y27.2-
    - ~ in bathtub X11.0-
    - ~ running X11.1-
    - ~ stated as undetermined whether accidental or intentional Y27.1-
  - ■ toaster X15.1-
  - ■ tool X17.-
  - ■ vapors X13.1-
    - ~ inhalation X13.0-
  - ■ water (tap) X11.8-
    - ~ boiling X12.-
    - ◊ stated as undetermined whether accidental or intentional Y27.2-
    - ~ heated on stove X12.-
    - ◊ stated as undetermined whether accidental or intentional Y27.2-
    - ~ in bathtub X11.0-

Contact (accidental), *continued*

- ~ running X11.1-
- ~ stated as undetermined whether accidental or intentional Y27.1-
- hotplate X15.2-
- ice-pick W27.4-
- insect (nonvenomous) NEC W57.-
- kettle (hot) X15.8-
- knife W26.0-
  - ■ assault X99.1-
  - ■ electric W29.1-
  - ■ stated as undetermined whether accidental or intentional Y28.1-
  - ■ suicide (attempt) X78.1-
- lathe (metalworking) W31.1-
  - ■ turnings W45.8-
  - ■ woodworking W31.2-
- lawnmower (powered) (ridden) W28.-
  - ■ causing electrocution W86.8-
  - ■ unpowered W27.1-
- lift, lifting (devices) W24.0-
  - ■ agricultural operations W30.89-
  - ■ shaft W24.0-
- liquefied gas—*see* Exposure, cold, man-made
- liquid air, hydrogen, nitrogen—*see* Exposure, cold, man-made
- lizard (nonvenomous) W59.09-
  - ■ bite W59.01-
  - ■ strike W59.02-
- llama W55.39-
- macaw W61.1-
- machine, machinery W31.9-
  - ■ abrasive wheel W31.1-
  - ■ agricultural including animal-powered W30.-
  - ■ band or bench or circular saw W31.2-
  - ■ commercial NEC W31.82-
  - ■ drilling, metal (industrial) W31.1-
  - ■ earth-drilling W31.0-
  - ■ earthmoving or scraping W31.89-
  - ■ excavating W31.89-
  - ■ forging machine W31.1-
  - ■ gas turbine W31.3-
  - ■ hot X17.-
  - ■ internal combustion engine W31.3-
  - ■ land drill W31.0-
  - ■ lathe W31.1-
  - ■ lifting (devices) W24.0-
  - ■ metal drill W31.1-
  - ■ metalworking (industrial) W31.1-
  - ■ milling, metal W31.1-
  - ■ mining W31.0-
  - ■ molding W31.2-
  - ■ overhead plane W31.2-
  - ■ power press, metal W31.1-
  - ■ prime mover W31.3-
  - ■ printing W31.89-
  - ■ radial saw W31.2-
  - ■ recreational W31.81-
  - ■ roller-coaster W31.81-
  - ■ rolling mill, metal W31.1-
  - ■ sander W31.2-
  - ■ seabed drill W31.0-
  - ■ shaft
    - ~ hoist W31.0-
    - ~ lift W31.0-
  - ■ specified NEC W31.89-
  - ■ spinning W31.89-
  - ■ steam engine W31.3-
  - ■ transmission W24.1-
  - ■ undercutter W31.0-
  - ■ water driven turbine W31.3-
  - ■ weaving W31.89-
  - ■ woodworking or forming (industrial) W31.2-
- mammal (feces) (urine) W55.89-
  - ■ marine W56.39- (refer to specific animal by name)
    - ~ specified NEC W56.3-
  - ■ specified NEC W55.8-
- marine
  - ■ animal W56.8- (refer to specific animal by name)
- meat
  - ■ grinder (domestic) W29.0-
    - ~ industrial W31.82-
  - ■ nonpowered W27.4-

ICD-10-CM EXTERNAL CAUSE OF INJURIES INDEX

Contact (accidental), *continued*

- ■ slicer (domestic) W29.0-
  - industrial W31.82-
- merry go round W31.81-
- metal, hot (liquid) (molten) NEC X18.-
- millipede W57.-
- nail W45.0-
  - ■ gun W29.4-
- needle (sewing) W27.3-
  - ■ hypodermic W46.0-
    - contaminated W46.1-
- object (blunt) NEC
  - ■ hot NEC X19.-
  - ■ sharp NEC W26.8-
    - inflicted by other person NEC W26.8-
    - self-inflicted X78.9-
- orca W56.2-
- overhead plane W31.2-
- paper (as sharp object) W26.2-
- paper-cutter W27.5-
- parrot W61.0-
- pig W55.4-
- pipe, hot X16.-
- pitchfork W27.1-
- plane (metal) (wood) W27.0-
  - ■ overhead W31.2-
- plant thorns, spines, sharp leaves or other mechanisms W60.-
- powered
  - ■ garden cultivator W29.3-
  - ■ household appliance, implement, or machine W29.8-
- saw (industrial) W31.2-
  - hand W29.8-
- printing machine W31.89-
- pulley (block) (transmission) W24.0-
  - ■ agricultural operations W30.89-
- raccoon W55.5-
- radial-saw (industrial) W31.2-
- radiator (hot) X16.-
- rake W27.1-
- rattlesnake X58.-
- reaper W30.0-
- reptile W59.8- (refer to specific reptile by name)
- rivet gun (powered) W29.4-
- rodent (feces) (urine) W53.8-
  - ■ mouse W53.0-
  - ■ rat W53.1-
  - ■ specified NEC W53.8-
  - ■ squirrel W53.2-
- roller coaster W31.81-
- rope NEC W24.0-
  - ■ agricultural operations W30.89-
- saliva—*see* Contact, with, by type of animal
- sander W29.8-
  - ■ industrial W31.2-
- saucepan (hot) (glass) (metal) X15.3-
- saw W27.0-
  - ■ band (industrial) W31.2-
  - ■ bench (industrial) W31.2-
  - ■ chain W29.3-
  - ■ hand W27.0-
- sawing machine, metal W31.1-
- scissors W27.2-
- scorpion X58.-
- screwdriver W27.0-
  - ■ powered W29.8-
- sea
  - ■ anemone, cucumber or urchin (spine) X58.-
  - ■ lion W56.1-
- sewing-machine (electric) (powered) W29.2-
  - ■ not powered W27.8-
- shaft (hoist) (lift) (transmission) NEC W24.0-
  - ■ agricultural W30.89-
- shark W56.4-
- shears (hand) W27.2-
  - ■ powered (industrial) W31.1-
    - domestic W29.2-
- sheep W55.3-
- shovel W27.8-
- snake (nonvenomous) W59.11-
- spade W27.1-
- spider (venomous) X58.-

Contact (accidental), *continued*

- spin-drier W29.2-
- spinning machine W31.89-
- splinter W45.8-
- sports equipment W21.9-
- staple gun (powered) W29.8-
- steam X13.1-
  - ■ engine W31.3-
  - ■ inhalation X13.0-
  - ■ pipe X16.-
  - ■ shovel W31.89-
- stove (hot) (kitchen) X15.0-
- substance, hot NEC X19.-
  - ■ molten (metal) X18.-
- sword W26.1-
  - ■ assault X99.2-
  - ■ stated as undetermined whether accidental or intentional Y28.2-
- tarantula X58.-
- thresher W30.0-
- tin can lid W26.8-
- toad W62.1-
- toaster (hot) X15.1-
- tool W27.8-
  - ■ hand (not powered) W27.8-
    - auger W27.0-
    - axe W27.0-
    - can opener W27.4-
    - chisel W27.0-
    - fork W27.4-
    - garden W27.1-
    - handsaw W27.0-
    - hoe W27.1-
    - ice-pick W27.4-
    - kitchen utensil W27.4-
    - manual
    - ◊ lawn mower W27.1-
    - ◊ sewing machine W27.8-
    - meat grinder W27.4-
    - needle (sewing) W27.3-
    - ◊ hypodermic W46.0-
      - » contaminated W46.1-
    - paper cutter W27.5-
    - pitchfork W27.1-
    - rake W27.1-
    - scissors W27.2-
    - screwdriver W27.0-
    - specified NEC W27.8-
    - workbench W27.0-
  - ■ hot X17.-
  - ■ powered W29.8-
    - blender W29.0-
    - ◊ commercial W31.82-
    - can opener W29.0-
    - ◊ commercial W31.82-
    - chainsaw W29.3-
    - clothes dryer W29.2-
    - ◊ commercial W31.82-
    - dishwasher W29.2-
    - ◊ commercial W31.82-
    - edger W29.3-
    - electric fan W29.2-
    - ◊ commercial W31.82-
    - electric knife W29.1-
    - food processor W29.0-
    - ◊ commercial W31.82-
    - garbage disposal W29.0-
    - ◊ commercial W31.82-
    - garden tool W29.3-
    - hedge trimmer W29.3-
    - ice maker W29.0-
    - ◊ commercial W31.82-
    - kitchen appliance W29.0-
    - ◊ commercial W31.82-
    - lawn mower W28.-
    - ◊ commercial W31.82-
    - meat grinder W29.0-
    - ◊ commercial W31.82-
    - mixer W29.0-
    - ◊ commercial W31.82-
    - rototiller W29.3-
    - sewing machine W29.2-
    - ◊ commercial W31.82-

Contact (accidental), *continued*

- washing machine W29.2-
  - ◊ commercial W31.82-
- transmission device (belt, cable, chain, gear, pinion, shaft) W24.1-
  - ■ agricultural operations W30.89-
- turbine (gas) (water-driven) W31.3-
- turkey W61.4-
- turtle (nonvenomous) W59.2-
  - ■ terrestrial W59.8-
- under-cutter W31.0-
- vehicle
  - ■ agricultural use (transport)—*see* Accident, transport, agricultural vehicle
    - not on public highway W30.81-
  - ■ industrial use (transport)—*see* Accident, transport, industrial vehicle
    - not on public highway W31.83-
  - ■ off-road use (transport)—*see* Accident, transport, all-terrain or off-road vehicle
    - not on public highway W31.83-
- venomous animal/plant X58.-
  - viper X58.-
- washing-machine (powered) W29.2-
- wasp X58.-
- weaving-machine W31.89-
- winch W24.0-
  - ■ agricultural operations W30.89-
- wire NEC W24.0-
  - ■ agricultural operations W30.89-
- wood slivers W45.8-
- yellow jacket X58.-
- zebra W55.39-

Coup de soleil X32.-

Crash

- aircraft (in transit) (powered) V95.9-
  - balloon V96.01-
  - fixed wing NEC (private) V95.21-
    - ■ commercial V95.31-
  - glider V96.21-
    - ■ hang V96.11-
    - ■ powered V95.11-
  - helicopter V95.01-
  - microlight V95.11-
  - nonpowered V96.9-
    - ■ specified NEC V96.8-
  - powered NEC V95.8-
  - stated as
    - ■ homicide (attempt) Y08.81-
    - ■ suicide (attempt) X83.0-
  - ultralight V95.11-
- transport vehicle NEC (*see also* Accident, transport) V89.9-

Crushed (accidentally) X58.-

- between objects (moving) (stationary and moving) W23.0-
  - stationary W23.1-
- by
  - alligator W58.03-
  - avalanche NEC—*see* Landslide
  - cave-in W20.0-
    - ■ caused by cataclysmic earth surface movement—*see* Landslide
  - crocodile W58.13-
  - crowd or human stampede W52.-
  - falling
    - ■ aircraft V97.39-
    - ■ earth, material W20.0-
      - caused by cataclysmic earth surface movement—*see* Landslide
    - ■ object NEC W20.8-
  - landslide NEC—*see* Landslide
  - lizard (nonvenomous) W59.09-
  - machinery—*see* Contact, with, by type of machine
  - reptile NEC W59.89-
  - snake (nonvenomous) W59.13-
- in
  - machinery—*see* Contact, with, by type of machine

Cut, cutting (any part of body) (accidental)—*see also* Contact, with, by object or machine

Cut, cutting (any part of body) (accidental) *continued*

- during medical or surgical treatment as misadventure—*see* Index to Diseases and Injuries, Complications
- inflicted by other person—*see* Assault, cutting or piercing instrument
- machine NEC (*see also* Contact, with, by type of machine) W31.9-
- self-inflicted—*see* Suicide, cutting or piercing instrument
- suicide (attempt)—*see* Suicide, cutting or piercing instrument

Cyclone (any injury) X37.1-

D

Dehydration from lack of water X58.-

Deprivation X58.-

Derailment (accidental)

- railway (rolling stock) (train) (vehicle) (without antecedent collision) V81.7-
  - with antecedent collision—*see* Accident, transport, railway vehicle occupant
- streetcar (without antecedent collision) V82.7-
  - with antecedent collision—*see* Accident, transport, streetcar occupant

Descent

- parachute (voluntary) (without accident to aircraft) V97.29-
  - due to accident to aircraft—*see* Accident, transport, aircraft

Desertion X58.-

Destitution X58.-

Disability, late effect or sequela of injury—*see* Sequelae

Discharge (accidental)

- airgun W34.010-
  - assault X95.01-
  - stated as undetermined whether accidental or intentional Y24.0-
- BB gun—*see* Discharge, airgun
- firearm (accidental) W34.00-
  - assault X95.9-
  - handgun (pistol) (revolver) W32.0-
    - assault X93.-
    - stated as undetermined whether accidental or intentional Y22.-
  - homicide (attempt) X95.9-
  - hunting rifle W33.02-
    - assault X94.1-
    - stated as undetermined whether accidental or intentional Y23.1-
  - larger W33.00-
    - hunting rifle—*see* Discharge, firearm, hunting rifle
    - shotgun—*see* Discharge, firearm, shotgun
    - specified NEC W33.09-
      - ~ stated as undetermined whether accidental or intentional Y23.8-
    - stated as undetermined whether accidental or intentional Y23.9-
    - using rubber bullet
      - ~ injuring
        - ◊ bystander Y35.042-
        - ◊ law enforcement personnel Y35.041-
        - ◊ suspect Y35.043-
  - machine gun W33.03-
    - stated as undetermined whether accidental or intentional Y23.3-
  - pellet gun—*see* Discharge, airgun
  - shotgun W33.01-
    - stated as undetermined whether accidental or intentional Y23.0-
  - specified NEC W34.09-
    - assault X95.8-
    - stated as undetermined whether accidental or intentional Y24.8-
  - stated as undetermined whether accidental or intentional Y24.9-
  - Very pistol W34.09-
    - assault X95.8-
    - stated as undetermined whether accidental or intentional Y24.8-

Discharge (accidental), *continued*

- firework(s) W39.-
  - stated as undetermined whether accidental or intentional Y25.-
- gas-operated gun NEC W34.018-
  - airgun—*see* Discharge, airgun
  - assault X95.09-
  - paintball gun—*see* Discharge, paintball gun
  - stated as undetermined whether accidental or intentional Y24.8-
- gun NEC—*see also* Discharge, firearm NEC
  - air—*see* Discharge, airgun
  - BB—*see* Discharge, airgun
  - for single hand use—*see* Discharge, firearm, handgun
  - hand—*see* Discharge, firearm, handgun
  - machine—*see* Discharge, firearm, machine gun
  - other specified—*see* Discharge, firearm NEC
  - paintball—*see* Discharge, paintball gun
  - pellet—*see* Discharge, airgun
- handgun—*see* Discharge, firearm, handgun
- machine gun—*see* Discharge, firearm, machine gun
- paintball gun W34.011-
  - assault X95.02-
  - stated as undetermined whether accidental or intentional Y24.8-
- rifle (hunting)—*see* Discharge, firearm, hunting rifle
- shotgun—*see* Discharge, firearm, shotgun
- spring-operated gun NEC W34.018-
  - assault / homicide (attempt) X95.09-
  - stated as undetermined whether accidental or intentional Y24.8-

Diver's disease, palsy, paralysis, squeeze—*see* Air, pressure

Diving (into water)—*see* Accident, diving

Dog bite W54.0-

Dragged by transport vehicle NEC (*see also* Accident, transport) V09.9-

Drinking poison (accidental)—*see* Table of Drugs and Chemicals

Dropped (accidentally) while being carried or supported by other person W04.-

Drowning (accidental) W74.-

- assault X92.9-
- due to
  - accident (to)
    - machinery—*see* Contact, with, by type of machine
    - watercraft V90.89-
      - ~ burning V90.29-
        - ◊ powered V90.2-
        - ◊ unpowered V90.2-
      - ~ crushed V90.39-
        - ◊ powered V90.3-
        - ◊ unpowered V90.3-
      - ~ overturning V90.09-
        - ◊ powered V90.0-
        - ◊ unpowered V90.0-
      - ~ sinking V90.19-
        - ◊ powered V90.1-
        - ◊ unpowered V90.1-
      - ~ specified type NEC V90.89-
        - ◊ powered V90.8-
        - ◊ unpowered V90.8-
  - avalanche—*see* Landslide
  - cataclysmic
    - earth surface movement NEC—*see* Forces of nature, earth movement
    - storm—*see* Forces of nature, cataclysmic storm
  - cloudburst X37.8-
  - cyclone X37.1-
  - fall overboard (from) V92.09-
    - powered craft V92.0-
    - resulting from
      - accident to watercraft—*see* Drowning, due to, accident to, watercraft
      - being washed overboard (from) V92.29-
        - ◊ powered craft V92.2-
        - ◊ unpowered craft V92.2-
    - ~ motion of watercraft V92.19-
      - ◊ powered craft V92.1-
      - ◊ unpowered craft V92.1-

Drowning (accidental), *continued*

- unpowered craft V92.0-
- hurricane X37.0-
- jumping into water from watercraft (involved in accident)—*see also* Drowning, due to, accident to, watercraft
  - without accident to or on watercraft W16.711-
- torrential rain X37.8-
- following
  - fall
    - into
      - ~ bathtub W16.211-
      - ~ bucket W16.221-
      - ~ fountain—*see* Drowning, following, fall, into, water, specified NEC
      - ~ quarry—*see* Drowning, following, fall, into, water, specified NEC
      - ~ reservoir—*see* Drowning, following, fall, into, water, specified NEC
      - ~ swimming-pool W16.011-
        - ◊ striking
          - » bottom W16.021-
          - » wall W16.031-
        - ◊ stated as undetermined whether accidental or intentional Y21.3-
      - ~ water NOS W16.41-
        - ◊ natural (lake) (open sea) (river) (stream) (pond) W16.111-
          - » striking
            - ♦ bottom W16.121-
            - ♦ side W16.131-
        - ◊ specified NEC W16.311-
          - » striking
            - ♦ bottom W16.321-
            - ♦ wall W16.331-
    - overboard NEC—*see* Drowning, due to, fall overboard
  - jump or dive
    - from boat W16.711-
      - ~ striking bottom W16.721-
    - into
      - ~ fountain—*see* Drowning, following, jump or dive, into, water, specified NEC
      - ~ quarry—*see* Drowning, following, jump or dive, into, water, specified NEC
      - ~ reservoir—*see* Drowning, following, jump or dive, into, water, specified NEC
      - ~ swimming-pool W16.511-
        - ◊ striking
          - » bottom W16.521-
          - » wall W16.531-
      - ~ water NOS W16.91-
        - ◊ natural (lake) (open sea) (river) (stream) (pond) W16.611-
        - ◊ specified NEC W16.811-
          - » striking
            - ♦ bottom W16.821-
            - ♦ wall W16.831-
        - ◊ striking bottom W16.621-
- in
  - bathtub (accidental) W65.-
    - assault X92.0-
    - following fall W16.211-
      - stated as undetermined whether accidental or intentional Y21.1-
    - stated as undetermined whether accidental or intentional Y21.0-
  - lake—*see* Drowning, in, natural water
  - natural water (lake) (open sea) (river) (stream) (pond) W69.-
    - assault X92.3-
    - following
      - ~ dive or jump W16.611-
        - ◊ striking bottom W16.621-
      - ~ fall W16.111-
        - ◊ striking
          - » bottom W16.121-
          - » side W16.131-
    - stated as undetermined whether accidental or intentional Y21.4-
  - quarry—*see* Drowning, in, specified place NEC
  - quenching tank—*see* Drowning, in, specified place NEC

Drowning (accidental), *continued*

- reservoir—*see* Drowning, in, specified place NEC
- river—*see* Drowning, in, natural water
- sea—*see* Drowning, in, natural water
- specified place
  - ■ assault X92.8-
  - ■ following
    - ~ dive or jump W16.811-
      - ◊ striking
        - » bottom W16.821-
        - » wall W16.831-
    - ~ fall W16.311-
      - ◊ striking
        - » bottom W16.321-
        - » wall W16.331-
  - ■ stated as undetermined whether accidental or intentional Y21.8-
- stream—*see* Drowning, in, natural water
- swimming-pool W67.-
  - ■ assault X92.1-
    - ~ following fall X92.2-
  - ■ following
    - ~ dive or jump W16.511-
      - ◊ striking
        - » bottom W16.521-
        - » wall W16.531-
    - ~ fall W16.011-
      - ◊ striking
        - » bottom W16.021-
        - » wall W16.031-
  - ■ stated as undetermined whether accidental or intentional Y21.2-
    - ~ following fall Y21.3-
    - ~ following fall X71.2-
- resulting from accident to watercraft *see* Drowning, due to, accident, watercraft
- self-inflicted X71.9-
- stated as undetermined whether accidental or intentional Y21.9-

E

Earth falling (on) W20.0-

- caused by cataclysmic earth surface movement or eruption—*see* Landslide

Earth (surface) movement NEC—*see* Forces of nature, earth movement

Earthquake (any injury) X34.-

Effect(s) (adverse) of

- air pressure (any)—*see* Air, pressure
- cold, excessive (exposure to)—*see* Exposure, cold
- heat (excessive)—*see* Heat
- hot place (weather)—*see* Heat
- insolation X30.-
- late—*see* Sequelae
- motion—*see* Motion
- radiation—*see* Radiation
- travel—*see* Travel

Electric shock (accidental) (by) (in)—*see* Exposure, electric current

Electrocution (accidental)—*see* Exposure, electric current

Endotracheal tube wrongly placed during anesthetic procedure

Entanglement

- in
  - bed linen, causing suffocation—*see* category T71
  - wheel of pedal cycle V19.88-

Entry of foreign body or material—*see* Foreign body

Environmental pollution related condition—*see* Z57

Exhaustion

- cold—*see* Exposure, cold
- due to excessive exertion—*see* category Y93
- heat—*see* Heat

Explosion (accidental) (of) (with secondary fire) W40.9-

- acetylene W40.1-
- aerosol can W36.1-
- air tank (compressed) (in machinery) W36.2-
- aircraft (in transit) (powered) NEC V95.9
  - balloon V96.05-

Explosion (accidental) (of) (with secondary fire), *continued*

- fixed wing NEC (private) V95.25-
  - ■ commercial V95.35-
- glider V96.25-
  - ■ hang V96.15-
  - ■ powered V95.15-
- helicopter V95.05-
- microlight V95.15-
- nonpowered V96.9-
  - ■ specified NEC V96.8-
- powered NEC V95.8-
- ultralight V95.15-
- anesthetic gas in operating room W40.1-
- bicycle tire W37.0-
- blasting (cap) (materials) W40.0-
- boiler (machinery), not on transport vehicle W35.-
  - on watercraft—*see* Explosion, in, watercraft
- butane W40.1-
- caused by other person X96.9-
- coal gas W40.1-
- detonator W40.0-
- dump (munitions) W40.8-
- dynamite W40.0-
  - in
    - ■ assault X96.8-
- explosive (material) W40.9-
  - gas W40.1-
  - specified NEC W40.8-
    - ■ in
- factory (munitions) W40.8-
- firearm (parts) NEC W34.19
  - airgun W34.110-
  - BB gun W34.110-
  - gas, air or spring-operated gun NEC W34.118-
  - handgun W32.1
  - hunting rifle W33.12-
  - larger firearm W33.10-
    - ■ specified NEC W33.19-
  - machine gun W33.13-
  - paintball gun W34.111-
  - pellet gun W34.110-
  - shotgun W33.11-
  - Very pistol [flare] W34.19-
- fire-damp W40.1-
- fireworks W39.-
- gas (coal) (explosive) W40.1-
  - cylinder W36.9-
    - ■ aerosol can W36.1-
    - ■ air tank W36.2-
    - ■ pressurized W36.3-
    - ■ specified NEC W36.8-
- gasoline (fumes) (tank) not in moving motor vehicle W40.1-
  - in motor vehicle—*see* Accident, transport, by type of vehicle
- grain store W40.8-
- handgun (parts)—*see* Explosion, firearm, handgun (parts)
- homicide (attempt) X96.9-
  - specified NEC X96.8-
- hose, pressurized W37.8-
- hot water heater, tank (in machinery) W35.-
  - on watercraft—*see* Explosion, in, watercraft
- in, on
  - dump W40.8-
  - factory W40.8-
  - watercraft V93.59-
    - ■ powered craft V93.53-
    - ~ ferry boat V93.51-
    - ~ fishing boat V93.52-
    - ~ jet skis V93.53-
    - ~ liner V93.51-
    - ~ merchant ship V93.50-
    - ~ passenger ship V93.51-
    - ~ sailboat V93.54-
- machinery—*see also* Contact, with, by type of machine
  - on board watercraft—*see* Explosion, in, watercraft
  - pressure vessel—*see* Explosion, by type of vessel
- methane W40.1-
- missile NEC W40.8-
- munitions (dump) (factory) W40.8-
- pipe, pressurized W37.8-
- pressure, pressurized

Explosion (accidental) (of) (with secondary fire), *continued*

- cooker W38.-
- gas tank (in machinery) W36.3-
- hose W37.8-
- pipe W37.8-
- specified device NEC W38.-
- tire W37.8-
  - ■ bicycle W37.0-
- vessel (in machinery) W38.-
- propane W40.1-
- self-inflicted X75.-
- stated as undetermined whether accidental or intentional Y25.-
- steam or water lines (in machinery) W37.8-
- stove W40.9-
- tire, pressurized W37.8-
  - bicycle W37.0-
- undetermined whether accidental or intentional Y25.-
- vehicle tire NEC W37.8-
  - bicycle W37.0-

Exposure (to) X58

- air pressure change—*see* Air, pressure
- cold (accidental) (excessive) (extreme) (natural) (place) X31.-
  - assault Y08.89-
  - due to
    - ■ man-made conditions W93.8-
    - ~ dry ice (contact) W93.01-
      - ◊ inhalation W93.02-
    - ~ liquid air (contact) (hydrogen) (nitrogen) W93.11-
      - ◊ inhalation W93.12-
    - ~ refrigeration unit (deep freeze) W93.2-
    - ■ weather (conditions) X31.-
  - self-inflicted X83.2-
- due to abandonment or neglect X58.-
- electric current W86.8-
  - appliance (faulty) W86.8-
    - ■ domestic W86.0-
  - caused by other person Y08.89-
  - conductor (faulty) W86.1-
  - control apparatus (faulty) W86.1-
  - electric power generating plant, distribution station W86.1-
  - electroshock gun—*see* Exposure, electric current, taser
  - lightning—*see* subcategory T75.0-
  - live rail W86.8-
  - misadventure in medical or surgical procedure in electroshock therapy Y63.4-
  - motor (electric) (faulty) W86.8-
    - ■ domestic W86.0-
  - self-inflicted X83.1-
  - specified NEC W86.8-
    - ■ domestic W86.0-
  - stun gun—*see* Exposure, electric current, taser
  - taser W86.8-
    - ■ assault Y08.89-
    - ■ self-harm (intentional) X83.8-
    - ■ undetermined intent Y33.-
  - third rail W86.8-
  - transformer (faulty) W86.1-
- environmental tobacco smoke X58.-
- excessive
  - cold—*see* Exposure, cold
  - heat (natural) NEC X30.-
- factor(s) NOS X58.-
  - environmental NEC X58.-
    - ■ natural NEC—*see* Forces of nature
    - ■ specified NEC X58.-
- fire, flames (accidental) X08.8
  - assault X97.-
  - campfire—*see* Exposure, fire, controlled, not in building
  - controlled (in)
    - ■ with ignition (of) clothing (*see also* Ignition, clothes) X06.2-
      - ~ nightwear X05.-
    - ■ bonfire—*see* Exposure, fire, controlled, not in building

Exposure (to), *continued*

- ■ brazier (in building or structure)—*see also* Exposure, fire, controlled, building
  - ~ not in building or structure—*see* Exposure, fire, controlled, not in building
- ■ building or structure X02.0-
  - ~ with
    - ◊ fall from building X02.3-
    - ◊ injury due to building collapse X02.2-
    - ◊ from building X02.5-
    - ◊ smoke inhalation X02.1-
  - ~ hit by object from building X02.4-
  - ~ specified mode of injury NEC X02.8-
- ■ fireplace, furnace or stove—*see* Exposure, fire, controlled, building
- ■ not in building or structure X03.0-
  - ~ with
    - ◊ fall X03.3
    - ◊ smoke inhalation X03.1-
  - ~ hit by object X03.4-
  - ~ specified mode of injury NEC X03.8-
- ■ trash—*see* Exposure, fire, controlled, not in building
- ~ fireplace—*see* Exposure, fire, controlled, building
- ~ fittings or furniture (in building or structure) (uncontrolled)—*see* Exposure, fire, uncontrolled, building
- ~ forest (uncontrolled)—*see* Exposure, fire, uncontrolled, not in building
- ~ grass (uncontrolled)—*see* Exposure, fire, uncontrolled, not in building
- ~ hay (uncontrolled)—*see* Exposure, fire, uncontrolled, not in building
- ~ ignition of highly flammable material X04.-
- ~ in, of, on, starting in
  - ■ machinery—*see* Contact, with, by type of machine
  - ■ motor vehicle (in motion) (*see also* Accident, transport, occupant by type of vehicle) V87.8-
    - ~ with collision—*see* Collision
  - ■ railway rolling stock, train, vehicle V81.81-
    - ~ with collision—*see* Accident, transport, railway vehicle occupant
  - ■ streetcar (in motion) V82.8-
    - ~ with collision—*see* Accident, transport, streetcar occupant
  - ■ transport vehicle NEC—*see also* Accident, transport
    - ~ with collision—*see* Collision
  - ■ watercraft (in transit) (not in transit) V91.09-
    - ~ localized—*see* Burn, on board watercraft, due to, fire on board
    - ~ powered craft V91.03-
      - ◊ ferry boat V91.01-
      - ◊ fishing boat V91.02-
      - ◊ jet skis V91.03-
      - ◊ liner V91.01-
      - ◊ merchant ship V91.00-
      - ◊ passenger ship V91.01-
    - ~ unpowered craft V91.08-
      - ◊ canoe V91.05-
      - ◊ inflatable V91.06-
      - ◊ kayak V91.05-
      - ◊ sailboat V91.04-
      - ◊ surf-board V91.08-
      - ◊ waterskis V91.07-
      - ◊ windsurfer V91.08-
- ~ lumber (uncontrolled)—*see* Exposure, fire, uncontrolled, not in building
- ~ prairie (uncontrolled)—*see* Exposure, fire, uncontrolled, not in building
- ~ resulting from
  - ■ explosion—*see* Explosion
  - ■ lightning X08.8-
- ~ self-inflicted X76.-
- ~ specified NEC X08.8-
- ~ started by other person X97.-
  - stated as undetermined whether accidental or intentional Y26.-
- ~ stove—*see* Exposure, fire, controlled, building
- ~ tunnel (uncontrolled)—*see* Exposure, fire, uncontrolled, not in building

Exposure (to), *continued*

- ~ uncontrolled
  - ■ in building or structure X00.0-
    - ~ with
      - ◊ fall from building X00.3-
      - ◊ injury due to building collapse X00.2-
      - ◊ jump from building X00.5-
      - ◊ smoke inhalation X00.1-
    - ~ bed X08.00-
      - ◊ due to
        - » cigarette X08.01-
        - » specified material NEC X08.09-
    - ~ furniture NEC X08.20-
      - ◊ due to
        - » cigarette X08.21-
        - » specified material NEC X08.29-
    - ~ hit by object from building X00.4-
    - ~ sofa X08.10-
      - ◊ due to
        - » cigarette X08.11-
        - » specified material NEC X08.19-
    - ~ specified mode of injury NEC X00.8-
  - ■ not in building or structure (any) X01.0-
    - ~ with
      - ◊ fall X01.3-
      - ◊ smoke inhalation X01.1-
    - ~ hit by object X01.4-
    - ~ specified mode of injury NEC X01.8-
    - ~ undetermined whether accidental or intentional Y26.-
- forces of nature NEC—*see* Forces of nature
- G-forces (abnormal) W49.9-
- gravitational forces (abnormal) W49.9-
- heat (natural) NEC—*see* Heat
- high-pressure jet (hydraulic) (pneumatic) W49.9-
- hydraulic jet W49.9-
- inanimate mechanical force W49.9-
- jet, high-pressure (hydraulic) (pneumatic) W49.9-
- lightning—*see* subcategory T75.0-
  - ~ causing fire—*see* Exposure, fire
- mechanical forces NEC W49.9-
  - ~ inanimate NEC W49.9-
- noise W42.9-
  - ~ supersonic W42.0-
- noxious substance—*see* Table of Drugs and Chemicals
- pneumatic jet W49.9-
- prolonged in deep-freeze unit or refrigerator W93.2-
- radiation—*see* Radiation
- smoke—*see also* Exposure, fire
  - ~ tobacco, second hand Z77.22
- specified factors NEC X58.-
- sunlight X32.-
- supersonic waves W42.0-
- vibration W49.9-
- waves
  - ~ infrasound W49.9-
  - ~ sound W42.9-
    - ~ supersonic W42.0-
- weather NEC—*see* Forces of nature

External cause status Y99.9

- child assisting in compensated work for family Y99.8
- civilian activity done for financial or other compensation Y99.0
- civilian activity done for income or pay Y99.0
- family member assisting in compensated work for other family member Y99.8
- hobby not done for income Y99.8
- leisure activity Y99.8
- off-duty activity of military personnel Y99.8
- recreation or sport not for income or while a student Y99.8
- specified NEC Y99.8
- student activity Y99.8
- volunteer activity Y99.2

F

Factors, supplemental

- alcohol
  - ~ blood level Y90.-
- environmental-pollution-related condition—*see* Z57
- nosocomial condition Y95.-
- work-related condition Y99.0

Failure

- in suture or ligature during surgical procedure Y65.2-
- mechanical, of instrument or apparatus (any) (during any medical or surgical procedure) Y65.8-
- sterile precautions (during medical and surgical care)—*see* Misadventure, failure, sterile precautions, by type of procedure
- to
  - ~ introduce tube or instrument Y65.4-
    - ■ endotracheal tube during anesthesia Y65.3-
  - ~ make curve (transport vehicle) NEC—*see* Accident, transport
  - ~ remove tube or instrument Y65.4-

Fall, falling (accidental) W19.-

- building W20.1-
  - ~ burning (uncontrolled fire) X00.3-
- down
  - ~ embankment W17.81-
  - ~ escalator W10.0-
  - ~ hill W17.81-
  - ~ ladder W11.-
  - ~ ramp W10.2-
  - ~ stairs, steps W10.9-
- due to
  - ~ bumping against
    - ■ object W18.00-
      - ~ sharp glass W18.02-
      - ~ specified NEC W18.09-
    - ~ sports equipment W18.01-
    - ■ person W03.-
      - ~ due to ice or snow W00.0-
      - ~ on pedestrian conveyance—*see* Accident, transport, pedestrian, conveyance
  - ~ collision with another person W03.-
    - ~ due to ice or snow W00.0-
    - ■ involving pedestrian conveyance—*see* Accident, transport, pedestrian, conveyance
  - ~ grocery cart tipping over W17.82-
  - ~ ice or snow W00.9-
  - ■ from one level to another W00.2-
    - ~ on stairs or steps W00.1-
    - ■ involving pedestrian conveyance—*see* Accident, transport, pedestrian, conveyance
  - ■ on same level W00.0-
  - ~ slipping (on moving sidewalk) W01.0-
  - ~ with subsequent striking against object W01.10-
    - ~ furniture W01.190-
      - ~ sharp object W01.119-
        - ◊ glass W01.110-
        - ◊ power tool or machine W01.111-
        - ◊ specified NEC W01.118-
      - ~ specified NEC W01.198-
  - ~ striking against
    - ■ object W18.00-
      - ~ sharp glass W18.02-
      - ~ specified NEC W18.09-
    - ~ sports equipment W18.01-
    - ■ person W03.-
      - ~ due to ice or snow W00.0-
      - ~ on pedestrian conveyance—*see* Accident, transport, pedestrian, conveyance
- earth (with asphyxia or suffocation (by pressure))—*see* Earth, falling
- from, off, out of
  - ~ aircraft NEC (with accident to aircraft NEC) V97.0-
    - ■ while boarding or alighting V97.1-
  - ~ balcony W13.0-
  - ~ bed W06.-
  - ~ boat, ship, watercraft NEC (with drowning or submersion)—*see* Drowning, due to, fall overboard
    - ■ with hitting bottom or object V94.0-
  - ~ bridge W13.1-
  - ~ building W13.9-
    - ■ burning (uncontrolled fire) X00.3-
  - ~ cavity W17.2-
  - ~ chair W07.-
  - ~ cherry picker W17.89-
  - ~ cliff W15.-
  - ~ dock W17.4-
  - ~ embankment W17.81-
  - ~ escalator W10.0-
  - ~ flagpole W13.8-
  - ~ furniture NEC W08.-

ICD-10-CM EXTERNAL CAUSE OF INJURIES INDEX

Fall, falling (accidental), *continued*

- grocery cart W17.82-
- haystack W17.89-
- high place NEC W17.89-
  - stated as undetermined whether accidental or intentional Y30.-
- hole W17.2-
- incline W10.2-
- ladder W11.-
- lifting device W17.89-
- machine, machinery—*see also* Contact, with, by type of machine
  - not in operation W17.89-
- manhole W17.1-
- mobile elevated work platform [MEWP] W17.89-
- motorized mobility scooter W05.2-
- one level to another W17.89-
  - intentional, purposeful, suicide (attempt) X80.-
  - stated as undetermined whether accidental or intentional Y30.-
- pit W17.2-
- playground equipment W09.8-
  - jungle gym W09.2-
  - slide W09.0-
  - swing W09.1-
- quarry W17.89-
- railing W13.9-
- ramp W10.2-
- roof W13.2-
- scaffolding W12.-
- scooter (nonmotorized) W05.1-
  - motorized mobility W05.2-
- sky lift W17.89-
- stairs, steps W10.9-
  - curb W10.1-
  - due to ice or snow W00.1-
  - escalator W10.0-
  - incline W10.2-
  - ramp W10.2-
  - sidewalk curb W10.1-
  - specified NEC W10.8-
  - standing
    - electric scooter V00.841-
    - micro-mobility pedestrian conveyance V00.848-
- stepladder W11.-
- storm drain W17.1-
- streetcar NEC V82.6-
  - with antecedent collision—*see* Accident, transport, streetcar occupant
  - while boarding or alighting V82.4-
- structure NEC W13.8-
  - burning (uncontrolled fire) X00.3-
- table W08.-
- toilet W18.11-
  - with subsequent striking against object W18.12-
- train NEC V81.6-
  - during derailment (without antecedent collision) V81.7-
    - with antecedent collision—*see* Accident, transport, railway vehicle occupant
  - while boarding or alighting V81.4-
- transport vehicle after collision—*see* Accident, transport, by type of vehicle, collision
- tree W14.-
- vehicle (in motion) NEC (*see also* Accident, transport) V89.9-
  - motor NEC (*see also* Accident, transport, occupant, by type of vehicle) V87.8-
  - stationary W17.89-
    - while boarding or alighting—*see* Accident, transport, by type of vehicle, while boarding or alighting
- viaduct W13.8-
- wall W13.8-
- watercraft—*see also* Drowning, due to, fall overboard
  - with hitting bottom or object V94.0-
- well W17.0-
- wheelchair, non-moving W05.0-
  - powered—*see* Accident, transport, pedestrian, conveyance occupant, specified type NEC
- window W13.4-

Fall, falling (accidental), *continued*

- in, on
  - aircraft NEC V97.0-
    - with accident to aircraft V97.0-
    - while boarding or alighting V97.1-
  - bathtub (empty) W18.2-
    - filled W16.212-
      - causing drowning W16.211-
  - escalator W10.0-
  - incline W10.2-
  - ladder W11.-
  - machine, machinery—*see* Contact, with, by type of machine
  - object, edged, pointed or sharp (with cut)—*see* Fall, by type
  - playground equipment W09.8-
    - jungle gym W09.2-
    - slide W09.0-
    - swing W09.1-
  - ramp W10.2-
  - scaffolding W12.-
  - shower W18.2-
    - causing drowning W16.211-
  - staircase, stairs, steps W10.9-
    - curb W10.1-
    - due to ice or snow W00.1-
    - escalator W10.0-
    - incline W10.2-
    - specified NEC W10.8-
  - streetcar (without antecedent collision) V82.5-
    - with antecedent collision—*see* Accident, transport, streetcar occupant
    - while boarding or alighting V82.4-
  - train (without antecedent collision) V81.5-
    - with antecedent collision—*see* Accident, transport, railway vehicle occupant
    - during derailment (without antecedent collision) V81.7-
      - with antecedent collision—*see* Accident, transport, railway vehicle occupant
    - while boarding or alighting V81.4-
  - transport vehicle after collision—*see* Accident, transport, by type of vehicle, collision
  - watercraft V93.39-
    - due to
      - accident to craft V91.29-
        - ◊ powered craft V91.2-
        - ◊ unpowered craft V91.2-
      - powered craft V93.3-
      - unpowered craft V93.3-
- into
  - cavity W17.2-
  - dock W17.4-
  - fire—*see* Exposure, fire, by type
  - haystack W17.89-
  - hole W17.2-
  - lake—*see* Fall, into, water
  - manhole W17.1-
  - moving part of machinery—*see* Contact, with, by type of machine
  - ocean—*see* Fall, into, water
  - opening in surface NEC W17.89-
  - pit W17.2-
  - pond—*see* Fall, into, water
  - quarry W17.89-
  - river—*see* Fall, into, water
  - shaft W17.89-
  - storm drain W17.1-
  - stream—*see* Fall, into, water
  - swimming pool—*see also* Fall, into, water, in, swimming pool
    - empty W17.3-
  - tank W17.89-
  - water W16.42-
    - causing drowning W16.41-
    - from watercraft—*see* Drowning, due to, fall overboard
    - hitting diving board W21.4-
    - in
      - bathtub W16.212-
        - ◊ causing drowning W16.211-
      - bucket W16.222-
        - ◊ causing drowning W16.221-

Fall, falling (accidental), *continued*

- natural body of water W16.112-
  - ◊ causing drowning W16.111-
  - ◊ striking
    - ▸ bottom W16.122-
      - ✦ causing drowning W16.121-
    - ▸ side W16.132-
      - ✦ causing drowning W16.131-
- specified water NEC W16.312-
  - ◊ causing drowning W16.311-
  - ◊ striking
    - ▸ bottom W16.322-
      - ✦ causing drowning W16.321-
    - ▸ wall W16.332-
      - ✦ causing drowning W16.331-
- swimming pool W16.012-
  - ◊ causing drowning W16.011-
  - ◊ striking
    - ▸ bottom W16.022-
      - ✦ causing drowning W16.021-
    - ▸ wall W16.032-
      - ✦ causing drowning W16.031-
- utility bucket W16.222-
  - ◊ causing drowning W16.221-
- well W17.0-
- involving
  - bed W06.-
  - chair W07.-
  - furniture NEC W08.-
  - glass—*see* Fall, by type
  - playground equipment W09.8-
    - jungle gym W09.2-
    - slide W09.0-
    - swing W09.1-
  - roller blades—*see* Accident, transport, pedestrian, conveyance
  - skateboard(s)—*see* Accident, transport, pedestrian, conveyance
  - skates (ice) (in line) (roller)—*see* Accident, transport, pedestrian, conveyance
  - skis—*see* Accident, transport, pedestrian, conveyance
  - table W08.-
  - wheelchair, non-moving W05.0-
    - powered—*see* Accident, transport, pedestrian, conveyance, specified type NEC
- object—*see* Struck by, object, falling
- off
  - toilet W18.11-
    - with subsequent striking against object W18.12-
- on same level W18.30-
  - due to
    - specified NEC W18.39-
    - stepping on an object W18.31-
- out of
  - bed W06.-
  - building NEC W13.8-
  - chair W07.-
  - furniture NEC W08.-
  - wheelchair, non-moving W05.0-
    - powered—*see* Accident, transport, pedestrian, conveyance, specified type NEC
  - window W13.4-
- over
  - animal W01.0-
  - cliff W15.-
  - embankment W17.81-
  - small object W01.0-
- rock W20.8-
- same level W18.30-
  - from
    - being crushed, pushed, or stepped on by a crowd or human stampede W52.-
    - collision, pushing, shoving, by or with other person W03.-
    - slipping, stumbling, tripping W01.0-
  - involving ice or snow W00.0-
    - involving skates (ice) (roller), skateboard, skis—*see* Accident, transport, pedestrian, conveyance
- snowslide (avalanche)—*see* Landslide
- stone W20.8-

Fall, falling (accidental), *continued*

- structure W20.1-
  - burning (uncontrolled fire) X00.3-
- through
  - bridge W13.1-
  - floor W13.3-
  - roof W13.2-
  - wall W13.8-
  - window W13.4-
- timber W20.8-
- tree (caused by lightning) W20.8-
- while being carried or supported by other person(s) W04.-

Fallen on by

- animal (not being ridden) NEC W55.89-

Felo-de-se—*see* Suicide

Fight (hand) (fists) (foot)—*see* Assault, fight

Fire (accidental)—*see* Exposure, fire

Firearm discharge—*see* Discharge, firearm

Fireworks (explosion) W39.-

Flail chest associated with chest compression M96.A4

Flash burns from explosion—*see* Explosion

Flood (any injury) (caused by) X38.-

- collapse of man-made structure causing earth movement X36.0-
- tidal wave—*see* Forces of nature, tidal wave

Food (any type) in

- air passages (with asphyxia, obstruction, or suffocation) (*see* categories T17 and) T18
- alimentary tract causing asphyxia (due to compression of trachea) (*see* categories T17 and) T18

Forces of nature X39.8-

- avalanche X36.1-
  - causing transport accident—*see* Accident, transport, by type of vehicle
- blizzard X37.2-
- cataclysmic storm X37.9-
  - with flood X38.-
  - blizzard X37.2-
  - cloudburst X37.8-
  - cyclone X37.1-
  - dust storm X37.3-
  - hurricane X37.0-
  - specified storm NEC X37.8-
  - storm surge X37.0-
  - tornado X37.1-
  - twister X37.1-
  - typhoon X37.0-
- cloudburst X37.8-
- cold (natural) X31.-
- cyclone X37.1-
- dam collapse causing earth movement X36.0-
- dust storm X37.3-
- earth movement X36.1-
  - caused by dam or structure collapse X36.0-
  - earthquake X34.-
- earthquake X34.-
- flood (caused by) X38.-
  - dam collapse X36.0-
  - tidal wave—*see* Forces of nature, tidal wave
- heat (natural) X30.-
- hurricane X37.0-
- landslide X36.1-
  - causing transport accident—*see* Accident, transport, by type of vehicle
- lightning—*see* subcategory T75.0-
  - causing fire—*see* Exposure, fire
- mudslide X36.1-
  - causing transport accident—*see* Accident, transport, by type of vehicle
- specified force NEC X39.8-
- storm surge X37.0-
- structure collapse causing earth movement X36.0-
- sunlight X32.-
- tidal wave X37.41-
  - due to
    - earthquake X37.41-
    - landslide X37.43-
    - storm X37.42-
- volcanic eruption X37.41-

Forces of nature, *continued*

- tornado X37.1-
- tsunami X37.41-
- twister X37.1-
- typhoon X37.0-
- volcanic eruption X35.-

Foreign body

- aspiration—*see* Index to Diseases and Injuries, Foreign body, respiratory tract
- entering through skin W45.8-
  - can lid W26.8-
  - nail W45.0-
  - paper W26.2-
  - specified NEC W45.8-
  - splinter W45.8-

Forest fire (exposure to)—*see* Exposure, fire, uncontrolled, not in building

Found injured X58.-

- from exposure (to)—*see* Exposure
- on
  - highway, road (way), street V89.9-
  - railway right of way V81.9-

Fracture

- associated with chest compression
  - multiple ribs M96.A3
  - one rib M96.A2
  - other M96.A9
  - sternum M96.A1
- circumstances unknown or unspecified X58.-
- due to specified cause NEC X58.-

Frostbite X31.-

- due to man-made conditions—*see* Exposure, cold, man-made

Frozen—*see* Exposure, cold

G

Gunshot wound W34.00-

H

Hailstones, injured by X39.8-

Hanged herself or himself—*see* Hanging, self-inflicted

Hanging (accidental) (*see also* category) T71

Heat (effects of) (excessive) X30.-

- due to
  - man-made conditions
    - on board watercraft V93.29-
      - fishing boat V93.22-
      - merchant ship V93.20-
      - passenger ship V93.21-
      - sailboat V93.24-
      - specified powered craft NEC V93.23-
  - weather (conditions) X30.-
- from
  - electric heating apparatus causing burning X16.-
  - inappropriate in local application or packing in medical or surgical procedure Y63.5-

Hemorrhage

- delayed following medical or surgical treatment without mention of misadventure—*see* Index to Diseases and Injuries, Complication(s)
- during medical or surgical treatment as misadventure—*see* Index to Diseases and Injuries, Complication(s)

High

- altitude (effects)—*see* Air, pressure, low
- level of radioactivity, effects—*see* Radiation
- pressure (effects)—*see* Air, pressure, high
- temperature, effects—*see* Heat

Hit, hitting (accidental) by—*see* Struck by

Hitting against—*see* Striking against

Hot

- place, effects—*see also* Heat
- weather, effects X30.-

House fire (uncontrolled)—*see* Exposure, fire, uncontrolled, building

Humidity, causing problem X39.8-

Hunger X58.-

Hurricane (any injury) X37.0-

Hypobarism, hypobaropathy—*see* Air, pressure, low

I

Ictus

- caloris—*see also* Heat
- solaris X30.-

Ignition (accidental) (*see also* Exposure, fire) X08.8-

- anesthetic gas in operating room W40.1-
- apparel X06.2-
  - from highly flammable material X04.-
  - nightwear X05.-
- bed linen (sheets) (spreads) (pillows) (mattress)—*see* Exposure, fire, uncontrolled, building, bed
- benzine X04.-
- clothes, clothing NEC (from controlled fire) X06.2-
  - from
    - highly flammable material X04.-
  - ether X04.-
  - in operating room W40.1-
  - explosive material—*see* Explosion
  - gasoline X04.-
  - jewelry (plastic) (any) X06.0-
  - kerosene X04.-
  - material
    - explosive—*see* Explosion
    - highly flammable with secondary explosion X04.-
  - nightwear X05.-
  - paraffin X04.-
  - petrol X04.-

Immersion (accidental)—*see also* Drowning

- hand or foot due to cold (excessive) X31.-

Implantation of quills of porcupine W55.89-

Inanition (from) (hunger) X58.-

- thirst X58.-

Inappropriate operation performed

- correct operation on wrong side or body part (wrong side) (wrong site) Y65.53-
- operation intended for another patient done on wrong patient Y65.52-
- wrong operation performed on correct patient Y65.51-

Incident, adverse

- device
  - anesthesiology Y70.-
  - cardiovascular Y71.-
  - gastroenterology Y73.-
  - general
    - hospital Y74.-
    - surgical Y81.-
  - gynecological Y76.-
  - medical Y82.9-
    - specified type NEC Y82.8-
  - neurological Y75.-
  - obstetrical Y76.-
  - ophthalmic Y77.-
  - orthopedic Y79.-
  - otorhinolaryngological Y72.-
  - personal use Y74.-
  - physical medicine Y80.-
  - plastic surgical Y81.-
  - radiological Y78.-
  - urology Y73.-

Incineration (accidental)—*see* Exposure, fire

Infanticide—*see* Assault

Infrasound waves (causing injury) W49.9-

Ingestion

- foreign body (causing injury) (with obstruction) T17 or T18
- poisonous
  - plant(s) X58.-
  - substance NEC—*see* Table of Drugs and Chemicals

Inhalation

- excessively cold substance, man-made—*see* Exposure, cold, man-made
- food (any type) (into respiratory tract) (with asphyxia, obstruction respiratory tract, suffocation) (*see* categories T17 and) T18
- foreign body—*see* Foreign body, aspiration

ICD-10-CM EXTERNAL CAUSE OF INJURIES INDEX

Inhalation, *continued*

- gastric contents (with asphyxia, obstruction respiratory passage, suffocation) T17.81-
- liquid air, hydrogen, nitrogen W93.12-
- steam X13.0-
  - assault X98.0-
  - stated as undetermined whether accidental or intentional Y27.0-
- toxic gas—*see* Table of Drugs and Chemicals
- vomitus (with asphyxia, obstruction respiratory passage, suffocation) T17.81-

Injury, injured (accidental(ly)) NOS X58.-

- by, caused by, from
  - assault—*see* Assault
- homicide (*see also* Assault) Y09.-
- inflicted (by)
  - other person
    - stated as
      - accidental X58.-
      - undetermined whether accidental or intentional Y33.-
  - purposely (inflicted) by other person(s)—*see* Assault
  - self-inflicted X83.8-
    - stated as accidental X58.-
    - specified cause NEC X58.-
    - undetermined whether accidental or intentional Y33.-

Insolation, effects X30.-

Insufficient nourishment X58.-

Interruption of respiration (by)

- food (lodged in esophagus) (*see* categories T17 and) T18
- vomitus (lodged in esophagus) T17.81-

Intoxication

- drug—*see* Table of Drugs and Chemicals
- poison—*see* Table of Drugs and Chemicals

J

Jammed (accidentally)

- between objects (moving) (stationary and moving) W23.0-
  - stationary W23.1-

Jumped, jumping

- before moving object NEC X81.8-
  - motor vehicle X81.0-
  - subway train X81.1-
  - train X81.1-
  - undetermined whether accidental or intentional Y31
- from
  - boat (into water) voluntarily, without accident (to or on boat) W16.712-
  - with
    - accident to or on boat—*see* Accident, watercraft
    - drowning or submersion W16.711-
    - striking bottom W16.722-
      - causing drowning W16.721-
  - building (*see also* Jumped, from, high place) W13.9-
    - burning (uncontrolled fire) X00.5-
    - high place NEC W17.89-
      - suicide (attempt) X80.-
      - undetermined whether accidental or intentional Y30.-
  - structure (*see also* Jumped, from, high place) W13.9-
    - burning (uncontrolled fire) X00.5-
- into water W16.92-
  - causing drowning W16.91-
  - from, off watercraft—*see* Jumped, from, boat
  - in
    - natural body W16.612-
      - causing drowning W16.611-
      - striking bottom W16.622-
        - ◊ causing drowning W16.621-
    - specified place NEC W16.812-
      - causing drowning W16.811-
      - striking
        - ◊ bottom W16.822-
          - » causing drowning W16.821-
        - ◊ wall W16.832-
          - » causing drowning W16.831-

Jumped, jumping, *continued*

- swimming pool W16.512-
  - causing drowning W16.511-
  - striking
    - ◊ bottom W16.522-
      - » causing drowning W16.521-
    - ◊ wall W16.532-
      - » causing drowning W16.531-

K

Kicked by

- animal NEC W55.82-
- person(s) (accidentally) W50.1-
  - with intent to injure or kill Y04.0-
  - as, or caused by, a crowd or human stampede (with fall) W52.-
  - assault Y04.0-
  - in
    - fight Y04.0-

Kicking against

- object W22.8-
  - sports equipment W21.9-
  - stationary W22.09-
    - sports equipment W21.89-
- person—*see* Striking against, person
- sports equipment W21.9-

Knocked down (accidentally) (by) NOS X58.-

- animal (not being ridden) NEC—*see also* Struck by, by type of animal
- crowd or human stampede W52.-
- person W51.-
  - in brawl, fight Y04.0-
- transport vehicle NEC (*see also* Accident, transport) V09.9-

L

Laceration NEC—*see* Injury

Lack of

- care (helpless person) (infant) (newborn) X58.-
- food except as result of abandonment or neglect X58.-
  - due to abandonment or neglect X58.-
- water except as result of transport accident X58.-
  - due to transport accident—*see* Accident, transport, by type
  - helpless person, infant, newborn X58.-

Landslide (falling on transport vehicle) X36.1-

- caused by collapse of man-made structure X36.0-

Late effect—*see* Sequelae

Lightning (shock) (stroke) (struck by)—*see* subcategory T75.0-

- causing fire—*see* Exposure, fire

Long term use (current)

- alkylating agent Z79.630
- antimetabolite agent Z79.631
- antitumor antibiotic Z79.632
- calcineurin inhibitor Z79.621
- immunomodulator Z79.61
- immunosuppressive biologic Z79.620
- inhibitors of nucleotide synthesis Z79.624
- injectable non-insulin antidiabetic drugs Z79.85
- Janus kinase inhibitor Z79.622
- mammalian target of rapamycin (mTOR) inhibitor Z79.623
- mitotic inhibitor Z79.633
- myelosuppressive agent Z79.64
- other immunomodulators and immunosuppressants Z79.69
- topoisomerase inhibitor Z79.634
- unspecified immunomodulators and immunosuppressants Z79.60

Loss of control (transport vehicle) NEC—*see* Accident, transport

Lying before train, vehicle or other moving object X81.8-

- subway train X81.1-
- train X81.1-
- undetermined whether accidental or intentional Y31

M

Malfunction (mechanism or component) (of)

- firearm W34.10-
  - airgun W34.110-
  - BB gun W34.110-
  - gas, air or spring-operated gun NEC W34.118-
  - handgun W32.1-
  - hunting rifle W33.12-
  - larger firearm W33.10-
    - specified NEC W33.19-
    - machine gun W33.13-
  - paintball gun W34.111-
  - pellet gun W34.110-
  - shotgun W33.11-
  - specified NEC W34.19-
  - Very pistol [flare] W34.19-
- handgun—*see* Malfunction, firearm, handgun

Maltreatment—*see* Perpetrator

Mangled (accidentally) NOS X58.-

Manhandling (in brawl, fight) Y04.0-

Manslaughter (nonaccidental)—*see* Assault

Mauled by animal NEC W55.89-

Medical procedure, complication of (delayed or as an abnormal reaction without mention of misadventure)—*see* Complication of or following, by specified type of procedure

- due to or as a result of misadventure—*see* Misadventure

Melting (due to fire)—*see also* Exposure, fire

- apparel NEC X06.3-
- clothes, clothing NEC X06.3-
  - nightwear X05.-
- fittings or furniture (burning building) (uncontrolled fire) X00.8-
  - nightwear X05.-
- plastic jewelry X06.1-

Mental cruelty X58.-

Military operations (injuries to military and civilians occurring during peacetime on military property and during routine military exercises and operations) (by) (from) (involving)—*Refer to ICD-10-CM Manual*

Misadventure(s) to patient(s) during surgical or medical care Y69.-

- contaminated medical or biological substance (blood, drug, fluid) Y64.9-
  - administered (by) NEC Y64.9-
    - immunization Y64.1-
    - infusion Y64.0-
    - injection Y64.1-
    - specified means NEC Y64.8-
    - transfusion Y64.0-
    - vaccination Y64.1-
- excessive amount of blood or other fluid during transfusion or infusion Y63.0-
- failure
  - in dosage Y63.9-
    - electroshock therapy Y63.4-
    - inappropriate temperature (too hot or too cold) in local application and packing Y63.5-
    - infusion
      - excessive amount of fluid Y63.0-
      - incorrect dilution of fluid Y63.1-
    - insulin-shock therapy Y63.4-
    - nonadministration of necessary drug or biological substance Y63.6-
    - overdose—*see* Table of Drugs and Chemicals
      - radiation, in therapy Y63.2-
      - radiation
      - overdose Y63.2-
    - specified procedure NEC Y63.8-
    - transfusion
      - excessive amount of blood Y63.0-
  - mechanical, of instrument or apparatus (any) (during any procedure) Y65.8-
  - sterile precautions (during procedure) Y62.9-
    - aspiration of fluid or tissue (by puncture or catheterization, except heart) Y62.6-
    - biopsy (except needle aspiration) Y62.8-
      - needle (aspirating) Y62.6-
    - blood sampling Y62.6-

Misadventure(s) to patient(s) during surgical or medical care, *continued*

- ■ catheterization Y62.6-
  - heart Y62.5-
- ■ dialysis (kidney) Y62.2-
- ■ endoscopic examination Y62.4-
- ■ enema Y62.8-
- ■ immunization Y62.3-
- ■ infusion Y62.1-
- ■ injection Y62.3-
- ■ needle biopsy Y62.6-
- ■ paracentesis (abdominal) (thoracic) Y62.6-
- ■ perfusion Y62.2-
- ■ puncture (lumbar) Y62.6-
- ■ removal of catheter or packing Y62.8-
- ■ specified procedure NEC Y62.8-
- ■ surgical operation Y62.0-
- ■ transfusion Y62.1-
- ■ vaccination Y62.3-
- suture or ligature during surgical procedure Y65.2-
- to introduce or to remove tube or instrument—*see* Failure, to
- hemorrhage—*see* Index to Diseases and Injuries, Complication(s)
- inadvertent exposure of patient to radiation Y63.3-
- inappropriate
  - operation performed—*see* Inappropriate operation performed
  - temperature (too hot or too cold) in local application or packing Y63.5-
- infusion (*see also* Misadventure, by type, infusion) Y69.-
  - excessive amount of fluid Y63.0-
  - incorrect dilution of fluid Y63.1-
  - wrong fluid Y65.1-
- nonadministration of necessary drug or biological substance Y63.6-
- overdose—*see* Table of Drugs and Chemicals
  - radiation (in therapy) Y63.2-
- perforation—*see* Index to Diseases and Injuries, Complication(s)
- performance of inappropriate operation—*see* Inappropriate operation performed
- puncture—*see* Index to Diseases and Injuries, Complication(s)
- specified type NEC Y65.8-
  - failure
    - ■ suture or ligature during surgical operation Y65.2-
    - ■ to introduce or to remove tube or instrument—*see* Failure, to
  - infusion of wrong fluid Y65.1-
  - performance of inappropriate operation—*see* Inappropriate operation performed
  - transfusion of mismatched blood Y65.0-
  - wrong
    - ■ fluid in infusion Y65.1-
    - ■ placement of endotracheal tube during anesthetic procedure Y65.3-
- transfusion—*see* Misadventure, by type, transfusion
  - excessive amount of blood Y63.0-
  - mismatched blood Y65.0-
- wrong
  - drug given in error—*see* Table of Drugs and Chemicals
  - fluid in infusion Y65.1-
  - placement of endotracheal tube during anesthetic procedure Y65.3-

Mismatched blood in transfusion Y65.0-

Motion sickness T75.3-

Mountain sickness W94.11-

Mudslide (of cataclysmic nature)—*see* Landslide

N

Nail, contact with W45.0-
- gun W29.4-

Noise (causing injury) (pollution) W42.9-
- supersonic W42.0-

Nonadministration (of)
- drug or biological substance (necessary) Y63.6-
- surgical and medical care Y66.-

Noncollision—*see* Accident, transport
- nontraffic accident
  - electric (assisted) bicycle driver V28.01-
  - electric (assisted) bicycle passenger V28.11-
  - other motorcycle driver V28.09-
  - other motorcycle passenger V28.19-
  - unspecified electric (assisted) bicycle rider V28.21-
  - unspecified rider of other motorcycle V28.29-
- person boarding, alighting an electric (assisted) bicycle V28.31-
- person boarding, alighting other motorcycle V28.39-
- traffic accident
  - electric (assisted) bicycle driver V28.41-
  - electric (assisted) bicycle passenger V28.51-
  - other motorcycle driver V28.49-
  - other motorcycle passenger V28.59-
  - unspecified electric (assisted) bicycle rider V28.91-
  - unspecified rider of other motorcycle V28.99-

Nosocomial condition Y95.-

O

Object
- falling
  - from, in, on, hitting
    - ■ machinery—*see* Contact, with, by type of machine
- set in motion by
  - accidental explosion or rupture of pressure vessel W38.-
  - firearm—*see* Discharge, firearm, by type
  - machine(ry)—*see* Contact, with, by type of machine

Overdose (drug)—*see* Table of Drugs and Chemicals
- radiation Y63.2-

Overexertion
- due to
  - other or unspecified movement X50.9-
  - prolonged static or awkward postures X50.1-
  - repetitive movements X50.3-
  - strenuous movement X50.0-

Overexposure (accidental) (to)
- cold (*see also* Exposure, cold) X31.-
  - due to man-made conditions—*see* Exposure, cold, man-made
- heat (*see also* Heat) X30.-
- radiation—*see* Radiation
- sun (sunburn) X32.-
- weather NEC—*see* Forces of nature
- wind NEC—*see* Forces of nature

Overheated—*see* Heat

Overturning (accidental)
- machinery—*see* Contact, with, by type of machine
- transport vehicle NEC (*see also* Accident, transport) V89.9-
- watercraft (causing drowning, submersion)—*see also* Drowning, due to, accident to, watercraft, overturning
  - causing injury except drowning or submersion—*see* Accident, watercraft, causing, injury NEC

P

Parachute descent (voluntary) (without accident to aircraft) V97.29-
- due to accident to aircraft—*see* Accident, transport, aircraft

Pecked by bird W61.99-

Perforation during medical or surgical treatment as misadventure—*see* Index to Diseases and Injuries, Complication(s)

Perpetrator, perpetration, of assault, maltreatment and neglect (by) Y07.-

Piercing—*see* Contact, with, by type of object or machine

Pinched
- between objects (moving) (stationary and moving) W23.0-
  - stationary W23.1-

Pinned under machine(ry)—*see* Contact, with, by type of machine

Place of occurrence Y92.9
- abandoned house Y92.89
- airplane Y92.813

Place of occurrence, *continued*
- airport Y92.520
- ambulatory health services establishment NEC Y92.538
- ambulatory surgery center Y92.530
- amusement park Y92.831
- apartment (co-op) Y92.039
  - bathroom Y92.031
  - bedroom Y92.032
  - kitchen Y92.030
  - specified NEC Y92.038
- assembly hall Y92.29
- bank Y92.510
- barn Y92.71
- baseball field Y92.320
- basketball court Y92.310
- beach Y92.832
- boat Y92.814
- bowling alley Y92.39
- bridge Y92.89
- building under construction Y92.61
- bus Y92.811
  - station Y92.521
- cafe Y92.511
- campsite Y92.833
- campus—*see* Place of occurrence, school
- canal Y92.89
- car Y92.810
- casino Y92.59
- church Y92.22
- cinema Y92.26
- clubhouse Y92.29
- coal pit Y92.64
- college (community) Y92.214
- condominium—*see* apartment
- construction area—Y92.6-
- convalescent home—Y92.129
- court-house Y92.240
- cricket ground Y92.328
- cultural building Y92.25-
- dancehall Y92.252
- day nursery Y92.210
- dentist office Y92.531
- derelict house Y92.89
- desert Y92.820
- dock NOS Y92.89
- dockyard Y92.62
- doctor's office Y92.531
- dormitory—*see* institutional, school dormitory
- dry dock Y92.62
- factory (building) (premises) Y92.63
- farm (land under cultivation) (outbuildings) Y92.7-
- football field Y92.321
- forest Y92.821
- freeway Y92.411
- gallery Y92.250
- garage (commercial) Y92.59 (refer to specific residence)
- gas station Y92.524
- gasworks Y92.69
- golf course Y92.39
- gravel pit Y92.64
- grocery Y92.512
- gymnasium Y92.39
- handball court Y92.318
- harbor Y92.89
- harness racing course Y92.39
- healthcare provider office Y92.531
- highway (interstate) Y92.411
- hill Y92.828
- hockey rink Y92.330
- home—*see* residence
- hospice—Y92.129
- hospital Y92.23-
  - patient room Y92.23-
- hotel Y92.59
- house—*see also* residence
  - abandoned Y92.89
  - under construction Y92.61
- industrial and construction area (yard) Y92.6-
- kindergarten Y92.211
- lacrosse field Y92.328
- lake Y92.828
- library Y92.241
- mall Y92.59

ICD-10-CM EXTERNAL CAUSE OF INJURIES INDEX

Place of occurrence, *continued*

- market Y92.512
- marsh Y92.828
- mosque Y92.22
- motel Y92.59
- motorway (interstate) Y92.411
- mountain Y92.828
- movie-house Y92.26
- museum Y92.251
- music-hall Y92.252
- not applicable Y92.9
- nuclear power station Y92.69
- nursing home—Y92.129
- office building Y92.59
- offshore installation Y92.65
- opera-house Y92.253
- orphanage—Y92.11-
- outpatient surgery center Y92.530
- park (public) Y92.830
  - amusement Y92.831
- parking garage Y92.89
  - lot Y92.481
- pavement Y92.480
- physician office Y92.531
- polo field Y92.328
- pond Y92.828
- post office Y92.242
- power station Y92.69
- prairie Y92.828
- public
  - administration building Y92.24-
  - building NEC Y92.29
  - hall Y92.29
  - place NOS Y92.89
- race course Y92.39
- railway line (bridge) Y92.85
- ranch (outbuildings) Y92.7-
- recreation area Y92.838 (refer to specific sites)
- religious institution Y92.22
- reform school—*see* institutional, reform school
- residence (non-institutional) (private) Y92.009
  - apartment Y92.039
    - bathroom Y92.031
    - bedroom Y92.032
    - kitchen Y92.030
    - specified NEC Y92.038
  - boarding house Y92.04-
  - home, unspecified Y92.009
    - bathroom Y92.002
    - bedroom Y92.003
    - dining room Y92.001
    - garden Y92.007
    - kitchen Y92.000
  - house, single family Y92.019
    - bathroom Y92.012
    - bedroom Y92.013
    - dining room Y92.011
    - driveway Y92.014
    - garage Y92.015
    - garden Y92.017
    - kitchen Y92.010
    - specified NEC Y92.018
    - swimming pool Y92.016
    - yard Y92.017
  - institutional Y92.10-
    - hospice Y92.12-
    - nursing home Y92.12-
    - orphanage Y92.119
      - bathroom Y92.111
      - bedroom Y92.112
      - driveway Y92.113
      - garage Y92.114
      - garden Y92.116
      - kitchen Y92.110
      - specified NEC Y92.118
      - swimming pool Y92.115
      - yard Y92.116
    - reform school Y92.15-
    - school dormitory Y92.169
      - bathroom Y92.162
      - bedroom Y92.163
      - dining room Y92.161

Place of occurrence, *continued*

  - kitchen Y92.160
  - specified NEC Y92.168
- specified NEC Y92.19-
- mobile home Y92.029
  - bathroom Y92.022
  - bedroom Y92.023
  - dining room Y92.021
  - driveway Y92.024
  - garage Y92.025
  - garden Y92.027
  - kitchen Y92.020
  - specified NEC Y92.028
  - swimming pool Y92.026
  - yard Y92.027
- specified place in residence NEC Y92.008
- specified residence type NEC Y92.09-
- restaurant Y92.511
- riding school Y92.39
- river Y92.828
- road Y92.410
- rodeo ring Y92.39
- rugby field Y92.328
- same day surgery center Y92.530
- sand pit Y92.64
- school (private) (public) (state) Y92.219
  - college Y92.214
  - daycare center Y92.210
  - elementary school Y92.211
  - high school Y92.213
  - kindergarten Y92.211
  - middle school Y92.212
  - specified NEC Y92.218
  - trade school Y92.215
  - university Y92.214
  - vocational school Y92.215
- sea (shore) Y92.832
- senior citizen center Y92.29
- service area (refer to specific site)
- shipyard Y92.62
- shop (commercial) Y92.513
- sidewalk Y92.480
- skating rink (roller) Y92.331
  - ice Y92.330
- soccer field Y92.322
- specified place NEC Y92.89
- sports area Y92.39 (also refer to specific sites)
  - athletic
    - court Y92.31-
    - field Y92.32-
  - golf course Y92.39
  - gymnasium Y92.39
  - riding school Y92.39
  - stadium Y92.39
  - swimming pool Y92.34
- squash court Y92.311
- stadium Y92.39
- steeple chasing course Y92.39
- store Y92.512
- stream Y92.828
- street and highway Y92.410
  - bike path Y92.482
  - freeway Y92.411
  - highway ramp Y92.415
  - interstate highway Y92.411
  - local residential or business street Y92.414
  - motorway Y92.411
  - parking lot Y92.481
  - parkway Y92.412
  - sidewalk Y92.480
  - specified NEC Y92.488
  - state road Y92.413
- subway car Y92.816
- supermarket Y92.512
- swamp Y92.828
- swimming pool (public) Y92.34
  - private (at) Y92.095 (refer to specific residence)
- synagogue Y92.22
- tennis court Y92.312
- theater Y92.254
- trade area Y92.59 (refer to specific site)
- trailer park, residential—*see* mobile home
- trailer site NOS Y92.89

Place of occurrence, *continued*

- train Y92.815
  - station Y92.522
- truck Y92.812
- tunnel under construction Y92.69
- urgent (health) care center Y92.532
- university Y92.214
- vehicle (transport) Y92.818
  - airplane Y92.813
  - boat Y92.814
  - bus Y92.811
  - car Y92.810
  - specified NEC Y92.818
  - subway car Y92.816
  - train Y92.815
  - truck Y92.812
- warehouse Y92.59
- water reservoir Y92.89
- wilderness area Y92.82-
- workshop Y92.69
- yard, private Y92.096 (refer to specific residence)
- youth center Y92.29
- zoo (zoological garden) Y92.834

Poisoning (accidental) (by)—*see also* Table of Drugs and Chemicals

- by plant, thorns, spines, sharp leaves or other mechanisms NEC X58.-
- carbon monoxide
  - generated by
    - motor vehicle—*see* Accident, transport
    - watercraft (in transit) (not in transit) V93.8-
- caused by injection of poisons into skin by plant thorns, spines, sharp leaves X58.-
- marine or sea plants (venomous) X58.-
- exhaust gas
  - generated by
    - motor vehicle—*see* Accident, transport
    - watercraft (in transit) (not in transit) V93.89-
      - ferry boat V93.81-
      - fishing boat V93.82-
      - jet skis V93.83-
      - liner V93.81-
      - merchant ship V93.80-
      - passenger ship V93.81-
      - powered craft NEC V93.83-
- fumes or smoke due to
  - explosion (*see also* Explosion) W40.9-
  - fire—*see* Exposure, fire
  - ignition—*see* Ignition

Powder burn (by) (from)

- airgun W34.110-
- BB gun W34.110-
- firearm NEC W34.19-
- gas, air or spring-operated gun NEC W34.118-
- handgun W32.1-
- hunting rifle W33.12-
- larger firearm W33.10-
  - specified NEC W33.19-
- machine gun W33.13-
- paintball gun W34.111-
- pellet gun W34.110-
- shotgun W33.11-
- Very pistol [flare] W34.19-

Premature cessation (of) surgical and medical care Y66.-

Privation (food) (water) X58.-

Procedure (operation)

- correct, on wrong side or body part (wrong side) (wrong site) Y65.53-
- intended for another patient done on wrong patient Y65.52-
- performed on patient not scheduled for surgery Y65.52-
- performed on wrong patient Y65.52-
- wrong, performed on correct patient Y65.51-

Prolonged

- sitting in transport vehicle—*see* Travel, by type of vehicle
- stay in
  - high altitude as cause of anoxia, barodontalgia, barotitis or hypoxia W94.11-

Pulling, excessive—*see* category Y93

Puncture, puncturing—*see also* Contact, with, by type of object or machine
- by
  - plant thorns, spines, sharp leaves or other mechanisms NEC W60.-
- during medical or surgical treatment as misadventure—*see* Index to Diseases and Injuries, Complication(s)

Pushed, pushing (accidental) (injury in) (overexertion)—*see* category Y93
- by other person(s) (accidentally) W51.-
  - with fall W03.-
    - due to ice or snow W00.0-
  - as, or caused by, a crowd or human stampede (with fall) W52.-
  - before moving object NEC Y02.8-
    - motor vehicle Y02.0-
    - subway train Y02.1-
    - train Y02.1-
  - from
    - high place NEC
      - in accidental circumstances W17.89-
      - stated as
        - ◊ intentional, homicide (attempt) Y01.-
        - ◊ undetermined whether accidental or intentional Y30.-
    - transport vehicle NEC (*see also* Accident, transport) V89.9-

R

Radiation (exposure to) (refer to *ICD-10-CM* manual for more)
- light sources (man-made visible and ultraviolet)
  - natural X32.-
- misadventure in medical or surgical procedure Y63.2-
- natural NEC X39.08-
- overdose (in medical or surgical procedure) Y63.2-
- sun X32.-
- ultraviolet (light) (man-made)
  - natural X32.-

Range disease W94.11-

Rape (attempted) (confirmed) T74.2-
- suspected T76.2-

Rat bite W53.11

Reaction, abnormal to medical procedure (*see also* Complication of or following, by type of procedure) Y84.9
- with misadventure—*see* Misadventure
- biologicals or drugs or vaccine—*see* Table of Drugs and Chemicals

Recoil
- airgun W34.110-
- BB gun W34.110-
- firearm NEC W34.19-
- gas, air or spring-operated gun NEC W34.118-
- handgun W32.1-
- hunting rifle W33.12-
- larger firearm W33.10-
  - specified NEC W33.19-
- machine gun W33.13-
- paintball gun W34.111-
- pellet T34.110-
- shotgun W33.11-
- Very pistol [flare] W34.19-

Reduction in
- atmospheric pressure—*see* Air, pressure, change

Rock falling on or hitting (accidentally) (person) W20.8-
- in cave-in W20.0-

Run over (accidentally) (by)
- animal (not being ridden) NEC W55.89-
- machinery—*see* Contact, with, by specified type of machine
- transport vehicle NEC (*see also* Accident, transport) V09.9-
  - motor NEC V09.20-

Running
- before moving object X81.8-
  - motor vehicle X81.0-

Running off, away
- animal (being ridden) (*see also* Accident, transport) V80.918-
  - not being ridden W55.89-
- animal-drawn vehicle NEC (*see also* Accident, transport) V80.928-
- highway, road (way), street
  - transport vehicle NEC (*see also* Accident, transport) V89.9-

Rupture pressurized devices—*see* Explosion, by type of device

S

Saturnism—*see* Table of Drugs and Chemicals, lead

Scald, scalding (accidental) (by) (from) (in) X19.-
- liquid (boiling) (hot) NEC X12.-
  - stated as undetermined whether accidental or intentional Y27.2-
- local application of externally applied substance in medical or surgical care Y63.5-
- metal (molten) (liquid) (hot) NEC X18.-
- self-inflicted X77.9-
  - stated as undetermined whether accidental or intentional Y27.8-
- steam X13.1-
  - assault X98.0-
  - stated as undetermined whether accidental or intentional Y27.0-
- vapor (hot) X13.1-
  - assault X98.0-
  - stated as undetermined whether accidental or intentional Y27.0-

Scratched by
- cat W55.03-
- person(s) (accidentally) W50.4-
  - with intent to injure or kill Y04.0-
  - as, or caused by, a crowd or human stampede (with fall) W52.-
  - assault Y04.0-
  - in
    - fight Y04.0-

Seasickness T75.3-

Self-harm NEC—*see also* External cause by type, undetermined whether accidental or intentional
- intentional—*see* Suicide
- poisoning NEC—*see* Table of Drugs and Chemicals

Self-inflicted (injury) NEC—*see also* External cause by type, undetermined whether accidental or intentional
- intentional—*see* Suicide
- poisoning NEC—*see* Table of Drugs and Chemicals

Sequelae (of)
Use original code to define how the injury occurred with 7th character S

Shock
- electric—*see* Exposure, electric current
- from electric appliance (any) (faulty) W86.8-
  - domestic W86.0-

Shooting, shot (accidental(ly))—*see also* Discharge, firearm, by type
- herself or himself—*see* Discharge, firearm by type, self-inflicted
- inflicted by other person—*see* Discharge, firearm by type, homicide
  - accidental—*see* Discharge, firearm, by type of firearm
- self-inflicted—*see* Discharge, firearm by type, suicide
  - accidental—*see* Discharge, firearm, by type of firearm
- suicide (attempt)—*see* Discharge, firearm by type, suicide

Shoving (accidentally) by other person—*see* Pushed, by other person

Sickness
- alpine W94.11-
- motion—*see* Motion
- mountain W94.11-

Sinking (accidental)
- watercraft (causing drowning, submersion)—*see also* Drowning, due to, accident to, watercraft, sinking
  - causing injury except drowning or submersion—*see* Accident, watercraft, causing, injury NEC

Siriasis X32.-

Slashed wrists—*see* Cut, self-inflicted

Slipping (accidental) (on same level) (with fall) W01.0-
- on
  - ice W00.0-
    - with skates—*see* Accident, transport, pedestrian, conveyance
  - mud W01.0-
  - oil W01.0-
  - snow W00.0-
    - with skis—*see* Accident, transport, pedestrian, conveyance
  - surface (slippery) (wet) NEC W01.0-
- without fall W18.40-
  - due to
    - specified NEC W18.49-
    - stepping from one level to another W18.43-
    - stepping into hole or opening W18.42-
    - stepping on object W18.41-

Sliver, wood, contact with W45.8-

Smoldering (due to fire)—*see* Exposure, fire

Sodomy (attempted) by force T74.2-

Sound waves (causing injury) W42.9-
- supersonic W42.0-

Splinter, contact with W45.8-

Stab, stabbing—*see* Cut

Starvation X58.-

Status of external cause Y99.-

Stepped on
- by
  - animal (not being ridden) NEC W55.89-
  - crowd or human stampede W52.-
  - person W50.0-

Stepping on
- object W22.8-
  - with fall W18.31-
  - sports equipment W21.9-
  - stationary W22.09-
    - sports equipment W21.89-
- person W51.-
  - by crowd or human stampede W52.-
  - sports equipment W21.9-

Sting
- arthropod, nonvenomous W57.-
- insect, nonvenomous W57.-

Storm (cataclysmic)—*see* Forces of nature, cataclysmic storm

Straining, excessive—*see* category Y93

Strangling—*see* Strangulation

Strangulation (accidental)—*see* category T71

Strenuous movements—*see* category Y93

Striking against
- airbag (automobile) W22.10-
  - driver side W22.11-
  - front passenger side W22.12-
  - specified NEC W22.19-
- bottom when
  - diving or jumping into water (in) W16.822-
    - causing drowning W16.821-
  - from boat W16.722-
    - causing drowning W16.721-
  - natural body W16.622-
    - causing drowning W16.821-
  - swimming pool W16.522-
    - causing drowning W16.521-
  - falling into water (in) W16.322-
    - causing drowning W16.321-
  - fountain—*see* Striking against, bottom when, falling into water, specified NEC
  - natural body W16.122-
    - causing drowning W16.121-
  - reservoir—*see* Striking against, bottom when, falling into water, specified NEC

Striking against, *continued*

- ■ specified NEC W16.322-
  - ~ causing drowning W16.321-
  - ■ swimming pool W16.022-
    - ~ causing drowning W16.021-
- diving board (swimming-pool) W21.4-
- object W22.8-
  - with
    - ■ drowning or submersion—*see* Drowning
    - ■ fall—*see* Fall, due to, bumping against, object
  - caused by crowd or human stampede (with fall) W52.-
  - furniture W22.03-
  - lamppost W22.02-
  - sports equipment W21.9-
  - stationary W22.09-
    - ■ sports equipment W21.89-
  - wall W22.01-
- person(s) W51.-
  - with fall W03.-
    - ■ due to ice or snow W00.0-
    - ■ sports equipment W21.9-
  - as, or caused by, a crowd or human stampede (with fall) W52.-
  - assault Y04.2-
- sports equipment W21.9-
- wall (when) W22.01-
  - diving or jumping into water (in) W16.832-
    - ■ causing drowning W16.831-
    - ■ swimming pool W16.532-
      - ~ causing drowning W16.531-
  - falling into water (in) W16.332-
    - ■ causing drowning W16.331-
    - ■ fountain—*see* Striking against, wall when, falling into water, specified NEC
    - ■ natural body W16.132-
      - ~ causing drowning W16.131-
    - ■ reservoir—*see* Striking against, wall when, falling into water, specified NEC
    - ■ specified NEC W16.332-
      - ~ causing drowning W16.331-
    - ■ swimming pool W16.032-
      - ~ causing drowning W16.031-
  - swimming pool (when) W22.042-
    - ■ causing drowning W22.041-
    - ■ diving or jumping into water W16.532-
      - ~ causing drowning W16.531-
    - ■ falling into water W16.032-
      - ~ causing drowning W16.031-

Struck (accidentally) by

- airbag (automobile) W22.10-
  - driver side W22.11-
  - front passenger side W22.12-
  - specified NEC W22.19-
- alligator W58.02-
- animal (not being ridden) NEC W55.89-
- avalanche—*see* Landslide
- ball (hit) (thrown) W21.00-
  - assault Y08.09-
  - baseball W21.03-
  - basketball W21.05-
  - golf ball W21.04-
  - football W21.01-
  - soccer W21.02-
  - softball W21.07-
  - specified NEC W21.09-
  - volleyball W21.06-
- bat or racquet
  - baseball bat W21.11-
    - ■ assault Y08.02-
  - golf club W21.13-
    - ■ assault Y08.09-
  - specified NEC W21.19-
    - ■ assault Y08.09-
  - tennis racquet W21.12-
    - ■ assault Y08.09-
- bullet—*see also* Discharge, firearm by type
- crocodile W58.12-
- dog W54.1-
- flare, Very pistol—*see* Discharge, firearm NEC
- hailstones X39.8-

Struck (accidentally) by, *continued*

- hockey (ice)
  - field
    - ■ puck W21.221-
    - ■ stick W21.211-
  - puck W21.220-
  - stick W21.210-
    - ■ assault Y08.01-
- landslide—*see* Landslide
- lightning—*see* subcategory T75.0-
  - causing fire—*see* Exposure, fire
- machine—*see* Contact, with, by type of machine
- mammal NEC W55.89-
  - marine W56.32-
- marine animal W56.82-
- object W22.8-
  - blunt W22.8-
    - ■ assault Y00.-
    - ■ undetermined whether accidental or intentional Y29.-
  - falling W20.8-
    - ■ from, in, on
      - ~ building W20.1-
        - ◊ burning (uncontrolled fire) X00.4-
      - ~ cataclysmic
        - ◊ earth surface movement NEC—*see* Landslide
        - ◊ storm—*see* Forces of nature, cataclysmic storm
      - ~ cave-in W20.0-
      - ~ earthquake X34.-
      - ~ machine (in operation)—*see* Contact, with, by type of machine
      - ~ structure W20.1-
        - ◊ burning X00.4-
      - ~ transport vehicle (in motion)—*see* Accident, transport, by type of vehicle
      - ~ watercraft V93.49-
        - ◊ due to
          - » accident to craft V91.39-
            - ✦ powered craft V91.3-
            - ✦ unpowered craft V91.3-
          - ◊ powered craft V93.4-
          - ◊ unpowered craft V93.4-
  - moving NEC W20.8-
  - projected W20.8-
    - ■ assault Y00.-
    - ■ in sports W21.9-
      - ~ assault Y08.09-
      - ~ ball W21.00-
        - ◊ baseball W21.03-
        - ◊ basketball W21.05-
        - ◊ football W21.01-
        - ◊ golf ball W21.04-
        - ◊ soccer W21.02-
        - ◊ softball W21.07-
        - ◊ specified NEC W21.09-
        - ◊ volleyball W21.06-
      - ~ bat or racquet
        - ◊ baseball bat W21.11-
          - » assault Y08.02-
        - ◊ golf club W21.13-
          - » assault Y08.09-
        - ◊ specified NEC W21.19-
          - » assault Y08.09-
        - ◊ tennis racquet W21.12-
          - » assault Y08.09-
      - ~ hockey (ice)
        - ◊ field
          - » puck W21.221-
          - » stick W21.211-
        - ◊ puck W21.220-
        - ◊ stick W21.210-
          - » assault Y08.01-
      - ~ specified NEC W21.89-
  - set in motion by explosion—*see* Explosion
  - thrown W20.8-
    - ■ assault Y00.-
    - ■ in sports W21.9-
      - ~ assault Y08.09-
      - ~ ball W21.00-
        - ◊ baseball W21.03-
        - ◊ basketball W21.05-
        - ◊ football W21.01-

Struck (accidentally) by, *continued*

- ◊ golf ball W21.04-
- ◊ soccer W21.02-
- ◊ soft ball W21.07-
- ◊ specified NEC W21.09-
- ◊ volleyball W21.06-
- ~ bat or racquet
  - ◊ baseball bat W21.11-
    - » assault Y08.02-
  - ◊ golf club W21.13-
    - » assault Y08.09-
  - ◊ specified NEC W21.19-
    - » assault Y08.09-
  - ◊ tennis racquet W21.12-
    - » assault Y08.09-
- ~ hockey (ice)
  - ◊ field
    - » puck W21.221-
    - » stick W21.211-
  - ◊ puck W21.220-
  - ◊ stick W21.210-
    - » assault Y08.01-
- ~ specified NEC W21.89-
- other person(s) W50.0-
  - with
    - ■ blunt object W22.8-
      - ~ intentional, homicide (attempt) Y00.-
      - ~ sports equipment W21.9-
      - ~ undetermined whether accidental or intentional Y29.-
    - ■ fall W03.-
      - ~ due to ice or snow W00.0-
  - as, or caused by, a crowd or human stampede (with fall) W52.-
  - assault Y04.2-
  - sports equipment W21.9-
- sports equipment W21.9-
  - assault Y08.09-
  - ball W21.00-
    - ■ baseball W21.03-
    - ■ basketball W21.05-
    - ■ football W21.01-
    - ■ golf ball W21.04-
    - ■ soccer W21.02-
    - ■ soft ball W21.07-
    - ■ specified NEC W21.09-
    - ■ volleyball W21.06-
  - bat or racquet
    - ■ baseball bat W21.11-
      - ~ assault Y08.02-
    - ■ golf club W21.13-
      - ~ assault Y08.09-
    - ■ specified NEC W21.19-
    - ■ tennis racquet W21.12-
      - ~ assault Y08.09-
  - cleats (shoe) W21.31-
  - foot wear NEC W21.39-
  - football helmet W21.81-
  - hockey (ice)
    - ■ field
      - ~ puck W21.221-
      - ~ stick W21.211-
    - ■ puck W21.220-
    - ■ stick W21.210-
      - ~ assault Y08.01-
  - skate blades W21.32-
  - specified NEC W21.89-
    - ■ assault Y08.09-
- thunderbolt—*see* subcategory T75.0-
  - causing fire—*see* Exposure, fire
- transport vehicle NEC (*see also* Accident, transport) V09.9-
  - intentional, homicide (attempt) Y03.0-
  - motor NEC (*see also* Accident, transport) V09.20-
- vehicle (transport) NEC—*see* Accident, transport, by type of vehicle
  - stationary (falling from jack, hydraulic lift, ramp) W20.8-

Stumbling

- over
  - animal NEC W01.0-
    - ■ with fall W18.09-

Stumbling, *continued*
- carpet, rug or (small) object W22.8-
  - ■ with fall W18.09-
- person W51.-
  - ■ with fall W03.-
    - due to ice or snow W00.0-
- without fall W18.40-
  - due to
    - ■ specified NEC W18.49-
    - ■ stepping from one level to another W18.43-
    - ■ stepping into hole or opening W18.42-
    - ■ stepping on object W18.41-

Submersion (accidental)—*see* Drowning

Suffocation (accidental) (by external means) (by pressure) (mechanical) (*see also* category) T71
- due to, by
  - avalanche—*see* Landslide
  - explosion—*see* Explosion
  - fire—*see* Exposure, fire
  - food, any type (aspiration) (ingestion) (inhalation) (see categories T17 and) T18
  - ignition—*see* Ignition
  - landslide—*see* Landslide
  - machine(ry)—*see* Contact, with, by type of machine
  - vomitus (aspiration) (inhalation) T17.81-
- in
  - burning building X00.8-

Suicide, suicidal (attempted) (by) X83.8-
- blunt object X79.-
- burning, burns X76.-
  - hot object X77.9-
    - ■ fluid NEC X77.2-
    - ■ household appliance X77.3-
    - ■ specified NEC X77.8-
    - ■ steam X77.0-
    - ■ tap water X77.1-
    - ■ vapors X77.0-
- caustic substance—*see* Table of Drugs and Chemicals
- cold, extreme X83.2-
- collision of motor vehicle with
  - motor vehicle X82.0-
  - specified NEC X82.8-
  - train X82.1-
  - tree X82.2-
- cut (any part of body) X78.9-
- cutting or piercing instrument X78.9-
  - dagger X78.2-
  - glass X78.0-
  - knife X78.1-
  - specified NEC X78.8-
  - sword X78.2-
- drowning (in) X71.9-
  - bathtub X71.0-
  - natural water X71.3-
  - specified NEC X71.8-
  - swimming pool X71.1-
    - ■ following fall X71.2-
- electrocution X83.1-
- explosive(s) (material) X75.-
- fire, flames X76.-
- firearm X74.9-
  - airgun X74.01-
  - handgun X72.-
  - hunting rifle X73.1-
  - larger X73.9-
    - ■ specified NEC X73.8-
  - machine gun X73.2-
  - paintball gun X74.02-
  - shotgun X73.0-
  - specified NEC X74.8-

Suicide, suicidal (attempted) (by), *continued*
- hanging X83.8-
- hot object—*see* Suicide, burning, hot object
- jumping
  - before moving object X81.8-
    - ■ motor vehicle X81.0-
    - ■ subway train X81.1-
    - ■ train X81.1-
  - from high place X80.-
- lying before moving object, train, vehicle X81.8-
- poisoning—*see* Table of Drugs and Chemicals
- puncture (any part of body)—*see* Suicide, cutting or piercing instrument
- scald—*see* Suicide, burning, hot object
- sharp object (any)—*see* Suicide, cutting or piercing instrument
- shooting—*see* Suicide, firearm
- specified means NEC X83.8-
- stab (any part of body)—*see* Suicide, cutting or piercing instrument
- steam, hot vapors X77.0-
- strangulation X83.8-
- submersion—*see* Suicide, drowning
- suffocation X83.8-
- wound NEC X83.8-

Sunstroke X32.-

Supersonic waves (causing injury) W42.0-

Surgical procedure, complication of (delayed or as an abnormal reaction without mention of misadventure)—*see also* Complication of or following, by type of procedure
- due to or as a result of misadventure—*see* Misadventure

Swallowed, swallowing
- foreign body T18.-
- poison—*see* Table of Drugs and Chemicals
- substance
  - caustic or corrosive—*see* Table of Drugs and Chemicals
  - poisonous—*see* Table of Drugs and Chemicals

T

Tackle in sport W03.-

Terrorism (involving) Y38.8-

Thirst X58.-

Thrown (accidentally)
- against part (any) of or object in transport vehicle (in motion) NEC—*see also* Accident, transport
- from
  - high place, homicide (attempt) Y01.-
  - machinery—*see* Contact, with, by type of machine
  - transport vehicle NEC (*see also* Accident, transport) V89.9-
- off—*see* Thrown, from

Thunderbolt—*see* subcategory T75.0-
- causing fire—*see* Exposure, fire

Tidal wave (any injury) NEC—*see* Forces of nature, tidal wave

Took
- overdose (drug)—*see* Table of Drugs and Chemicals
- poison—*see* Table of Drugs and Chemicals

Tornado (any injury) X37.1-

Torrential rain (any injury) X37.8-

Torture X58.-

Trampled by animal NEC W55.89-

Trapped (accidentally)
- between objects (moving) (stationary and moving)—*see* Caught
- by part (any) of
  - motorcycle V29.88-
  - pedal cycle V19.88-
  - transport vehicle NEC (*see also* Accident, transport) V89.9-

Travel (effects) (sickness) T75.3-

Tree falling on or hitting (accidentally) (person) W20.8-

Tripping
- over
  - animal W01.0-
  - carpet, rug or (small) object W22.8-
    - ■ with fall W18.09-
  - person W51.-
    - ■ with fall W03.-
      - due to ice or snow W00.0-
- without fall W18.40-
  - due to
    - ■ specified NEC W18.49-
    - ■ stepping from one level to another W18.43-
    - ■ stepping into hole or opening W18.42-
    - ■ stepping on object W18.41-

Twisted by person(s) (accidentally) W50.2-
- with intent to injure or kill Y04.0-
  - as, or caused by, a crowd or human stampede (with fall) W52.-
- assault Y04.0-
- in fight Y04.0-

Twisting, excessive—*see* category Y93

U

Underdosing of necessary drugs, medicaments or biological substances Y63.6-

V

Vibration (causing injury) W49.9-

Volcanic eruption (any injury) X35.-

Vomitus, gastric contents in air passages (with asphyxia, obstruction or suffocation) T17.81-

W

Walked into stationary object (any) W22.09-
- furniture W22.03-
- lamppost W22.02-
- wall W22.01-

War operations (injuries to military personnel and civilians during war, civil insurrection and peacekeeping missions) (by) (from) (involving)—*Refer to ICD-10-CM Manual*

Washed
- away by flood—*see* Flood
- off road by storm (transport vehicle)—*see* Forces of nature, cataclysmic storm

Weather exposure NEC—*see* Forces of nature

Work related condition Y99.0

Wound (accidental) NEC (*see also* Injury) X58.-
- battle (*see also* War operations) Y36.90-
- gunshot—*see* Discharge, firearm by type

Wrong
- device implanted into correct surgical site Y65.51-
- fluid in infusion Y65.1-
- procedure (operation) on correct patient Y65.51-
- patient, procedure performed on Y65.52-

Table of Drugs and Chemicals

The following table is a quick reference for all poisonings (accidental/unintentional, intentional/self-harm, assault), adverse effects, and underdosing as a result of a specific drug or chemical. The drugs/chemicals are listed alphabetically with their respective subcategory code. Every code is listed with a dash (-) to indicate that the next character is missing and should be reported with the fifth or sixth character as follows:

1	**Poisoning, accidental, unintentional**
2	**Poisoning, intentional, self-harm**
3	**Poisoning, assault**
4	**Poisoning, undetermined**
5	**Adverse effect**
6	**Underdosing**

DO NOT CODE FROM THE TABLE—ALWAYS REFER TO THE TABULAR. If the code requires an "encounter type," please refer to the tabular for more details.

EXAMPLE

Accidental Poisoning From Lysol—Initial Encounter
Lysol is listed as T54.1X-.
Lysol accidental poisoning would be T54.1X1-.
Lysol accidental poisoning, initial encounter, would be T54.1X1A.

Underdosing of Barbiturate—Follow-up Encounter
Barbiturate is listed as T42.3X-.
Underdosing of barbiturate would be T42.3X6-.
Underdosing of barbiturate, subsequent encounter, would be T42.3X6D.

Drug/Chemical	Code	Drug/Chemical	Code
1-propanol	T51.3X-	**Acetomorphine**	T40.1X-
2-propanol	T51.2X-	**Acetone (oils)**	T52.4X-
2,4-D (dichlorophen-oxyacetic acid)	T60.3X-	**Acetonitrile**	T52.8X-
2,4-toluene diisocyanate	T65.0X-	**Acetophenazine**	T43.3X-
2,4,5-T (trichloro-phenoxyacetic acid)	T60.1X-	**Acetophenetedin**	T39.1X-
14-hydroxydihydro-morphinone	T40.2X-	**Acetophenone**	T52.4X-
ABOB	T37.5X-	**Acetorphine**	T40.2X-
Abrine	T62.2X-	**Acetosulfone (sodium)**	T37.1X-
Abrus (seed)	T62.2X-	**Acetrizoate (sodium)**	T50.8X-
Absinthe (beverage)	T51.0X-	**Acetrizoic acid**	T50.8X-
Acaricide	T60.8X-	**Acetyl (bromide) (chloride)**	T53.6X-
Acebutolol	T44.7X-	**Acetylcarbromal**	T42.6X-
Acecarbromal	T42.6X-	**Acetylcholine (chloride)**	T44.1X-
Aceclidine	T44.1X-	derivative	T44.1X-
Acedapsone	T37.0X-	**Acetylcysteine**	T48.4X-
Acefylline piperazine	T48.6X-	**Acetyldigitoxin**	T46.0X-
Acemorphan	T40.2X-	**Acetyldigoxin**	T46.0X-
Acenocoumarin/Acenocoumarol	T45.51-	**Acetyldihydrocodeine**	T40.2X-
Acepifylline	T48.6X-	**Acetyldihydrocodeinone**	T40.2X-
Acepromazine	T43.3X-	**Acetylene (gas)**	T59.89-
Acesulfamethoxypyridazine	T37.0X-	dichloride	T53.6X-
Acetal	T52.8X-	incomplete combustion of	T58.1-
Acetaldehyde (vapor)	T52.8X-	industrial	T59.89-
liquid	T65.89-	tetrachloride	T53.6X-
P-Acetamidophenol	T39.1X-	vapor	T53.6X-
Acetaminophen	T39.1X-	**Acetylpheneturide**	T42.6X-
Acetaminosalol	T39.1X-	**Acetylphenylhydrazine**	T39.8X-
Acetanilide	T39.1X-	**Acetylsalicylic acid (salts)**	T39.01-
Acetarsol	T37.3X-	enteric coated	T39.01-
Acetazolamide	T50.2X-	**Acetylsulfamethoxypyridazine**	T37.0X-
Acetiamine	T45.2X-	**Achromycin**	T36.4X-
Acetic		ophthalmic preparation	T49.5X-
acid	T54.2X-	topical NEC	T49.0X-
w/sodium acetate (ointment)	T49.3X-	**Aciclovir**	T37.5X-
ester (solvent) (vapor)	T52.8X-	**Acid (corrosive) NEC**	T54.2X-
irrigating solution	T50.3X-	**Acidifying agent NEC**	T50.90-
medicinal (lotion)	T49.2X-	**Acipimox**	T46.6X-
anhydride	T65.89-	**Acitretin**	T50.99-
ether (vapor)	T52.8X-	**Aclarubicin**	T45.1X-
Acetohexamide	T38.3X-	**Aclatonium napadisilate**	T48.1X-
Acetohydroxamic acid	T50.99-	**Aconite (wild)**	T46.99-
Acetomenaphthone	T45.7X-	**Aconitine**	T46.99-

TABLE OF DRUGS AND CHEMICALS

Drug/Chemical	Code
Aconitum ferox	T46.99-
Acridine	T65.6X-
vapor	T59.89-
Acriflavine	T37.9-
Acriflavinium chloride	T49.0X-
Acrinol	T49.0X-
Acrisorcin	T49.0X-
Acrivastine	T45.0X-
Acrolein (gas)	T59.89-
liquid	T54.1X-
Acrylamide	T65.89-
Acrylic resin	T49.3X-
Acrylonitrile	T65.89-
Actaea spicata	T62.2X-
berry	T62.1X-
Acterol	T37.3X-
ACTH	T38.81-
Actinomycin C	T45.1X-
Actinomycin D	T45.1X-
Activated charcoal—*see also Charcoal, medicinal*	T47.6X-
Acyclovir	T37.5X-
Adenine	T45.2X-
arabinoside	T37.5X-
Adenosine (phosphate)	T46.2X-
ADH	T38.89-
Adhesive NEC	T65.89-
Adicillin	T36.0X-
Adiphenine	T44.3X-
Adipiodone	T50.8X-
Adjunct, pharmaceutical	T50.90-
Adrenal (extract, cortex or medulla) (gluco or mineral corticoids) (hormones)	T38.0X-
ENT agent	T49.6X-
ophthalmic preparation	T49.5X-
topical NEC	T49.0X-
Adrenaline / Adrenalin	T44.5X-
Adrenergic NEC	T44.90-
blocking agent NEC	T44.8X-
beta, heart	T44.7X-
specified NEC	T44.99-
Adrenochrome	
(mono)semicarbazone	T46.99-
derivative	T46.99-
Adrenocorticotrophic hormone	T38.81-
Adrenocorticotrophin	T38.81-
Adriamycin	T45.1X-
Aerosol spray NEC	T65.9-
Aerosporin	T36.8X-
ENT agent	T49.6X-
ophthalmic preparation	T49.5X-
topical NEC	T49.0X-
Aethusa cynapium	T62.2X-
Afghanistan black	T40.71-
Aflatoxin	T64.0-
Afloqualone	T42.8X-

Drug/Chemical	Code
African boxwood	T62.2X-
Agar	T47.4X-
Agonist (predominantly)	
alpha-adrenoreceptor	T44.4X-
beta-adrenoreceptor	T44.5X-
Agricultural agent NEC	T65.9-
Agrypnal	T42.3X-
AHLG	T50.Z1-
Air contaminant(s) type NOS	T65.9-
Ajmaline	T46.2X-
Akee	T62.1X-
Akrinol	T49.0X-
Akritoin	T37.8X-
Alacepril	T46.4X-
Alantolactone	T37.4X-
Albamycin	T36.8X-
Albendazole	T37.4X-
Albumin	T45.8X-
Albuterol	T48.6X-
Albutoin	T42.0X-
Alclometasone	T49.0X-
Alcohol	T51.9-
allyl	T51.8X-
amyl / butyl / propyl	T51.3X-
antifreeze / methyl	T51.1X-
beverage (grain, ethyl)	T51.0X-
dehydrated / denatured	T51.0X-
deterrent NEC	T50.6X-
diagnostic (gastric function)	T50.8X-
industrial	T51.0X-
isopropyl	T51.2X-
preparation for consumption	T51.0X-
radiator	T51.1X-
rubbing	T51.2X-
specified type NEC	T51.8X-
surgical	T51.0X-
vapor (any type of Alcohol)	T59.89-
wood	T51.1X-
Alcuronium (chloride)	T48.1X-
Aldactone	T50.0X-
Aldesulfone sodium	T37.1X-
Aldicarb	T60.0X-
Aldomet	T46.5X-
Aldosterone	T50.0X-
Aldrin (dust)	T60.1X-
Alexitol sodium	T47.1X-
Alfacalcidol	T45.2X-
Alfadolone	T41.1X-
Alfaxalone	T41.1X-
Alfentanil	T40.4X-
Alfuzosin (hydrochloride)	T44.8X-
Algae (harmful) (toxin)	T65.821
Algeldrate	T47.1X-
Algin	T47.8X-
Alglucerase	T45.3X-

TABLE OF DRUGS AND CHEMICALS

Drug/Chemical	Code
Alidase	T45.3X-
Alimemazine	T43.3X-
Aliphatic thiocyanates	T65.0X-
Alizapride	T45.0X-
Alkali (caustic)	T54.3X-
Alkaline antiseptic solution (aromatic)	T49.6X-
Alkalinizing agents (medicinal)	T50.90-
Alkalizing agent NEC	T50.90-
Alka-seltzer	T39.01-
Alkavervir	T46.5X-
Alkonium (bromide)	T49.0X-
Alkylating drug NEC	T45.1X-
antimyeloproliferative or lymphatic	T45.1X-
Alkylisocyanate	T65.0X-
Allantoin	T49.4X-
Allegron	T43.01-
Allethrin	T49.0X-
Allobarbital	T42.3X-
Allopurinol	T50.4X-
Allyl	
Alcohol	T51.8X-
disulfide	T46.6X-
Allylestrenol	T38.5X-
Allylisopropylacetylurea	T42.6X-
Allylisopropylmalonylurea	T42.3X-
Allylthiourea	T49.3X-
Allyltribromide	T42.6X-
Allypropymal	T42.3X-
Almagate	T47.1X-
Almasilate	T47.1X-
Almitrine	T50.7X-
Aloes	T47.2X-
Aloglutamol	T47.1X-
Aloin	T47.2X-
Aloxidone	T42.2X-
Alpha	
acetyldigoxin	T46.0X-
adrenergic blocking drug	T44.6X-
amylase	T45.3X-
tocoferol (acetate) toco	T45.2X-
tocopherol	T45.2X-
Alphadolone	T41.1X-
Alphaprodine	T40.4X-
Alphaxalone	T41.1X-
Alprazolam	T42.4X-
Alprenolol	T44.7X-
Alprostadil	T46.7X-
Alsactide	T38.81-
Alseroxylon	T46.5X-
Alteplase	T45.61-
Altizide	T50.2X-
Altretamine	T45.1X-
Alum (medicinal)	T49.4X-
nonmedicinal (ammonium) (potassium)	T56.89-
Aluminium, aluminum	
acetate / chloride	T49.2X-
solution	T49.0X-
aspirin / bis (acetylsalicylate)	T39.01-
carbonate (gel, basic)	T47.1X-
chlorhydroxide-complex	T47.1X-
clofibrate	T46.6X-
diacetate	T49.2X-
glycinate	T47.1X-
hydroxide (gel)	T47.1X-
hydroxide-magn. carb. gel	T47.1X-
magnesium silicate	T47.1X-
nicotinate	T46.7X-
ointment (surgical) (topical)	T49.3X-
phosphate / silicate (sodium)	T47.1X-
salicylate	T39.09-
subacetate	T49.2X-
sulfate	T49.0X-
tannate	T47.6X-
Alurate	T42.3X-
Alverine	T44.3X-
Alvodine	T40.2X-
Amanita phalloides	T62.0X-
Amanitine	T62.0X-
Amantadine	T42.8X-
Ambazone	T49.6X-
Ambenonium (chloride)	T44.0X-
Ambroxol	T48.4X-
Ambuphylline	T48.6X-
Ambutonium bromide	T44.3X-
Amcinonide	T49.0X-
Amdinocilline	T36.0X-
Ametazole	T50.8X-
Amethocaine (regional, spinal)	T41.3X-
Amethopterin	T45.1X-
Amezinium metilsulfate	T44.99-
Amfebutamone	T43.29-
Amfepramone	T50.5X-
Amfetamine	T43.62-
Amfetaminil	T43.62-
Amfomycin	T36.8X-
Amidefrine mesilate	T48.5X-
Amidone	T40.3X-
Amidopyrine	T39.2X-
Amidotrizoate	T50.8X-
Amiflamine	T43.1X-
Amikacin	T36.5X-
Amikhelline	T46.3X-
Amiloride	T50.2X-
Aminacrine	T49.0X-
Amineptine	T43.01-
Aminitrozole	T37.3X-
Amino acids	T50.3X-
Aminoacetic acid (derivatives)	T50.3X-
Aminoacridine	T49.0X-

TABLE OF DRUGS AND CHEMICALS

Drug/Chemical	Code
Aminobenzoic acid (-p)	T49.3X-
4-Aminobutyric acid	T43.8X-
Aminocaproic acid	T45.62-
Aminoethylisothiourium	T45.8X-
Aminofenazone	T39.2X-
Aminoglutethimide	T45.1X-
Aminohippuric acid	T50.8X-
Aminomethylbenzoic acid	T45.69-
Aminometradine	T50.2X-
Aminopentamide	T44.3X-
Aminophenazone	T39.2X-
Aminophenol	T54.0X-
4-Aminophenol derivatives	T39.1X-
Aminophenylpyridone	T43.59-
Aminophylline	T48.6X-
Aminopterin sodium	T45.1X-
Aminopyrine	T39.2X-
8-Aminoquinoline drugs	T37.2X-
Aminorex	T50.5X-
Aminosalicylic acid	T37.1X-
Aminosalylum	T37.1X-
Amiodarone	T46.2X-
Amiphenazole	T50.7X-
Amiquinsin	T46.5X-
Amisometradine	T50.2X-
Amisulpride	T43.59-
Amitriptyline	T43.01-
Amitriptylinoxide	T43.01-
Amlexanox	T48.6X-
Ammonia (fumes/vapor) (gas)	T59.89-
aromatic spirit	T48.99-
liquid (household)	T54.3X-
Ammoniated mercury	T49.0X-
Ammonium	
acid tartrate	T49.5X-
bromide	T42.6X-
carbonate	T54.3X-
chloride	T50.99-
expectorant	T48.4X-
compounds (household) NEC	T54.3X-
fumes (any usage)	T59.89-
industrial	T54.3X-
ichthyosulronate	T49.4X-
mandelate	T37.9-
sulfamate	T60.3X-
sulfonate resin	T47.8X-
Amobarbital (sodium)	T42.3X-
Amodiaquine	T37.2X-
Amopyroquin (e)	T37.2X-
Amoxapine	T43.01-
Amoxicillin	T36.0X-
Amperozide	T43.59-
Amphenidone	T43.59-
Amphetamine NEC	T43.62-
Amphomycin	T36.8X-

Drug/Chemical	Code
Amphotalide	T37.4X-
Amphotericin B	T36.7X-
topical	T49.0X-
Ampicillin	T36.0X-
Amprotropine	T44.3X-
Amsacrine	T45.1X-
Amygdaline	T62.2X-
Amyl	
acetate	T52.8X-
vapor	T59.89-
alcohol	T51.3X-
chloride	T53.6X-
formate	T52.8X-
nitrite	T46.3X-
propionate	T65.89-
Amylase	T47.5X-
Amyleine, regional	T41.3X-
Amylene	
dichloride	T53.6X-
hydrate	T51.3X-
Amylmetacresol	T49.6X-
Amylobarbitone	T42.3X-
Amylocaine, regional (infiltration) (subcutaneous) (nerve block) (spinal) (topical)	T41.3X-
Amylopectin	T47.6X-
Amytal (sodium)	T42.3X-
Anabolic steroid	T38.7X-
Analeptic NEC	T50.7X-
Analgesic	T39.9-
anti-inflammatory NEC	T39.9-
propionic acid derivative	T39.31-
antirheumatic NEC	T39.4X-
aromatic NEC	T39.1X-
narcotic NEC	T40.60-
non-narcotic NEC	T39.9-
pyrazole	T39.2X-
specified NEC	T39.8X-
Analgin	T39.2X-
Anamirta cocculus	T62.1X-
Ancillin	T36.0X-
Ancrod	T45.69-
Androgen	T38.7X-
Androgen-estrogen mixture	T38.7X-
Androstalone	T38.7X-
Androstanolone	T38.7X-
Androsterone	T38.7X-
Anemone pulsatilla	T62.2X-
Anesthesia	
caudal	T41.3X-
endotracheal	T41.0X-
epidural	T41.3X-
inhalation	T41.0X-
local (nerve or plexus blocking)	T41.3X-
mucosal	T41.3X-
muscle relaxation	T48.1X-

TABLE OF DRUGS AND CHEMICALS

Drug/Chemical	Code	Drug/Chemical	Code
Anesthesia, continued		**Antagonist, continued**	
potentiated	T41.20-	pyrimidine	T45.1X-
rectal (general)	T41.20-	serotonin	T46.5X-
local	T41.3X-	**Antazolin (e)**	T45.0X-
regional	T41.3X-	**Anterior pituitary hormone NEC**	T38.81-
surface	T41.3X-	**Anthelmintic NEC**	T37.4X-
Anesthetic NEC	T41.41	**Anthiolimine**	T37.4X-
with muscle relaxant	T41.20-	**Anthralin**	T49.4X-
general	T41.20-	**Anthramycin**	T45.1X-
local	T41.3X-	**Antiadrenergic NEC**	T44.8X-
gaseous NEC	T41.0X-	**Antiallergic NEC**	T45.0X-
general NEC	T41.20-	**Anti-anemic (drug) (preparation)**	T45.8X-
halogenated hydrocarbon derivatives NEC	T41.0X-	**Antiandrogen NEC**	T38.6X-
infiltration NEC	T41.3X-	**Antianxiety drug NEC**	T43.50-
intravenous NEC	T41.1X-	**Antiaris toxicaria**	T65.89-
local NEC	T41.3X-	**Antiarteriosclerotic drug**	T46.6X-
rectal (general)	T41.20-	**Antiasthmatic drug NEC**	T48.6X-
local	T41.3X-	**Antibiotic NEC**	T36.9-
regional NEC / spinal NEC	T41.3X-	aminoglycoside	T36.5X-
thiobarbiturate	T41.1X-	anticancer	T45.1X-
topical	T41.3X-	antifungal	T36.7X-
Aneurine	T45.2X-	antimycobacterial	T36.5X-
Angio-Conray	T50.8X-	antineoplastic	T45.1X-
Angiotensin	T44.5X-	cephalosporin (group)	T36.1X-
Angiotensinamide	T44.99-	chloramphenicol (group)	T36.2X-
Anhydrohydroxy-progesterone	T38.5X-	ENT	T49.6X-
Anhydron	T50.2X-	eye	T49.5X-
Anileridine	T40.4X-	fungicidal (local)	T49.0X-
Aniline (dye) (liquid)	T65.3X-	intestinal	T36.8X-
analgesic	T39.1X-	b-lactam NEC	T36.1X-
derivatives, therapeutic NEC	T39.1X-	local	T49.0X-
vapor	T65.3X-	macrolides	T36.3X-
Aniscoropine	T44.3X-	polypeptide	T36.8X-
Anise oil	T47.5X-	specified NEC	T36.8X-
Anisidine	T65.3X-	tetracycline (group)	T36.4X-
Anisindione	T45.51-	throat	T49.6X-
Anisotropine methyl-bromide	T44.3X-	**Anticancer agents NEC**	T45.1X-
Anistreplase	T45.61-	**Anticholesterolemic drug NEC**	T46.6X-
Anorexiant (central)	T50.5X-	**Anticholinergic NEC**	T44.3X-
Anorexic agents	T50.5X-	**Anticholinesterase**	T44.0X-
Ansamycin	T36.6X-	organophosphorus	T44.0X-
Ant (bite) (sting)	T63.421	insecticide	T60.0X-
Antabuse	T50.6X-	nerve gas	T59.89-
Antacid NEC	T47.1X-	reversible	T44.0X-
Antagonist		ophthalmological	T49.5X-
Aldosterone	T50.0X-	**Anticoagulant NEC**	T45.51-
alpha-adrenoreceptor	T44.6X-	Antagonist	T45.7X-
anticoagulant	T45.7X-	**Anti-common-cold drug NEC**	T48.5X-
beta-adrenoreceptor	T44.7X-	**Anticonvulsant**	T42.71
extrapyramidal NEC	T44.3X-	barbiturate	T42.3X-
folic acid	T45.1X-	combination (with barbiturate)	T42.3X-
H2 receptor	T47.0X-	hydantoin	T42.0X-
heavy metal	T45.8X-	hypnotic NEC	T42.6X-
narcotic analgesic	T50.7X-	oxazolidinedione	T42.2X-
opiate	T50.7X-	pyrimidinedione	T42.6X-

TABLE OF DRUGS AND CHEMICALS

Drug/Chemical	Code	Drug/Chemical	Code
Anticonvulsant, continued		**Antihookworm drug**	T37.4X-
specified NEC	T42.6X-	**Anti-human lymphocytic globulin**	T50.Z1-
succinimide	T42.2X-	**Antihyperlipidemic drug**	T46.6X-
Anti-D immunoglobulin (human)	T50.Z1-	**Antihypertensive drug NEC**	T46.5X-
Antidepressant	T43.20-	**Anti-infective NEC**	T37.9-
monoamine oxidase inhibitor	T43.1X-	anthelmintic	T37.4X-
SSNRI	T43.21-	antibiotics	T36.9-
SSRI	T43.22-	specified NEC	T36.8X-
specified NEC	T43.29-	antimalarial	T37.2X-
tetracyclic	T43.02-	antimycobacterial NEC	T37.1X-
triazolopyridine	T43.21-	antibiotics	T36.5X-
tricyclic	T43.01-	antiprotozoal NEC	T37.3X-
Antidiabetic NEC	T38.3X-	blood	T37.2X-
biguanide	T38.3X-	antiviral	T37.5X-
and sulfonyl combined	T38.3X-	arsenical	T37.8X-
combined	T38.3X-	bismuth, local	T49.0X-
sulfonylurea	T38.3X-	ENT	T49.6X-
Antidiarrheal drug NEC	T47.6X-	eye NEC	T49.5X-
absorbent	T47.6X-	heavy metals NEC	T37.8X-
Antidiphtheria serum	T50.Z1-	local NEC	T49.0X-
Antidiuretic hormone	T38.89-	specified NEC	T49.0X-
Antidote NEC	T50.6X-	mixed	T37.9-
heavy metal	T45.8X-	ophthalmic preparation	T49.5X-
Antidysrhythmic NEC	T46.2X-	topical NEC	T49.0X-
Antiemetic drug	T45.0X-	**Anti-inflammatory drug NEC**	T39.39-
Antiepilepsy agent	T42.71	local	T49.0X-
combination or mixed	T42.5X-	nonsteroidal NEC	T39.39-
specified, NEC	T42.6X-	propionic acid derivative	T39.31-
Antiestrogen NEC	T38.6X-	specified NEC	T39.39-
Antifertility pill	T38.4X-	**Antikaluretic**	T50.3X-
Antifibrinolytic drug	T45.62-	**Antiknock (tetraethyl lead)**	T56.0X-
Antifilarial drug	T37.4X-	**Antilipemic drug NEC**	T46.6X-
Antiflatulent	T47.5X-	**Antimalarial**	T37.2X-
Antifreeze	T65.9-	prophylactic NEC	T37.2X-
alcohol	T51.1X-	pyrimidine derivative	T37.2X-
ethylene glycol	T51.8X-	**Antimetabolite**	T45.1X-
Antifungal		**Antimitotic agent**	T45.1X-
antibiotic (systemic)	T36.7X-	**Antimony (compounds) (vapor) NEC**	T56.89-
anti-infective NEC	T37.9-	anti-infectives	T37.8X-
disinfectant, local	T49.0X-	dimercaptosuccinate	T37.3X-
nonmedicinal (spray)	T60.3X-	hydride	T56.89-
topical	T49.0X-	pesticide (vapor)	T60.8X-
Anti-gastric-secretion drug NEC	T47.1X-	potassium (sodium)tartrate	T37.8X-
Antigonadotrophin NEC	T38.6X-	sodium dimercaptosuccinate	T37.3X-
Antihallucinogen	T43.50-	tartrated	T37.8X-
Antihelmintics	T37.4X-	**Antimuscarinic NEC**	T44.3X-
Antihemophilic		**Antimycobacterial drug NEC**	T37.1X-
factor	T45.8X-	antibiotics	T36.5X-
fraction	T45.8X-	combination	T37.1X-
globulin concentrate	T45.7X-	**Antinausea drug**	T45.0X-
human plasma	T45.8X-	**Antinematode drug**	T37.4X-
plasma, dried	T45.7X-	**Antineoplastic NEC**	T45.1X-
Antihemorrhoidal preparation	T49.2X-	alkaloidal	T45.1X-
Antiheparin drug	T45.7X-	antibiotics	T45.1X-
Antihistamine	T45.0X-	combination	T45.1X-

TABLE OF DRUGS AND CHEMICALS

Drug/Chemical	Code	Drug/Chemical	Code
Antineoplastic NEC, continued	T45.1X-	**Apresoline**	T46.5X-
estrogen	T38.5X-	**Aprindine**	T46.2X-
steroid	T38.7X-	**Aprobarbital**	T42.3X-
Antiparasitic drug (systemic)	T37.9-	**Apronalide**	T42.6X-
local	T49.0X-	**Aprotinin**	T45.62-
specified NEC	T37.8X-	**Aptocaine**	T41.3X-
Antiparkinsonism drug NEC	T42.8X-	**Aqua fortis**	T54.2X-
Antiperspirant NEC	T49.2X-	**Ara-A**	T37.5X-
Antiphlogistic NEC	T39.4X-	**Ara-C**	T45.1X-
Antiplatyhelmintic drug	T37.4X-	**Arachis oil**	T49.3X-
Antiprotozoal drug NEC	T37.3X-	cathartic	T47.4X-
blood	T37.2X-	**Aralen**	T37.2X-
local	T49.0X-	**Arecoline**	T44.1X-
Antipruritic drug NEC	T49.1X-	**Arginine**	T50.99-
Antipsychotic drug	T43.50-	glutamate	T50.99-
specified NEC	T43.59-	**Argyrol**	T49.0X-
Antipyretic	T39.9-	ENT agent	T49.6X-
specified NEC	T39.8X-	ophthalmic preparation	T49.5X-
Antipyrine	T39.2X-	**Aristocort**	T38.0X-
Antirabies hyperimmune serum	T50.Z1-	ENT agent	T49.6X-
Antirheumatic NEC	T39.4X-	ophthalmic preparation	T49.5X-
Antirigidity drug NEC	T42.8X-	topical NEC	T49.0X-
Antischistosomal drug	T37.4X-	**Aromatics, corrosive**	T54.1X-
Antiscorpion sera	T50.Z1-	disinfectants	T54.1X-
Antiseborrheics	T49.4X-	**Arsenate of lead**	T57.0X-
Antiseptics (external) (medicinal)	T49.0X-	herbicide	T57.0X-
Antistine	T45.0X-	**Arsenic, arsenicals (compounds) (dust) (vapor) NEC**	T57.0X-
Antitapeworm drug	T37.4X-	anti-infectives	T37.8X-
Antitetanus immunoglobulin	T50.Z1-	pesticide (dust) (fumes)	T57.0X-
Antithrombotic	T45.52-	**Arsine (gas)**	T57.0X-
Antithyroid drug NEC	T38.2X-	**Arsphenamine (silver)**	T37.8X-
Antitoxin	T50.Z1-	**Arsthinol**	T37.3X-
Antitrichomonal drug	T37.3X-	**Artane**	T44.3X-
Antituberculars	T37.1X-	**Arthropod (venomous) NEC**	T63.481
antibiotics	T36.5X-	**Articaine**	T41.3X-
Antitussive NEC	T48.3X-	**Asbestos**	T57.8X-
codeine mixture	T40.2X-	**Ascaridole**	T37.4X-
opiate	T40.2X-	**Ascorbic acid**	T45.2X-
Antivaricose drug	T46.8X-	**Asiaticoside**	T49.0X-
Antivenin, antivenom (sera)	T50.Z1-	**Asparaginase**	T45.1X-
crotaline	T50.Z1-	**Aspidium (oleoresin)**	T37.4X-
spider bite	T50.Z1-	**Aspirin (aluminum) (soluble)**	T39.01-
Antivertigo drug	T45.0X-	**Aspoxicillin**	T36.0X-
Antiviral drug NEC	T37.5X-	**Astemizole**	T45.0X-
eye	T49.5X-	**Astringent (local)**	T49.2X-
Antiwhipworm drug	T37.4X-	specified NEC	T49.2X-
		Astromicin	T36.5X-
Antrol—*see also specific chemical*	T60.9-	**Ataractic drug NEC**	T43.50-
fungicide	T60.9-	**Atenolol**	T44.7X-
ANTU (alpha naphthylthiourea)	T60.4X-	**Atonia drug, intestinal**	T47.4X-
Apalcillin	T36.0X-	**Atophan**	T50.4X-
APC	T48.5X-	**Atracurium besilate**	T48.1X-
Aplonidine	T44.4X-	**Atropine**	T44.3X-
Apomorphine	T47.7X-	derivative	T44.3X-
Appetite depressants, central	T50.5X-	methonitrate	T44.3X-
Apraclonidine (hydrochloride)	T44.4X-		

TABLE OF DRUGS AND CHEMICALS

Drug/Chemical	Code
Attapulgite	T47.6X-
Auramine	T65.89-
dye	T65.6X-
fungicide	T60.3X-
Auranofin	T39.4X-
Aurantiin	T46.99-
Aureomycin	T36.4X-
ophthalmic preparation	T49.5X-
topical NEC	T49.0X-
Aurothioglucose	T39.4X-
Aurothioglycanide	T39.4X-
Aurothiomalate sodium	T39.4X-
Aurotioprol	T39.4X-
Automobile fuel	T52.0X-
Autonomic nervous system agent NEC	T44.90-
Avlosulfon	T37.1X-
Avomine	T42.6X-
Axerophthol	T45.2X-
Azacitidine	T45.1X-
Azacyclonol	T43.59-
Azadirachta	T60.2X-
Azanidazole	T37.3X-
Azapetine	T46.7X-
Azapropazone	T39.2X-
Azaribine	T45.1X-
Azaserine	T45.1X-
Azatadine	T45.0X-
Azatepa	T45.1X-
Azathioprine	T45.1X-
Azelaic acid	T49.0X-
Azelastine	T45.0X-
Azidocillin	T36.0X-
Azidothymidine	T37.5X-
Azinphos (ethyl) (methyl)	T60.0X-
Aziridine (chelating)	T54.1X-
Azithromycin	T36.3X-
Azlocillin	T36.0X-
Azobenzene smoke	T65.3X-
acaricide	T60.8X-
Azosulfamide	T37.0X-
AZT	T37.5X-
Aztreonam	T36.1X-
Azulfidine	T37.0X-
Azuresin	T50.8X-
Bacampicillin	T36.0X-
Bacillus	
lactobacillus	T47.8X-
subtilis	T47.6X-
Bacimycin	T49.0X-
ophthalmic preparation	T49.5X-
Bacitracin zinc	T49.0X-
with neomycin	T49.0X-
ENT agent	T49.6X-
ophthalmic preparation	T49.5X-
topical NEC	T49.0X-

Drug/Chemical	Code
Baclofen	T42.8X-
Baking soda	T50.99-
BAL	T45.8X-
Bambuterol	T48.6X-
Bamethan (sulfate)	T46.7X-
Bamifylline	T48.6X-
Bamipine	T45.0X-
Baneberry—*see Actaea spicata*	
Banewort—*see Belladonna*	
Barbenyl	T42.3X-
Barbexaclone	T42.6X-
Barbital (sodium)	T42.3X-
Barbitone	T42.3X-
Barbiturate NEC	T42.3X-
with tranquilizer	T42.3X-
anesthetic (intravenous)	T41.1X-
Barium (carbonate) (chloride) (sulfite)	T57.8X-
diagnostic agent	T50.8X-
pesticide / rodenticide	T60.4X-
sulfate (medicinal)	T50.8X-
Barrier cream	T49.3X-
Basic fuchsin	T49.0X-
Battery acid or fluid	T54.2X-
Bay rum	T51.8X-
BCG (vaccine)	T50.A9-
BCNU	T45.1X-
Bearsfoot	T62.2X-
Beclamide	T42.6X-
Beclomethasone	T44.5X-
Bee (sting) (venom)	T63.441
Befunolol	T49.5X-
Bekanamycin	T36.5X-
Belladonna—*see Nightshade*	T44.3X-
Bemegride	T50.7X-
Benactyzine	T44.3X-
Benadryl	T45.0X-
Benaprizine	T44.3X-
Benazepril	T46.4X-
Bencyclane	T46.7X-
Bendazol	T46.3X-
Bendrofluazide	T50.2X-
Bendroflumethiazide	T50.2X-
Benemid	T50.4X-
Benethamine penicillin	T36.0X-
Benexate	T47.1X-
Benfluorex	T46.6X-
Benfotiamine	T45.2X-
Benisone	T49.0X-
Benomyl	T60.0X-
Benoquin	T49.8X-
Benoxinate	T41.3X-
Benperidol	T43.4X-
Benproperine	T48.3X-
Benserazide	T42.8X-
Bentazepam	T42.4X-

TABLE OF DRUGS AND CHEMICALS

Drug/Chemical	Code
Bentiromide	T50.8X-
Bentonite	T49.3X-
Benzalbutyramide	T46.6X-
Benzalkonium (chloride)	T49.0X-
ophthalmic preparation	T49.5X-
Benzamidosalicylate (calcium)	T37.1X-
Benzamine	T41.3X-
lactate	T49.1X-
Benzamphetamine	T50.5X-
Benzapril hydrochloride	T46.5X-
Benzathine benzylpenicillin	T36.0X-
Benzathine penicillin	T36.0X-
Benzatropine	T42.8X-
Benzbromarone	T50.4X-
Benzcarbimine	T45.1X-
Benzedrex	T44.99-
Benzedrine (amphetamine)	T43.62-
Benzenamine	T65.3X-
Benzene	T52.1X-
homologues (acetyl) (dimethyl) (methyl) (solvent)	T52.2X-
Benzethonium (chloride)	T49.0X-
Benzfetamine	T50.5X-
Benzhexol	T44.3X-
Benzhydramine (chloride)	T45.0X-
Benzidine	T65.89-
Benzilonium bromide	T44.3X-
Benzimidazole	T60.3X-
Benziodarone	T46.3X-
Benznidazole	T37.3X-
Benzocaine	T41.3X-
Benzodiapin	T42.4X-
Benzodiazepine NEC	T42.4X-
Benzoic acid	T49.0X-
with salicylic acid	T49.0X-
Benzoin (tincture)	T48.5X-
Benzol (benzene)	T52.1X-
vapor	T52.0X-
Benzomorphan	T40.2X-
Benzonatate	T48.3X-
Benzophenones	T49.3X-
Benzopyrone	T46.99-
Benzothiadiazides	T50.2X-
Benzoxonium chloride	T49.0X-
Benzoyl peroxide	T49.0X-
Benzoylpas calcium	T37.1X-
Benzperidin	T43.59-
Benzperidol	T43.59-
Benzphetamine	T50.5X-
Benzpyrinium bromide	T44.1X-
Benzquinamide	T45.0X-
Benzthiazide	T50.2X-
Benztropine	
anticholinergic	T44.3X-
antiparkinson	T42.8X-
Benzydamine	T49.0X-
Benzyl	
acetate	T52.8X-
alcohol	T49.0X-
benzoate	T49.0X-
Benzoic acid	T49.0X-
morphine	T40.2X-
nicotinate	T46.6X-
penicillin	T36.0X-
Benzylhydrochlorthiazide	T50.2X-
Benzylpenicillin	T36.0X-
Benzylthiouracil	T38.2X-
Bephenium hydroxy-naphthoate	T37.4X-
Bepridil	T46.1X-
Bergamot oil	T65.89-
Bergapten	T50.99-
Berries, poisonous	T62.1X-
Beryllium (compounds)	T56.7X-
b-acetyldigoxin	T46.0X-
beta adrenergic blocking agent, heart	T44.7X-
b-benzalbutyramide	T46.6X-
Betacarotene	T45.2X-
b-eucaine	T49.1X-
Beta-Chlor	T42.6X-
b-galactosidase	T47.5X-
Betahistine	T46.7X-
Betaine	T47.5X-
Betamethasone	T49.0X-
topical	T49.0X-
Betamicin	T36.8X-
Betanidine	T46.5X-
b-Sitosterol(s)	T46.6X-
Betaxolol	T44.7X-
Betazole	T50.8X-
Bethanechol	T44.1X-
chloride	T44.1X-
Bethanidine	T46.5X-
Betoxycaine	T41.3X-
Betula oil	T49.3X-
Bevantolol	T44.7X-
Bevonium metilsulfate	T44.3X-
Bezafibrate	T46.6X-
Bezitramide	T40.4X-
BHA	T50.99-
Bhang	T40.71-
BHC (medicinal)	T49.0X-
nonmedicinal (vapor)	T53.6X-
Bialamicol	T37.3X-
Bibenzonium bromide	T48.3X-
Bibrocathol	T49.5X-
Bichloride of mercury—*see Mercury, chloride*	
Bichromates (calcium) (potassium) (sodium) (crystals)	T57.8X-
fumes	T56.2X-
Biclotymol	T49.6X-

TABLE OF DRUGS AND CHEMICALS

Drug/Chemical	Code
Bicucculine	T50.7X-
Bifemelane	T43.29-
Biguanide derivatives, oral	T38.3X-
Bile salts	T47.5X-
Biligrafin	T50.8X-
Bilopaque	T50.8X-
Binifibrate	T46.6X-
Binitrobenzol	T65.3X-
Bioflavonoid(s)	T46.99-
Biological substance NEC	T50.90-
Biotin	T45.2X-
Biperiden	T44.3X-
Bisacodyl	T47.2X-
Bisbentiamine	T45.2X-
Bisbutiamine	T45.2X-
Bisdequalinium (salts) (diacetate)	T49.6X-
Bishydroxycoumarin	T45.51-
Bismarsen	T37.8X-
Bismuth salts	T47.6X-
aluminate	T47.1X-
anti-infectives	T37.8X-
formic iodide	T49.0X-
glycolylarsenate	T49.0X-
nonmedicinal (compounds) NEC	T65.9-
subcarbonate	T47.6X-
subsalicylate	T37.8X-
sulfarsphenamine	T37.8X-
Bisoprolol	T44.7X-
Bisoxatin	T47.2X-
Bisulepin (hydrochloride)	T45.0X-
Bithionol	T37.8X-
anthelminthic	T37.4X-
Bitolterol	T48.6X-
Bitoscanate	T37.4X-
Bitter almond oil	T62.8X-
Bittersweet	T62.2X-
Black	
flag	T60.9-
henbane	T62.2X-
leaf (40)	T60.9-
widow spider (bite)	T63.31-
antivenin	T50.Z1-
Blast furnace gas (carbon monoxide)	T58.8X-
Bleach	T54.9-
Bleaching agent (medicinal)	T49.4X-
Bleomycin	T45.1X-
Blockain (infiltration) (topical) (subcutaneous) (nerve block)	T41.3X-
Blockers, calcium channel	T46.1X-
Blood (derivatives) (natural) (plasma) (whole) (substitute)	T45.8X-
dried	T45.8X-
drug affecting NEC	T45.9-
expander NEC	T45.8X-
fraction NEC	T45.8X-

Drug/Chemical	Code
Blue velvet	T40.2X-
Bone meal	T62.8X-
Bonine	T45.0X-
Bopindolol	T44.7X-
Boracic acid	T49.0X-
ENT agent	T49.6X-
ophthalmic preparation	T49.5X-
Borane complex	T57.8X-
Borate(s)	T57.8X-
buffer	T50.99-
cleanser	T54.9-
sodium	T57.8X-
Borax (cleanser)	T54.9-
Bordeaux mixture	T60.3X-
Boric acid	T49.0X-
ENT agent	T49.6X-
ophthalmic preparation	T49.5X-
Bornaprine	T44.3X-
Boron	T57.8X-
hydride NEC	T57.8X-
fumes or gas	T57.8X-
trifluoride	T59.89-
Botox	T48.29-
Botulinus anti-toxin (type A, B)	T50.Z1-
Brake fluid vapor	T59.89-
Brallobarbital	T42.3X-
Bran (wheat)	T47.4X-
Brass (fumes)	T56.89-
Brasso	T52.0X-
Bretylium tosilate	T46.2X-
Brevital (sodium)	T41.1X-
Brinase	T45.3X-
British antilewisite	T45.8X-
Brodifacoum	T60.4X-
Bromal (hydrate)	T42.6X-
Bromazepam	T42.4X-
Bromazine	T45.0X-
Brombenzylcyanide	T59.3X-
Bromelains	T45.3X-
Bromethalin	T60.4X-
Bromhexine	T48.4X-
Bromide salts	T42.6X-
Bromindione	T45.51-
Bromine	
compounds (medicinal)	T42.6X-
sedative	T42.6X-
vapor	T59.89-
Bromisoval	T42.6X-
Bromisovalum	T42.6X-
Bromobenzylcyanide	T59.3X-
Bromochlorosalicylanilide	T49.0X-
Bromocriptine	T42.8X-
Bromodiphenhydramine	T45.0X-
Bromoform	T42.6X-
Bromophenol blue reagent	T50.99-

TABLE OF DRUGS AND CHEMICALS

Drug/Chemical	Code
Bromopride	T47.8X-
Bromosalicylchloranitide	T49.0X-
Bromosalicylhydroxamic acid	T37.1X-
Bromo-seltzer	T39.1X-
Bromoxynil	T60.3X-
Bromperidol	T43.4X-
Brompheniramine	T45.0X-
Bromsulfophthalein	T50.8X-
Bromural	T42.6X-
Bromvaletone	T42.6X-
Bronchodilator NEC	T48.6X-
Brotizolam	T42.4X-
Brovincamine	T46.7X-
Brown recluse spider (bite) (venom)	T63.33-
Brown spider (bite) (venom)	T63.39-
Broxaterol	T48.6X-
Broxuridine	T45.1X-
Broxyquinoline	T37.8X-
Bruceine	T48.29-
Brucia	T62.2X-
Brucine	T65.1X-
Bryonia	T47.2X-
Buclizine	T45.0X-
Buclosamide	T49.0X-
Budesonide	T44.5X-
Budralazine	T46.5X-
Bufferin	T39.01-
Buflomedil	T46.7X-
Buformin	T38.3X-
Bufotenine	T40.99-
Bufrolin	T48.6X-
Bufylline	T48.6X-
Bulk filler	T50.5X-
cathartic	T47.4X-
Bumetanide	T50.1X-
Bunaftine	T46.2X-
Bunamiodyl	T50.8X-
Bunazosin	T44.6X-
Bunitrolol	T44.7X-
Buphenine	T46.7X-
Bupivacaine (infiltration) (Nerve block) (spinal)	T41.3X-
Bupranolol	T44.7X-
Buprenorphine	T40.4X-
Bupropion	T43.29-
Burimamide	T47.1X-
Buserelin	T38.89-
Buspirone	T43.59-
Busulfan, busulphan	T45.1X-
Butabarbital (sodium)	T42.3X-
Butabarbitone	T42.3X-
Butabarpal	T42.3X-
Butacaine	T41.3X-
Butalamine	T46.7X-
Butalbital	T42.3X-
Butallylonal	T42.3X-
Butamben	T41.3X-
Butamirate	T48.3X-
Butane (distributed in mobile container or through pipes)	T59.89-
incomplete combustion	T58.1-
Butanilicaine	T41.3X-
Butanol	T51.3X-
Butanone, 2-butanone	T52.4X-
Butantrone	T49.4X-
Butaperazine	T43.3X-
Butazolidin	T39.2X-
Butetamate	T48.6X-
Butethal	T42.3X-
Butethamate	T44.3X-
Buthalitone (sodium)	T41.1X-
Butisol (sodium)	T42.3X-
Butizide	T50.2X-
Butobarbital (sodium)	T42.3X-
Butobarbitone	T42.3X-
Butoconazole (nitrate)	T49.0X-
Butorphanol	T40.4X-
Butriptyline	T43.01-
Butropium bromide	T44.3X-
Buttercups	T62.2X-
Butyl	
acetate (secondary)	T52.8X-
alcohol	T51.3X-
aminobenzoate	T41.3X-
butyrate	T52.8X-
carbinol or carbitol	T51.3X-
cellosolve	T52.3X-
chloral (hydrate)	T42.6X-
formate or lactate or propionate	T52.8X-
scopolamine bromide	T44.3X-
thiobarbital sodium	T41.1X-
Butylated hydroxy-anisole	T50.99-
Butylchloral hydrate	T42.6X-
Butyltoluene	T52.2X-
Butyn	T41.3X-
Butyrophenone (-based tranquilizers)	T43.4X-
Cabergoline	T42.8X-
Cacodyl, cacodylic acid	T57.0X-
Cactinomycin	T45.1X-
Cade oil	T49.4X-
Cadexomer iodine	T49.0X-
Cadmium (chloride) (fumes) (oxide)	T56.3X-
sulfide (medicinal) NEC	T49.4X-
Cadralazine	T46.5X-
Caffeine	T43.61-
Calabar bean	T62.2X-
Caladium seguinum	T62.2X-
Calamine (lotion)	T49.3X-
Calcifediol	T45.2X-
Calciferol	T45.2X-
Calcitonin	T50.99-

TABLE OF DRUGS AND CHEMICALS

Drug/Chemical	Code
Calcitriol	T45.2X-
Calcium	T50.3X-
actylsalicylate	T39.01-
benzamidosalicylate	T37.1X-
bromide or bromolactobionate	T42.6X-
carbaspirin	T39.01-
carbimide	T50.6X-
carbonate	T47.1X-
chloride (anhydrous)	T50.99-
cyanide	T57.8X-
dioctyl sulfosuccinate	T47.4X-
disodium edathamil	T45.8X-
disodium edetate	T45.8X-
dobesilate	T46.99-
EDTA	T45.8X-
ferrous citrate	T45.4X-
folinate	T45.8X-
glubionate	T50.3X-
gluconate or – gluconogalactogluconate	T50.3X-
hydrate, hydroxide	T54.3X-
hypochlorite	T54.3X-
iodide	T48.4X-
ipodate	T50.8X-
lactate	T50.3X-
leucovorin	T45.8X-
mandelate	T37.9-
oxide	T54.3X-
pantothenate	T45.2X-
phosphate	T50.3X-
salicylate	T39.09-
salts	T50.3X-
Calculus-dissolving drug	T50.99-
Calomel	T49.0X-
Caloric agent	T50.3X-
Calusterone	T38.7X-
Camazepam	T42.4X-
Camomile	T49.0X-
Camoquin	T37.2X-
Camphor	
insecticide	T60.2X-
medicinal	T49.8X-
Camylofin	T44.3X-
Cancer chemo drug regimen	T45.1X-
Candeptin	T49.0X-
Candicidin	T49.0X-
Cannabinoids, synthetic	T40.72-
Cannabinol	T40.71-
Cannabis (derivatives)	T40.71-
Canned heat	T51.1X-
Canrenoic acid	T50.0X-
Canrenone	T50.0X-
Cantharides, cantharidin, cantharis	T49.8X-
Canthaxanthin	T50.99-
Capillary-active drug NEC	T46.90-
Capreomycin	T36.8X-

Drug/Chemical	Code
Capsicum	T49.4X-
Captafol	T60.3X-
Captan	T60.3X-
Captodiame, captodiamine	T43.59-
Captopril	T46.4X-
Caramiphen	T44.3X-
Carazolol	T44.7X-
Carbachol	T44.1X-
Carbacrylamine (resin)	T50.3X-
Carbamate (insecticide)	T60.0X-
Carbamate (sedative)	T42.6X-
herbicide or insecticide	T60.0X-
Carbamazepine	T42.1X-
Carbamide	T47.3X-
peroxide	T49.0X-
topical	T49.8X-
Carbamylcholine chloride	T44.1X-
Carbaril	T60.0X-
Carbarsone	T37.3X-
Carbaryl	T60.0X-
Carbaspirin	T39.01-
Carbazochrome (salicylate) (sodium sulfonate)	T49.4X-
Carbenicillin	T36.0X-
Carbenoxolone	T47.1X-
Carbetapentane	T48.3X-
Carbethyl salicylate	T39.09-
Carbidopa (with levodopa)	T42.8X-
Carbimazole	T38.2X-
Carbinol	T51.1X-
Carbinoxamine	T45.0X-
Carbiphene	T39.8X-
Carbitol	T52.3X-
Carbo medicinalis	T47.6X-
Carbocaine (infiltration) (topical) (subcutaneous) (nerve block)	T41.3X-
Carbocisteine	T48.4X-
Carbocromen	T46.3X-
Carbol fuchsin	T49.0X-
Carbolic acid—*see also Phenol*	T54.0X-
Carbolonium (bromide)	T48.1X-
Carbomycin	T36.8X-
Carbon	
bisulfide (liquid) or vapor	T65.4X-
dioxide (gas)	T59.7X-
medicinal	T41.5X-
nonmedicinal	T59.7X-
snow	T49.4X-
disulfide (liquid) or vapor	T65.4X-
monoxide (from incomplete combustion)	T58.9-
blast furnace gas	T58.8X-
butane (distributed in mobile container or through pipes)	T58.1-
charcoal fumes or coal	T58.2X-
coke (in domestic stoves, fireplaces)	T58.2X-
gas (piped)	T58.1-

TABLE OF DRUGS AND CHEMICALS

Drug/Chemical	Code
Carbon, continued	
solid (in domestic stoves, fireplaces)	T58.2X-
exhaust gas (motor)not in transit	T58.0-
combustion engine, any not in watercraft	T58.0-
farm tractor, not in transit	T58.0-
gas engine / motor pump	T58.01
motor vehicle, not in transit	T58.0-
fuel (in domestic use)	T58.2X-
gas (piped) (natural) or in mobile container	T58.1-
utility	T58.1-
in mobile container	T58.1-
illuminating gas	T58.1-
industrial fuels or gases, any	T58.8X-
kerosene (in domestic stoves, fireplaces)	T58.2X-
kiln gas or vapor	T58.8X-
motor exhaust gas, not in transit	T58.0-
piped gas (manufactured) (natural)	T58.1-
producer gas	T58.8X-
propane (distributed in mobile container)	T58.1-
distributed through pipes	T58.1-
specified source NEC	T58.8X-
stove gas (piped) / utility gas (piped) / water gas	T58.1-
wood (in domestic stoves, fireplaces)	T58.2X-
tetrachloride (vapor) NEC	T53.0X-
Carbonic acid gas	T59.7X-
anhydrase inhibitor NEC	T50.2X-
Carbophenothion	T60.0X-
Carboplatin	T45.1X-
Carboprost	T48.0X-
Carboquone	T45.1X-
Carbowax	T49.3X-
Carboxymethyl-cellulose	T47.4X-
S-Carboxymethyl-cysteine	T48.4X-
Carbrital	T42.3X-
Carbromal	T42.6X-
Carbutamide	T38.3X-
Carbuterol	T48.6X-
Cardiac medications (depressants) (rhythm regulater) NEC	T46.2X-
Cardiografin	T50.8X-
Cardio-green	T50.8X-
Cardiotonic (glycoside) NEC	T46.0X-
Cardiovascular drug NEC	T46.90-
Cardrase	T50.2X-
Carfecillin	T36.0X-
Carfenazine	T43.3X-
Carfusin	T49.0X-
Carindacillin	T36.0X-
Carisoprodol	T42.8X-
Carmellose	T47.4X-
Carminative	T47.5X-
Carmofur	T45.1X-
Carmustine	T45.1X-
Carotene	T45.2X-
Carphenazine	T43.3X-

Drug/Chemical	Code
Carpipramine	T42.4X-
Carprofen	T39.31-
Carpronium chloride	T44.3X-
Carrageenan	T47.8X-
Carteolol	T44.7X-
Carter's Little Pills	T47.2X-
Cascara (sagrada)	T47.2X-
Cassava	T62.2X-
Castellani's paint	T49.0X-
Castor (bean) (oil)	T62.2X-
Catalase	T45.3X-
Caterpillar (sting)	T63.431
Catha (edulis) (tea)	T43.69-
Cathartic NEC	T47.4X-
anthacene derivative	T47.2X-
bulk	T47.4X-
contact	T47.2X-
emollient NEC	T47.4X-
irritant NEC	T47.2X-
mucilage	T47.4X-
saline	T47.3X-
vegetable	T47.2X-
Cathine	T50.5X-
Cathomycin	T36.8X-
Cation exchange resin	T50.3X-
Caustic(s) NEC	T54.9-
alkali	T54.3X-
hydroxide	T54.3X-
potash	T54.3X-
soda	T54.3X-
specified NEC	T54.9-
Ceepryn	T49.0X-
ENT agent	T49.6X-
lozenges	T49.6X-
Cefacetrile	T36.1X-
Cefaclor	T36.1X-
Cefadroxil	T36.1X-
Cefalexin	T36.1X-
Cefaloglycin	T36.1X-
Cefaloridine	T36.1X-
Cefalosporins	T36.1X-
Cefalotin	T36.1X-
Cefamandole	T36.1X-
Cefamycin antibiotic	T36.1X-
Cefapirin	T36.1X-
Cefatrizine	T36.1X-
Cefazedone	T36.1X-
Cefazolin	T36.1X-
Cefbuperazone	T36.1X-
Cefetamet	T36.1X-
Cefixime	T36.1X-
Cefmenoxime	T36.1X-
Cefmetazole	T36.1X-
Cefminox	T36.1X-
Cefonicid	T36.1X-

TABLE OF DRUGS AND CHEMICALS

Drug/Chemical	Code	Drug/Chemical	Code
Cefoperazone	T36.1X-	**Cephalexin**	T36.1X-
Ceforanide	T36.1X-	**Cephaloglycin**	T36.1X-
Cefotaxime	T36.1X-	**Cephaloridine**	T36.1X-
Cefotetan	T36.1X-	**Cephalosporins**	T36.1X-
Cefotiam	T36.1X-	N (adicillin)	T36.0X-
Cefoxitin	T36.1X-	**Cephalothin**	T36.1X-
Cefpimizole	T36.1X-	**Cephalotin**	T36.1X-
Cefpiramide	T36.1X-	**Cephradine**	T36.1X-
Cefradine	T36.1X-	**Cerbera (odallam)**	T62.2X-
Cefroxadine	T36.1X-	**Cerberin**	T46.0X-
Cefsulodin	T36.1X-	**Cerebral stimulants**	T43.60-
Ceftazidime	T36.1X-	psychotherapeutic	T43.60-
Cefteram	T36.1X-	specified NEC	T43.69-
Ceftezole	T36.1X-	**Cerium oxalate**	T45.0X-
Ceftizoxime	T36.1X-	**Cerous oxalate**	T45.0X-
Ceftriaxone	T36.1X-	**Ceruletide**	T50.8X-
Cefuroxime	T36.1X-	**Cetalkonium (chloride)**	T49.0X-
Cefuzonam	T36.1X-	**Cethexonium chloride**	T49.0X-
Celestone	T38.0X-	**Cetiedil**	T46.7X-
topical	T49.0X-	**Cetirizine**	T45.0X-
Celiprolol	T44.7X-	**Cetomacrogol**	T50.99-
Cell stimulants and proliferants	T49.8X-	**Cetotiamine**	T45.2X-
Cellosolve	T52.9-	**Cetoxime**	T45.0X-
Cellulose		**Cetraxate**	T47.1X-
cathartic	T47.4X-	**Cetrimide**	T49.0X-
hydroxyethyl	T47.4X-	**Cetrimonium (bromide)**	T49.0X-
nitrates (topical)	T49.3X-	**Cetylpyridinium chloride**	T49.0X-
oxidized	T49.4X-	ENT agent or lozenges	T49.6X-
Centipede (bite)	T63.41-	**Cevitamic acid**	T45.2X-
Central nervous system		**Chalk, precipitated**	T47.1X-
depressants	T42.71	**Chamomile**	T49.0X-
anesthetic (general) NEC	T41.20-	**Ch'an su**	T46.0X-
gases NEC	T41.0X-	**Charcoal**	T47.6X-
intravenous	T41.1X-	activated—*see also Charcoal, medicinal*	T47.6X-
barbiturates	T42.3X-	fumes (Carbon monoxide)	T58.2X-
benzodiazepines	T42.4X-	industrial	T58.8X-
bromides	T42.6X-	medicinal (activated)	T47.6X-
cannabis sativa	T40.71-	antidiarrheal	T47.6X-
chloral hydrate	T42.6X-	poison control	T47.8X-
ethanol	T51.0X-	specified use other than for diarrhea	T47.8X-
hallucinogenics	T40.90-	topical	T49.8X-
hypnotics	T42.71	**Chaulmosulfone**	T37.1X-
specified NEC	T42.6X-	**Chelating agent NEC**	T50.6X-
muscle relaxants	T42.8X-	**Chelidonium majus**	T62.2X-
paraldehyde	T42.6X-	**Chemical substance NEC**	T65.9-
sedatives; sedative-hypnotics	T42.71	**Chenodeoxycholic acid**	T47.5X-
mixed NEC	T42.6X-	**Chenodiol**	T47.5X-
specified NEC	T42.6X-	**Chenopodium**	T37.4X-
muscle-tone depressants	T42.8X-	**Cherry laurel**	T62.2X-
stimulants	T43.60-	**Chinidin (e)**	T46.2X-
amphetamines	T43.62-	**Chiniofon**	T37.8X-
analeptics	T50.7X-	**Chlophedianol**	T48.3X-
antidepressants	T43.20-	**Chloral**	T42.6X-
opiate antagonists	T50.7X-	derivative	T42.6X-
specified NEC	T43.69-	hydrate	T42.6X-

TABLE OF DRUGS AND CHEMICALS

Drug/Chemical	Code
Chloralamide	T42.6X-
Chloralodol	T42.6X-
Chloralose	T60.4X-
Chlorambucil	T45.1X-
Chloramine	T57.8X-
topical	T49.0X-
Chloramphenicol	T36.2X-
ENT agent	T49.6X-
ophthalmic preparation	T49.5X-
topical NEC	T49.0X-
Chlorate (potassium) (sodium) NEC	T60.3X-
herbicide	T60.3X-
Chlorazanil	T50.2X-
Chlorbenzene, chlorbenzol	T53.7X-
Chlorbenzoxamine	T44.3X-
Chlorbutol	T42.6X-
Chlorcyclizine	T45.0X-
Chlordan (e) (dust)	T60.1X-
Chlordantoin	T49.0X-
Chlordiazepoxide	T42.4X-
Chlordiethyl benzamide	T49.3X-
Chloresium	T49.8X-
Chlorethiazol	T42.6X-
Chlorethyl—*see Ethyl, chloride*	
Chloretone	T42.6X-
Chlorex	T53.6X-
insecticide	T60.1X-
Chlorfenvinphos	T60.0X-
Chlorhexadol	T42.6X-
Chlorhexamide	T45.1X-
Chlorhexidine	T49.0X-
Chlorhydroxyquinolin	T49.0X-
Chloride of lime (bleach)	T54.3X-
Chlorimipramine	T43.01-
Chlorinated	
camphene	T53.6X-
diphenyl	T53.7X-
hydrocarbons NEC (solvents)	T53.9-
lime (bleach)	T54.3X-
and boric acid solution	T49.0X-
naphthalene (insecticide)	T60.1X-
industrial (non-pesticide)	T53.7X-
pesticide NEC	T60.8X-
solution	T49.0X-
Chlorine (fumes) (gas)	T59.4X-
bleach	T54.3X-
compound gas NEC	T59.4X-
disinfectant	T59.4X-
releasing agents NEC	T59.4X-
Chlorisondamine chloride	T46.99-
Chlormadinone	T38.5X-
Chlormephos	T60.0X-
Chlormerodrin	T50.2X-
Chlormethiazole	T42.6X-
Chlormethine	T45.1X-
Chlormethylenecycline	T36.4X-
Chlormezanone	T42.6X-
Chloroacetic acid	T60.3X-
Chloroacetone	T59.3X-
Chloroacetophenone	T59.3X-
Chloroaniline	T53.7X-
Chlorobenzene, chlorobenzol	T53.7X-
Chlorobromomethane (fire extinguisher)	T53.6X-
Chlorobutanol	T49.0X-
Chlorocresol	T49.0X-
Chlorodehydro-methyltestosterone	T38.7X-
Chlorodinitrobenzene	T53.7X-
Chlorodiphenyl	T53.7X-
Chloroethane—*see Ethyl, chloride*	
Chloroethylene	T53.6X-
Chlorofluorocarbons	T53.5X-
Chloroform (fumes) (vapor)	T53.1X-
anesthetic	T41.0X-
solvent	T53.1X-
water, concentrated	T41.0X-
Chloroguanide	T37.2X-
Chloromycetin	T36.2X-
ENT agent or otic solution	T49.6X-
ophthalmic preparation	T49.5X-
topical NEC	T49.0X-
Chloronitrobenzene	T53.7X-
Chlorophacinone	T60.4X-
Chlorophenol	T53.7X-
Chlorophenothane	T60.1X-
Chlorophyll	T50.99-
Chloropicrin (fumes)	T53.6X-
fumigant / pesticide	T60.8X-
fungicide	T60.3X-
Chloroprocaine (infiltration) (topical) (subcutaneous) (nerve block) (spinal)	T41.3X-
Chloroptic	T49.5X-
Chloropurine	T45.1X-
Chloropyramine	T45.0X-
Chloropyrifos	T60.0X-
Chloropyrilene	T45.0X-
Chloroquine	T37.2X-
Chlorothalonil	T60.3X-
Chlorothen	T45.0X-
Chlorothiazide	T50.2X-
Chlorothymol	T49.4X-
Chlorotrianisene	T38.5X-
Chlorovinyldichloro-arsine	T57.0X-
Chloroxine	T49.4X-
Chloroxylenol	T49.0X-
Chlorphenamine	T45.0X-
Chlorphenesin	T42.8X-
topical (antifungal)	T49.0X-
Chlorpheniramine	T45.0X-
Chlorphenoxamine	T45.0X-
Chlorphentermine	T50.5X-

TABLE OF DRUGS AND CHEMICALS

Drug/Chemical	Code
Chlorproguanil	T37.2X-
Chlorpromazine	T43.3X-
Chlorpropamide	T38.3X-
Chlorprothixene	T43.4X-
Chlorquinaldol	T49.0X-
Chlorquinol	T49.0X-
Chlortalidone	T50.2X-
Chlortetracycline	T36.4X-
Chlorthalidone	T50.2X-
Chlorthion	T60.0X-
Chlorthiophos	T60.0X-
Chlortrianisene	T38.5X-
Chlor-Trimeton	T45.0X-
Chlorzoxazone	T42.8X-
Choke damp	T59.7X-
Cholagogues	T47.5X-
Cholebrine	T50.8X-
Cholecalciferol	T45.2X-
Cholecystokinin	T50.8X-
Cholera vaccine	T50.A9-
Choleretic	T47.5X-
Cholesterol-lowering agents	T46.6X-
Cholestyramine (resin)	T46.6X-
Cholic acid	T47.5X-
Choline	T48.6X-
chloride	T50.99-
dihydrogen citrate	T50.99-
salicylate	T39.09-
theophyllinate	T48.6X-
Cholinergic (drug) NEC	T44.1X-
muscle tone enhancer	T44.1X-
organophosphorus	T44.0X-
insecticide	T60.0X-
nerve gas	T59.89-
trimethyl ammonium propanediol	T44.1X-
Cholinesterase reactivator	T50.6X-
Cholografin	T50.8X-
Chorionic gonadotropin	T38.89-
Chromate	T56.2X-
dust or mist	T56.2X-
lead—*see also lead*	T56.0X-
paint	T56.0X-
Chromic	
acid	T56.2X-
dust or mist	T56.2X-
phosphate 32P	T45.1X-
Chromium	T56.2X-
compounds—*see Chromate*	
sesquioxide	T50.8X-
Chromomycin A3	T45.1X-
Chromonar	T46.3X-
Chromyl chloride	T56.2X-
Chrysarobin	T49.4X-
Chrysazin	T47.2X-

Drug/Chemical	Code
Chymar	T45.3X-
ophthalmic preparation	T49.5X-
Chymopapain	T45.3X-
Chymotrypsin	T45.3X-
ophthalmic preparation	T49.5X-
Cianidanol	T50.99-
Cianopramine	T43.01-
Cibenzoline	T46.2X-
Ciclacillin	T36.0X-
Ciclobarbital—*see Hexobarbital*	
Ciclonicate	T46.7X-
Ciclopirox (olamine)	T49.0X-
Ciclosporin	T45.1X-
Cicuta maculata or virosa	T62.2X-
Cicutoxin	T62.2X-
Cigarette lighter fluid	T52.0X-
Cigarettes (tobacco)	T65.22-
Ciguatoxin	T61.0-
Cilazapril	T46.4X-
Cimetidine	T47.0X-
Cimetropium bromide	T44.3X-
Cinchocaine	T41.3X-
Cinchona	T37.2X-
Cinchonine alkaloids	T37.2X-
Cinchophen	T50.4X-
Cinepazide	T46.7X-
Cinnamedrine	T48.5X-
Cinnarizine	T45.0X-
Cinoxacin	T37.8X-
Ciprofibrate	T46.6X-
Ciprofloxacin	T36.8X-
Cisapride	T47.8X-
Cisplatin	T45.1X-
Citalopram	T43.22-
Citanest (infiltration) (topical) (subcutaneous) (nerve block)	T41.3X-
Citric acid	T47.5X-
Citrovorum (factor)	T45.8X-
Claviceps purpurea	T62.2X-
Clavulanic acid	T36.1X-
Cleaner, cleansing agent, type not specified	T65.89-
of paint or varnish	T52.9-
specified type NEC	T65.89-
Clebopride	T47.8X-
Clefamide	T37.3X-
Clemastine	T45.0X-
Clematis vitalba	T62.2X-
Clemizole (penicillin)	T45.0X-
Clenbuterol	T48.6X-
Clidinium bromide	T44.3X-
Clindamycin	T36.8X-
Clinofibrate	T46.6X-
Clioquinol	T37.8X-
Cliradon	T40.2X-
Clobazam	T42.4X-

TABLE OF DRUGS AND CHEMICALS

Drug/Chemical	Code
Clobenzorex	T50.5X-
Clobetasol	T49.0X-
Clobetasone	T49.0X-
Clobutinol	T48.3X-
Clocortolone	T38.0X-
Clodantoin	T49.0X-
Clodronic acid	T50.99-
Clofazimine	T37.1X-
Clofedanol	T48.3X-
Clofenamide	T50.2X-
Clofenotane	T49.0X-
Clofezone	T39.2X-
Clofibrate	T46.6X-
Clofibride	T46.6X-
Cloforex	T50.5X-
Clomethiazole	T42.6X-
Clometocillin	T36.0X-
Clomifene	T38.5X-
Clomiphene	T38.5X-
Clomipramine	T43.01-
Clomocycline	T36.4X-
Clonazepam	T42.4X-
Clonidine	T46.5X-
Clonixin	T39.8X-
Clopamide	T50.2X-
Clopenthixol	T43.4X-
Cloperastine	T48.3X-
Clophedianol	T48.3X-
Cloponone	T36.2X-
Cloprednol	T38.0X-
Cloral betaine	T42.6X-
Cloramfenicol	T36.2X-
Clorazepate (dipotassium)	T42.4X-
Clorexolone	T50.2X-
Clorfenamine	T45.0X-
Clorgiline	T43.1X-
Clorotepine	T44.3X-
Clorox (bleach)	T54.9-
Clorprenaline	T48.6X-
Clortermine	T50.5X-
Clotiapine	T43.59-
Clotiazepam	T42.4X-
Clotibric acid	T46.6X-
Clotrimazole	T49.0X-
Cloxacillin	T36.0X-
Cloxazolam	T42.4X-
Cloxiquine	T49.0X-
Clozapine	T42.4X-
Coagulant NEC	T45.7X-
Coal (carbon monoxide from)—*see also Carbon, monoxide, coal*	T58.2X-
oil—*see Kerosene*	
tar	T49.1X-
fumes	T59.89-
Coal (carbon monoxide from), continued	T58.2X-
medicinal (ointment)	T49.4X-
analgesics NEC	T39.2X-
naphtha (solvent)	T52.0X-
Cobalamine	T45.2X-
Cobalt (nonmedicinal) (fumes) (industrial)	T56.89-
medicinal (trace) (chloride)	T45.8X-
Cobra (venom)	T63.041
Coca (leaf)	T40.5X-
Cocaine	T40.5X-
topical anesthetic	T41.3X-
Cocarboxylase	T45.3X-
Coccidioidin	T50.8X-
Cocculus indicus	T62.1X-
Cochineal	T65.6X-
medicinal products	T50.99-
Codeine	T40.2X-
Cod-liver oil	T45.2X-
Coenzyme A	T50.99-
Coffee	T62.8X-
Cogalactoiso-merase	T50.99-
Cogentin	T44.3X-
Coke fumes or gas (carbon monoxide)	T58.2X-
industrial use	T58.8X-
Colace	T47.4X-
Colaspase	T45.1X-
Colchicine	T50.4X-
Colchicum	T62.2X-
Cold cream	T49.3X-
Colecalciferol	T45.2X-
Colestipol	T46.6X-
Colestyramine	T46.6X-
Colimycin	T36.8X-
Colistimethate	T36.8X-
Colistin	T36.8X-
sulfate (eye preparation)	T49.5X-
Collagen	T50.99-
Collagenase	T49.4X-
Collodion	T49.3X-
Colocynth	T47.2X-
Colophony adhesive	T49.3X-
Colorant—*see also Dye*	T50.99-
Combustion gas (after combustion)—*see Carbon, monoxide*	
prior to combustion	T59.89-
Compazine	T43.3X-
Compound	
42 (warfarin)	T60.4X-
269 (endrin)	T60.1X-
497 (dieldrin)	T60.1X-
1080 (sodium fluoroacetate)	T60.4X-
3422 (parathion)	T60.0X-
3911 (phorate)	T60.0X-
3956 (toxaphene)	T60.1X-
4049 (malathion)	T60.0X-

TABLE OF DRUGS AND CHEMICALS

Drug/Chemical	Code
Compound, continued	
4069 (malathion)	T60.0X-
4124 (dicapthon)	T60.0X-
E (cortisone)	T38.0X-
F (hydrocortisone)	T38.0X-
Congener, anabolic	T38.7X-
Congo red	T50.8X-
Coniine, conine	T62.2X-
Conium (maculatum)	T62.2X-
Conjugated estrogenic substances	T38.5X-
Contac	T48.5X-
Contact lens solution	T49.5X-
Contraceptive (oral)	T38.4X-
vaginal	T49.8X-
Contrast medium, radiography	T50.8X-
Convallaria glycosides	T46.0X-
Convallaria majalis	T62.2X-
berry	T62.1X-
Copper (dust) (fumes) (nonmedicinal) NEC	T56.4X-
arsenate, arsenite	T57.0X-
insecticide	T60.2X-
emetic	T47.7X-
fungicide	T60.3X-
gluconate	T49.0X-
insecticide	T60.2X-
medicinal (trace)	T45.8X-
oleate	T49.0X-
sulfate	T56.4X-
cupric	T56.4X-
fungicide	T60.3X-
medicinal	
ear	T49.6X-
emetic	T47.7X-
eye	T49.5X-
cuprous	T56.4X-
fungicide	T60.3X-
medicinal	
ear	T49.6X-
emetic	T47.7X-
eye	T49.5X-
Copperhead snake (bite) (venom)	T63.06-
Coral (sting)	T63.69-
snake (bite) (venom)	T63.02-
Corbadrine	T49.6X-
Cordite	T65.89-
vapor	T59.89-
Cordran	T49.0X-
Corn cures	T49.4X-
Corn starch	T49.3X-
Cornhusker's lotion	T49.3X-
Coronary vasodilator NEC	T46.3X-
Corrosive NEC	T54.9-
acid NEC	T54.2X-
aromatics	T54.1X-
disinfectant	T54.1X-

Drug/Chemical	Code
Corrosive NEC, continued	T54.9-
fumes NEC	T54.9-
specified NEC	T54.9-
sublimate	T56.1X-
Cortate	T38.0X-
Cort-Dome	T38.0X-
ENT agent	T49.6X-
ophthalmic preparation	T49.5X-
topical NEC	T49.0X-
Cortef	T38.0X-
ENT agent	T49.6X-
ophthalmic preparation	T49.5X-
topical NEC	T49.0X-
Corticosteroid	T38.0X-
ENT agent	T49.6X-
mineral	T50.0X-
ophthalmic	T49.5X-
topical NEC	T49.0X-
Corticotropin	T38.81-
Cortisol	T49.0X-
ENT agent	T49.6X-
ophthalmic preparation	T49.5X-
topical NEC	T49.0X-
Cortisone (acetate)	T38.0X-
ENT agent	T49.6X-
ophthalmic preparation	T49.5X-
topical NEC	T49.0X-
Cortivazol	T38.0X-
Cortogen	T38.0X-
ENT agent	T49.6X-
ophthalmic preparation	T49.5X-
Cortone	T38.0X-
ENT agent	T49.6X-
ophthalmic preparation	T49.5X-
Cortril	T38.0X-
ENT agent	T49.6X-
ophthalmic preparation	T49.5X-
topical NEC	T49.0X-
Corynebacterium parvum	T45.1X-
Cosmetic preparation	T49.8X-
Cosmetics	T49.8X-
Cosyntropin	T38.81-
Cotarnine	T45.7X-
Co-trimoxazole	T36.8X-
Cottonseed oil	T49.3X-
Cough mixture (syrup)	T48.4X-
containing opiates	T40.2X-
expectorants	T48.4X-
Coumadin	T45.51-
rodenticide	T60.4X-
Coumaphos	T60.0X-
Coumarin	T45.51-
Coumetarol	T45.51-
Cowbane	T62.2X-
Cozyme	T45.2X-

TABLE OF DRUGS AND CHEMICALS

Drug/Chemical	Code	Drug/Chemical	Code
Crack	T40.5X-	**Cyclamate**	T50.99-
Crataegus extract	T46.0X-	**Cyclamen europaeum**	T62.2X-
Creolin	T54.1X-	**Cyclandelate**	T46.7X-
disinfectant	T54.1X-	**Cyclazocine**	T50.7X-
Creosol (compound)	T49.0X-	**Cyclizine**	T45.0X-
Creosote (coal tar) (beechwood)	T49.0X-	**Cyclobarbital**	T42.3X-
medicinal (expectorant) (syrup)	T48.4X-	**Cyclobarbitone**	T42.3X-
Cresol(s)	T49.0X-	**Cyclobenzaprine**	T48.1X-
and soap solution	T49.0X-	**Cyclodrine**	T44.3X-
Cresyl acetate	T49.0X-	**Cycloguanil embonate**	T37.2X-
Cresylic acid	T49.0X-	**Cyclohexane**	T52.8X-
Crimidine	T60.4X-	**Cyclohexanol**	T51.8X-
Croconazole	T37.8X-	**Cyclohexanone**	T52.4X-
Cromoglicic acid	T48.6X-	**Cycloheximide**	T60.3X-
Cromolyn	T48.6X-	**Cyclohexyl acetate**	T52.8X-
Cromonar	T46.3X-	**Cycloleucin**	T45.1X-
Cropropamide	T39.8X-	**Cyclomethycaine**	T41.3X-
with crotethamide	T50.7X-	**Cyclopentamine**	T44.4X-
Crotamiton	T49.0X-	**Cyclopenthiazide**	T50.2X-
Crotethamide	T39.8X-	**Cyclopentolate**	T44.3X-
with cropropamide	T50.7X-	**Cyclophosphamide**	T45.1X-
Croton (oil)	T47.2X-	**Cycloplegic drug**	T49.5X-
chloral	T42.6X-	**Cyclopropane**	T41.29-
Crude oil	T52.0X-	**Cyclopyrabital**	T39.8X-
Cryogenine	T39.8X-	**Cycloserine**	T37.1X-
Cryolite (vapor)	T60.1X-	**Cyclosporin**	T45.1X-
insecticide	T60.1X-	**Cyclothiazide**	T50.2X-
Cryptenamine (tannates)	T46.5X-	**Cycrimine**	T44.3X-
Crystal violet	T49.0X-	**Cyhalothrin**	T60.1X-
Cuckoopint	T62.2X-	**Cymarin**	T46.0X-
Cumetharol	T45.51-	**Cypermethrin**	T60.1X-
Cupric		**Cyphenothrin**	T60.2X-
acetate	T60.3X-	**Cyproheptadine**	T45.0X-
acetoarsenite	T57.0X-	**Cyproterone**	T38.6X-
arsenate	T57.0X-	**Cysteamine**	T50.6X-
gluconate	T49.0X-	**Cytarabine**	T45.1X-
oleate	T49.0X-	**Cytisus**	T62.2X-
sulfate	T56.4X-	**Cytochrome C**	T47.5X-
Cuprous sulfate—*see also Copper, sulfate*	T56.4X-	**Cytomel**	T38.1X-
Curare, curarine	T48.1X-	**Cytosine arabinoside**	T45.1X-
Cyamemazine	T43.3X-	**Cytoxan**	T45.1X-
Cyamopsis tetragono-loba	T46.6X-	**Cytozyme**	T45.7X-
Cyanacetyl hydrazide	T37.1X-	**2,4-D**	T60.3X-
Cyanic acid (gas)	T59.89-	**Dacarbazine**	T45.1X-
Cyanide(s) (compounds) (potassium) (sodium) NEC	T65.0X-	**Dactinomycin**	T45.1X-
dust or gas (inhalation) NEC	T57.3X-	**DADPS**	T37.1X-
fumigant	T65.0X-	**Dakin's solution**	T49.0X-
hydrogen	T57.3X-	**Dalapon (sodium)**	T60.3X-
mercuric—see Mercury		**Dalmane**	T42.4X-
pesticide (dust) (fumes)	T65.0X-	**Danazol**	T38.6X-
Cyanoacrylate adhesive	T49.3X-	**Danilone**	T45.51-
Cyanocobalamin	T45.8X-	**Danthron**	T47.2X-
Cyanogen (chloride) (gas) NEC	T59.89-	**Dantrolene**	T42.8X-
Cyclacillin	T36.0X-	**Dantron**	T47.2X-
Cyclaine	T41.3X-		

TABLE OF DRUGS AND CHEMICALS

Drug/Chemical	Code
Daphne (gnidium) (mezereum)	T62.2X-
berry	T62.1X-
Dapsone	T37.1X-
Daraprim	T37.2X-
Darnel	T62.2X-
Darvon	T39.8X-
Daunomycin	T45.1X-
Daunorubicin	T45.1X-
DBI	T38.3X-
D-Con	T60.9-
insecticide	T60.2X-
rodenticide	T60.4X-
DDAVP	T38.89-
DDE (bis [chlorophenyl]-dichloroethylene)	T60.2X-
DDS	T37.1X-
DDT (dust)	T60.1X-
Deadly nightshade	T62.2X-
berry	T62.1X-
Deamino-D-arginine vasopressin	T38.89-
Deanol (aceglumate)	T50.99-
Debrisoquine	T46.5X-
Decaborane	T57.8X-
fumes	T59.89-
Decadron	T38.0X-
topical NEC	T49.0X-
Decahydronaphthalene	T52.8X-
Decalin	T52.8X-
Decamethonium (bromide)	T48.1X-
Decholin	T47.5X-
Declomycin	T36.4X-
Decongestant, nasal (mucosa)	T48.5X-
Deet	T60.8X-
Deferoxamine	T45.8X-
Deflazacort	T38.0X-
Deglycyrrhizinized extract of licorice	T48.4X-
Dehydrocholic acid	T47.5X-
Dehydroemetine	T37.3X-
Dekalin	T52.8X-
Delalutin	T38.5X-
Delorazepam	T42.4X-
Delphinium	T62.2X-
Deltamethrin	T60.1X-
Deltasone	T38.0X-
Deltra	T38.0X-
Delvinal	T42.3X-
Demecarium (bromide)	T49.5X-
Demeclocycline	T36.4X-
Demecolcine	T45.1X-
Demegestone	T38.5X-
Demelanizing agents	T49.8X-
Demephion -0 and -S	T60.0X-
Demerol	T40.2X-
Demethylchlortetracycline	T36.4X-
Demethyltetracycline	T36.4X-

Drug/Chemical	Code
Demeton -0 and -S	T60.0X-
Demulcent (external)	T49.3X-
Demulen	T38.4X-
Denatured alcohol	T51.0X-
Dendrid	T49.5X-
Dental drug, topical application NEC	T49.7X-
Dentifrice	T49.7X-
Deodorant spray (feminine hygiene)	T49.8X-
Deoxycortone	T50.0X-
2-Deoxy-5-fluorouridine	T45.1X-
5-Deoxy-5-fluorouridine	T45.1X-
Deoxyribonuclease (pancreatic)	T45.3X-
Depilatory	T49.4X-
Deprenalin	T42.8X-
Deprenyl	T42.8X-
Depressant, appetite	T50.5X-
Depressant	
appetite (central)	T50.5X-
cardiac	T46.2X-
central nervous system (anesthetic)—*see also Central nervous system, depressants*	T42.7-
general anesthetic	T41.20-
muscle tone	T42.8X-
muscle tone, central	T42.8X-
psychotherapeutic	T43.50-
Deptropine	T45.0X-
Dequalinium (chloride)	T49.0X-
Derris root	T60.2X-
Deserpidine	T46.5X-
Desferrioxamine	T45.8X-
Desipramine	T43.01-
Deslanoside	T46.0X-
Desloughing agent	T49.4X-
Desmethylimipramine	T43.01-
Desmopressin	T38.89-
Desocodeine	T40.2X-
Desogestrel	T38.5X-
Desomorphine	T40.2X-
Desonide	T49.0X-
Desoximetasone	T49.0X-
Desoxycorticosteroid	T50.0X-
Desoxycortone	T50.0X-
Desoxyephedrine	T43.65-
Detaxtran	T46.6X-
Detergent	T49.2X-
external medication	T49.2X-
local	T49.2X-
medicinal	T49.2X-
nonmedicinal	T55.1X-
specified NEC	T55.1X-
Deterrent, alcohol	T50.6X-
Detoxifying agent	T50.6X-
Detrothyronine	T38.1X-
Dettol (external medication)	T49.0X-

TABLE OF DRUGS AND CHEMICALS

Drug/Chemical	Code	Drug/Chemical	Code
Dexamethasone	T38.0X-	**Dibekacin**	T36.5X-
ENT agent	T49.6X-	**Dibenamine**	T44.6X-
ophthalmic preparation	T49.5X-	**Dibenzepin**	T43.01-
topical NEC	T49.0X-	**Dibenzheptropine**	T45.0X-
Dexamfetamine	T43.62-	**Dibenzyline**	T44.6X-
Dexamphetamine	T43.62-	**Diborane (gas)**	T59.89-
Dexbrompheniramine	T45.0X-	**Dibromochloropropane**	T60.8X-
Dexchlorpheniramine	T45.0X-	**Dibromodulcitol**	T45.1X-
Dexedrine	T43.62-	**Dibromoethane**	T53.6X-
Dexetimide	T44.3X-	**Dibromomannitol**	T45.1X-
Dexfenfluramine	T50.5X-	**Dibromopropamidine isethionate**	T49.0X-
Dexpanthenol	T45.2X-	**Dibrompropamidine**	T49.0X-
Dextran (40) (70) (150)	T45.8X-	**Dibucaine**	T41.3X-
Dextriferron	T45.4X-	**Dibunate sodium**	T48.3X-
Dextro calcium pantothenate	T45.2X-	**Dibutoline sulfate**	T44.3X-
Dextro pantothenyl alcohol	T45.2X-	**Dicamba**	T60.3X-
Dextroamphetamine	T43.62-	**Dicapthon**	T60.0X-
Dextromethorphan	T48.3X-	**Dichlobenil**	T60.3X-
Dextromoramide	T40.4X-	**Dichlone**	T60.3X-
topical	T49.8X-	**Dichloralphenozone**	T42.6X-
Dextropropoxyphene	T40.4X-	**Dichlorbenzidine**	T65.3X-
Dextrorphan	T40.2X-	**Dichlorhydrin**	T52.8X-
Dextrose	T50.3X-	**Dichlorhydroxyquinoline**	T37.8X-
concentrated solution, intravenous	T46.8X-	**Dichlorobenzene**	T53.7X-
Dextrothyroxin	T38.1X-	**Dichlorobenzyl alcohol**	T49.6X-
Dextrothyroxine sodium	T38.1X-	**Dichlorodifluoromethane**	T53.5X-
DFP	T44.0X-	**Dichloroethane**	T52.8X-
DHE	T37.3X-	**Sym-Dichloroethyl ether**	T53.6X-
45	T46.5X-	**Dichloroethyl sulfide, not in war**	T59.89-
Diabinese	T38.3X-	**Dichloroethylene**	T53.6X-
Diacetone alcohol	T52.4X-	**Dichloroformoxine, not in war**	T59.89-
Diacetyl monoxime	T50.99-	**Dichlorohydrin, alpha-dichlorohydrin**	T52.8X-
Diacetylmorphine	T40.1X-	**Dichloromethane (solvent) (vapor)**	T53.4X-
Diachylon plaster	T49.4X-	**Dichloronaphthoquinone**	T60.3X-
Diaethylstilboestrolum	T38.5X-	**Dichlorophen**	T37.4X-
Diagnostic agent NEC	T50.8X-	**2,4-Dichlorophenoxyacetic acid**	T60.3X-
Dial (soap)	T49.2X-	**Dichloropropene**	T60.3X-
sedative	T42.3X-	**Dichloropropionic acid**	T60.3X-
Dialkyl carbonate	T52.9-	**Dichlorphenamide**	T50.2X-
Diallylbarbituric acid	T42.3X-	**Dichlorvos**	T60.0X-
Diallymal	T42.3X-	**Diclofenac**	T39.39-
Dialysis solution (intraperitoneal)	T50.3X-	**Diclofenamide**	T50.2X-
Diaminodiphenylsulfone	T37.1X-	**Diclofensine**	T43.29-
Diamorphine	T40.1X-	**Diclonixine**	T39.8X-
Diamox	T50.2X-	**Dicloxacillin**	T36.0X-
Diamthazole	T49.0X-	**Dicophane**	T49.0X-
Dianthone	T47.2X-	**Dicoumarol, dicoumarin, dicumarol**	T45.51-
Diaphenylsulfone	T37.0X-	**Dicrotophos**	T60.0X-
Diasone (sodium)	T37.1X-	**Dicyanogen (gas)**	T65.0X-
Diastase	T47.5X-	**Dicyclomine**	T44.3X-
Diatrizoate	T50.8X-	**Dicycloverine**	T44.3X-
Diazepam	T42.4X-	**Dideoxycytidine**	T37.5X-
Diazinon	T60.0X-	**Dideoxyinosine**	T37.5X-
Diazomethane (gas)	T59.89-	**Dieldrin (vapor)**	T60.1X-
Diazoxide	T46.5X-	**Diemal**	T42.3X-

TABLE OF DRUGS AND CHEMICALS

Drug/Chemical	Code
Dienestrol	T38.5X-
Dienoestrol	T38.5X-
Dietetic drug NEC	T50.90-
Diethazine	T42.8X-
Diethyl	
barbituric acid / carbinol	T42.3X-
carbamazine	T37.4X-
carbonate / oxide	T52.8X-
ether (vapor)—see also ether	T41.0X-
propion	T50.5X-
stilbestrol	T38.5X-
toluamide (nonmedicinal)	T60.8X-
medicinal	T49.3X-
Diethylcarbamazine	T37.4X-
Diethylene	
dioxide	T52.8X-
glycol (monoacetate) (monobutyl ether) (monoethyl ether)	T52.3X-
Diethylhexylphthalate	T65.89-
Diethylpropion	T50.5X-
Diethylstilbestrol	T38.5X-
Diethylstilboestrol	T38.5X-
Diethylsulfone-diethylmethane	T42.6X-
Diethyltoluamide	T49.0X-
Diethyltryptamine (DET)	T40.99-
Difebarbamate	T42.3X-
Difencloxazine	T40.2X-
Difenidol	T45.0X-
Difenoxin	T47.6X-
Difetarsone	T37.3X-
Diffusin	T45.3X-
Diflorasone	T49.0X-
Diflos	T44.0X-
Diflubenzuron	T60.1X-
Diflucortolone	T49.0X-
Diflunisal	T39.09-
Difluoromethyldopa	T42.8X-
Difluorophate	T44.0X-
Digestant NEC	T47.5X-
Digitalin (e)	T46.0X-
Digitalis (leaf) (glycoside)	T46.0X-
Digitoxin	T46.0X-
Digitoxose	T46.0X-
Digoxin	T46.0X-
Digoxine	T46.0X-
Dihydralazine	T46.5X-
Dihydrazine	T46.5X-
Dihydrocodeine	T40.2X-
Dihydrocodeinone	T40.2X-
Dihydroergocornine	T46.7X-
Dihydroergocristine (mesilate)	T46.7X-
Dihydroergokryptine	T46.7X-
Dihydroergotamine	T46.5X-
Dihydroergotoxine (mesilate)	T46.7X-
Dihydrohydroxycodeinone	T40.2X-
Dihydrohydroxymorphinone	T40.2X-
Dihydroisocodeine	T40.2X-
Dihydromorphine	T40.2X-
Dihydromorphinone	T40.2X-
Dihydrostreptomycin	T36.5X-
Dihydrotachysterol	T45.2X-
Dihydroxyaluminum aminoacetate	T47.1X-
Dihydroxyaluminum sodium carbonate	T47.1X-
Dihydroxyanthraquinone	T47.2X-
Dihydroxycodeinone	T40.2X-
Dihydroxypropyl theophylline	T50.2X-
Diiodohydroxyquin	T37.8X-
topical	T49.0X-
Diiodohydroxyquinoline	T37.8X-
Diiodotyrosine	T38.2X-
Diisopromine	T44.3X-
Diisopropylamine	T46.3X-
Diisopropylfluorophos-phonate	T44.0X-
Dilantin	T42.0X-
Dilaudid	T40.2X-
Dilazep	T46.3X-
Dill	T47.5X-
Diloxanide	T37.3X-
Diltiazem	T46.1X-
Dimazole	T49.0X-
Dimefline	T50.7X-
Dimefox	T60.0X-
Dimemorfan	T48.3X-
Dimenhydrinate	T45.0X-
Dimercaprol (British anti-lewisite)	T45.8X-
Dimercaptopropanol	T45.8X-
Dimestrol	T38.5X-
Dimetane	T45.0X-
Dimethicone	T47.1X-
Dimethindene	T45.0X-
Dimethisoquin	T49.1X-
Dimethisterone	T38.5X-
Dimethoate	T60.0X-
Dimethocaine	T41.3X-
Dimethoxanate	T48.3X-
Dimethyl	
arsine, arsinic acid	T57.0X-
carbinol	T51.2X-
carbonate	T52.8X-
diguanide	T38.3X-
ketone (vapor)	T52.4X-
meperidine	T40.2X-
parathion	T60.0X-
phthalate	T49.3X-
polysiloxane	T47.8X-
sulfate (fumes)	T59.89-
liquid	T65.89-
sulfoxide (nonmedicinal)	T52.8X-
medicinal	T49.4X-

TABLE OF DRUGS AND CHEMICALS

Drug/Chemical	Code
Dimethyl, continued	
tryptamine	T40.99-
tubocurarine	T48.1X-
Dimethylamine sulfate	T49.4X-
Dimethylformamide	T52.8X-
Dimethyltubocurarinium chloride	T48.1X-
Dimeticone	T47.1X-
Dimetilan	T60.0X-
Dimetindene	T45.0X-
Dimetotiazine	T43.3X-
Dimorpholamine	T50.7X-
Dimoxyline	T46.3X-
Dinitrobenzene	T65.3X-
vapor	T59.89-
Dinitrobenzol	T65.3X-
vapor	T59.89-
Dinitrobutylphenol	T65.3X-
Dinitro (-ortho-) cresol (pesticide) (spray)	T65.3X-
Dinitrocyclohexylphenol	T65.3X-
Dinitrophenol	T65.3X-
Dinoprost	T48.0X-
Dinoprostone	T48.0X-
Dinoseb	T60.3X-
Dioctyl sulfosuccinate (calcium) (sodium)	T47.4X-
Diodone	T50.8X-
Diodoquin	T37.8X-
Dionin	T40.2X-
Diosmin	T46.99-
Dioxane	T52.8X-
Dioxathion	T60.0X-
Dioxin	T53.7X-
Dioxopromethazine	T43.3X-
Dioxyline	T46.3X-
Dipentene	T52.8X-
Diperodon	T41.3X-
Diphacinone	T60.4X-
Diphemanil	T44.3X-
metilsulfate	T44.3X-
Diphenadione	T45.51-
rodenticide	T60.4X-
Diphenhydramine	T45.0X-
Diphenidol	T45.0X-
Diphenoxylate	T47.6X-
Diphenylamine	T65.3X-
Diphenylbutazone	T39.2X-
Diphenylchloroarsine, not in war	T57.0X-
Diphenylhydantoin	T42.0X-
Diphenylmethane dye	T52.1X-
Diphenylpyraline	T45.0X-
Diphtheria	
antitoxin	T50.Z1-
vaccine—*See also Vaccines*	T50.A9-
Diphylline	T50.2X-
Dipipanone	T40.4X-
Dipivefrine	T49.5X-

Drug/Chemical	Code
Diplovax	T50.B9-
Diprophylline	T50.2X-
Dipropyline	T48.29-
Dipyridamole	T46.3X-
Dipyrone	T39.2X-
Diquat (dibromide)	T60.3X-
Disinfectant	T65.89-
alkaline	T54.3X-
aromatic	T54.1X-
intestinal	T37.8X-
Disipal	T42.8X-
Disodium edetate	T50.6X-
Disoprofol	T41.29-
Disopyramide	T46.2X-
Distigmine (bromide)	T44.0X-
Disulfamide	T50.2X-
Disulfanilamide	T37.0X-
Disulfiram	T50.6X-
Disulfoton	T60.0X-
Dithiazanine iodide	T37.4X-
Dithiocarbamate	T60.0X-
Dithranol	T49.4X-
Diucardin	T50.2X-
Diupres	T50.2X-
Diuretic NEC	T50.2X-
benzothiadiazine	T50.2X-
carbonic acid anhydrase inhibitors	T50.2X-
furfuryl NEC	T50.2X-
loop (high-ceiling)	T50.1X-
mercurial NEC or osmotic	T50.2X-
purine or saluretic NEC	T50.2X-
sulfonamide	T50.2X-
thiazide NEC or xanthine	T50.2X-
Diurgin	T50.2X-
Diuril	T50.2X-
Diuron	T60.3X-
Divalproex	T42.6X-
Divinyl ether	T41.0X-
Dixanthogen	T49.0X-
Dixyrazine	T43.3X-
D-lysergic acid diethylamide	T40.8X-
DMCT	T36.4X-
DMSO—*see Dimethyl, sulfoxide*	
DNBP	T60.3X-
DNOC	T65.3X-
Dobutamine	T44.5X-
DOCA	T38.0X-
Docusate sodium	T47.4X-
Dodicin	T49.0X-
Dofamium chloride	T49.0X-
Dolophine	T40.3X-
Doloxene	T39.8X-
Domestic gas (after combustion)—*see Gas, utility*	
prior to combustion	T59.89-
Domiodol	T48.4X-

TABLE OF DRUGS AND CHEMICALS

Drug/Chemical	Code
Domiphen (bromide)	T49.0X-
Domperidone	T45.0X-
Dopa	T42.8X-
Dopamine	T44.99-
Doriden	T42.6X-
Dormiral	T42.3X-
Dormison	T42.6X-
Dornase	T48.4X-
Dorsacaine	T41.3X-
Dosulepin	T43.01-
Dothiepin	T43.01-
Doxantrazole	T48.6X-
Doxapram	T50.7X-
Doxazosin	T44.6X-
Doxepin	T43.01-
Doxifluridine	T45.1X-
Doxorubicin	T45.1X-
Doxycycline	T36.4X-
Doxylamine	T45.0X-
Dramamine	T45.0X-
Drano (drain cleaner)	T54.3X-
Dressing, live pulp	T49.7X-
Drocode	T40.2X-
Dromoran	T40.2X-
Dromostanolone	T38.7X-
Dronabinol	T40.71-
Droperidol	T43.59-
Dropropizine	T48.3X-
Drostanolone	T38.7X-
Drotaverine	T44.3X-
Drotrecogin alfa	T45.51-
Drug NEC	T50.90-
specified NEC	T50.99-
DTaP	T50.A1
DTIC	T45.1X-
Duboisine	T44.3X-
Dulcolax	T47.2X-
Duponol (C) (EP)	T49.2X-
Durabolin	T38.7X-
Dyclone	T41.3X-
Dyclonine	T41.3X-
Dydrogesterone	T38.5X-
Dye NEC	T65.6X-
antiseptic	T49.0X-
diagnostic agents	T50.8X-
pharmaceutical NEC	T50.90-
Dyflos	T44.0X-
Dymelor	T38.3X-
Dynamite	T65.3X-
fumes	T59.89-
Dyphylline	T44.3X-
Ear drug NEC	T49.6X-
Ear preparations	T49.6X-
Echothiophate, echothiopate, ecothiopate	T49.5X-
Econazole	T49.0X-
Ecothiopate iodide	T49.5X-
Ecstasy	T43.64-
Ectylurea	T42.6X-
Edathamil disodium	T45.8X-
Edecrin	T50.1X-
Edetate, disodium (calcium)	T45.8X-
Edoxudine	T49.5X-
Edrophonium	T44.0X-
chloride	T44.0X-
EDTA	T50.6X-
Eflornithine	T37.2X-
Efloxate	T46.3X-
Elase	T49.8X-
Elastase	T47.5X-
Elaterium	T47.2X-
Elcatonin	T50.99-
Elder	T62.2X-
berry, (unripe)	T62.1X-
Electrolyte balance drug	T50.3X-
Electrolytes NEC	T50.3X-
Electrolytic agent NEC	T50.3X-
Elemental diet	T50.90-
Elliptinium acetate	T45.1X-
Embramine	T45.0X-
Emepronium (salts) (bromide)	T44.3X-
Emetic NEC	T47.7X-
Emetine	T37.3X-
Emollient NEC	T49.3X-
Emorfazone	T39.8X-
Emylcamate	T43.59-
Enalapril	T46.4X-
Enalaprilat	T46.4X-
Encainide	T46.2X-
Endocaine	T41.3X-
Endosulfan	T60.2X-
Endothall	T60.3X-
Endralazine	T46.5X-
Endrin	T60.1X-
Enflurane	T41.0X-
Enhexymal	T42.3X-
Enocitabine	T45.1X-
Enovid	T38.4X-
Enoxacin	T36.8X-
Enoxaparin (sodium)	T45.51-
Enpiprazole	T43.59-
Enprofylline	T48.6X-
Enprostil	T47.1X-
ENT preparations (anti-infectives)	T49.6X-
Enterogastrone	T38.89-
Enviomycin	T36.8X-
Enzodase	T45.3X-
Enzyme NEC	T45.3X-
depolymerizing	T49.8X-
fibrolytic	T45.3X-
gastric / intestinal	T47.5X-

TABLE OF DRUGS AND CHEMICALS

Drug/Chemical	Code	Drug/Chemical	Code
Enzyme NEC, continued	T45.3X-	**Esmolol**	T44.7X-
local action / proteolytic	T49.4X-	**Estanozolol**	T38.7X-
thrombolytic	T45.3X-	**Estazolam**	T42.4X-
EPAB	T41.3X-	**Estradiol**	T38.5X-
Epanutin	T42.0X-	with testosterone	T38.7X-
Ephedra	T44.99-	benzoate	T38.5X-
Ephedrine	T44.99-	**Estramustine**	T45.1X-
Epichlorhydrin, epichlorohydrin	T52.8X-	**Estriol**	T38.5X-
Epicillin	T36.0X-	**Estrogen**	T38.5X-
Epiestriol	T38.5X-	**Estrone**	T38.5X-
Epilim—*see Sodium, valproate*	T42.6X-	**Estropipate**	T38.5X-
Epimestrol	T38.5X-	**Etacrynate sodium**	T50.1X-
Epinephrine	T44.5X-	**Etacrynic acid**	T50.1X-
Epirubicin	T45.1X-	**Etafedrine**	T48.6X-
Epitiostanol	T38.7X-	**Etafenone**	T46.3X-
Epitizide	T50.2X-	**Etambutol**	T37.1X-
EPN	T60.0X-	**Etamiphyllin**	T48.6X-
EPO	T45.8X-	**Etamivan**	T50.7X-
Epoetin alpha	T45.8X-	**Etamsylate**	T45.7X-
Epomediol	T50.99-	**Etebenecid**	T50.4X-
Epoprostenol	T45.521	**Ethacridine**	T49.0X-
Epoxy resin	T65.89-	**Ethacrynic acid**	T50.1X-
Eprazinone	T48.4X-	**Ethadione**	T42.2X-
Epsilon amino-caproic acid	T45.62-	**Ethambutol**	T37.1X-
Epsom salt	T47.3X-	**Ethamide**	T50.2X-
Eptazocine	T40.4X-	**Ethamivan**	T50.7X-
Equanil	T43.59-	**Ethamsylate**	T45.7X-
Equisetum	T62.2X-	**Ethanol (beverage)**	T51.0X-
diuretic	T50.2X-	**Ethanolamine oleate**	T46.8X-
Ergobasine	T48.0X-	**Ethaverine**	T44.3X-
Ergocalciferol	T45.2X-	**Ethchlorvynol**	T42.6X-
Ergoloid mesylates	T46.7X-	**Ethebenecid**	T50.4X-
Ergometrine	T48.0X-	**Ether (vapor)**	T41.0X-
Ergonovine	T48.0X-	anesthetic	T41.0X-
Ergot NEC	T64.81	divinyl	T41.0X-
derivative or medicinal (alkaloids) or prepared	T48.0X-	ethyl (medicinal)	T41.0X-
Ergotamine	T46.5X-	nonmedicinal	T52.8X-
Ergotocine	T48.0X-	solvent	T52.8X-
Ergotrate	T48.0X-	**Ethiazide**	T50.2X-
Eritrityl tetranitrate	T46.3X-	**Ethidium chloride (vapor)**	T59.89-
Erythrityl tetranitrate	T46.3X-	**Ethinamate**	T42.6X-
Erythrol tetranitrate	T46.3X-	**Ethinylestradiol, ethinyloestradiol**	T38.5X-
Erythromycin (salts)	T36.3X-	with	
ophthalmic preparation	T49.5X-	levonorgestrel or norethisterone	T38.4X-
topical NEC	T49.0X-	**Ethiodized oil (131 I)**	T50.8X-
Erythropoietin	T45.8X-	**Ethion**	T60.0X-
human	T45.8X-	**Ethionamide**	T37.1X-
Escin	T46.99-	**Ethioniamide**	T37.1X-
Esculin	T45.2X-	**Ethisterone**	T38.5X-
Esculoside	T45.2X-	**Ethobral**	T42.3X-
ESDT (ether-soluble tar distillate)	T49.1X-	**Ethocaine (infiltration) (topical) (nerve block) (spinal)**	T41.3X-
Eserine	T49.5X-	**Ethoheptazine**	T40.4X-
Esflurbiprofen	T39.31-	**Ethopropazine**	T44.3X-
Eskabarb	T42.3X-	**Ethosuximide**	T42.2X-
Eskalith	T43.8X-	**Ethotoin**	T42.0X-

TABLE OF DRUGS AND CHEMICALS

Drug/Chemical	Code
Ethoxazene	T37.9-
Ethoxazorutoside	T46.99-
2-Ethoxyethanol	T52.3X-
Ethoxzolamide	T50.2X-
Ethyl	
acetate	T52.8X-
alcohol (beverage)	T51.0X-
aldehyde (vapor)	T59.89-
liquid	T52.8X-
aminobenzoate	T41.3X-
aminophenothiazine	T43.3X-
benzoate	T52.8X-
biscoumacetate	T45.51-
bromide (anesthetic)	T41.0X-
carbamate	T45.1X-
carbinol	T51.3X-
carbonate	T52.8X-
chaulmoograte	T37.1X-
chloride (anesthetic)	T41.0X-
anesthetic (local)	T41.3X-
inhaled	T41.0X-
local	T49.4X-
solvent	T53.6X-
dibunate	T48.3X-
dichloroarsine (vapor)	T57.0X-
estranol	T38.7X-
ether—*see also ether*	T52.8X-
formate NEC (solvent)	T52.0X-
fumarate	T49.4X-
hydroxyisobutyrate NEC (solvent)	T52.8X-
iodoacetate	T59.3X-
lactate NEC (solvent)	T52.8X-
loflazepate	T42.4X-
mercuric chloride	T56.1X-
methylcarbinol	T51.8X-
morphine	T40.2X-
noradrenaline	T48.6X-
oxybutyrate NEC (solvent)	T52.8X-
Ethylene (gas)	T59.89-
anesthetic (general)	T41.0X-
chlorohydrin	T52.8X-
vapor	T53.6X-
dichloride	T52.8X-
vapor	T53.6X-
dinitrate	T52.3X-
glycol(s)	T52.8X-
dinitrate	T52.3X-
monobutyl ether	T52.3X-
imine	T54.1X-
oxide (fumigant) (nonmedicinal)	T59.89-
medicinal	T49.0X-
Ethylenediamine theophylline	T48.6X-
Ethylenediaminetetra-acetic acid	T50.6X-
Ethylenedinitrilotetra-acetate	T50.6X-
Ethylestrenol	T38.7X-

Drug/Chemical	Code
Ethylhydroxycellulose	T47.4X-
Ethylidene	
chloride NEC	T53.6X-
diacetate	T60.3X-
dicoumarin / dicoumarol	T45.51-
diethyl ether	T52.0X-
Ethylmorphine	T40.2X-
Ethylnorepinephrine	T48.6X-
Ethylparachlorophen-oxyisobutyrate	T46.6X-
Ethynodiol	T38.4X-
with mestranol diacetate	T38.4X-
Etidocaine (infiltration) (subcutaneous) (nerve block)	T41.3X-
Etidronate	T50.99-
Etidronic acid (disodium salt)	T50.99-
Etifoxine	T42.6X-
Etilefrine	T44.4X-
Etilfen	T42.3X-
Etinodiol	T38.4X-
Etiroxate	T46.6X-
Etizolam	T42.4X-
Etodolac	T39.39-
Etofamide	T37.3X-
Etofibrate	T46.6X-
Etofylline	T46.7X-
clofibrate	T46.6X-
Etoglucid	T45.1X-
Etomidate	T41.1X-
Etomide	T39.8X-
Etomidoline	T44.3X-
Etoposide	T45.1X-
Etorphine	T40.2X-
Etoval	T42.3X-
Etozolin	T50.1X-
Etretinate	T50.99-
Etryptamine	T43.69-
Etybenzatropine	T44.3X-
Etynodiol	T38.4X-
Eucaine	T41.3X-
Eucalyptus oil	T49.7X-
Eucatropine	T49.5X-
Eucodal	T40.2X-
Euneryl	T42.3X-
Euphthalmine	T44.3X-
Eurax	T49.0X-
Euresol	T49.4X-
Euthroid	T38.1X-
Evans blue	T50.8X-
Evipal	T42.3X-
sodium	T41.1X-
Evipan	T42.3X-
sodium	T41.1X-
Exalamide	T49.0X-
Exalgin	T39.1X-
Excipients, pharmaceutical	T50.90-
Exhaust gas (engine) (motor vehicle)	T58.0-

TABLE OF DRUGS AND CHEMICALS

Drug/Chemical	Code
Ex-Lax (phenolphthalein)	T47.2X-
Expectorant NEC	T48.4X-
Extended insulin zinc suspension	T38.3X-
External medications (skin) (mucous membrane)	T49.9-
dental agent	T49.7X-
ENT agent	T49.6X-
ophthalmic preparation	T49.5X-
specified NEC	T49.8X-
Extrapyramidal antagonist NEC	T44.3X-
Eye agents (anti-infective)	T49.5X-
Eye drug NEC	T49.5X-
FAC (fluorouracil + doxorubicin + cyclophosphamide)	T45.1X-
Factor	
I (fibrinogen)	T45.8X-
III (thromboplastin)	T45.8X-
VIII (antihemophilic Factor) (concentrate)	T45.8X-
IX complex	T45.7X-
human	T45.8X-
Famotidine	T47.0X-
Fat suspension, intravenous	T50.99-
Fazadinium bromide	T48.1X-
Febarbamate	T42.3X-
Fecal softener	T47.4X-
Fedrilate	T48.3X-
Felodipine	T46.1X-
Felypressin	T38.89-
Femoxetine	T43.22-
Fenalcomine	T46.3X-
Fenamisal	T37.1X-
Fenazone	T39.2X-
Fenbendazole	T37.4X-
Fenbutrazate	T50.5X-
Fencamfamine	T43.69-
Fendiline	T46.1X-
Fenetylline	T43.69-
Fenflumizole	T39.39-
Fenfluramine	T50.5X-
Fenobarbital	T42.3X-
Fenofibrate	T46.6X-
Fenoprofen	T39.31-
Fenoterol	T48.6X-
Fenoverine	T44.3X-
Fenoxazoline	T48.5X-
Fenproporex	T50.5X-
Fenquizone	T50.2X-
Fentanyl	T40.4X-
Fentanyl/fentanyl analogs	T40.41-
Fentazin	T43.3X-
Fenthion	T60.0X-
Fenticlor	T49.0X-
Fenylbutazone	T39.2X-
Feprazone	T39.2X-
Fer de lance (bite) (venom)	T63.06-

Drug/Chemical	Code
Ferric—*see also Iron*	
chloride	T45.4X-
citrate	T45.4X-
hydroxide	T45.4X-
pyrophosphate	T45.4X-
Ferritin	T45.4X-
Ferrocholinate	T45.4X-
Ferrodextrane	T45.4X-
Ferropolimaler	T45.4X-
Ferrous—*see also Iron*	T45.4X-
Ferrous fumerate, gluconate, lactate, salt NEC, sulfate (medicinal)	T45.4X-
Ferrovanadium (fumes)	T59.89-
Ferrum—*see Iron*	
Fertilizers NEC	T65.89-
with herbicide mixture	T60.3X-
Fetoxilate	T47.6X-
Fiber, dietary	T47.4X-
Fiberglass	T65.831
Fibrinogen (human)	T45.8X-
Fibrinolysin (human)	T45.69-
Fibrinolysis	
affecting drug	T45.60-
inhibitor NEC	T45.62-
Fibrinolytic drug	T45.61-
Filix mas	T37.4X-
Filtering cream	T49.3X-
Fiorinal	T39.01-
Firedamp	T59.89-
Fish, noxious, nonbacterial	T61.9-
ciguatera	T61.0-
scombroid	T61.1-
shell	T61.781-
specified NEC	T61.771-
Flagyl	T37.3X-
Flavine adenine dinucleotide	T45.2X-
Flavodic acid	T46.99-
Flavoxate	T44.3X-
Flaxedil	T48.1X-
Flaxseed (medicinal)	T49.3X-
Flecainide	T46.2X-
Fleroxacin	T36.8X-
Floctafenine	T39.8X-
Flomax	T44.6X-
Flomoxef	T36.1X-
Flopropione	T44.3X-
Florantyrone	T47.5X-
Floraquin	T37.8X-
Florinef	T38.0X-
ENT agent	T49.6X-
ophthalmic preparation	T49.5X-
topical NEC	T49.0X-
Flowers of sulfur	T49.4X-
Floxuridine	T45.1X-
Fluanisone	T43.4X-

TABLE OF DRUGS AND CHEMICALS

Drug/Chemical	Code
Flubendazole	T37.4X-
Fluclorolone acetonide	T49.0X-
Flucloxacillin	T36.0X-
Fluconazole	T37.8X-
Flucytosine	T37.8X-
Fludeoxyglucose (18F)	T50.8X-
Fludiazepam	T42.4X-
Fludrocortisone	T50.0X-
ENT agent	T49.6X-
ophthalmic preparation	T49.5X-
topical NEC	T49.0X-
Fludroxycortide	T49.0X-
Flufenamic acid	T39.39-
Fluindione	T45.51-
Flumequine	T37.8X-
Flumethasone	T49.0X-
Flumethiazide	T50.2X-
Flumidin	T37.5X-
Flunarizine	T46.7X-
Flunidazole	T37.8X-
Flunisolide	T48.6X-
Flunitrazepam	T42.4X-
Fluocinolone (acetonide)	T49.0X-
Fluocinonide	T49.0X-
Fluocortin (butyl)	T49.0X-
Fluocortolone	T49.0X-
Fluohydrocortisone	T38.0X-
ENT agent	T49.6X-
ophthalmic preparation	T49.5X-
topical NEC	T49.0X-
Fluonid	T49.0X-
Fluopromazine	T43.3X-
Fluoracetate	T60.8X-
Fluorescein	T50.8X-
Fluorhydrocortisone	T50.0X-
Fluoride (nonmedicinal) (pesticide) (sodium) NEC	T60.8X-
medicinal NEC	T50.99-
dental use	T49.7X-
not pesticide NEC	T54.9-
stannous	T49.7X-
Fluorinated corticosteroids	T38.0X-
Fluorine (gas)	T59.5X-
Fluoristan	T49.7X-
Fluormetholone	T49.0X-
Fluoroacetate	T60.8X-
Fluorocarbon monomer	T53.6X-
Fluorocytosine	T37.8X-
Fluorodeoxyuridine	T45.1X-
Fluorometholone	T49.0X-
ophthalmic preparation	T49.5X-
Fluorophosphate insecticide	T60.0X-
Fluorosol	T46.3X-
Fluorouracil	T45.1X-
Fluorphenylalanine	T49.5X-
Fluothane	T41.0X-
Fluoxetine	T43.22-
Fluoxymesterone	T38.7X-
Flupenthixol	T43.4X-
Flupentixol	T43.4X-
Fluphenazine	T43.3X-
Fluprednidene	T49.0X-
Fluprednisolone	T38.0X-
Fluradoline	T39.8X-
Flurandrenolide	T49.0X-
Flurandrenolone	T49.0X-
Flurazepam	T42.4X-
Flurbiprofen	T39.31-
Flurobate	T49.0X-
Fluroxene	T41.0X-
Fluspirilene	T43.59-
Flutamide	T38.6X-
Flutazolam	T42.4X-
Fluticasone propionate	T38.0X-
Flutoprazepam	T42.4X-
Flutropium bromide	T48.6X-
Fluvoxamine	T43.22-
Folacin	T45.8X-
Folic acid	T45.8X-
with ferrous salt	T45.2X-
antagonist	T45.1X-
Folinic acid	T45.8X-
Folium stramoniae	T48.6X-
Follicle-stimulating hormone, human	T38.81-
Folpet	T60.3X-
Fominoben	T48.3X-
Food, foodstuffs, noxious, nonbacterial, NEC	T62.9-
berries	T62.1X-
mushrooms	T62.0X-
plants	T62.2X-
seafood	T61.9-
specified NEC	T61.8X-
seeds	T62.2X-
shellfish	T61.781
specified NEC	T62.8X-
Fool's parsley	T62.2X-
Formaldehyde (solution), gas or vapor	T59.2X-
fungicide	T60.3X-
Formalin	T59.2X-
fungicide	T60.3X-
vapor	T59.2X-
Formic acid	T54.2X-
vapor	T59.89-
Foscarnet sodium	T37.5X-
Fosfestrol	T38.5X-
Fosfomycin	T36.8X-
Fosfonet sodium	T37.5X-
Fosinopril	T46.4X-
sodium	T46.4X-
Fowler's solution	T57.0X-
Foxglove	T62.2X-

TABLE OF DRUGS AND CHEMICALS

Drug/Chemical	Code
Framycetin	T36.5X-
Frangula	T47.2X-
extract	T47.2X-
Frei antigen	T50.8X-
Freon	T53.5X-
Fructose	T50.3X-
Frusemide	T50.1X-
FSH	T38.81-
Ftorafur	T45.1X-
Fuel	
automobile	T52.0X-
exhaust gas, not in transit	T58.0-
vapor NEC	T52.0X-
gas (domestic use) / utility / in mobile container / piped	T59.89-
industrial, incomplete combustion	T58.8X-
Fugillin	T36.8X-
Fulminate of mercury	T56.1X-
Fulvicin	T36.7X-
Fumadil	T36.8X-
Fumagillin	T36.8X-
Fumaric acid	T49.4X-
Fumes (from)	T59.9-
corrosive NEC	T54.9-
freons	T53.5X-
hydrocarbons (all types)	T59.89-
nitrogen dioxide	T59.0X-
pesticides—see Pesticide	T60.9-
petroleum (liquefied) (distributed)	T59.89-
polyester	T59.89-
specified source NEC	T59.89-
sulfur dioxide	T59.1X-
Fumigant NEC	T60.9-
Fungi, noxious, used as food	T62.0X-
Fungicide NEC (nonmedicinal)	T60.3X-
Fungizone	T36.7X-
topical	T49.0X-
Furacin	T49.0X-
Furadantin	T37.9-
Furazolidone	T37.8X-
Furazolium chloride	T49.0X-
Furfural	T52.8X-
Furnace (coal burning) (domestic), gas from	T58.2X-
industrial	T58.8X-
Furniture polish	T65.89-
Furosemide	T50.1X-
Furoxone	T37.9-
Fursultiamine	T45.2X-
Fusafungine	T36.8X-
Fusel oil (any) (amyl) (butyl) (propyl), vapor	T51.3X-
Fusidate (ethanolamine) (sodium)	T36.8X-
Fusidic acid	T36.8X-
Fytic acid, nonasodium	T50.6X-
GABA	T43.8X-
Gadolinium	T56.82-

Drug/Chemical	Code
Gadopentetic acid	T50.8X-
Galactose	T50.3X-
b-Galactosidase	T47.5X-
Galantamine	T44.0X-
Gallamine (triethiodide)	T48.1X-
Gallium citrate	T50.99-
Gallopamil	T46.1X-
Gamboge	T47.2X-
Gamimune	T50.Z1-
Gamma globulin	T50.Z1-
Gamma-aminobutyric acid	T43.8X-
Gamma-benzene hexachloride (medicinal)	T49.0X-
nonmedicinal, vapor	T53.6X-
Gamma-BHC (medicinal)	T49.0X-
Gamulin	T50.Z1-
Ganciclovir (sodium)	T37.5X-
Ganglionic blocking drug NEC	T44.2X-
specified NEC	T44.2X-
Ganja	T40.71-
Garamycin	T36.5X-
ophthalmic preparation	T49.5X-
topical NEC	T49.0X-
Gardenal	T42.3X-
Gardepanyl	T42.3X-
Gas NEC	T59.91
acetylene	T59.89-
incomplete combustion of	T58.1-
air contaminants, source or type not specified	T59.9-
anesthetic	T41.0X-
blast furnace	T58.8X-
chlorine	T59.4X-
coal	T58.2X-
cyanide	T57.3X-
dicyanogen	T65.0X-
exhaust	T58.0-
prior to combustion	T59.89-
from wood- or coal-burning stove or fireplace	T58.2X-
industrial use	T58.8X-
prior to combustion	T59.89-
utility (in mobile container or piped)	T59.89-
garage	T58.0-
hydrocarbon NEC (piped)	T59.89-
hydrocyanic acid	T65.0X-
illuminating (after combustion)	T58.1-
prior to combustion	T59.89-
incomplete combustion of—see Carbon, monoxide, fuel, utility	T58.1-
kiln	T58.8X-
lacrimogenic	T59.3X-
marsh	T59.89-
motor exhaust, not in transit	T58.0-
natural	T59.89-
oil	T52.0X-
petroleum (liquefied) (distributed in mobile containers) (piped)	T59.89-

TABLE OF DRUGS AND CHEMICALS

Drug/Chemical	Code
Gas NEC, continued	T59.9-
producer	T58.8X-
refrigerant (chlorofluoro-carbon)	T53.5X-
not chlorofluoro-carbon	T59.89-
sewer	T59.9-
specified source NEC	T59.9-
stove (after combustion)	T58.1-
prior to combustion	T59.89-
tear	T59.3X-
therapeutic	T41.5X-
utility (for cooking, heating, or lighting) (piped) (mobile container) NEC	T59.89-
water	T58.1-
Gasoline	T52.0X-
vapor	T52.0X-
Gastric enzymes	T47.5X-
Gastrografin	T50.8X-
Gastrointestinal drug	T47.9-
biological	T47.8X-
specified NEC	T47.8X-
Gaultheria procumbens	T62.2X-
Gefarnate	T44.3X-
Gelatin (intravenous)	T45.8X-
absorbable (sponge)	T45.7X-
Gelfilm	T49.8X-
Gelfoam	T45.7X-
Gelsemine	T50.99-
Gelsemium (sempervirens)	T62.2X-
Gemeprost	T48.0X-
Gemfibrozil	T46.6X-
Gemonil	T42.3X-
Gentamicin	T36.5X-
ophthalmic preparation	T49.5X-
topical NEC	T49.0X-
Gentian	T47.5X-
violet	T49.0X-
Gepefrine	T44.4X-
Gestonorone caproate	T38.5X-
Gexane	T49.0X-
Gila monster (venom)	T63.11-
Ginger	T47.5X-
Gitalin	T46.0X-
Gitaloxin	T46.0X-
Gitoxin	T46.0X-
Glafenine	T39.8X-
Glandular extract (medicinal) NEC	T50.Z9-
Glaucarubin	T37.3X-
Glibenclamide	T38.3X-
Glibornuride	T38.3X-
Gliclazide	T38.3X-
Glimidine	T38.3X-
Glipizide	T38.3X-
Gliquidone	T38.3X-
Glisolamide	T38.3X-
Glisoxepide	T38.3X-

Drug/Chemical	Code
Globin zinc insulin	T38.3X-
Globulin (antilymphocytic) (antirhesus) (antivenin) (antiviral)	T50.Z1-
Glucagon	T38.3X-
Glucocorticoids	T38.0X-
Glucocorticosteroid	T38.0X-
Gluconic acid	T50.99-
Glucosamine sulfate	T39.4X-
Glucose	T50.3X-
with sodium chloride	T50.3X-
Glucosulfone sodium	T37.1X-
Glucurolactone	T47.8X-
Glue NEC	T52.8X-
Glutamic acid	T47.5X-
Glutaral (medicinal)	T49.0X-
nonmedicinal	T65.89-
Glutaraldehyde (nonmedicinal)	T65.89-
medicinal	T49.0X-
Glutathione	T50.6X-
Glutethimide	T42.6X-
Glyburide	T38.3X-
Glycerin	T47.4X-
Glycerol	T47.4X-
borax	T49.6X-
intravenous	T50.3X-
iodinated	T48.4X-
Glycerophosphate	T50.99-
Glyceryl	
gualacolate	T48.4X-
nitrate	T46.3X-
triacetate (topical)	T49.0X-
trinitrate	T46.3X-
Glycine	T50.3X-
Glyclopyramide	T38.3X-
Glycobiarsol	T37.3X-
Glycols (ether)	T52.3X-
Glyconiazide	T37.1X-
Glycopyrrolate	T44.3X-
Glycopyrronium (bromide)	T44.3X-
Glycoside, cardiac (stimulant)	T46.0X-
Glycyclamide	T38.3X-
Glycyrrhiza extract	T48.4X-
Glycyrrhizic acid	T48.4X-
Glycyrrhizinate potassium	T48.4X-
Glymidine sodium	T38.3X-
Glyphosate	T60.3X-
Glyphylline	T48.6X-
Gold	
colloidal (l98Au)	T45.1X-
salts	T39.4X-
Golden sulfide of antimony	T56.89-
Goldylocks	T62.2X-
Gonadal tissue extract	T38.90-
female	T38.5X-
male	T38.7X-

TABLE OF DRUGS AND CHEMICALS

Drug/Chemical	Code	Drug/Chemical	Code
Gonadorelin	T38.89-	**Harmonyl**	T46.5X-
Gonadotropin	T38.89-	**Hartmann's solution**	T50.3X-
chorionic	T38.89-	**Hashish**	T40.71-
pituitary	T38.81-	**Hawaiian Woodrose seeds**	T40.99-
Goserelin	T45.1X-	**HCB**	T60.3X-
Grain alcohol	T51.0X-	**HCH**	T53.6X-
Gramicidin	T49.0X-	medicinal	T49.0X-
Granisetron	T45.0X-	**HCN**	T57.3X-
Gratiola officinalis	T62.2X-	**Headache cures, drugs, powders NEC**	T50.90-
Grease	T65.89-	**Heavenly Blue (morning glory)**	T40.99-
Green hellebore	T62.2X-	**Heavy metal antidote**	T45.8X-
Green soap	T49.2X-	**Hedaquinium**	T49.0X-
Grifulvin	T36.7X-	**Hedge hyssop**	T62.2X-
Griseofulvin	T36.7X-	**Heet**	T49.8X-
Growth hormone	T38.81-	**Helenin**	T37.4X-
Guaiac reagent	T50.99-	**Helium (nonmedicinal) NEC**	T59.89-
Guaiacol derivatives	T48.4X-	medicinal	T48.99-
Guaifenesin	T48.4X-	**Hellebore (black) (green) (white)**	T62.2X-
Guaimesal	T48.4X-	**Hematin**	T45.8X-
Guaiphenesin	T48.4X-	**Hematinic preparation**	T45.8X-
Guamecycline	T36.4X-	**Hematological agent**	T45.9-
Guanabenz	T46.5X-	specified NEC	T45.8X-
Guanacline	T46.5X-	**Hemlock**	T62.2X-
Guanadrel	T46.5X-	**Hemostatic**	T45.62-
Guanatol	T37.2X-	drug, systemic	T45.62-
Guanethidine	T46.5X-	**Hemostyptic**	T49.4X-
Guanfacine	T46.5X-	**Henbane**	T62.2X-
Guano	T65.89-	**Heparin (sodium)**	T45.51-
Guanochlor	T46.5X-	action reverser	T45.7X-
Guanoclor	T46.5X-	**Heparin-fraction**	T45.51-
Guanoctine	T46.5X-	**Heparinoid (systemic)**	T45.51-
Guanoxabenz	T46.5X-	**Hepatic secretion stimulant**	T47.8X-
Guanoxan	T46.5X-	**Hepatitis B**	
Guar gum (medicinal)	T46.6X-	immune globulin	T50.Z1-
Hachimycin	T36.7X-	vaccine	T50.B9-
Hair		**Hepronicate**	T46.7X-
dye	T49.4X-	**Heptabarb**	T42.3X-
preparation NEC	T49.4X-	**Heptabarbital**	T42.3X-
Halazepam	T42.4X-	**Heptabarbitone**	T42.3X-
Halcinolone	T49.0X-	**Heptachlor**	T60.1X-
Halcinonide	T49.0X-	**Heptalgin**	T40.2X-
Halethazole	T49.0X-	**Heptaminol**	T46.3X-
Hallucinogen NOS	T40.90-	**Herbicide NEC**	T60.3X-
specified NEC	T40.99-	**Heroin**	T40.1X-
Halofantrine	T37.2X-	**Herplex**	T49.5X-
Halofenate	T46.6X-	**HES**	T45.8X-
Halometasone	T49.0X-	**Hesperidin**	T46.99-
Haloperidol	T43.4X-	**Hetacillin**	T36.0X-
Haloprogin	T49.0X-	**Hetastarch**	T45.8X-
Halotex	T49.0X-	**HETP**	T60.0X-
Halothane	T41.0X-	**Hexachlorobenzene (vapor)**	T60.3X-
Haloxazolam	T42.4X-	**Hexachlorocyclohexane**	T53.6X-
Halquinols	T49.0X-	**Hexachlorophene**	T49.0X-
Hamamelis	T49.2X-	**Hexadiline**	T46.3X-
Haptendextran	T45.8X-	**Hexadimethrine (bromide)**	T45.7X-

TABLE OF DRUGS AND CHEMICALS

Drug/Chemical	Code
Hexadylamine	T46.3X-
Hexaethyl tetraphosphate	T60.0X-
Hexafluorenium bromide	T48.1X-
Hexafluronium (bromide)	T48.1X-
Hexa-germ	T49.2X-
Hexahydrobenzol	T52.8X-
Hexahydrocresol(s)	T51.8X-
arsenide	T57.0X-
arseniurated	T57.0X-
cyanide	T57.3X-
gas	T59.89-
Fluoride (liquid)	T57.8X-
vapor	T59.89-
phophorated	T60.0X-
sulfate	T57.8X-
sulfide (gas)	T59.6X-
arseniurated	T57.0X-
sulfurated	T57.8X-
Hexahydrophenol	T51.8X-
Hexalen	T51.8X-
Hexamethonium bromide	T44.2X-
Hexamethylene	T52.8X-
Hexamethylmelamine	T45.1X-
Hexamidine	T49.0X-
Hexamine (mandelate)	T37.8X-
Hexanone, 2-hexanone	T52.4X-
Hexanuorenium	T48.1X-
Hexapropymate	T42.6X-
Hexasonium iodide	T44.3X-
Hexcarbacholine bromide	T48.1X-
Hexemal	T42.3X-
Hexestrol	T38.5X-
Hexethal (sodium)	T42.3X-
Hexetidine	T37.8X-
Hexobarbital	T42.3X-
rectal	T41.29-
sodium	T41.1X-
Hexobendine	T46.3X-
Hexocyclium (metilsulfate)	T44.3X-
Hexoestrol	T38.5X-
Hexone	T52.4X-
Hexoprenaline	T48.6X-
Hexylcaine	T41.3X-
Hexylresorcinol	T52.2X-
HGH (human growth hormone)	T38.81-
Hinkle's pills	T47.2X-
Histalog	T50.8X-
Histamine (phosphate)	T50.8X-
Histoplasmin	T50.8X-
Holly berries	T62.2X-
Homatropine	T44.3X-
methylbromide	T44.3X-
Homochlorcyclizine	T45.0X-
Homosalate	T49.3X-

Drug/Chemical	Code
Homo-tet	T50.Z1-
Hormone	T38.80-
adrenal cortical steroids	T38.0X-
androgenic	T38.7X-
anterior pituitary NEC	T38.81-
antidiabetic agents	T38.3X-
antidiuretic	T38.89-
cancer therapy	T45.1X-
follicle stimulating	T38.81-
gonadotropic	T38.89-
pituitary	T38.81-
growth	T38.81-
luteinizing	T38.81-
ovarian	T38.5X-
oxytocic	T48.0X-
parathyroid (derivatives)	T50.99-
pituitary (posterior) NEC	T38.89-
anterior	T38.81-
specified, NEC	T38.89-
thyroid	T38.1X-
Hornet (sting)	T63.451
Horse anti-human lymphocytic serum	T50.Z1-
Horticulture agent NEC	T65.9-
with pesticide	T60.9-
Human	
albumin	T45.8X-
growth hormone (HGH)	T38.81-
immune serum	T50.Z1-
Hyaluronidase	T45.3X-
Hyazyme	T45.3X-
Hycodan	T40.2X-
Hydantoin derivative NEC	T42.0X-
Hydeltra	T38.0X-
Hydergine	T44.6X-
Hydrabamine penicillin	T36.0X-
Hydralazine	T46.5X-
Hydrargaphen	T49.0X-
Hydrargyri amino-chloridum	T49.0X-
Hydrastine	T48.29-
Hydrazine	T54.1X-
monoamine oxidase inhibitors	T43.1X-
Hydrazoic acid, azides	T54.2X-
Hydriodic acid	T48.4X-
Hydrocarbon gas	T59.89-
Hydrochloric acid (liquid)	T54.2X-
medicinal (digestant)	T47.5X-
vapor	T59.89-
Hydrochlorothiazide	T50.2X-
Hydrocodone	T40.2X-
Hydrocortisone (derivatives)	T49.0X-
aceponate	T49.0X-
ENT agent	T49.6X-
ophthalmic preparation	T49.5X-
topical NEC	T49.0X-

HEXADYLAMINE–HYDROCORTISONE (DERIVATIVES)

TABLE OF DRUGS AND CHEMICALS

Drug/Chemical	Code	Drug/Chemical	Code
Hydrocortone	T38.0X-	**Hypaque**	T50.8X-
ENT agent	T49.6X-	**Hypertussis**	T50.Z1-
ophthalmic preparation	T49.5X-	**Hypnotic**	T42.71
topical NEC	T49.0X-	anticonvulsant	T42.71
Hydrocyanic acid (liquid)	T57.3X-	specified NEC	T42.6X-
gas	T65.0X-	**Hypochlorite**	T49.0X-
Hydroflumethiazide	T50.2X-	**Hypophysis, posterior**	T38.89-
Hydrofluoric acid (liquid)	T54.2X-	**Hypotensive NEC**	T46.5X-
vapor	T59.89-	**Hypromellose**	T49.5X-
Hydrogen	T59.89-	**Ibacitabine**	T37.5X-
arsenide	T57.0X-	**Ibopamine**	T44.99-
arseniureted	T57.0X-	**Ibufenac**	T39.31-
chloride	T57.8X-	**Ibuprofen**	T39.31-
cyanide (salts) (gas)	T57.3X-	**Ibuproxam**	T39.31-
Fluoride (vapor)	T59.5X-	**Ibuterol**	T48.6X-
peroxide	T49.0X-	**Ichthammol**	T49.0X-
phosphureted	T57.1X-	**Ichthyol**	T49.4X-
sulfide (sulfureted)	T59.6X-	**Idarubicin**	T45.1X-
arseniureted	T57.0X-	**Idrocilamide**	T42.8X-
Hydromethylpyridine	T46.7X-	**Ifenprodil**	T46.7X-
Hydromorphinol	T40.2X-	**Ifosfamide**	T45.1X-
Hydromorphinone	T40.2X-	**Iletin**	T38.3X-
Hydromorphone	T40.2X-	**Ilex**	T62.2X-
Hydromox	T50.2X-	**Illuminating gas (after combustion)**	T58.1-
Hydrophilic lotion	T49.3X-	prior to combustion	T59.89-
Hydroquinidine	T46.2X-	**Ilopan**	T45.2X-
Hydroquinone	T52.2X-	**Iloprost**	T46.7X-
vapor	T59.89-	**Ilotycin**	T36.3X-
Hydrosulfuric acid (gas)	T59.6X-	ophthalmic preparation	T49.5X-
Hydrotalcite	T47.1X-	topical NEC	T49.0X-
Hydrous wool fat	T49.3X-	**Imidazole-4-carboxamide**	T45.1X-
Hydroxide, caustic	T54.3X-	**Iminostilbene**	T42.1X-
Hydroxocobalamin	T45.8X-	**Imipenem**	T36.0X-
Hydroxyamphetamine	T49.5X-	**Imipramine**	T43.01-
Hydroxycarbamide	T45.1X-	**Immu-G**	T50.Z1-
Hydroxychloroquine	T37.8X-	**Immuglobin**	T50.Z1-
Hydroxydihydrocodeinone	T40.2X-	**Immune (globulin) (serum)**	T50.Z1-
Hydroxyestrone	T38.5X-	**Immunoglobin human (intravenous) (normal)**	T50.Z1-
Hydroxyethyl starch	T45.8X-	**Immunosuppressive drug**	T45.1X-
Hydroxymethylpenta-none	T52.4X-	**Immu-tetanus**	T50.Z1-
Hydroxyphenamate	T43.59-	**Indalpine**	T43.22-
Hydroxyphenylbutazone	T39.2X-	**Indanazoline**	T48.5X-
Hydroxyprogesterone	T38.5X-	**Indandione (derivatives)**	T45.51-
caproate	T38.5X-	**Indapamide**	T46.5X-
Hydroxyquinoline (derivatives) NEC	T37.8X-	**Indendione (derivatives)**	T45.51-
Hydroxystilbamidine	T37.3X-	**Indenolol**	T44.7X-
Hydroxytoluene (nonmedicinal)	T54.0X-	**Inderal**	T44.7X-
medicinal	T49.0X-	**Indian**	
Hydroxyurea	T45.1X-	hemp	T40.71-
Hydroxyzine	T43.59-	tobacco	T62.2X-
antiallergic	T45.0X-	**Indigo carmine**	T50.8X-
Hyoscine	T44.3X-	**Indobufen**	T45.521
Hyoscyamine	T44.3X-	**Indocin**	T39.2X-
Hyoscyamus	T44.3X-	**Indocyanine green**	T50.8X-
dry extract	T44.3X-	**Indometacin**	T39.39-

TABLE OF DRUGS AND CHEMICALS

Drug/Chemical	Code
Indomethacin	T39.39-
farnesil	T39.4X-
Indoramin	T44.6X-
Industrial	
alcohol	T51.0X-
fumes	T59.89-
solvents (fumes) (vapors)	T52.9-
Influenza vaccine	T50.B9-
Ingested substance NEC	T65.9-
INH	T37.1X-
Inhibitor	
angiotensin-converting enzyme	T46.4X-
carbonic anhydrase	T50.2X-
fibrinolysis	T45.62-
monoamine oxidase NEC	T43.1X-
hydrazine	T43.1X-
postsynaptic	T43.8X-
prothrombin synthesis	T45.51-
Ink	T65.89-
Inorganic substance NEC	T57.9-
Inosine pranobex	T37.5X-
Inositol	T50.99-
nicotinate	T46.7X-
Inproquone	T45.1X-
Insect (sting), venomous	T63.481
ant	T63.421
bee	T63.441
caterpillar	T63.431
hornet	T63.451
wasp	T63.461
Insecticide NEC	T60.9-
carbamate	T60.0X-
chlorinated	T60.1X-
mixed	T60.9-
organochlorine	T60.1X-
organophosphorus	T60.0X-
Insular tissue extract	T38.3X-
Insulin (amorphous) (globin) (isophane) (Lente) (NPH) (Semilente) (Ultralente)	T38.3X-
defalan	T38.3X-
human	T38.3X-
injection, soluble (biphasic)	T38.3X-
intermediate acting	T38.3X-
protamine zinc	T38.3X-
slow acting	T38.3X-
zinc protamine injection/suspension (amorphous) (crystalline)	T38.3X-
Interferon (alpha) (beta) (gamma)	T37.5X-
Intestinal motility control drug	T47.6X-
biological	T47.8X-
Intranarcon	T41.1X-
Intravenous	
amino acids or fat suspensions	T50.99-
Inulin	T50.8X-
Invert sugar	T50.3X-

Drug/Chemical	Code
Iobenzamic acid	T50.8X-
Iocarmic acid	T50.8X-
Iocetamic acid	T50.8X-
Iodamide	T50.8X-
Iodide NEC—*see also Iodine*	T49.0X-
mercury (ointment)	T49.0X-
methylate	T49.0X-
potassium (expectorant) NEC	T48.4X-
Iodinated	
contrast medium	T50.8X-
glycerol	T48.4X-
human serum albumin (131I)	T50.8X-
Iodine (antiseptic, external) (tincture) NEC	T49.0X-
125—*see also Radiation sickness, and Exposure to radioactive isotopes*	T50.8X-
therapeutic	T50.99-
131—*see also Radiation sickness, and Exposure to radioactive isotopes*	T50.8X-
therapeutic	T38.2X-
diagnostic	T50.8X-
for thyroid conditions (antithyroid)	T38.2X-
solution	T49.0X-
vapor	T59.89-
Iodipamide	T50.8X-
Iodized (poppy seed) oil	T50.8X-
Iodobismitol	T37.8X-
Iodochlorhydroxyquin	T37.8X-
topical	T49.0X-
Iodochlorhydroxyquinoline	T37.8X-
Iodocholesterol (131I)	T50.8X-
Iodoform	T49.0X-
Iodohippuric acid	T50.8X-
Iodopanoic acid	T50.8X-
Iodophthalein (sodium)	T50.8X-
Iodopyracet	T50.8X-
Iodoquinol	T37.8X-
Iodoxamic acid	T50.8X-
Iofendylate	T50.8X-
Ioglycamic acid	T50.8X-
Iohexol	T50.8X-
Ion exchange resin	
anion	T47.8X-
cation	T50.3X-
cholestyramine	T46.6X-
intestinal	T47.8X-
Iopamidol	T50.8X-
Iopanoic acid	T50.8X-
Iophenoic acid	T50.8X-
Iopodate, sodium	T50.8X-
Iopodic acid	T50.8X-
Iopromide	T50.8X-
Iopydol	T50.8X-
Iotalamic acid	T50.8X-
Iothalamate	T50.8X-
Iothiouracil	T38.2X-

TABLE OF DRUGS AND CHEMICALS

Drug/Chemical	Code
Iotrol	T50.8X-
Iotrolan	T50.8X-
Iotroxate	T50.8X-
Iotroxic acid	T50.8X-
Ioversol	T50.8X-
Ioxaglate	T50.8X-
Ioxaglic acid	T50.8X-
Ioxitalamic acid	T50.8X-
Ipecac	T47.7X-
Ipecacuanha	T48.4X-
Ipodate, calcium	T50.8X-
Ipral	T42.3X-
Ipratropium (bromide)	T48.6X-
Ipriflavone	T46.3X-
Iprindole	T43.01-
Iproclozide	T43.1X-
Iprofenin	T50.8X-
Iproheptine	T49.2X-
Iproniazid	T43.1X-
Iproplatin	T45.1X-
Iproveratril	T46.1X-
Iron (compounds) (medicinal) NEC	T45.4X-
ammonium/dextran injection/salts/sorbitex/sorbitol citric acid complex	T45.4X-
nonmedicinal	T56.89-
Irrigating fluid (vaginal)	T49.8X-
eye	T49.5X-
Isepamicin	T36.5X-
Isoaminile (citrate)	T48.3X-
Isoamyl nitrite	T46.3X-
Isobenzan	T60.1X-
Isobutyl acetate	T52.8X-
Isocarboxazid	T43.1X-
Isoconazole	T49.0X-
Isocyanate	T65.0X-
Isoephedrine	T44.99-
Isoetarine	T48.6X-
Isoethadione	T42.2X-
Isoetharine	T44.5X-
Isoflurane	T41.0X-
Isoflurophate	T44.0X-
Isomaltose, ferric complex	T45.4X-
Isometheptene	T44.3X-
Isoniazid	T37.1X-
with	
rifampicin	T36.6X-
thioacetazone	T37.1X-
Isonicotinic acid hydrazide	T37.1X-
Isonipecaine	T40.4X-
Isopentaquine	T37.2X-
Isophane insulin	T38.3X-
Isophorone	T65.89-
Isophosphamide	T45.1X-
Isopregnenone	T38.5X-
Isoprenaline	T48.6X-
Isopromethazine	T43.3X-
Isopropamide	T44.3X-
iodide	T44.3X-
Isopropanol	T51.2X-
Isopropyl	
acetate	T52.8X-
alcohol	T51.2X-
medicinal	T49.4X-
ether	T52.8X-
Isopropylaminophenazone	T39.2X-
Isoproterenol	T48.6X-
Isosorbide dinitrate	T46.3X-
Isothipendyl	T45.0X-
Isotretinoin	T50.99-
Isoxazolyl penicillin	T36.0X-
Isoxicam	T39.39-
Isoxsuprine	T46.7X-
Ispagula	T47.4X-
husk	T47.4X-
Isradipine	T46.1X-
I-thyroxine sodium	T38.1X-
Itraconazole	T37.8X-
Itramin tosilate	T46.3X-
Ivermectin	T37.4X-
Izoniazid	T37.1X-
with thioacetazone	T37.1X-
Jalap	T47.2X-
Jamaica	
dogwood (bark)	T39.8X-
ginger	T65.89-
root	T62.2X-
Jatropha	T62.2X-
curcas	T62.2X-
Jectofer	T45.4X-
Jellyfish (sting)	T63.62-
Jequirity (bean)	T62.2X-
Jimson weed (stramonium)	T62.2X-
Josamycin	T36.3X-
Juniper tar	T49.1X-
Kallidinogenase	T46.7X-
Kallikrein	T46.7X-
Kanamycin	T36.5X-
Kantrex	T36.5X-
Kaolin	T47.6X-
light	T47.6X-
Karaya (gum)	T47.4X-
Kebuzone	T39.2X-
Kelevan	T60.1X-
Kemithal	T41.1X-
Kenacort	T38.0X-
Keratolytic drug NEC	T49.4X-
anthracene	T49.4X-
Keratoplastic NEC	T49.4X-

TABLE OF DRUGS AND CHEMICALS

Drug/Chemical	Code
Kerosene, kerosine (fuel) (solvent) NEC	T52.0X-
insecticide	T52.0X-
vapor	T52.0X-
Ketamine	T41.29-
Ketazolam	T42.4X-
Ketazon	T39.2X-
Ketobemidone	T40.4X-
Ketoconazole	T49.0X-
Ketols	T52.4X-
Ketone oils	T52.4X-
Ketoprofen	T39.31-
Ketorolac	T39.8X-
Ketotifen	T45.0X-
Khat	T43.69-
Khellin	T46.3X-
Khelloside	T46.3X-
Kiln gas or vapor (carbon monoxide)	T58.8X-
Kitasamycin	T36.3X-
Konsyl	T47.4X-
Kosam seed	T62.2X-
Krait (venom)	T63.09-
Kwell (insecticide)	T60.1X-
anti-infective (topical)	T49.0X-
Labetalol	T44.8X-
Laburnum (seeds)	T62.2X-
leaves	T62.2X-
Lachesine	T49.5X-
Lacidipine	T46.5X-
Lacquer	T65.6X-
Lacrimogenic gas	T59.3X-
Lactated potassic saline	T50.3X-
Lactic acid	T49.8X-
Lactobacillus (all forms or compounds)	T47.6X-
Lactoflavin	T45.2X-
Lactose (as excipient)	T50.90-
Lactuca (virosa) (extract)	T42.6X-
Lactucarium	T42.6X-
Lactulose	T47.3X-
Laevo—*see Levo-*	
Lanatosides	T46.0X-
Lanolin	T49.3X-
Largactil	T43.3X-
Larkspur	T62.2X-
Laroxyl	T43.01-
Lasix	T50.1X-
Lassar's paste	T49.4X-
Latamoxef	T36.1X-
Latex	T65.81-
Lathyrus (seed)	T62.2X-
Laudanum	T40.0X-
Laudexium	T48.1X-
Laughing gas	T41.0X-
Laurel, black or cherry	T62.2X-
Laurolinium	T49.0X-

Drug/Chemical	Code
Lauryl sulfoacetate	T49.2X-
Laxative NEC	T47.4X-
osmotic	T47.3X-
saline	T47.3X-
stimulant	T47.2X-
L-dopa	T42.8X-
Lead (dust) (fumes) (vapor) NEC	T56.0X-
acetate	T49.2X-
alkyl (fuel additive)	T56.0X-
anti-infectives	T37.8X-
antiknock compound (tetraethyl)	T56.0X-
arsenate, arsenite (dust) (herbicide) (insecticide) (vapor)	T57.0X-
carbonate (paint)	T56.0X-
chromate (paint)	T56.0X-
dioxide	T56.0X-
inorganic	T56.0X-
iodide (pigment) (paint)	T56.0X-
monoxide (dust) (paint)	T56.0X-
organic	T56.0X-
oxide (paint)	T56.0X-
salts	T56.0X-
specified compound NEC	T56.0X-
tetra-ethyl	T56.0X-
Lebanese red	T40.71-
Lefetamine	T39.8X-
Lenperone	T43.4X-
Lente lietin (insulin)	T38.3X-
Leptazol	T50.7X-
Leptophos	T60.0X-
Leritine	T40.2X-
Letosteine	T48.4X-
Letter	T38.1X-
Lettuce opium	T42.6X-
Leucinocaine	T41.3X-
Leucocianidol	T46.99-
Leucovorin (factor)	T45.8X-
Leukeran	T45.1X-
Leuprolide	T38.89-
Levalbuterol	T48.6X-
Levallorphan	T50.7X-
Levamisole	T37.4X-
Levanil	T42.6X-
Levarterenol	T44.4X-
Levdropropizine	T48.3X-
Levobunolol	T49.5X-
Levocabastine (hydrochloride)	T45.0X-
Levocarnitine	T50.99-
Levodopa (w carbidopa)	T42.8X-
Levo-dromoran	T40.2X-
Levoglutamide	T50.99-
Levoid	T38.1X-
Levo-iso-methadone	T40.3X-
Levomepromazine	T43.3X-
Levonordefrin	T49.6X-

TABLE OF DRUGS AND CHEMICALS

Drug/Chemical	Code
Levonorgestrel	T38.4X-
with ethinylestradiol	T38.5X-
Levopromazine	T43.3X-
Levoprome	T42.6X-
Levopropoxyphene	T40.4X-
Levopropylhexedrine	T50.5X-
Levoproxyphylline	T48.6X-
Levorphanol	T40.4X-
Levothyroxine	T38.1X-
sodium	T38.1X-
Levsin	T44.3X-
Levulose	T50.3X-
Lewisite (gas), not in war	T57.0X-
Librium	T42.4X-
Lidex	T49.0X-
Lidocaine	T41.3X-
regional	T41.3X-
spinal	T41.3X-
Lidofenin	T50.8X-
Lidoflazine	T46.1X-
Lighter fluid	T52.0X-
Lignin hemicellulose	T47.6X-
Lignocaine	T41.3X-
regional	T41.3X-
spinal	T41.3X-
Ligroin (e) (solvent)	T52.0X-
vapor	T59.89-
Ligustrum vulgare	T62.2X-
Lily of the valley	T62.2X-
Lime (chloride)	T54.3X-
Limonene	T52.8X-
Lincomycin	T36.8X-
Lindane (insecticide) (nonmedicinal) (vapor)	T53.6X-
medicinal	T49.0X-
Liniments NEC	T49.9-
Linoleic acid	T46.6X-
Linolenic acid	T46.6X-
Linseed	T47.4X-
Liothyronine	T38.1X-
Liotrix	T38.1X-
Lipancreatin	T47.5X-
Lipo-alprostadil	T46.7X-
Lipo-Lutin	T38.5X-
Lipotropic drug NEC	T50.90-
Liquefied petroleum gases	T59.89-
piped (pure or mixed with air)	T59.89-
Liquid	
paraffin	T47.4X-
petrolatum	T47.4X-
topical	T49.3X-
specified NEC	T65.89-
substance	T65.9-
Liquor creosolis compositus	T65.89-
Liquorice	T48.4X-
extract	T47.8X-
Lisinopril	T46.4X-
Lisuride	T42.8X-
Lithane	T43.8X-
Lithium	T56.89-
gluconate	T43.59-
salts (carbonate)	T43.59-
Lithonate	T43.8X-
Liver	
extract	T45.8X-
for parenteral use	T45.8X-
fraction 1	T45.8X-
hydrolysate	T45.8X-
Lizard (bite) (venom)	T63.121
LMD	T45.8X-
Lobelia	T62.2X-
Lobeline	T50.7X-
Local action drug NEC	T49.8X-
Locorten	T49.0X-
Lofepramine	T43.01-
Lolium temulentum	T62.2X-
Lomotil	T47.6X-
Lomustine	T45.1X-
Lonidamine	T45.1X-
Loperamide	T47.6X-
Loprazolam	T42.4X-
Lorajmine	T46.2X-
Loratidine	T45.0X-
Lorazepam	T42.4X-
Lorcainide	T46.2X-
Lormetazepam	T42.4X-
Lotions NEC	T49.9-
Lotusate	T42.3X-
Lovastatin	T46.6X-
Lowila	T49.2X-
Loxapine	T43.59-
Lozenges (throat)	T49.6X-
LSD	T40.8X-
L-Tryptophan—*see amino acid*	
Lubricant, eye	T49.5X-
Lubricating oil NEC	T52.0X-
Lucanthone	T37.4X-
Luminal	T42.3X-
Lung irritant (gas) NEC	T59.9-
Luteinizing hormone	T38.81-
Lutocylol	T38.5X-
Lutromone	T38.5X-
Lututrin	T48.29-
Lye (concentrated)	T54.3X-
Lygranum (skin test)	T50.8X-
Lymecycline	T36.4X-
Lymphogranuloma venereum antigen	T50.8X-
Lynestrenol	T38.4X-
Lyovac Sodium Edecrin	T50.1X-
Lypressin	T38.89-
Lysergic acid diethylamide	T40.8X-

TABLE OF DRUGS AND CHEMICALS

Drug/Chemical	Code
Lysergide	T40.8X-
Lysine vasopressin	T38.89-
Lysol	T54.1X-
Lysozyme	T49.0X-
Lytta (vitatta)	T49.8X-
Mace	T59.3X-
Macrogol	T50.99-
Macrolide	
anabolic drug	T38.7X-
antibiotic	T36.3X-
Mafenide	T49.0X-
Magaldrate	T47.1X-
Magic mushroom	T40.99-
Magnamycin	T36.8X-
Magnesia magma	T47.1X-
Magnesium NEC	T56.89-
carbonate	T47.1X-
citrate	T47.4X-
hydroxide (oxide)	T47.1X-
peroxide	T49.0X-
salicylate	T39.09-
silicofluoride	T50.3X-
sulfate	T47.4X-
thiosulfate	T45.0X-
trisilicate	T47.1X-
Malathion (medicinal) (insecticide)	T49.0X-
insecticide	T60.0X-
Male fern extract	T37.4X-
M-AMSA	T45.1X-
Mandelic acid	T37.8X-
Manganese (dioxide) (salts)	T57.2X-
medicinal	T50.99-
Mannitol	T47.3X-
hexanitrate	T46.3X-
Mannomustine	T45.1X-
MAO inhibitors	T43.1X-
Mapharsen	T37.8X-
Maphenide	T49.0X-
Maprotiline	T43.02-
Marcaine (infiltration) (subcutaneous) (nerve block)	T41.3X-
Marezine	T45.0X-
Marijuana/Marihuana	T40.71-
Marine (sting)	T63.69-
animals (sting)	T63.69-
plants (sting)	T63.71-
Marplan	T43.1X-
Marsh gas	T59.89-
Marsilid	T43.1X-
Matulane	T45.1X-
Mazindol	T50.5X-
MCPA	T60.3X-
MDMA	T43.64-
Meadow saffron	T62.2X-
Measles virus vaccine (attenuated)	T50.B9-
Meat, noxious	T62.8X-
Meballymal	T42.3X-
Mebanazine	T43.1X-
Mebaral	T42.3X-
Mebendazole	T37.4X-
Mebeverine	T44.3X-
Mebhydrolin	T45.0X-
Mebumal	T42.3X-
Mebutamate	T43.59-
Mecamylamine	T44.2X-
Mechlorethamine	T45.1X-
Mecillinam	T36.0X-
Meclizine (hydrochloride)	T45.0X-
Meclocycline	T36.4X-
Meclofenamate	T39.39-
Meclofenamic acid	T39.39-
Meclofenoxate	T43.69-
Meclozine	T45.0X-
Mecobalamin	T45.8X-
Mecoprop	T60.3X-
Mecrilate	T49.3X-
Mecysteine	T48.4X-
Medazepam	T42.4X-
Medicament NEC	T50.90-
Medinal	T42.3X-
Medomin	T42.3X-
Medrogestone	T38.5X-
Medroxalol	T44.8X-
Medroxyprogesterone acetate (depot)	T38.5X-
Medrysone	T49.0X-
Mefenamic acid	T39.39-
Mefenorex	T50.5X-
Mefloquine	T37.2X-
Mefruside	T50.2X-
Megahallucinogen	T40.90-
Megestrol	T38.5X-
Meglumine	
antimoniate	T37.8X-
diatrizoate	T50.8X-
iodipamide	T50.8X-
iotroxate	T50.8X-
MEK (methyl ethyl ketone)	T52.4X-
Meladinin	T49.3X-
Meladrazine	T44.3X-
Melaleuca alternifolia oil	T49.0X-
Melanizing agents	T49.3X-
Melanocyte-stimulating hormone	T38.89-
Melarsonyl potassium	T37.3X-
Melarsoprol	T37.3X-
Melia azedarach	T62.2X-
Melitracen	T43.01-
Mellaril	T43.3X-
Meloxine	T49.3X-
Melperone	T43.4X-
Melphalan	T45.1X-
Memantine	T43.8X-

TABLE OF DRUGS AND CHEMICALS

Drug/Chemical	Code
Menadiol (sodium sulfate)	T45.7X-
Menadione	T45.7X-
sodium bisulfite	T45.7X-
Menaphthone	T45.7X-
Menaquinone	T45.7X-
Menatetrenone	T45.7X-
Meningococcal vaccine	T50.A9-
Menningovax (-AC) (-C)	T50.A9-
Menotropins	T38.81-
Menthol	T48.5X-
Mepacrine	T37.2X-
Meparfynol	T42.6X-
Mepartricin	T36.7X-
Mepazine	T43.3X-
Mepenzolate	T44.3X-
bromide	T44.3X-
Meperidine	T40.4X-
Mephebarbital	T42.3X-
Mephenamin (e)	T42.8X-
Mephenesin	T42.8X-
Mephenhydramine	T45.0X-
Mephenoxalone	T42.8X-
Mephentermine	T44.99-
Mephenytoin	T42.0X-
with phenobarbital	T42.3X-
Mephobarbital	T42.3X-
Mephosfolan	T60.0X-
Mepindolol	T44.7X-
Mepiperphenidol	T44.3X-
Mepitiostane	T38.7X-
Mepivacaine (epidural)	T41.3X-
Meprednisone	T38.0X-
Meprobam	T43.59-
Meprobamate	T43.59-
Meproscillarin	T46.0X-
Meprylcaine	T41.3X-
Meptazinol	T39.8X-
Mepyramine	T45.0X-
Mequitazine	T43.3X-
Meralluride	T50.2X-
Merbaphen	T50.2X-
Merbromin	T49.0X-
Mercaptobenzothiazole salts	T49.0X-
Mercaptomerin	T50.2X-
Mercaptopurine	T45.1X-
Mercumatilin	T50.2X-
Mercuramide	T50.2X-
Mercurochrome	T49.0X-
Mercurophylline	T50.2X-
Mercury, mercurial, mercuric, mercurous (compounds) (cyanide) (fumes) (nonmedicinal) (vapor) NEC	T56.1X-
ammoniated	T49.0X-
anti-infective	
local	T49.0X-
systemic	T37.8X-

Drug/Chemical	Code
Mercury, mercurial, mercuric, mercurous (compounds) (cyanide) (fumes) (nonmedicinal) (vapor) NEC, continued	
topical	T49.0X-
chloride (ammoniated)	T49.0X-
diuretic NEC	T50.2X-
fungicide (organic)	T56.1X-
oxide, yellow	T49.0X-
Mersalyl	T50.2X-
Merthiolate	T49.0X-
ophthalmic preparation	T49.5X-
Meruvax	T50.B9-
Mesalazine	T47.8X-
Mescal buttons	T40.99-
Mescaline	T40.99-
Mesna	T48.4X-
Mesoglycan	T46.6X-
Mesoridazine	T43.3X-
Mestanolone	T38.7X-
Mesterolone	T38.7X-
Mestranol	T38.5X-
Mesulergine	T42.8X-
Mesulfen	T49.0X-
Mesuximide	T42.2X-
Metabutethamine	T41.3X-
Metactesylacetate	T49.0X-
Metacycline	T36.4X-
Metaldehyde (snail killer) NEC	T60.8X-
Metals (heavy) (nonmedicinal)	T56.9-
dust, fumes, or vapor NEC	T56.9-
light NEC	T56.9-
dust, fumes, or vapor NEC	T56.9-
specified NEC	T56.89-
thallium	T56.81-
Metamfetamine	T43.65-
Metamizole sodium	T39.2X-
Metampicillin	T36.0X-
Metamucil	T47.4X-
Metandienone	T38.7X-
Metandrostenolone	T38.7X-
Metaphen	T49.0X-
Metaphos	T60.0X-
Metapramine	T43.01-
Metaproterenol	T48.29-
Metaraminol	T44.4X-
Metaxalone	T42.8X-
Metenolone	T38.7X-
Metergoline	T42.8X-
Metescufylline	T46.99-
Metetoin	T42.0X-
Metformin	T38.3X-
Methacholine	T44.1X-
Methacycline	T36.4X-
Methadone	T40.3X-
Methallenestril	T38.5X-
Methallenoestril	T38.5X-

TABLE OF DRUGS AND CHEMICALS

Drug/Chemical	Code	Drug/Chemical	Code
Methamphetamine	T43.65-	8-Methoxypsoralen (8-MOP)	T50.99-
Methampyrone	T39.2X-	Methscopolamine bromide	T44.3X-
Methandienone	T38.7X-	Methsuximide	T42.2X-
Methandriol	T38.7X-	Methylclothiazide	T50.2X-
Methandrostenolone	T38.7X-	**Methyl**	
Methane	T59.89-	acetate	T52.4X-
Methanethiol	T59.89-	acetone	T52.4X-
Methaniazide	T37.1X-	acrylate	T65.89-
Methanol (vapor)	T51.1X-	alcohol	T51.1X-
Methantheline	T44.3X-	aminophenol	T65.3X-
Methanthelinium bromide	T44.3X-	amphetamine	T43.65-
Methaphenilene	T45.0X-	androstanolone	T38.7X-
Methapyrilene	T45.0X-	atropine	T44.3X-
Methaqualone (compound)	T42.6X-	benzene	T52.2X-
Metharbital	T42.3X-	benzoate	T52.8X-
Methazolamide	T50.2X-	benzol	T52.2X-
Methdilazine	T43.3X-	bromide (gas)	T59.89-
Methedrine	T43.65-	fumigant	T60.8X-
Methenamine (mandelate)	T37.8X-	butanol	T51.3X-
Methenolone	T38.7X-	carbinol	T51.1X-
Methergine	T48.0X-	carbonate	T52.8X-
Methetoin	T42.0X-	CCNU	T45.1X-
Methiacil	T38.2X-	cellosolve	T52.9-
Methicillin	T36.0X-	cellulose	T47.4X-
Methimazole	T38.2X-	chloride (gas)	T59.89-
Methiodal sodium	T50.8X-	chloroformate	T59.3X-
Methionine	T50.99-	cyclohexane	T52.8X
Methisazone	T37.5X-	cyclohexanol	T51.8X-
Methisoprinol	T37.5X-	cyclohexanone	T52.8X-
Methitural	T42.3X-	cyclohexyl acetate	T52.8X-
Methixene	T44.3X-	demeton	T60.0X-
Methobarbital, methobarbitone	T42.3X-	dihydromorphinone	T40.2X-
Methocarbamol	T42.8X-	ergometrine	T48.0X-
skeletal muscle relaxant	T48.1X-	ergonovine	T48.0X-
Methohexital	T41.1X-	ethyl ketone	T52.4X-
Methohexitone	T41.1X-	glucamine antimonate	T37.8X-
Methoin	T42.0X-	hydrazine	T65.89-
Methopholine	T39.8X-	iodide	T65.89-
Methopromazine	T43.3X-	isobutyl ketone	T52.4X-
Methorate	T48.3X-	isothiocyanate	T60.3X-
Methoserpidine	T46.5X-	mercaptan	T59.89-
Methotrexate	T45.1X-	morphine NEC	T40.2X-
Methotrimeprazine	T43.3X-	nicotinate	T49.4X-
Methoxa-Dome	T49.3X-	paraben	T49.0X-
Methoxamine	T44.4X-	parafynol	T42.6X-
Methoxsalen	T50.99-	parathion	T60.0X-
Methoxyaniline	T65.3X-	peridol	T43.4X-
Methoxybenzyl penicillin	T36.0X-	phenidate	T43.631
Methoxychlor	T53.7X-	ENT agent	T49.6X-
Methoxy-DDT	T53.7X-	ophthalmic preparation	T49.5X-
2-Methoxyethanol	T52.3X-	topical NEC	T49.0X-
Methoxyflurane	T41.0X-	propylcarbinol	T51.3X-
Methoxyphenamine	T48.6X-	rosaniline NEC	T49.0X-
Methoxypromazine	T43.3X-	salicylate	T49.2X-
5-Methoxypsoralen (5-MOP)	T50.99-	sulfate (fumes)	T59.89-

TABLE OF DRUGS AND CHEMICALS

Drug/Chemical	Code
Methyl, continued	
liquid	T52.8X-
sulfonal	T42.6X-
testosterone	T38.7X-
thiouracil	T38.2X-
Methylamphetamine	T43.65-
Methylated spirit	T51.1X-
Methylatropine nitrate	T44.3X-
Methylbenactyzium bromide	T44.3X-
Methylbenzethonium chloride	T49.0X-
Methylcellulose	T47.4X-
laxative	T47.4X-
Methylchlorophenoxy-acetic acid	T60.3X-
Methyldopa	T46.5X-
Methyldopate	T46.5X-
Methylene	
blue	T50.6X-
chloride or dichloride (solvent) NEC	T53.4X-
Methylenedioxyamphetamine	T43.62-
Methylenedioxymethamphetamine	T43.64-
Methylergometrine	T48.0X-
Methylergonovine	T48.0X-
Methylestrenolone	T38.5X-
Methylethyl cellulose	T50.99-
Methylhexabital	T42.3X-
Methylmorphine	T40.2X-
Methylparaben (ophthalmic)	T49.5X-
Methylparafynol	T42.6X-
Methylpentynol, methylpenthynol	T42.6X-
Methylphenidate	T43.631
Methylphenobarbital	T42.3X-
Methylpolysiloxane	T47.1X-
Methylprednisolone	T38.0X-
Methylrosaniline	T49.0X-
Methylrosanilinium chloride	T49.0X-
Methyltestosterone	T38.7X-
Methylthionine chloride	T50.6X-
Methylthioninium chloride	T50.6X-
Methylthiouracil	T38.2X-
Methyprylon	T42.6X-
Methysergide	T46.5X-
Metiamide	T47.1X-
Meticillin	T36.0X-
Meticrane	T50.2X-
Metildigoxin	T46.0X-
Metipranolol	T49.5X-
Metirosine	T46.5X-
Metisazone	T37.5X-
Metixene	T44.3X-
Metizoline	T48.5X-
Metoclopramide	T45.0X-
Metofenazate	T43.3X-
Metofoline	T39.8X-
Metolazone	T50.2X-
Metopon	T40.2X-
Metoprine	T45.1X-
Metoprolol	T44.7X-
Metrifonate	T60.0X-
Metrizamide	T50.8X-
Metrizoic acid	T50.8X-
Metronidazole	T37.8X-
Metycaine (infiltration) (topical) (subcutaneous) (nerve block)	T41.3X-
Metyrapone	T50.8X-
Mevinphos	T60.0X-
Mexazolam	T42.4X-
Mexenone	T49.3X-
Mexiletine	T46.2X-
Mezereon	T62.2X-
berries	T62.1X-
Mezlocillin	T36.0X-
Mianserin	T43.02-
Micatin	T49.0X-
Miconazole	T49.0X-
Micronomicin	T36.5X-
Midazolam	T42.4X-
Midecamycin	T36.3X-
Mifepristone	T38.6X-
Milk of magnesia	T47.1X-
Millipede (tropical) (venomous)	T63.41-
Miltown	T43.59-
Milverine	T44.3X-
Minaprine	T43.29-
Minaxolone	T41.29-
Mineral	
acids	T54.2X-
oil (laxative) (medicinal)	T47.4X-
emulsion	T47.2X-
nonmedicinal	T52.0X-
topical	T49.3X-
salt NEC	T50.3X-
spirits	T52.0X-
Mineralocorticosteroid	T50.0X-
Minocycline	T36.4X-
Minoxidil	T46.7X-
Miokamycin	T36.3X-
Miotic drug	T49.5X-
Mipafox	T60.0X-
Mirex	T60.1X-
Mirtazapine	T43.02-
Misonidazole	T37.3X-
Misoprostol	T47.1X-
Mithramycin	T45.1X-
Mitobronitol	T45.1X-
Mitoguazone	T45.1X-
Mitolactol	T45.1X-
Mitomycin	T45.1X-
Mitopodozide	T45.1X-
Mitotane	T45.1X-
Mitoxantrone	T45.1X-

TABLE OF DRUGS AND CHEMICALS

Drug/Chemical	Code
Mivacurium chloride	T48.1X-
Miyari bacteria	T47.6X-
MMR vaccine	T50.B9-
Moclobemide	T43.1X-
Moderil	T46.5X-
Mofebutazone	T39.2X-
Molindone	T43.59-
Molsidomine	T46.3X-
Mometasone	T49.0X-
Monistat	T49.0X-
Monkshood	T62.2X-
Monoamine oxidase inhibitor NEC	T43.1X-
hydrazine	T43.1X-
Monobenzone	T49.4X-
Monochloroacetic acid	T60.3X-
Monochlorobenzene	T53.7X-
Monoethanolamine (oleate)	T46.8X-
Monooctanoin	T50.99-
Monophenylbutazone	T39.2X-
Monosodium glutamate	T65.89-
Monosulfiram	T49.0X-
Monoxidine hydrochloride	T46.1X-
Monuron	T60.3X-
Moperone	T43.4X-
Mopidamol	T45.1X-
MOPP (mechloreth-amine + vincristine + prednisone + procarbazine)	T45.1X-
Morfin	T40.2X-
Morinamide	T37.1X-
Morning glory seeds	T40.99-
Moroxydine	T37.5X-
Morphazinamide	T37.1X-
Morphine	T40.2X-
antagonist	T50.7X-
Morpholinylethylmorphine	T40.2X-
Morsuximide	T42.2X-
Mosapramine	T43.59-
Moth balls (naphthalene)—*see also Pesticide*	T60.2X-
paradichlorobenzene	T60.1X-
Motor exhaust gas	T58.0-
Mouthwash (antiseptic)	T49.6X-
Moxastine	T45.0X-
Moxaverine	T44.3X-
Moxisylyte	T46.7X-
Mucilage, plant	T47.4X-
Mucolytic drug	T48.4X-
Mucomyst	T48.4X-
Mucous membrane agents (external)	T49.9-
specified NEC	T49.8X-
Multiple unspec drugs	T50.91-
Mumps	
immune globulin (human)	T50.Z1-
skin test antigen	T50.8X-
Mupirocin	T49.0X-

Drug/Chemical	Code
Muromonab-CD3	T45.1X-
Muscle-action drug NEC	T48.20-
Muscle affecting agents NEC	T48.20-
oxytocic	T48.0X-
relaxants	T48.20-
central nervous system	T42.8X-
skeletal	T48.1X-
smooth	T44.3X-
Mushroom, noxious	T62.0X-
Mussel, noxious	T61.781
Mustard (emetic) (black)	T47.7X-
gas, not in war	T59.9-
nitrogen	T45.1X-
Mustine	T45.1X-
M-vac	T45.1X-
Mycifradin	T36.5X-
topical	T49.0X-
Mycitracin	T36.8X-
ophthalmic preparation	T49.5X-
Mycostatin	T36.7X-
topical	T49.0X-
Mycotoxins (NEC)	T64.81
aflatoxin	T64.0-
Mydriacyl	T44.3X-
Mydriatic drug	T49.5X-
Myelobromal	T45.1X-
Myleran	T45.1X-
Myochrysin (e)	T39.2X-
Myoneural blocking agents	T48.1X-
Myralact	T49.0X-
Myristica fragrans	T62.2X-
Myristicin	T65.89-
Mysoline	T42.3X-
Nabilone	T40.71-
Nabumetone	T39.39-
Nadolol	T44.7X-
Nafcillin	T36.0X-
Nafoxidine	T38.6X-
Naftazone	T46.99-
Naftidrofuryl (oxalate)	T46.7X-
Naftifine	T49.0X-
Nail polish remover	T52.9-
Nalbuphine	T40.4X-
Naled	T60.0X-
Nalidixic acid	T37.8X-
Nalorphine	T50.7X-
Naloxone	T50.7X-
Naltrexone	T50.7X-
Namenda	T43.8X-
Nandrolone	T38.7X-
Naphazoline	T48.5X-
Naphtha (painters') (petroleum)	T52.0X-
solvent	T52.0X-
vapor	T52.0X-

TABLE OF DRUGS AND CHEMICALS

Drug/Chemical	Code
Naphthalene (non-chlorinated)	T60.2X-
chlorinated	T60.1X-
vapor	T60.1X-
insecticide or moth repellent	T60.2X-
chlorinated	T60.1X-
vapor	T60.2X-
chlorinated	T60.1X-
Naphthol	T65.89-
Naphthylamine	T65.89-
Naphthylthiourea (ANTU)	T60.4X-
Naproxen (Naprosyn)	T39.31-
Narcotic (drug)	T40.60-
analgesic NEC	T40.60-
antagonist	T50.7X-
specified NEC	T40.69-
synthetic (other)	T40.49-
Narcotine	T48.3X-
Nardil	T43.1X-
Nasal drug NEC	T49.6X-
Natamycin	T49.0X-
Natural	
blood (product)	T45.8X-
gas (piped)	T59.89-
incomplete combustion	T58.1-
Nealbarbital	T42.3X-
Nectadon	T48.3X-
Nedocromil	T48.6X-
Nefopam	T39.8X-
Nematocyst (sting)	T63.69-
Nembutal	T42.3X-
Nemonapride	T43.59-
Neoarsphenamine	T37.8X-
Neocinchophen	T50.4X-
Neomycin (derivatives)	T36.5X-
with bacitracin	T49.0X-
with neostigmine	T44.0X-
ENT agent	T49.6X-
ophthalmic preparation	T49.5X-
topical NEC	T49.0X-
Neonal	T42.3X-
Neoprontosil	T37.0X-
Neosalvarsan	T37.8X-
Neosilversalvarsan	T37.8X-
Neosporin	T36.8X-
ENT agent	T49.6X-
opthalmic preparation	T49.5X-
topical NEC	T49.0X-
Neostigmine bromide	T44.0X-
Neraval	T42.3X-
Neravan	T42.3X-
Nerium oleander	T62.2X-
Nerve gas, not in war	T59.9-
Nesacaine (infiltration) (subcutaneous) (nerve block)	T41.3X-
Netilmicin	T36.5X-
Neurobarb	T42.3X-

Drug/Chemical	Code
Neuroleptic drug NEC	T43.50-
Neuromuscular blocking drug	T48.1X-
Neutral insulin injection	T38.3X-
Neutral spirits (beverage)	T51.0X-
Niacin	T46.7X-
Niacinamide	T45.2X-
Nialamide	T43.1X-
Niaprazine	T42.6X-
Nicametate	T46.7X-
Nicardipine	T46.1X-
Nicergoline	T46.7X-
Nickel (carbonyl) (tetra-carbonyl) (fumes) (vapor)	T56.89-
Nickelocene	T56.89-
Niclosamide	T37.4X-
Nicofuranose	T46.7X-
Nicomorphine	T40.2X-
Nicorandil	T46.3X-
Nicotiana (plant)	T62.2X-
Nicotinamide	T45.2X-
Nicotine (insecticide) (spray) (sulfate) NEC	T60.2X-
from tobacco	T65.29-
cigarettes	T65.22-
not insecticide	T65.29-
Nicotinic acid	T46.7X-
Nicotinyl alcohol	T46.7X-
Nicoumalone	T45.51-
Nifedipine	T46.1X-
Nifenazone	T39.2X-
Nifuraldezone	T37.9-
Nifuratel	T37.8X-
Nifurtimox	T37.3X-
Nifurtoinol	T37.8X-
Nightshade, deadly (solanum)	T62.2X-
berry	T62.1X-
Nikethamide	T50.7X-
Nilstat	T36.7X-
topical	T49.0X-
Nilutamide	T38.6X-
Nimesulide	T39.39-
Nimetazepam	T42.4X-
Nimodipine	T46.1X-
Nimorazole	T37.3X-
Nimustine	T45.1X-
Niridazole	T37.4X-
Nisentil	T40.2X-
Nisoldipine	T46.1X-
Nitramine	T65.3X-
Nitrate, organic	T46.3X-
Nitrazepam	T42.4X-
Nitrefazole	T50.6X-
Nitrendipine	T46.1X-
Nitric	
acid (liquid)	T54.2X-
vapor	T59.89-
oxide (gas)	T59.0X-

TABLE OF DRUGS AND CHEMICALS

Drug/Chemical	Code
Nitrimidazine	T37.3X-
Nitrite, amyl (medicinal) (vapor)	T46.3X-
Nitroaniline	T65.3X-
vapor	T59.89-
Nitrobenzene, nitrobenzol (vapor)	T65.3X-
Nitrocellulose	T65.89-
lacquer	T65.89-
Nitrodiphenyl	T65.3X-
Nitrofural	T49.0X-
Nitrofurantoin	T37.8X-
Nitrofurazone	T49.0X-
Nitrogen	T59.0X-
mustard	T45.1X-
Nitroglycerin, nitro-glycerol (medicinal)	T46.3X-
nonmedicinal	T65.5X-
fumes	T65.5X-
Nitroglycol	T52.3X-
Nitrohydrochloric acid	T54.2X-
Nitromersol	T49.0X-
Nitronaphthalene	T65.89-
Nitrophenol	T54.0X-
Nitropropane	T52.8X-
Nitroprusside	T46.5X-
Nitrosodimethylamine	T65.3X-
Nitrothiazol	T37.4X-
Nitrotoluene, nitrotoluol	T65.3X-
vapor	T65.3X-
Nitrous	
acid (liquid)	T54.2X-
fumes	T59.89-
ether spirit	T46.3X-
oxide	T41.0X-
Nitroxoline	T37.8X-
Nitrozone	T49.0X-
Nizatidine	T47.0X-
Nizofenone	T43.8X-
Noctec	T42.6X-
Noludar	T42.6X-
Nomegestrol	T38.5X-
Nomifensine	T43.29-
Nonoxinol	T49.8X-
Nonylphenoxy (polyethoxy-ethanol)	T49.8X-
Noptil	T42.3X-
Noradrenaline	T44.4X-
Noramidopyrine	T39.2X-
methanesulfonate sodium	T39.2X-
Norbormide	T60.4X-
Nordazepam	T42.4X-
Norepinephrine	T44.4X-
Norethandrolone	T38.7X-
Norethindrone	T38.4X-
Norethisterone (acetate) (enantate)	T38.4X-
with ethinylestradiol	T38.5X-
Noretynodrel	T38.5X-
Norfenefrine	T44.4X-
Norfloxacin	T36.8X-
Norgestrel	T38.4X-
Norgestrienone	T38.4X-
Norlestrin	T38.4X-
Norlutin	T38.4X-
Normal serum albumin (human), salt-poor	T45.8X-
Normethandrone	T38.5X-
Normorphine	T40.2X-
Norpseudoephedrine	T50.5X-
Nortestosterone (furanpropionate)	T38.7X-
Nortriptyline	T43.01-
Noscapine	T48.3X-
Nose preparations	T49.6X-
Novobiocin	T36.5X-
Novocain (infiltration) (topical) (spinal)	T41.3X-
Noxious foodstuff	T62.9-
specified NEC	T62.8X-
Noxiptiline	T43.01-
Noxytiolin	T49.0X-
NPH Iletin (insulin)	T38.3X-
Numorphan	T40.2X-
Nunol	T42.3X-
Nupercaine (spinal anesthetic)	T41.3X-
topical (surface)	T41.3X-
Nutmeg oil (liniment)	T49.3X-
Nutritional supplement	T50.90-
Nux vomica	T65.1X-
Nydrazid	T37.1X-
Nylidrin	T46.7X-
Nystatin	T36.7X-
topical	T49.0X-
Nytol	T45.0X-
Obidoxime chloride	T50.6X-
Octafonium (chloride)	T49.3X-
Octamethyl pyrophos-phoramide	T60.0X-
Octanoin	T50.99-
Octatropine methyl-bromide	T44.3X-
Octotiamine	T45.2X-
Octoxinol (9)	T49.8X-
Octreotide	T38.99-
Octyl nitrite	T46.3X-
Oestradiol	T38.5X-
Oestriol	T38.5X-
Oestrogen	T38.5X-
Oestrone	T38.5X-
Ofloxacin	T36.8X-
Oil (of)	T65.89-
bitter almond	T62.8X-
cloves	T49.7X-
colors	T65.6X-
fumes	T59.89-
lubricating	T52.0X-
Niobe	T52.8X-

TABLE OF DRUGS AND CHEMICALS

Drug/Chemical	Code	Drug/Chemical	Code
Oil (of), continued	T65.89-	**Ouabain (e)**	T46.0X-
vitriol (liquid)	T54.2X-	**Ovarian (hormone) (stimulant)**	T38.5X-
fumes	T54.2X-	**Ovral**	T38.4X-
wintergreen (bitter) NEC	T49.3X-	**Ovulen**	T38.4X-
Oily preparation (for skin)	T49.3X-	**Oxacillin**	T36.0X-
Ointment NEC	T49.3X-	**Oxalic acid**	T54.2X-
Olanzapine	T43.59-	ammonium salt	T50.99-
Oleander	T62.2X-	**Oxamniquine**	T37.4X-
Oleandomycin	T36.3X-	**Oxanamide**	T43.59-
Oleandrin	T46.0X-	**Oxandrolone**	T38.7X-
Oleic acid	T46.6X-	**Oxantel**	T37.4X-
Oleovitamin A	T45.2X-	**Oxapium iodide**	T44.3X-
Oleum ricini	T47.2X-	**Oxaprotiline**	T43.02-
Olive oil (medicinal) NEC	T47.4X-	**Oxaprozin**	T39.31-
Olivomycin	T45.1X-	**Oxatomide**	T45.0X-
Olsalazine	T47.8X-	**Oxazepam**	T42.4X-
Omeprazole	T47.1X-	**Oxazimedrine**	T50.5X-
OMPA	T60.0X-	**Oxazolam**	T42.4X-
Oncovin	T45.1X-	**Oxazolidine derivatives**	T42.2X-
Ondansetron	T45.0X-	**Oxazolidinedione (derivative)**	T42.2X-
Ophthaine	T41.3X-	**Oxcarbazepine**	T42.1X-
Ophthetic	T41.3X-	**Oxedrine**	T44.4X-
Opiate NEC	T40.60-	**Oxeladin (citrate)**	T48.3X-
antagonists	T50.7X-	**Oxendolone**	T38.5X-
Opioid NEC	T40.2X-	**Oxetacaine**	T41.3X-
Opipramol	T43.01-	**Oxethazine**	T41.3X-
Opium alkaloids (total)	T40.0X-	**Oxetorone**	T39.8X-
Oracon	T38.4X-	**Oxiconazole**	T49.0X-
Oragrafin	T50.8X-	**Oxidizing agent NEC**	T54.9-
Oral contraceptives	T38.4X-	**Oxipurinol**	T50.4X-
Oral rehydration salts	T50.3X-	**Oxitriptan**	T43.29-
Orazamide	T50.99-	**Oxitropium bromide**	T48.6X-
Orciprenaline	T48.29-	**Oxodipine**	T46.1X-
Organidin	T48.4X-	**Oxolamine**	T48.3X-
Organonitrate NEC	T46.3X-	**Oxolinic acid**	T37.8X-
Organophosphates	T60.0X-	**Oxomemazine**	T43.3X-
Orimune	T50.B9-	**Oxophenarsine**	T37.3X-
Orinase	T38.3X-	**Oxprenolol**	T44.7X-
Ormeloxifene	T38.6X-	**Oxsoralen**	T49.3X-
Ornidazole	T37.3X-	**Oxtriphylline**	T48.6X-
Ornithine aspartate	T50.99-	**Oxybate sodium**	T41.29-
Ornoprostil	T47.1X-	**Oxybuprocaine**	T41.3X-
Orphenadrine (hydrochloride)	T42.8X-	**Oxybutynin**	T44.3X-
Ortal (sodium)	T42.3X-	**Oxychlorosene**	T49.0X-
Orthoboric acid	T49.0X-	**Oxycodone**	T40.2X-
ENT agent	T49.6X-	**Oxyfedrine**	T46.3X-
ophthalmic preparation	T49.5X-	**Oxygen**	T41.5X-
Orthocaine	T41.3X-	**Oxylone**	T49.0X-
Orthodichlorobenzene	T53.7X-	ophthalmic preparation	T49.5X-
Ortho-Novum	T38.4X-	**Oxymesterone**	T38.7X-
Orthotolidine (reagent)	T54.2X-	**Oxymetazoline**	T48.5X-
Osmic acid (liquid) (fumes)	T54.2X-	**Oxymetholone**	T38.7X-
Osmotic diuretics	T50.2X-	**Oxymorphone**	T40.2X-
Otilonium bromide	T44.3X-	**Oxypertine**	T43.59-
Otorhinolaryngological drug NEC	T49.6X-	**Oxyphenbutazone**	T39.2X-

TABLE OF DRUGS AND CHEMICALS

Drug/Chemical	Code
Oxyphencyclimine	T44.3X-
Oxyphenisatine	T47.2X-
Oxyphenonium bromide	T44.3X-
Oxypolygelatin	T45.8X-
Oxyquinoline (derivatives)	T37.8X-
Oxytetracycline	T36.4X-
Oxytocic drug NEC	T48.0X-
Oxytocin (synthetic)	T48.0X-
Ozone	T59.89-
PABA	T49.3X-
Packed red cells	T45.8X-
Padimate	T49.3X-
Paint NEC	T65.6X-
cleaner	T52.9-
fumes NEC	T59.89-
lead (fumes)	T56.0X-
solvent NEC	T52.8X-
stripper	T52.8X-
Palfium	T40.2X-
Palm kernel oil	T50.99-
Paludrine	T37.2X-
PAM (pralidoxime)	T50.6X-
Pamaquine (naphthoute)	T37.2X-
Panadol	T39.1X-
Pancreatic	
digestive secretion stimulant	T47.8X-
dornase	T45.3X-
Pancreatin	T47.5X-
Pancrelipase	T47.5X-
Pancuronium (bromide)	T48.1X-
Pangamic acid	T45.2X-
Panthenol	T45.2X-
topical	T49.8X-
Pantopon	T40.0X-
Pantothenic acid	T45.2X-
Panwarfin	T45.51-
Papain (digestant)	T47.5X-
Papaveretum	T40.0X-
Papaverine	T44.3X-
Para-acetamidophenol	T39.1X-
Para-aminobenzoic acid	T49.3X-
Para-aminophenol derivatives	T39.1X-
Para-aminosalicylic acid	T37.1X-
Paracetaldehyde	T42.6X-
Paracetamol	T39.1X-
Parachlorophenol (camphorated)	T49.0X-
Paracodin	T40.2X-
Paradione	T42.2X-
Paraffin(s) (wax)	T52.0X-
liquid (medicinal)	T47.4X-
nonmedicinal	T52.0X-
Paraformaldehyde	T60.3X-
Paraldehyde	T42.6X-
Paramethadione	T42.2X-

Drug/Chemical	Code
Paramethasone	T38.0X-
acetate	T49.0X-
Paraoxon	T60.0X-
Paraquat	T60.3X-
Parasympatholytic NEC	T44.3X-
Parasympathomimetic drug NEC	T44.1X-
Parathion	T60.0X-
Parathormone	T50.99-
Parathyroid extract	T50.99-
Paratyphoid vaccine	T50.A9-
Paredrine	T44.4X-
Paregoric	T40.0X-
Pargyline	T46.5X-
Paris green (insecticide)	T57.0X-
Parnate	T43.1X-
Paromomycin	T36.5X-
Paroxypropione	T45.1X-
Parzone	T40.2X-
PAS	T37.1X-
Pasiniazid	T37.1X-
PBB (polybrominated biphenyls)	T65.89-
PCB	T65.89-
PCP	
meaning pentachlorophenol	T60.1X-
fungicide / herbicide	T60.3X-
insecticide	T60.1X-
meaning phencyclidine	T40.99-
Peach kernel oil (emulsion)	T47.4X-
Peanut oil (emulsion) NEC	T47.4X-
topical	T49.3X-
Pearly Gates (morning glory seeds)	T40.99-
Pecazine	T43.3X-
Pectin	T47.6X-
Pefloxacin	T37.8X-
Pegademase, bovine	T50.Z9-
Pelletierine tannate	T37.4X-
Pemirolast (potassium)	T48.6X-
Pemoline	T50.7X-
Pempidine	T44.2X-
Penamecillin	T36.0X-
Penbutolol	T44.7X-
Penethamate	T36.0X-
Penfluridol	T43.59-
Penflutizide	T50.2X-
Pengitoxin	T46.0X-
Penicillamine	T50.6X-
Penicillin (any)	T36.0X-
Penicillinase	T45.3X-
Penicilloyl polylysine	T50.8X-
Penimepicycline	T36.4X-
Pentachloroethane	T53.6X-
Pentachloronaphthalene	T53.7X-
Pentachlorophenol (pesticide)	T60.1X-
fungicide / herbicide	T60.3X-
insecticide	T60.1X-

TABLE OF DRUGS AND CHEMICALS

Drug/Chemical	Code
Pentaerythritol	T46.3X-
chloral	T42.6X-
tetranitrate NEC	T46.3X-
Pentaerythrityl tetranitrate	T46.3X-
Pentagastrin	T50.8X-
Pentalin	T53.6X-
Pentamethonium bromide	T44.2X-
Pentamidine	T37.3X-
Pentanol	T51.3X-
Pentapyrrolinium (bitartrate)	T44.2X-
Pentaquine	T37.2X-
Pentazocine	T40.4X-
Pentetrazole	T50.7X-
Penthienate bromide	T44.3X-
Pentifylline	T46.7X-
Pentobarbital (sodium)	T42.3X-
Pentobarbitone	T42.3X-
Pentolonium tartrate	T44.2X-
Pentosan polysulfate (sodium)	T39.8X-
Pentostatin	T45.1X-
Pentothal	T41.1X-
Pentoxifylline	T46.7X-
Pentoxyverine	T48.3X-
Pentrinat	T46.3X-
Pentylenetetrazole	T50.7X-
Pentylsalicylamide	T37.1X-
Pentymal	T42.3X-
Peplomycin	T45.1X-
Peppermint (oil)	T47.5X-
Pepsin (digestant)	T47.5X-
Pepstatin	T47.1X-
Peptavlon	T50.8X-
Perazine	T43.3X-
Percaine (spinal)	T41.3X-
topical (surface)	T41.3X-
Perchloroethylene	T53.3X-
medicinal	T37.4X-
vapor	T53.3X-
Percodan	T40.2X-
Percogesic	T45.0X-
Percorten	T38.0X-
Pergolide	T42.8X-
Pergonal	T38.81-
Perhexilene	T46.3X-
Perhexiline (maleate)	T46.3X-
Periactin	T45.0X-
Periciazine	T43.3X-
Periclor	T42.6X-
Perindopril	T46.4X-
Perisoxal	T39.8X-
Peritoneal dialysis solution	T50.3X-
Peritrate	T46.3X-
Perlapine	T42.4X-
Permanganate	T65.89-
Permethrin	T60.1X-

Drug/Chemical	Code
Pernocton	T42.3X-
Pernoston	T42.3X-
Peronine	T40.2X-
Perphenazine	T43.3X-
Pertofrane	T43.01-
Pertussis immune serum (human)	T50.Z1-
Peruvian balsam	T49.0X-
Peruvoside	T46.0X-
Pesticide (dust) (fumes) (vapor) NEC	T60.9-
arsenic	T57.0X-
chlorinated	T60.1X-
cyanide / kerosene	T65.0X-
mixture (of compounds)	T60.9-
naphthalene	T60.2X-
organochlorine (compounds)	T60.1X-
petroleum (distillate) (products) NEC	T60.8X-
specified ingredient NEC	T60.8X-
strychnine	T65.1X-
thallium	T60.4X-
Pethidine	T40.4X-
Petrichloral	T42.6X-
Petrol	T52.0X-
vapor	T52.0X-
Petrolatum	T49.3X-
hydrophilic	T49.3X-
liquid	T47.4X-
topical	T49.3X-
nonmedicinal	T52.0X-
red veterinary	T49.3X-
white	T49.3X-
Petroleum (products) NEC	T52.0X-
jelly	T49.3X-
pesticide	T60.8X-
solids	T52.0X-
solvents	T52.0X-
vapor	T52.0X-
Peyote	T40.99-
Phanodorm, phanodorn	T42.3X-
Phanquinone	T37.3X-
Phanquone	T37.3X-
Pharmaceutical (adjunct) (excipient) (sweetner) NEC	T50.90-
Phemitone	T42.3X-
Phenacaine	T41.3X-
Phenacemide	T42.6X-
Phenacetin	T39.1X-
Phenadoxone	T40.2X-
Phenaglycodol	T43.59-
Phenantoin	T42.0X-
Phenaphthazine reagent	T50.99-
Phenazocine	T40.4X-
Phenazone	T39.2X-
Phenazopyridine	T39.8X-
Phenbenicillin	T36.0X-
Phenbutrazate	T50.5X-
Phencyclidine	T40.99-

TABLE OF DRUGS AND CHEMICALS

Drug/Chemical	Code
Phendimetrazine	T50.5X-
Phenelzine	T43.1X-
Phenemal	T42.3X-
Phenergan	T42.6X-
Pheneticillin	T36.0X-
Pheneturide	T42.6X-
Phenformin	T38.3X-
Phenglutarimide	T44.3X-
Phenicarbazide	T39.8X-
Phenindamine	T45.0X-
Phenindione	T45.51-
Pheniprazine	T43.1X-
Pheniramine	T45.0X-
Phenisatin	T47.2X-
Phenmetrazine	T50.5X-
Phenobal	T42.3X-
Phenobarbital	T42.3X-
with mephenytoin	T42.3X-
with phenytoin	T42.3X-
sodium	T42.3X-
Phenobarbitone	T42.3X-
Phenobutiodil	T50.8X-
Phenoctide	T49.0X-
Phenol	T49.0X-
disinfectant	T54.0X-
in oil injection	T46.8X-
medicinal	T49.1X-
nonmedicinal NEC	T54.0X-
pesticide	T60.8X-
red	T50.8X-
Phenolic preparation	T49.1X-
Phenolphthalein	T47.2X-
Phenolsulfonphthalein	T50.8X-
Phenomorphan	T40.2X-
Phenonyl	T42.3X-
Phenoperidine	T40.4X-
Phenopyrazone	T46.99-
Phenoquin	T50.4X-
Phenothiazine (psychotropic) NEC	T43.3X-
insecticide	T60.2X-
Phenothrin	T49.0X-
Phenoxybenzamine	T46.7X-
Phenoxyethanol	T49.0X-
Phenoxymethyl penicillin	T36.0X-
Phenprobamate	T42.8X-
Phenprocoumon	T45.51-
Phensuximide	T42.2X-
Phentermine	T50.5X-
Phenthicillin	T36.0X-
Phentolamine	T46.7X-
Phenyl	
butazone	T39.2X-
enediamine	T65.3X-
Phenyl, continued	
hydrazine	T65.3X-
antineoplastic	T45.1X-
salicylate	T49.3X-
Phenylalanine mustard	T45.1X-
Phenylbutazone	T39.2X-
Phenylenediamine	T65.3X-
Phenylephrine	T44.4X-
Phenylethylbiguanide	T38.3X-
Phenylmercuric (acetate) (borate) (nitrate)	T49.0X-
Phenylmethylbarbitone	T42.3X-
Phenylpropanol	T47.5X-
Phenylpropanolamine	T44.99-
Phenylsulfthion	T60.0X-
Phenyltoloxamine	T45.0X-
Phenyramidol, phenyramidon	T39.8X-
Phenytoin	T42.0X-
with Phenobarbital	T42.3X-
pHisoHex	T49.2X-
Pholcodine	T48.3X-
Pholedrine	T46.99-
Phorate	T60.0X-
Phosdrin	T60.0X-
Phosfolan	T60.0X-
Phosgene (gas)	T59.89-
Phosphamidon	T60.0X-
Phosphate	T65.89-
laxative	T47.4X-
organic	T60.0X-
solvent	T52.9-
tricresyl	T65.89-
Phosphine (fumigate)	T57.1X-
Phospholine	T49.5X-
Phosphoric acid	T54.2X-
Phosphorus (compound) NEC	T57.1X-
pesticide	T60.0X-
Phthalates	T65.89-
Phthalic anhydride	T65.89-
Phthalimidoglutarimide	T42.6X-
Phthalylsulfathiazole	T37.0X-
Phylloquinone	T45.7X-
Physeptone	T40.3X-
Physostigma venenosum	T62.2X-
Physostigmine	T49.5X-
Phytolacca decandra	T62.2X-
berries	T62.1X-
Phytomenadione	T45.7X-
Phytonadione	T45.7X-
Picoperine	T48.3X-
Picosulfate (sodium)	T47.2X-
Picric (acid)	T54.2X-
Picrotoxin	T50.7X-
Piketoprofen	T49.0X-
Pilocarpine	T44.1X-
Pilocarpus (jaborandi) extract	T44.1X-

TABLE OF DRUGS AND CHEMICALS

Drug/Chemical	Code
Pilsicainide (hydrochloride)	T46.2X-
Pimaricin	T36.7X-
Pimeclone	T50.7X-
Pimelic ketone	T52.8X-
Pimethixene	T45.0X-
Piminodine	T40.2X-
Pimozide	T43.59-
Pinacidil	T46.5X-
Pinaverium bromide	T44.3X-
Pinazepam	T42.4X-
Pindolol	T44.7X-
Pindone	T60.4X-
Pine oil (disinfectant)	T65.89-
Pinkroot	T37.4X-
Pipadone	T40.2X-
Pipamazine	T45.0X-
Pipamperone	T43.4X-
Pipazetate	T48.3X-
Pipemidic acid	T37.8X-
Pipenzolate bromide	T44.3X-
Piperacetazine	T43.3X-
Piperacillin	T36.0X-
Piperazine	T37.4X-
estrone sulfate	T38.5X-
Piper cubeba	T62.2X-
Piperidione	T48.3X-
Piperidolate	T44.3X-
Piperocaine (all types)	T41.3X-
Piperonyl butoxide	T60.8X-
Pipethanate	T44.3X-
Pipobroman	T45.1X-
Pipotiazine	T43.3X-
Pipoxizine	T45.0X-
Pipradrol	T43.69-
Piprinhydrinate	T45.0X-
Pirarubicin	T45.1X-
Pirazinamide	T37.1X-
Pirbuterol	T48.6X-
Pirenzepine	T47.1X-
Piretanide	T50.1X-
Piribedil	T42.8X-
Piridoxilate	T46.3X-
Piritramide	T40.4X-
Piromidic acid	T37.8X-
Piroxicam	T39.39-
beta-cyclodextrin complex	T39.8X-
Pirozadil	T46.6X-
Piscidia (bark) (erythrina)	T39.8X-
Pitch	T65.89-
Pitkin's solution	T41.3X-
Pitocin	T48.0X-
Pitressin (tannate)	T38.89-
Pituitary extracts (posterior)	T38.89-
anterior	T38.81-
Pituitrin	T38.89-

Drug/Chemical	Code
Pivampicillin	T36.0X-
Pivmecillinam	T36.0X-
Placental hormone	T38.89-
Placidyl	T42.6X-
Plague vaccine	T50.A9-
Plant	
food or fertilizer NEC	T65.89-
containing herbicide	T60.3X-
noxious, used as food	T62.2X-
berries	T62.1X-
seeds	T62.2X-
specified type NEC	T62.2X-
Plasma	T45.8X-
Plasmanate	T45.8X-
Plasminogen (tissue) activator	T45.61-
Plaster dressing	T49.3X-
Plastic dressing	T49.3X-
Plegicil	T43.3X-
Plicamycin	T45.1X-
Podophyllotoxin	T49.8X-
Podophyllum (resin)	T49.4X-
Poison NEC	T65.9-
Poisonous berries	T62.1X-
Pokeweed (any part)	T62.2X-
Poldine metilsulfate	T44.3X-
Polidexide (sulfate)	T46.6X-
Polidocanol	T46.8X-
Poliomyelitis vaccine	T50.B9-
Polish (car) (floor) (furniture) (metal) (porcelain) (silver)	T65.89-
Poloxalkol	T47.4X-
Poloxamer	T47.4X-
Polyaminostyrene resins	T50.3X-
Polycarbophil	T47.4X-
Polychlorinated biphenyl	T65.89-
Polycycline	T36.4X-
Polyester fumes	T59.89-
Polyester resin hardener	T52.9-
fumes	T59.89-
Polyestradiol phosphate	T38.5X-
Polyethanolamine alkyl sulfate	T49.2X-
Polyethylene adhesive	T49.3X-
Polyferose	T45.4X-
Polygeline	T45.8X-
Polymyxin	T36.8X-
B	T36.8X-
ENT agent	T49.6X-
ophthalmic preparation	T49.5X-
topical NEC	T49.0X-
E sulfate (eye preparation)	T49.5X-
Polynoxylin	T49.0X-
Polyoestradiol phosphate	T38.5X-
Polyoxymethyleneurea	T49.0X-
Polysilane	T47.8X-
Polytetrafluoroethylene (inhaled)	T59.89-

TABLE OF DRUGS AND CHEMICALS

Drug/Chemical	Code
Polythiazide	T50.2X-
Polyvidone	T45.8X-
Polyvinylpyrrolidone	T45.8X-
Pontocaine (hydrochloride) (infiltration) (topical)	T41.3X-
Porfiromycin	T45.1X-
Posterior pituitary hormone NEC	T38.89-
Pot	T40.71-
Potash (caustic)	T54.3X-
Potassic saline injection (lactated)	T50.3X-
Potassium (salts) NEC	T50.3X-
aminobenzoate	T45.8X-
aminosalicylate	T37.1X-
antimony ' tartrate'	T37.8X-
arsenite (solution)	T57.0X-
bichromate	T56.2X-
bisulfate	T47.3X-
bromide	T42.6X-
canrenoate	T50.0X-
carbonate	T54.3X-
chlorate NEC	T65.89-
chloride	T50.3X-
citrate	T50.99-
cyanide	T65.0X-
ferric hexacyanoferrate (medicinal)	T50.6X-
nonmedicinal	T65.89-
Fluoride	T57.8X-
glucaldrate	T47.1X-
hydroxide	I54.3X-
iodate	T49.0X-
iodide	T48.4X-
nitrate	T57.8X-
oxalate	T65.89-
perchlorate (nonmedicinal) NEC	T65.89-
antithyroid	T38.2X-
medicinal	T38.2X-
Permanganate (nonmedicinal)	T65.89-
medicinal	T49.0X-
sulfate	T47.2X-
Potassium-removing resin	T50.3X-
Potassium-retaining drug	T50.3X-
Povidone	T45.8X-
iodine	T49.0X-
Practolol	T44.7X-
Prajmalium bitartrate	T46.2X-
Pralidoxime (iodide) (chloride)	T50.6X-
Pramiverine	T44.3X-
Pramocaine	T49.1X-
Pramoxine	T49.1X-
Prasterone	T38.7X-
Pravastatin	T46.6X-
Prazepam	T42.4X-
Praziquantel	T37.4X-
Prazitone	T43.29-
Prazosin	T44.6X-
Prednicarbate	T49.0X-

Drug/Chemical	Code
Prednimustine	T45.1X-
Prednisolone	T38.0X-
ENT agent	T49.6X-
ophthalmic preparation	T49.5X-
steaglate	T49.0X-
topical NEC	T49.0X-
Prednisone	T38.0X-
Prednylidene	T38.0X-
Pregnandiol	T38.5X-
Pregneninolone	T38.5X-
Preludin	T43.69-
Premarin	T38.5X-
Premedication anesthetic	T41.20-
Prenalterol	T44.5X-
Prenoxdiazine	T48.3X-
Prenylamine	T46.3X-
Preparation H	T49.8X-
Preparation, local	T49.4X-
Preservative (nonmedicinal)	T65.89-
medicinal	T50.90-
wood	T60.9-
Prethcamide	T50.7X-
Pride of China	T62.2X-
Pridinol	T44.3X-
Prifinium bromide	T44.3X-
Prilocaine	T41.3X-
Primaquine	T37.2X-
Primidone	T42.6X-
Primula (veris)	T62.2X-
Prinadol	T40.2X-
Priscol, Priscoline	T44.6X-
Pristinamycin	T36.3X-
Privet	T62.2X-
berries	T62.1X-
Privine	T44.4X-
Pro-Banthine	T44.3X-
Probarbital	T42.3X-
Probenecid	T50.4X-
Probucol	T46.6X-
Procainamide	T46.2X-
Procaine	T41.3X-
benzylpenicillin	T36.0X-
nerve block (periphreal) (plexus)	T41.3X-
penicillin G	T36.0X-
regional / spinal	T41.3X-
Procalmidol	T43.59-
Procarbazine	T45.1X-
Procaterol	T44.5X-
Prochlorperazine	T43.3X-
Procyclidine	T44.3X-
Producer gas	T58.8X-
Profadol	T40.4X-
Profenamine	T44.3X-
Profenil	T44.3X-
Proflavine	T49.0X-

TABLE OF DRUGS AND CHEMICALS

Drug/Chemical	Code
Progabide	T42.6X-
Progesterone	T38.5X-
Progestin	T38.5X-
oral contraceptive	T38.4X-
Progestogen NEC	T38.5X-
Progestone	T38.5X-
Proglumide	T47.1X-
Proguanil	T37.2X-
Prolactin	T38.81-
Prolintane	T43.69-
Proloid	T38.1X-
Proluton	T38.5X-
Promacetin	T37.1X-
Promazine	T43.3X-
Promedol	T40.2X-
Promegestone	T38.5X-
Promethazine (teoclate)	T43.3X-
Promin	T37.1X-
Pronase	T45.3X-
Pronestyl (hydrochloride)	T46.2X-
Pronetalol	T44.7X-
Prontosil	T37.0X-
Propachlor	T60.3X-
Propafenone	T46.2X-
Propallylonal	T42.3X-
Propamidine	T49.0X-
Propane (in mobile container)	T59.89-
distributed through pipes	T59.89-
incomplete combustion	T58.1-
Propanidid	T41.29-
Propanil	T60.3X-
1-Propanol	T51.3X-
2-Propanol	T51.2X-
Propantheline (bromide)	T44.3X-
Proparacaine	T41.3X-
Propatylnitrate	T46.3X-
Propicillin	T36.0X-
Propiolactone	T49.0X-
Propiomazine	T45.0X-
Propionaldehyde (medicinal)	T42.6X-
Propionate (calcium) (sodium)	T49.0X-
Propion gel	T49.0X-
Propitocaine	T41.3X-
Propofol	T41.29-
Propoxur	T60.0X-
Propoxycaine (infiltration) (spinal) (subcutaneous) (nerve block) (topical)	T41.3X-
Propoxyphene	T40.4X-
Propranolol	T44.7X-
Propyl	
alcohol	T51.3X-
carbinol	T51.3X-
hexadrine	T44.4X-
iodone	T50.8X-
thiouracil	T38.2X-
Propylaminopheno-thiazine	T43.3X-
Propylene	T59.89-
Propylhexedrine	T48.5X-
Propyliodone	T50.8X-
Propylparaben (ophthalmic)	T49.5X-
Propylthiouracil	T38.2X-
Propyphenazone	T39.2X-
Proquazone	T39.39-
Proscillaridin	T46.0X-
Prostacyclin	T45.521
Prostaglandin (I2)	T45.521
E1	T46.7X-
E2	T48.0X-
F2 alpha	T48.0X-
Prostigmin	T44.0X-
Prosultiamine	T45.2X-
Protamine sulfate	T45.7X-
zinc insulin	T38.3X-
Protease	T47.5X-
Protectant, skin NEC	T49.3X-
Protein hydrolysate	T50.99-
Prothiaden—*see Dothiepin hydrochloride*	
Prothionamide	T37.1X-
Prothipendyl	T43.59-
Prothoate	T60.0X-
Prothrombin	
activator	T45.7X-
synthesis inhibitor	T45.51-
Protionamide	T37.1X-
Protirelin	T38.89-
Protokylol	T48.6X-
Protopam	T50.6X-
Protoveratrine(s) (A) (B)	T46.5X-
Protriptyline	T43.01-
Provera	T38.5X-
Provitamin A	T45.2X-
Proxibarbal	T42.3X-
Proxymetacaine	T41.3X-
Proxyphylline	T48.6X-
Prozac—*see Fluoxetine hydrochloride*	
Prunus	
laurocerasus	T62.2X-
virginiana	T62.2X-
Prussian blue	
commercial	T65.89-
therapeutic	T50.6X-
Prussic acid	T65.0X-
vapor	T57.3X-
Pseudoephedrine	T44.99-
Psilocin	T40.99-
Psilocybin	T40.99-
Psilocybine	T40.99-
Psoralene (nonmedicinal)	T65.89-
Psoralens (medicinal)	T50.99-
PSP (phenolsulfonphthalein)	T50.8X-

TABLE OF DRUGS AND CHEMICALS

Drug/Chemical	Code
Psychodysleptic drug NOS	T40.90-
specified NEC	T40.99-
Psychostimulant	T43.60-
amphetamine	T43.62-
caffeine	T43.61-
methylphenidate	T43.631
specified NEC	T43.69-
Psychotherapeutic drug NEC	T43.9-
antidepressants	T43.20-
specified NEC	T43.8X-
tranquilizers NEC	T43.50-
Psychotomimetic agents	T40.90-
Psychotropic drug NEC	T43.9-
specified NEC	T43.8X-
Psyllium hydrophilic mucilloid	T47.4X-
Pteroylglutamic acid	T45.8X-
Pteroyltriglutamate	T45.1X-
PTFE—*see Polytetrafluoroethylene*	
Pulp	
devitalizing paste	T49.7X-
dressing	T49.7X-
Pulsatilla	T62.2X-
Pumpkin seed extract	T37.4X-
Purex (bleach)	T54.9-
Purgative NEC—*see also Cathartic*	T47.4X-
Purine analogue (antineoplastic)	T45.1X-
Purine diuretics	T50.2X-
Purinethol	T45.1X-
PVP	T45.8X-
Pyrabital	T39.8X-
Pyramidon	T39.2X-
Pyrantel	T37.4X-
Pyrathiazine	T45.0X-
Pyrazinamide	T37.1X-
Pyrazinoic acid (amide)	T37.1X-
Pyrazole (derivatives)	T39.2X-
Pyrazolone analgesic NEC	T39.2X-
Pyrethrin, pyrethrum (nonmedicinal)	T60.2X-
Pyrethrum extract	T49.0X-
Pyribenzamine	T45.0X-
Pyridine	T52.8X-
aldoxime methiodide	T50.6X-
aldoxime methyl chloride	T50.6X-
vapor	T59.89-
Pyridium	T39.8X-
Pyridostigmine bromide	T44.0X-
Pyridoxal phosphate	T45.2X-
Pyridoxine	T45.2X-
Pyrilamine	T45.0X-
Pyrimethamine (w/ sulfadoxine)	T37.2X-
Pyrimidine antagonist	T45.1X-
Pyriminil	T60.4X-
Pyrithione zinc	T49.4X-
Pyrithyldione	T42.6X-
Pyrogallic acid	T49.0X-

Drug/Chemical	Code
Pyrogallol	T49.0X-
Pyroxylin	T49.3X-
Pyrrobutamine	T45.0X-
Pyrrolizidine alkaloids	T62.8X-
Pyrvinium chloride	T37.4X-
PZI	T38.3X-
Quaalude	T42.6X-
Quarternary ammonium	
anti-infective	T49.0X-
ganglion blocking	T44.2X-
parasympatholytic	T44.3X-
Quazepam	T42.4X-
Quicklime	T54.3X-
Quillaja extract	T48.4X-
Quinacrine	T37.2X-
Quinaglute	T46.2X-
Quinalbarbital	T42.3X-
Quinalbarbitone sodium	T42.3X-
Quinalphos	T60.0X-
Quinapril	T46.4X-
Quinestradiol	T38.5X-
Quinestradol	T38.5X-
Quinestrol	T38.5X-
Quinethazone	T50.2X-
Quingestanol	T38.4X-
Quinidine	T46.2X-
Quinine	T37.2X-
Quiniobine	T37.8X-
Quinisocaine	T49.1X-
Quinocide	T37.2X-
Quinoline (derivatives) NEC	T37.8X-
Quinupramine	T43.01-
Quotane	T41.3X-
Rabies	
immune globulin (human)	T50.Z1-
vaccine	T50.B9-
Racemoramide	T40.2X-
Racemorphan	T40.2X-
Racepinefrin	T44.5X-
Raclopride	T43.59-
Radiator alcohol	T51.1X-
Radioactive drug NEC	T50.8X-
Radio-opaque (drugs) (materials)	T50.8X-
Ramifenazone	T39.2X-
Ramipril	T46.4X-
Ranitidine	T47.0X-
Ranunculus	T62.2X-
Rat poison NEC	T60.4X-
Rattlesnake (venom)	T63.01-
Raubasine	T46.7X-
Raudixin	T46.5X-
Rautensin	T46.5X-
Rautina	T46.5X-
Rautotal	T46.5X-
Rauwiloid	T46.5X-

TABLE OF DRUGS AND CHEMICALS

Drug/Chemical	Code
Rauwoldin	T46.5X-
Rauwolfia (alkaloids)	T46.5X-
Razoxane	T45.1X-
Realgar	T57.0X-
Recombinant (R)—see specific protein	
Red blood cells, packed	T45.8X-
Red squill (scilliroside)	T60.4X-
Reducing agent, industrial NEC	T65.89-
Refrigerant gas (CFC)	T53.5X-
not chlorofluoro-carbon	T59.89-
Regroton	T50.2X-
Rehydration salts (oral)	T50.3X-
Rela	T42.8X-
Relaxant, muscle	
anesthetic	T48.1X-
central nervous system	T42.8X-
skeletal NEC	T48.1X-
smooth NEC	T44.3X-
Remoxipride	T43.59-
Renese	T50.2X-
Renografin	T50.8X-
Replacement solution	T50.3X-
Reproterol	T48.6X-
Rescinnamine	T46.5X-
Reserpin (e)	T46.5X-
Resorcin, resorcinol (nonmedicinal)	T65.89-
medicinal	T49.4X-
Respaire	T48.4X-
Respiratory drug NEC	T48.90-
antiasthmatic NEC	T48.6X-
anti-common-cold NEC	T48.5X-
expectorant NEC	T48.4X-
stimulant	T48.90-
Retinoic acid	T49.0X-
Retinol	T45.2X-
Rh (D) immune globulin (human)	T50.Z1-
Rhodine	T39.01-
RhoGAM	T50.Z1-
Rhubarb	
dry extract	T47.2X-
tincture, compound	T47.2X-
Ribavirin	T37.5X-
Riboflavin	T45.2X-
Ribostamycin	T36.5X-
Ricin	T62.2X-
Ricinus communis	T62.2X-
Rickettsial vaccine NEC	T50.A9-
Rifabutin	T36.6X-
Rifamide	T36.6X-
Rifampicin	T36.6X-
with isoniazid	T37.1X-
Rifampin	T36.6X-
Rifamycin	T36.6X-
Rifaximin	T36.6X-
Rimantadine	T37.5X-
Rimazolium metilsulfate	T39.8X-
Rimifon	T37.1X-
Rimiterol	T48.6X-
Ringer (lactate) solution	T50.3X-
Ristocetin	T36.8X-
Ritalin	T43.631
Ritodrine	T44.5X-
Rociverine	T44.3X-
Rocky Mtn spotted fever vaccine	T50.A9-
Rodenticide NEC	T60.4X-
Rohypnol	T42.4X-
Rokitamycin	T36.3X-
Rolaids	T47.1X-
Rolitetracycline	T36.4X-
Romilar	T48.3X-
Ronifibrate	T46.6X-
Rosaprostol	T47.1X-
Rose bengal sodium (131I)	T50.8X-
Rose water ointment	T49.3X-
Rosoxacin	T37.8X-
Rotenone	T60.2X-
Rotoxamine	T45.0X-
Rough-on-rats	T60.4X-
Roxatidine	T47.0X-
Roxithromycin	T36.3X-
Rt-PA	T45.61-
Rubbing alcohol	T51.2X-
Rubefacient	T49.4X-
Rubidium chloride Rb82	T50.8X-
Rubidomycin	T45.1X-
Rue	T62.2X-
Rufocromomycin	T45.1X-
Russel's viper venin	T45.7X-
Ruta (graveolens)	T62.2X-
Rutinum	T46.99-
Rutoside	T46.99-
Sabadilla (plant) (pesticide)	T62.2X-
Saccharated iron oxide	T45.8X-
Saccharin	T50.90-
Saccharomyces boulardii	T47.6X-
Safflower oil	T46.6X-
Safrazine	T43.1X-
Salazosulfapyridine	T37.0X-
Salbutamol	T48.6X-
Salicylamide	T39.09-
Salicylate NEC	T39.09-
methyl	T49.3X-
theobromine calcium	T50.2X-
Salicylazosulfapyridine	T37.0X-
Salicylhydroxamic acid	T49.0X-
Salicylic acid	T49.4X-
with benzoic acid	T49.4X-
congeners/derivatives/salts	T39.09-
Salinazid	T37.1X-
Salmeterol	T48.6X-

TABLE OF DRUGS AND CHEMICALS

Drug/Chemical	Code
Salol	T49.3X-
Salsalate	T39.09-
Salt substitute	T50.90-
Salt-replacing drug	T50.90-
Salt-retaining mineralocorticoid	T50.0X-
Saluretic NEC	T50.2X-
Saluron	T50.2X-
Salvarsan 606 (neosilver) (silver)	T37.8X-
Sambucus canadensis	T62.2X-
berry	T62.1X-
Sandril	T46.5X-
Sanguinaria canadensis	T62.2X-
Saniflush (cleaner)	T54.2X-
Santonin	T37.4X-
Santyl	T49.8X-
Saralasin	T46.5X-
Sarcolysin	T45.1X-
Sarkomycin	T45.1X-
Saroten	T43.01-
Savin (oil)	T49.4X-
Scammony	T47.2X-
Scarlet red	T49.8X-
Scheele's green	T57.0X-
insecticide	T57.0X-
Schizontozide (blood) (tissue)	T37.2X-
Schradan	T60.0X-
Schweinfurth green	T57.0X-
insecticide	T57.0X-
Scilla, rat poison	T60.4X-
Scillaren	T60.4X-
Sclerosing agent	T46.8X-
Scombrotoxin	T61.1-
Scopolamine	T44.3X-
Scopolia extract	T44.3X-
Scouring powder	T65.89-
Sea	
anemone (sting)	T63.631
cucumber (sting)	T63.69-
snake (bite) (venom)	T63.09-
urchin spine (puncture)	T63.69-
Seafood	T61.9-
specified NEC	T61.8X-
Secbutabarbital	T42.3X-
Secbutabarbitone	T42.3X-
Secnidazole	T37.3X-
Secobarbital	T42.3X-
Seconal	T42.3X-
Secretin	T50.8X-
Sedative NEC	T42.71
mixed NEC	T42.6X-
Sedormid	T42.6X-
Seed disinfectant or dressing	T60.8X-
Seeds (poisonous)	T62.2X-
Selegiline	T42.8X-
Selenium NEC (fumes)	T56.89-
disulfide or sulfide	T49.4X-
Selenomethionine (75Se)	T50.8X-
Selsun	T49.4X-
Semustine	T45.1X-
Senega syrup	T48.4X-
Senna	T47.2X-
Sennoside A+B	T47.2X-
Septisol	T49.2X-
Seractide	T38.81-
Serax	T42.4X-
Serenesil	T42.6X-
Serenium (hydrochloride)	T37.9-
Serepax—*see Oxazepam*	
Sermorelin	T38.89-
Sernyl	T41.1X-
Serotonin	T50.99-
Serpasil	T46.5X-
Serrapeptase	T45.3X-
Serum	
antibotulinus	T50.Z1-
anticytotoxic	T50.Z1-
antidiphtheria	T50.Z1-
antimeningococcus	T50.Z1-
anti-Rh	T50.Z1-
anti-snake-bite	T50.Z1-
antitetanic	T50.Z1-
antitoxic	T50.Z1-
complement (inhibitor)	T45.8X-
convalescent	T50.Z1-
hemolytic complement	T45.8X-
immune (human)	T50.Z1-
protective NEC	T50.Z1-
Setastine	T45.0X-
Setoperone	T43.59-
Sewer gas	T59.9-
Shampoo	T55.0X-
Shellfish, noxious, nonbacterial	T61.781
Sildenafil	T46.7X-
Silibinin	T50.99-
Silicone NEC	T65.89-
medicinal	T49.3X-
Silvadene	T49.0X-
Silver	T49.0X-
anti-infectives	T49.0X-
arsphenamine	T37.8X-
colloidal	T49.0X-
nitrate	T49.0X-
ophthalmic preparation	T49.5X-
toughened (keratolytic)	T49.4X-
nonmedicinal (dust)	T56.89-
protein	T49.5X-
salvarsan	T37.8X-
sulfadiazine	T49.4X-
Silymarin	T50.99-

TABLE OF DRUGS AND CHEMICALS

Drug/Chemical	Code
Simaldrate	T47.1X-
Simazine	T60.3X-
Simethicone	T47.1X-
Simfibrate	T46.6X-
Simvastatin	T46.6X-
Sincalide	T50.8X-
Sinequan	T43.01-
Singoserp	T46.5X-
Sintrom	T45.51-
Sisomicin	T36.5X-
Sitosterols	T46.6X-
Skeletal muscle relaxants	T48.1X-
Skin	
agents (external)	T49.9-
specified NEC	T49.8X-
test antigen	T50.8X-
Sleep-eze	T45.0X-
Sleeping draught, pill	T42.71
Smallpox vaccine	T50.B1-
Smelter fumes NEC	T56.9-
Smog	T59.1X-
Smoke NEC	T59.81-
Smooth muscle relaxant	T44.3X-
Snail killer NEC	T60.8X-
Snake venom or bite	T63.00-
hemocoagulase	T45.7X-
Snuff	T65.21-
Soap (powder) (product)	T55.0X-
enema	T47.4X-
medicinal, soft	T49.2X-
superfatted	T49.2X-
Sobrerol	T48.4X-
Soda (caustic)	T54.3X-
bicarb	T47.1X-
Sodium	
acetosulfone	T37.1X-
acetrizoate	T50.8X-
acid phosphate	T50.3X-
alginate	T47.8X-
amidotrizoate	T50.8X-
aminopterin	T45.1X-
amylosulfate	T47.8X-
amytal	T42.3X-
antimony gluconate	T37.3X-
arsenate	T57.0X-
aurothiomalate	T39.4X-
aurothiosulfate	T39.4X-
barbiturate	T42.3X-
basic phosphate	T47.4X-
bicarbonate	T47.1X-
bichromate	T57.8X-
biphosphate	T50.3X-
bisulfate	T65.89-
borate	

Drug/Chemical	Code
Sodium, continued	
cleanser	T57.8X-
eye	T49.5X-
therapeutic	T49.8X-
bromide	T42.6X-
cacodylate (nonmedicinal) NEC	T50.8X-
anti-infective	T37.8X-
herbicide	T60.3X-
calcium edetate	T45.8X-
carbonate NEC	T54.3X-
chlorate NEC	T65.89-
herbicide	T54.9-
chloride	T50.3X-
with glucose	T50.3X-
chromate	T65.89-
citrate	T50.99-
cromoglicate	T48.6X-
cyanide	T65.0X-
cyclamate	T50.3X-
dehydrocholate	T45.8X-
diatrizoate	T50.8X-
dibunate	T48.4X-
dioctyl sulfosuccinate	T47.4X-
dipantoyl ferrate	T45.8X-
edetate	T45.8X-
ethacrynate	T50.1X-
feredetate	T45.8X-
fluoride—*see Fluoride*	
fluoroacetate (dust) (pesticide)	T60.4X-
free salt	T50.3X-
fusidate	T36.8X-
glucaldrate	T47.1X-
glucosulfone	T37.1X-
glutamate	T45.8X-
hydrogen carbonate	T50.3X-
hydroxide	T54.3X-
hypochlorite (bleach) NEC	T54.3X-
disinfectant	T54.3X-
medicinal (anti-infective) (external)	T49.0X-
vapor	T54.3X-
hyposulfite	T49.0X-
indigotin disulfonate	T50.8X-
iodide	T50.99-
I-131	T50.8X-
therapeutic	T38.2X-
iodohippurate (131I)	T50.8X-
iopodate	T50.8X-
iothalamate	T50.8X-
iron edetate	T45.4X-
lactate (compound solution)	T45.8X-
lauryl (sulfate)	T49.2X-
L-triiodothyronine	T38.1X-
magnesium citrate	T50.99-
mersalate	T50.2X-
metasilicate	T65.89-

TABLE OF DRUGS AND CHEMICALS

Drug/Chemical	Code
Sodium, continued	
metrizoate	T50.8X-
monofluoroacetate (pesticide)	T60.1X-
morrhuate	T46.8X-
nafcillin	T36.0X-
nitrate (oxidizing agent)	T65.89-
nitrite	T50.6X-
nitroferricyanide	T46.5X-
nitroprusside	T46.5X-
oxalate	T65.89-
oxide/peroxide	T65.89-
oxybate	T41.29-
para-aminohippurate	T50.8X-
perborate (nonmedicinal) NEC	T65.89-
medicinal	T49.0X-
soap	T55.0X-
percarbonate—see Sodium, perborate	
pertechnetate Tc99m	T50.8X-
phosphate	
cellulose	T45.8X-
dibasic	T47.2X-
monobasic	T47.2X-
phytate	T50.6X-
picosulfate	T47.2X-
polyhydroxyaluminium monocarbonate	T47.1X-
polystyrene sulfonate	T50.3X-
propionate	T49.0X-
propyl hydroxybenzoate	T50.99-
psylliate	T46.8X-
removing resins	T50.3X-
salicylate	T39.09-
salt NEC	T50.3X-
selenate	T60.2X-
stibogluconate	T37.3X-
sulfate	T47.4X-
sulfoxone	T37.1X-
tetradecyl sulfate	T46.8X-
thiopental	T41.1X-
thiosalicylate	T39.09-
thiosulfate	T50.6X-
tolbutamide	T38.3X-
(L)-triiodothyronine	T38.1X-
tyropanoate	T50.8X-
valproate	T42.6X-
versenate	T50.6X-
Sodium-free salt	T50.90-
Sodium-removing resin	T50.3X-
Soft soap	T55.0X-
Solanine	T62.2X-
berries	T62.1X-
Solanum dulcamara	T62.2X-
berries	T62.1X-
Solapsone	T37.1X-
Solar lotion	T49.3X-
Solasulfone	T37.1X-

Drug/Chemical	Code
Soldering fluid	T65.89-
Solid substance	T65.9-
specified NEC	T65.89-
Solvent, industrial NEC	T52.9-
naphtha	T52.0X-
petroleum	T52.0X-
specified NEC	T52.8X-
Soma	T42.8X-
Somatorelin	T38.89-
Somatostatin	T38.99-
Somatotropin	T38.81-
Somatrem	T38.81-
Somatropin	T38.81-
Sominex	T45.0X-
Somnos	T42.6X-
Somonal	T42.3X-
Soneryl	T42.3X-
Soothing syrup	T50.90-
Sopor	T42.6X-
Soporific	T42.71
Soporific drug	T42.71
specified type NEC	T42.6X-
Sorbide nitrate	T46.3X-
Sorbitol	T47.4X-
Sotalol	T44.7X-
Sotradecol	T46.8X-
Soysterol	T46.6X-
Spacoline	T44.3X-
Spanish fly	T49.8X-
Sparine	T43.3X-
Sparteine	T48.0X-
Spasmolytic	
anticholinergics	T44.3X-
autonomic	T44.3X-
bronchial NEC	T48.6X-
quaternary ammonium	T44.3X-
skeletal muscle NEC	T48.1X-
Spectinomycin	T36.5X-
Speed	T43.65-
Spermicide	T49.8X-
Spider (bite) (venom)	T63.39-
antivenin	T50.Z1-
Spigelia (root)	T37.4X-
Spindle inactivator	T50.4X-
Spiperone	T43.4X-
Spiramycin	T36.3X-
Spirapril	T46.4X-
Spirilene	T43.59-
Spirit(s) (neutral) NEC	T51.0X-
beverage / industrial/ mineral/surgical	T51.0X-
Spironolactone	T50.0X-
Spiroperidol	T43.4X-
Sponge, absorbable (gelatin)	T45.7X-
Sporostacin	T49.0X-

SODIUM-SPOROSTACIN

TABLE OF DRUGS AND CHEMICALS

Drug/Chemical	Code	Drug/Chemical	Code
Spray (aerosol)	T65.91-	**Streptozocin**	T45.1X-
cosmetic	T65.89-	**Streptozotocin**	T45.1X-
medicinal NEC	T50.90-	**Stripper (paint) (solvent)**	T52.8X-
pesticides—*see Pesticide*	T60.9-	**Strobane**	T60.1X-
Spurge flax	T62.2X-	**Strofantina**	T46.0X-
Spurges	T62.2X-	**Strophanthin (g) (k)**	T46.0X-
Sputum viscosity-lowering drug	T48.4X-	**Strophanthus**	T46.0X-
Squill	T46.0X-	**Strophantin**	T46.0X-
rat poison	T60.4X-	**Strophantin-g**	T46.0X-
Squirting cucumber (cathartic)	T47.2X-	**Strychnine (nonmedicinal) (pesticide) (salts)**	T65.1X-
Stains	T65.6X-	medicinal	T48.29-
Stannous fluoride	T49.7X-	**Styramate**	T42.8X-
Stanolone	T38.7X-	**Styrene**	T65.89-
Stanozolol	T38.7X-	**Succinimide, antiepileptic or anticonvulsant**	T42.2X-
Staphisagria or stavesacre (pediculicide)	T49.0X-	**Succinylcholine**	T48.1X-
Starch	T50.90-	**Succinylsulfathiazole**	T37.0X-
Stelazine	T43.3X-	**Sucralfate**	T47.1X-
Stemetil	T43.3X-	**Sucrose**	T50.3X-
Stepronin	T48.4X-	**Sufentanil**	T40.4X-
Sterculia	T47.4X-	**Sulbactam**	T36.0X-
Sternutator gas	T59.89-	**Sulbenicillin**	T36.0X-
Steroid	T38.0X-	**Sulbentine**	T49.0X-
anabolic	T38.7X-	**Sulfacetamide**	T49.0X-
androgenic	T38.7X-	ophthalmic preparation	T49.5X-
antineoplastic, hormone	T38.7X-	**Sulfachlorpyridazine**	T37.0X-
estrogen	T38.5X-	**Sulfacitine**	T37.0X-
ENT agent	T49.6X-	**Sulfadiasulfone sodium**	T37.0X-
ophthalmic preparation	T49.5X-	**Sulfadiazine**	T37.0X-
topical NEC	T49.0X-	silver (topical)	T49.0X-
Stibine	T56.89-	**Sulfadimethoxine**	T37.0X-
Stibogluconate	T37.3X-	**Sulfadimidine**	T37.0X-
Stibophen	T37.4X-	**Sulfadoxine**	T37.0X-
Stilbamidine (isetionate)	T37.3X-	with pyrimethamine	T37.2X-
Stilbestrol	T38.5X-	**Sulfaethidole**	T37.0X-
Stilboestrol	T38.5X-	**Sulfafurazole**	T37.0X-
Stimulant		**Sulfaguanidine**	T37.0X-
central nervous system	T43.60-	**Sulfalene**	T37.0X-
analeptics / opiate antagonist	T50.7X-	**Sulfaloxate**	T37.0X-
psychotherapeutic NEC	T43.60-	**Sulfaloxic acid**	T37.0X-
specified NEC	T43.69-	**Sulfamazone**	T39.2X-
respiratory	T48.90-	**Sulfamerazine**	T37.0X-
Stone-dissolving drug	T50.90-	**Sulfameter**	T37.0X-
Storage battery (cells) (acid)	T54.2X-	**Sulfamethazine**	T37.0X-
Stovaine (infiltration) (topical) (subcutaneous) (nerve block) (spinal)	T41.3X-	**Sulfamethizole**	T37.0X-
		Sulfamethoxazole	T37.0X-
Stovarsal	T37.8X-	with trimethoprim	T36.8X-
Stoxil	T49.5X-	**Sulfamethoxydiazine**	T37.0X-
Stramonium	T48.6X-	**Sulfamethoxypyridazine**	T37.0X-
natural state	T62.2X-	**Sulfamethylthiazole**	T37.0X-
Streptodornase	T45.3X-	**Sulfametoxydiazine**	T37.0X-
Streptoduocin	T36.5X-	**Sulfamidopyrine**	T39.2X-
Streptokinase	T45.61-	**Sulfamonomethoxine**	T37.0X-
Streptomycin (derivative)	T36.5X-	**Sulfamoxole**	T37.0X-
Streptonivicin	T36.5X-	**Sulfamylon**	T49.0X-
Streptovarycin	T36.5X-	**Sulfan blue (diagnostic dye)**	T50.8X-

TABLE OF DRUGS AND CHEMICALS

Drug/Chemical	Code
Sulfanilamide	T37.0X-
Sulfanilylguanidine	T37.0X-
Sulfaperin	T37.0X-
Sulfaphenazole	T37.0X-
Sulfaphenylthiazole	T37.0X-
Sulfaproxyline	T37.0X-
Sulfapyridine	T37.0X-
Sulfapyrimidine	T37.0X-
Sulfarsphenamine	T37.8X-
Sulfasalazine	T37.0X-
Sulfasuxidine	T37.0X-
Sulfasymazine	T37.0X-
Sulfated amylopectin	T47.8X-
Sulfathiazole	T37.0X-
Sulfatostearate	T49.2X-
Sulfinpyrazone	T50.4X-
Sulfiram	T49.0X-
Sulfisomidine	T37.0X-
Sulfisoxazole	T37.0X-
ophthalmic preparation	T49.5X-
Sulfobromophthalein (sodium)	T50.8X-
Sulfbromphthalein	T50.8X-
Sulfogaiacol	T48.4X-
Sulfomyxin	T36.8X-
Sulfonal	T42.6X-
Sulfonamide NEC	T37.0X-
eye	T49.5X-
Sulfonazide	I37.1X-
Sulfones	T37.1X-
Sulfonethylmethane	T42.6X-
Sulfonmethane	T42.6X-
Sulfonphthal, sulfonphthol	T50.8X-
Sulfonylurea derivatives, oral	T38.3X-
Sulforidazine	T43.3X-
Sulfoxone	T37.1X-
Sulfur, sulfurated, sulfuric, (compounds NEC) (medicinal)	T49.4X-
acid	T54.2X-
dioxide (gas)	T59.1X-
hydrogen	T59.6X-
ointment	T49.0X-
pesticide (vapor)	T60.9-
vapor NEC	T59.89-
Sulfuric acid	T54.2X-
Sulglicotide	T47.1X-
Sulindac	T39.39-
Sulisatin	T47.2X-
Sulisobenzone	T49.3X-
Sulkowitch's reagent	T50.8X-
Sulmetozine	T44.3X-
Suloctidil	T46.7X-
Sulphadiazine	T37.0X-
Sulphadimethoxine	T37.0X-
Sulphadimidine	T37.0X-
Sulphadione	T37.1X-
Sulphafurazole	T37.0X-
Sulphamethizole	T37.0X-
Sulphamethoxazole	T37.0X-
Sulphan blue	T50.8X-
Sulphaphenazole	T37.0X-
Sulphapyridine	T37.0X-
Sulphasalazine	T37.0X-
Sulphinpyrazone	T50.4X-
Sulpiride	T43.59-
Sulprostone	T48.0X-
Sulpyrine	T39.2X-
Sultamicillin	T36.0X-
Sulthiame	T42.6X-
Sultiame	T42.6X-
Sultopride	T43.59-
Sumatriptan	T39.8X-
Sunflower seed oil	T46.6X-
Superinone	T48.4X-
Suprofen	T39.31-
Suramin (sodium)	T37.4X-
Surfacaine	T41.3X-
Surital	T41.1X-
Sutilains	T45.3X-
Suxamethonium (chloride)	T48.1X-
Suxethonium (chloride)	T48.1X-
Suxibuzone	T39.2X-
Sweet niter spirit	T46.3X-
Sweet oil (birch)	T49.3X-
Sweetener	T50.90-
Sym-dichloroethyl ether	T53.6X-
Sympatholytic NEC	T44.8X-
haloalkylamine	T44.8X-
Sympathomimetic NEC	T44.90-
anti-common-cold	T48.5X-
bronchodilator	T48.6X-
specified NEC	T44.99-
Synagis	T50.B9-
Synalar	T49.0X-
Synthetic cannabinoids	T40.72-
Synthetic narcotics (other)	T40.49-
Synthroid	T38.1X-
Syntocinon	T48.0X-
Syrosingopine	T46.5X-
Systemic drug	T45.9-
specified NEC	T45.8X-
2,4,5-T	T60.3X-
Tablets—*see also specified substance*	T50.90-
Tace	T38.5X-
Tacrine	T44.0X-
Tadalafil	T46.7X-
Talampicillin	T36.0X-
Talbutal	T42.3X-
Talc powder	T49.3X-
Talcum	T49.3X-
Taleranol	T38.6X-

TABLE OF DRUGS AND CHEMICALS

Drug/Chemical	Code	Drug/Chemical	Code
Tamoxifen	T38.6X-	**Tessalon**	T48.3X-
Tamsulosin	T44.6X-	**Testolactone**	T38.7X-
Tandearil, tanderil	T39.2X-	**Testosterone**	T38.7X-
Tannic acid (Tannin)	T49.2X-	**Tetanus toxoid or vaccine**	T50.A9-
medicinal (astringent)	T49.2X-	antitoxin	T50.Z1-
Tansy	T62.2X-	immune globulin (human)	T50.Z1-
TAO	T36.3X-	toxoid	T50.A9-
Tapazole	T38.2X-	with diphtheria toxoid	T50.A2-
Tar NEC	T52.0X-	with pertussis	T50.A1-
camphor	T60.1X-	**Tetrabenazine**	T43.59-
distillate	T49.1X-	**Tetracaine**	T41.3X-
fumes	T59.89-	**Tetrachlorethylene—*see Tetrachloroethylene***	
medicinal (ointment)	T49.1X-	**Tetrachlormethiazide**	T50.2X-
Taractan	T43.59-	**2,3,7,8-Tetrachlorodibenzo-p-dioxin**	T53.7X-
Tarantula (venomous)	T63.321	**Tetrachloroethane**	T53.6X-
Tartar emetic	T37.8X-	vapor	T53.6X-
Tartaric acid	T65.89-	paint or varnish	T53.6X-
Tartrate, laxative	T47.4X-	**Tetrachloroethylene (liquid)**	T53.3X-
Tartrated antimony (anti-infective)	T37.8X-	medicinal	T37.4X-
Tauromustine	T45.1X-	vapor	T53.3X-
TCA—*see Trichloroacetic acid*		**Tetracosactide**	T38.81-
TCDD	T53.7X-	**Tetracosactrin**	T38.81-
TDI (vapor)	T65.0X-	**Tetracycline**	T36.4X-
Teclothiazide	T50.2X-	ophthalmic preparation	T49.5X-
Teclozan	T37.3X-	topical NEC	T49.0X-
Tegafur	T45.1X-	**Tetradifon**	T60.8X-
Tegretol	T42.1X-	**Tetradotoxin**	T61.771
Teicoplanin	T36.8X-	**Tetraethyl**	
Telepaque	T50.8X-	lead	T56.0X-
Tellurium	T56.89-	pyrophosphate	T60.0X-
TEM	T45.1X-	**Tetraethylammonium chloride**	T44.2X-
Temazepam	T42.4X-	**Tetraethylthiuram disulfide**	T50.6X-
Temocillin	T36.0X-	**Tetrahydroaminoacridine**	T44.0X-
Tenamfetamine	T43.62-	**Tetrahydrocannabinol**	T40.71-
Teniposide	T45.1X-	**Tetrahydrofuran**	T52.8X-
Tenitramine	T46.3X-	**Tetrahydronaphthalene**	T52.8X-
Tenoglicin	T48.4X-	**Tetrahydrozoline**	T49.5X-
Tenonitrozole	T37.3X-	**Tetralin**	T52.8X-
Tenoxicam	T39.39-	**Tetramethrin**	T60.2X-
TEPA	T45.1X-	**Tetramethylthiuram (disulfide) NEC**	T60.3X-
TEPP	T60.0X-	medicinal	T49.0X-
Teprotide	T46.5X-	**Tetramisole**	T37.4X-
Terazosin	T44.6X-	**Tetranicotinoyl fructose**	T46.7X-
Terbufos	T60.0X-	**Tetrazepam**	T42.4X-
Terbutaline	T48.6X-	**Tetronal**	T42.6X-
Terconazole	T49.0X-	**Tetryl**	T65.3X-
Terfenadine	T45.0X-	**Tetrylammonium chloride**	T44.2X-
Teriparatide (acetate)	T50.99-	**Tetryzoline**	T49.5X-
Terizidone	T37.1X-	**Thalidomide**	T45.1X-
Terlipressin	T38.89-	**Thallium (compounds) (dust) NEC**	T56.81-
Terodiline	T46.3X-	pesticide	T60.4X-
Teroxalene	T37.4X-	**THC**	T40.71-
Terpin (cis)hydrate	T48.4X-	**Thebacon**	T48.3X-
Terramycin	T36.4X-	**Thebaine**	T40.2X-
Tertatolol	T44.7X-	**Thenoic acid**	T49.6X-

TABLE OF DRUGS AND CHEMICALS

Drug/Chemical	Code
Thenyldiamine	T45.0X-
Theobromine (calcium salicylate)	T48.6X-
sodium salicylate	T48.6X-
Theophyllamine	T48.6X-
Theophylline	T48.6X-
Thiabendazole	T37.4X-
Thialbarbital	T41.1X-
Thiamazole	T38.2X-
Thiambutosine	T37.1X-
Thiamine	T45.2X-
Thiamphenicol	T36.2X-
Thiamylal (sodium)	T41.1X-
Thiazesim	T43.29-
Thiazides (diuretics)	T50.2X-
Thiazinamium metilsulfate	T43.3X-
Thiethylperazine	T43.3X-
Thimerosal	T49.0X-
ophthalmic preparation	T49.5X-
Thioacetazone	T37.1X-
Thiobarbital sodium	T41.1X-
Thiobarbiturate anesthetic	T41.1X-
Thiobismol	T37.8X-
Thiobutabarbital sodium	T41.1X-
Thiocarbamate (insecticide)	T60.0X-
Thiocarbamide	T38.2X-
Thiocarbarsone	T37.8X-
Thiocarlide	T37.1X-
Thioctamide	T50.99-
Thioctic acid	T50.99-
Thiofos	T60.0X-
Thioglycolate	T49.4X-
Thioglycolic acid	T65.89-
Thioguanine	T45.1X-
Thiomercaptomerin	T50.2X-
Thiomerin	T50.2X-
Thiomersal	T49.0X-
Thionazin	T60.0X-
Thiopental (sodium)	T41.1X-
Thiopentone (sodium)	T41.1X-
Thiopropazate	T43.3X-
Thioproperazine	T43.3X-
Thioridazine	T43.3X-
Thiosinamine	T49.3X-
Thiotepa	T45.1X-
Thiothixene	T43.4X-
Thiouracil (benzyl) (methyl) (propyl)	T38.2X-
Thiourea	T38.2X-
Thiphenamil	T44.3X-
Thiram	T60.3X-
medicinal	T49.2X-
Thonzylamine (systemic)	T45.0X-
mucosal decongestant	T48.5X-
Thorazine	T43.3X-
Thorium dioxide suspension	T50.8X-
Thornapple	T62.2X-

Drug/Chemical	Code
Throat drug NEC	T49.6X-
Thrombin	T45.7X-
Thrombolysin	T45.61-
Thromboplastin	T45.7X-
Thurfyl nicotinate	T46.7X-
Thymol	T49.0X-
Thymopentin	T37.5X-
Thymoxamine	T46.7X-
Thymus extract	T38.89-
Thyreotrophic hormone	T38.81-
Thyroglobulin	T38.1X-
Thyroid (hormone)	T38.1X-
Thyrolar	T38.1X-
Thyrotrophin	T38.81-
Thyrotropic hormone	T38.81-
Thyroxine	T38.1X-
Tiabendazole	T37.4X-
Tiamizide	T50.2X-
Tianeptine	T43.29-
Tiapamil	T46.1X-
Tiapride	T43.59-
Tiaprofenic acid	T39.31-
Tiaramide	T39.8X-
Ticarcillin	T36.0X-
Ticlatone	T49.0X-
Ticlopidine	T45.521
Ticrynafen	T50.1X-
Tidiacic	T50.99-
Tiemonium	T44.3X-
iodide	T44.3X-
Tienilic acid	T50.1X-
Tifenamil	T44.3X-
Tigan	T45.0X-
Tigloidine	T44.3X-
Tilactase	T47.5X-
Tiletamine	T41.29-
Tilidine	T40.4X-
Timepidium bromide	T44.3X-
Timiperone	T43.4X-
Timolol	T44.7X-
Tin (chloride) (dust) (oxide) NEC	T56.6X-
anti-infectives	T37.8X-
Tindal	T43.3X-
Tinidazole	T37.3X-
Tinoridine	T39.8X-
Tiocarlide	T37.1X-
Tioclomarol	T45.51-
Tioconazole	T49.0X-
Tioguanine	T45.1X-
Tiopronin	T50.99-
Tiotixene	T43.4X-
Tioxolone	T49.4X-
Tipepidine	T48.3X-
Tiquizium bromide	T44.3X-
Tiratricol	T38.1X-

TABLE OF DRUGS AND CHEMICALS

Drug/Chemical	Code
Tisopurine	T50.4X-
Titanium (compounds) (vapor)	T56.89-
dioxide/ointment/oxide	T49.3X-
tetrachloride	T56.89-
Titanocene	T56.89-
Titroid	T38.1X-
Tizanidine	T42.8X-
TMTD	T60.3X-
TNT (fumes)	T65.3X-
Toadstool	T62.0X-
Tobacco NEC	T65.29-
cigarettes	T65.22-
Indian	T62.2X-
smoke, second-hand	T65.22-
Tobramycin	T36.5X-
Tocainide	T46.2X-
Tocoferol	T45.2X-
Tocopherol (acetate)	T45.2X-
Tocosamine	T48.0X-
Todralazine	T46.5X-
Tofisopam	T42.4X-
Tofranil	T43.01-
Toilet deodorizer	T65.89-
Tolamolol	T44.7X-
Tolazamide	T38.3X-
Tolazoline	T46.7X-
Tolbutamide (sodium)	T38.3X-
Tolciclate	T49.0X-
Tolmetin	T39.39-
Tolnaftate	T49.0X-
Tolonidine	T46.5X-
Toloxatone	T42.6X-
Tolperisone	T44.3X-
Tolserol	T42.8X-
Toluene (liquid)	T52.2X-
diisocyanate	T65.0X-
Toluidine (vapor)	T65.89-
Toluol (liquid)	T52.2X-
vapor	T52.2X-
Toluylenediamine	T65.3X-
Tolylene-2,4-diisocyanate	T65.0X-
Tonic NEC	T50.90-
Topical action drug NEC	T49.9-
ear, nose or throat	T49.6X-
eye	T49.5X-
skin	T49.9-
specified NEC	T49.8X-
Toquizine	T44.3X-
Toremifene	T38.6X-
Tosylchloramide sodium	T49.8X-
Toxaphene (dust) (spray)	T60.1X-
Toxin, diphtheria (Schick Test)	T50.8X-
Tractor fuel NEC	T52.0X-
Tragacanth	T50.99-
Tramadol	T40.42-

Drug/Chemical	Code
Tramazoline	T48.5X-
Tranexamic acid	T45.62-
Tranilast	T45.0X-
Tranquilizer NEC	T43.50-
with hypnotic or sedative	T42.6X-
benzodiazepine NEC	T42.4X-
butyrophenone NEC	T43.4X-
carbamate	T43.59-
dimethylamine / ethylamine	T43.3X-
hydroxyzine	T43.59-
major NEC	T43.50-
penothiazine NEC / piperazine NEC	T43.3X-
piperidine / propylamine	T43.3X-
specified NEC	T43.59-
thioxanthene NEC	T43.59-
Tranxene	T42.4X-
Tranylcypromine	T43.1X-
Trapidil	T46.3X-
Trasentine	T44.3X-
Travert	T50.3X-
Trazodone	T43.21-
Trecator	T37.1X-
Treosulfan	T45.1X-
Tretamine	T45.1X-
Tretinoin	T49.0X-
Tretoquinol	T48.6X-
Triacetin	T49.0X-
Triacetoxyanthracene	T49.4X-
Triacetyloleandomycin	T36.3X-
Triamcinolone	T38.0X-
ENT agent	T49.6X-
hexacetonide	T49.0X-
ophthalmic preparation	T49.5X-
topical NEC	T49.0X-
Triampyzine	T44.3X-
Triamterene	T50.2X-
Triazine (herbicide)	T60.3X-
Triaziquone	T45.1X-
Triazolam	T42.4X-
Triazole (herbicide)	T60.3X-
Tribenoside	T46.99-
Tribromacetaldehyde	T42.6X-
Tribromoethanol, rectal	T41.29-
Tribromomethane	T42.6X-
Trichlorethane	T53.2X-
Trichlorethylene	T53.2X-
Trichlorfon	T60.0X-
Trichlormethiazide	T50.2X-
Trichlormethine	T45.1X-
Trichloroacetic acid, Trichloracetic acid	T54.2X-
medicinal	T49.4X-
Trichloroethane	T53.2X-
Trichloroethanol	T42.6X-
Trichloroethyl phosphate	T42.6X-

TABLE OF DRUGS AND CHEMICALS

Drug/Chemical	Code	Drug/Chemical	Code
Trichloroethylene (liquid) (vapor)	T53.2X-	**Trional**	T42.6X-
anesthetic (gas)	T41.0X-	**Triorthocresyl phosphate**	T65.89-
Trichlorofluoromethane NEC	T53.5X-	**Trioxide of arsenic**	T57.0X-
Trichloronate	T60.0X-	**Trioxysalen**	T49.4X-
2,4,5-Trichlorophen-oxyacetic acid	T60.3X-	**Tripamide**	T50.2X-
Trichloropropane	T53.6X-	**Triparanol**	T46.6X-
Trichlorotriethylamine	T45.1X-	**Tripelennamine**	T45.0X-
Trichomonacides NEC	T37.3X-	**Triperiden**	T44.3X-
Trichomycin	T36.7X-	**Triperidol**	T43.4X-
Triclobisonium chloride	T49.0X-	**Triphenylphosphate**	T65.89-
Triclocarban	T49.0X-	**Triple bromides**	T42.6X-
Triclofos	T42.6X-	**Triple carbonate**	T47.1X-
Triclosan	T49.0X-	**Triprolidine**	T45.0X-
Tricresyl phosphate	T65.89-	**Trisodium hydrogen edetate**	T50.6X-
solvent	T52.9-	**Trisoralen**	T49.3X-
Tricyclamol chloride	T44.3X-	**Trisulfapyrimidines**	T37.0X-
Tridesilon	T49.0X-	**Trithiozine**	T44.3X-
Tridihexethyl iodide	T44.3X-	**Tritiozine**	T44.3X-
Tridione	T42.2X-	**Tritoqualine**	T45.0X-
Trientine	T45.8X-	**Trofosfamide**	T45.1X-
Triethanolamine NEC	T54.3X-	**Troleandomycin**	T36.3X-
Triethanomelamine	T45.1X-	**Trolnitrate (phosphate)**	T46.3X-
Triethylenemelamine	T45.1X-	**Tromantadine**	T37.5X-
Triethylenephosphoramide	T45.1X-	**Trometamol**	T50.2X-
Triethylenethiophosphoramide	T45.1X-	**Tromethamine**	T50.2X-
Trifluoperazine	T43.3X-	**Tronothane**	T41.3X-
Trifluoroethyl vinyl ether	T41.0X-	**Tropacine**	T44.3X-
Trifluperidol	T43.4X-	**Tropatepine**	T44.3X-
Triflupromazine	T43.3X-	**Tropicamide**	T44.3X-
Trifluridine	T37.5X-	**Trospium chloride**	T44.3X-
Triflusal	T45.521	**Troxerutin**	T46.99-
Trihexyphenidyl	T44.3X-	**Troxidone**	T42.2X-
Triiodothyronine	T38.1X-	**Tryparsamide**	T37.3X-
Trilene	T41.0X-	**Trypsin**	T45.3X-
Trilostane	T38.99-	**Tryptizol**	T43.01-
Trimebutine	T44.3X-	**TSH**	T38.81-
Trimecaine	T41.3X-	**Tuaminoheptane**	T48.5X-
Trimeprazine (tartrate)	T44.3X-	**Tuberculin (PPD)**	T50.8X-
Trimetaphan camsilate	T44.2X-	**Tubocurare**	T48.1X-
Trimetazidine	T46.7X-	**Tubocurarine (chloride)**	T48.1X-
Trimethadione	T42.2X-	**Tulobuterol**	T48.6X-
Trimethaphan	T44.2X-	**Turpentine (spirits of)**	T52.8X-
Trimethidinium	T44.2X-	vapor	T52.8X-
Trimethobenzamide	T45.0X-	**Tybamate**	T43.59-
Trimethoprim (w/ sulfamethoxazole)	T37.8X-	**Tyloxapol**	T48.4X-
Trimethylcarbinol	T51.3X-	**Tymazoline**	T48.5X-
Trimethylpsoralen	T49.3X-	**Tyropanoate**	T50.8X-
Trimeton	T45.0X-	**Tyrothricin**	T49.6X-
Trimetrexate	T45.1X-	ENT agent	T49.6X-
Trimipramine	T43.01-	ophthalmic preparation	T49.5X-
Trimustine	T45.1X-	**Ufenamate**	T39.39-
Trinitrine	T46.3X-	**Ultraviolet light protectant**	T49.3X-
Trinitrobenzol	T65.3X-	**Undecenoic acid**	T49.0X-
Trinitrophenol	T65.3X-	**Undecoylium**	T49.0X-
Trinitrotoluene (fumes)	T65.3X-	**Undecylenic acid (derivatives)**	T49.0X-

TABLE OF DRUGS AND CHEMICALS

Drug/Chemical	Code	Drug/Chemical	Code
Unna's boot	T49.3X-	Vaccine NEC, continued	
Unsaturated fatty acid	T46.6X-	viral NEC	
Unspecified drug or substance	T50.90-	yellow fever	
Unspecified drug or substance, multiple	T50.91-	**Vaccinia immune globulin**	
Uracil mustard	T45.1X-	**Vaginal contraceptives**	
Uramustine	T45.1X-	**Valerian (root) (tincture)**	T4
Urapidil	T46.5X-	tincture	T42.
Urari	T48.1X-	**Valethamate bromide**	T44.3.
Urate oxidase	T50.4X-	**Valisone**	T49.0X-
Urea	T47.3X-	**Valium**	T42.4X-
peroxide	T49.0X-	**Valmid**	T42.6X-
stibamine	T37.4X-	**Valnoctamide**	T42.6X-
topical	T49.8X-	**Valproate (sodium)**	T42.6X-
Urethane	T45.1X-	**Valproic acid**	T42.6X-
Uric acid metabolism drug NEC	T50.4X-	**Valpromide**	T42.6X-
Uricosuric agent	T50.4X-	**Vanadium**	T56.89-
Urinary anti-infective	T37.8X-	**Vancomycin**	T36.8X-
Urofollitropin	T38.81-	**Vapor**—*see also Gas*	T59.9-
Urokinase	T45.61-	kiln (carbon monoxide)	T58.8X-
Urokon	T50.8X-	specified source NEC	T59.89-
Ursodeoxycholic acid	T50.99-	**Vardenafil**	T46.7X-
Ursodiol	T50.99-	**Varicose reduction drug**	T46.8X-
Urtica	T62.2X-	**Varnish**	T65.4X-
Vaccine NEC	T50.Z9-	cleaner	T52.9-
antineoplastic	T50.Z9-	**Vaseline**	T49.3X-
bacterial NEC	T50.A9-	**Vasodilan**	T46.7X-
with		**Vasodilator**	
other bacterial component	T50.A2-	coronary NEC	T46.3X-
pertussis component	T50.A1-	peripheral NEC	T46.7X-
viral-rickettsial component	T50.A2-	**Vasopressin**	T38.89-
mixed NEC	T50.A2-	**Vasopressor drugs**	T38.89-
BCG	T50.A9-	**Vecuronium bromide**	T48.1X-
cholera	T50.A9-	**Vegetable extract, astringent**	T49.2X-
diphtheria	T50.A9-	**Venlafaxine**	T43.21-
with tetanus	T50.A2-	**Venom, venomous (bite) (sting)**	T63.9-
and pertussis	T50.A1-	amphibian NEC	T63.831
influenza	T50.B9-	animal NEC	T63.89-
measles, mumps and rubella (MMR)	T50.B9-	ant	T63.421
meningococcal	T50.A9-	arthropod NEC	T63.481
paratyphoid	T50.A9-	bee	T63.441
plague	T50.A9-	centipede	T63.41-
poliomyelitis	T50.B9-	fish	T63.59-
rabies	T50.B9-	frog	T63.81-
respiratory syncytial virus	T50.B9-	hornet	T63.451
rickettsial NEC	T50.A9-	insect NEC	T63.481
with		lizard	T63.121
bacterial component	T50.A2-	marine	
Rocky Mountain spotted fever	T50.A9-	animals	T63.69-
sabin oral	T50.B9-	bluebottle	T63.61-
smallpox	T50.B1-	jellyfish NEC	T63.62-
TAB	T50.A9-	Portugese Man-o-war	T63.61-
tetanus	T50.A9-	sea anemone	T63.631
typhoid	T50.A9-	specified NEC	T63.69-
typhus	T50.A9-	fish	T63.59-
		plants	T63.71-

TABLE OF DRUGS AND CHEMICALS

Drug/Chemical	Code
White, continued	
lotion (keratolytic)	T49.4X-
spirit	T52.0X-
Whitewash	T65.89-
Whole blood (human)	T45.8X-
Wild (black cherry) (poisonous plants NEC)	T62.2X-
Window cleaning fluid	T65.89-
Wintergreen (oil)	T49.3X-
Wisterine	T62.2X-
Witch hazel	T49.2X-
Wood alcohol or spirit	T51.1X-
Wool fat (hydrous)	T49.3X-
Woorali	T48.1X-
Wormseed, American	T37.4X-
Xamoterol	T44.5X-
Xanthine diuretics	T50.2X-
Xanthinol nicotinate	T46.7X-
Xanthotoxin	T49.3X-
Xantinol nicotinate	T46.7X-
Xantocillin	T36.0X-
Xenon (127Xe) (133Xe)	T50.8X-
Xenysalate	T49.4X-
Xibornol	T37.8X-
Xigris	T45.51-
Xipamide	T50.2X-
Xylene (vapor)	T52.2X-
Xylocaine (infiltration) (topical)	T41.3X-
Xylol (vapor)	T52.2X-
Xylometazoline	T48.5X-
Yeast (dried)	T45.2X-
Yellow (jasmine)	T62.2X-
phenolphthalein	T47.2X-
Yew	T62.2X-
Yohimbic acid	T40.99-
Zactane	T39.8X-
Zalcitabine	T37.5X-

Drug/Chemical	Code
Zaroxolyn	T50.2X-
Zephiran (topical)	T49.0X-
ophthalmic preparation	T49.5X-
Zeranol	T38.7X-
Zerone	T51.1X-
Zidovudine	T37.5X-
Zimeldine	T43.22-
Zinc (compounds) (fumes) (vapor) NEC	T56.5X-
anti-infectives (bacitracin)	T49.0X-
antivaricose	T46.8X-
chloride (mouthwash)	T49.6X-
chromate	T56.5X-
gelatin or oxide (plaster)	T49.3X-
peroxide	T49.0X-
pesticides	T56.5X-
phosphide or pyrithionate	T60.4X-
stearate	T49.3X-
sulfate	T49.5X-
ENT agent	T49.6X-
ophthalmic solution	T49.5X-
topical NEC	T49.0X-
undecylenate	T49.0X-
Zineb	T60.0X-
Zinostatin	T45.1X-
Zipeprol	T48.3X-
Zofenopril	T46.4X-
Zolpidem	T42.6X-
Zomepirac	T39.39-
Zopiclone	T42.6X-
Zorubicin	T45.1X-
Zotepine	T43.59-
Zovant	T45.51-
Zoxazolamine	T42.8X-
Zuclopenthixol	T43.4X-
Zygadenus (venenosus)	T62.2X-
Zyprexa	T43.59-

NEW! 2025 Coding Resources From the AAP

Coding for Pediatrics 2025

A Manual for Pediatric Documentation and Payment, 30th Edition

The 30th edition of the AAP cornerstone coding publication has been completely updated to include all pediatric changes in CPT® codes for 2025—complete with expert guidance on their application. This year's edition includes a new chapter discussing telemedicine code changes, immunization coding updates; the addition of codes for reporting contraception services, and more.

Spiral-bound, November 2024—544 pages
MA1150
Book ISBN 978-1-61002-749-6
eBook ISBN 978-1-61002-750-2
Price: $141.95 **Member Price: $113.95**

Pediatric ICD-10-CM 2025

A Manual for Provider-Based Coding, 10th Edition

This completely updated 10th edition condenses the vast ICD-10-CM code set into only pediatric-centered guidelines and codes. New codes have been added in the following categories: Anal fistulas; Blood type; Body mass index; Eating disorders; Epilepsy and recurrent seizures, plus more.

Spiral-bound, October 2024—571 pages
MA1151
Book ISBN 978-1-61002-751-9
eBook ISBN 978-1-61002-752-6
Price: $121.95 **Member Price: $97.95**

AAP Pediatric Coding Newsletter™

This information-packed monthly publication brings you proven coding strategies, tips, and techniques you won't see in any other periodical. Available in print and online formats, each issue presents ways to help your practice reduce errors, avoid overcoding and undercoding, and get payment approved more quickly.

FOR INDIVIDUAL (SINGLE-USER) ITEM#: sub1005
1 year, $255 **Member Price:** $205
2 year: ~~$510~~ $434 **Member Price:** ~~$410~~ $349 **SAVE 15%!**

Pediatric Telehealth Coding

Expert Guidance for Your Practice

This handy resource is filled with expert guidance to help prepare for the changes coming to telehealth coding under *Current Procedural Terminology* (CPT®) in 2025. Contents include: Relevant chapters of *Coding for Pediatrics* 2025; an appendix composed of articles from the AAP *Pediatric Coding Newsletter*; additional content from the AAP coding team, and a quiz for CEUs.

Paperback, available January 2025—130 pages
MA1159
Book ISBN 978-61002-760-1
eBook ISBN 978-1-61002-761-8
Price: $69.95 **Member Price: $55.95**

2025 Quick Reference Coding Tools for Pediatrics

2025 Coding Card Toolbox

Buy this package and SAVE 15%

This package includes all 8 of the 2025 quick reference coding tools for pediatrics.

MA1168
Price ~~$199~~ $169 **Member Price:** ~~$159~~ **$135**

Order at **aap.org/shopaap** or call toll-free **866-843-2271** to order today.

shopAAP
aap.org/shopaap

American Academy of Pediatrics
DEDICATED TO THE HEALTH OF ALL CHILDREN®